TENTH EDITION

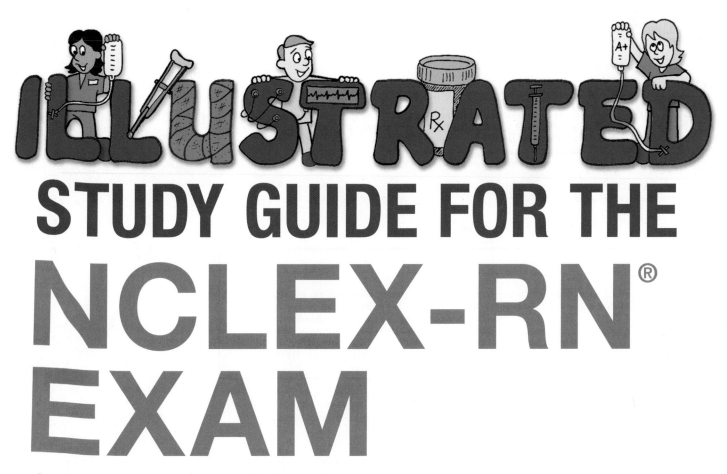

# STUDY GUIDE FOR THE
# NCLEX-RN® EXAM

## JoAnn Zerwekh, EdD, MSN, RN

President/CEO
Nursing Education Consultants, Inc.
Chandler, AZ

Upper Iowa University
Adjunct Faculty
Mesa, AZ

ELSEVIER

**ELSEVIER**

3251 Riverport Lane
St. Louis, Missouri 63043

ILLUSTRATED STUDY GUIDE FOR THE NCLEX-RN® EXAM,
TENTH EDITION

ISBN: 978-0-323-53097-2

---

**Notices**

Practitioners and researchers must always rely on their own experience and knowledge in evaluating and using any information, methods, compounds or experiments described herein. Because of rapid advances in the medical sciences, in particular, independent verification of diagnoses and drug dosages should be made. To the fullest extent of the law, no responsibility is assumed by Elsevier, authors, editors or contributors for any injury and/or damage to persons or property as a matter of products liability, negligence or otherwise, or from any use or operation of any methods, products, instructions, or ideas contained in the material herein.

---

NCLEX®, NCLEX-RN®, and NCLEX-PN® are registered trademarks of the National Council of State Boards of Nursing, Inc.

**Library of Congress Control Number:  2018960008**

*Executive Content Strategist:* Jamie Blum
*Content Development Manager:* Lisa Newton
*Content Development Specialists:* Danielle Frazier and Melissa Rawe
*Publishing Services Manager:* Shereen Jameel
*Book Production Specialist:* Anitha Rajarathnam
*Book Designer:* Amy Buxton
*Marketing Manager:* Megan Richter

Printed in Canada.

Last digit is the print number:  9  8  7  6  5  4  3  2  1

# Contributors

**Mary Boyce, MSN, RN, CCRN, CNE**
Nursing Faculty
Mesa Community College
Mesa, AZ

**Ellen Cummings, MSN, RN, CNE**
Nursing Faculty
GateWay Community College
Phoenix, AZ

**Mary Alice Estes, RN, MSN, CNE**
Instructor, Associate Degree Nursing
Alvin Community College
Alvin, TX

**Cindy Farris, PhD, MSN, MPH, BSN, CNE**
Director of Undergraduate Nursing/Assistant Professor
Indiana Purdue University Fort Wayne
Fort Wayne, IN

**Debra L. Fontenot, DNP, RN, CPNP, CNE**
Director, Nursing Programs
Alvin Community College
Alvin, TX

**Shirley A. Greenway, MSN, RN**
Associate Degree Nursing Professor
Grayson College
Denison, TX

**Tiffanie Hoffmeyer, PhD, MSN Ed, RN**
Associate Professor
Chaminade University
Honolulu, HI

**Sharon Johns, MSN, RN, CNE**
Nurse Educator
Nursing Education Consultants, Inc.
Chandler, AZ
Sherman, TX

**Denise McEnroe-Petitte, PhD, MSN, BSN, AS, RN**
Associate Professor, Nursing
Kent State University Tuscarawas
New Philadelphia, OH

**Karin J. Sherrill, RN, MSN, CNE, ANEF**
Nursing Faculty
Maricopa Community Colleges
Phoenix, AZ

**Renee Spellacy, MSN, MA, RN, CMSRN, CRC**
Nursing Faculty
GateWay Community College
Phoenix, AZ

**Ashley White, MSN, RN, OCN**
Nursing Instructor
Alvin Community College
Alvin, TX

**Tyler Zerwekh, BA, MPH, DrPH, REHS**
Administrator
Environmental Health Services Bureau
Shelby County Health Department
Memphis, TN

**Ashley Zerwekh Garneau, PhD, RN**
Nursing Faculty
GateWay Community College
Phoenix, AZ

## ITEM WRITER

**Mary Boyce, MSN, RN, CCRN, CNE**
Nursing Faculty
Mesa Community College
Mesa, AZ

# Preface

The tenth edition of *Illustrated Study Guide for the NCLEX-RN® Exam* continues to provide an up-to-date review book illustrated with graphics, pictures, and cartoon images to enhance your review and retention of critical nursing information. The book contains information specifically designed to assist you in preparing for the National Council Licensure Examination for Registered Nurses (NCLEX-RN®). This text emphasizes the integrated approach to nursing practice that the NCLEX-RN is designed to test. The book's primary purpose is to assist you to thoroughly review facts, principles, and applications of the nursing process. It should alleviate many of the concerns you may have about what, how, and when to study.

I have spent a great deal of time studying the NCLEX-RN test format and have incorporated that information into this book. Discussion and examples of the alternate format questions are included. In my review courses, which I have taught across the country, I have identified specific student needs and correlated this information with the test plan to develop this study guide. Study questions are at the end of each chapter to help you check your level of comprehension. In addition, there is a companion Evolve website (https://evolve.elsevier.com/Zerwekh/studyguide/) that contains questions for practicing your testing skills.

Graphics highlighting important information make the book more visually appealing. They include:

## PRIORITY CONCEPTS

Priority Concepts added to the beginning of each chapter assist you in concept-based nursing programs by focusing on priority concepts for each chapter

**ALERT** Alert identifies important concepts that are reflected on the RN Practice Analysis from the National Council of State Boards of Nursing, Inc.

Nursing Priority assists to distinguish priorities of nursing care.

Adult disease conditions are easily located by this design element.

Pediatric disease conditions are easily located by this design element.

Self-Care and Home Care can be found under the Nursing Interventions section.

Medication information is easily found in chapter appendixes.

▲ High-Alert Medications identified by The Joint Commission and the Institute for Safe Medication Practices are noted by this symbol.

The comments from my review course participants and extensive content reviews have helped shape the development of this tenth edition. I hope this text will prove to be even more beneficial to nursing faculty, students, and graduate nurses. Thank you for allowing me to be part of your success in nursing.

**JoAnn Zerwekh**

# Acknowledgments

I truly appreciate the continuing support of my children and stepchildren—Tyler Zerwekh, Ashley Zerwekh Garneau, Carrie Parks, and Matt Masog—who have given me my wonderful grandchildren who lighten my day and make me smile—Maddie and Harper Zerwekh, Ben Garneau, Brooklyn Parks, and Owen, Emmett, and Cole Masog.

To John Masog, my husband, thank you for your tolerance, love, and willingness to continue to share and support me in the midst of our busy lives. Thanks also for the awesome lemon drops (you are the consummate mixologist) and the excellent meals you prepare for us.

A special note of thanks to C. J. Miller, RN, BSN, cartoonist, who has worked with me from the beginning of the *Memory Notebooks of Nursing* and the many editions of *Nursing Today: Transition and Trends*, and more recently with the *Mosby's Memory Notecard* series. She continues to bring to all of my books images and cartoons that are unique and humorous.

This edition offers the opportunity to be responsive to nursing faculty and students who have utilized the book. Their comments and suggestions for the production of this tenth edition have been incorporated in the revision.

It is my pleasure to acknowledge the individuals who assisted me in the technical preparation and production of this edition. My sincere appreciation to the following:

Elaine Nokes, my chief of operations, who keeps everything with Nursing Education Consultants, Inc., my review business, and my publishing company organized and running smoothly.

Jamie Blum, senior content strategist with whom I have worked on many editions of the *Nursing Today: Transition and Trends* book—it has been so easy to work with you on the *Illustrated Study Guide for the NCLEX-RN® Exam* review book.

Melissa Rawe and Danielle Frazier, content development specialists who provided helpful assistance to me and the contributors from the beginning of the revision process through the entire production cycle of the book.

Anitha Rajarathnam, book production specialist who monitored the production of this book and kept me on schedule. It is always a pleasure to work with you!

Thank you to all!

# Contents

# CHAPTER ONE

# Testing Strategies for the NCLEX-RN® Examination

One of the first steps to being successful on the NCLEX® (National Council Licensure Examination) is to understand how the test is developed. An important step in preparing for the examination is to find out as much as possible about the test. This will help reduce stress and anxiety. During each of your nursing classes, you were given a syllabus with course objectives and provided with presentations to guide you through the information that would be included on course examinations. In most academic settings, the faculty member who teaches the course is also responsible for the development and construction of examinations; thus you are being taught by the same person who prepares the tests, which can be a great advantage. As you begin to prepare for the NCLEX, it is important to consider who determines the content of the test plan and constructs the questions based on the test plan.

The National Council of State Boards of Nursing (NCSBN) is responsible for the development of the content and the construction of questions or items for the NCLEX examination. A practice analysis is conducted by the NCSBN every 3 years to validate the test plan and to determine currency of nursing practice. Content experts are consulted to assist in the creation of the practice analysis. The activity performances and knowledge identified by the content experts are analyzed with consideration given to frequency and importance of the nursing activity. The percentage of test items on the test plan does not specifically address specialty areas. However, on review of the nursing activities, many of the test plan areas address specialty areas of nursing practice. This analysis provides the basis for development of the content to be included in the NCLEX test plan.

The content experts are practicing nurses who work with or supervise new graduates in the practice setting. These content experts represent all geographic areas and are selected according to their area of practice; therefore all areas of nursing practice are addressed in the development of the test plan. Item writers are selected to create questions based on the content identified in the test plan. All new test items or questions are reviewed by item reviewers who are also nurses in current practice and who have been directly involved with supervision of new graduate nurses. Content experts and item reviewers not only create new items; they are also involved in the continual review of items in the NCLEX test pool to ensure all items reflect current practice.

So what does all this mean? It means that nurses in current practice and nursing faculty work together to identify the content and to develop questions for the NCLEX-RN. All geographic areas and all areas of nursing practice are included. The purpose of the examination is to assure the public that each candidate who passes the examination can practice safely and effectively as a newly licensed, entry-level registered nurse (RN).

Every US state uses the NCLEX-RN to determine entry into nursing practice as an RN. Each state is responsible for the testing requirements, retesting procedures, and entry into practice within that state. Each state requires the same competency level or passing standard on the NCLEX. There is no variation in the passing standard from state to state.

## TEST PLAN

The test plan is based on research conducted by the NCSBN every 3 years. The purpose of this research is to determine the most important and frequent activities of nurses who were successful on the NCLEX and who have been working after successful completion of the NCLEX. The research indicates that the majority of graduate nurses are working in an acute care environment and are responsible for caring for adult and older adult clients. Each question reflects a level of the nursing process or an area of client needs, and each question is categorized according to a validated level of difficulty. The examination consists of questions that are designed to test the candidate's ability to apply the nursing process, prioritize client care, and determine appropriate nursing responses and interventions to provide safe nursing care.

### Integrated Processes

Integrated throughout the test plan are principles that are fundamental to the practice of nursing.

#### Nursing Process

The nursing process is a scientific approach to problem solving; it has been a common thread in your nursing curriculum since the beginning of school. There is nothing new about the nursing process on the NCLEX. Assessment data are obtained, the data are analyzed, a plan is formulated, nursing actions are implemented, and the results of that intervention are evaluated. It is important to keep the steps of the nursing process in mind when you are critically evaluating an NCLEX question. See Box 1-1, Key Words for Identifying the Nursing Process.

#### Caring

The interaction of the client and the nurse occurs in an atmosphere of mutual respect and trust. To achieve the desired outcome, the nurse provides hope, support, and compassion to the client.

The following words and phrases have the same meaning and are often interchangeable. The words are associated with activities in the practice analysis.

- **Assessment:** gather objective and subjective, determine, observe, identify findings, recognize changes, notice, detect, find data, verify data, gather information, describe status, assess client
- **Analysis:** interpret data, identify a nursing diagnosis, collect additional data, examine client data, consider nursing data, examine client data for priority
- **Planning:** establish goals, plan interventions, create plan, generate goals, prioritize outcomes of client care, arrange priorities and interventions, formulate short-term goal or long-term goals, prepare list of client outcomes, develop and modify nursing plan of care
- **Implementation:** implement nursing interventions, delegate nursing care, offer alternatives, teach, give, administer, chart, document, explain, inform, encourage, advise, provide, prepare, counsel, teach, perform or assist with client care and needs
- **Evaluation:** evaluate nursing care, question results, monitor findings, repeat assessment, compare outcomes with expected nursing care outcomes, reestablish, consider alternatives, determine changes and response, appraise findings, modify plan of care, evaluate plan of care based on client compliance

### Communication and Documentation

Events and activities—both verbal and nonverbal—that involve the client, the client's significant others, and the health care team are documented in handwritten or electronic records. These records reflect quality and accountability in the provision of client care. Principles of documentation and provision of client confidentiality are important considerations in any area of nursing practice.

### Teaching and Learning

Nurses provide or facilitate knowledge, skills, and attitudes that promote a change in clients' behavior through teaching and learning. Nurses provide education to clients and to their significant others in a variety of settings. Identifying critical learning needs for clients and their significant others and providing information in a manner that promotes the health and safety of clients are important across all levels of nursing practice.

### Culture and Spirituality

The interaction between the nurse and the client (individual, family, or group, including significant others and population), which recognizes and considers the client-reported, self-identified, unique, and individual preferences to client care relates to the integrated processes of culture and spirituality.

### Areas of Client Needs

The National Council Examination Committee has identified four primary areas of client needs, which provide a structure to define nursing actions and competencies across

all practice settings and for all clients. These areas reflect an integrated approach to the testing content; no predetermined number of questions or percentage of questions pertain to any particular area of practice (e.g., medical–surgical, pediatric, obstetric).

Table 1-1 lists the areas of client needs along with the subcategories and the specific percentages associated with each subcategory. The range of percentages for each category reflects how important that area is on the test plan. Management of care, pharmacologic and parenteral therapies, and reduction of risk potential are the subcategories with the highest emphasis on the test plan. When you are studying for the NCLEX, these are concepts that should be identified across the scope of nursing practice. This table has been adapted and summarized; it does not reflect the entire test plan content. The National Council's Detailed Test Plan for the NCLEX-RN may be obtained from the NCSBN, Inc. (https://www.ncsbn.org). What was great new information in last month's nursing journals will not be immediately reflected on the NCLEX. New information or new practices must be established as a standard of practice across the nation before being included on the NCLEX. Throughout this book are ALERT boxes that call your attention to areas of the test plan. Pay attention to these boxes and think about how each concept or principle can apply to different types of clients.

**TEST ALERT:** The NCLEX-RN is a test that requires utilization of the nursing process and application of nursing concepts and principles across the life span.

As client conditions or nursing principles are presented, the NURSING PRIORITY boxes call your attention to critical information regarding a client with a specific condition or situation being presented.

**⊞ NURSING PRIORITY:** This is critical information to consider in providing safe nursing care for a client with a specific problem.

### Classification of Questions

The majority of questions on the NCLEX are written at the level of application or a higher level of cognitive ability. This means a candidate must have the knowledge and understand concepts to be able to apply the nursing process to the client situation presented in the question. NCLEX questions are based on critical thinking concepts that demonstrate a candidate's ability to make decisions and solve problems. NCLEX questions are not fact, recall, or memory-level questions. Nurses who have taken the NCLEX have stated that the NCLEX questions were not like any questions they had on nursing school examinations; however, the nursing content and principles needed to determine the answer were provided in their nursing school curriculum. The questions and answers have been thoroughly researched and validated. The standardization of information is important, because the NCLEX is administered nationwide to determine entry level into nursing practice. This ensures that regional differences in nursing care will not be a factor in the examination.

**Table 1-1   NCLEX-RN TEST PLAN—EFFECTIVE APRIL 2019 TO MARCH 2022ª**

**Safe and Effective Care Environment**

| | |
|---|---|
| Management of Care (17%–23%) | Concepts of management of nursing care—assignment, delegation, supervision, establishing priorities in client care; legal and ethical responsibilities; client rights; confidentiality; information technology |
| Safety and Infection Control (9%–15%) | Prevention of errors and accidents, implementation of standard precautions, asepsis, use of restraints, disaster planning, handling hazardous materials, emergency response plan |

**Health Promotion and Maintenance**
(6%–12%)
Aging process and developmental stages, lifestyle choices, high-risk behaviors; principles of learning and teaching; ante-, intra-, postpartum and newborn; health promotion and disease prevention, techniques of physical assessment

**Psychosocial Integrity**
(6%–12%)
Mental health concepts and interventions; end-of-life care; grief and loss; sensory and perceptual alterations; cultural, religious, and spiritual influences; behavioral intervention/crisis intervention; chemical and substance use dependency; abuse and neglect; therapeutic communication

**Physiologic Integrity**

| | |
|---|---|
| Basic Care and Comfort (6%–12%) | Assistive devices, mobility/immobility, nutrition and oral hydration, personal hygiene, elimination, nonpharmacologic comfort measures, rest and sleep |
| Pharmacologic and Parenteral Therapies (12%–18%) | Medication administration; expected medication actions, adverse effects/contraindication; nursing implications; dosage calculation; blood administration, parenteral/IV therapy, central venous access devices, pain control, parenteral nutrition |
| Reduction of Risk Potential (9%–15%) | Pathophysiology, nursing implications for and nursing care to minimize potential complications of diagnostic tests/procedures/surgery; potential for alterations in body systems (tubes, pacemakers, hyper-/hypoglycemia, specimens, bleeding, wounds, positions); laboratory values; changes in and/or abnormal vital signs; system specific assessments |
| Physiologic Adaptation (11%–17%) | Pathophysiology/alterations in body systems: fluid and electrolyte imbalances, hemodynamics, medical emergencies (CPR, airway, hemorrhage), unexpected response to therapies (seizures, changes in vital signs); nursing management of illness |

*CPR,* Cardiopulmonary resuscitation; *IV,* intravenous.
ªThis is the *proposed test plan* as presented at the annual NCSBN meeting, August 2018. Test plan information is presented as examples only and is not intended to be a complete or thorough representation of information included in any specific category.
Adapted from the NCLEX-RN® Test Plan for the National Council Licensure Examination for Registered Nurses. (2019). Chicago, National Council of State Boards of Nursing.

All questions presented to a candidate taking the NCLEX have been developed according to the test plan and the integrated processes fundamental to nursing practice and have been categorized according to their level of difficulty. The questions have been researched and documented as pertaining to entry-level nursing behaviors.

## WHAT IS COMPUTER ADAPTIVE TESTING?

Computer adaptive testing (CAT) provides a method for generating an examination according to each candidate's ability. Each time a candidate answers a question, the computer then selects the next question based on the candidate's answer to the previous question. The examination continues to present test items based on the test plan and identified level of difficulty and provides an opportunity for each candidate to demonstrate competency. The NCLEX-RN is graded in a manner different from the grading of conventional school examinations. A candidate's score is not based on the number of questions answered correctly but on the standard of competency as established by the NCSBN (Figure 1-1).

A test bank of questions is loaded into the candidate's computer at the beginning of the examination. With CAT, each candidate's test is unique. Different candidates receive different sets of questions, but all test banks contain questions that are developed according to the same test plan. For example, standard precautions are a critical element of the test plan. Many situations and clients can be presented to test this concept. One candidate may have a question based on

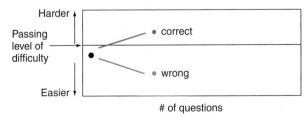

**Computer Adaptive Testing**

**FIGURE 1-1** Competency level.

**Decision: Fail**

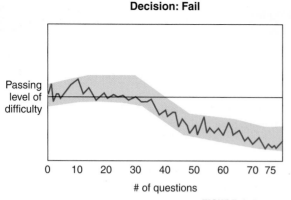

**Decision: Pass**

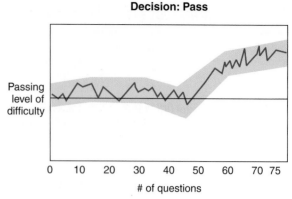

**FIGURE 1-2** Plateau to establish pass or fail.

standard precautions required for a client in labor; someone else, a situation with implications for a client with a respiratory problem; and still someone else, a situation involving a newborn. All the questions are different, but they are all based on the test plan's critical element of standard precautions.

The questions to be presented to the candidate are determined by the candidate's response to the previous questions. When a question is answered correctly, the next question presented to the candidate may have a higher level of difficulty. The more higher-level questions a candidate answers correctly, the closer he or she is to passing (Figure 1-2). A candidate cannot skip questions or go back to previously answered questions. As the examination progresses, it is interactively assembled. As questions are answered correctly, the next question is selected to test another area of the test plan, and it may be at a higher level of difficulty. When a question is answered incorrectly, the computer will select an easier question. This helps prevent a candidate from being bombarded with difficult questions and becoming increasingly frustrated. The computer will continue to present questions that are based on the test plan and on the level of ability of the candidate until a level of competency has been established (see Figure 1-2).

## TAKING THE NCLEX EXAMINATION

### Application

An application must be submitted to the state board of nursing in the state in which the candidate wants to be licensed. The contact information for the state boards of nursing is available on the NCSBN website. After the candidate's application and registration fees have been received and approved by the state, the candidate will receive an authorization to test (ATT) from the NCSBN. After the examination fee has been paid, it will not be refunded regardless of how the candidate registered. The candidate may register for the NCLEX at the NCLEX Candidate website (listed in the ATT) or by regular mail or by telephone (also listed in the ATT). The Candidate Bulletin (CB) is available on the NCSBN website; be sure to print this bulletin for future reference. The CB provides critical information, including addresses and phone numbers for registration and specific details regarding the registration process.

## SCHEDULING THE EXAMINATION

After you have been declared eligible to take the NCLEX and have received an ATT via email, you may schedule an examination date. You *must have an ATT* before you can schedule your examination. The CB lists the phone number to call to schedule the examination. Once the ATT has been emailed to the candidate, the state stipulates a period of time within which you must take the examination. This ranges from 60 to 365 days, with the average being 90 days; this period *cannot* be extended. You must test within the validity dates noted on your ATT. The paper copy of the ATT letter is no longer necessary for test admittance. You are encouraged to schedule the appointment to take the examination as soon as possible after receiving the ATT, even if you do not plan to take the test immediately. This will increase the probability of getting the testing date you want.

Pearson Vue is the company that provides the testing facility and computers for the examination. A tutorial on how to use the computer on NCLEX is available at http://www.pearsonvue.com/nclex/. Go to the site and review the tutorial. It should be familiar to you when you see it on NCLEX. This same tutorial will be presented to you at the beginning of your examination.

### Testing Center Identification

An acceptable form of identification is required at the testing site. If you arrive without your identification, you will be turned away and required to reregister and pay the $200 examination fee again. The first and last name printed on your identification must match exactly the first and last name provided when registering (name printed on the Authorization to Test email). If the name with which you have registered is different from the name on your identification, you must bring legal name change documentation with you to the test center on the day of your test. The only acceptable forms of legal documentation are a marriage license, divorce decree, and/or a court action legal name change document. Identification must be in English, cannot be expired, and must contain your signature. Acceptable forms of identification are a US driver's license, a passport, a US state-issued identification, permanent residence card, or a US military issued identification. At the testing site, each candidate is digitally fingerprinted, a photo is taken, and a signature and palm vein reader scan are required before testing.

## Day of the Examination

You should plan to arrive at the center about 30 minutes before the scheduled testing time. If you arrive more than 30 minutes late, the scheduled testing time will be canceled, and you may have to reapply and pay the examination fee again. An erasable note board will be available at your computer terminal. You are not allowed to take any type of books, personal belongings, hats, coats, blank tablets, or scratch paper into the testing area. Cell/mobile/smart phones, pagers, or other electronic devices may not be accessed during the examination, including during breaks. Candidates will be provided a plastic bag to store their cell/mobile/smart phones and electronic devices, which will be collected by the testing center agent and sealed. Upon completion of the examination, the testing center agent will break the seal on the plastic bag and return the devices to the candidate.

## Testing

You will have a maximum of 6 hours to complete the examination. After 2 hours of testing, you have a preprogrammed break; another optional break occurs after 3.5 hours of testing. If you need a break before that time, raise your hand to notify one of the attendants at the testing center. The computer will automatically signal when a scheduled break begins. All of the break times and the tutorial are considered part of the total 6 hours of testing time. A palm vein scan will be taken when you leave the testing area and will be taken to reenter the testing area after each break.

The examination will stop when one of the following occurs:

1. Seventy-five questions have been answered and a minimum level of competency has been established, or a lack of minimum competency has been established (see Figure 1-2).
2. The candidate has answered the maximum number of 265 questions.
3. The candidate has been testing for 6 hours, regardless of the number of questions answered.

Each candidate will receive between 75 and 265 questions. The number of questions on the NCLEX is not indicative of the level of competency. The majority of candidates who complete all 265 questions will have demonstrated a level of minimum competency and therefore pass the NCLEX. A mouse is used for selecting answers, so candidates should not worry about different computer keyboard function keys. An onscreen calculator is also available to use for math problems. If any problems occur with the environment or with the equipment, someone will be available to provide assistance.

In each candidate's examination, there are 15 pretest or unscored items or questions. The statistics on these items are evaluated to determine whether the item is a valid test item to be included in future NCLEX test banks. All of the items that are scored or counted on a candidate's examination have been pretested and validated. It is impossible to determine which questions or items are scored items and which are pretest items. It is important to treat each question as a scored item.

The CB from the NCSBN is important; read it carefully and keep it until the results from the NCLEX have been received. This bulletin will provide directions and will answer more of your questions regarding the NCLEX. The CB is available online (from the NCSBN at https://www.ncsbn.org or from Pearson Vue at http://www.pearsonvue.com/nclex/).

## Test Results

Each examination is scored twice, once at the testing center and again at the testing service. The test results are electronically transferred to the state boards of nursing. Test results are *not* available at the testing center, from Pearson Vue, or from the NCSBN. Check the information received from the appropriate state board of nursing to determine how and when your results will be available. Test results may be available online. In some states, results may be available within 2 to 3 days; in others, the results will be mailed, which will require a longer notification period. Do *not* call the Pearson Professional Center, NCLEX Candidate Services, the National Council, or the individual state board of nursing for test results. Follow the procedure found in the information from the state board of nursing where the license will be issued.

## NCLEX TEST-TAKING STRATEGIES

> **TEST ALERT:** Practicing test-taking skills is critical if a candidate is going to be able to use them effectively on the NCLEX. Practice test taking should be a component of NCLEX preparation.

Being able to apply test-taking strategies effectively on an examination is almost as important as having the basic knowledge required to answer the questions correctly. Everyone has taken an examination only to find, on review of the examination, that questions were missed because of poor test-taking skills. Nursing education provides the graduate with a comprehensive base of knowledge; how effectively the graduate can *demonstrate* the use of this knowledge is a major factor in the successful completion of the examination.

The NCLEX-RN is designed to evaluate minimum levels of competency. The examination does not test total knowledge, knowledge of specialty areas, or any degree of professionalism. The purpose of the examination is to determine whether a candidate has the knowledge, skills, and ability required for safe and effective entry-level nursing practice. Throughout the examination, questions are described as being based on clinical situations common in nursing; uncommon situations are not emphasized. NCLEX questions are not fact, recall, or memory-level questions; they are questions that require critical thinking to determine the correct answer. Critical thinking requires an analysis of client data, an understanding of the client's condition or disease, and the ability to determine the best action or nursing judgment that will most effectively meet the client's needs.

Practice testing is an excellent method of studying for the NCLEX. After taking a practice test, use the results to determine whether you need additional review in certain areas or whether you are missing questions because of poor test-taking strategies.

The NCLEX questions are different from those used in nursing schools. One of the biggest problems candidates encounter is that two or more answers may appear to be correct. Sometimes a candidate believes that more information is necessary to answer the question, but the answer must be determined from the information provided. No one is going to clarify or provide additional information regarding a specific question or content. The following strategies are critical in evaluating and successfully answering NCLEX questions.

- **The NCLEX Hospital:** What a great place to work! Remember, on the NCLEX, all clients are being cared for in an ideal environment—the NCLEX Hospital. Questions ask for nursing care and decisions based on situations in which everything is available for client care. *NCLEX questions are based on textbook practices, not necessarily on the real world.* It must be assumed that clients will respond just as the textbooks indicate they will. Candidates who have a lot of clinical experience will have problems on the test if they answer questions based on the possibility that there may not be adequate staff or equipment or if they believe the option for the nursing care presented is not "realistic." Nursing care provided on the examination is performed in the NCLEX Hospital, where the nurse always has adequate staff, supplies, and anything else required to provide the safest care for the client. This approach is necessary because this is a nationally standardized examination.
- **Calling the Doctor (or anyone else):** Be cautious about passing the responsibility for care of the client to someone else. This is an examination on nursing care; evaluate the question carefully and see what nursing action should be taken before consulting or calling someone else. This includes the social worker, respiratory therapist, hospital chaplain, and the physician. After you have carefully evaluated the question, if the client's condition is such that the nurse cannot do anything to resolve the problem, then calling for assistance may be the best answer. Frequently there is a nursing action to be taken before contacting someone for assistance. A specific item on the test plan states that the nurse will identify client data that must be reported immediately.
- **Doctor's Orders:** It should be assumed that a doctor's order is available to provide the nursing care in the options presented in the question. If the question asks for administration of a specific medication for the client's problem, then assume that there is an order for it. If the focus of a question is to determine whether a nursing action is a dependent or an independent nursing action, then it will be stated in the stem of the question. For example, the question may ask what would be an independent nursing action to provide pain relief for a specific client.
- **Focus on the Client:** Look for answers that focus on the client. Identify the significant or central person in the question. Most often, this is going to be the client. Wrong choices would be those that focus on maintaining hospital rules and policies, dealing with equipment, or solving the nurse's problems. Evaluate the status of the client first, and then deal with the equipment problems or concerns. Other questions may ask the nurse to respond to a client's family or significant others. Determine the person to whom the question is directed.
- **Client's Age:** Consider a client to be an adult unless otherwise stated. If the age of a client is important to the question, it will be stated in years or in months. Descriptions such as "elderly adult" and "geriatric client" are not commonly used. These terms have been established as negative descriptors of older clients. The description of such a client may be "older adult" or a specific age may be given.
- **Laboratory Values:** It is important to know normal values for the common laboratory tests. Be able to identify laboratory values and/or diagnostic procedures that indicate a client's progress or lack of progress or indicate whether a client's status is getting better or worse. Determine whether specific nursing actions are required based on the abnormal values or diagnostic results. For example, when a client's blood glucose level is 50 mg/mL (2.8 mmol/L) and he or she is awake and alert, the client will need something to eat, preferably a complex carbohydrate. If a client has a hemoglobin value of 8.5 g/dL (85 mmol/L), nursing care will involve avoidance of unnecessary physical activities, and the client will need to be kept warm.
- **Positions:** Positioning a client may be an option to consider in the implementation of care. If a specific position for the client appears in the stem of the question, then consider whether the position is for comfort, for treatment, or to prevent a complication. Evaluate the question: What is to be accomplished by placing the client in the position, and why is the position important for this client? Sometimes a client position will appear in the options. Consider whether positioning is important to the care of the client presented. For example, the semi-Fowler's position is very important to a client who is having difficulty breathing, and the supine position or low Fowler's position may provide the most comfort for a client after surgery. Determine why a client is placed in a specific position and then determine whether this is a priority in planning or intervention. See Appendix 3-1 for a further description of positions.
- **Mathematic Computations:** Mathematic computations may include calculations of intravenous (IV) rate and drip factors, calculations of medication dosages, conversion of units of measurement, and calculation of intake and output. You should be able to apply the appropriate formula to the situation. Some of the questions may call for two computations, as in a question in which all items must be converted to one unit of measurement before a dosage is calculated. There will be an onscreen calculator; find the "calculator" button when you do the NCLEX Tutorial. The mathematic calculations may be presented in a multiple-choice format or in an alternate-format question in which you are asked to fill in the blank. For fill-in-the-blank questions, calculate your answer and then type the answer in the box provided. The unit of measurement will be provided in the box.

## Management of Client Care

As the role of the RN has expanded, management of client care has become increasingly important. Nursing care assignments should take into consideration the nurse who is educationally prepared, experienced, and most capable of caring for the client. Unlicensed assistive personnel (UAP), patient care attendants (PCA), and/or nursing assistants (CNAs) must be directly supervised in the provision of safe nursing care. Licensed practical nurses (LPNs) or licensed vocational nurses (LVNs) have more independence in providing nursing care. They may direct the care of the nursing assistants; however, LPNs are ultimately under the supervision of a registered nurse. Don't panic and pull out all your management textbooks to review. Evaluate such questions in terms of general guidelines for delegation and supervision. Pay close attention to the person to whom the nurse is assigning the care or nursing activity: Is it to another RN, is it to a less qualified person (LVN or LPN), or is a specific activity (bathing, ambulating, etc.) being delegated to a UAP?

- **Don't assign steps of the nursing process or nursing judgment to anyone except an RN.** The implementation of the nursing process and the judgments based on the nursing process must be performed by an RN.
- **Don't delegate teaching assignments to anyone except another RN.** This is another area that is the primary responsibility of the RN.
- **Keep in mind the NCLEX Hospital.** Adequate staff is available to provide client care; don't worry about staff shortages. Focus on the needs of the client in the question; what is happening in the rest of the unit is not a consideration unless it is part of the actual question. The only client to consider in each question is the one involved in that question, not the other clients the nurse may have been assigned.
- **Identify the most stable client.** The most stable client is the one who has the *most predictable outcome* and is *least likely* to have abrupt changes in condition that would require critical nursing judgments. For stable clients, some nursing care activities can be delegated to a certified nursing assistant or assigned to an LPN. When determining the stability of clients, consider Maslow's hierarchy of needs (see Chapter 3, Figure 3-1). Carefully assess and identify clients who are in a changing, unstable situation, especially those clients with a potential for respiratory compromise. These are clients for whom an RN should provide the care.
- **Delegate tasks that have specific guidelines.** Those tasks that have specific guidelines that are unchanging and are used in the care of a stable client can often be delegated. Bathing, collecting urine samples, feeding, providing personal hygiene, and assisting with ambulation are just a few examples of these activities. Remember you are in the NCLEX Hospital, so carefully evaluate the question and select an answer that has the RN delegating tasks to the assistive personnel and making appropriate assignments for other licensed health care personnel.
- **Identify your priority client.** The priority client is the one who is most likely to experience problems or ill effects if not taken care of first. Priority clients include those with respiratory compromise, those whose conditions are unstable and changing, and those who are at high risk for

developing complications. NCLEX questions may present a typical nursing care assignment and ask which client the nurse would care for first; or a situation with a client may be presented and you will be asked to select the first nursing action. Review the testing strategies regarding priority questions. It is important to identify the most unstable client, to see him or her first, and to determine what is necessary to do first for this client.

### Establishing Nursing Priorities

Almost all nurses will agree that the NCLEX is full of priority questions. These questions may be worded in a variety of ways:

"What is the priority nursing action?"
"What should the nurse do first?"
"What is the best nursing action?"

In other words, the NCLEX wants to know whether the nurse can identify the most important nursing action to be taken to provide safe care for the client in the situation presented. In such cases, three or four of the options are frequently correct actions; however, one of the actions needs to be performed before the others. This is where critical thinking is necessary—*think like a nurse!* There are three areas to consider when determining priority nursing actions: Maslow's hierarchy of needs, the nursing process, and client safety.

- **Maslow's Hierarchy of Needs:** And you thought this was just for fundamentals! *Always consider Maslow's hierarchy of needs and remember that physiologic needs must come first.* When evaluating options, identify client needs that are physiologic and those that are psychosocial. Physiologic needs are a higher priority than psychosocial or teaching needs. A client's physical needs must be met before his or her psychosocial or teaching needs are considered. Also remember that the ABCs (airway, breathing, and circulation) are the critical physiologic needs because these are at the base of Maslow's pyramid. However, be cautious; don't always select "airway" as the best answer. Sometimes the client does not have an airway problem, so don't read into the question and give the client an airway problem! Maslow's hierarchy of needs also applies to psychosocial questions (see the section in this chapter regarding answering psychosocial questions).
- **Nursing Process:** The first step in the nursing process is *assessment.* However, do not automatically select an option that includes the word *assess* or an option that involves assessment. Assessment must be done to analyze and construct a nursing diagnosis, to develop a plan of care, and to determine the priority of nursing care implementation. If the assessment data are provided in the stem of the question, then it will be important to consider Maslow's hierarchy of needs when planning or selecting the best nursing action or implementation. If a nursing action has been implemented, then the question may focus on evaluating the effectiveness of the nursing action. Read the question carefully and determine what is being asked.
- **Safety Issues:** These issues may include situations in the hospital or in the client's home environment. The first issue to consider is meeting basic needs of survival: oxygen,

hydration, nutrition, elimination. Reduction of environmental hazards is also a concern and may include prevention of falls, accidents, and medication errors. Environmental safety also includes the prevention and spread of disease. This may include how to avoid contagious diseases or even activities such as handwashing. When you are critically evaluating questions that involve a client's safety and multiple options appear to be correct, determine which activity will be of most benefit to the client.

### Example Questions for Management and Priority Setting

#### Question 1

An RN who has been working in the labor and delivery area has been reassigned to a step-down telemetry unit for the afternoon shift. Which clients would reflect the most appropriate assignment for this nurse?

1. Client who has undergone cardioversion and a client who was admitted during the night for possible myocardial infarction (MI).
2. Client who had a cardiac catheterization this morning and a client admitted for 24-hour observation for first-degree heart block.
3. Client who is currently in third-degree heart block and a client who had a hypertensive crisis with congestive heart failure 48 hours ago.
4. Client who had an MI 72 hours ago and is experiencing an increase in premature ventricular contractions (PVCs) and a newly admitted client with paroxysmal onset of atrial fibrillation.

*Answer: 2. The labor and delivery RN needs to be assigned the most stable clients and the ones with the most predictable prognoses; these are the clients in option 2. Do not read into the situation and give the client who has had cardiac catheterization more problems. In option 1, the client who had a possible MI 16 hours ago is at risk for complications, as is the client who underwent cardioversion. In option 3, the client with third-degree heart block is most likely very unstable and may need a pacemaker. In option 4, the client who has had an MI is demonstrating signs of ventricular irritability, and the client with atrial fibrillation will need to be evaluated.*

#### Question 2

The nurse is assigned a group of clients for care. Which client would the nurse assess first?

1. A client who had surgery 2 days ago and who is complaining of pain.
2. An older adult client reported to have increasing confusion and lethargy.
3. A newly admitted client with a serum blood urea nitrogen (BUN) level of 32 mg/dL (11.43 mmol/L).
4. A hypertensive client complaining of epigastric discomfort and midsternum chest pain.

*Answer: 4. The client with chest pain is at greatest risk of experiencing immediate problems. This client needs to be evaluated immediately. Option 1, the client who had surgery, is experiencing pain. This is important but not alarming. Pain control needs to be addressed as soon as possible. In option 2, the client with increased*

lethargy and confusion needs to be evaluated. The confusion and lethargy are increasing; therefore, they were present before this time. These are psychosocial needs that need to be addressed; however, with the information presented, they do not represent an immediate physical problem. The newly admitted client in option 3 has a slightly elevated BUN level. This could be related to hydration problems, but the client is not presented in an unstable situation.*

#### Question 3

A cardiac client turns on his call light and tells the nurse he is experiencing chest pain. What is the first nursing action?

1. Administer oxygen to the client at 4 L/min through a nasal cannula.
2. Assess heart sounds for the presence of ectopic beats.
3. Auscultate breath sounds and maintain airway.
4. Determine what the client was doing before the onset of pain.

*Answer: 1. When a client complains of chest pain, oxygen should be started immediately and then vital signs should be further assessed. In the stem of the question, a cardiac client with chest pain is presented; that is enough critical assessment information for a nursing action. It is assumed that the nurse has an order for the oxygen. Further assessment will determine the status of the vital signs, and options 2 and 4 can be completed. Listening for ectopic beats and determining breath sounds are assessment activities; however, this does not provide further definitive information for determining immediate nursing care. In option 4, whether physical exertion was a factor in the occurrence of the chest pain can be determined later, but this is not an immediate concern. Option 3 gives this client airway problems, and there is no indication in the stem that the airway is an issue at this time.*

#### Question 4

A client has returned from abdominal surgery, and the nurse is assessing the incisional area. The dressing has some bright red blood on it, and on closer inspection, the nurse determines that there is a loop of bowel protruding. What is the best nursing action?

1. Remove the dressing and place a sterile dressing soaked in saline on the wound with dry reinforcement dressings on top.
2. Remove the dressing and with sterile gloves apply gentle pressure to replace the exposed bowel.
3. Leave the dressing in place and apply an abdominal pressure dressing to prevent further exposure of the bowel.
4. Immediately notify the health care provider and then cleanse the wound area with sterile saline solution and replace the dressing.

*Answer: 1. The best nursing action is to cover the exposed bowel with a sterile dressing soaked in saline to prevent drying and tissue damage to the exposed bowel; then the surgeon or health care provider should be notified. Option 2 should not be done, because there may be vascular impairment to the bowel below the surface. In option 3, the dressing needs to be replaced with a moist one to protect the bowel. In option 4, the wound needs to be covered with the moist dressing before notifying the doctor. The wound should not be cleansed because it is not a dirty wound.*

**Check Out the Question!**
- Read the question from beginning to end.
- Check for words that establish the question as asking for a priority: *first action, priority nursing action, most important,* or *best.*
- Is the answer going to be a true or positive statement? Or is the question asking for an answer that is a negative or false statement? Words such as *not working, contraindication,* and *avoid* indicate answers that are giving negative or false statements.
- Rephrase the question in your own words. Do you understand what the question is asking?

**Now Go for the Options**
- Look at option 1: Is it true or false? Does it answer what the question is asking?
- Go through every option: Eliminate it if it is not a correct answer; keep it around if it is a possible right answer.
- If option 2 is a good option, but option 3 is better, then eliminate option 2! After all options have been evaluated, what is left? If you are left with only one option, great—that's the answer!
- If you are left with two options, go back and reread the question; decide which of the two options is best, select it, and move on.

## Strategies for Evaluating Multiple-Choice Questions

Test-taking strategies are beneficial during nursing school and on the NCLEX. Start using them on current examinations. Implementing testing strategies now will help increase test scores in school in addition to being one more step toward success on the NCLEX (Box 1-2).

### Question Characteristics

The majority of questions on the NCLEX and on nursing school examinations are multiple-choice format. This is the type of test question that is the most familiar to candidates.

### Stem of the Question

The *stem* presents information or describes a client situation. The part of the stem that asks the question will present a problem or situation. The question may be presented as a complete or an incomplete sentence. One of the options presented will most correctly answer the question or complete the sentence (Figure 1-3).

### Options

There are four options from which to choose an answer.

- Three options are distracters; they are designed to create a distraction from the correct answer.
- One option correctly answers the question asked in the stem.
- There is only one correct response; no partial credit is given for another answer.

## SPECIFIC STRATEGIES AND EXAMPLES OF MULTIPLE-CHOICE QUESTIONS

### Read the Question Carefully, Without Reading Into It

- *Read the question carefully before ever looking at or considering the options.* If you glance through the options before understanding the question, you may pick up key words that will affect the way you perceive the question.

  It is important to understand the question and not formulate an opinion about the answer before you understand the question. On a paper-and-pencil test, cover the answers with your hand or a note card. If you practice this strategy before taking the NCLEX, you will be able to focus on the question without physically covering the answers when taking a test on the computer.
- *Do not read extra meaning into the question.* The question is asking for specific information; if it appears to be simple "common sense," then assume it is simple. Do not look for a hidden meaning in a question. Avoid asking yourself, "what if . . . ?" or speculating about the future ("maybe the client will . . ."). Don't make the client any sicker than he or she already is!

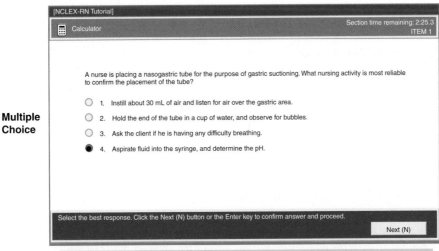

**FIGURE 1-3** Multiple-choice question.

*Example:* A bronchoscopy was performed on a client at 7:00 a.m. The client returns to his room, and the nurse plans to assist him with his morning care. The client refuses the morning care. What is the best nursing action regarding the morning care for this client?

1. Perform all of his morning care to prevent him from becoming short of breath.
2. Avoid morning care and continue to monitor vital signs and assess swallowing reflexes.
3. Postpone the morning care until the client is more comfortable and can participate.
4. Cancel all of the morning care because it is not necessary to perform it after a bronchoscopy.

*The correct answer is 3. The question is asking for a nursing judgment regarding morning care. Do not read into the question and make it more difficult by trying to put in information relating to respiratory care, such as checking for gag and swallowing reflexes.*

## Make Sure You Know What the Question Is Asking

- *Make sure you understand exactly what information the question is asking.* Determine whether the question is stated in a positive (true) or negative (false) format.
- *Watch for words that provide direction to the question.* A positive or true stem may include the following: "indicates the client understands," "the best nursing action is," "the preoperative teaching would include," or "the best nursing assignment is." Also watch for words in the stem that have a negative meaning so that the question is asking for a response that is *not* accurate or is false. Phrases such as "is contraindicated," "the client should *avoid*," "indicate the client *does not understand*," "does not occur," and "indicates (medication, equipment, nursing action) is *not working*" are negative indicators. The question is asking for information that is not accurate or actions the nurse would not take. The following words or phrases change the direction of the question: *except, never, avoid, least, contraindicated, would not occur.* It may help to rephrase the question in your own words to better understand what information is being requested.

*Example:* Clients with coronary artery disease (CAD) go through several stages before becoming severely compromised. In considering the pathophysiology of CAD, the nurse would identify what physical response that does not occur in the early stages of CAD?

1. Decreased urine output.
2. Dyspnea on exercise.
3. Anginal pain relieved by rest.
4. Increased serum triglyceride levels.

*Rephrase the question: What is not a characteristic finding in the early stages of CAD? It is important to identify the key point "early stages of CAD" and the key words "does not occur." If you miss these essential points, you do not understand the question, and chances are you will not choose the correct answer. The correct answer is option 1; a decrease in urine output occurs when cardiac disease is advanced enough to cause a severe decrease in*
cardiac output and renal perfusion. All the other options occur earlier in CAD.*

## Consider Information About Timing

- *Watch where the client is in the disease process or condition he or she is experiencing.* Examples of this are phrases such as "immediately postoperatively," "the first postoperative day," and "experienced a myocardial infarction this morning."

*Example:* A client had a cardiac catheterization through the left femoral artery. During the first few hours after the cardiac catheterization procedure, which nursing action would be most important?
*Rewording: What is the most important nursing care in the first few hours after a cardiac catheterization?*

1. Check his temperature every 2 hours and monitor catheter insertion site for inflammation.
2. Elevate the head of his bed 90 degrees and keep the affected extremity straight.
3. Evaluate his blood pressure and respiratory status every 15 minutes for 4 to 6 hours.
4. Check his pedal and femoral pulses every 15 minutes for the first hour and then every 30 minutes.

*The correct answer is 4. The phrase "during the first few hours after the procedure" is important in answering this question correctly. The danger of hemorrhage and hematoma at the puncture site is greatest during this time. The question also asks for the most important nursing care. In option 3, it is important to evaluate vital signs, but it is not required that they be evaluated every 15 minutes for 4 to 6 hours if client is stable. Option 4 is critical in the first few hours after a cardiac catheterization.*

## Consider Characteristics of the Condition

- *Before considering the options, think about the characteristics of the condition and critical nursing concepts.* What are the nursing priorities in caring for a client with this condition/procedure/medication/problem?

*Example:* A woman who gave birth 3 days ago returns to the clinic with complaints of soreness and fullness in her breasts and states that she wants to stop breastfeeding her infant until her breasts feel better. What is the best nursing response?
*This is a positive question. The answer will be a true statement. Think about breastfeeding and the common discomforts and problems the client encounters. Don't look at the options yet. Think, "Is it normal to have fullness and soreness in the breasts during the first 3 days of lactation, and what happens if she stops breastfeeding the infant?" Now evaluate the options:*

1. Show the client how to apply a breast binder to decrease the discomfort and the production of milk.
2. Tell the client that breast fullness may be a sign of infection and she will not be able to continue breastfeeding.
3. Suggest to the client that she decrease her fluid intake for the next 24 hours to temporarily suppress lactation.
4. Explain to the client that the breast discomfort is normal and that the infant's sucking will promote the flow of milk.

*In this question, option 4 is correct. Initially, breast soreness may occur for about 2 to 3 minutes at the beginning of each feeding until the letdown reflex is established. Options 1, 2, and 3 would decrease her milk production; the question did not state that she wanted to quit breastfeeding permanently.*

## Identify the Step in the Nursing Process

• *Identify the step in the nursing process being tested.* Remember that you must have adequate *assessment* data before you move through the steps of the nursing process. Is there adequate information presented in the stem of the question to determine appropriate nursing planning or intervention? Is the correct nursing action to obtain further assessment data? Look for key words that can assist you in determining what type of information is being requested.

*Example:* An 85-year-old client from a residential care facility is brought into the emergency department. Numerous bruises and abrasions in various stages of healing are present on the client's face and arms. The attendant from the residential facility explains that the client fell down. What is the priority nursing action?

1. Call the residential facility and ask for an incident report.
2. Put ice on the bruises and cover the abrasions with protective gauze.
3. Notify the supervisor regarding the possibility of an abusive situation.
4. Perform a head-to-toe assessment and determine the extent of the injuries.

*The correct answer is option 4, to determine or assess the extent of injuries. The stem of the question did not present adequate information with which to make a nursing judgment, and the client's physiologic needs are the priority. Option 1 does not immediately alleviate pain or assist the client. Options 2 and 3 relate to nursing actions that may be done after the immediate injuries and needs have been assessed. Focus on the client; priority setting and physiologic needs must be addressed first.*

## What to Do If You're Confused

• *Confused at this point?* What if, after reading the question, you aren't sure what the question is even asking? Take a deep breath, reread the question, and ask yourself, "What is the main topic of the question?" Now read the option choices, not to eliminate options or select a correct answer, but to get a clue as to the *direction* of the question. It might be helpful to read the options from the bottom up (start with option 4, rather than option 1) to help your brain focus on the options.

*Example:* A mother brings in a toddler with pediculosis capitis. A prescription of 1% permethrin is given to her. What is important for the nurse to teach the mother?
*Ask yourself: Is the question asking about prevention of pediculosis, complications, prevention of spread of the disease, or treatment? Check out the options. Is there an indication in the options as to the direction of the question?*

1. Medication should be applied daily for 1 week with an additional follow-up treatment in 7 days.

2. Clothing, toys, and personal belongings of other family members do not require any special care.
3. Solution should be applied today and applied again if nits are still visible in 24 hours.
4. Allow the medication to remain in contact with the scalp for 10 minutes and then thoroughly rinse.

*After checking out the options, it appears that the question is asking for teaching implications for the mother regarding the use of the medication, 1% permethrin. Now that you have determined what you need to identify, you can begin the process of elimination of the options until you have found the correct answer.*

The correct answer is option 4. The 1% permethrin solution needs to remain on the scalp for 10 minutes before the hair is rinsed. Option 1 is too frequent for the medication to be used. Option 2 is incorrect, because the child's clothing and toys, as well as clothing and toys of the siblings, will need to be treated. Option 3 is not correct because medication should be reapplied in 7 days.

## Focus on the Options

• *Don't focus on predicting a right answer! Frequently, the answer you anticipate is not going to be an option!* Keep in mind the characteristics and concepts of nursing care for a client with the condition or problem in the situation presented. Eliminate options: Every time you eliminate an option, you increase your chance of selecting a correct answer. If all of the options are plausible, then rank the options. The first one is the highest priority, and the fourth one is the lowest priority. Which one is the first action or answers the question?

*Example:* A client has an ulcer 2 in × 2 in (5 cm × 5 cm) on the calf of his right leg. The area around the ulcer is inflamed, and the ulcer is draining purulent fluid. The vital signs are pulse, 114 beats/min; respiration, 22 breaths/min; temperature, 101°F (38.3°C). Which order will the nurse implement first?
*Reword the question: The client has an infection in the ulcer on his leg. His temperature is elevated, and so is his pulse; this is a normal response to infection. Of the orders listed here, what nursing actions do I need to do first?*

1. Administer ceftriaxone, 1 g, intravenously every 4 hours.
2. Perform blood cultures ×2, 20 minutes apart and drawn from different sites.
3. Apply bacitracin ointment topically to leg ulcer three times a day.
4. Administer acetaminophen, 650 mg suppository, every 4 hours for temperature greater than 101.8°F (38.7°C).

*Rank the options:*

*1st—Option 2; blood cultures must be obtained before antibiotic is administered.*

*2nd—Option 1 needs to done after the blood cultures have been drawn.*

*3rd—Option 4 will not produce any immediate response or assistance in treating the problem, although it will make the client more comfortable.*

*4th—Option 3 will help reduce the infection, but the priority is to obtain the culture and then for the antibiotic to be started.*

Here is another approach to the options:

*Consider option 1—This is an antibiotic that will begin to fight the infection.*

*Consider option 2—This is important to do to identify the causative bacteria. This is more important now than option 1; eliminate option 1.*

*Consider option 3—This is treating the infection topically. It will cause a decrease in the surface bacteria, but the blood cultures are still a priority. Eliminate this option because both options 1 and 2 are more important.*

*Consider option 4—This is treating the symptoms rather than the cause of the problem, which is not as important as option 1 or option 2; eliminate it.*

*All of these options are feasible for treating this; however, obtaining the blood culture is the most important (option 2). If you had approached this question with a specific answer in mind (give an antibiotic), you would have found that answer; however, it would have been wrong.*

## Evaluate the Options

- *Evaluate all of the options in a systematic manner.* After you understand the question, read all options carefully. Remember, distracters are designed to be plausible to the situation and thus to "distract" you from the correct answer. All the options may be correct, but only one will be the best answer.

*Example:* A client has just returned to his room from the recovery room after a lumbar laminectomy and is in stable condition. In considering possible complications the client might experience in the next few hours, what nursing action is most important?

1. Monitor vital signs every 4 hours.
2. Assess breath sounds every 2 hours.
3. Evaluate every 2 hours for urinary retention.
4. Check when he last had a bowel movement.

*All of these options are plausible for the situation. However, consider that this is the client's operative day, he is currently stable, and the question is asking for complications he might encounter in the next few hours after lumbar laminectomy. Options 1 and 4 are not appropriate at this period of postoperative recovery; vital signs should be checked more often, and constipation can be more effectively addressed at a later time—eliminate these from consideration. Option 2 would be appropriate if respiratory problems were anticipated; however, there is no indication of respiratory compromise. (Remember, don't always select airway-related answers.) The correct answer is option 3, because urinary retention is a common problem in the immediate postoperative period after a lumbar laminectomy.*

## True or False

- *As you read the options, eliminate those that you know are not correct. Consider each option as true or false.* This will help narrow the field of choice. When you select an answer or

eliminate an option, you should have a specific reason for doing so. Correctly eliminating options will increase your chances of selecting the correct answer.

*Example:* A client is in her third trimester of pregnancy and is scheduled for an abdominal ultrasonogram. The nurse explains to the client that results of this examination will reveal *what* information regarding the fetus?

1. Maturity of the fetus's lungs. *(No, this is false; the ultrasound does not show any evidence of surfactant or maturity level of the lungs.)*
2. Presence of congenital heart defect. *(No, this is false; the ultrasound is not specific enough to reveal congenital heart defects, but it will show fetal cardiac movement.)*
3. Gestational age. *(Yes, this is true; ultrasonography gives an overall picture of bone formation [biparietal diameter (BPD)], thereby indicating gestational age.)*
4. Rh factor antibody level. *(No, this is false; this level must be determined by a blood test to evaluate for isoimmunization or hemolytic disease of the newborn.)*

*After a systematic evaluation of the options, option 3 is the correct answer.*

## Identify Similarities

- *Identify similarities in the options.* Frequently the options will contain similar information, and sometimes you can eliminate similar options. If three options are similar, the different one may be the correct answer. When two of the options are similar and one of those options is not any better than the other, both of them are probably wrong, so start looking for another answer. Sometimes three of the options have similar characteristics; the option that is different may be the correct answer.

*Example:* The nurse is assisting a client to identify foods that would meet the requirements for a high-protein, low-residue diet. Which foods would represent correct choices for this diet?

1. Roast beef, slice of white bread.
2. Fried chicken, green peas.
3. Broiled fish, green beans.
4. Cottage cheese, tomatoes.

*The correct answer is option 1, for both high-protein and low-residue qualities. Options 1, 2, and 3 all contain a meat or fish that would be needed for a high-protein diet, therefore option 4 can be eliminated. Options 2, 3, and 4 all contain a vegetable that has a skin, making these high-residue choices. Note that the NCLEX will not focus on dishes that contain a mixture of foods, in which you would need to know the recipe to answer correctly. Also, unless specified, do not attribute special characteristics to a food; if a food has a special characteristic, it will be stated (e.g., "low-sodium" soup or "low-fat" yogurt).*

## Identify Qualifiers

- *Look for words in the options that are "qualifiers." Every, none, all, always, never,* and *only* are words that have no exceptions. Options containing these words are frequently incorrect. Seldom in health care is anything absolute with no exceptions; thus, you can often eliminate these options. In some situations, the qualifiers are correct, especially when a principle or policy is described. For example, the nurse *always* establishes positive client identification before administering medications. This would be a correct statement. Carefully evaluate qualifiers; they are clues to the correct answer.

*Example:* The nurse is obtaining a specimen from a client's incisional area for a wound culture and sensitivity. What client information will the sensitivity part of the procedure reflect?

1. Presence and characteristics of all bacteria present in the client's wound.
2. Which antibiotics will effectively treat the bacteria present.
3. Differentiation of the bacteria and viruses present in the wound.
4. All the treatments to which the bacteria are responsive.

*Options 1 and 4 contain the word "all." If you did not know the answer, you could eliminate options 1 and 4. Identifying all the bacteria and all the treatments is not feasible from a culture and sensitivity. This would give you a 50% chance of finding the right answer, which is option 2. Although a part of option 3 is correct (differentiating the bacteria present [not viruses]), all of the options must be correct for it to be a correct answer, which is why it is incorrect.*

## Select the Comprehensive Answer

- *Choose the most comprehensive answer.* All of the options may be correct, but one option may *include* the other three options or need to be considered first.

*Example:* The nurse is planning to teach a client with diabetes about his condition. Before the nurse provides instruction, what is most important to evaluate? The client's:

1. Required dietary modifications.
2. Understanding of carbohydrate counting.
3. Ability to administer insulin.
4. Present understanding of diabetes.

*Options 1, 2, and 3 are certainly important considerations in diabetic education; however, they cannot be initiated until the nurse evaluates the client's knowledge of his or her disease state, which is the reason that option 4 is the correct answer. When two options appear to say the same thing but in different words, then look for another answer; that is, eliminate the options that you know are incorrect. Options 1 and 2 both refer to the client's understanding of nutrition.*

## Consider All Information in the Options

- *Some questions may have options that contain several items to consider.* After you are sure you understand what information the question is requesting, evaluate each part of the option. Is the option appropriate to what the question is asking? If an option contains one incorrect item,

the entire option is incorrect. All of the items listed in the option must be correct if that option is to be the correct answer to the question.

*Example:* In evaluating the laboratory data of a client experiencing renal failure, the nurse would identify what findings as indicative of increasing renal failure?

1. Increased BUN level, hyperkalemia, decreased creatinine clearance.
2. Increased hemoglobin, hyponatremia, increased urine electrolytes.
3. High fasting blood glucose level, increased prothrombin time.
4. Increased platelets, increased urine specific gravity, proteinuria.

*Option 1 is correct. In a methodic evaluation of the items in the options, you can eliminate options. The item "increased hemoglobin and urine electrolytes" in option 2 and the item "increased urine specific gravity" in option 4 make these two options incorrect, because they are not typical symptoms seen in renal failure. Option 3 has nothing to do with renal failure; the blood glucose level is associated more with diabetes and endocrine problems. Prothrombin time measures anticoagulation.*

## Reread the Question

- *After you have selected an answer, reread the question.* Does the answer you chose give the information the question is asking for? Sometimes the options are correct but do not answer the question.

*Example:* An 88-year-old client has previously been alert, oriented, and active. The nursing assistant reports that on awakening this morning, the client was disoriented and confused. What initial action would the nurse take to determine the possible cause of this change in the client's behavior?

1. Review the history for any previous episodes of this type of behavior.
2. Call the health care provider and discuss the changes in the client's behavior.
3. Do a thorough neurologic evaluation to evaluate the specific changes in behavior.
4. Evaluate for the presence of a urinary tract infection and for adequate hydration.

*Option 4 is the only answer that supplies what the question asked for ("determine the possible cause of this change"). The most common cause of a sudden change in the behavior of an older adult client is a significant physiologic change, often an infection (commonly in the urinary tract) or dehydration. Options 1 and 3 relate more to the gradual behavior changes seen in the progression of dementia and do nothing "to determine the possible cause." Option 2 also does not provide any assistance in determining the cause of the behavior change; further nursing assessment needs to be conducted before calling for assistance.*

## Alternate Format Questions

In an effort to improve and more effectively assess the entry-level nurse, the NCSBN has introduced "alternate format questions" to the examination. These questions were included on the NCLEX beginning in April 2003. There is no established percentage of alternate-format items a candidate will receive. The alternate-format questions that have been previously validated are placed in the test item pools and are randomly selected to meet the items on the test plan and the established level of difficulty. The NCSBN has not specified a number of alternate format questions that will be included in a candidate's test bank. A candidate should expect several alternate format questions. It is important to consider that there will be 15 pretest or unscored items in the first 75 questions on every candidate's examination. Within those 15 items, there may be several unscored alternate format items. It is important to answer all the questions to the best of your ability because you do not know which questions are scored items and which are unscored items.

The alternate-format questions should not have any effect on what or how you study. The content on the alternate-format questions is from the same test plan as the other questions. The test-taking strategies are essentially the same with minor modifications. In other words, there is no reason to be alarmed about the alternate format questions; they are testing the same information, just in a different type of question. Types of alternate format questions include:

- Multiple-response
- Fill-in-the-blank
- Hot spot
- Ordered response (drag and drop)
- Chart or exhibit
- Graphic options
- Audio

Examples of each type of question, screenshots displaying how these questions appear on the companion Evolve site, and test strategies for each type of question are included in the following pages. *All item types may include multimedia such as charts, tables, graphics, sound, and video.*

## Multiple Response

Multiple-response items require you to select all of the options that apply to the question. The items have more than four options from which to select and will clearly state "Select all that apply." Using the mouse, you will select each item to be included in the answer; consider each item and make a decision whether it is to be included in the correct answer. The options are preceded by square boxes, and you can check more than one box. You must select all the answers to the question that are correct. If you do not select all of the correct options that apply to the question, the answer will be considered wrong.

**Testing Strategy:** Think about the question presented in Figure 1-4. Standard plus droplet precautions will be used for this client. What is added to standard precautions when droplet precautions are included? Go through all of the options and decide which options are true and are something the nurse should do; then select all of the true options that apply to this client.

*Answer: Options 1, 4, and 5. In option 1, yes (true), the nurse is going to provide morning care and have direct contact with the client, therefore, gloves should be worn. Option 2, no (false), the suctioning supplies should be left in the room. Option 3, no (false), the gown and mask are disposed of in the client's room. Option 4, yes (true), a mask is necessary if the nurse is to come within 3 feet of the client, which the nurse can expect to do when providing or assisting with morning care. Option 5, yes (true), a gown should be worn because the nurse is going to be close to and have direct contact with the client. Option 6, no (false), the stethoscope should not be taken into the client's room; if it is taken into the room, it should be left in the room.*

## Fill-in-the-Blank

Fill-in-the-blank questions are frequently presented for medication dosage calculations, IV drip calculations, or intake and output calculations, just to name a few (Figure 1-5). A drop-down calculator is provided on the computer screen.

**Multiple Response**

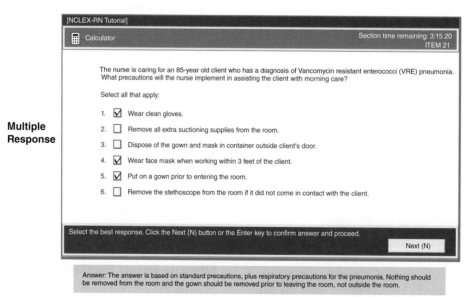

**FIGURE 1-4** Alternate item format question—multiple response.

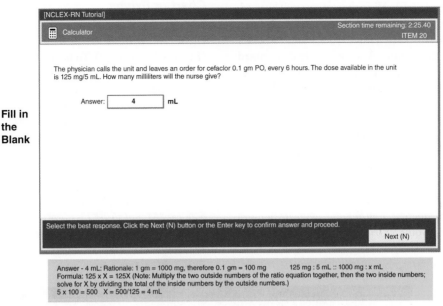

Answer - 4 mL: Rationale: 1 gm = 1000 mg, therefore 0.1 gm = 100 mg      125 mg : 5 mL :: 1000 mg : x mL
Formula: 125 x X = 125X (Note: Multiply the two outside numbers of the ratio equation together, then the two inside numbers;
solve for X by dividing the total of the inside numbers by the outside numbers.)
5 x 100 = 500    X = 500/125 = 4 mL

**FIGURE 1-5** Alternate item format question—fill in the blank.

With calculation questions, the final unit of measurement is always provided. Only the number is placed in the answer box. Check the items necessary to make this calculation. For example, is it necessary to make conversions from grams to milligrams or from liters to milliliters? Make sure all of the units of measure needed in the final answer are in the same system of measurement.

Memorize the formulas necessary to calculate the drug dosages and conversions. The number of decimal places to be included in the answer is indicated in the question. Do not round any numbers until you have the final answer. You should not enter any other characters except those necessary to form a number.

## Hot Spot

In a hot-spot question (Figure 1-6), you will be presented with a graphic and asked to identify a specific item, area, or location on the graphic by clicking on it with the mouse.

*Answer: The "hot spot" (in this case, the correct area to assess the apical heart rate) is at the point of maximum impulse (PMI), which is located at the fifth intercostal space, just to the left of the sternal border. In this situation, you would place the mouse over the area and click on that area.*

## Ordered Response (Drag and Drop)

In an ordered response or drag-and-drop question, several steps or actions are listed, and your job is to place them in a

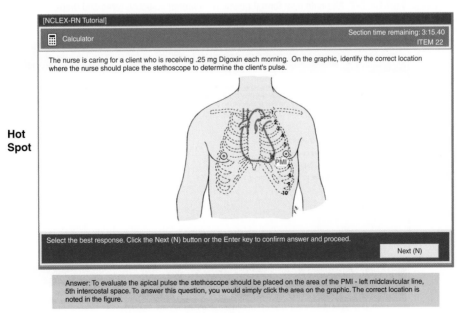

Answer: To evaluate the apical pulse the stethoscope should be placed on the area of the PMI - left midclavicular line, 5th intercostal space. To answer this question, you would simply click the area on the graphic. The correct location is noted in the figure.

**FIGURE 1-6** Alternate item format question—hot spot.

correct sequence (Figure 1-7). All of the options will be used, but you must place them in the correct order. The first thing to do is to decide in what order you want to place the options or rank the actions. After you have determined your answer, click on the option you want to place first, "drag" that option over, and place it in the first box. Then select the option you want to place second, drag that option over, and place it in the next box. Continue this process until you have used all of the options present. Practice by considering how you would answer the question in Figure 1-7.

*Answer: The client should be placed in a semi-Fowler's position before oxygen administration is started; an antipyretic medication should then be given. This action addresses current needs. Next, encourage intake of clear liquids to decrease viscosity of secretions. Finally, provide instruction regarding risk factors (psychosocial need).*

## Chart or Exhibit

In this type of question, a client situation or problem and client information are provided in a chart or an exhibit (Figures 1-8 to 1-12). To begin, click on the tab on the bottom of the screen to see the exhibit; then click on the tabs within the exhibit to find the information needed to answer the question. There may be several tabs to click on; check the information included within each tab and determine whether it is pertinent to the situation.

*Interpretation of information: Client received morphine 10 mg IM at 11:00 a.m., became lethargic, and slept for the next 5 hours. He received hydrocodone PO at 4:00 p.m. and was comfortable for the next 4 hours. The doctor's orders are current for both the IM and the PO medication for pain.*

*Answer: 4. Give the hydrocodone, PO, for pain at this time. It is preferable to give a client a PO pain medication than a*

**Drag and Drop**

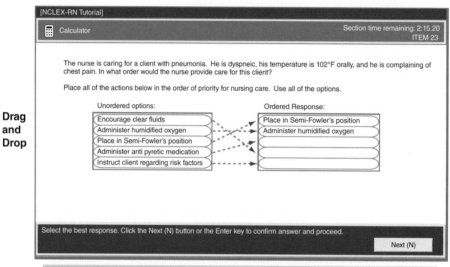

**FIGURE 1-7** Alternate item format question—ordered response (drag and drop).

**Chart or Exhibit**

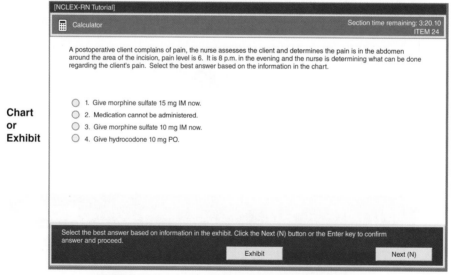

**FIGURE 1-8** Alternate item format question—exhibit item.

**Chart
or
Exhibit**

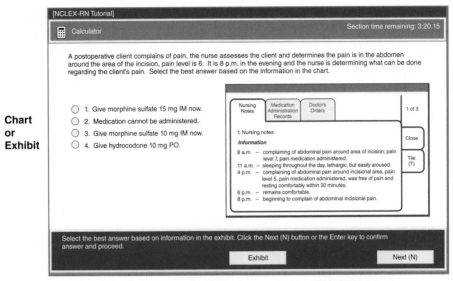

**FIGURE 1-9** Alternate item format question—exhibit item with first tab open.

**Chart
or
Exhibit**

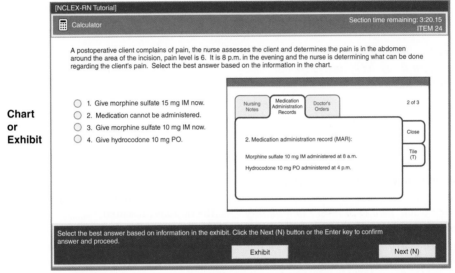

**FIGURE 1-10** Alternate item format question—second tab on exhibit item.

**Chart
or
Exhibit**

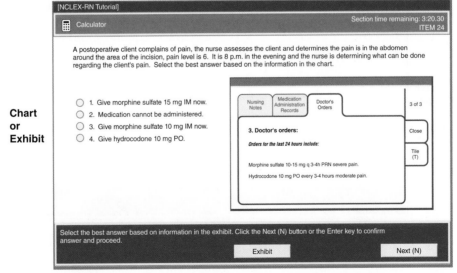

**FIGURE 1-11** Alternate item format question—third tab on exhibit item.

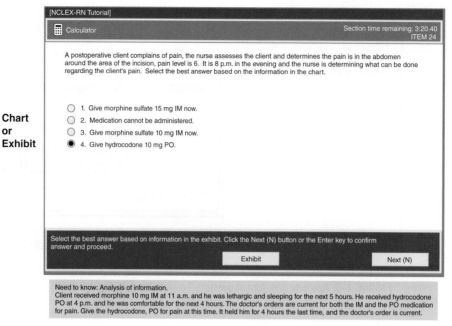

**FIGURE 1-12** Alternate item format question—analysis and selection of an answer for exhibit item.

parenteral pain medication. *The hydrocodone provided effective pain relief for 4 hours when it was administered the last time, and the doctor's order is current.*

### Graphic Options

In this type of question, graphics instead of text are used for the answer options (Figure 1-13). You will need to select the appropriate graphic answer. This is similar to a multiple-choice question; the only difference is viewing graphics as the answer options.

*Answer: 4. The nurse would need to intervene immediately if a client demonstrates ventricular fibrillation, which is indicative of a life-threatening dysrhythmia. The priority for this client will be defibrillation and cardiopulmonary resuscitation*

(CPR). *Option 1 is normal sinus rhythm with multifocal premature ventricular contractions (PVCs). Option 2 is sinus tachycardia. Option 3 is sinus bradycardia.*

### Audio

Audio questions will tell you to put on the headphones to listen to the audio clip of information (Figure 1-14). You will need to click on the "play" button to hear the information. The information may be replayed if necessary. After listening to the information, you will select an answer from the options presented.

*Answer: 1. Bowel sounds are noted on the audio clip, which means that peristalsis has returned to the gastrointestinal tract, and the client can begin a clear liquid diet. If bowel*

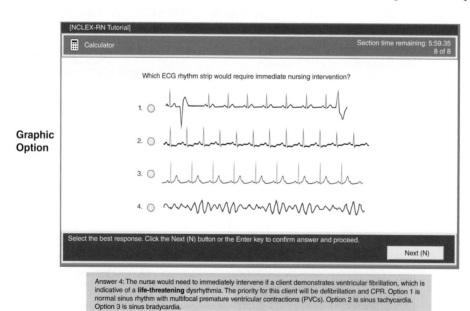

**FIGURE 1-13** Alternate item format question—graphic options.

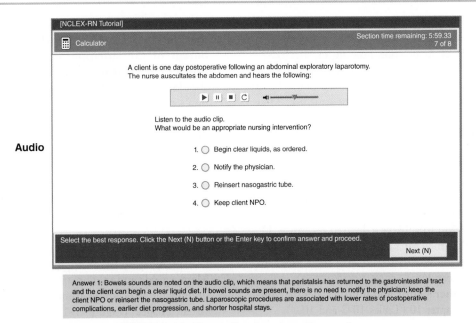

FIGURE 1-14 Alternate item format question—audio.

*sounds are present, there is no need to notify the physician, keep the client NPO, or reinsert the nasogastric tube. Laparoscopic procedures are associated with lower rates of post-operative complications, earlier diet progression, and shorter hospital stays.*

## Therapeutic Nursing Process: Principles of Communication

Throughout the examination, there will be questions requiring use of the principles of therapeutic communication. In therapeutic communication questions, do not assume the client is being manipulative or is in control of how he or she feels. Psychosocial problems or mental health problems are most often not under the conscious control of the client.

**TEST ALERT:** Use therapeutic communication techniques to provide support to client and the family; establish a trusting nurse–client relationship; assess psychosocial, spiritual, cultural, and occupational factors affecting care; allow time to communicate with client/family and significant others; provide therapeutic environment.

- **Situations requiring use of therapeutic communication are not always centered on a psychiatric client.** Frequently these questions are centered on the client experiencing stress and anxiety. There may be questions relating to therapeutic communication in the care of clients experiencing stress, anxiety related to a specific client situation, or a change in body image as a result of physiologic problems.
- **Look for responses that focus on the concerns of the client.** Do not focus on the concerns of the nurse, hospital, or physician. Determine whether the client is the central focus of the question or whether the question pertains to a spouse or significant other.

- **Watch for responses that are open ended and encourage the client to express how he or she feels.** Clients frequently experience difficulty in expressing their feelings. Focus on responses that encourage a client to describe how he or she feels. These are frequently open-ended statements made by the nurse.
- **Eliminate responses that are not honest and direct.** To build trust and promote a positive relationship, it is important to be honest with the client. Options that include telling the client "don't worry," or "everything is going to be all right," or "your doctor knows best" are wrong answers.
- **Look for responses that indicate acceptance of the client.** Regardless of whether the client's views or moral values are in agreement with yours, it is important to respect his or her views and beliefs. Responses that involve telling clients what they *should* or *should not* be doing are often wrong answers (e.g., telling an alcoholic that she should quit drinking or telling a depressed client that he should not feel that way).
- **Be careful about responses that give opinions or advice on the client's situation.** Do not assume an authoritarian position. You should not insist that the client follow your advice (e.g., quit drinking, exercise more, quit smoking).
- **Do not select options or responses that block further interaction.** These options are frequently presented as closed statements or questions that encourage a yes-or-no answer from the client. Better responses are those that indicate an expectation of a more revealing verbal response from the client. *Examples:* "Are you feeling better today?" The client can just answer no to this question. It is better to ask, "How are you feeling today compared with yesterday?" Likewise, it is better to ask, "How did you feel when your family visited today?" rather than "Did your family visit today?"

- **Look for responses that reflect, restate, or paraphrase feelings the client expressed.** Look for responses that encourage the client to describe how he or she feels—responses that reflect, restate, or paraphrase feelings the client expresses. An option such as "You should not feel that way" is bound to be a wrong answer. It is better to ask, "How did that make you feel?"
- **Do not ask "why" a client feels the way he or she does.** Most of the time, if a client understood why he or she felt a certain way, the client would be able to do something about it. The most common answer when a nurse asks a client why he or she feels a certain way is "I don't know," which does not help anyone.
- **Do not use coercion to achieve a desired response.** Do not tell clients that they can't have their lunch until they get out of bed or bribe children to take their medicine with a promise of candy.
- **See examples of therapeutic and nontherapeutic communication in** Chapter 10 (Tables 10-3 and 10-4).

## TIPS FOR TEST-TAKING SUCCESS

- **Do not indiscriminately change answers.** On a paper-and-pencil test, if you go back and change an answer, you should have a specific reason for doing so. Sometimes you do remember information and realize you answered the question incorrectly. However, students often talk themselves out of the correct answer and change it to the incorrect one. The good news is that you cannot go back to previously answered questions on the NCLEX. At the point at which the examination asks you to confirm your answer, review the strategies used to answer the question, confirm your answer, and move on to the next question.
- **Watch your timing. Do not spend too much time on one question.** It is important to track your timing on practice examinations. This will help you be more comfortable with timing on computer testing. The NCLEX will allow you a total of 6 hours to complete the examination. When you are taking a practice test, plan to spend about a minute on each question. Some questions you will answer quickly; others may take some time. Do not spend more than 2 minutes deliberating the answer to a question. If you do not have a good direction for the right answer in 2 minutes, then you probably don't know the answer. Eliminate all of the options you can, pick the best one, and move on. (Remember, you are not supposed to know *all* of the right answers.) Plan for an hour of practice testing, select 60 questions, and answer the questions using testing strategies. After answering the questions, review the correct answers and focus on what questions you missed and why. Practice your timing and application of test strategies so you will be comfortable with timing and the progression of questions on the NCLEX.
- **The NCLEX is a nursing competency examination, and the correct answer will focus on nursing knowledge, safety, and the provision of nursing care.** The examination does not focus on medical management or making a medical diagnosis.

- **Eliminate distracters that include the assumption that the client would not understand or would be ignorant of the situation and those distracters that protect clients from worry.** For example, "The client should not be told she has cancer because it would upset her too much" would almost certainly be an incorrect answer.
- **There is no pattern of correct answers.** The examination is compiled by a computer, and the position of the correct answers is selected at random. So do not believe those who say to pick option 3 when you are guessing.

## STUDY HABITS

### Study Effectively

1. **Use memory aids, mind mapping, and mnemonics.** Memory aids and mind mapping are tools that assist you in drawing associations from other ideas with the use of visual images (Figure 1-15). Mnemonics are words, phrases, or other techniques that help you remember information. Images, pictures, and mnemonics will stay with you longer than written text information.
2. **Develop 3 × 5 cards with critical information.** Do not overload the card; put a statement or question on one side and answers or follow-up information on the other side. For example, on one side you might write "low potassium," and on the other side you would list the relevant values. Another card might say "nursing care for hypokalemia" on the front, and on the back, you could list the nursing care. These cards are much easier for you to carry than a load of books or class notes. When you have developed and studied your set of cards with priority information, trade them with friends and see what they have put on their cards. Sets of cards can be used whenever you have only 15 to 20 minutes of study time. Take 20 cards with you to soccer practice, the doctor's office, or anywhere you are going where you will have to sit and wait for a few minutes. This is quick, easy, and effective.
3. **Review class notes the next day.** An effective study habit to develop during school is to review your class notes the day after the class. Set aside time after the class and spend about 30 to 45 minutes reviewing the notes from class. Do the notes make sense to you, or are you unclear on the meaning of some of the areas? Correlate the notes and the visuals the instructor presented with the information in the textbook. It is important to take the time now to understand the information presented the previous day because it is fresher in your mind and you are more receptive to learning. By reviewing the information after the class presentation, you more effectively and positively reinforce the learning process.
4. **Plan your study time when you are most receptive to learning.** Do not wait until the end of the day when you have finished everything else. It is difficult to get up at 6:00 a.m., work all day, deal with family activities, and finally realize at 10:30 p.m. that you are just too tired to study. You may feel guilty that you were not able to study

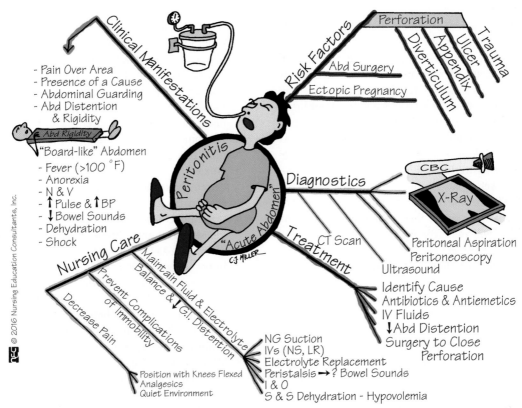

**FIGURE 1-15** Peritonitis. (From Zerwekh, J., Garneau, A., & Miller, C. J. [2017]. *Digital collection of the memory notebooks of nursing* [4th ed.]. Chandler, AZ: Nursing Education Consultants, Inc.)

for the intended 2 hours that evening. Schedule your study time; it may be easier for you to study for 2 hours before leaving school than it may be to study for 2 hours when you get home.

5. **Set a schedule and let everyone know the schedule.** For example, when you set aside 1 hour for review on the day after your class, make sure everyone knows this is your study time. Do not expect your family to leave you alone while you study; this is frequently too much to ask, especially of children or a spouse. Go to the library, nursing school, or someone's house where there are no disturbances.

6. **Start planning your NCLEX preparation at the beginning of your last semester in school or 2 to 3 months before you will take the NCLEX.** Do not wait until the week before the examination to start preparing. Even if you were an A student, you still need to review. Information that was presented at the beginning of school, last year, or even last semester may not be current in your knowledge base.

### Set a Study Goal

1. Decide on a study method.
2. Divide the review material into segments.
3. Prioritize the segments; review first the areas in which you feel you are deficient or weak. Leave those areas you

are the most comfortable with and most knowledgeable about for last.

4. Practice testing or an end of the semester assessment examination will help you identify areas in which you need additional review. Review this information in an NCLEX review book, and then if it is not clear or if you need further explanation and information, consult your nursing textbooks.

5. Establish a realistic schedule and follow it. Planning for 8 hours of studying on your day off does not work. Instead, plan for 2 to 4 hours each day (in 20- to 30-minute chunks of time) and maybe 3 to 4 hours on your days off. Let everyone know when you are planning to study and how important it is for you to study.

6. Plan on achieving your study goal several days before the examination.

### Group Study

1. Limit the group to four or five people.
2. Group members should be mature and serious about studying.
3. The group should agree on the planned study schedule.
4. If the group makes you anxious or you do not feel it meets your study needs, do not continue to participate.
5. Group study is effective with the right mix of participants.

## Testing Practice

1. Include testing practice in your schedule.
2. Structure your practice testing.
   - Plan to answer one question per minute. Set aside 10 questions and answer them in 10 minutes; then review the answer and rationale for the question. This will allow you to focus on testing strategies and not break your train of thought by checking the right answers.
   - Evaluate your comfortable pace for answering questions; this will keep you on target with your timing as you practice answering test questions.
   - Do not answer a question and then stop to look up the correct answer. Answer all of the questions in the section you have set aside; then review the correct answers. This will reinforce your test-taking strategies and your test timing.
3. Try to answer the questions as if you were taking the real examination.
4. Use the testing strategies and practice on the questions included at the end of each chapter in the book and on the CD that accompanies this book.
5. Evaluate your practice examinations for problem areas.
   - Test-taking skills: Did you know the material but answer the question incorrectly? In this case, a test-taking strategy can be applied; go back and review the strategies. Can you identify what strategy you should have used to identify the correct answer? By becoming aware of your test-taking habits, you will become more aware of the strategies you need to implement and you can begin to practice them more effectively.
   - Knowledge base: You did not know the material. Make a note of these areas and see whether the content begins to show trends or clusters of information in areas you need to study/review.
6. Evaluate the questions you answered incorrectly. Review the rationale for the right answer and understand why you missed it.
7. Reuse the questions at a later point to review the information again.
8. A CD with additional practice questions can be found in the back of this book. The more questions you practice answering, the more effectively you will implement test-taking strategies.

## DECREASE ANXIETY

Your activities on the day of the examination will strongly influence your level of anxiety. By carefully planning ahead, you can eliminate some anxiety-provoking situations.

1. Review the NCLEX tutorial at the Pearson Vue website. This same tutorial will be your orientation to the computer and the testing process. It should seem like an old friend when you see it.
2. Visit the examination site before the day of the examination. Consider travel time, parking, and time to get to the designated area. Get an early start to allow extra time; you need to arrive at the site 30 minutes before your scheduled testing time.
3. If you have to travel some distance to the examination site, try to spend the night in the immediate vicinity. Don't cram four or five people in one room. Everyone needs his or her own space!
4. Do something pleasant the evening before the examination. This is not the time to cram.
5. Anxiety is contagious. If those around you are extremely anxious, avoid contact with them before the examination.
6. Carefully consider whether you want to go to the testing site with anyone else. If the other person finishes before you do, will it put increased pressure on you to hurry up and finish? You don't need any additional pressures on the day of the examination or while you are taking it.
7. Make sure your meal before the test is a light, healthy one. Avoid eating highly spiced or different foods. This is not the time for a gastrointestinal upset.
8. Wear comfortable clothes. This is not a good time to wear tight clothing or new shoes.
9. Wear clothing of moderate weight. It is difficult to control the temperature to keep everyone comfortable. Wear layers of clothes that can be removed if you get too warm.
10. Wear soft-soled shoes; this decreases the noise in the testing area.
11. Make sure you have the ATT papers and photo ID that are required to gain admission to the examination site.
12. Do not take study material to the examination site. You are not allowed to take it into the testing area, and it is too late to study.
13. Do not panic when you encounter a clinical situation you have not heard of or a situation that increases your anxiety. Take a deep breath, close your eyes, and take a "mini" vacation to one of your favorite places. Give yourself about 30 to 45 seconds and then return to the question. You may have gained a different perspective. Use good test-taking strategies, select an answer, and move on.
14. Reaffirm to yourself that you know the material. This is not the time for self-defeating behavior or negative self-talk. **YOU WILL PASS!** Build your confidence by visualizing yourself in 6 months as an RN working in the area you desire. Create that mental picture of where you want to be and who you want to be—an RN. Use your past successes to bring positive energy and "vibes" to your NCLEX examination. **WE KNOW YOU CAN DO IT!**

# CHAPTER TWO

# Health Implications Across the Life Span

**2**

Development, Family Dynamics, Health Promotion, Nutrition

## GROWTH AND DEVELOPMENT

A. Normal growth and development progresses in a steady, predictable pattern across the life span.
B. When assessing the growth and development of a child or an adult, it is important to consider the characteristics of the developmental stage.
   1. Development progresses in a cephalocaudal (head to toe) manner.
   2. Development progresses from proximal to distal, with a progression from gross to fine motor skills.
C. Psychosocial, cognitive, moral, and spiritual development can be observed to occur in specific patterns as an infant matures.
D. The developmental age of a client is critical to the planning of care in the hospital.
   1. Nurses need to be aware of the major developmental milestones.
   2. Nursing care is planned around the child's developmental level, not his or her chronologic age.
   3. If an infant displays head lag at 6 months or cannot sit with support at 9 months, this is considered a significant developmental lag, and the infant needs to have further developmental/neurologic evaluation (Table 2-1).

**TEST ALERT:** Assess developmental stage of client. Evaluate client and/or family achievement of expected developmental level, especially with consideration to the developmental milestones.

### Anticipatory Guidance for the Family of an Infant

A. Use an infant car seat, facing backward.
B. Put the baby on his or her back to sleep; keep items such as pillows, quilts, bumper pads, stuffed toys, and positional devices out of crib.
C. By 3 to 4 months, infants sleep approximately 15 hours per day.
D. Safety.
   1. Keep one hand on the baby when he or she is on a high surface; baby rolls over around age 3 to 4 months.
   2. Never leave the baby alone with young children or pets.
   3. Baby-proof your home: prevent access to stairs and cabinets; practice pool and tub water safety; avoid exposure to secondhand smoke.
   4. After feeding, place infant on his or her right side.

E. Immunization schedule (Figure 2-1).

**⚠ NURSING PRIORITY:** General contraindications to receiving an immunization include a severe febrile and/or an anaphylactic reaction to a previously administered immunization or to a substance in the immunization.

F. Talk and read to infant; provide visual and auditory stimulation; toys should stimulate hand–eye coordination and provide sensory stimulation; provide 30 to 60 minutes of tummy time per day.
G. To prevent bottle tooth decay, do not put infant to bed with a bottle; offer water in a cup when infant can put his or her lips to the rim of the cup.
H. For colds, fevers, and reactions to immunizations, administer appropriate weight-based dose of acetaminophen and/or ibuprofen; increase fluids; do not administer aspirin products. Tepid baths also help reduce fever.
I. Separation anxiety is a major stress for the hospitalized child from middle infancy through the preschool years.
   1. Protest: loud crying and screaming for parent; child refuses attention from anyone else.
   2. Despair: crying stops, and there is less activity; child is not interested in play and withdraws.
   3. Detachment (denial): child appears to have adjusted to hospitalization. Behavior is due to resignation; it is not a sign of contentment. This is not a positive reaction to hospitalization.

**TEST ALERT:** Assist client/family to identify and participate in activities fitting the child's age, preference, physical capacity, and developmental level. Provide care that meets the special needs of the preschool client ages 1 month to 4 years.

### Anticipatory Guidance for the Family of a Toddler

A. Continue to emphasize safety; discuss medications, poisons, car seats, latches on doors, falls, and water safety.
B. Toilet training usually begins around 2 years; accidents are common.
C. Sibling rivalry is common if there is a new baby in the family.
D. Temper tantrums are attention-seeking behavior and are not uncommon for a toddler.
E. Start regular dental checkups.
F. Establish and maintain consistency in discipline.
G. Toddler enjoys motion toys such as pull toys, riding toys, and wagons.

## Table 2-1 GROWTH AND DEVELOPMENT

| | | |
|---|---|---|
| Birth–4 months | Consistently gains weight (5–7 oz; 142–198 g per week) <br> Posterior fontanel closes <br> Responds to sounds and begins vocalizing <br> Gains head control → lifts chest → rolls over one way <br> Smiles responsively → smiles when spoken to | Teething may begin <br> Coordination progresses from jerky movement to grasping objects <br> Provide toys that increase hand–eye coordination |
| 4–9 months | Doubles birth weight (gains 3–5 oz; 85–142 g per week) <br> Teething begins with lower incisors <br> Sits with support; begins crawling <br> Turns over in both directions <br> Laughs aloud | Reaches for objects and grasps them <br> Begins "stranger anxiety" <br> Begins vocalizing with single consonants <br> Provide brightly colored toys that are easy to grasp <br> Enjoys noisemakers and mirrors; plays pat-a-cake |
| 9–12 months | Birth weight triples <br> Head and chest circumferences are equal <br> Anterior fontanel begins to close <br> Teething: has 6–8 teeth <br> Sits alone → moves from prone to sitting position <br> Crawling → pulling up → walks holding on to furniture | May stand alone <br> Has developed crude to fine pincer grasp <br> Transfers objects from one hand to another <br> Recognizes own name <br> Enjoys playing alone (solitary) <br> Explores objects by putting them in mouth |
| Toddler <br> (12–24 months) | 50% of height at 2 years <br> Exaggerated lumbar curve <br> Mobile: walks, runs, jumps <br> Walks up and down stairs, one foot at a time <br> Begins using eating utensils <br> Obeys simple commands <br> Begins to develop vocabulary | Speech becomes understandable <br> Thumb sucking may be at peak <br> Solitary play at 12 months; parallel play at 18 months <br> Beginning to develop bladder and bowel control <br> Attention-seeking behavior: temper tantrums <br> Enjoys activities that provide mobility: riding vehicles, wagons, pull toys |
| Preschool <br> (3–5 years) | Birth length doubles at 4 years <br> Coordination continues to improve <br> Rides tricycle, throws a ball <br> Walks up and down stairs with alternating feet | Begins to demonstrate self-care abilities <br> Knows own name <br> Good verbalization: talks about activities <br> Plays "dress up"; plays with cars, dolls, grooming aids |
| School-age <br> (6–10 years) | Growth spurts begin <br> Increasingly active <br> Very concerned with body image <br> Need for conformity: rules and rituals | Increasing importance of peer groups <br> Plays with groups of same sex <br> Competes for attention |
| Adolescence <br> (11–17 years) | Beginning and completing puberty <br> Girls mature earlier than boys <br> Very conscious of changes in body <br> Rapid growth | Moves from concrete to abstract thinking <br> Increased independence <br> Strong peer group association <br> Increased interest in opposite sex |
| Young adult <br> (18–30 years) | Physical maturity <br> Full mental capacity <br> Assumes responsibility for own learning <br> Adult relationship with parents | Launches career <br> Selects a mate, begins own family <br> Begins involvement in community |
| Adult <br> (30–60 years) | Physiologic processes begin slow decline <br> Cognitive skills peak <br> Creativity at maximum <br> Increase in community involvement <br> Increase in concern for future of society | Family tasks <br> Assist children to responsible adulthood <br> Role reversal with aging parents <br> Defines role of grandparenting |
| Older adult <br> (60+ years) | Decline of physiologic status <br> Demineralization of bones <br> ↓ Cardiac output <br> ↓ Respiratory vital capacity <br> ↓ Glomerular filtration rate <br> ↓ Serum albumin <br> ↓ Glucose tolerance | Maintains reasoning ability and abstract thinking <br> Thinking slows <br> Restructure in family roles <br> Retirement <br> Reorganization of activities <br> Continues with community involvement and politics |

H. Finger paints, interlocking blocks, and large-piece puzzles increase fine motor skills; read to child.

I. May regress to previous level of development in time of stress and illness, especially with toilet training.

J. Has no concept of death; primary reaction is to separation and loss.

K. See separation anxiety under anticipatory guidance for the infant.

**TEST ALERT:** Identify expected physical, cognitive, psychosocial, and moral stages of development.

**Figure 1. Recommended immunization schedule for persons aged 0 through 18 years – United States, 2018.**
**(FOR THOSE WHO FALL BEHIND OR START LATE, SEE THE CATCH-UP SCHEDULE AT THE CDC WEBSITE).**
These recommendations must be read with the footnotes that follow. For those who fall behind or start late, provide catch-up vaccination at the earliest opportunity as indicated by the green bars in Figure 1. To determine minimum intervals between doses, see the catch-up schedule (Figure 2), which can be obtained at https://www.cdc.gov/vaccines/schedules/downloads/child/0-18yrs-child-combined-schedule.pdf. School entry and adolescent vaccine age groups are shaded.

| Vaccine | Birth | 1 mo | 2 mos | 4 mos | 6 mos | 9 mos | 12 mos | 15 mos | 18 mos | 19-23 mos | 2-3 yrs | 4-6 yrs | 7-10 yrs | 11-12 yrs | 13-15 yrs | 16 yrs | 17-18 yrs |
|---|---|---|---|---|---|---|---|---|---|---|---|---|---|---|---|---|---|
| Hepatitis B[1] (HepB) | 1st dose | ◄------2nd dose-----► | | | ◄----------3rd dose----------► | | | | | | | | | | | | |
| Rotavirus[2] (RV) RV1 (2-dose series); RV5 (3-dose series) | | | 1st dose | 2nd dose | See footnote 2 | | | | | | | | | | | | |
| Diphtheria, tetanus, & acellular pertussis[3] (DTaP: <7 yrs) | | | 1st dose | 2nd dose | 3rd dose | | | ◄------4th dose------► | | | | 5th dose | | | | | |
| *Haemophilus influenzae* type b[4] (Hib) | | | 1st dose | 2nd dose | See footnote 4 | | ◄---3rd or 4th dose, See footnote 4---► | | | | | | | | | | |
| Pneumococcal conjugate[5] (PCV13) | | | 1st dose | 2nd dose | 3rd dose | | ◄-----4th dose-----► | | | | | | | | | | |
| Inactivated poliovirus[6] (IPV: <18 yrs) | | | 1st dose | 2nd dose | ◄----------3rd dose----------► | | | | | | | 4th dose | | | | | |
| Influenza[7] (IIV) | | | | | Annual vaccination (IIV) 1 or 2 doses | | | | | | | | Annual vaccination (IIV) 1 dose only | | | | |
| Measles, mumps, rubella[8] (MMR) | | | | | See footnote 8 | | ◄----- 1st dose-----► | | | | | 2nd dose | | | | | |
| Varicella[9] (VAR) | | | | | | | ◄----- 1st dose-----► | | | | | 2nd dose | | | | | |
| Hepatitis A[10] (HepA) | | | | | | | ◄------2-dose series, See footnote 10------► | | | | | | | | | | |
| Meningococcal[11] (MenACWY-D ≥9 mos; MenACWY-CRM ≥2 mos) | | | See footnote 11 | | | | | | | | | | | 1st dose | | 2nd dose | |
| Tetanus, diphtheria, & acellular pertussis[13] (Tdap: ≥7 yrs) | | | | | | | | | | | | | | Tdap | | | |
| Human papillomavirus[14] (HPV) | | | | | | | | | | | | | | See footnote 14 | | | |
| Meningococcal B[12] | | | | | | | | | | | | | | | | See footnote 12 | |
| Pneumococcal polysaccharide[5] (PPSV23) | | | | | | | | | | | See footnote 5 | | | | | | |

Legend: Range of recommended ages for all children; Range of recommended ages for catch-up immunization; Range of recommended ages for certain high-risk groups; Range of recommended ages for non-high-risk groups that may receive vaccine, subject to individual clinical decision making; No recommendation

This schedule includes recommendations in effect as of January 1, 2018. Any dose not administered at the recommended age should be administered at a subsequent visit, when indicated and feasible. The use of a combination vaccine generally is preferred over separate injections of its equivalent component vaccines. Vaccination providers should consult the relevant Advisory Committee on Immunization Practices (ACIP) statement for detailed recommendations, available online at http://www.cdc.gov/vaccines/hcp/acip-recs/index.html. Clinically significant adverse events that follow vaccination should be reported to the Vaccine Adverse Event Reporting System (VAERS) online (http://www.vaers.hhs.gov) or by telephone (800-822-7967). Suspected cases of vaccine-preventable diseases should be reported to the state or local health department.

This schedule is approved by the Advisory Committee on Immunization Practices (http//www.cdc.gov/vaccines/acip), the American Academy of Pediatrics (http://www.aap.org), the American Academy of Family Physicians (http://www.aafp.org), and the American College of Obstetricians and Gynecologists (http://www.acog.org).

**NOTE: The above recommendations must be read along with the footnotes of this schedule. Please visit https://www.cdc.gov/vaccines/schedules/downloads/child/0-18yrs-child-combined-schedule.pdf for a listing of the footnotes.**

**FIGURE 2-1 Recommended Immunization Schedule for Persons Aged 0 to 18 Years, 2018.** For recent updates and a full explanation of footnotes, refer to the Centers for Disease Control and Prevention website, https://www.cdc.gov/vaccines/schedules/hcp/child-adolescent.html#note (From Centers for Disease Control and Prevention, Advisory Committee on Immunization Practices [ACIP], United States. [2018]. Available at https://www.cdc.gov/.)

## Anticipatory Guidance for the Family of a Preschooler

A. Safety: discuss use of car seat/seat belts and booster seats, precautions for swimming pools, pedestrian and street safety skills, and proper use of playground equipment.
B. Preschool activities: reading, puzzles, and coloring large pictures; toys: building blocks, cars, and dolls.
C. Control time spent watching TV; screen programs for suitability; limit screen time to 1 to 2 hours per day.
D. Encourage socialization with other children.
E. Household chores: picking up clothes, straightening room, and so on.
F. Structured learning environment: Mother's Day Out, Head Start, Sunday school.
G. School readiness (attention span, easy separation from mother) begins around 5 years.
H. Should know full name and address by 5 years of age.
I. Curious about fire, matches, and firearms; keep such items out of reach and locked up.
J. Sees death as temporary and reversible, much like going to sleep; may view death as a punishment; fears the separation and abandonment.
K. Can tolerate brief periods of hospitalization; may trust other significant adults. Stress of illness may cause regression of previously attained levels of behavior, and separation anxiety may become an issue.

**TEST ALERT:** Provide care that meets the needs of the school-age client who is 5–12 years of age.

## Anticipatory Guidance for the Family of a School-Age Child

A. Safety: water, seat belts, skateboard, bicycle, fire safety; establish a plan for child if approached by stranger (stranger danger).
B. Encourage good dental hygiene habits.
C. Encourage good eating habits.
D. Encourage regular physical activity (group and team activities); make sure child wears protective sports gear.
E. Encourage peer relationships and communication.
F. Maintain consistency in limit setting.
G. Parental role-model behaviors: using seat belts, avoiding tobacco, eating properly, exercising regularly.
H. Teaching: avoid drugs, alcohol, and tobacco.
I. Provide age-appropriate sex education materials.
J. Injury prevention: around 8 to 10 years of age, a child may begin to engage in dangerous risk-taking behavior (dares, smoking, drinking).
K. Maintain yearly health checkups and immunizations as indicated (see Figure 2-1).
L. Develop independence: give allowance, choice of when to complete household chores; child tests rules and questions authority.
M. Avoid high noise levels (e.g., music headsets).
N. Physical development and puberty changes may begin in girls as early as 10 years.
O. Strong influence and dependence on peer group.
P. Spends less time with family.
Q. In early childhood, begins to see death as irreversible; may interpret it as destructive, scary, and/or violent.
R. In later childhood, views death as final and irreversible; may become interested in details regarding biological death and funerals.
S. The hospitalized child fears being away from the family, peers, and usual activities and may exhibit feelings of loneliness, boredom, and isolation.

> **TEST ALERT:** Evaluate the client/family's incorporation of healthy behaviors (screening examinations, immunizations, limiting risk-taking behaviors) into their lifestyle.

## Anticipatory Guidance for the Family of an Adolescent

A. Establish realistic expectations for family rules.
B. Minimize criticism, nagging, and derogatory or demeaning comments.
C. Respect the child's need for privacy.
D. Recognize positive behavior and achievement.
E. Establish clear limits: curfew, work hours.
F. Strives for independence from parents and acceptance by peers.
G. Begins to exhibit a mature understanding of death but may deny own mortality by increased risk taking; may have difficulty coping with death of significant other.
H. Maintain yearly physical checkups and immunizations as indicated (see Figure 2-1).
I. Hospitalized adolescents may exhibit rejection, uncooperativeness, or withdrawal because of the loss of control.

Caregivers frequently label them as difficult, unmanageable clients.

> **TEST ALERT:** Modify approaches to care in accordance with client developmental stage. Provide care that meets the special needs of the adult client ages 19–64 years.

## Anticipatory Guidance for the Adolescent

A. Learn techniques to protect self from physical, emotional, and sexual abuse, including rape.
B. Seek help if physically or sexually abused.
C. If sexually active, obtain information about safe sex and pregnancy prevention (e.g., condoms, sexually transmitted diseases, contraceptives).
D. Avoid smoking, drugs, and alcohol.
E. Review safety: firearms; automobile (as a driver and passenger); hearing (loud noises and head phones).

## Health Implications and Guidance for Adults and Older Adults (Box 2-1)

> **TEST ALERT:** Provide care to meet the special needs of older clients aged 65–85 years and adult clients older than 85 years.

A. Assist in identifying healthcare resources within community.
B. Encourage health screening (blood pressure, mammography, depression, vision/hearing testing, and colonoscopy), regular physical examination, regular dental visits, and immunizations as indicated (Figure 2-2).
C. Encourage a healthy living style: exercise, good nutrition (low-fat, well-balanced diet), weight reduction if overweight, decreased stress, decreased alcohol intake, and no tobacco use.
D. Safety concerns: risk for falls related to health status (impaired vision, postural hypotension, mobility issues, altered bladder function, and cognitive impairment) and environmental hazards (poor lighting, slippery floors,

### Box 2-1   OLDER ADULT CARE FOCUS

**Age-Related Factors Influencing Older Adult Care**
- Frequent absence of social and financial support
  *Examples:* Disease and/or loss of spouse, inadequate income from pension
- Presence of significant concurrent illness
  *Examples:* Dementia, chronic obstructive pulmonary disease, congestive heart failure, depression, diabetes, hypertension
- Altered pain perception
  *Examples:* Increased incidence of referred pain
- Impaired homeostatic mechanisms
  *Examples:* Increased problems with dehydration, incontinence, decreased lymphocyte production, altered immune status
- Impaired mobility
  *Examples:* Dependence on assistive devices (e.g., walkers and canes), need for assistance with bed transferring, change in use of transportation, presence of Parkinsonism or degenerative joint disease
- Increased frequency of adverse reactions to drugs
- Impaired equilibrium, resulting in falls

**Figure 1. Recommended immunization schedule for adults aged 19 years or older by age group, United States, 2018**

This figure should be reviewed with the accompanying footnotes. This figure and the footnotes describe indications for which vaccines, if not previously administered, should be administered unless noted otherwise.

| Vaccine | 19–21 years | 22–26 years | 27–49 years | 50–64 years | ≥65 years |
|---|---|---|---|---|---|
| Influenza[1] | 1 dose annually | | | | |
| Tdap[2] or Td[2] | 1 dose Tdap, then Td booster every 10 yrs | | | | |
| MMR[3] | 1 or 2 doses depending on indication (if born in 1957 or later) | | | | |
| VAR[4] | 2 doses | | | | |
| RZV[5] (preferred) | | | | | 2 doses RZV (preferred) |
| - - - or - - - | | | | | - - - or - - - |
| ZVL[5] | | | | | 1 dose ZVL |
| HPV–Female[6] | 2 or 3 doses depending on age at series initiation | | | | |
| HPV–Male[6] | 2 or 3 doses depending on age at series initiation | | | | |
| PCV13[7] | | | | 1 dose | |
| PPSV23[7] | 1 or 2 doses depending on indication | | | 1 dose | |
| HepA[8] | 2 or 3 doses depending on vaccine | | | | |
| HepB[9] | 3 doses | | | | |
| MenACWY[10] | 1 or 2 doses depending on indication, then booster every 5 yrs if risk remains | | | | |
| MenB[10] | 2 or 3 doses depending on vaccine | | | | |
| Hib[11] | 1 or 3 doses depending on indication | | | | |

▢ Recommended for adults who meet the age requirement, lack documentation of vaccination, or lack evidence of past infection    ▢ Recommended for adults with other indications    ▢ No recommendation

**Figure 2. Recommended immunization schedule for adults aged 19 years or older by medical condition and other indications, United States, 2018**

This figure should be reviewed with the accompanying footnotes. This figure and the footnotes describe indications for which vaccines, if not previously administered, should be administered unless noted otherwise.

| Vaccine | Pregnancy[1-6] | Immuno-compromised (excluding HIV infection)[3-7,11] | HIV infection CD4+ count (cells/μL)[3-7,9-10] <200 | ≥200 | Asplenia, complement deficiencies[7,10,11] | End-stage renal disease, on hemodialysis[7,9] | Heart or lung disease, alcoholism[7] | Chronic liver disease[7-9] | Diabetes[7,9] | Health care personnel[3,4,9] | Men who have sex with men[6,8,9] |
|---|---|---|---|---|---|---|---|---|---|---|---|
| Influenza[1] | 1 dose annually | | | | | | | | | | |
| Tdap[2] or Td[2] | 1 dose Tdap each pregnancy | 1 dose Tdap, then Td booster every 10 yrs | | | | | | | | | |
| MMR[3] | contraindicated | | | | 1 or 2 doses depending on indication | | | | | | |
| VAR[4] | contraindicated | | | | 2 doses | | | | | | |
| RZV[5] (preferred) | | | | | 2 doses RZV at age ≥50 yrs (preferred) | | | | | | |
| - - - or - - - | | | | | - - - or - - - | | | | | | |
| ZVL[5] | contraindicated | | | | 1 dose ZVL at age ≥60 yrs | | | | | | |
| HPV–Female[6] | | 3 doses through age 26 yrs | | | 2 or 3 doses through age 26 yrs | | | | | | |
| HPV–Male[6] | | 3 doses through age 26 yrs | | | 2 or 3 doses through age 21 yrs | | | | | | 2 or 3 doses through age 26 yrs |
| PCV13[7] | | 1 dose | | | | | | | | | |
| PPSV23[7] | | 1, 2, or 3 doses depending on indication | | | | | | | | | |
| HepA[8] | | 2 or 3 doses depending on vaccine | | | | | | | | | |
| HepB[9] | | 3 doses | | | | | | | | | |
| MenACWY[10] | | 1 or 2 doses depending on indication, then booster every 5 yrs if risk remains | | | | | | | | | |
| MenB[10] | | 2 or 3 doses depending on vaccine | | | | | | | | | |
| Hib[11] | | 3 doses HSCT recipients only | | | 1 dose | | | | | | |

▢ Recommended for adults who meet the age requirement, lack documentation of vaccination, or lack evidence of past infection    ▢ Recommended for adults with other indications    ▢ Contraindicated    ▢ No recommendation

NOTE: In February 2018, the *Recommended Immunization Schedule for Adults Aged 19 Years or Older, United States, 2018* became effective, as recommended by the Advisory Committee on Immunization Practices (ACIP) and approved by the Centers for Disease Control and Prevention (CDC). The adult immunization schedule was also approved by the American College of Physicians, the American Academy of Family Physicians, the American College of Obstetricians and Gynecologists, and the American College of Nurse-Midwives.

Please visit https://www.cdc.gov/vaccines/schedules/downloads/adult/adult-combined-schedule.pdf for a listing of the footnotes.

**FIGURE 2-2 Recommended Adult Immunization Schedule, 2018.** For recent updates and a full explanation of footnotes, refer to the Centers for Disease Control and Prevention website, http://www.cdc.gov/vaccines/schedules/hcp/adult.html (From Centers for Disease Control and Prevention, Advisory Committee on Immunization Practices [ACIP], United States. [2018]. Available at https://www.cdc.gov/.)

stairs, shoes in poor repair, and household items that are trip hazards, like rugs and extension cords).

E. Response to hospitalization will reflect moral and cultural values.

F. Hospitalization causes increased stress because of family and job responsibilities, as well as being a threat to the client's well-being.

G. Direct nursing interventions to stabilize chronic conditions, promote health, and promote independence in basic and instrumental activities of daily living.

H. Concepts of death follow common sequence.
   1. Shock, anger, denial, disbelief.
   2. Development of an awareness, bargaining; may experience depression.
   3. Acceptance, reorganization, restitution.

I. Adults 18 to 65 years of age tend to have an abstract and realistic concept of death.

J. Older adult clients (aged 65 and older) have frequently lost a spouse, a child, or close friends. Attitudes toward death are realistic, but older adults tend to have a more philosophic concept of death.

# COMMUNICABLE DISEASES

> **TEST ALERT:** Understand communicable diseases and modes of organism transmission (airborne, droplet, contact). Apply principles of infection control.

A. Incubation period: time from exposure to the pathogen until clinical symptoms occur.

B. Communicability: period in which an infected person is most likely to pass the pathogens to another person.

C. Prodromal period: begins with early manifestations of the disease or infection and continues until there are overt clinical symptoms characteristic of the disease.

D. Vaccinations for healthcare workers (Table 2-2).

## 🍦 Varicella (Chicken Pox)

### Characteristics

A. Herpes virus: varicella zoster; highly contagious, usually occurs in children under 15 years of age.

B. Maculopapular rash with vesicular scabs in multiple stages of healing.

C. Incubation period: 14 to 16 days.

D. Transmission: contact, airborne.

E. Communicability: 1 day before lesions appear to time when all lesions have formed crusts.

### Assessment

A. Prodromal: low-grade fever, malaise.

B. Acute phase: red maculopapular rash, which turns almost immediately to vesicles, each with an erythematous base; vesicles ooze and crust.

C. New crops of vesicles continue to form for 3 to 5 days, spreading from trunk to extremities.

D. All three stages are usually present in varying degrees at one time; pruritus.

E. Complications: secondary infection may lead to sepsis, abscess, cellulitis, or pneumonia.

### Health Care Interventions

A. Preventive: varicella immunization (see Figures 2-1 and 2-2; Table 2-2).

B. Skin care to decrease itching.
   1. Antihistamines, antipruritics, calamine lotion, and acetaminophen and/or ibuprofen for fever.
   2. Acyclovir decreases the number of lesions and shortens duration of clinical symptoms; may be used for immunocompromised children.
   3. Cool baths.
   4. A paste of baking soda and/or calamine lotion may decrease irritation.

| Table 2-2  CENTERS FOR DISEASE CONTROL (CDC) AND PREVENTION HEALTH CARE PERSONNEL (HCP) VACCINE RECOMMENDATIONS | |
|---|---|
| **Vaccine** | **Recommendations in Brief** |
| Hepatitis B | If you don't have documented evidence of a complete hepB vaccine series, or if you don't have an up-to-date blood test that shows you are immune to hepatitis B (i.e., no serologic evidence of immunity or prior vaccination) then you should:<br>• Get 3-dose series (dose #1 now, #2 in 1 month, #3 approximately 5 months after #2). Give IM.<br>• Obtain anti-HBs serologic testing 1–2 months after dose #3. |
| Influenza | Get 1 dose of influenza vaccine annually. |
| Tetanus /diphtheria/ pertussis (Tdap) | Get a one-time dose of Tdap (regardless of when previous dose of Td was received) as soon as possible for all healthcare personnel (HCP) who have not received Tdap previously and to pregnant HCP with each pregnancy (see website). Give Td boosters every 10 years thereafter. Administer IM. |
| Measles/ mumps/ rubella (MMR) | For HCP born in 1957 or later without serologic evidence of immunity or prior vaccination, give 2 doses of MMR, 4 weeks apart. For HCP born before 1957, see website. Give SC. |
| Varicella (chickenpox) | For HCP who have no serologic proof of immunity, prior vaccination, or history of varicella disease, give 2 doses of varicella vaccine, 4 weeks apart. Give SC. |
| Meningococcal | Those who are routinely exposed to isolates of *N. meningitidis* should get one dose. |

From Centers for Disease Control and Prevention. (2017). *Healthcare personnel vaccine recommendations.* Atlanta, GA: Center for Disease Control and Prevention. Retrieved update from https://www.cdc.gov/vaccines/adults/rec-vac/hcw.html

C. Keep child's fingernails short; apply mittens if necessary.

D. Isolate affected child from other children until vesicles have crusted.

E. Provide quiet activities to keep child occupied to lessen pruritus and prevent scratching.

F. Avoid use of aspirin.

G. Check with health care provider before administering vaccine to immunocompromised children. Vaccine should not be given to pregnant women.

## Parotitis (Mumps)

### Characteristics

A. An acute viral disease characterized by tenderness and swelling of one or both of the parotid glands and/or the other salivary glands.

B. Incubation period: 14 to 21 days.

C. Transmission: direct contact and droplet.

D. Communicability: most commonly occurs immediately before and after swelling begins.

### Assessment

A. Prodromal: headache, fever, malaise.

B. Acute phase: swelling of salivary glands (peaks in 3 days), leading to difficulty in swallowing, earache.

C. Complications.
  1. Postinfectious encephalitis.
  2. Sensorineural deafness.
  3. Orchitis, epididymitis.

### Health Care Interventions

A. Preventive: MMR immunization (see Figures 2-1 and 2-2; Table 2-2); MMR vaccine should not be given to pregnant or severely immunocompromised clients.

B. Bed rest until swelling subsides.

C. Droplet precautions indicated until 9 days after onset of parotid swelling.

D. Fluids and soft, bland food.

E. Avoid aspirin.

F. Orchitis: warm or cold packs; light support to scrotum.

G. Cool compresses applied to swollen neck area.

## Rubeola (Measles, Hard Measles, Red Measles)

### Characteristics

A. An acute viral disease characterized by fever and a rash.

B. Incubation: 10 to 20 days.

C. Transmission: direct contact with respiratory droplet.

D. Communicability: 4 days before rash to 5 days after rash appears.

### Assessment

A. Prodromal: fever, malaise, coldlike symptoms.

B. Koplik spots: small, irregular red spots noticed on the buccal mucosa opposite the molars; usually appear 2 days before rash.

C. Acute phase: begins 3 to 4 days after prodromal symptoms; maculopapular rash begins on face and gradually spreads downward from head to feet.

D. Photophobia, conjunctivitis, and bronchitis.

E. Complications: otitis media, pneumonia, laryngotracheitis, and encephalitis.

### Health Care Interventions

A. Preventive: MMR immunization (see Figures 2-1 and 2-2; Table 2-2); MMR should not be given to pregnant or severely immunocompromised clients.

B. Vitamin A supplementation reduces morbidity and mortality.

C. Bed rest until fever subsides, acetaminophen or ibuprofen for fever control; isolation (airborne precautions) until day 5 of rash.

D. Dim lights to decrease photophobia.

E. Tepid baths and lotion to relieve itching.

F. Encourage intake of fluids to maintain hydration; temperature may spike 2 to 3 days after rash appears.

## Rubella (German Measles)

### Characteristics

A. An acute, mild systemic viral disease that produces a distinctive 3-day rash and lymphadenopathy.

B. Incubation: 14 to 21 days.

C. Transmission: nasopharyngeal secretions, direct contact.

D. Communicability: from up to 7 days before rash until 5 days after rash.

### Assessment

A. Prodromal: low-grade fever, headache, malaise, and symptoms of a cold.

B. Rash first appears on face and spreads down to neck, arms, trunk, and then legs.

C. Diagnostics: persistent rubella antibody titer of 1:8 usually indicates immunity.

D. Complications: can have teratogenic effects on fetus.

### Health Care Interventions

A. Primarily symptomatic; bed rest until fever subsides; droplet precautions.

B. Preventive: MMR immunization (see Figures 2-1 and 2-2; Table 2-2); MMR should not be given to severely immunosuppressed clients.

C. Pregnant women should avoid contact with children who have rubella. If not immunized before pregnancy, vaccination should not be given until completion of pregnancy.

## Roseola Infantum (Exanthema Subitum)

### Characteristics

A. A common, acute benign viral infection, usually occurring in infants and young children (ages 6 months to 3 years), characterized by sudden onset of a high temperature followed by a rash.

B. Incubation period: usually 5 to 15 days.

C. Transmission: unknown, generally limited to children age 6 months to 3 years.

D. Communicability: unknown.

### Assessment

A. Sudden onset of high fever—103° F (39.5° C).

B. As fever drops, a maculopapular, nonpruritic rash appears abruptly; rash blanches or fades under pressure and disappears in 1 to 2 days.

C. Complications: febrile seizures.

### Health Care Interventions

A. Symptomatic: provide tepid baths, offer fluids frequently, dress child in cool clothing.

B. Acetaminophen and/or ibuprofen for fever control.

## Diphtheria

### Characteristics

A. An infection caused by Corynebacterium diphtheriae.

B. Incubation period: 2 to 5 days.

C. Transmission: direct contact, contaminated articles (fomites).

D. Communicability: variable, usually 2 weeks, or after 4 days of antibiotics; three negative cultures required.

### Assessment

A. Nasal discharge, anorexia, sore throat, low-grade fever.

B. Smooth white or gray membrane over tonsillar region; hoarseness and potential airway obstruction.

C. Frequently, tachypnea, dyspnea, stridor, or airway obstruction may occur if condition goes untreated.

D. Complications: cardiomyopathy, neuropathy.

### Health Care Interventions

A. Maintain isolation from other children.

B. Antibiotic and IV diphtheria antitoxin are common medications.

C. Humidified oxygen with respiratory problems; have tracheostomy set available.

D. Provide adequate humidification to allow for liquefaction of secretions.

E. Preventive: DTaP immunization (see Figures 2-1 and 2-2; Table 2-2).

## Pertussis (Whooping Cough)

### Characteristics

A. An acute inflammation of the respiratory tract caused by *Bordetella pertussis*, most severe in children under 2 years of age.

B. Incubation period: 6 to 20 days; average, 7 days.

C. Transmission: droplet and direct contact.

D. Communicability: highly contagious; greatest during the catarrhal stage before the onset of paroxysms of coughing and lasting until 5 days of effective antibiotics.

### Assessment

A. Catarrhal stage: usually begins with symptoms of an upper respiratory tract infection, fever.

B. Paroxysmal stage.
   1. Cough occurs primarily at night; it consists of a series of short rapid coughs, followed by a sudden inspiration that is a high-pitched, crowing sound or a "whoop."
   2. Paroxysms of coughing may continue until a thick mucous plug is expelled.

C. Convalescent stage: paroxysms of coughing are less frequent.

D. Diagnostics: culture and sensitivity of nasopharyngeal secretions; identification of organism.

E. Complications: pneumonia, atelectasis, convulsions.

F. Preventive: DTaP immunization (see Figure 2-1); adults (19–64 years of age) should receive one dose Tdap booster to reduce transmission of pertussis to infants (see Figure 2-2).

### Health Care Interventions

A. Droplet precautions are recommended during catarrhal stage; continue bed rest as long as fever is present.

B. Administer antibiotic therapy (clarithromycin, erythromycin, or azithromycin [used with caution]).

C. Provide oxygen and humidification and observe for signs of increasing respiratory distress.

D. Avoid exposure to environmental precipitants of paroxysms of coughing, such as cold air, smoke, and dust.

E. Maintain nutrition with small frequent feedings.

F. Avoid use of cough suppressants and sedatives.

G. Report cases to local public health department.

## Tetanus (Lockjaw)

### Characteristics

A. An acute, serious, potentially fatal disease characterized by painful muscle spasms and convulsions caused by the anaerobic gram-positive bacillus *Clostridium tetani*.

B. Incubation period: generally from 2 days to 2 months; average is 10 days.

C. Transmission: through a puncture wound that is contaminated by soil, dust, or excreta that contain *Clostridium tetani* or by way of burns and minor wounds (e.g., infection of the umbilicus of a newborn).

### Assessment

A. Progressive stiffness and tenderness in the muscles of the neck and jaw (trismus or lockjaw).

B. Progressive involvement of trunk muscles causes opisthotonos positioning.

C. Paroxysmal contractions occur in response to stimuli (noise, touch, light).

D. Client remains alert; mental status is not affected.

E. Complications: laryngospasm and tetany of the respiratory muscles cause contractions that may precipitate atelectasis and pneumonia.

### Health Care Interventions

A. Preventive.
   1. Careful cleansing and debridement of wounds.
   2. Immunization: DTaP for child (see Figures 2-1 and 2-2); adult tetanus toxoid (Td) every 10 years (see Figure 2-2).

B. Administration of tetanus immune globulin and tetanus toxoid for inadequate immunization in child who receives a tetanus-prone injury/wound.

C. Maintain seizure precautions: quiet, nonstimulating environment; monitor vital signs, muscle tone, etc.

## Poliomyelitis

### Characteristics

A. An acute, contagious disease affecting the central nervous system.

B. Incubation period: 5 to 35 days; average, 7 to 14 days.

C. Transmission: fecal–oral or pharyngeal–oropharyngeal contact.

D. Communicability: virus in throat for 1 week after onset; in feces, intermittently for 4 to 6 weeks.

### Assessment

A. Abortive or inapparent type.
1. Fever, sore throat, headache, malaise, nausea, vomiting, abdominal pain.
2. Lasts a few hours to a few days.

B. Nonparalytic type: same symptoms as abortive type but more severe, with pain and stiffness in the neck, back, and legs.

C. Paralytic type: initial symptoms are similar to those of nonparalytic poliomyelitis, followed by recovery, then signs of central nervous system paralysis.

### Health Care Interventions

A. Preventive: inactivated polio virus vaccine (see Figures 2-1 and 2-2).

B. Bed rest during acute phase; standard and droplet precautions.

C. Physical therapy with warm moist packs and range of motion.

D. Position to maintain body alignment.

E. Complications: teach family and client early symptoms of respiratory distress.

## Scarlet Fever

### Characteristics

A. Group A beta-hemolytic streptococcal infection that often follows acute streptopharyngitis.

B. Incubation period: 1 to 7 days; average 3 days.

C. Transmission: direct contact or droplet of nasopharyngeal secretions; indirect contact with contaminated objects or ingestion of contaminated food.

D. Communicability: variable, approximately 10 days.

### Assessment

A. Sudden onset of high fever and tachycardia.

B. Enlarged edematous tonsils covered with exudate; nausea, vomiting; "strawberry" tongue.

C. Diffuse, fine erythematous rash that resembles a sunburn with goose bumps; rash is more intense in folds and joints but is often absent from the face.

D. Desquamation of the skin, which usually begins by end of first week and is often seen on the palms and soles of the feet during the convalescent period.

E. Diagnostics: history of a recent streptococcal infection, positive antistreptolysin-O (ASO) titer, and a throat culture positive for group A beta-hemolytic streptococci.

F. Complications: otitis media, tonsillar abscess, glomerulonephritis, acute rheumatic fever.

### Health Care Interventions

A. Administration of a full course of penicillin (or erythromycin in penicillin-sensitive clients).

B. Administration of antipyretics and anesthetic throat sprays or gargles to relieve sore throat.

C. Encourage intake of fluids to prevent dehydration during febrile phase.

D. Assess for—and teach family to observe for—early symptoms of complications.

E. Discuss prevention of spread: discard toothbrush; avoid sharing eating and drinking utensils.

## Infectious Mononucleosis

### Characteristics

A. An acute, self-limiting infectious disease caused by the Epstein–Barr virus; member of the herpes group of viruses, occurring most often among young persons under 25 years of age; often called the "kissing disease."

B. Incubation period: 30 to 50 days.

C. Transmission: direct or indirect contact with oral secretions—intimate contact, sharing same drinking cup, hand to mouth; probably oropharyngeal route.

### Assessment

A. Onset of symptoms occurs anytime from 10 days to 6 weeks after exposure; it may be acute or insidious.

B. Malaise, sore throat, fever with generalized lymphadenopathy, splenomegaly.

C. Diagnostic: a positive heterophile antibody test (titer of 1:160 is considered diagnostic); positive monospot test result.

D. Complications: spleen involvement; pneumonitis, pericarditis, and neurologic involvement.

### Health Care Interventions

A. Bed rest, anesthetic throat gargles, antipyretics.

B. Provide adequate nutrition: soft foods, fluids.

**TEST ALERT:** Provide information about health maintenance (e.g., physician visits, immunizations, screening examinations).

## Zika Virus

### Characteristics

A. Incubation estimated to be several days to a week.

B. Most infections are asymptomatic.

### Assessment

A. Acute onset of fever, maculopapular rash, joint pain, and/or conjunctivitis (Figure 2-3).

B. Zika virus infection in pregnant women might lead to microcephaly in offspring.

C. Diagnostics: serology for Zika virus–specific IgM (ELISA).

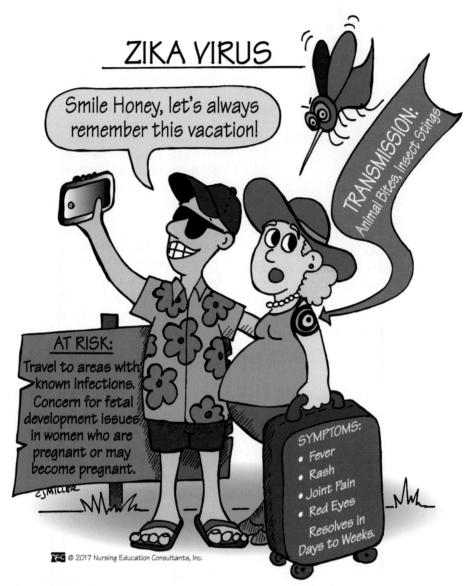

**FIGURE 2-3 Zika Virus.** (From Zerwekh, J., Garneau, A., & Miller, C. J. [2017]. *Digital collection of the memory notebooks of nursing* [4th ed.]. Chandler, AZ: Nursing Education Consultants, Inc.)

### *Nursing Interventions*

A. No vaccine or antiviral therapy is available.

B. Prevention via insect repellents/mosquito control and clothing that minimizes skin exposure, especially during daylight hours.

C. Pregnant women should consider avoiding travel to areas with ongoing Zika virus outbreaks.

D. Male partners exposed to, or infected with, Zika virus should use condoms consistently or refrain from sex with pregnant women.

E. Cases should be reported to state health department.

## POISONING

### General Principles (Remember *SIRES*)

A. **S**tabilize the client's condition.
   1. Assess the condition and provide respiratory support; obtain IV access site.

   2. Terminate exposure to the toxic substance: remove pills from mouth, flush eyes, remove contaminated clothing, etc.

B. **I**dentify the toxic substance.
   1. Obtain accurate history and retrieve any available poison.
   2. Notify local poison control center, emergency facility, or physician for immediate care and advice regarding treatment.

C. **R**emove the substance to decrease absorption.
   1. Shower or wash off radioactive substances.
   2. Antidotes: for heroin or other drug overdose.
   3. Ingested substances: lavage, absorbents (activated charcoal), or cathartics.

D. **E**liminate the substance from the client's body.
   1. Activated charcoal may be administered to absorb the toxic substance. Inducing emesis by administering syrup of ipecac is no longer routinely recommended for home or emergency treatment.

E. **S**upport the client both physically and psychologically.
  1. If overdose is intentional or a suicide attempt, refer for psychiatric evaluation.
  2. If accidental poisoning occurs with a child, parents often demonstrate guilt and self-reproach in regard to their parenting role.

> **TEST ALERT:** Educate client/family on home safety issues.

## Salicylate Poisoning

A. Toxic dose levels: 300 to 500 mg/kg (1086–2172 μmol/L) of body weight. For a 30 lb child (13.6 kg), 12 adult-strength aspirin or 48 baby aspirin would be toxic.
B. In severe toxic overdose, metabolic activity increases; this results in an increased consumption of oxygen, increased temperature, and increased production of carbon dioxide. Metabolic acidosis eventually occurs as a result of the change in body processes.
C. Chronic use causes a deficiency in platelets, leading to bleeding tendencies.

### Assessment

A. Clinical manifestations.
  1. Hyperventilation, nausea, vomiting.
  2. Increased temperature, tinnitus.
  3. Altered consciousness, oliguria.
  4. Metabolic acidosis, seizures (severe toxicity).
  5. Diaphoresis and dehydration.
  6. Bleeding tendencies in chronic poisoning.
B. Diagnostics.
  1. Serum salicylate level.
  2. Electrolytes.

### Treatment

A. Administer activated charcoal.
B. Administer vitamin K to decrease bleeding tendencies.
C. Provide oxygen and ventilatory support for respiratory depression; provide IV fluids and sodium bicarbonate to treat the acidosis.
D. Administer cooling activities and treatments for hyperthermia.
E. In severe cases, hemodialysis may be performed.

### Nursing Interventions

**Goal:** To provide initial stabilization of the child.

A. Administer activated charcoal to reduce systemic absorption. Dose of charcoal should be 10 times the amount of drug ingested; it is frequently difficult to get this amount down the child.
B. Administer a cathartic (magnesium sulfate) with charcoal to hasten elimination of the drug.
C. Ongoing assessment of vital signs, level of consciousness, and urine output.

**Goal:** To prevent salicylate poisoning and provide teaching to family.

A. Educate family regarding safe storage of medications: childproof caps, locked medicine cabinets, etc.
B. Teach parents to read labels on medications; other medications frequently contain salicylate.
C. Advise parents that activated charcoal will cause the child's stool to be black.

## Acetaminophen Poisoning

A. Definition of toxicity in children is 150 mg/kg or greater.
B. Primary toxic effects are on the liver.
C. Antidote: *N*-acetylcysteine.
D. Most common poisoning in children.

### Assessment

A. Clinical manifestations: four stages.
  1. Stage 1 (2–4 hours).
    a. Nausea and vomiting.
    b. Sweating and pallor.
  2. Stage 2 (latent stage, 24–36 hours); child improves.
  3. Stage 3 (hepatic involvement).
    a. Right upper quadrant pain.
    b. Coagulation defects.
    c. Jaundice.
  4. Stage 4 (recovery if hepatic damage is not severe).

### Treatment

A. Early administration of activated charcoal—preferably within 30 minutes to 1 hour after ingestion.
B. *N*-acetylcysteine: one loading dose and multiple maintenance doses.

### Nursing Interventions

See Salicylate Poisoning.

## Lead Poisoning

A. Ingestion of lead from hand to mouth and exposure to lead-contaminated dust, eating from improperly glazed glassware (leaded glass) or lead-based pottery, or chewing on furniture with lead-based paint.
B. Increased risk in children under 6 years of age because they absorb 40% to 50% of lead, whereas adults absorb only 5% to 10%.

### Assessment

A. Clinical manifestations.
  1. Renal: problem in adults with occupational exposure; renal impairment will delay excretion of the lead from the body.
  2. Hematologic.
    a. Anemia.
    b. Iron deficiencies increase lead absorption; serum ferritin level is sensitive indicator of iron status.
    c. Chronic: blue lead line on gums and "lead lines" on x-rays of the long bones.
  3. Neurologic.
    a. Hyperactivity.
    b. Increased distractibility.
    c. Possible encephalopathy to mental retardation.
    d. Seizures.

B. Diagnostics.
   1. Blood lead level (BLL) is used for screening and for diagnosis. A BLL >10 mcg/dL (0.48 μmol/L) requires follow-up investigation; a BLL >20 mcg/dL (0.97 μmol/L) requires treatment.

### Treatment

A. Chelation therapy process for removing lead from the circulating blood; aids in secretion by the kidneys.
   1. Succimer: an oral chelator for lead level of 35 to 45 mcg/dL.
   2. Edetate calcium disodium (EDTA) administered by deep intramuscular injection or by IV for lead level of >70 mcg/dL; do not give in absence of adequate urine output.
   3. Dimercaprol (BAL): administered by deep intramuscular injection, along with EDTA.

### Nursing Interventions

**Goal:** To identify lead poisoning and assist with the elimination of lead from the body.

A. Identify high-risk groups such as children who engaged in pica or those living in an environment containing old lead-based paint.
   1. Monitor children with lead levels >10 mcg/dL (0.48 μmol/L).
   2. Treat children at 6 to 12 months of age.
B. Administer chelating agents: compliance is critical; it is important to support the child who will be receiving multiple injections.
C. Encourage high fluid intake.
D. Seizure precautions.

**Goal:** To educate parents and child as to the nature of the disease and provide instruction in ways to maintain homeostasis and reduce lead exposure.

A. Educate parents about the dangers and sources of lead ingestion, including 12 to 24 months being the age of greatest risk.
B. Assist parents in identifying measures to prevent occurrence or recurrence of the problem.

## LONG-TERM CARE

Long-term care includes those services provided in institutional settings, such as a nursing home, rehabilitation center, or adult day care program after the acute phase of an illness has passed. This often involves restorative care for clients with chronic health care problems.

A. Types of long-term care facilities.
   1. Nursing home: provides services ranging from maintenance to restorative care with skilled nursing, use of certified nursing assistants, licensed practical nurses, and registered nurses.
   2. Adult day care facility: the client lives at home during the evening and night and spends the day in a facility that provides a range of care from skilled nursing to restorative care.

3. Hospice care: end-of-life care provided in the home and/or client care settings. (See End-of-Life Care, Chapter 3).
4. Respite care: a type of short-term care provided to give the primary caregiver (often a family member), a rest from the daily responsibilities of taking care of the client.
5. Rehabilitation center: a facility that provides multiple services for the client and family to make adjustments to daily living. It assists the client in achieving as much independence as possible in activities of daily living (ADLs).
6. Home care: nursing care provided in the home to clients who do not need hospitalization but do need additional assistance with medical problems.
7. Adult housing or assisted living centers: facilities for clients to live as independently as possible but still receive supervision, meals, and other services.

## CHRONIC ILLNESS

A chronic illness may be defined as an illness or condition that is present for more than 3 months in a year and interferes with daily function and lifestyle. As medical technology continues to increase the life spans of individuals with chronic illnesses, the nurse's role continues to expand, including providing initial health care and assisting with planning and providing long-term care.

> **TEST ALERT:** Help the client cope with life transitions. Help the client and significant others adjust to role changes; assess the family's emotional reaction to the client's illness; determine the ability of the family/support system to provide care for client.

### Nursing Considerations

A. The majority of clients with extended health care needs have at least two chronic health conditions. These conditions may or may not be interrelated.
B. The focus of care for chronically ill clients is on assisting them to control their health problems and disease symptoms and manage their lifestyle.
   1. Prevention and management of medical crises.
   2. The control of disease symptoms, which may focus on pain control and comfort measures.
   3. Implementation of the prescribed therapeutic regimens.
   4. Psychosocial implications and adjustments to lifestyle; frequently, client must deal with social isolation.
   5. Adjustments to lifestyle as disease or condition changes.
   6. Financial strain caused by paying for medical care and supplies.
   7. Coping with strain on marriage and family structure.
C. The majority of clients with chronic health care needs are older than 65 years of age. The developmental level of these individuals, according to Erikson, is ego integrity versus despair. The feeling of powerlessness is a common problem in the older adult.
D. The nursing process is directed toward identification of nursing actions to assist the older adult to maintain independence and be as functional as possible.

**NURSING PRIORITY:** In planning home health care for a client with a chronic disease, remember that the goal is to *assist the client in maintaining control* over his or her condition and lifestyle. Frequently, health care providers and family tend to take control of the situation, thus increasing the feeling of powerlessness in the individual.

### Chronically Ill Pediatric Client

The diagnosis of a child's chronic illness is a major situational crisis in the family. Available support systems, perception of the problem, and coping mechanisms will ultimately determine the resolution of the crisis.

A. Focus care on the child's developmental age rather than chronologic age. Emphasis should be placed on the child's strengths rather than disabilities.
B. Assist the child and the family in returning to or establishing a normal pattern of living.
C. Promote the child's maximum level of growth and development. The current trend is to promote education within child's peer group.
D. Assess the family's response to the child's illness and evaluate for parental overprotection. Overprotection by the parents prevents the child from developing self-esteem, independence, and self-control over the disease and ADLs. Observe for the following parental characteristics that will impede development:
   1. Inconsistency in discipline; disciplinary measures often differ from those used with other children in the family.
   2. Attempts to protect the child from every discomfort, both physical and psychosocial. Frequently restricts play with peers based on fear of injury and/or rejection by peers.
   3. Makes decisions for the child without involving the child.
   4. Does not allow the child the opportunity to learn self-care; frequently is afraid the child cannot handle the requirements for self-care (e.g., a child with diabetes becoming responsible for administration of his or her own insulin).
   5. Continues to do things for the child, even when child is capable of doing them on his or her own.
   6. Self-sacrifice and isolation of family from social interactions.

**NURSING PRIORITY:** Determine the needs of the family regarding ability to provide home care after discharge. A pediatric situation may include questions regarding the parents' or family's response to the child's chronic illness.

It is frequently the nurse who assesses the family and the client regarding their immediate needs. The appropriateness of the nurse's response depends on the nurse–client–family relationship and the environment. Priorities of care must be established, with goals and nursing interventions to meet the client's immediate health care needs. In an acute care environment, it is difficult even to *attempt* to meet long-term needs of the client and family. It is important to assist them in identifying community resources and to determine the availability of counseling and home health care to meet the ever-changing needs encountered in dealing with a chronic health condition.

## REHABILITATION

**TEST ALERT:** Assist and intervene in client's performance of instrumental ADLs. Provide support to client and/or family in coping with life changes. Determine the client's ability to perform self-care (ADLs, hygiene, resources); plan with the client to meet self-care needs.

Rehabilitation means the restoration of an individual to his or her optimal level of functioning. This includes physical, mental, social, vocational, and economic parameters.

### Goals of Rehabilitation

**NURSING PRIORITY:** Rehabilitation is an area that affects all levels of nursing care. Primary goals in planning any client's care are prevention of complications and promotion of independence.

For the client undergoing rehabilitation to achieve the highest level of productivity, the rehabilitation process must begin when the condition becomes evident or when the disease is diagnosed.

A. Prevention of deformities and complications.
   1. Maintain function and prevent deterioration of unaffected organs or areas.
   2. Prevent further injury to affected area or organ.
   3. Prevent or reduce complications of immobility.
B. Assist client in performing ADLs with minimum or no assistance, depending on his or her level of disability. *Examples of ADLs:* eating, dressing, bathing.
C. Assist client with independent activities of daily living (IADLs). *Examples of IADLs:* shopping for groceries, paying bills, lawn care.
D. Promote continuity of care when the client is discharged or transferred.
   1. Consult with other rehabilitation team members to determine appropriate placement.
   2. Assist client and family through the transitional process.

**NURSING PRIORITY:** The client needs to be actively involved in setting goals for his or her care.

### Psychological Responses to Disability

Not every client will progress through all stages of grief in an orderly fashion. Clients will fluctuate between emotional crises.

A. Initial responses of confusion, disorganization, and denial represent a state of internal conflict.

B. A period of depression may occur as the client mourns for the loss of or change in body function.

C. An anger stage may occur as the client projects blame and hostility on family and health care providers.

D. Adaptation and adjustment will come as the client begins to redirect his or her energy toward coping with the disability.

E. New situations (going home, new job, etc.) may precipitate emotional outbursts and trauma.

F. Some clients will refuse to accept their disability and will not put forth any effort to adapt to everyday living.

## HOME HEALTH CARE

Home health care is the provision of health care to clients in the home environment.

A. Levels of home health care.
  1. Intensive: clients with serious health care problems requiring the expertise of skilled nursing care.
  2. Intermediate: clients with stable health care problems who require a professional level of care to promote rehabilitation through restorative nursing.
  3. Maintenance: clients who require assistance with ADLs; the underlying health care problem is stable.

B. Guidelines for home health care personnel.
  1. Respect client's religious, cultural, and ethnic background.
  2. As a caregiver/guest in the client's home, your behavior should reflect sensitivity to the client and family; a pleasant attitude and sense of humor are helpful.
  3. Develop family members and significant others as your advocates.
  4. Communication with other health care team members is vital to the maintenance of the client's well-being.
  5. Working with more autonomy without immediate hospital support is challenging and requires an increased level of nursing competence for decision making.
  6. A Patient's Bill of Rights is applicable in the home health care setting (e.g., client has the right to disclosure of information concerning his or her condition and care and the right to refuse or stop treatment, etc.).

## NUTRITION

> **TEST ALERT:** Monitor the client's nutritional and hydration status.

### Dietary Considerations Throughout the Life Span
*Infant*

> **! NURSING PRIORITY:** A newborn will lose weight for the first few days but should not lose more than 10% of his or her birth weight or take longer than 10–14 days to regain it.

A. Growth.
  1. Birth weight doubles by 6 months, and triples by 1 year.
  2. Infant gains only another 4 to 6 lb until 2 years of age.

*Birth weight 7 lb (3.17kg); at 6 months, should be 14 lb (6.36 kg); at 1 year, another 7 lb (3.17 kg) gained = 21 lb (9.54 kg) (birth weight tripled).*

B. Diet
  1. Ideal food is breast milk because it is nutritionally superior to alternatives, is easier to digest, and contains maternal antibodies.
  2. Bottle-fed infants need to be on a formula that is iron fortified.
  3. Breastfed infants do not need additional water.

> **! NURSING PRIORITY:** A newborn has a higher fluid requirement in relation to body size than an adult.

  4. Breastfed infants should receive 400 international units of vitamin D as a daily supplement.
  5. Bottle-fed infants should receive 400 IU of vitamin D until the infant is consuming greater than 1 L/day (or 1 quart) of vitamin D–fortified formula.
  6. Whole cow's milk, low-fat cow's milk, skim milk, and imitation milks are not recommended for infants younger than 12 months of age.
  7. Iron fortified cereal, usually rice, is the first solid food introduced and is recommended around age 4 to 6 months.
  8. Strained vegetables and fruits are introduced one at a time to determine infant's tolerance of each food.
  9. Chopped foods are introduced at 6 to 9 months.
  10. Strained meats are usually added last because of the difficulty the infant may encounter swallowing.

> **! NURSING PRIORITY:** Breastfed infants may gain weight at a slower rate than formula-fed infants. Breastfed infants are leaner and often have less body fat than formula fed infants.

  11. Formula consumption.
    a. 1 month old: up to 22 oz (650 mL) per day.
    b. 4 months old: up to 30 oz (887 mL) per day.
    c. 6 months old: up to 28 oz (828 mL) per day; solid foods are introduced.
    d. 12 months old: up to 23 oz (680 mL) per day with intake of solid food.

C. Implications for family teaching.

> **TEST ALERT:** Assist client with infant feeding. Provide discharge instructions (postpartum and newborn care).

  1. Newborns cannot swallow voluntarily until 10 to 12 weeks of age.
  2. Extrusion reflex (pushing food out of mouth with tongue) lasts until 4 months, therefore solids are not introduced until around 6 months.
  3. When solids are being introduced, offer only one new food per week; avoid multigrain cereals until tolerance is established.
  4. Usual progression of food textures is strained to mashed to minced to chopped to cut-up table foods.

5. Increase the use of small-sized finger foods as pincer grasp develops (9 months). Be alert for choking hazard.
6. Texture of food becomes increasingly important from 6 months to 1 year, but the food must be easily dissolved (e.g., crackers or zwiebacks).
7. Teach parents *not* to warm frozen breast milk in the microwave; this may change the composition of the milk.

### Toddler

A. Diet.
1. Needs 16 oz (473 mL) of milk daily; more than 24 oz (709 mL) can lead to refusal of other foods and development of a milk anemia (peak incidence at 18 months).
2. Whole milk is recommended between 1 to 2 years; switch to 2% milk after age 2.
3. Prefers finger foods (e.g., vegetables he or she can pick up, crackers, macaroni).
4. Tends to refuse casseroles, salads, and mixed dishes.
5. Use of 100% fruit juice in limited quantities.
6. Struggle for autonomy may be manifested by refusal of food, mealtime negativism, and ritualism.
7. Bribery and rewards for eating should be avoided.
8. Around 18 months of age, a decreased appetite is normal; toddler may become a picky eater. Don't mix foods on plate or overfill the plate.
9. Ritualistic behavior frequently carries over into eating habits (e.g., same dish, same spoon, etc.).

### Preschooler

A. Diet.
1. *Food jags* are common; the child may refuse to eat anything except one food at each meal.
2. Three meals and two snacks/day; begin to encourage five servings of fruits and vegetables.
3. Finger foods remain popular.
4. Do not bribe the child to eat or tell him or her to "clean your plate." Serve smaller portions; if sufficient amounts are not eaten during mealtimes, eliminate snacks; limit visits to fast food restaurants.
5. Recognize that refusing to eat is a way to attract attention.

### School-Age Child

A. Diet.
1. Food intake is more varied.
2. Child enjoys most foods, with vegetables being the least favorite.
B. Implications for family teaching.
1. After-school snack: encourage healthy choices such as fruits, raw vegetable sticks, and peanut butter sandwiches.
2. Appetite is usually good, but a child often does not want to take the time to eat. Sometimes it is helpful to spend a specific amount of time at the table (15–20 minutes) to prevent the child from forming the habit of gulping food down.
3. Avoid using food as a reward for behavior.

4. Influence of media and peers regarding fast food is increased.
5. Begin teaching child to recognize high-fat foods.

### Adolescent

A. Rapid growth rate and maturation changes make the adolescent vulnerable to nutritional deficiencies. Diets in general are deficient in iron, calcium, and vitamin C.
B. Girls' peak growth occurs between 10 and 14 years of age.
C. Boys' peak growth occurs between 12 and 15 years of age.
D. Six out of 10 girls eat only two-thirds of the nutrients required. Girls tend to be deficient in iron, whereas boys tend to be deficient in thiamine (Table 2-3).

### Adult

A. Diet.
1. Energy requirements decrease with age.
   *Example:* A 55-year-old man requires 2400 kcal; at age 76, he requires only 2050 kcal.
   *Example:* A 55-year-old woman requires 1800 kcal; at age 76, she requires only 1600 kcal.
2. Improved financial status during middle adulthood tends to promote an increased intake of rich foods and frequency of dining out.
B. Nursing implications.
1. Adherence to a prudent diet pattern.
2. Promotion and continued maintenance of a regular exercise program.
3. Reduce sodium intake to 2300 mg daily.
4. Maintain serum cholesterol level <200 mg/dL (5.20 mmol/L).

### Older Adult

A. Diet.
1. Encourage a diet low in fat and high in fiber, iron, vitamin C, and thiamine with adequate sources of calcium (see Table 2-3).
2. If bed rest is prescribed, fluid intake should be as high as 3 to 4 L/day to prevent kidney stones, unless client has fluid restrictions (e.g., client with heart failure).
3. Because the older adult often has impaired renal function, protein and potassium intake should be evaluated.
B. Nursing implications.
1. Alteration in taste and reduced digestive function occur.
2. Logical sequence of eating food is biting, chewing, and swallowing. New denture wearers should be encouraged to reverse this order: swallow a liquid diet first, then chew soft foods, and finally bite into regular foods.
3. The older adult may intentionally restrict fluids because of nocturia or stress incontinence.
4. Constipation is a chronic problem caused by decreased peristalsis; encourage increased intake of fluids and a high-fiber diet.
5. Loneliness and depression are often associated with poor appetite.

## Table 2-3   VITAMINS AND MINERALS

| Name | Function | Food Sources | Nursing Implications |
|---|---|---|---|
| **Vitamins: Fat-Soluble** | | | |
| Vitamin A: Retinol | Vision adaptation, night vision, normal bone and tooth formation | Liver, whole milk, egg yolk, yellow/green vegetables | If child eats excessive amounts of yellow vegetables, he or she may have yellow skin color. Important in preterm infants. Children with reduced fat absorption may have deficiency (CF, hepatitis, etc.) |
| Vitamin D: Cholecalciferol | Promotes normal absorption of calcium and phosphorus | Fish, direct sunlight, enriched foods (e.g., milk products, cereals) | All infants need 400 IU supplement every day, starting soon after birth. Expose infant to short periods of mild sunlight. |
| Vitamin E: Tocopherol | Production of normal red blood cells, antioxidant | Milk, meat, egg yolks, whole grains, legumes, spinach, broccoli | Preterm infant may need supplement. |
| Vitamin K: Aqua-Mephyton | Necessary for production of clotting factors | Pork, liver, green leafy vegetables, tomatoes, egg yolks, cheese | Administer vitamin K prophylactically to newborns. Intake may be decreased in clients receiving warfarin and dicumarol anticoagulants. |
| **Vitamins: Water-Soluble** | | | |
| Vitamin $B_1$: Thiamine | Necessary for healthy nervous system, coenzyme for carbohydrate metabolism | Pork, beef, legumes, whole grains, enriched cereals, green vegetables | Clients with increased metabolic rate need more vitamin $B_1$ (e.g., clients with fever, clients who are pregnant, clients receiving long-term IV therapy). Increase intake in alcoholic clients. |
| Vitamin $B_6$: Pyridoxine | Stimulates heme production for red blood cells, necessary for antibody formation | Organ meats, wheat and corn cereal grains, soybeans, tuna, chicken, salmon | Be aware of drug-induced deficiencies: isoniazid, oral contraceptives. |
| Vitamin $B_{12}$: Cobalamin | Formation of normal red blood cells, nerve function | Meat, liver, fish, poultry, milk, eggs, cheese | Supplement necessary for clients with gastric resection; must have intrinsic factor for normal absorption. |
| Vitamin C: Ascorbic acid | Increases absorption of iron for hemoglobin formation, necessary for collagen formation, antioxidant | Citrus fruits, tomatoes, strawberries, potatoes, cabbage, broccoli, melons, spinach | Cook vegetables with a lid and minimum water added. Need is increased during growth or conditions that cause an increase in metabolism. |
| **Minerals** | | | |
| Iron (Fe) | Normal formation of hemoglobin, essential part of enzymes | Red meat such as liver, pork, and beef; poultry; beans; whole grains; enriched infant formula; enriched cereals and bread | Administer iron between meals with citrus juices to increase absorption; avoid use of antacids; stool will be black. Increase iron intake for clients with iron-deficiency anemias, those on vegetarian diets, pregnant women, infants consuming excessive amounts of milk. |
| Calcium (Ca) | Normal formation of bone and teeth; muscle contraction, especially the heart; clotting factors; normal nerve conduction | Dairy products, dark-green leafy vegetables, fortified grains and cereal, sardines | Adequate intake is needed for normal bone and tooth formation. Administer IV preparations with caution because of effects on heart. Increase supplements during pregnancy and lactation and after menopause. |
| Potassium (K) | Acid–base balance, nerve conduction, cardiac muscle contraction | Dried fruits, bananas, citrus fruits, tomatoes | Supplement when client is taking diuretics. Decreased potassium increases effects of digitalis. |
| Sodium (Na) | Acid–base balance, fluid balance | Table salt, processed foods | Sodium deficiency is rare; focus is on decreasing intake except in situations of significant sodium loss (e.g., CF, diaphoresis). |

*CF,* cystic fibrosis; *IU,* international unit; *IV,* intravenous.

**❗ OLDER ADULT PRIORITY:** It usually takes more time for an older person to eat, and satiety is reached more quickly. Encourage frequent small meals rather than three large meals; providing liquid supplements is also beneficial.

## Nutritional Assessment

A. Assess nutritional needs.
B. Create client profile: age, sex, height, weight, socioeconomic status, and culture.
C. Determine nutritional status: note food habits; observe for physical signs indicative of nutritional status.
D. Determine disease or pathophysiologic process.
E. Be alert to high-risk clients: those who are overweight or underweight; those with congenital anomalies of GI tract; those who have had surgery of the GI tract; those who have problems with ingestion, digestion, and/or absorption; and those receiving IV therapy for 10 days or more.

**TEST ALERT:** Intervene with the client who has an alteration in nutritional intake (adjust diet, change delivery to include method, time, and food preferences).

## Diet Therapy for High-Level Wellness

A. MyPlate (Figure 2-4).
B. Prudent diet.
   1. Increased amounts of fresh fruits, vegetables, and whole grains.
   2. Reduced amounts of animal fats, cholesterol, refined sugar, salt, and alcohol.
   3. Adaptations to MyPlate (see Figure 2-4).
      a. Meat: includes fish, chicken, turkey, beef, legumes, eggs, nuts, and seeds as a source of protein (select lean or low-fat meat and poultry).
      b. Milk: includes milk, soymilk, yogurt, and cheese (select no-fat or low-fat).
      c. Oils: use selected fish, nut, and vegetable oils; limit butter, margarine, shortening, and lard (select oils with no trans fats).
      d. Fruits and vegetables: eat a variety; 100% fruit juice is acceptable; eat more dark green and orange vegetables. (Fruits and vegetables should make up half your plate.)
      e. Grains, breads, and cereals: whole-grain products should make up half the daily grain.
   4. Drink water instead of sugary drinks.
C. Body mass index (BMI) measures weight as corrected for height.
   1. Divide the client's weight in kilograms by height in meters squared.
   2. A client who weighs 165 lb (75 kg) and is 5 ft 9 in tall (1.8 m) has a BMI of 23.15 (75 divided by $1.8^2$ = 23.15).
   3. A client is considered overweight if the BMI is 25 to 30. A BMI greater than 30 is considered as obese.

**TEST ALERT:** Apply knowledge of mathematics to client nutrition (e.g., BMI). Evaluate and monitor client height and weight.

## Therapeutic Meal Plans

A therapeutic meal plan or prescription diet is a modification of an individual's normal nutritional requirements based on the changes in his or her physiologic needs as a result of an illness or disease state (Table 2-4).

**TEST ALERT:** Consider client choices regarding meeting nutritional requirements and/or maintaining dietary restrictions, including mention of specific food items. Provide/maintain special diets based on the client diagnosis/nutritional needs and cultural considerations.

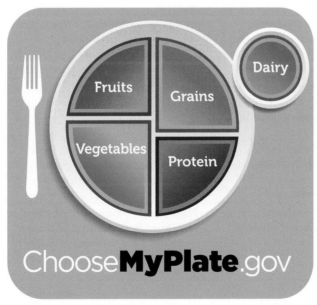

**FIGURE 2-4  MyPlate Food Guide.** (From the U.S. Department of Agriculture. ChooseMyPlate.gov. Available at https://www.choosemyplate.gov/.)

**Table 2-4   THERAPEUTIC MEAL PLANS**

| Diet | Purpose/Use | Foods Allowed | Foods Restricted |
|---|---|---|---|
| Clear liquid | To begin introduction of food after removal of NG tube, after GI surgery, and/or before GI diagnostics | Liquids that are clear, such as tea and coffee without cream, apple juice, ice pops, broth, clear sodas | Milk products, juice with pulp, any solid food; anything that is not liquid at room temperature |
| Full liquid | To begin introduction of food; used after removal of NG tube or after GI surgery | Any food that is liquid at room temperature | Any solid food |
| Soft diet | To progress diet as tolerated; food should be easy to chew and swallow | Soft, tender foods easy to swallow and digest; eggs | Highly seasoned foods, whole grains, fruits, vegetables, nuts, fried foods |
| Mechanical soft diet | To assist clients who cannot chew effectively | Soft foods that are easy to chew and swallow | Tough foods that are difficult to digest and swallow; steak |
| Bland diet | To eliminate foods irritating to the digestive system; used in clients after GI surgery and those with peptic ulcer disease and GI inflammatory problems | Milk, custards, refined cereals, creamed soups, potatoes (baked or broiled); all foods are white; no bright-colored food | Highly seasoned or strong-flavored foods; tea, colas, coffee, fruits, whole grains, raw fruit |
| Low-residue diet | To decrease fiber or stool in GI tract; acute episodes of enteritis, diarrhea; before and/or after GI surgery | Clear liquids, meats, fats, eggs, refined cereals, white bread, peeled white potatoes, small amount of milk | Cheeses; whole grains; raw fruits and vegetables; high-carbohydrate foods, which are usually high in residue and fiber |
| High-residue diet (also known as high-fiber) | To prevent constipation and acute diverticulitis; recommended for clients with irritable bowel syndrome (IBS) | Raw fruits and vegetables; whole grains; high-carbohydrate foods, which are high in residue and fiber | Indigestible fibers: celery, whole corn; seeds such as sesame and poppy; foods with small seeds |
| Lactose-free diet | To prevent GI effects of lactose intolerance | Nonmilk products, yogurt | Milk and milk products, processed foods that may have dried milk as filler |
| PKU diet | To control intake of phenylalanine, an essential acid; affected children cannot metabolize it | Specially prepared infant formula if infant is not breastfed, vegetables, fruits, juices, some cereals, and breads; may allow 20–30 mg of phenylalanine per kilogram of body weight to fulfill normal growth needs | Most high-protein foods, including meat and dairy products, are significantly reduced |
| Low-fat/low-cholesterol diet | To prevent gall bladder spasms, clients with increased cholesterol levels, or problems with malabsorption of fat (cystic fibrosis) | Low-fat or fat-free milk, fruits, vegetables, breads, cereals, reduced amounts of red meat | Egg yolks, whole milk, fried foods, processed cheese, shrimp, avocados, pastries, butter |
| Low-sodium diet | To reduce sodium intake to decrease retention of fluids, especially in clients with cardiac disease or hypertension | Salt-free preparations, fresh fruits, vegetables with no added salt | Processed foods, smoked or salted meats, prepared foods, frozen and canned vegetables, breads and pastries |
| High-potassium diet | To replace lost potassium in clients taking diuretics and/or digitalis | Dried fruits, fruit juices, fresh fruits (e.g., bananas, apricots, grapefruit, oranges, and tomatoes); sweet potatoes, legumes | No specific restrictions |
| Renal diet | Control potassium, sodium, and protein levels in clients with renal problems | High biologic protein (limited intake): eggs, milk, meat; decreased sodium products and decreased potassium (cabbage, peas, cucumbers are low in potassium) | High-potassium foods (dried fruits), high-sodium foods (processed foods), salt substitutes with high-potassium content |
| Low-purine diet | To decrease serum levels of uric acid; prescribed for clients with gout and high levels of uric acid | Vegetables, fruits, cereals, eggs, fat-free milk, cottage cheese | Glandular meats, fish, poultry, nuts, beans, oatmeal, whole wheat, cauliflower |

*GI*, Gastrointestinal; *NG*, nasogastric; *PKU*, phenylketonuria.

Appendix 2.1   DEVELOPMENTAL TASKS

| Stage of Development | Erikson's Developmental Tasks | Play/Social Activities | Health Promotion/Maintenance |
|---|---|---|---|
| Infancy (birth to 1 year) | *Trust versus mistrust.* Parent–child bonding is crucial to the foundation for building a basic sense of trust. It is essential for primary needs to be gratified promptly. | Involved in solitary play activities. Provide toys that are soft, cuddly, and colorful; mobiles are popular. | Encourage routine immunizations. Teach safety precautions related to burns, poisonings, accidents, and drowning. |
| Toddler (1–3 years) | *Autonomy versus shame and doubt.* Child relies heavily on parental responses for support. | Toilet training is the major developmental accomplishment. Involved in parallel play activities. Provide toys that can be pulled, stacked together. | Continue to monitor safety by "childproofing" the home. Increased incidence of respiratory tract and ear infections. |
| Early childhood (3–6 years) | *Initiative versus guilt.* Child uses imagination and creativeness. | Follows rules, compares self to others. | Progresses from solitary play to more cooperative play with others in a group. |
| Middle childhood (6–12 years) | *Industry versus inferiority.* "Chum" period; progresses from self-centered to more other-directed behavior. Reality testing improves. | Younger child plays by assuming roles as a fireman, doctor, nurse, teacher, etc. Older child involved with bicycle riding, table games, sports, etc. | Respiratory tract infections are common illnesses as child goes to school. Booster immunizations are important. |
| Adolescence (12–18 years) | *Identity versus role confusion.* Completion of previous tasks successfully will lead to a secure sense of self. | Peer groups are most important, with behavior being defined more by group members. Social activities include dating. | Mood swings common. Accidents associated with driving cars and motorcycles become more common. |
| Young adulthood (18–44 years) | *Intimacy versus isolation.* Disturbances in sex role identity may occur because of inadequate resolution of identity crisis. | Involvement with social network of peers from community, work, etc. Appraisals by others affects sense of identity and self. | Stress-related illnesses and drug and alcohol abuse are common during this period. Another health issue is pregnancy. |
| Middle adulthood (45–64 years) | *Generativity versus stagnation.* Reassessment of life goals. Mutuality among peers. | Leisure time becomes more of a concern. Key socializing agents are lovers, spouses, and close friends. Retirement occurs. | Menopause and chronic health problems occur (e.g., diabetes, cancer). |
| Older adulthood (65 years and older) | *Ego integrity versus despair.* If person viewed life as worthwhile, will be better equipped to deal with aging. | Central process is introspection with the favorable outcome of wisdom along with a detached yet active concern with life in the face of death. | Safety concerns reoccur because of impaired sensory input. Alterations in all major body systems occur. |

## Study Questions
## Health Implications Across the Life Span

More questions on

1. Which behavior indicates that an 18-month-old infant is developing a nonadaptive reaction to hospitalization?
   1. Cries when the mother leaves.
   2. Ignores mother when she arrives to visit.
   3. Eats using fingers rather than utensils.
   4. Is afraid of the dark.

2. An 8-month-old infant is sitting contentedly on the mother's lap. The nurse is preparing to perform a well-baby checkup. Which of the following steps should the nurse do first?
   1. Measure the head circumference.
   2. Obtain body weight and height.
   3. Auscultate heart and lung sounds.
   4. Check pupil response to light.

3. When obtaining a health history from an older client, the nurse must take which characteristics of the older client into consideration?
   1. The older client responds to pain sensation with the same intensity as a young client.
   2. Auditory acuity is the most common sensory loss in the older adult population and may hinder the interview.
   3. The older client requires a lot of repetition because the IQ declines with the aging process.
   4. An older client's response time to answering a question is just as quick as that of a young client.

4. Which of the following actions would the nurse recommend providing to a 12-month-old infant with nutrients for growth?
   1. Exclude milk from the infant's diet until he or she begins to like other foods.
   2. Offer the infant small amounts of meat and vegetables before offering milk.
   3. Withhold desserts until the infant has eaten his or her vegetables.
   4. Mix strained meat and vegetables into the milk given to the infant.

5. What are appropriate toys for an 18-month-old infant to have for play while in isolation?
   1. Rattles
   2. Stacking rings
   3. Crayons and coloring book
   4. Soap bubbles

6. The nurse is discussing nutrition with a woman who is 50 years old, perimenopausal, and has a history of hypertension. What food choices would be best to help meet the dietary needs of this client?
   1. Cheese and macaroni, fresh fruit, and milk shake
   2. Cottage cheese, glass of skim milk, and fresh spinach salad
   3. Roast beef with whole wheat bread, potato, and lettuce salad
   4. Cheeseburger, French fries, and milk shake

7. The nurse is serving a food tray to a client who has glomerulonephritis and azotemia. Which food selection would the nurse question?
   1. Bread and rice
   2. Dried peaches and apricots
   3. Bran muffin and eggs
   4. Apples and cucumbers

8. Planning anticipatory guidance is an important nursing function. Considering the teaching for the family of an 18-month-old girl, which comment by the mother indicates she understands safety concerns?
   1. "I will keep an eye on her all of the time; I will not let her out of my sight."
   2. "When she says 'no-no,' then she understands right and wrong."
   3. "I will need to be sure that the locks on the medicine cabinet are secure."
   4. "I'll be sure to give her syrup of ipecac if she swallows any poison."

9. The nurse is assisting in the discharge preparation of a new mother and her infant. The mother asks when the immunizations will begin for her infant. What is the best nursing response?
   1. The first series of the DTaP vaccine will be given before her discharge.
   2. DTaP and varicella vaccines will be administered around 3 months of age.
   3. The series of infant immunizations will begin around 6 months of age.
   4. Immunizations are recommended to begin as early as after birth.

10. The nurse is assessing an infant on the first office visit after birth. The mother asks the nurse when the chickenpox vaccination should be given. What is the best nursing response?
    1. The infant received this vaccination at the hospital when he was born.
    2. The varicella vaccination will be given at the infant's 1-month checkup.
    3. The infant should receive the immunization immediately if he is exposed to varicella.
    4. The varicella vaccination is administered after 12 months.

11. A mother brings her 5-year-old daughter to the wellness clinic complaining of a rash covering the child's body. The nurse recognizes the rash as chickenpox (varicella), which is characterized by:
    1. Clusters of small blisters
    2. Raised, reddened areas on the upper trunk
    3. A maculopapular rash
    4. Petechiae

12. A client comes to the emergency department with a deep, penetrating wound he received in his garden. What is an important nursing action?
    1. Rinse the wound with antibiotic solution.
    2. Administer gamma globulin intramuscularly.
    3. Anticipate notifying poison control for plant toxicology.
    4. Determine when the client received his last tetanus injection.

13. A toddler is admitted after taking an unknown number of acetaminophen tablets. Which of the following early symptoms would the nurse expect to find on her assessment? Select all that apply.
    1. Pallor
    2. Hot, dry skin
    3. Pain in the upper right quadrant
    4. Severe burning pain in stomach
    5. Nausea, vomiting
    6. Coughing and inability to clear secretions

14. An infant with a diagnosis of acquired immunodeficiency syndrome (AIDS) has a nursing diagnosis of altered growth and development on the nursing care plan. Which nursing measure would enhance growth and development in the infant?
    1. Provide opportunities for the family to participate in the infant's care.
    2. Stimulate the infant with a mobile in the crib.
    3. Weigh the infant daily and count diapers for estimation of fluid loss.
    4. Provide nutritional supplements throughout the day.

15. In clients 65 years of age and older, how is death most commonly viewed?
    1. As a romanticized situation
    2. As a time of disassociation
    3. As a part of life
    4. As a time of denial

16. A child is diagnosed with a severe case of rubeola. The nurse would question which of the following orders?
    1. Administer an oral dose of 200,000 IU of vitamin A.
    2. Administer antipyretics.
    3. Administer oral fluids as tolerated.
    4. Administer intravenous immune globulin (IVIG) after exposure.

17. A client who is scheduled for a colonoscopy is instructed to take nothing except clear liquids for 6 hours before the procedure. What comment by the client would indicate to the nurse that the client does not understand the concept of clear liquids?
    1. "I can have beef or chicken broth."
    2. "Lemon-, orange-, or lime-flavored gelatin is okay."
    3. "I can have a small amount of vanilla ice cream."
    4. "I can have tea and coffee with sugar."

18. Which of the following is a priority teaching topic for the parents of a school-age child?
    1. Using a nightlight to allay night terrors
    2. Encouraging the child to dress without help
    3. Explaining the components of a healthy diet
    4. Reviewing information about accident prevention

19. A preschool-age child is admitted to the hospital for treatment of pneumonia. The mother is embarrassed because the child has voided in the bed, which the child has not done since he was toilet-trained. Which of the following statements by the nurse would be appropriate?
    1. "This happens quite often with children when they are admitted to the hospital. When he feels better, his toileting skills will return to normal."
    2. "My, how embarrassing for you to have your child do this. Don't worry. We see this all the time."
    3. "Bedwetting is often a side effect of the antibiotic medication that your child is receiving. When the medicine is finished, his toileting skills will return to normal."
    4. "I will be sure to report the bedwetting to the physician because it may require additional tests to determine the cause."

20. A preschool child has a history of an appendectomy and is scheduled for an open reduction and internal fixation of the femur. What would be appropriate for preoperative teaching?
    1. Have the mother read the child a favorite story to reduce anxiety before the surgery.
    2. Ask the child how she felt after the last surgery.
    3. Provide appropriate materials and involve the child in role-playing.
    4. Tell the child that she will return with just a cast on and that it won't hurt.

21. The nurse is caring for an older adult client who is on bed rest. What considerations should be made for the client's nutritional intake?
    1. Intake of breads, rice, and pasta is increased.
    2. Bran, whole grains, and fresh green vegetables are increased.
    3. Fish and poultry should be increased, with a decrease in beef.
    4. Milk and milk products are increased.

22. What would the nurse expect to find when exploring a 9-year-old's concept of death?
    1. Knows that death is a final process.
    2. Regards death as a temporary state of sleep.
    3. Believes death is something that "just happens."
    4. Thinks death results from being bad.

# Answers to Study Questions

**1.** *2*
Usually, the toddler clings to the mother. As separation anxiety becomes intolerable, the child ignores the parent. At this stage, the child relates better to the staff and doesn't mind the absence of the parent. Eating with his fingers and being afraid of the dark are normal for an infant at this age. (Hockenberry & Wilson, 10 ed., pp. 864–867)

**2.** *3*
While the infant is quiet, it is important to auscultate the heart and lungs. Placing a tape measure on the infant's head, shining a light in the eyes, or undressing the infant before weighing may cause distress, which could make auscultating the heart and lungs, as well as the rest of the examination, more difficult. (Hockenberry & Wilson, 10 ed., pp. 112–118)

**3.** *2*
When interviewing an older client, auditory acuity is the most common age-related aspect to take into consideration. It is important to make sure the client hears and understands the questions. If the client does not hear the question correctly, the response time cannot be determined. The IQ may decline with dementia. (Potter & Perry, 9 ed., p. 178)

**4.** *2*
Children at this age are prone to anemia, especially when milk is offered frequently; therefore holding liquids until after solid food is offered prevents the child from filling up on liquids. (Hockenberry & Wilson, 10 ed., p. 1385)

**5.** *2*
Stacking rings are a good toy to promote fine motor skills for a toddler. Because 18-month-old infants tend to put objects in their mouth, crayons and soap bubbles would not be appropriate. (Hockenberry & Wilson, 10 ed., p. 497)

**6.** *2*
Because the woman is perimenopausal, she needs increased calcium intake (1500 mg/day). With a diagnosis of hypertension, she also needs a decreased-sodium diet. Foods high in calcium include milk products, leafy green vegetables, and dried beans. Yellow vegetables are not high in calcium. Pasta and breads are a source of sodium. (Lewis, Dirksen, Heitkemper et al., 10 ed., pp. 688)

**7.** *2*
The increased potassium found in dried peaches and apricots is contraindicated for a client with increased potassium and blood urea nitrogen (BUN) levels. Dried fruit is high in potassium. (Lewis, Dirksen, Heitkemper et al., 10 ed., p. 1083)

**8.** *3*
Having medications and other dangerous cleaning materials and chemicals locked away in secure areas is an important safety issue for toddlers. It is not advisable to induce vomiting (giving syrup of ipecac) without calling the local poison control center first to be sure that it is okay to do so. Ingested materials may be corrosive, and inducing vomiting would not be an appropriate nursing action. (Hockenberry & Wilson, 10 ed., pp. 516–517)

**9.** *4*
Immunizations are started as early as birth to 1 month (first dose of hepatitis B vaccine is recommended to be given before discharge from the hospital). The diphtheria, tetanus, and pertussis (DTaP) vaccine and inactivated poliovirus vaccine (IPV) series, pneumococcal vaccine (PCV), and *Haemophilus influenzae* (Hib) series are started at 2 months. (Hockenberry & Wilson, 10 ed., pp. 195–206)

**10.** *4*
The varicella vaccine (chicken pox) can be administered any time after 12 months of age. It is not given before this age because the infant's immune system has not yet matured. (Hockenberry & Wilson, 10 ed., p. 195–206.)

**11.** *3*
Varicella is an acute viral disease characterized by a maculopapular rash with vesicular scabs in multiple stages of healing. Most erythematous rashes start on the face and progress to the rest of the body. (Hockenberry & Wilson, 10 ed., p. 204)

**12.** *4*
Deep, penetrating wounds that are contaminated by soil, dust, or excreta containing *Clostridium tetani* are the cause of tetanus, or lockjaw. First, the wound should be thoroughly cleansed, but not with antibiotic solution. The nurse should determine when the client received his last tetanus immunization. As a rule, clients will receive a tetanus booster as a safeguard. (Hockenberry & Wilson, 10 ed., p. 202)

**13.** *1, 5*
Pallor, sweating, nausea, and vomiting are symptoms seen in the first stage of acetaminophen poisoning followed by a latent period (24–36 hours) where the child improves. Pain in the upper right quadrant is indicative of hepatic involvement, which is considered the third stage or later symptom of acetaminophen poisoning. There is no indication that acetaminophen causes burning pain in the stomach, as does aspirin. The drug does not cause coughing or difficulty with handling secretions. (Hockenberry & Wilson, 10 ed., p. 545)

**14.** *4*
Nutrition is the key to adequate growth and development for an infant who is immunocompromised. Supplements will support normal nutrition and should be considered as part of the care for an infant with this nursing diagnosis. The family should be encouraged to participate in care, but that does not necessarily promote nutrition. (Hockenberry & Wilson, 10 ed., p. 714–716.)

**15.** *3*
The older adult finds meaning in life and adjusts to the death of a spouse or loved one. He or she is aware of death as an inevitable part of living and often reacts to dying as a time of reflection, rest, and peace. (Potter & Perry, 9 ed., p. 183)

16. *4*

The nurse would question the order for intravenous immune globulin (IVIG) because it is associated with varicella (chickenpox) and is administered after exposure to high-risk children. The child with rubeola or measles will be receiving antipyretics to reduce fever during the febrile period and should be encouraged to increase fluids. Supplementation with vitamin A decreases morbidity and mortality in measles. (Hockenberry & Wilson, 10 ed., p. 203)

17. *3*

Ice cream is not a clear liquid. The gelatins are okay, but red-colored gelatin is often prohibited. Coffee and tea are both acceptable with sugar, but no cream is allowed. (Potter & Perry, 9 ed., p. 1074)

18. *4*

In this instance all of these responses would be appropriate to teach, but accidents are the leading cause of death and disability in the school-age child, which makes this information a priority teaching topic. (Hockenberry & Wilson, 10 ed., pp. 3–6)

19. *1*

Children often regress during a hospitalization, so behavior such as toilet training may be temporarily lost but will return when the child feels better and returns home to a normal routine. Antibiotics do not typically cause incontinence. The other responses do not involve therapeutic communication. (Hockenberry & Wilson, 10 ed., p. 832)

20. *3*

School-age children need concrete experiences; hence, a pediatric orientation program would be most appropriate in this situation. Having materials or props with which to role-play would be beneficial in the preoperative care for this child. Role-playing is appropriate with children who can verbalize and talk about their activities. Never lie to the child about what is going to happen. (Hockenberry & Wilson,10 ed., p. 892)

21. *2*

Increase intake of fiber. Foods high in vitamins and low carbohydrate foods are increased. There is a decrease in metabolism, so carbohydrates and fats are decreased. The client should have an adequate, not necessarily increased, protein intake. Concern is with constipation and adequate vitamin intake. (Potter & Perry, 9 ed., p. 1061)

22. *1*

By the age of 9 or 10 years, the child has developed the mental and emotional security to express an understanding of death as a final and inevitable outcome of life. The preschooler sees death as temporary or as a punishment. (Hockenberry & Wilson, 10 ed., pp. 798–800)

# 3 Concepts of Nursing Practice

Health Promotion, Mobility, Pain, Patient Education

## BASIC HUMAN NEEDS

A. Maslow's hierarchy of basic human needs.
  1. Human behavior is motivated by a system of needs.
  2. Clients will focus on or attempt to satisfy needs at the base of the pyramid before focusing on those higher up in the pyramid (Figure 3-1).
  3. Human needs are *universal,* but some may be modified by cultural influence.
  4. The nursing process is always concerned with physiologic needs first; it then progresses to safety, teaching, decreasing anxiety, etc. This is also true for the client with psychosocial needs; the client's physiologic and safety needs must be met before he or she can progress to the next level.

> **NURSING PRIORITY:** Maslow's hierarchy of needs is useful in answering test questions related to setting priorities. Always remember that the physiologic needs at the base of the pyramid must be satisfied before turning to focus on other needs—and remember that oxygenation is always the first physiologic need or priority.

## Maslow's Hierarchy of Basic Human Needs

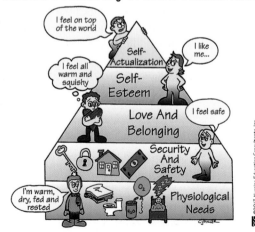

**FIGURE 3-1  Maslow's Hierarchy of Needs.** (From Zerwekh, J., Garneau, A., & Miller, C. J. [2017]. *Digital collection of the memory notebooks of nursing* [4th ed.]. Chandler, AZ: Nursing Education Consultants, Inc.)

## HEALTH ASSESSMENT

### Patient Health Interview

> **TEST ALERT:** Obtain a health history; perform a comprehensive health assessment; complete a focused health assessment.

> **NURSING PRIORITY:** Ensure proper identification of client when providing care, using a minimum of two identifiers (e.g., full name and date of birth). Maintain client confidentiality and privacy.

### *Health History*

A. Demographic data.
  1. Name, address, phone, age, sex, marital status.
  2. Race, religion, usual source of medical care.
B. Chief complaint/reason for visit.
  1. Chief complaint: main reason client sought health care.
  2. Chief complaint is recorded in client's own words.
  *Example:* "I have been vomiting blood since this morning."
C. History of the present illness.
  1. Chronologic narrative.
  2. Areas of investigation to evaluate the symptoms.
    a. Sequence, chronology, and frequency.
    b. Bodily location and radiation.
    c. Character of the symptoms: intensity or severity.
    d. Associated phenomena or manifestations.
    e. Aggravating or alleviating factors.
  3. Includes relevant family history.
D. Medical history.
  1. Perception of illness.
  2. Previous illnesses: hospitalization, surgery, chronic illnesses.
  3. Allergies, status of immunizations.
  4. Accidents and injuries.
  5. Current medications—prescribed and nonprescribed, over-the-counter medications, including herbs and any complementary therapies.
  6. Prenatal, labor and delivery, or neonatal history (recorded for all children under age 5 and older children with a congenital or developmental problem).
  7. Psychosocial history: sources of stress, coping mechanisms.
  8. Activities of daily living.
    a. Nutrition and elimination routine.
    b. Rest/sleep.

c. Personal habits (alcohol, smoking, exercise, illicit drugs, etc.)
9. Developmental level: school/education, work, family activities, social activities.
   a. The Denver Developmental Screening Test (Denver II): a developmental screening test for toddlers and preschool children; not an IQ test but a test to identify developmental delay in toddlers and young children by determining their behavioral and cognitive function.
   b. Mental status exam: the purpose is to evaluate the client's current cognitive processes (see Chapter 12).

**TEST ALERT:** Perform a mental status assessment on the nonpsychiatric client (see Chapter 12 for mental status exam).

E. Review of systems.
   1. Brief account from the client regarding any recent signs or symptoms associated with the body systems.
   2. Contains subjective data given by the client; *does not* contain objective data from the physical examination.
   3. When a symptom or problem is encountered in the review of systems, the following information should be determined:
      a. Location: In what area of the body does the symptom occur?
      b. Character: Quality of the problem, feeling, or sensation. Is pain sharp or dull, constant or intermittent?
      c. Intensity: Severity of symptom or feeling. Does it interfere with activities of daily living?
      d. Timing: When does the problem occur (onset, duration, frequency)? Does anything precipitate the problem?
      e. Aggravating/alleviating factors: What activities make the problem better or worse?
   4. Review of system progresses from head to toe. The pertinent information to include is located in the assessment section at the beginning of each system.

## Nursing Assessment
*Comprehensive Health Assessment*

**TEST ALERT:** Perform comprehensive health assessment—physical, psychosocial, and health history. Choose physical assessment equipment and technique appropriate for client.

A. General guidelines.
   1. If the examiner is right-handed, the examination should be conducted from the right side of the bed.
   2. Position bed or examining table at appropriate height.
   3. Adequately expose areas being examined.
   4. Explain each part of the examination to the client as the examination proceeds.
   5. Establish rapport by asking nonpersonal and/or general health questions before the physical examination.

B. Techniques of physical assessment.
   1. Inspection.
      a. Careful examination and observation are important parts of the assessment.
      b. Each anatomic area is inspected *before* it is touched by examiner's hands or instruments.
   2. Palpation.
      a. Parts of the hand used during palpation.
         (1) Fingertips for fine, tactile discrimination (e.g., lymph nodes, skin texture).
         (2) Dorsa of hands for skin temperature (dorsal skin is thinner and more sensitive).
         (3) Palmar and ulnar surfaces for vibratory sensation.
         (4) Grasping position (pinching) of fingers for tissue consistency.
      b. Light palpation identifies areas of tenderness and muscle resistance.
      c. Deep palpation is essentially the same as light palpation, but the examiner uses two hands to press more deeply into the client's body region. If there is any tenderness present, perform deep palpation last.
   3. Percussion.
      a. Technique of striking body surface lightly but sharply to produce sounds.
      b. Indirect percussion.
         (1) Middle finger of the nondominant hand *(pleximeter)* is placed against the body surface with palm and other fingers raised off the skin. Tip of middle finger of dominant hand *(plexor)* strikes the base of the distal phalanx of the pleximeter in a quick, sharp stroke.
      c. Direct percussion.
         (1) Gentle, direct striking of the body with one or more fingers or with the ulnar surface of the clenched fist.
         (2) Useful in assessing sinuses, kidneys, or the liver.
      d. Percussion sounds.
         (1) Resonance: loud, low note heard over normal lung tissue.
         (2) Hyperresonance: louder, lower, and longer note heard over emphysematous lung.
         (3) Tympany: loud, musical note with drumlike quality; heard over air-filled viscera (e.g., stomach or bowel).
         (4) Flat: soft, high-pitched, short note heard, for example, over the thigh.
         (5) Dull: medium-pitched note of intensity and duration heard over the liver.
   4. Auscultation.
      a. Bell of stethoscope is used for low-pitched sounds, such as murmurs and bruits.
      b. Diaphragm of stethoscope is used for high-pitched sounds such as wheezes and crackles.

C. Sequence of the physical examination (Table 3-1)
D. When a client indicates a problem or symptom during the physical examination, that area should be investigated (see review of systems earlier in chapter).

## Table 3-1 SEQUENCE OF PHYSICAL EXAMINATION

| Client Position | Areas Assessed |
| --- | --- |
| Supine, sitting, and standing | Vital signs and pulse oximetry |
| Supine | Breasts, heart, abdomen, inguinal region, female genitourinary system (lithotomy position), hips, knees, ankles, feet |
| Sitting | Head, face, eyes, ears, nose, mouth, neck, chest, heart, lungs, breasts, reflexes, hands, arms, shoulders (muscle strength), cerebellum (rapid, alternating movements, sensory function [stereognosis]) |
| Standing | Spine, ROM, varicose veins, cerebellum, gait, balance, male genitourinary system |

*ROM*, Range of motion.

E. Detailed assessment findings for each body system are discussed at the beginning of each chapter.

### *Focused Assessment*

> **TEST ALERT:** Perform a focused assessment (gastrointestinal [GI], respiratory, sensory, etc.). Perform a risk assessment (falls, mobility, skin, and activities of daily living [ADLs]).

A. A focused assessment is limited to the particular need, health care problem, or health risk the client is experiencing.
B. Frequently used for bedside assessments.
 1. Assess the specific characteristics of the problem.
 2. Determine what type of nursing intervention is necessary.
 3. Determine when the intervention should be done: immediately, later in shift, before client's discharge, etc.
C. An initial assessment is frequently focused on a client's current health problems. This type of assessment is most often done at the beginning of each shift by the nurse responsible for the care of the client. *Reassessments are performed throughout the shift, as warranted by any change in the client's status.*
 1. Focus on client's current status; determine whether it correlates with the report the nurse received.
 2. Monitor or determine the client's response to previous nursing interventions.
 3. Evaluate client's response to current plan of care and determine whether any changes are necessary.
 4. Evaluate for any evidence of complications developing. (A systems focused assessment is found at the beginning of each of the system chapters.)

> **TEST ALERT:** Implement measures to manage/prevent/lessen complications of the client's condition.

5. Determine whether there are any other problems the client is experiencing that have not been addressed.

## HEALTH PROMOTION

### Levels of Prevention

Preventive health care is more dynamic than health maintenance; it focuses on health enhancement and health promotion, whereas health maintenance is concerned with maintaining the status quo.
A. Primary: prevention of disease.
 1. The goal is to achieve maximum functioning in each health potential area.
 *Examples:* Stop smoking, practice safe sex, maintain body weight, limit alcohol intake, follow a regular exercise program and a healthy diet.
B. Secondary: early diagnosis and treatment.
 1. Emphasis is on determining intervention priorities.
 *Examples:* Screening for tuberculosis, glaucoma test, Pap smear, colorectal cancer, and testicular self-examination.
C. Tertiary: prevention of complications and maximize functional capabilities.
 1. The focus is on the prevention of complications and rehabilitation after the disease or condition has already occurred.
 *Examples:* Have blood drawn for a complete blood count before chemotherapy; initiate speech therapy after a cerebrovascular accident; start cardiac rehabilitation after a heart attack.

> **TEST ALERT:** Provide information regarding health maintenance recommendations, teach client actions to maintain health and prevent disease (immunizations, screening, etc.)

## HEALTH TEACHING

### Principles of Client Education (Box 3-1)

> **Box 3-1 TEPS IN CLIENT EDUCATION**
>
> - **Assessment**—What needs to be taught? Assess the client's knowledge of the condition, what the client most wants to learn about the condition, and what needs to be taught. How does the client perceive the need to learn? Are there any physical or psychosocial learning barriers? Consider the client's age and developmental level.
> - **Planning**—Establish learning objectives and content to be discussed. Determine how it will best be delivered (handouts, video, pictures).
> - **Implementation**—Determine whether the client is comfortable (physiologic needs are always first). Present the information in a manner the client can understand; provide opportunity for client feedback; provide written information and review it with the client; provide positive feedback.
> - **Evaluation**—Plan for a return demonstration if skill was taught; follow up with family; plan home visits, etc. to determine client's use of information.

> **⚠ NURSING PRIORITY:** Consider client's background, culture, and developmental stage when preparing teaching materials and determine when client is ready to learn.

A. Common characteristics of the adult learner.
  1. Self-directed.
  2. The client's background of experience, skills, attitudes, and culture form the basis for any new information received.
  3. The level of psychosocial development affects the client's readiness to learn.
  4. The client wants to apply the learning immediately.

> **⚠ OLDER ADULT PRIORITY:** Older clients tend to be solitary learners; the nurse needs to consider chronic health conditions and sensory deficits that may affect learning (e.g., provide large-print books for reading); encourage wearing prescription eyeglasses and hearing aids.

B. Factors contributing to the teaching–learning process.
  1. Readiness to learn.
    a. Belief that material is relevant.
    b. Mental capacity to learn and physical ability to perform the skills.
    c. Must have physical and safety needs met.
    d. Comfort.
      (1) Physical comfort: discomforts such as pain, nausea, hunger, and the need to void are distractions that affect the learning process.
      (2) Psychological comfort: anger, frustration, fear, and guilt severely hamper the learning process.

> **⚠ NURSING PRIORITY:** The first step in the education process is to make sure the client's physiologic needs are met; then determine what the client already knows about his or her condition.

    e. Client and nurse need to discuss and agree on specific long-term and short-term goals.
C. Factors relating to the presentation.

> **TEST ALERT:** Assess readiness to learn, learning preferences, and barriers to learning. Use age- and cognitive-appropriate explanations of procedures and treatments. Evaluate and document client understanding and willingness to comply with the information presented.

  1. State the specific objective of each teaching session; identify exactly what the client is to gain.
  2. Use vocabulary and terminology appropriate to the client's understanding and to his or her developmental level. Use correct terms for body parts.
  3. Try to stimulate as many senses as possible. Use visual aids (pictures and handouts) and pieces of equipment when appropriate.
  4. Repetition is an integral part of learning.
  5. The more active the client is in the process, the better he or she will retain the information.
  6. Plan short sessions; do not overwhelm the client with too much information at one time.
  7. Actively involve the family and significant others when appropriate.
  8. Be generous with positive reinforcement.
D. Pediatric factors influencing the learning process.
  1. Intellectual development moves from the concrete to the abstract.
  2. The nurse needs to assess the developmental level of a child before planning the educational approach.

> **⚠ NURSING PRIORITY:** A typical "no" response from a toddler being taught a new activity (e.g., combing hair) is usually an assertion of the child's independence, not an indication that he or she will not learn.

    a. Preschooler.
      (1) Frequently experiences fear of injury.
      (2) If under 4 years:
        (a) Generally does not benefit from anatomy and physiology information.
        (b) Needs clarification of reality and fantasy.
        (c) Separation anxiety is a problem; include the parents in the teaching session.
      (3) Preschoolers are aware of the physical and mechanical causes of problems they can see and are unaware of physical and mechanical forces they cannot see.

> **⚠ NURSING PRIORITY:** It is important to emphasize to the preschooler that treatment is not punishment.

    b. School-age child.
      (1) Benefits from tours, drawings, and anatomically correct dolls.
      (2) Cooperates with treatment and expresses feelings in words.
      (3) Learns well from dolls, role-playing, and puppets.
      (4) Needs to have parents included in teaching session for reinforcement and consistency.
    c. Adolescent.
      (1) Needs to be as independent as possible in management of health problem.
      (2) Present information with a scientific rationale rather than by giving specific directions.
      (3) Needs assistance in coping with loss of independence and self-direction.
      (4) Focus programs to deal with changes in body image and maintaining ego.
E. Special needs of the older client.
  1. Determine functional losses (e.g., hearing or vision impairment, memory loss).
  2. Identify social support to aid the older adult; this often increases compliance with instructions.

## END-OF-LIFE CARE

A. Provide psychosocial support to client and family.

1. Assist the client and family to participate in treatment decisions and prepare advance directives.
2. Promote spiritual comfort—encourage/assist client to contact spiritual advisors.
3. Protect client from feeling abandoned or isolated—respond quickly to call lights, check on client often, and tell the client when the nurse or health care provider will return.
4. Encourage family to participate in care—assisting with food, hygiene measures, physical contact.
5. Common symptoms: anxiety, depression, withdrawal, anger, hopelessness, powerlessness, fear, unusual communication around unresolved issues, vision-like experiences, resignation, acceptance, peace.

B. Promote culturally competent care—acknowledge and respect cultural differences and needs.
C. Assist client to understand end-of-life options and related terminology.

1. Do not resuscitate (DNR) or allow natural death (AND): maintain comfort measures, hygiene, and pain control; order must be written on chart.
2. Full code: full cardiopulmonary resuscitation (CPR) actions, including medications.
3. Modified code: reflects individual decisions, such as medications but no CPR.
4. Hospice care or palliative care.
   a. *Hospice* does not refer to a place but to a concept of care that provides support for the client who is dying.
   b. Care may be provided in a long-term care facility, hospital, a hospice center, or at home.
   c. Criteria for hospice care include the client's desire for the service and a physician's statement that the client will probably not survive beyond the next 6 months (the allowed time frame is somewhat flexible because the actual amount of time cannot be predicted).

### Physical Management of Symptoms

A. Physical symptoms of impending death.
1. Sensory.
   a. Hearing is usually the last sense to disappear.
   b. Taste and smell are diminished.
   c. Vision is often blurred; blink reflex may be absent.
2. Integumentary: skin is often cool and clammy; mottling occurs on extremities; cyanosis occurs around mouth and nose and on nail beds.
3. Respiratory.
   a. Respirations become shallow and irregular; Cheyne–Stokes respiration—periods of apnea alternating with deep, rapid breathing.

   b. Increased mucus in upper airway causing gurgling, noisy respirations.
   c. Inability to cough or clear airway.
4. Cardiovascular.
   a. Heart rate may vary from a regular, increased rate to a slowing and irregular heartbeat before death.
   b. Decreased blood pressure and tissue perfusion.
5. Elimination.
   a. Urinary: output decreases, incontinence occurs.
   b. Bowel: monitor for constipation; bowel incontinence may occur.
6. Musculoskeletal.
   a. Gradual loss of ability to move, loss of facial muscle tone.
   b. Difficulty speaking, unaware of body position.
7. Neurologic.
   a. Decreased level of consciousness.
   b. Decreased reflexes: gag, cough, swallow.

B. Nursing interventions.
1. Provide palliative pain management—the prevention or relief of pain when a cure for the client's illness is not feasible.

   a. Pain medication is frequently administered on an around-the-clock schedule to maintain therapeutic levels of medication; do not delay or deny pain relief measures to a dying client.
   b. Moderate to large amounts of opioids may be required to maintain client's comfort.
   c. Administer analgesics on the basis of client's level of pain; medication is increased as client's pain increases.
   d. Adjuvant medications to increase effectiveness of analgesics—antiemetics, antidepressants, corticosteroids.
   e. A nurse's or family's fear that the client will become dependent on, addicted to, or tolerant to the pain medication is inappropriate in provision of pain control in palliative care.
2. Dehydration: maintain oral hygiene; do not force the client to eat or drink. The option to withhold artificial nutrition or hydration should be made by the client in the advance directive or by the person designated in the advance directive.
3. Respiratory distress: elevate the head of the bed, offer oxygen, and provide medications to decrease apprehension.
4. Elimination.
   a. Utilize incontinence pads, prevent skin irritation, and follow facility protocol for indwelling catheters.
   b. Monitor bowel function, assess for impaction, and promote normal function within client limitations.

5. Anorexia, nausea, and vomiting.
   a. Assess for precipitating cause and administer medications to decrease nausea.
   b. Offer small, frequent meals, but do not focus on client's need to eat.
6. Determine client's personal preferences and cultural implications regarding death. Provide family care regarding cultural needs.

## Postmortem Care

**TEST ALERT:** Provide postmortem care.

A. Determine whether there are any tissues or organs to be donated.
B. Determine whether the client's death should be reported and whether the client's death necessitates an autopsy and/or release from autopsy.
C. Determine legal implications/indications requiring an autopsy in the state of residence or in the state in which the client died.
   1. Death resulting from foul play, homicide, suicide, or accident.
   2. Unattended death; death occurring at a workplace or during incarceration.
   3. Determine legal implications in the state of residence or in the state in which the client died.
D. Perform postmortem care as soon as possible.
   1. Determine whether family wants to participate in postmortem care.
   2. Unless client is to have an autopsy, remove all equipment according to facility policy.
   3. Cleanse the body and cover with a clean sheet. Place a pillow under the head and leave the arms on the outside of the sheet. Deodorize room if necessary.
   4. Offer the family an opportunity to be with the client. Provide privacy in an unrushed atmosphere.
   5. Return all personal belongings to the family. Document what items were taken and by whom.
   6. Attach identification to the body and to the shroud. Shroud the body according to facility policy.

## BASIC NURSING SKILLS

### Body Alignment and Range of Motion

A. Characteristics of correct body alignment in bed.
   1. Head up with eyes looking straight forward.
   2. Neck and back straight.
   3. Arms relaxed and supported at sides.
   4. Legs parallel to hips with knees slightly flexed.
   5. Feet separated and parallel to the legs with the toes pointed upward and slightly outward.

**TEST ALERT:** Perform a risk assessment for problems with mobility and skin. Maintain correct body alignment.

B. Range of motion (ROM) (Figure 3-2).
   1. Active ROM.
      a. Client performs exercise without assistance.
      b. Used for client who independently performs ADLs but for some reason is immobilized or limited in terms of activity.
      c. Purpose is to maintain muscle tone, decrease venous stasis, prevent muscle atrophy, and prevent contracture.
   2. Passive ROM.
      a. Client cannot actively move.
      b. Client cannot contract muscles; therefore muscle strengthening *cannot* be accomplished.
      c. Purpose is to maintain joint flexibility, prevent contractures, and promote venous return.
C. Principles of ROM exercises.
   1. Stretch muscles by moving the body part; avoid movement to the point of discomfort.
   2. Perform ROM at least twice daily for immobile clients, with a minimum of four to five repetitions of each exercise.
   3. Always support extremity above and below the joint when performing passive ROM on extremities.
   4. Involve the client in planning the exercise program.
D. Client positions (see Appendix 3-1).

## Asepsis

**TEST ALERT:** Always apply principles of infection control (handwashing/hand hygiene, room assignment, isolation, aseptic/sterile technique, standard precautions).

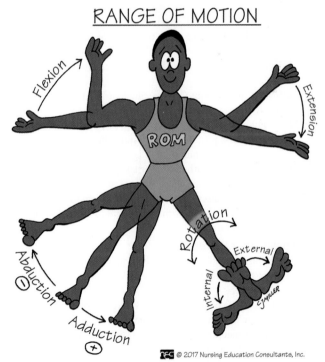

**FIGURE 3-2 Range of Motion.** (From Zerwekh, J., Garneau, A., & Miller, C. J. [2017]. *Digital collection of the memory notebooks of nursing* [4th ed.]. Chandler, AZ: Nursing Education Consultants, Inc.)

A. Medical asepsis.
1. Designed to reduce the number of pathogens in an area and decrease the likelihood of their transfer (e.g., by handwashing/hand hygiene).
2. Often referred to as *clean technique;* wash hands between visits with individual clients.
3. Included in this category are daily hygiene practices and administration of oral medications, enemas, and tube feedings.
B. Surgical asepsis.
1. Designed not simply to *reduce* the number of pathogens but to make the object *free* of all microorganisms.
2. Also known as *sterile technique.*
3. Surgical asepsis is reserved primarily for sterile dressing changes, sterile catheterizations, and surgical procedures in the operating room (Box 3-2).

> **TEST ALERT:** Set up a sterile field. Use appropriate supplies to maintain asepsis (gloves, mask, sterile supplies); evaluate whether aseptic techniques are performed correctly.

## Wound Care

A wound is a disruption in normal tissue caused by traumatic injury or created surgically.

> **TEST ALERT:** Provide wound care (irrigations, dressings). Monitor wounds for signs of infection.

### Box 3-2 STERILE TECHNIQUE: PROCEDURES AND GUIDELINES

**Procedures Requiring Sterile Technique**
- Surgical procedures in the operating room (e.g., transurethral prostatectomy [TURP], appendectomy)
- Biopsies in the operating room, treatment room, or client's room
- Catheterizations of the heart, bladder, or other body cavities
- Injections: intramuscular (IM), subcutaneous (subQ), intradermal
- Infusions: intravenous (IV), instillations or infusions of medication or radioactive isotopes into body cavities
- Dressing changes:
  - Usually, first postoperative dressing change done by using sterile technique
  - Dressings over catheters inserted into body cavities (e.g., Hickman catheter, subclavian lines, dialysis access sites, peripherally inserted central venous catheter [PICC])
  - Dressings of clients with burns, immunologic disorders, and skin grafts

**Guidelines for Sterile Field**
- Never turn your back on or reach across a sterile field. The front of the sterile gown is considered sterile.
- Avoid talking.
- Keep all sterile objects within view (e.g., below waist and above shoulders are not within sterile field; the outer 1-inch perimeter is not considered sterile; avoid placing objects in this area).
- Moisture will carry bacteria across/through a cloth or paper barrier.
- Transfer of objects from sterile to contaminated (not sterile) = contaminated.

A. Primary goals.
1. Promote healing.
2. Prevent further damage.
3. Prevent infection.
B. Types of wounds.
1. Black wounds.
a. Necrotic devitalized tissue; high risk for infection.
b. Frequently require debridement of necrotic tissue for healing to occur.
2. Yellow wounds.
a. Contain devitalized tissue; require cleaning for healing to occur.
b. Mechanical debridement requires irrigations and dressing changes. A soft 19-gauge angiocatheter on a 35-mL syringe provides safe pressure for irrigation and removal of devitalized tissue.
c. Wet-to-dry dressings, wet-to-moist dressings, wound packing, and enzymatic debridement may be used to cleanse yellow wounds.
d. Hydrocolloidal dressings to retain moisture.
3. Red wounds.
a. Require protection of fragile granulation tissue.
b. Topical antibiotic ointment and nonadhering dressings may be used on shallow wounds.
c. Wounds should be kept moist (moisture-retention dressings); dry dressings will damage the new granulation tissue when removed.
C. Wound healing.
1. Primary intention: wound margins are well approximated, as in a surgical incision or a repaired laceration.
2. Secondary intention.
a. Traumatic, infected wounds with exudate and wide, irregular margins and extensive tissue loss.
b. Healing occurs by granulation from the edges inward and/or from the bottom up.
c. Larger scar formation than with primary healing.
3. Tertiary intention.
a. Delayed suturing of the wound after infection is cleared and granulation tissue has been established.
b. Occurs when a primary wound is infected and left open to heal by secondary intention; then the wound is sutured.
D. Wound healing affected by:
1. Nutritional status.
a. Adequate calories; protein; vitamins A, C, and E; zinc; and fluids are necessary for tissue healing.
b. The obese client is at increased risk for poor wound healing and ineffective wound approximation.
2. Tissue perfusion and oxygenation to wound.
3. Excessive wound drainage impairs tissue regeneration and will harbor bacteria.
4. Diseases such as cancer, renal disease, diabetes, and hepatic disease can delay wound healing.
5. Medications such as corticosteroids delay wound healing.
6. Aging: slowing of tissue repair.
7. Infection prolongs inflammation and delays wound granulation.

# WOUND CLEANSING

- Cleanse from top to bottom
- Middle of wound to outside
- Inside or center of wound to the outside (using a circular motion)

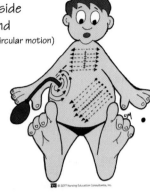

- Remember to cleanse from the cleanest part of the wound (suture area) to the dirtiest (surrounding skin)

FIGURE 3-3 **Wound Cleansing.** (From Zerwekh, J., Garneau, A., & Miller, C. J. [2017]. *Digital collection of the memory notebooks of nursing* [4th ed.]. Chandler, AZ: Nursing Education Consultants, Inc.)

> **TEST ALERT:** Promote client wound healing (proper nutrition, prevention of infection); identify factors that result in delayed wound healing.

> **TEST ALERT:** Monitor and maintain devices and equipment used for drainage. Manage wound care (irrigations, dressings, wound suction devices).

E. Nursing intervention.

> **! NURSING PRIORITY:** When cleansing an area, always start at the cleanest area and work away from that area. Never return to an area you have previously cleaned; discard cleansing swab after each horizontal or vertical stroke.

1. Cleansing of wound (Figure 3-3).
   a. Horizontal wound: cleansed from center of incision outward, then laterally.
   b. Vertical wound: cleansed from top to bottom, then laterally.
   c. Drain or stab wound: cleansed in a circular motion (Figure 3-3).
2. Penrose drain: a soft, flexible drain inserted in an open wound to prevent the accumulation of secretions and exudate; frequent dressing changes are preferable to reinforcement of the same dressing (Figure 3-4).

> **! NURSING PRIORITY:** Avoid pooling of excessive drainage under saturated dressing; this can lead to skin irritation and infection.

3. Montgomery straps are used when frequent dressing changes are needed; they help prevent skin irritation that could occur with tape removal.
4. Elasticized abdominal binders provide support to large incisions.
5. Jackson–Pratt catheter or drainage system: bulb must be compressed to allow air to escape and then recapped to maintain suction (Figure 3-5).
6. Hemovac: evacuator must be compressed at least every 4 hours to provide suction; be sure to empty drainage from pouring spout; keep drainage spout sterile when emptying.

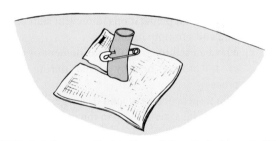

FIGURE 3-4 **Penrose Drain.** (From Potter, P., & Perry, A. [2017]. *Fundamentals of nursing* [9th ed.]. St. Louis, MO: Mosby.)

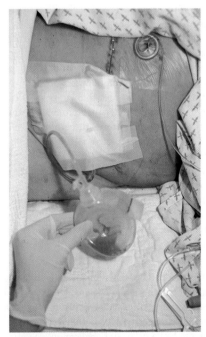

FIGURE 3-5 **Jackson–Pratt Drain.** (From Perry, A., & Potter, P. [2017]. *Fundamentals of nursing* [9th ed.]. St. Louis, MO: Mosby.)

7. In negative-pressure wound therapy, a device (vacuum-assisted closure [VAC] system) is used to apply localized negative pressure to the wound to assist in closing the wound.
   a. Measure appropriate size foam to cover the wound.
   b. Apply transparent dressing over foam, sealing the wound.
   c. Secure tubing from the vacuum source to the port on the transparent dressing.
   d. Dressing and foam are changed every 24 hours to several days.
8. Wet-to-dry dressings.
   a. The purpose is to trap necrotic or nonviable tissue in the dressing as it dries.
   b. Dressing should be moist when applied and allowed to dry for 4 to 6 hours.
   c. When dressing is changed, the packed dressing should be gently removed along with absorbed drainage and nonviable tissue. Do not soak packing before removal; this will decrease the removal of nonviable tissue.
9. Moisture retention dressings.
   a. Maintain moisture to promote healing and prevent damage to healing tissue.
   b. Dressing is coated with hydrogel, colloids, or antibacterial preparations to prevent skin maceration and promote healing.
   c. May be used to assist in debridement of wounds or to protect healthy tissue during healing process.
10. Obtain a specimen of wound drainage.
    a. Gently roll a sterile swab in the purulent drainage.

b. Obtain wound specimen before any medication or antimicrobial agent is applied to wound area or administered to client.

## Specimen Collection

A. General principles.
   1. Use sterile equipment.
   2. Use the correct container for each specimen; preservatives, anticoagulants, or chemicals may be required.
   3. Always observe standard precautions when obtaining specimens; keep outside of container clean to prevent contamination in transfer to the laboratory.
   4. Properly label the specimen. Collect the correct amount at the correct time.

> **TEST ALERT:** Obtain specimens for diagnostic testing (e.g., wound cultures, stool, urine).

B. Types of specimen (refer to appendices in chapters listed).
   1. Urine (see Chapter 25).
   2. Stool (see Chapter 20).
   3. Sputum and throat (see Chapter 17).
   4. Blood (see Chapter 16).

> **TEST ALERT:** Obtain blood specimens peripherally or through a central line.

   5. Wound specimen.

## Heat and Cold Applications

A. Heat applications (Box 3-3).
   1. Purposes: to soften exudate, increase vasodilation, promote healing, decrease pain.

---

### Box 3-3   KEY POINTS AND SAFETY TIPS FOR APPLYING HEAT OR COLD THERAPY

**General**
- Understand that some areas of the body, such as the neck, inner part of the wrist and forearm, and perineal area, are more sensitive to temperature changes and that the foot and hand are less sensitive.
- Keep in mind the very young and the very old are most sensitive to heat and cold applications.
- Be aware that clients are able to tolerate short exposure to temperature extremes better than prolonged exposure.
- Teach the client to report any discomfort or change in sensation during or after the application.
- Keep the client's call light within reach.
- Have some type of method or timer to monitor the time for the application.
- Explain to the client not to adjust any temperature settings.
- Maintain close monitoring with clients who are unable to sense temperature changes or move away from the temperature source.

**Heat**
- Promotes vasodilation, which improves blood flow, promotes exchange of nutrients and waste products by increasing capillary permeability, and reduces venous congestion in injured tissue.
- Reduces blood viscosity, which facilitates movement of leukocytes (white blood cells) and medications to an injured area.

- Reduces muscle relaxation and diminished pain from spasm and stiffness.
- Heat should not be applied over an area that is being treated with radiation therapy, is bleeding, has localized inflammation (abscessed tooth or appendicitis), has been injured within the past 24 hours, or has decreased sensation.

**Cold**
- Promotes vasoconstriction, which reduces blood flow to an injured area, reduces inflammation, and prevents edema formation.
- Reduces oxygen needs by decreasing cell metabolic rate.
- Increases blood viscosity, which promotes clotting of blood at injured area.
- Relieves pain by decreasing muscle tension and providing a local anesthesia effect.
- Cold should be avoided when edema is present at an injured area, as it will slow circulation and prevent absorption of interstitial fluid.
- Cold should not be applied if the client has neuropathy, due to the client's inability to determine whether the area becomes too cold from the application.
- Avoid cold applications when a client is shivering, as shivering raises body temperature.

Adapted from Potter, P. A., Perry, A. G., Stocker, P. A., & Hall, A. M. (2017). *Fundamentals of nursing* (9th ed., p. 1216–1219). St. Louis, MO: Elsevier Mosby.

2. General principles.
   a. Moist heat penetrates more deeply than dry heat.
   b. Unless a physician orders continuous heat applications, treatment time is usually 20 minutes.
   c. Caution client regarding hot baths and vasodilating effect that may cause postural hypotension.
3. Types of heat application.
   a. Moist heat pack.
   b. Pad that circulates warmed water to distribute dry heat to body parts. Cover the source to protect the skin.
   c. Sitz bath. Partial submersion of the body (only to the pelvic region) in a warmed solution. Commonly used following rectal surgery and episiotomies.
   d. Warm soak. Affected area is submerged in a warmed solution.
B. Cold applications.
1. Purposes: to promote vasoconstriction, decrease edema or temperature, stop bleeding, or stop pain by numbing pain receptors.
2. Types of cold applications.
   a. Ice bag, ice collar, cold soak, cold compress, or cold pack.
   b. Hypothermia blanket.
   c. Always cover the source with a cloth or towel to protect the skin.
3. Reduces edema, if applied immediately after an injury.

**NURSING PRIORITY:** Do not use hot or cold applications with conditions of impaired circulation (e.g., peripheral vascular disease or diabetes).

## Vital Signs

**TEST ALERT:** Assess client's vital signs. Intervene when vital signs are abnormal (hypotension, hypertension, bradycardia, etc.) Be able to compare client's current vital signs with baseline and know the range of normal for vital signs at different age levels. This is critical in identifying abnormal findings and in evaluating response to treatment and specific criteria for medication administration.

A. Normal values (Table 3-2).
B. Assessment.
1. Respirations.
   a. Evaluate an infant's respiratory pattern before stimulating him or her.
   b. Check thoracic cavity for symmetric excursion.
   c. Breath sounds: evaluate the adult client in sitting position.
   d. Compare breath sounds on each side of the client's chest.
2. Pulse.
   a. Irregular radial pulse, weak volume, or low rate should be assessed by taking an apical pulse for a full minute.

### Table 3-2 NORMAL VITAL SIGNS

| Neonate | |
|---|---|
| Respiration | 30–60 breaths/min |
| Pulse | 120–140 beats/min |
| Temperature | 36.5°–37.6°C (97.7°–99.7°F) |
| Blood pressure | 65/41 mmHg |
| **Child 2–4 years** | |
| Respiration | 24–32 breaths/min |
| Pulse | 90–130 beats/min |
| Temperature | 37°–37.5°C (98.6°–99.5°F) |
| Blood pressure | 89/46–112/72 mmHg |
| **Child 6–10 years** | |
| Respiration | 15–26 breaths/min |
| Pulse | 70–110 beats/min |
| Temperature | 37°–37.5°C (98.6°–99.5°F) |
| Blood pressure | 90/40–110/60 mmHg |
| **Adult** | |
| Respiration | 12–20 breaths/min |
| Pulse | 60–100 beats/min |
| Temperature | 36°–38°C (96.8°–100.4°F) |
| Blood pressure | Systolic <120 mmHg Diastolic <80 mmHg |

b. Apical pulse: auscultated at the fifth intercostal space at the midclavicular line (point of maximal impulse).
c. Apical–radial pulse: determined by two people counting both the apical and radial pulses at the same time; provides the *pulse deficit*, which is the difference in the two values.
d. Weak peripheral pulse: evaluate by means of Doppler ultrasonography.
e. Check apical pulse in neonates, infants, and small children.
3. Temperature.
   a. Temperature is affected by mouth breathing and temperature of oral intake.
   b. Oral temperature is taken unless otherwise indicated.
4. Blood pressure assessment (Box 3-4).

**TEST ALERT:** Apply knowledge of client's pathophysiology when measuring and assessing vital signs.

## IMMOBILITY

Immobility is the therapeutic or unavoidable restriction of a client's physical activity.

A. Causes of restricted movement.
1. Spinal cord injury or neurologic damage.
2. Presence of severe pain (e.g., from arthritis, surgery, or injury).

**Box 3-4  BLOOD PRESSURE ASSESSMENT**

**Procedure:** Client should be in a sitting position without legs crossed. Place the lower edge of the cuff 1 inch (2.5 cm) above the antecubital space, allowing room for positioning the stethoscope bell or diaphragm. The inflatable cuff is wrapped snugly around the upper half of the arm. The cuff is inflated 20–30 mmHg above the point at which radial pulsation disappears. As the cuff is deflated, a sound is produced within the brachial artery and is audible with the stethoscope. The sounds (Korotkoff sounds) coincide with each pulse beat. Usually, when the cuff pressure is below diastolic, the sounds will cease or become muffled.

**Nursing Implications:** The size of the cuff should be 20% wider than the diameter of the limb. If the cuff is too large (e.g., on a child's arm), the BP obtained will be substantially lower than the true BP. If the cuff is too small (e.g., on an obese person's arm), the BP obtained will be higher than the true BP. Cloth or disposable vinyl compression cuffs contain an inflatable bladder and come in different sizes. The size selected is proportional to the circumference of the limb being assessed. The difference in BP between the right and left arms is normally 5–10 mmHg.

B. Therapeutic reasons for restricted movement.
   1. To decrease pain.
   2. To immobilize a wound or bone.
   3. To limit exercise and activity for clients with cardiac problems.
   4. To reduce effects of gravity on the vascular bed and reduce edema formation.

## Adverse Physical Effects of Immobility

**TEST ALERT:** Identify complications of immobility. Provide measures to prevent complications of immobility.

**Goal:** To prevent complications.

A. Cardiovascular system.
   1. Assessment of physical effects.
      a. Orthostatic hypotension.
      b. Decrease in cardiac reserve.
      c. Venous stasis.
      d. Formation of thrombi.
      e. Increase in cardiac workload.
   2. Nursing implications.
      a. Position body to decrease venous stasis.
      b. Change position frequently.
      c. Passive and active ROM.
      d. Begin activity gradually; allow client to sit before standing and to rise slowly to standing position.
      e. Have client use bedside commode when possible to decrease effects of Valsalva maneuver.
B. Respiratory system.
   1. Assessment of physical effects.
      a. Decrease in thoracic excursion.
      b. Decrease in ability to mobilize secretions.
      c. Decrease in oxygen/carbon dioxide exchange.
      d. Increase in pulmonary infections.
   2. Nursing implications.
      a. Elevate head of bed.
      b. Maintain adequate hydration: 2400 to 3000 mL/day if tolerated.
      c. Have client turn, cough, and breathe deeply at regular intervals (every 2 hours while awake); use incentive spirometry.
      d. Promote increase in activity as soon as possible; have client sit up in chair at bedside.
      e. Evaluate pulmonary secretions for infection.
C. Urinary system.
   1. Assessment of physical effects.
      a. Urinary stasis.
      b. Increased calcium level, stasis, and infection precipitate stone formation.
      c. Urinary tract infections.
   2. Nursing implications.
      a. Have client sit or stand to void if possible.
      b. Establish and maintain a voiding schedule.
D. Musculoskeletal system.
   1. Assessment of physical effects.
      a. Demineralization of bones: decrease in bone strength.
      b. Muscle weakness and atrophy.
      c. Loss of motion in joints leads to fibrosis and contractures.
   2. Nursing implications.
      a. Perform ROM exercises.
      b. Active contraction and relaxation of large muscles.
      c. Position body to maintain proper alignment.
      d. Encourage daily weight-bearing exercise when possible.
E. Gastrointestinal system.
   1. Assessment of physical effects.

**TEST ALERT:** Identify factors that interfere with elimination.

      a. Anorexia.
      b. Ineffective movement of feces through colon: constipation and fecal impaction.
      c. Diarrhea caused by impaction.
   2. Nursing implications.
      a. Establish bowel program: every other day or three times a week.
      b. Encourage diet with adequate protein, fiber, and fluids.
      c. Check for fecal impaction.
F. Integumentary system.
   1. Assessment of physical effects.

**TEST ALERT:** Identify client with potential for skin breakdown; maintain client skin integrity; manage client with impaired skin integrity.

      a. Decrease in tissue perfusion leading to pressure ulcer development.

b. Decrease in sensation in area of increased pressure.
2. Nursing implications.
   a. Maintain cleanliness.
   b. Promote circulation through frequent repositioning.
   c. Protect bony prominences when turning.
   d. Prevent creation of pressure areas by tight clothing, cast, or braces.
   e. Perform frequent visual inspection of pressure prone areas.

## Adverse Psychological Effects of Immobility

A. Assessment of psychological effects.
   1. Depression, increased anxiety.
   2. Feelings of helplessness.
   3. Intellectual and sensory deprivation.
   4. Change in body image.
B. Nursing implications.
   1. Maintain sensory stimulation.
   2. Encourage family, social contact.
   3. Promote reality orientation.
   4. Encourage family to bring items from home such as pictures, bed clothes, toys.
   5. Encourage verbalization of feelings.
   6. Provide opportunities for client to make choices and participate in care.
   7. Arrange counseling—vocational, sexual, financial—as appropriate.

> **TEST ALERT:** Evaluate client's response to immobility and response to interventions to prevent complications of immobility.

# PAIN

- Clients have the right to appropriate assessment and pain management.
- Physiologic and behavioral signs of pain should not replace the client's ability to report the pain unless client is unable to communicate.
- Pain can exist even when there is no identifiable cause; pain is always a subjective personal experience.
- Different clients experience different pain levels even in response to the same type of pain stimulus.
- Pain is an early warning system; its presence triggers awareness that something is wrong in the body.
- Unrelieved pain causes adverse physical and psychological responses.

> **TEST ALERT:** Plan measures to care for clients with anticipated or actual alterations in comfort.

## Classification of Pain

- *Acute pain:* has an identifiable cause; is protective; short, predictable duration (lasting less than 3 months); immediate onset; reversible or controllable with treatment. It most often has an identifiable source such as postoperative pain that disappears as the surgical site heals.

- *Chronic pain:* lasts more than 6 months; continual or persistent and recurrent. Pain may not go away; periods of decreased and increased pain. Origin of pain may not be known.
- *Cancer pain:* pain arising from cancer (tumor compressing on nerve[s] or organ involvement) and treatments (chemotherapy, surgery, radiation) associated with treating cancer.
- *Breakthrough pain:* pain experienced in individuals with cancer and chronic pain. Pain medication that normally controls the cancer or chronic pain does not relieve breakthrough pain. Therefore, the client may experience intense pain that requires additional pain relief measures.
- *Nociceptive pain:* somatic pain that affects skeletal muscles, joints, and ligaments; generally diffuse and less localized; *visceral* pain arises from internal organs and may be caused by a tumor or obstruction.
- *Neuropathic pain:* caused by damage to peripheral nerves or to the central nervous system; can result from trauma, metabolic disease, or neurologic disease.
- *Referred pain:* pain that does not occur at the site of injury. For example, pain related to myocardial ischemia may be felt in the left arm or shoulder only; cholecystitis may be felt as shoulder pain.
- *Phantom pain:* pain that follows the amputation of a body part; it may be described as throbbing, cramping, or burning in the body part amputated.

## Pain Characteristics

> **TEST ALERT:** Assess and document client's discomfort and pain levels.

A. Pattern of pain (Box 3-5).
   1. Pain onset and duration: when it started, precipitating causes, and how long it lasts.
   2. Pain pattern: continuous, intermittent, and timing of when pain occurs (morning, evening, after activity).
B. Area of pain.
   1. Ask the client to identify the pain site.
   2. Pain may be referred from the precipitating site to another location—shoulder pain with cholecystitis, left arm pain with myocardial infarction (MI).
   3. Radiating pain involves pain traveling along a nerve pathway from the pain origination site to another region of the body. Sciatica pain follows a nerve pathway

| Box 3-5 | MNEMONIC TO EVALUATE PAIN |
|---------|---------------------------|
| **O:** | Onset |
| **P:** | Provoking or palliative factors |
| **Q:** | Quality |
| **R:** | Region or radiation; relieving factors |
| **S:** | Severity |
| **T:** | Timing |

of the sciatic nerve, generally down the back of the thigh and inside the leg.

C. Intensity of pain: use a pain scale to help the client communicate the pain intensity.

D. Pain quality/type.
1. Neuropathic pain may be burning, numbing, electric shock-like, shooting.
2. Somatic pain may be superficial, sharp, throbbing, cramping.
3. Visceral pain may be sharp, dull, deep, aching.

E. Determine any activities and situations that increase the level of the pain—movement, ambulation, coughing.

F. Client responses to pain (Box 3-6).
1. Increased blood pressure, pulse, and respiration, diaphoresis, increased muscle tension, nausea and vomiting (acute pain).
2. Withdrawn, insomnia, decreased activity, hypersomnia, anxiety (chronic pain).
3. Client's interpretation and meaning of the pain experience.

**NURSING PRIORITY:** In addition to the pain and discomfort associated with a surgical procedure, it is important to assess other possible sources of discomfort, such as a full bladder, occluded catheter or tube, gas accumulation, intravenous infiltration, or compromised circulation caused by position or pressure.

## Cultural Implications of Pain

A. Cultural beliefs and values affect how a client responds to pain.

| Box 3-6   ASSESSING THE HARMFUL EFFECTS OF PAIN | |
|---|---|
| **ACUTE PAIN** | **CHRONIC PAIN** |
| Disturbs sleep | Fatigue |
| Appetite decreases | Weight gain |
| Fluid intake decreases | Poor concentration |
| Decreased diaphragmatic movement, decreased alveolar expansion and avoidance of coughing Increase pulse rate, increased systolic blood pressure, facial grimacing | Decreased use of thoracic muscles, decreased chest expansion, and avoidance of coughing |
| Nausea and vomiting | Job loss Divorce Depression |

**NURSING PRIORITY:** The nurse should administer pain medication to clients experiencing acute pain without fear of the client becoming addicted to the medication.

B. Assess attitudes and beliefs that may affect effective treatment of the pain. Some clients may believe that taking pain medications will cause "addiction"; other clients may believe that complaining of pain is a sign of weakness.

C. Avoid stereotyping clients by assuming that members of a specific cultural group will or will not exhibit more or less pain.

D. Nursing considerations of pain control associated with a client's culture.
1. Identify what the pain means to the client; for example, a woman in labor may perceive the pain differently from a client who experiences pain as an indication of advanced disease.
2. Identify cultural implications regarding how a client responds to or expresses pain; some clients moan and cry; others may be quiet and stoic.
3. Individualize pain control based on client's response to pain.
4. Establish a communication method for the client to express the level of pain and effectiveness of pain control (e.g., pain rating scale, FACES scale, pictures, images) (Box 3-7).
5. Expression of pain is subjective; accept the client's perception of pain and expression of pain and facilitate nursing care to meet the client's cultural needs when providing pain control.

**TEST ALERT:** Assess importance of client culture/ethnicity when planning, providing, and evaluating care.

## Nondrug Pain Relief Measures

A. Relaxation techniques.

**NURSING PRIORITY:** Low levels of anxiety or pain are easier to reduce or control than higher levels are. Consequently, pain relief measures should be used *before* pain becomes severe.

1. Relaxed muscles result in a decreased pain level.
2. Relaxation response requires quiet environment, comfortable position, and a focus of concentration.
3. Identify the relaxation method that is most effective for the client—music, guided imagery, and meditation for progressive muscle relaxation.
4. Meditation: focuses attention away from pain.

**TEST ALERT:** Assess client need for pain management and intervene using nonpharmacologic comfort measures. Recognize differences in client perception and response to pain. Evaluate client response to nonpharmacologic comfort measures.

B. Hypnosis produces a state of altered consciousness characterized by extreme responsiveness to suggestion.

C. Biofeedback provides client with information about changes in bodily functions of which he or she is usually unaware (e.g., blood pressure, pulse).

D. Cutaneous stimulation alleviates pain through stimulation of skin.

## Box 3-7   PAIN RATING SCALES FOR CHILDREN

FACES Pain Rating Scale consists of six cartoon faces ranging from smiling face for "no pain" to tearful face for "worst pain." FACES provides three scales in one: facial expressions, numbers, and words. The numbering system can be based on a 0–5 or a 0–10 pain scale. The nurse points to each face using the words to describe the pain intensity and then asks the child to choose the face that best describes his or her own pain and documents the appropriate number.

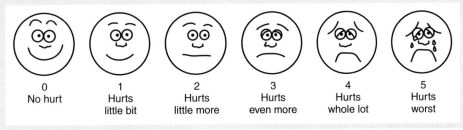

| 0 | 1 | 2 | 3 | 4 | 5 |
|---|---|---|---|---|---|
| No hurt | Hurts little bit | Hurts little more | Hurts even more | Hurts whole lot | Hurts worst |

From Hockenberry, M. J., & Wilson, D. (2015). *Wong's nursing care of infants and children* (10th ed.). St. Louis, MO: Mosby. Used with permission. Copyright 2015 Mosby.

1. Use of pressure, massage, bathing, and heat or cold therapy to promote relaxation.
   a. Applied to different areas of the body.
   b. Contralateral stimulation: when stimulation of the skin near the pain site is ineffective, the side *opposite* the painful area is stimulated for pain relief.
E. Therapeutic touch: holistic approach in which touch is used to realign energy fields (laying on of hands).
F. Transcutaneous electric nerve stimulation (TENS).
   1. Delivers an electrical current through electrodes applied to the skin surface of the painful region or to a peripheral nerve.
   2. Instruct client to adjust TENS unit intensity until it creates a pleasant sensation and relieves the pain.
G. Acupuncture is the most common complementary therapy.
   1. Requires insertion of thin metal needles into the body at designated points to relieve pain.
   2. Is effective in pain management and with nausea and vomiting associated with postoperative and chemotherapy.
   3. Encourage the client to review the credentials of the practitioner, who should have a master's degree in oriental medicine and be registered to practice in the state.
H. Nursing intervention for pain relief (nonpharmacologic).
   1. Change positions frequently and support body parts.
   2. Encourage early ambulation after surgery.
   3. Elevate swollen body parts.
   4. Check drainage tubes to ensure that they are not stretched, kinked, or pulled.
   5. Administering oral sucrose with and without nonnutritive sucking (pacifier) has a calming and pain-relieving effect for invasive procedure in neonates, such as heel sticks. Applying topical anesthetic creams (EMLA or LMX) is helpful in reducing the trauma of needlesticks and other painful procedures.

### Medications for Pain Relief

A. Nurse-administered as-needed (PRN) analgesic medications (see Appendix 3-2).

> **⚠ NURSING PRIORITY:** Plan pain medication administration schedule. Use a preventive approach to pain relief by giving analgesics before the pain occurs or before it reaches severe intensity.

1. Steps in administering PRN medications.
   a. Assess client to determine source, quality, and characteristics of pain (see Box 3-5).
   b. Analyze nursing assessment data; determine most appropriate nursing intervention.
   c. Check client's chart.
      (1) Determine the last medication received and how it was administered.
      (2) Determine the time administered.
      (3) Determine client's response to previous medication.
   d. Select appropriate medication.
      (1) Use nonopioid analgesics for mild to moderate pain.
      (2) Avoid combinations of opioids for older adults.
      (3) IV medications act more rapidly for acute pain relief.
      (4) Avoid intramuscular (IM) injections in older adults.
      (5) Sustained-release and extended-release oral medications work well for chronic pain management and will provide pain management over a longer period.
   e. Decrease stimuli in room (dim lights, adjust room temperature); determine other factors influencing discomfort.
   f. Assess client's response to pain intervention at regular intervals and document nursing actions.

> **TEST ALERT:** Determine client's need for PRN medications; review pertinent data before medication administration (vital signs, laboratory results, allergies, potential interactions); evaluate appropriateness/accuracy of medication order for client. Provide pharmacologic pain management appropriate for age and diagnosis; evaluate and document client's use of and response to pain medication following administration.

2. Types of medications.
   a. Narcotic analgesics (opioids) are used for relieving severe pain (see Appendix 3-2).
   b. Nonnarcotic analgesics act at peripheral sites to reduce pain (see Appendix 3-2).
B. Patient-controlled analgesia (PCA).
   1. Client controls pain by delivery of IV infusion of medication through a PCA pump.
   2. Assess and document pain relief, responses, and presence of adverse side effects to PCA at routine intervals.

> **! OLDER ADULT PRIORITY:** Analgesics tend to last longer in older adults; there is an increased risk for side effects and toxic effects. Recommendation from the American Geriatric Society is to "start low" and "go slow"—but provide adequate pain relief for older adults.

3. Surgical clients should be oriented to PCA procedure before surgery.
4. PCA is effective in pediatrics; the ability to comprehend the procedure is more important than the age.
5. Clients experiencing altered level of consciousness, confusion, or difficulty operating the PCA may have a nurse or family member operate the PCA based on specific criteria and agency guidelines; this is referred to as authorized agent–controlled analgesia (AACA).
6. PCA pump procedure.
   a. Pain should be under control when PCA is initiated.
   b. Delivers a specific amount of medication as controlled by client.
   c. Parameters for bolus dose of medication should be available for episodes of increased pain (dressing changes, chest tube insertion, etc.) and for the client who goes to sleep and awakens with severe pain unrelieved by PCA.
   d. Dose interval is usually 8 to 15 minutes with a lockout time of 1- to 4-hour dosage limits.
   e. Only one dose can be administered over 8 to 15 minutes for a lockout time of ordered dose in 1 hour. Even though the client may push the button several times in succession, only 1 dose will be given every 8 to 15 minutes and a total of prescribed dosage can be given in 1 hour.
   f. Example: PCA morphine sulfate 1 mg/1 mL, 1.5 mg of morphine sulfate every 8 minutes with a lockout of 10 mg over 1 hour.
   g. Monitor client's vital signs and level of sedation every 1 to 2 hours for the first 24 hours.
   h. Check the PCA pump per agency policy for correct settings and to determine how much pain medication is being used by the client.
   i. Instruct any family member or significant others *not* to administer medication (document that you have done this). Explain that PCA works on the principle that when the client is uncomfortable, he or she will use the PCA.

> **! NURSING PRIORITY:** PCA pumps are part of the High-Alert Medications ▲ and Patient Safety protocols from The Joint Commission. PCA protocols include a second RN to verify the prescriber's order, pump setting, medication, and dosage. Watch the decimals! An order for morphine sulfate 0.5 mg could be mistakenly entered in the PCA pump as 5 mg.

7. Advantages of PCA.
   a. More effective pain control.
   b. Decreased client anxiety (no waiting for medication).
   c. Increased client independence.
   d. Decreased level of sedation.
C. Patient-controlled epidural analgesia (PCEA).
   1. Injection of medication through a small catheter into the epidural space of the spinal cord; common pain medications are morphine sulfate and fentanyl.
      a. Relieves pain without causing sympathetic and motor nerve block.
      b. May be intermittent (patient- or nurse-controlled) or constant infusion.
      c. Client may experience numbness, tingling, and coolness when analgesia is initiated.
      d. Requires the use of High-Alert Medications.
   2. Complications.
      a. Opioid medications: nausea and vomiting, constipation, respiratory depression, and pruritus.
      b. Urinary retention may occur: palpate suprapubic area and perform bladder scan; client may require urinary catheterization.
      c. Catheter dislodgement and migration: client begins to experience pain even with additional medication; catheter should be securely taped and labeled.
      d. Lower extremity motor or sensory deficits can be the result of a hematoma or infection; notify the health care provider.
   3. Monitor every 15 minutes for initial response; then every hour after stabilization.
D. Perineural local anesthetic infusion.
   1. Utilizes an infusion pump, which provides local anesthetic (bupivacaine or ropivacaine) to a nerve root or a group of nerves.
      a. Catheter or tubing may be placed in a surgical wound and positioned near the nerve root; catheter is usually not sutured.
      b. May be continuous or on demand; usually left in place for about 48 hours.
   2. May be used in conjunction with oral analgesics.

## Barriers to Pain Management

A. Addiction: the need to take pain medication for reasons other than therapeutic relief of pain.
B. Physical dependence: the occurrence of withdrawal syndrome when the medication is abruptly decreased. When opioid medications are no longer needed for pain relief, a tapering schedule should be initiated to decrease the symptoms of the withdrawal syndrome.

C. Tolerance: characterized by the need to increase the medication dose to achieve the same reduction of pain. If opioid tolerance is suspected, use of another type of opioid is recommended.

> **OLDER ADULT PRIORITY:** Analgesics tend to last longer in older adults; this increases the risk for side effects and toxic effects.

### Palliative Pain Relief

A. The prevention or relief of pain when a cure for the client's illness is not feasible.

> **TEST ALERT:** Palliative/comfort care: assess client for nonverbal signs of pain/discomfort. Assess, intervene, and educate client/family about pain management.

B. Administer analgesics based on client's level of pain; medication is increased as client's pain increases.
C. Adjuvant medications are used to increase effectiveness of analgesics.
   1. Antiemetics, antidepressants.
   2. Corticosteroids.
   3. Nonsteroidal antiinflammatory drugs (NSAIDs).
D. Pain medication is frequently administered on an around-the-clock schedule rather than a PRN schedule to maintain therapeutic levels of medication. Pain medication is administered in the absence of pain.
E. A nurse's or client's fear that the client will become dependent on, addicted to, or tolerant to medication is inappropriate in the provision of pain control in palliative care.
F. Breakthrough pain occurs frequently in clients with cancer.
   1. Transient, moderate to severe pain that may occur with clients who have adequate pain control with dosing schedule.
   2. Develops quickly and intensifies rapidly.
   3. May occur spontaneously, may be precipitated by coughing, may occur at any time during the dosing interval, or may occur toward the end of the dose.
   4. Rescue medication should be available—a strong opioid with a rapid onset and short duration is preferred.
G. Fear that opioids will hasten death is unsubstantiated, even in clients at the very end of life. It is important that nurses provide adequate pain relief for the terminally ill client.

## PERIOPERATIVE CARE

### Preoperative Care

> **TEST ALERT:** Determine whether the client is prepared for a procedure or surgery.

A. Client profile.
   1. Age: older adult clients are more likely to have chronic health problems and age-related factors; infants have more difficulty maintaining homeostasis than adults and children (Box 3-8).

> **OLDER ADULT PRIORITY:** Older clients have less physiologic reserve (the ability of an organ to return to normal after a disturbance in its equilibrium) than younger clients.

   2. Obesity predisposes a client to postoperative complications of infection and wound dehiscence.
   3. Preoperative interview.
      a. Chronic health problems and previous surgical procedures and experiences.
      b. Past and current drug therapy, including over-the-counter medications (vitamins, herbal remedies, homeopathic medications).
      c. History of drug allergies and dietary restrictions.
      d. Client's perception of illness and impending surgery.
      e. Discomfort or symptoms client is currently experiencing.
      f. Religious affiliation.
      g. Family or significant others.

> **Box 3-8 OLDER ADULT CARE FOCUS**
>
> **Preoperative and Postoperative Considerations**
> Older clients are at increased risk for developing postoperative complications because of the decreased response of the immune system (which delays healing) and the increased incidence of chronic disease.
> 1. *Cardiovascular:* Decreased cardiac output and peripheral circulation, along with arrhythmias and increased incidence of arteriosclerosis and atherosclerosis, can lead to hypotension or hypertension, hypothermia, and cardiac problems.
> 2. *Respiratory:* Decreased vital capacity, reduced oxygenation, and decreased cough reflex can lead to an increased risk for atelectasis, pneumonia, and aspiration.
> 3. *Renal:* Decreased renal excretion of wastes and renal blood flow along with increased incidence of nocturia can lead to fluid overload, dehydration, electrolyte imbalance, and drug toxicity.
> 4. *Musculoskeletal:* Increased incidence of arthritis and osteoporosis can lead to bone and joint trauma with positioning in the operating room if pressure points and limbs are not padded.
> 5. *Sensory:* Decreased visual acuity and reaction time can lead to safety problems associated with falls and injuries.
> The older client may require repeated explanation, clarification, and additional time when providing teaching. Older clients often have reduced protein intake, which can delay wound healing and postoperative recovery.
>
> **GERIATRIC NURSING PRIORITY:** The nurse should monitor for adverse effects and toxicity of anesthetic agents and opioid analgesics in the older adult due to decreased metabolism by the liver.

4. Psychosocial needs: fear of the unknown is the primary cause of preoperative anxiety.

5. Medications may predispose client to operative complications.
   a. Antibiotics: aminoglycosides may cause respiratory depression if taken within 2 weeks of surgery.
   b. Anticoagulants potentiate bleeding.
   c. Antidepressants: monoamine oxidase inhibitors increase hypotensive effects of anesthetic agents.
   d. Tranquilizers increase the risk for hypotension; they may be used to enhance anesthetic agent.
   e. Loop and thiazide diuretics create electrolyte imbalance, particularly in potassium level.
   f. Steroids: prolonged use impairs the physiologic response of the body to stress and decreases wound healing and the inflammatory response necessary for wound healing.
6. Check results of routine diagnostic laboratory studies.
   a. Blood studies: complete blood count, serum electrolytes, coagulation studies, serum creatinine, blood urea nitrogen, and fasting glucose.
   b. Urinalysis.
   c. Chest x-ray.
   d. Electrocardiogram for clients over 40 years of age.
   e. Coagulation studies for clients with known problems or to establish a baseline.
B. Preoperative teaching: the goal is to decrease the client's anxiety and prevent postoperative complications.

1. Preoperative teaching content.
   a. Deep breathing and coughing exercises.
   b. Turning and extremity exercises.
   c. Pain medication administration policy.
   d. Adjunct equipment used for breathing: nebulizer, oxygen mask, spirometer.
   e. Explanation of NPO (nothing by mouth) policy.
   f. Antiembolism stockings and/or pneumatic compression device to decrease venous stasis.
2. Pediatric implications in preoperative teaching.
   a. Plan the teaching content around the child's developmental level and previous experiences.
   b. Use concrete terms and visual aids.
   c. Plan teaching session at a time in the child's schedule when he or she will be most receptive to learning.
   d. Use correct terms for body parts and clarify terms with which the child is unfamiliar.
   e. Introduce anxiety-provoking information last (increased anxiety may decrease comprehension).
   f. Use role-playing either to explain procedures to the child or to allow the child to do a return demonstration.
   g. Fear of anesthesia is common in children.
   h. Include the parents in the teaching process.
C. Physical preparation of client.
   1. Skin preparation: the purpose is to reduce bacteria on the skin (may be done in surgical suite or in the preoperative holding area).
      a. Area of preparation is always longer and wider than area of incision.
      b. Antiseptic soap/agent (2% chlorhexidine gluconate) is used to cleanse area.
      c. Assess for allergies before using, especially tape allergies.
   2. Gastrointestinal preparation.
      a. Food and fluid restriction: NPO orders may be individualized for each client. Client may be NPO for 6 to 8 hours before surgery or NPO from midnight on the night before surgery. Trend is to allow clear liquids up to 2 hours preoperatively. Always check prescriber orders and agency policy.
      b. Enemas or cathartics may be administered the evening before surgery to prevent fecal contamination in the peritoneal cavity.
   3. Promote sleep and rest: sleep-aid medication and antianxiety medication may be given to promote rest and reduce anxiety (e.g., benzodiazepine, alprazolam).
   4. In older adults, evaluate status of teeth, presence of bridges and dentures; in children, evaluate for presence of loose teeth.
D. Legal implications (see Chapter 6).
   1. Each surgical procedure must have the voluntary, informed, and written consent of the client or the person legally responsible for the client.

   2. Physician: gives the client a full explanation of the procedure, including complications, risks, and alternatives.
   3. Client's informed consent record (permit) must be signed by the client or guardian. A witness signs to validate this is the client's signature, that the client has voluntarily given consent, and that the client is competent to give consent. The witness is frequently a staff nurse. Depending on facility policy, the surgeon also may be required to sign the consent form.

4. The signed consent record (permit) is part of the permanent chart record and must accompany the client to the operating room.

## Day of Surgery

**TEST ALERT:** Monitor a client before, during, and after a procedure or surgery.

A. Nursing responsibilities (Figure 3-6).
1. Routine hygiene care.
2. Vital signs within 1 hour before "on call" to surgery or per agency policy.
3. Remove jewelry, including piercing jewelry; wedding bands may be taped on finger.
4. Remove contact lenses, fingernail polish, depending on agency policy.
5. Dress client in patient gown.
6. Determine whether dentures and removable bridgework need to be removed before surgery.
7. Instruct client and document disposition of glasses, dentures, bridgework, jewelry, and valuables before the administration of preoperative anesthetic.
8. Continue NPO status.
9. Check client's identification for two identifiers.
   a. The first identifier should reliably identify the client for whom service or treatment is intended, for example, the client's name.
   b. The second identifier is used to match the service or treatment to that individual, for example, the date of birth and/or client's hospital identification number.
10. Identify family and significant others who will be waiting for information regarding client's progress.
11. To decrease client anxiety, instruct client about what to expect in operating room, for example, skin preparation, cold room, availability of warm blankets, bright lights, and time-out procedure.
12. Check the chart for completeness regarding laboratory reports, consent form, significant client observations, history, and physical examination records (Figure 3-7).
13. Allow parent to accompany the child as far as possible.

B. Preoperative medications (see Appendix 3-2).

**NURSING PRIORITY:** Explain to client the purpose of preoperative medications and advise client not to get out of bed. Side rails should be up and the call light within reach.

1. Purpose.
   a. Induce anesthesia rapidly.
   b. Reduce anxiety.

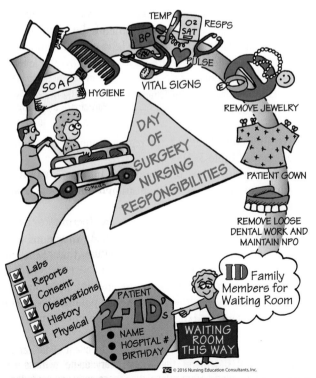

**FIGURE 3-6 Day of Surgery Nursing Responsibilities.** (From Zerwekh, J., Garneau, A., & Miller, C. J. [2017]. *Digital collection of the memory notebooks of nursing* [4th ed.]. Chandler, AZ: Nursing Education Consultants, Inc.)

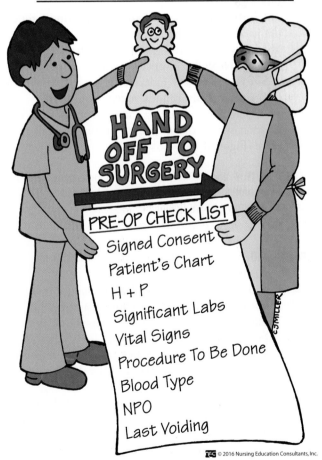

**FIGURE 3-7 Hand Off to Surgery.** (From Zerwekh, J., Garneau, A., & Miller, C. J. [2017]. *Digital collection of the memory notebooks of nursing* [4th ed.]. Chandler, AZ: Nursing Education Consultants, Inc.)

2. Nursing responsibilities.

> ⚠ **NURSING PRIORITY:** The operative permit or informed consent record must be signed before the client receives the preoperative medication.

    a. Confirm that all consent forms are signed and that the client understands the procedure.
    b. Ask client to void before administration of medication.
    c. Obtain baseline vital signs.
    d. Administer medication 45 minutes to 1 hour before surgery or as ordered.
    e. Raise the side rails and instruct the client not to get out of bed.
    f. Observe for side effects of medication.

C. The Joint Commission established Universal Protocol guidelines for preventing wrong site, wrong procedure or surgery, and wrong person must occur before the procedure or surgery.

    1. The Universal Protocol includes the following criteria: (1) preoperative verification of required documents (e.g., laboratory results, client chart, signed consent form); (2) marking the operative site with indelible ink; and (3) and a time-out just before the procedure.
    2. The surgical team is involved in conducting a time-out just before beginning the procedure.
    3. The time-out involves positive identification of the client, the intended procedure, and the site of the procedure is marked with indelible marker by the surgeon before entering the surgical suite.
    4. The operative site marking and time-out occur in the location where the procedure or surgery will take place (Figure 3-8).

> **TEST ALERT:** Prepare client for surgery or procedure; monitor client before, during, and after surgery or procedure; assess client's response to surgery and/or treatment.

## Anesthesia

A. General anesthesia.
    1. Intravenous anesthesia: used as an induction agent before the inhalation agent is administered.
    2. Inhalation anesthesia: used to progress the client from stage II to stage III of anesthesia.
B. Regional anesthesia: used to anesthetize one region of the body; client remains awake and alert throughout the procedure.
    1. Topical: anesthetizing medication applied to mucous membrane or skin; blocks peripheral nerve endings.
    2. Local infiltration: injection of anesthetic agent; only blocks peripheral nerves around area.
    3. Peripheral nerve block: anesthetizes individual nerves or nerve plexuses (digital, brachial plexus); it does not

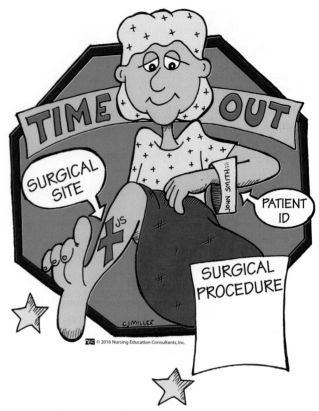

**FIGURE 3-8 Time Out.** (From Zerwekh, J., Garneau, A., & Miller, C. J. [2017]. *Digital collection of the memory notebooks of nursing* [4th ed.]. Chandler, AZ: Nursing Education Consultants, Inc.)

block the autonomic nerve fiber; medication is injected to block peripheral nerve fibers.
    4. Spinal anesthesia: local anesthetics are injected into the subarachnoid space; may be used with almost any type of major procedure performed below the level of the diaphragm.
    5. Epidural anesthesia: anesthetic agent is introduced into the epidural space; cerebral spinal fluid cannot be aspirated.
C. Nursing considerations for regional anesthesia (spinal/epidural) (Table 3-3).
D. Conscious sedation or monitored anesthesia care: the administration of an IV medication to produce sedation, analgesia, and amnesia.
    1. Characteristics.
       a. Client can respond to commands, maintains protective reflexes, and does not need assistance in maintaining an airway.
       b. Amnesia most often occurs after the procedure.
       c. Slurred speech and nystagmus indicate the end of conscious sedation.

> **TEST ALERT:** Determine that client and family understand relevant information before administration of conscious sedation. Assist with preparing client for conscious sedation. Monitor client physiologic response during and after conscious sedation.

## Table 3-3 NURSING CARE OF THE CLIENT UNDERGOING REGIONAL ANESTHESIA

| Problem | Nursing Interventions |
|---|---|
| Preparation for procedure | 1. Explain procedure.<br>2. Do preoperative preparation and have surgical client sign consent form.<br>3. Assess client for effectiveness as anesthesia is initiated.<br>4. Client will remain awake throughout the procedure. |
| Hypotension | 1. Report BP <100 mmHg systolic or any significant decrease.<br>2. Place client in a supine position. For clients undergoing spinal or epidural anesthesia, a supine position can only be done after the level of anesthesia is set.<br>3. Administer oxygen.<br>4. Increase IV rate if client is not prone to heart failure. |
| Respiratory paralysis | 1. Avoid extreme Trendelenburg position before level of anesthesia is set.<br>2. Evaluate client's respiratory status and oxygen saturation levels using pulse oximetry.<br>3. Have ventilatory support equipment available. |
| Nausea and vomiting | 1. Antiemetics<br>2. Anticipate nausea if client becomes hypotensive.<br>3. Suction the client or position the client to prevent aspiration. |
| Loss of bladder tone | 1. Evaluate for bladder distention. |
| Trauma to extremities | 1. Support extremity during movement.<br>2. Remove legs from stirrups simultaneously. |
| Headache | 1. Ensure adequate hydration before, during, and after procedure.<br>2. Maintain recumbent position 6–12 h after procedure.<br>3. Administer analgesics. |

*BP*, Blood pressure.

2. Nursing implications.
   a. Perform baseline assessment before procedure; implications for care are the same as those for a client receiving general anesthesia.
   b. Client is assessed continuously; vital signs are recorded every 5 to 15 minutes.
   c. Monitor level of consciousness; client should not be unconscious but relaxed and comfortable.
   d. Client should respond to physical and verbal stimuli; protective airway reflexes should remain intact.
   e. Potential complications include loss of gag reflex, aspiration, hypoxia, hypercapnia, and cardiopulmonary depression.
3. Does not require extensive postoperative recovery time.

## Immediate Postoperative Recovery

**TEST ALERT:** Provide postoperative care.

A. Admission of client to recovery area.
   1. Position client to promote patent airway and prevent aspiration.
   2. Perform baseline assessment.
      a. Vital signs, quality of respirations, pulse oximetry, pulse rate and rhythm, general skin color.
      b. Type and amount of fluid infusing.
      c. Special equipment; status of dressings.
   3. Determine specifics regarding the operation from the operating room nurse.
      a. Client's overall tolerance of surgery.
      b. Type of surgery performed, type of anesthetic agents used.
      c. Results of procedure: Was the condition corrected?
      d. Any specific complications to watch for.
      e. Status of fluid intake and urinary output.
      f. Common postoperative complications (Table 3-4).

**TEST ALERT:** Assess client's response to surgery; evaluate client's response to postoperative interventions to prevent complications; intervene to prevent aspiration.

B. Nursing management during recovery.

**Goal:** To maintain respiratory function.

**NURSING PRIORITY:** The client's respiratory status is a priority concern on admission to the postoperative recovery area and throughout the postoperative recovery period.

1. Leave airway in place until pharyngeal reflex (gag reflex) has returned.
2. Position client on side (lateral Sims' position) or on the back with the head turned to the side to prevent aspiration.
3. Suction excess secretions and prevent aspiration.
4. Encourage coughing and deep breathing.
5. Administer humidified oxygen.
6. Auscultate breath sounds.

**Goal:** To maintain cardiovascular stability.

**TEST ALERT:** Plan and implement interventions to prevent complications after surgery. Intervene to manage potential circulatory complications; monitor for signs of bleeding, hemorrhage, embolus, or shock.

1. Check vital signs every 15 minutes until condition is stable.
2. Report blood pressure that is continually dropping 5 to 10 mmHg with each reading.
3. Report increasing or persistent bradycardia or tachycardia.

### Table 3-4   COMMON POSTOPERATIVE COMPLICATIONS

| Complication | Signs and Symptoms | Nursing Intervention |
|---|---|---|
| Atelectasis | Dyspnea, decreased or absent breath sounds over affected area, asymmetric chest expansion, hypoxia | Prevention: have client turn, cough, and breathe deeply; provide adequate hydration; encourage ambulation and incentive spirometer use.<br>Position client on unaffected side.<br>Maintain humidification, oxygen (see Chapter 17). |
| Shock | Decreasing blood pressure, weak pulse, restless, confusion, oliguria | Initiate IV access, keep NPO, maintain bed rest.<br>Position supine with legs elevated and knees straight.<br>Monitor ventilation and vital signs frequently. |
| Wound infection | Poor wound healing, redness, tenderness, fever, tachycardia, leukocytosis, purulent drainage | Prevention: identify high-risk clients; maintain sterile technique with dressing changes.<br>Culture incision to determine organism.<br>Evaluate progress and prevent spread of infection. |

**TEST ALERT:** Monitor wounds for signs and symptoms of infection.

| Complication | Signs and Symptoms | Nursing Intervention |
|---|---|---|
| Wound dehiscence | Unintentional opening of the surgical incision | Evaluate for hemorrhage; use measures to prevent further pressure at incision site. |
| Wound evisceration | Protrusion of a loop bowel through the surgical wound | Cover bowel with sterile saline solution–soaked dressing.<br>Do not attempt to replace loop of bowel.<br>Notify physician; client will most likely return to surgery for further exploration. |
| Urinary retention | Inability to void after surgery; bladder may be palpable; voiding small amounts, dribbling | Determine preoperative risks: medications, length of surgery, history of prostate problems.<br>Determine amount of fluid intake and when to anticipate client to void—generally within 8 hr.<br>Palpate suprapubic area, run tap water, provide privacy.<br>Catheterize if necessary. |
| Gastric dilatation, paralytic ileus | Nausea, vomiting, abdominal distention, decreased bowel sounds | Prevention: Older adult clients are at increased risk; encourage activity as soon as possible; maintain NG tube suction and NPO status; if NG tube is not present, may begin early feeding of clear liquids to increase intestinal motility; maintain IV lines with hydrating solution. See Chapter 20. |

*IV,* Intravenous; *NPO,* nothing by mouth; *NG,* nasogastric.

4. Evaluate quality of pulse and presence of dysrhythmia.
5. Evaluate adequacy of cardiac output and tissue perfusion.

**Goal:** To maintain adequate fluid status.

> **NURSING PRIORITY:** Antidiuretic hormone secretion is increased in the immediate postoperative period. Administer fluids with caution; it is easy to cause fluid overload in a client.

1. Evaluate blood loss in surgery and response to fluid replacement.
2. Maintain rate of IV infusion; maintain intake and output (I&O) record.
3. Monitor urine output and possible bladder distention.
4. Evaluate hydration and electrolyte status.
5. Observe amount and character of drainage on dressings or drainage in collecting containers.
6. Assess amount and character of gastric drainage if nasogastric tube is in place.
7. Evaluate amount and characteristics of any emesis.

> **NURSING PRIORITY:** When a client is vomiting, prevent aspiration by positioning the client on the left side and suction, if not contraindicated.

**Goal:** To maintain incisional areas.

1. Evaluate amount and character of drainage from incision and drains.
2. Check and record status of Hemovac, Jackson–Pratt, Penrose, or any other wound drains.

**Goal:** To maintain psychological equilibrium.

1. Speak to client frequently in calm, unhurried manner.
2. Continually orient client; it is important to tell client that surgery is over and where he or she is.
3. Maintain quiet, restful atmosphere.
4. Promote comfort by maintaining proper body alignment.
5. Explain all procedures, even if client is not fully awake.
6. In the anesthetized client, sense of hearing is the last to be lost and the first to return.

**Goal:** Client meets criteria to return to room.

1. Vital signs are stable and within normal limits.
2. Client is awake and reflexes have returned.
3. Dressings are intact with no evidence of excessive drainage.
4. Client can maintain a patent airway without assistance.

## General Postoperative Care

> **TEST ALERT:** Anticipate situations with questions regarding basic postoperative nursing care and questions that are for a specific surgical condition or procedures. Nursing implications for specific surgical procedures may be found under the major systems in the care of the medical–surgical patient.

**Goal:** To maintain cardiovascular function and tissue perfusion.

1. Monitor vital signs every 4 hours.
2. Evaluate skin color and nail beds for pallor and cyanosis.
3. Monitor level of hematocrit.
4. Assess client's tolerance to increasing activity.
5. Encourage early activity and ambulation.

**Goal:** To maintain respiratory function.

1. Have client turn, cough, and breathe deeply every 2 hours.
2. Use incentive spirometry to promote deep breathing.
3. Administer small-volume nebulizer treatment and bronchodilator as needed.
4. Maintain adequate hydration to keep mucus secretions thin and easily mobilized.
5. Encourage deep breathing with ambulation.

**Goal:** To maintain adequate nutrition and elimination.

1. Assess for return of bowel sounds, normal peristalsis, and passage of flatus.
2. Assess client with a nasogastric tube for return of peristalsis.
3. Assess client's tolerance of oral fluids; usually begin with clear liquids.
4. Encourage intake of fluids unless contraindicated.
5. Progress diet as client's condition and appetite indicate or as ordered.
6. Record bowel movements; normal bowel function should return on the second or third postoperative day (provided that the client is eating).
7. Assess urinary output.
   a. Client should void within 8 to 10 hours after surgery.
   b. Assess urine output; should be at least 30 mL/hr.
   c. Promote voiding by allowing client to stand or use bedside commode.
   d. Avoid catheterization if possible.

**Goal:** To maintain fluid and electrolyte balance.

1. Assess for adequate hydration.
   a. Moist mucous membranes.
   b. Adequate urine output with normal urine specific gravity.
   c. Good skin turgor.
2. Assess laboratory reports of serum electrolytes.
3. Assess character and amount of gastric drainage through the nasogastric tube.
4. Assess urine output as it correlates with fluid intake; maintain I&O records.
5. Evaluate laboratory data for indications of decreased renal function.

**Goal:** To promote comfort.

1. Determine nonpharmacologic pain relief measures.
2. Administer analgesics and or monitor PCA.

## Appendix 3-1   POSITIONING AND BODY MECHANICS

| Position | Placement | Use |
| --- | --- | --- |
| Fowler's | Head of bed at 45- to 60-degree angle; hips flexed | The height may be determined by client preference or tolerance; frequently used for client with respiratory compromise |
| Semi-Fowler's | Head of bed at 30- to 45-degree angle; hips flexed | Used in cardiac, respiratory, neurosurgical conditions |
| Lateral (side-lying) | Head of bed lowered; pillows under arm and legs and behind back; flex knee of anterior side | For client comfort; increases uterine and renal perfusion in pregnancy and prevents supine vena cava syndrome during labor |
| Semiprone (Sims') | Head of bed lowered; client placed on side with dependent shoulder lifted out and lying partially on abdomen; place pillow under flexed arm and under upper flexed knees | Prevents pressure ulcer; used for administration of rectal enemas and suppositories (left Sims') |
| Lithotomy | On back with thigh flexed against abdomen and legs supported by stirrups | For examination of female reproductive tract and rectum, cystoscopy, and surgical procedures |

## Appendix 3-1  POSITIONING AND BODY MECHANICS—cont'd

| Position | Placement | Use |
|---|---|---|
| Prone | Head of bed flat, client on abdomen, head turned to side | To promote drainage after tonsillectomy; to prevent contractures in clients with above-the-knee amputation, to protect client with imperforate anus, or spina bifida |
| Supine | Bed in flat position, small pillow under head | For client comfort |
| Dorsal recumbent | Bed flat, small pillow under head, patient's knees flexed and soles of feet flat on bed | Used for a variety of procedures and examinations (Foley catheter insertion, perineal care, abdominal assessment) |
| Knee–chest | Variation of prone position; patient face down with head turned to side; chest, elbows, and knees rest on bed; thighs perpendicular to bed | Used for prolapsed cord during labor to prevent compression of the umbilical cord |

©Nursing Education Consultants, Inc.

**TEST ALERT:** Position client to prevent complications after tests, treatments, or procedures.

## Appendix 3-2  BODY MECHANICS—PREVENTION OF INJURY

- Use lift equipment and ask for adequate assistance.
- Manual lifting of a client should be avoided. If it is necessary to manually lift most or all of the client's weight, obtain adequate assistance or use safe client handling equipment.
- Ergonomics of lifting:
  1. Avoid twisting; keep your head and neck aligned with your spine.
  2. Place feet wide apart for good base of support; knees should be flexed.
  3. Position yourself close to the bed or close to the client.
  4. Use arms and legs to assist in lifting client, not your back.
- Use friction-reducing device and draw sheet to move client to side of bed and/or to move up in bed.

✓ **KEY POINTS: Assisting the Client to Move up in Bed**

- Lower the head of the bed so that it is flat or as low as the client can tolerate; raise the bed frame to a position that does not require leaning.

- If more than one person is needed for assistance, obtain a lifting device.
- Determine the client's strong side and have him or her assist with the move.
- Instruct the client to bend legs, put feet flat on bed, and push.
- Use a friction-reducing device and draw sheet.
- Never pull a client up in bed by his arms or by putting pressure under his arms.

✓ **KEY POINTS: Logrolling the Client**

- Spinal immobilization—use a team approach (three nurses).
- Maintain proper alignment on head and back areas while turning.
- Before moving client, place a pillow between client's knees and instruct client to cross arms over chest.
- Move client in one coordinated movement using a turn/lift sheet.

*Continued*

**Appendix 3-2   BODY MECHANICS—PREVENTION OF INJURY—cont'd**

## ✓ KEY POINTS: Moving From Bed to Chair

- Move client to the side of the bed (bed wheels locked) closest to the edge where the client will be getting up.
- Assist client out of bed on his strongest side.
- Raise head of bed to assist client in pivoting to the side of the bed.
- Move client to edge of bed and place hands under his legs and shift his weight forward; pivot his body so he is sitting position and his feet are flat on the floor.
- Have client reach across chair and grasp arm.
- Stabilize client by positioning your foot at the outside edge of client's foot.
- Pivot client into chair using your leg muscles instead of your back muscles.
- Assist client to move back and up in the chair for better position.

**TEST ALERT:** Maintain correct body alignment.

### Tips for Moving Clients

- Use a draw sheet to provide more support for client.
- Encourage client to assist in move by using the side rails and strong side of his or her body.
- No-lift policy: use of equipment and assistance whenever a client requires most of his weight to be supported or lifted by someone.
- Obtain additional assistance and/or use lift equipment to help in moving the client.
- Use trochanter roll made from bath blankets to align the client's hips to prevent external rotation.
- Use foam bolsters to maintain side-lying positions.
- Use folded towels, blankets, or small pillows to position client's hands and arms to prevent dependent edema.

**Appendix 3-3   MEDICATIONS: ANALGESICS, NSAIDS, AND PREOPERATIVE**

### Analgesics: General Nursing Implications

- Assess pain parameters, blood pressure, pulse, oxygen saturation, and respiratory status before and periodically after administration.
- Administer before pain is severe for better analgesic effect.
- Older or debilitated clients may require decreased dosage.

| *Medications* | *Side Effects* | *Nursing Implications* |
|---|---|---|

**Opioid Analgesics:** Bind to opiate receptors in the central nervous system (CNS), altering the perception of and emotional response to pain; controlled substances (Schedule II)

**Strong Opioid Analgesics**

| Medications | Side Effects | Nursing Implications |
|---|---|---|
| ▲ Morphine sulfate: PO, subQ, IM, IV, epidural, intrathecal, sublingual analgesia<br>Meperidine: PO, subQ, IM, IV<br>Fentanyl: IM, IV, transdermal, transmucosal, nasal spray | Respiratory depression<br>Orthostatic hypotension<br>Sedation, dizziness, lightheadedness, dysphoria<br>Constipation<br>Tolerance, physical and psychological dependence<br>May decrease awareness of bladder stimuli<br>Seizure with Demerol | 1. Morphine is most commonly administered drug for PCA.<br>2. Meperidine: The American Pain Society does not recommend use as an analgesic; use with caution in children and older adult clients because of increased risk for toxicity and seizures.<br>3. Morphine is not commonly used after biliary tract surgery.<br>4. All opioids: Use with caution in clients who have respiratory compromise.<br>5. Pediatric implications: Medication dosage is calculated according to body surface area and weight.<br>6. Assess voiding and encourage client to void every 4 hours.<br>7. Requires documentation as indicated by Controlled Substance Act.<br>8. Instruct client to change position slowly to minimize orthostatic hypotension. |

**❗ NURSING PRIORITY:** Advise clients using fentanyl patches not to expose patch to heat (hot tub, heating pad) because this will accelerate the release of the fentanyl.

**❗ OLDER ADULT PRIORITY:** Prevent problems with constipation.

**Appendix 3-3  MEDICATIONS: ANALGESICS, NSAIDS, AND PREOPERATIVE—cont'd**

| Medications | Side Effects | Nursing Implications |
|---|---|---|
| **Moderate to Strong Opioid Analgesics**<br>Codeine: PO, subQ, IM<br>Hydromorphone: PO, subQ, IM, IV<br>Oxycodone: PO (combination with ibuprofen; combination with acetaminophen)<br>Hydrocodone: PO (combination with acetaminophen; combination with ibuprofen) | Sedation, euphoria, respiratory depression, constipation, urinary retention, cough suppression<br><br>**⚠ NURSING PRIORITY:** Concurrent administration with nonnarcotic analgesics may enhance pain relief because they act at different sites. | 1. Usually administered by mouth.<br>2. Codeine is an extremely effective cough suppressant.<br>3. Do not confuse hydromorphone with morphine.<br>4. Warn client to avoid activities requiring alertness until effects of drug are known.<br>5. Medications are often in various strength combinations with acetaminophen and/or ibuprofen. Advise client not to take additional medication containing acetaminophen or ibuprofen. |
| **Moderate Opioids**<br>Butorphanol: IM, IV, nasal spray<br>Nalbuphine: subQ, IV, IM | Dizziness, drowsiness | 1. Monitor client for effective pain control.<br>2. Abrupt withdrawal after prolonged use may produce symptoms of withdrawal. |

**Opioid Antagonist:** Antagonist that competitively blocks the effect of opioids without producing analgesic effects

| Medications | Side Effects | Nursing Implications |
|---|---|---|
| Naloxone: IV, IM, subQ | Hypotension, hypertension, dysrhythmias | 1. Assess respiratory status, blood pressure, pulse, and level of consciousness until narcotic wears off. Repeat doses may be necessary if effect of opioid outlasts the effect of the opioid antagonist.<br>2. Remember that opioid antagonists reverse analgesia along with respiratory depression. Titrate dose accordingly and monitor pain level.<br>3. *Uses:* Used to reverse CNS and respiratory depression in opioid overdose.<br>4. *Contraindications and precautions:* Use with caution in opioid-dependent clients; may cause severe withdrawal symptoms. |

**Intravenous Anesthetic Agents:** Used alone or in combination with an inhalation anesthetic that permits a lower dose of inhalation agent or produces effects that cannot be achieved by inhalation agents.

| Medications | Side Effects | Nursing Implications |
|---|---|---|
| ▲ Propofol: IV | Unconsciousness develops within 60 seconds and lasts for 3–5 minutes<br>Cardiovascular and respiratory depression<br>Bacterial infections<br><br>**⚠ NURSING PRIORITY:** Rapid onset and short duration of action can lead to respiratory depression, so respiratory support should be immediately available. | 1. Monitor for adverse effects of profound respiratory depression (including apnea) and hypotension.<br>2. Administer only in settings where there is appropriate monitoring and resuscitation equipment available.<br>3. Monitor for infection, sepsis; discard open vials within 6 hours. |

**Nonsteroidal Antiinflammatory Drugs (NSAIDs) and Acetaminophen:** General Nursing Implications

- Give with a full glass of water, either with food or just after eating.
- Store in childproof containers and out of reach of small children.
- Do not exceed recommended doses.
- Discontinue 1–2 weeks before elective surgery.
- NSAIDs prolong bleeding time by decreasing platelet aggregation and may increase anticoagulant activity of warfarin products.
- Avoid in clients with history of peptic ulcer disease or bleeding problems.
- May compromise renal blood flow and precipitate renal impairment.
- Do not crush enteric-coated tablets; if available, administer as enteric or buffered tablets.
  **Uses:**
  **Fever:** acetaminophen, aspirin, ibuprofen; **Inflammation:** aspirin, naproxen, ketorolac; **Arthritis:** aspirin, ibuprofen, naproxen, piroxicam, sulindac; **Dysmenorrhea:** ibuprofen, naproxen

*Continued*

**Appendix 3-3   MEDICATIONS: ANALGESICS, NSAIDS, AND PREOPERATIVE—cont'd**

| Medications | Side Effects | Nursing Implications |
|---|---|---|

### Nonsteroidal Antiinflammatory Drugs (NSAIDs) and acetaminophen: Inhibit the enzyme cyclooxygenase, which is responsible for the synthesis of prostaglandins; suppress inflammation, relieve pain, and reduce fever

| Medications | Side Effects | Nursing Implications |
|---|---|---|
| Acetylsalicylic acid: PO | Salicylism: skin reactions, redness, rashes, ringing in the ears, GI upset, hyperventilation, sweating, and thirst<br>Long-term use: erosive gastritis with bleeding; increases anticoagulant properties of warfarin |  1. Most common agent responsible for accidental poisoning in small children.<br>2. Associated with Reye's syndrome in children.<br>3. Assess for bleeding tendencies.<br>4. Prophylactic use for colon cancer.<br>5. Prophylactic use for cardiovascular problems due to the antiplatelet aggregation properties. |

> ❗ **NURSING PRIORITY:** Advise client that the Centers for Disease Control and Prevention warns against giving aspirin to children or adolescents with a viral infection or influenza.

> ❗ **NURSING PRIORITY:** Aspirin is the only NSAID used to protects against MI and stroke.

| Medications | Side Effects | Nursing Implications |
|---|---|---|
| Ibuprofen: PO | Gastric ulceration<br>Dyspepsia (heartburn, nausea, epigastric distress)<br>Bleeding<br>Dizziness, rash, dermatitis | 1. Do not exceed 3.2 g per day in adults and older adult clients.<br>2. Avoid taking with aspirin.<br>3. Increased risk of myocardial infarction and stroke. |
| Naproxen: PO | Headache, dyspepsia, dizziness, drowsiness | 1. Avoid tasks requiring alertness until response is established.<br>2. Take with food to decrease GI irritation.<br>3. Primarily used for pain control. |
| Acetaminophen: PO<br><br>> ❗ **NURSING PRIORITY:** Frequently used in combination with OTC medications. Teach client to read labels to prevent overdosing. | Anorexia, nausea, diaphoresis<br>Toxicity: vomiting, right upper quadrant tenderness, elevated liver function tests<br>Antidote: acetylcysteine (Mucomyst, Acetadote) | 1. Maximum dose of acetaminophen, 3 g per day.<br>2. Does not have antiinflammatory properties.<br>3. Overdose can cause severe liver injury; client should consult physician if he or she drinks more than three alcoholic beverages every day.<br>4. Has not been conclusively linked to bleeding problems. |
| Piroxicam: PO<br>Sulindac: PO<br>Ketorolac: PO, IM, IV | Dyspepsia, nausea, dizziness, diarrhea, nephrotoxicity | 1. Piroxicam and sulindac are medications primarily indicated for clients who have rheumatoid and osteoarthritis.<br>2. Ketorolac: oral doses must be preceded by parenteral administration; given deep IM may cause pain at injection site; combined oral and parenteral treatment should not exceed 5 days. |

### Preoperative Medications
### Benzodiazepines: Decrease anxiety and promote amnesia before or during surgery

| Medications | Side Effects | Nursing Implications |
|---|---|---|
| ▲ Midazolam hydrochloride: PO, IM, IV | Respiratory depression; pain at IM or IV site; nausea, vomiting | 1. Commonly used for conscious sedation and amnesia before procedures.<br>2. Continuous cardiac and respiratory monitoring during parenteral administration.<br>3. Administer injection slowly over 2 minutes to minimize respiratory depression. |
| Lorazepam: PO, IM, IV | Drowsiness, ataxia, confusion, fatigue<br>May produce paradoxical effects in elderly | 1. Decrease stimuli in the room after administration.<br>2. Offer emotional support to the anxious client.<br>3. Maintain bed rest after administration to reduce effects of hypotension.<br>4. A schedule IV drug. |

## Appendix 3-3  MEDICATIONS: ANALGESICS, NSAIDS, AND PREOPERATIVE—cont'd

| Medications | Side Effects | Nursing Implications |
| --- | --- | --- |
| Diazepam: PO, IM, IV | Same as for Ativan | |

**Histamine (H₂ Receptor Antagonists):** Decrease gastric acid secretion by blocking the $H_2$ receptors on parietal cells, increase gastric pH, and reduce gastric volume

| Cimetidine<br>Famotidine<br>Ranitidine | See Appendix 20-2 | See Appendix 20-2 |
| --- | --- | --- |

**Anticholinergic:** Prevent bradycardia, decrease secretions

| Atropine: PO, IM, IV<br>Scopolamine: PO, IM<br>Glycopyrrolate: PO, IM, IV | Flushed face<br>Dilated pupils<br>Increased cardiac rate<br>Urinary retention | 1. Children and older adult clients are at increased risk for side effects.<br>2. Advise clients regarding atropine flush.<br>3. Administer with caution to clients with glaucoma, MI, or heart failure.<br>4. Postural hypotension may result if client ambulates after administration.<br>5. Monitor for urinary retention and decreased bowel sounds. |
| --- | --- | --- |

*CDC,* Centers for Disease Control and Prevention; *CNS,* central nervous system; *GI,* gastrointestinal; *IM,* intramuscular; *IV,* intravenous; *MI,* myocardial infarction; *PCA,* patient-controlled analgesia; *PO,* by mouth (orally); *OTC,* over the counter; *subQ,* subcutaneous.

## Study Questions
## Health Implications Across the Life Span

More questions on

1. The nurse is preparing to take blood pressure of a client who is obese. What is the most effective method for obtaining an accurate blood pressure reading from this client? (Select all that apply.)
   1. Obtain a cuff that covers the upper one-third of the client's arm.
   2. Obtain a cuff that is 20% wider than the diameter of the client's upper arm.
   3. Position the cuff approximately 4 inches above the antecubital space.
   4. Use a cuff that is wide enough to cover the upper two-thirds of the client's arm.
   5. Identify the Korotkoff sounds and take a systolic reading at 10 mmHg after the first sound.

2. The nurse is caring for a client who is dying. How will the nurse provide psychosocial comfort for the family and the client in the period before death?
   1. Encourage family to sit at the bedside, touch, and talk to the client.
   2. Discourage more than one family member at a time in the room.
   3. Discuss with the family the importance of not upsetting the client by talking to him.
   4. Administer pain medication so the client will not be upset by family grieving.

3. The nurse is preparing a client for surgery. Which of the following items on the client's presurgery laboratory results would indicate a need to contact the surgeon? (Select all that apply.)
   1. Platelet count of 125,000 mm3 (325 × 109/L)
   2. Total cholesterol of 325 mg/dL (8.41 mmol/L)
   3. Blood urea nitrogen (BUN) 17 mg/dL (6.07 mmol/L)
   4. Hemoglobin 12.5 g/dL (95 mmol/L)
   5. INR 4.5

4. The nurse has received shift report on assigned clients in the medical unit. In planning the initial assessment of each client, what is the best approach?
   1. A thorough history of the hospitalization should be reviewed for trends in care, responses to therapy, and currency of medication orders.
   2. A comprehensive assessment should be done to determine the client's current status, the development of complications, and whether any changes in nursing care are necessary.
   3. A focused assessment should be conducted with emphasis on current health care problems.
   4. All laboratory results for the past 24 hours should be reviewed to determine changes that have occurred in the client's condition and to plan effective nursing care.

5. Which of the following clients would be at an increased risk for the development of a pulmonary embolus?
   1. A man with a fractured femur who is in balanced skeletal traction
   2. An older adult woman with a fractured hip who is in physical therapy
   3. A woman who gave birth 2 days ago and is going home today
   4. A man who had a thoracotomy 2 days ago and has chest tubes

6. In the recovery room, the nurse notes that a postoperative client is suddenly presenting with increased restlessness and circumoral cyanosis. What is the priority nursing action?
   1. Begin administration of oxygen.
   2. Call for assistance.
   3. Determine airway patency.
   4. Insert an oral airway.

7. A 1-year-old infant is prescribed ibuprofen ordered 50 mg every 6 hours. It has been 6 hours since the last dose, and his parent has requested that the child receive his pain medication. When the nurse enters the room, the child is asleep. The parent requests that the pain medication be given because the child is still restless while sleeping. What is the best nursing action?
   1. Refuse to awaken the child.
   2. Wake the child and give the medication.
   3. Tell the parent to call as soon as the child awakens.
   4. Explain the purpose and use of pain medications to the parent.

8. The nurse is preparing the preoperative client for surgery. Which of the following statements indicate to the nurse that the client is knowledgeable about the upcoming surgery? (Select all that apply.)
   1. "After surgery, I will need to wear the pneumatic compression device while sitting in the chair."
   2. "My skin over the incision site will be cleaned with antiseptic soap."
   3. "I cannot have anything to drink or eat after midnight on the night before the surgery."
   4. "To ensure my safety, a time-out for identification will be conducted in the operating room before surgery."
   5. "I will be given the consent form, and I will sign it after I get to the operating room."

9. The nurse is designing a teaching plan for a 3-year-old in preparation for a surgical procedure. What teaching strategies should be included in the plan of care? (Select all that apply.)
   1. Include the child's parents in the teaching.
   2. Intellectual development moves from abstract to concrete.
   3. Prevent separation anxiety.
   4. Provide anatomy and physiology information.
   5. A "no" response from the child means he or she is not ready to learn.

10. A client is scheduled for major surgery. What is most important intervention for the nurse to implement prior to surgery?
   1. Remove all jewelry or tape wedding rings.
   2. Verify that all laboratory work is complete.
   3. Inform family or next of kin of recovery procedure.
   4. Check that consent forms are signed.

11. A client is admitted with a diagnosis of terminal cancer, and he is experiencing severe pain. The doctor has written a prescription for pain medication every 3 hours PRN. How should the nurse plan to manage the client's pain?
   1. Wait until the client complains of pain, then administer the medication.
   2. Evaluate the client and determine need for pain medication every 3 hours.
   3. Administer the pain medication every 3 hours.
   4. Try to increase time between injections during the night.

12. The nurse is caring for a first-day postoperative surgical client. Prioritize the client's desired dietary progression by numbering the following from 1 to 4 (with 1 being the first step and 4 being the last step).
   _____ Full liquid
   _____ NPO
   _____ Clear liquid
   _____ Light solid foods

13. What is the most effective method to initiate an admission interview with a 70-year-old client scheduled for a total hip replacement?
   1. Sit quietly until the client initiates the conversation.
   2. Start the interview with easy questions to build a rapport.
   3. Determine whether she has any family available to provide information.
   4. Focus on the diagnosis and its effect on the client.

14. At the beginning of the shift, the nurse receives a report on a client. He is receiving IV therapy at 125 mL/hr. The nasogastric tube is patent and draining green drainage at about 75 mL/hr. New prescriber orders include the following:
   Vancomycin 500 mg IV piggyback (PB) in 50 mL D5W over 60 minutes, every 8 hours
   Metoclopramide 10 mg IVPB in 50 mL D5W over 30 minutes, every 8 hours
   One unit of 250 mL of packed red blood cells to run concurrent with the IV; infuse unit over 4 hours
   Irrigate the nasogastric tube with 30 mL NS every 2 hours
   How many milliliters should the nurse document as the intake for the 8-hour shift?
   Answer: _____ mL

15. A postoperative patient receives a dinner tray with gelatin, pudding, and vanilla ice cream. Based on the foods on the client's tray, what would the nurse anticipate the client's current diet order to be?
   1. Bland diet
   2. Soft diet
   3. Full liquid diet
   4. Regular diet

# Answers to Study Questions

1. *2,4*
To obtain an accurate reading on any client, the blood pressure cuff should cover the upper two-thirds of the client's arm; it should be positioned approximately 1 inches (2.5 cm) above the antecubital space. This is applicable to the very thin client as well as the obese client. The blood pressure cuff should be approximately 20% wider than the diameter of the arm or leg. If it is too large or too small, it

will affect the accuracy of the reading. The systolic reading is obtained with the first of the Korotkoff sounds. (Potter & Perry, 9 ed., p. 506)

2. *1*
The family should be encouraged to sit with the dying client, touch him, and talk to him. This is a method of saying goodbye and acknowledging the impending death. Several members of the family

can be present at the same time, and if the client is comfortable, no pain medication is necessary. (Lewis et al., 10 ed., p. 137)

3. *1, 5*

The platelet level is low, and the INR value is high, indicating a risk for bleeding; the nurse needs to make sure the surgeon has the most recent laboratory values before surgery. This client's surgery may need to be rescheduled until the client is hemodynamically stable. The cholesterol is elevated, but this is not a concern before surgery. The hemoglobin level and the BUN are within normal limits. (Lewis et al., 10 ed., p. 308)

4. *2*

An initial comprehensive assessment should be conducted to determine the client's current status with regard to his primary health care needs. Does the assessment correlate with the information received in the shift report? Is the client experiencing any difficulties? Does the nursing care plan need to be changed? Other options presented do not reflect an evaluation of the current status of the client at the time the nurse begins the initial care for that shift. (Lewis et al., 10 ed., pp. 40–44)

5. *1*

The man with the fractured femur is in traction, which means he is immobilized. The immobilization is necessary to prevent rotation and/or further movement of the fracture site after the repair. The client who is immobilized is at the highest risk for venous stasis, particularly in the large pelvic veins in the abdomen. The other clients listed are all mobile—the client with the fractured hip is in physical therapy, postpartum client is going home, and the postthoracotomy client should be out of bed two or three times a day. Clients with chest tubes should be ambulated, when possible, to enhance pulmonary expansion. (Potter & Perry, 9 ed., p. 1290)

6. *3*

It is important to determine whether the airway is patent and whether the client is breathing. If a significant amount of mucus and gurgling are noted in the upper airway, the client should be suctioned. Insertion of an oral airway may be necessary to maintain an open airway, but the airway must be assessed before determining a course of action. Inserting an airway will not solve the problem if the client is not breathing. (Lewis et al., 10 ed., p. 335)

7. *2*

Frequently, the parent is the best judge of the young child's pain. Six hours have passed since the last dose, and it is appropriate to awaken the child and administer the medication. (Hockenberry & Wilson, 10 ed., pp. 158–159)

8. *2, 3, 4*

Verbalizing that the skin will be cleaned with an antiseptic soap, maintaining NPO status after midnight, and performing the time-out identification indicate a correct understanding of the preoperative teaching by the client. The pneumatic compression device is worn during bed rest and is removed when the client is out of bed or ambulating. The informed consent document should be signed before preoperative medication administration and before the client enters the operating room. Part of safety standards is to initiate a time-out in the operating room before the surgery is started. (Lewis et al., 10 ed., p. 308)

9. *1, 3*

Parents should be included in the teaching of the pediatric client, and separation anxiety should be minimized. If the client is younger than 4 years, he or she will generally not benefit from anatomy and physiology information; simple explanations are better. A "no" response from a toddler is usually an assertion of independence rather than an indication that the child is not ready to learn. Learning moves from concrete to abstract. (Hockenberry & Wilson, 10 ed., p. 864)

10. *4*

Consent forms must be signed by the client, family, or guardian with medical power of attorney before any procedure can be done. Consent forms also must be signed before the client receives any medications that would affect his reasoning. These medications are frequently in the preoperative medications ordered. (Lewis et al., 10 ed., p. 310)

11. *2*

Relief of pain in the client with terminal cancer is palliative. Medications should be available around the clock, and the client should be evaluated frequently to determine the level of pain control. The nurse should not wait until the client complains of pain but should assess the level of pain control frequently. The medication should not be administered every 3 hours; it is to be given on an as-needed basis. If the client is not achieving pain control with this schedule, the health care provider should be notified. (Lewis et al., 10 ed., p. 117)

12. *2, 3, 1, 4*

The client's status is NPO immediately after surgery. Desired diet progression advances next to clear liquid. Desired diet progression then advances to full liquid. Desired diet progression next advances to a light diet of solid foods and then finally to a regular diet as tolerated by the client. (Potter & Perry, 9 ed., p. 1073)

13. *2*

The best approach to a good interview is to start with the easy, less personal questions while building a rapport. Waiting for the client to initiate the conversation is not an efficient use of time; furthermore, the client will not know what information the nurse needs. Assume the client can provide an accurate health history unless there are indications that he or she cannot give accurate information. Information about the current health problem and its effects on the client can be assessed after rapport is established. (Potter & Perry, 9 ed., p. 319)

14. *1470 mL*

All of the listed IV fluids should be infused within the nurse's 8-hour shift. The nasogastric tube will have been irrigated four times.

IV @ 125 mL/h × 8 h = 1000 mL
Vancomycin IVPB = 50 mL
Metoclopramide IVPB = 50 mL
Packed RBCs = 250 mL
NG irrigation = 30 mL × 4 = 120 mL
Total = 1470 mL
(Potter & Perry, 9 ed., p. 949)

15. *3*

A full liquid diet includes liquids and foods that are liquid at room temperature, such as ice cream, custards, puddings, and some refined cereals. A bland diet consists of foods that are soft, not very spicy, and low in fiber. A soft or low-residue diet includes foods that are low fiber and easily digested, such as pastas, casseroles, canned fruits, and vegetables. A regular diet has no restrictions. (Potter & Perry, 9 ed., p. 1073)

# 4 Culture and Spiritual Awareness

## PRIORITY CONCEPTS

Culture, Health Promotion

## CULTURE

### Cultural Competence

A. The complex process and integration of acquiring specific knowledge, skills, and attitudes to ensure delivery of culturally congruent care, which involves cultural awareness (self-examination), knowledge, skills, encounters (cross-cultural interactions), and desire/motivation/commitment (Box 4-1).
  1. *Culturally congruent nursing care* is meaningful, supportive, and facilitative because it takes into consideration valued life patterns of clients from different cultures.
  2. *Cultural diversity* refers to the differences among people resulting from ethnic, racial, and cultural variations.
  3. *Transcultural nursing* is recognizing and understanding cultural diversity to identify specific and universal nursing care that is sensitive to the particular needs of the client and family.
  4. *Cultural humility* is the ability to recognize one's limitations in knowledge and cultural perspective and be open to new perspectives.
  5. *Cultural relativism* is the attitude that other ways of doing things are different but equally valid.
  6. *Acculturation* is the process by which a person from one culture adapts to another culture.
  7. *Cultural assimilation* happens when members of a minority group are absorbed by a dominant culture by taking on the characteristics of that dominant culture.
  8. *Ethnicity* is the person's identification with or membership in a particular racial, national, or cultural group and observation of the group's customs, beliefs, and language.
  9. *Race* is a group of people with biological similarities (e.g., similar physical characteristics, such as facial features, color of hair, eyes, and skin).
  10. *Ethnocentrism* is the belief that one ethnic or cultural group is superior to that of another group.
  11. A *stereotype* is a preconceived notion or fixed general idea or image, usually about a group of people; many stereotypes are racist, sexist, or homophobic.

B. A person's culture and life experiences shape his or her worldview about health, illness, and health care.

C. Informed consent materials need to be in the client's language whenever possible, and an interpreter should be available whenever discussing informed consent with a client (The Joint Commission, 2010).

## SPIRITUALITY

A. Spirituality is not the same as religion.
  1. Spirituality is a client's journey or awareness of one's inner self and a sense of connection to a higher being, nature, or some purpose greater than oneself.
  2. Religion is a set of institutionalized beliefs and rituals, which is one way that clients exercise spirituality.
    a. Often the term is used interchangeably with faith or belief system.
    b. There are numerous religions in the world (e.g., Christianity, Judaism, Islam, Buddhism, Hinduism).
  3. Religious and spiritual beliefs can influence interpersonal behaviors and expectations.

> **⚠ GERIATRIC NURSING PRIORITY:** Functional decline and dependence due to aging can threaten the older adult's sense of identity and connection with others and the world, which can cause spiritual distress.

B. Components of spirituality (Box 4-2).
C. Identification of spiritual distress.
  1. Inability to participate in spiritual rituals or religious activities.
  2. Life-threatening, chronic, or terminal illness.

### Box 4-1   CULTURE—A NURSING APPROACH

**C**onsider your own cultural biases and how these affect your nursing care.

**U**nderstand the need to recognize cultural implications in planning and implementing nursing care.

**L**earn how to use cultural assessment tools.

**T**reat patients with dignity and respect.

**U**se sensitivity in providing culturally competent care.

**R**ecognize opportunities to provide specific culturally based nursing care.

**E**valuate your own previous encounters with patients from other cultures and backgrounds.

Zerwekh, J. (2016). *CULTURE: A mnemonic for assessing and improving cultural competence.* Chandler, AZ: Nursing Education Consultants, Inc.

## Box 4-2  COMPONENTS OF SPIRITUALITY

- Spirituality is a universal concept relevant to all individuals.
- The uniqueness of the individual is paramount.
- Formal religious affiliation is not a prerequisite for spirituality.
- An individual may become more spiritually aware during a time of need.

From McSherry, W. (2008). *Making sense of spirituality in nursing practice: An integrative approach.* Edinburgh: Churchill Livingstone, p. 48.

3. Depression, cognitive impairment.
4. Loss of faith and interpersonal support.

D. A spiritual history must be taken and documented on clients admitted to a hospital, nursing home, or home health agency (Box 4-3).

**TEST ALERT:** Respect differences between client's and health care provider's cultural and spiritual practices.

## CULTURAL AND SPIRITUAL ASSESSMENT

### General Considerations

A. It is important to assess each client for cultural preferences because of the many variations among cultures and religions.
1. Giger and Davidhizar's Transcultural Assessment Model is a tool developed to assess cultural values of patients about health and disease behaviors and their effects (Figure 4-1).

## Box 4-3  SPIRITUAL ASSESSMENT

Examples of questions that could be but are not required in a spiritual assessment include the following questions directed to the patient or his/her family:
- Who or what provides the patient with strength and hope?
- Does the patient use prayer in their life?
- How does the patient express their spirituality?
- How would the patient describe their philosophy of life?
- What type of spiritual/religious support does the patient desire?
- What is the name of the patient's clergy, ministers, chaplains, pastor, rabbi?

- What does suffering mean to the patient?
- What does dying mean to the patient?
- What are the patient's spiritual goals?
- Is there a role of church/synagogue in the patient's life?
- How does your faith help the patient cope with illness?
- How does the patient keep going day after day?
- What helps the patient get through this health care experience?
- How has illness affected the patient and his/her family?

(The Joint Commission. *Medical Record – Spiritual Assessment.* Available at https://www.jointcommission.org/standards_information/jcfaqdetails.aspx? StandardsFaqId = 1492&ProgramId = 46)

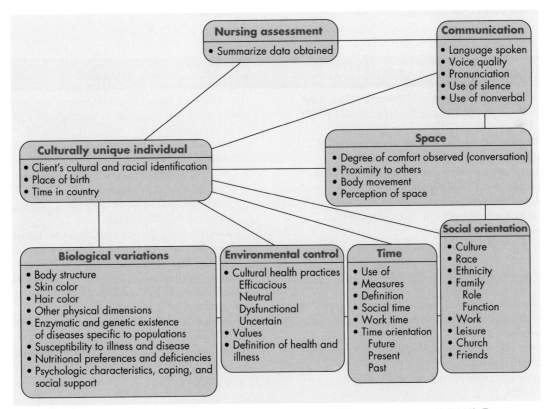

**FIGURE 4-1  Giger and Davidhizar's Transcultural Assessment Model.** (From Giger, J. N. [2016]. *Transcultural nursing: Assessment and intervention* (7th ed.). St. Louis: Mosby/Elsevier.)

2. The model contains six cultural dimensions: communication, space, social organizations, time, environmental control, and biological variations.

B. Identify various aspects of various cultures and world religions and the relevant beliefs that affect nursing care.

1. Definition of "illness or sickness" is based on the client's belief system.
2. Balance of "hot" and "cold" are factors needing to be kept in balance to remain well.
3. The role of pregnancy and birth events may have different meanings in various cultures.
4. Family and gender issues are important components of a cultural assessment.
   a. Promote sensitivity and understanding with lesbian, gay, bisexual, transsexual (LGBT) community (Box 4-4).
5. The experience of pain may be demonstrative or unemotional (uncommunicative).

C. Understand that how individuals respond to death or dying is directly related to their cultural and spiritual background.

D. Promote client's communication needs in all health care encounters.

1. Culturally oriented questions are by nature broad focused and require learning more about the client's personal history.
2. Use open-ended, focused, and contrasted questions.
3. Encourage clients to describe the values, beliefs, and practices that are significant to their care.
4. Use "teach back" and "show back" techniques to assess and ensure client understanding.

5. Provide information discussing only two or three important points at a time.
6. Use drawings, models, and illustrative devices to demonstrate key points and information.

> **TEST ALERT:** Include the client's cultural beliefs and practices in planning and providing nursing care.

## Assessment of Cultural Aspects

> **⚠ NURSING PRIORITY:** Avoid stereotyping. Clients are individuals who are unique, with beliefs, values, and traditions that deserve a personalized nursing assessment.

A. Communication styles.
1. Does the client speak English fluently? If not, what language is preferred?
   a. The absence of a language barrier does not preclude a cultural barrier.
   b. Consider individuals from English-speaking countries that have cultural diversity (e.g., India, American Samoa, South Africa).
   c. Use translated documents for frequently encountered languages to meet client communication needs.
2. What are considered signs of respect or disrespect? Attentiveness or nonattentiveness?
3. Is touch part of the communication process?
4. What practices are considered appropriate greetings or farewells?

---

### Box 4-4  CULTURAL SENSITIVITY WITH SEXUAL ORIENTATION AND GENDER IDENTITY

**Provision of Care, Treatment, and Services Checklist**

- Create a welcoming environment that is inclusive of LGBT patients.
  - Prominently post the hospital's nondiscrimination policy or patient bill of rights.
  - Waiting rooms and other common areas should reflect and be inclusive of LGBT patients and families.
  - Create or designate unisex or single-stall restrooms.
  - Ensure that visitation policies are implemented in a fair and nondiscriminatory manner.
  - Foster an environment that supports and nurtures all patients and families.
- Avoid assumptions about sexual orientation and gender identity.
  - Refrain from making assumptions about a person's sexual orientation or gender identity based on appearance.
  - Be aware of misconceptions, bias, stereotypes, and other communication barriers.
  - Recognize that self-identification and behaviors do not always align.

- Facilitate disclosure of sexual orientation and gender identity, but be aware that disclosure or "coming out" is an individual process.
  - Honor and respect the individual's decision and pacing in providing information.
  - All forms should contain inclusive, gender-neutral language that allows for self-identification.
  - Use neutral and inclusive language in interviews and when talking with patients.
  - Listen to and reflect patients' choice of language when they describe their own sexual orientation and how they refer to their relationship or partner.
- Provide information and guidance for the specific health concerns facing lesbian and bisexual women, gay and bisexual men, and transgender people.
  - Become familiar with online and local resources available for LGBT people.
  - Seek information and stay up to date on LGBT health topics. Be prepared with appropriate information and referrals.

From *Advancing effective communication, cultural competence, and patient- and family-centered care for the lesbian, gay, bisexual, and transgender (LGBT) community: A field guide.* (2011). Oak Brook, IL: The Joint Commission.

## Box 4-5 GUIDELINES FOR WORKING WITH INTERPRETERS

A. For those with limited English proficiency, a professional medical interpreter is needed whenever serious decisions are needed (e.g., end-of-life care, informed consent, treatment changes, discharge planning).

B. It is not recommended to use family, children, or support staff as interpreters.

C. Guidelines for working with interpreters:
1. Before an interview, instruct the interpreter to use the client's own words; avoid paraphrasing and inserting their ideas or omitting any information.
2. During the interview, look and speak with the client, not the interpreter.
3. Use brief, concise sentences and simple language—avoid technical terms and slang language.
4. If you feel an interpretation is not correct, stop and address the situation directly with the interpreter.
5. Watch and listen to the client's nonverbal communication when client is talking.

5. How is silence used in communication?
6. What is the use of nonverbal communication?
7. Is a medical interpreter needed? (Box 4-5)

**! NURSING PRIORITY:** Use a medical interpreter from the health care facility and avoid using family members.

B. Ethnic or religious group.
1. With what particular group does the client identify?
2. What cultural practices are important?
3. How closely does the client adhere to the traditional beliefs of the group?
4. Are there ethnic, cultural, or religious organizations that influence the client's approach or views about health care?
5. Are there specific times during the day to avoid scheduling tests or procedures with respect to religious or spiritual practices?

C. Nutrition.
1. What does the client and their family like to eat?
2. Are there certain ethnic or religious preferences about the selection or preparation of foods?
3. How is the food prepared? Who prepares it?
4. Are there foods to be encouraged (or avoided) when a person is ill?
5. Are there some fasting or requirements specific to beliefs or preferences concerning food items?
6. Are there any forbidden foods based on the client's culture or required for observance of a specific ceremony?

D. Family relationships.
1. Is the family matriarchal or patriarchal?
2. What role in the family does the client hold?
3. What is the role and attitude toward children and older family members (extended family)?

E. Health beliefs about health and illness.
1. How does the client define health and illness?
2. What does the client most fear about the illness?
3. What are the problems the illness has caused the client to experience?
4. Does the client rely on folk medicine practices or complementary and alternative therapies (e.g., acupuncture, healing touch, Ayurveda, etc.)?
5. Has the client been recently treated by any traditional healers?
6. Does the client take any herbal supplements or over-the-counter (OTC) medications?
7. Are there health topics that may be sensitive areas or considered taboo to discuss?

F. Health practices.
1. What are the strategies used to maintain health (e.g., hygiene, self-care)?
2. Who does the client contact when ill?
3. Does the client prefer to have a health professional of the same gender, age, ethnic, and/or racial background?
4. Are they any restrictions related to modesty that must be respected?
5. What examination procedures are considered immodest?
6. What is the client's way of responding to life events (e.g., birth, puberty, marriage, death)? Are there special events or ceremonies associated with the life event?

F. Time orientation.
1. What is the client's orientation to time? Are they future oriented, present oriented, or past oriented?
2. What are the client's views on being punctual and wasting time?

G. Personal space preferences.
1. What is the personal space preference?
   a. Territoriality or personal space is the distance that a client prefers to maintain from another. Large personal space is usually more than 18 inches.
   b. Various cultural groups have a wide variation in their perception of appropriate personal space.
2. What is the client's degree of comfort when talking or standing near others? (Figure 4-2).

H. End-of-life care.
1. What are the spiritual and religious practices that ease the client during end-of-life care?
2. Are there any garments, religious items, or rituals that are important during end-of-life care?
3. What are the practices about care of the body after death? How should the body be treated?
4. Does the client prefer a visit from a religious leader or clergy member?
   NOTE: The Joint Commission has a publication divided into two sections: cultures and religions, which is detailed and provides a handy resource for health care providers. (Galanti, G.A. [2018]. *Cultural and religious sensitivity: A pocket guide for health care professionals* [3rd ed.]. Oakbrook, IL: Joint Commission.)

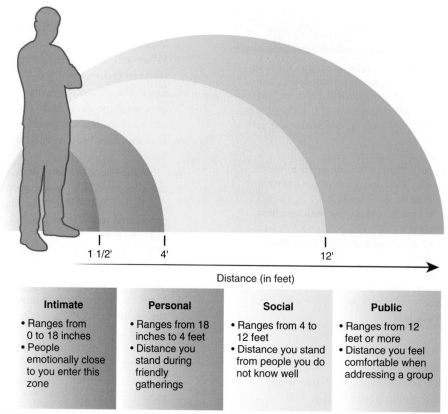

**FIGURE 4-2 Example of Personal Space Zones for European Americans.** (From Lewis, S. L., et al. [2017]. *Medical-surgical nursing: Assessment and management of clinical problems* [10th ed.]. St. Louis, MO: Mosby.)

## Study Questions
## Culture and Spirituality Awareness

More questions on

1. A nurse wants to improve cultural competence. What action shows progress toward this goal?
   1. Uses an evidence-based cultural assessment tool.
   2. Tries to treat all clients the same.
   3. Prioritizes care based on cultural needs.
   4. Wants to learn more about other ethnic groups.

2. What would be an appropriate spiritual nursing intervention for a client experiencing loneliness and social alienation?
   1. Assess client's ability to understand events.
   2. Asses client's level of functioning.
   3. Engage in active listening.
   4. Assist with both activities of daily living (ADLs) and instrumental activities of daily living (IADLs).

3. The nurse is caring for a client who is unconscious and is dying. The family has requested a priest to come. Which of the following sacraments would the family of a Catholic client request at this time?
   1. Reconciliation.
   2. Communion.
   3. Baptism.
   4. Anointing of the sick.

4. The clinic nurse answers a phone call from an Asian American client who is experiencing a fever. The client wants to self-treat first before taking an antipyretic medication. What would the nurse suggest to the client?
   1. Ingest yin foods.
   2. Meditate and pray.
   3. Have a massage.
   4. Ingest yang foods.

5. A client has identified that they are a practicing Orthodox Jew. The nurse understands the following about kosher diets. **Select all that apply.**
   1. Pork must be cooked in special "kosher" pots and pans.
   2. Fresh fruits should be avoided.
   3. Only meats allowed are those of vegetable eaters or cloven-hoofed animals (cattle, deer, goats, sheep) and animals that are ritually slaughtered.
   4. Fish that have scales and fins are allowed.
   5. No meat and milk combination is allowed; fish and milk eaten together are not allowed.

6. A family practices Buddhism and brings their 2-year-old child to the clinic for an annual well-child visit. The child is in the 60th percentile for both height and weight. The mother reports that she continues to breastfeed her child twice a day in the morning and at bedtime. She also states that the child eats most foods in their vegetarian diet. What would be an appropriate response by the nurse?
   1. "I am going to make a nutrition referral for you to speak with a dietitian about your child's diet to assist you with making better food choices for your child."
   2. "Because your child is in the 60th percentile for weight and height, I am going to refer you to home care services, so they can visit you at home while you are preparing a meal."
   3. "Can you tell me what your child typically eats for breakfast, lunch, and dinner?"
   4. "Your dietary Buddhism vegetarian practices are harming your child's growth and development and need to change."

7. A client is being admitted to a psychiatric unit for anxiety disorder. The nurse is conducting the admission interview and asks the client their religious preference. The client responds and states that they have not practiced their religion in many years and asks the nurse if religious practices would help decrease the symptoms of anxiety. What would be an appropriate therapeutic response?
   1. "Why haven't you practiced your religion?"
   2. "There are research study findings that have shown that religion and spiritual practice assist people to cope with anxiety."
   3. "I am not allowed to discuss religious or spiritual practices with the clients in our unit."
   4. "Would you like me to have our hospital chaplain come by and see you?"

8. What is ethnocentrism?
   1. The process by which a person from one culture adapts to another culture.
   2. A preconceived notion or fixed general idea or image about a group of people.
   3. The process when members of a minority group are absorbed by a dominant culture by taking on the characteristics of that dominant culture.
   4. The belief that one ethnic or cultural group is superior to that of another group.

9. What is the most effective approach to obtaining a cultural assessment on a client?
   1. Asking the client about their culture.
   2. Conferring with another nurse about the client's cultural preferences.
   3. Using a cultural assessment guide or tool.
   4. Observing the client's particular cultural preferences.

10. When you care for a client who does not speak English, it is necessary to call on a professional interpreter. Which of the following are proper principles for working with interpreters? **Select all that apply.**
   1. Expect the interpreter to interpret your statements word-for-word so there is no misunderstanding by the client.
   2. If you feel an interpretation is not correct, stop and address the situation directly with the interpreter.
   3. Pace a conversation so there is time for the client's response to be interpreted.
   4. Direct your questions to the interpreter.
   5. Ask the client for feedback and clarification at regular intervals.

## Answers to Study Questions

1. *1*
One action nurses can take to improve cultural competence is to learn how to use cultural assessment tools. The other actions are good steps but do not demonstrate progress to the stated goal as well as using an evidence-based tool does. (Zerwekh & Garneau, 9 ed., p. 486)

2. *3*
Active listening is an example of a spiritual nursing intervention. Other interventions include the following: prayer, presence, scripture reading, peaceful environment, meditation, music, pastoral care, inspiring hope, validation of the client's thoughts and feelings, values clarification, sensitive responses to client beliefs, and developing a trusting relationship. Identifying the level of functioning and ADLs and IADLs addresses basic human needs. Assessing cognitive function is identifying the client's ability to understand events. (Zerwekh & Garneau, 9 ed., pp. 494–495)

3. *4*
The sacrament or anointing of the sick may be administered along with other sacraments of reconciliation and communion, providing the client is conscious and can participate in reconciliation and communion. Because the client is Catholic, he or she would have already been baptized. (Zerwekh & Garneau, 9 ed., p. 491)

4. *1*
Yin foods are cold foods and yang foods are hot foods. A client experiencing a fever will want to eat yin foods or cold foods. Having a massage and meditating and praying are not part of the yin and yang approach to address symptoms of illness. (Zerwekh & Garneau, 9 ed., pp. 491–492)

5. *3, 4, 5*
The kosher diet only allows meats that are from vegetable eaters or cloven-hoofed animals (cattle, deer, goats, sheep) and animals that are ritually slaughtered. Fish that have scales and fins are allowed. No meat and milk combination is allowed; fish and milk eaten together are not allowed. Pork is prohibited. Fresh fruits are allowed. (Zerwekh & Garneau, 9 ed., pp. 491–492)

6. *3*
The nurse should assess and determine what foods the child is eating so the nurse can identify any dietary deficiencies and provide information to support nutrition for the child, so that improvement is noted in height and weight measurements. After an assessment is made by the nurse, the option to make a nutritional referral may be considered. Referral to home care services is not appropriate at this time. It is never appropriate to tell the family that they need to change their religious practices. (Zerwekh & Garneau, 9 ed., pp. 491–492)

7. *2*

The nurse's response of providing information about research studies supporting the reduction of stress and anxiety due to spiritual practices and religious beliefs is appropriate and directly addresses the client's question. Asking "why" questions tends to make the person justify their comment or belief. Nurses can and should discuss with the client when they have asked questions about religious and spiritual practices. The nurse calling the hospital chaplain does not answer the question. (Zerwekh & Garneau, 9 ed., pp. 491–492)

8. *4*

Ethnocentrism is the belief that one ethnic or cultural group is superior to that of another group. Acculturation is the process by which a person from one culture adapts to another culture. Cultural assimilation happens when members of a minority group are absorbed by a dominant culture by taking on the characteristics of that dominant culture. A stereotype is a preconceived notion or fixed general idea or image, usually about a group of people; many stereotypes are racist, sexist, or homophobic. (Zerwekh & Garneau, 9 ed., pp. 489–495)

9. *3*

The nurse should use a cultural assessment guide to obtain information during the admission assessment. This information can be included in the client's plan of care and is an objective and evidence-based approach. Although asking the client about their culture is not incorrect, a cultural assessment guide will direct the nurse in obtaining information that may not have readily been provided by asking the client or observing their behavior. (Zerwekh & Garneau, 9 ed., pp. 489–495)

10. *2, 3, 5*

There are helpful guidelines for working with interpreters, which include stopping and addressing the situation directly with the interpreter if you feel an interpretation is not correct. Pace a conversation so there is time for the client's response to be interpreted. Ask the client for feedback and clarification at regular intervals. During interview, look and speak with client, not interpreter. Watch and listen to client's nonverbal communication when client is talking. It is not recommended to use family, children, or support staff as interpreters. (Potter & Perry, 9 ed., p. 110)

# CHAPTER FIVE

# Nursing Management

**5**

Collaboration, Health Care Organizations, Health Care Quality, Leadership

## HEALTH CARE DELIVERY SYSTEMS

A. Managed care.
   1. Sought to change the fee-for-service approach.
   2. Early 1980s, Medicare introduced the prospective payment system as a way of reimbursing hospitals.
   3. A fixed fee was paid to the hospital according to a preset reimbursement rate for the diagnosis given at discharge.
   4. Impact of managed care on health care.
      a. Individual hospitals or physicians' offices merging into large-scale organizations.
      b. Nonprofit hospitals changing to for-profit status.
      c. Work environment likely to involve corporate culture.
B. Integrated health care delivery systems.
   1. Systems offer prevention services, acute- and long-term care facilities, home health care, and hospice services.
   2. They may offer high degree of continuity of care.
C. Case management.
   1. Ensures coordination of care while reducing costs.
   2. By assessing, planning, implementing, coordinating, monitoring, and evaluating options and services to meet a person's health needs.
   3. Effective in providing care, but not all clients need this intensity of interaction.
   4. Case managers are advocates who help clients understand their current health status, what they can do about it, and why those treatments are important.
      a. Guide clients through the health care delivery process and provide cohesion to other professionals on the health care delivery team.
      b. Case managers can be registered nurses, social workers, or therapists.

> **TEST ALERT:** Case management involves consultation, collaboration, communication, and attention to the transition between levels of nursing care.

D. Disease management.
   1. System of coordinated health care interventions and communications for populations with conditions in which client self-care efforts are helpful.
   2. Goal: support clients with chronic diseases who may receive services from various levels of care (acute care to home-based care).
   3. Teaches clients how to manage a particular chronic disease.
   4. Tools used to support case management are the clinical pathway (care map, critical pathway) or disease management protocol.
      a. Clinical pathway essential elements are:
         (1) Timeline outlining when specific care given.
         (2) Categories of care activities and interventions.
         (3) Intermediate and long-term outcomes to be achieved.
         (4) Variance record that compares specific client outcomes with expected outcomes noted on clinical pathway.
         (5) Do *not* replace individualized care.
      b. Disease-management protocols.
         (1) Supports physician/client relationship and plan of care.
         (2) Emphasizes prevention, uses evidence-based practice guidelines, empowers clients.
         (3) Evaluates clinical, humanistic, and economic outcomes—goal is to improve overall health.
      c. Both critical pathways and disease-management protocols are generally based on clinical guidelines that incorporate nationally acceptable ways to care for a specific disease.
         (1) Agency for Healthcare Research and Quality (AHRQ).
         (2) US Preventive Services Task Force (USPSTF).
         (3) Centers for Disease Control and Prevention (CDC).

## Nursing Care Delivery Systems

A. Total patient care or private duty model.
   1. When one nurse assumes responsibilities for the complete care of a group of clients on a 1:1 basis, providing total client care during the shift.
   2. Many nurses prefer this method.
B. Functional nursing.
   1. Breaks nursing care into a series of tasks performed by many people, e.g., LPN, CNA.
   2. Can result in fragmented, impersonal kind of care.
   3. Can lead to lack of accountability for the total client.
C. Team nursing.
   1. RN is a team leader who coordinates care for a group of designated patients.

2. Team leader assigns patient care to team members (LPN, CNA, UAP) based on level of acuity.
3. Team conference is important and promotes continuity of care.
D. Relationship-based practice (primary nursing).
   1. Nurse plans and directs care of client over 24-hour period.
   2. Registered nurse (RN) manages and coordinates client's care in hospital and client's discharge plan.
E. Patient-focused care.
   1. Traditional nursing interventions handled by ancillary workers under direction of RN.
   2. Moves RNs to higher level of functioning.

## Management and Leadership

A. Definitions.
   1. A **leader** selects and assumes a role; a **manager** is assigned or appointed to a role.
   2. **Management** is a problem-oriented process with similarities to the nursing process.
   3. **Leadership** is a way of behaving; it is the ability to cause others to respond, not because they have to but because they want to.
   4. Managers perform four functions: planning, organizing, directing, controlling.
B. Theories of management.
   1. Traditional (scientific) theory.
      a. Also known as bureaucratic theory.
      b. High productivity level expected from worker.
   2. Behavioral (human interaction) theory.
      a. Consider the workers' needs.
   3. Systems theory.
      a. Decisions based on how others will be affected.
      b. Considers the parts of a system as a whole.
   4. Contingency (motivational) theory.
      a. Examines what motivates workers to be productive and effective in completing the work.
C. Management style. (Figure 5-1)
   1. *Autocratic* manager uses authoritarian approach to direct activities of others.
   2. *Democratic* manager is people oriented and emphasizes effective group functioning.
   3. *Laissez-faire* manager maintains permissive climate with little direction or control exerted.
D. Theories of leadership. (Box 5-1)
E. Comparison of leadership and manager behaviors. (Box 5-2)
F. Types of managers.
   1. First level: nurse manager, head nurse.
   2. Middle level: supervisor, director.
   3. Upper level: executive, vice-president, president.
G. Power and authority.
   1. Power is having the ability to effect change and influence others.
      a. Power and responsibility always go hand in hand.
      b. Effective leaders use power to improve nursing care delivery and enhance the profession.
      c. Types of power. (Box 5-3)
   2. Authority relates to a specific position and the responsibility associated with that position.

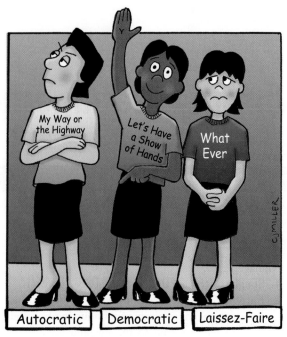

**FIGURE 5-1 Management.** (From Zerwekh, J. & Garneau, A. [2018]. *Nursing today: Transitions and trends* [9th ed.]. St. Louis: Elsevier Saunders.)

---

**Box 5-1   THEORIES OF LEADERSHIP**

**Desired Leadership Traits can be Learned through Education and Experience**

   **Contingency leadership**—leadership flexible enough to address varying situations.

   **Situational leadership**—situation is analyzed, leadership style is selected that will best address issue.

   **Interactional leadership**—development of trust in relationship; uses democratic concepts and views tasks from the standpoint of a team member.

   **Transactional leadership**—holds power and control over followers by providing incentives when followers respond in a positive way to leader's vision and actions needed to reach that vision.

   **Transformational leadership**—process in which leader and followers work together in a way that changes or transforms the organization, employees/followers, and leader.

   **Complexity theory leadership**—need to look at systems, such as those in health care organizations, as patterns of relationships and interactions that occur among those in the system.

From Wilcox, J. (2018). Challenges of nursing management and leadership. In J. Zerwekh & A. Garneau (Eds.), *Nursing today: Transitions and trends* (9th ed.). St. Louis, MO: Elsevier Saunders.

H. Comparison of the nursing process, problem solving, decision making. (Table 5-1)
   1. Nursing process and problem solving have similar steps.
   2. Problem solving involves obtaining information and using it to reach a solution to a problem.
   3. Decision making requires the definition of a clear objective to guide the process.

**Box 5-2 COMPARISON OF LEADERSHIP AND MANAGER BEHAVIORS**

- The manager administers; the leader innovates.
- The manager maintains; the leader develops.
- The manager focuses on systems and structure; the leader focuses on people.
- The manager relies on control; the leader inspires trust.
- The manager has a short-range view; the leader has a long-range perspective.
- The manager asks how and when; the leader asks what and why.
- The manager has their eye on the bottom line; the leader has their eye on the horizon.
- The manager imitates; the leader originates.
- The manager accepts the status quo; the leader challenges it.
- The manager is the classic good soldier; the leader is their own person.
- The manager does things right; the leader does the right thing.

From Bennis W. (1994). *On becoming a leader.* New York: Addison-Wesley, p. 45.

**Table 5-1 NURSING PROCESS, PROBLEM SOLVING, DECISION MAKING**

| Nursing Process | Problem Solving | Decision Making |
|---|---|---|
| Assessment | Data gathering | Awareness of problem |
| Analysis/nursing diagnosis | Definition of the problem | Set objective* |
| Development of plan | Identification of alternative solutions | Identify and evaluate alternative decisions |
| Implementation of plan | Selection of solution and implementation of plan | Make decision and implement |
| Evaluation/ assessment | Evaluation of solution and plan | Evaluate outcome |

*Decision making requires setting an objective, which is how it differs from problem solving.
Adapted from Wilcox, J. (2018). Challenges of nursing management and leadership. In J. Zerwekh & A. Garneau (Eds.), *Nursing today: Transitions and trends* (9th ed.). St. Louis, MO: Elsevier Saunders.

**Box 5-3 TYPES OF POWER**

- **Legitimate power** is power connected to a position of authority.
- **Reward power** comes about because the individual has the power to provide or withhold rewards.
- **Coercive power** is power derived from fear of consequences.
- **Expert power** is based on specialized knowledge, skills, or abilities that are recognized and respected by others.
- **Referent power** is power a person has because others closely identify with that person's personal characteristics; the person is liked and admired by others.
- **Information power** is knowledge a person possesses that is needed by others to function effectively.
  - This type of power is perhaps the most abused.
- **Leadership power** is being able to create stability and calmness out of the chaos created by conflict, problems, and disorder.

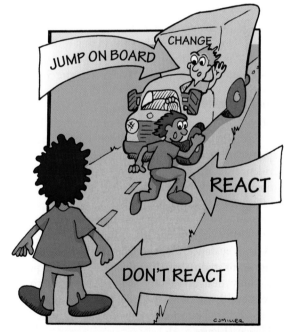

**FIGURE 5-2 Change: React, Don't React, or Jump on Board.** (From Zerwekh, J. & Garneau, A. [2018]. *Nursing today: Transitions and trends* [9th ed.]. St. Louis, MO: Elsevier Saunders.)

4. Decision making is values based, and problem solving is a more scientific process.
I. Change process. (Figure 5-2)
1. Change is inevitable, particularly in today's health care delivery system.
2. Lewin's change theory.
   a. Unfreezing phase.
      (1) In the unfreezing phase, all the factors that may cause resistance to change are considered.
      (2) Need to determine whether the environment of the organization is receptive to change.
   b. Moving phase.
      (1) This phase occurs once a group of individuals has been recruited to take on responsibilities for implementing the change.
      (2) Group identifies strategies and a plan to implement the change.
   c. Refreezing phase
      (1) This occurs when the plan is in place and everyone involved knows what is happening and what to expect.
      (2) Need to publicize the ongoing assessment of pros and cons of the planned change.

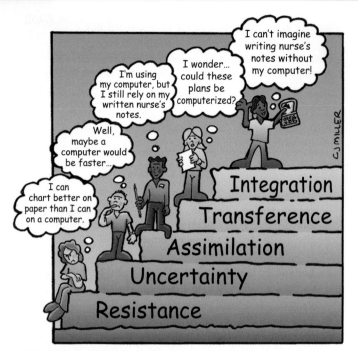

**FIGURE 5-3 Five Steps Toward Conquering Change.** (From Zerwekh, J. & Garneau, A. [2018]. *Nursing today: Transitions and trends* [9th ed.]. St. Louis, MO: Elsevier Saunders.)

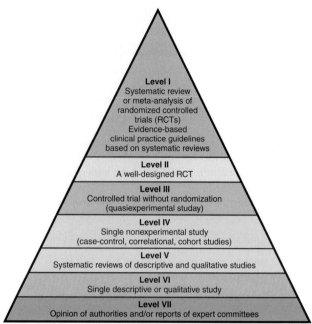

**FIGURE 5-4 Levels of Evidence; Evidence Hierarchy for Rating Levels of Evidence, Associated with a Study Design.** (From Zerwekh, J. & Garneau, A. [2018]. *Nursing today: Transitions and trends* [9th ed.]. St. Louis, MO: Elsevier Saunders.)

(3) Someone needs to be responsible for continuing to work on the plan so that it does not lose momentum.
3. Steps toward conquering change. (Figure 5-3)

## Evidenced-Based Practice

A. Evidence-based practice is the use of the current best practice research, client's values and preferences, and clinical expertise in the decision-making process for client care.
B. Evidence-based practice is one strategy to reduce the amount of time required to integrate new health care findings into practice.
C. Nurses should follow evidenced-based practice protocols and question approaches and rationales as needed.
D. Levels of evidence, also called hierarchy of evidence, are assigned to studies based on the methodologic quality of the study design, validity, and applicability to client care. Level 1 is the highest level, and when searching for evidence-based information, this level is the best possible evidence. (Figure 5-4)

## Quality Improvement

**TEST ALERT:** Participate in a quality (performance) improvement/quality assurance process (e.g., collect data or be a team member).

A. Continuous quality improvement (CQI): constantly and continuously looking for opportunities to improve client care.
1. Results from CQI audits are used to identify problem areas and to improve client care.
2. CQI evaluates all aspects of nursing care (e.g., nutrition services, radiology).

B. Quality assurance process.
1. Professional standards: use of general standards of care (e.g., American Nurses Association's *Standards of Nursing Practice*) along with the standards of each institution and each client care unit.
2. Determining criteria to meet standards.
   a. Provides a measurable indicator to evaluate performance: (e.g., "Nursing care plan is to be developed and written by an RN within 10 hours of admission.")
3. Evaluating performance or how well the criteria have been met.
   a. Usual method is reviewing documented records (chart) (e.g., checking the chart to see whether care plan is in place within the 10-hour period).
4. Following up on how effective changes were.
   a. Checking to see whether changes were made. For example, after the first audit of charts is done and suggested changes are made, a second audit of 20 charts determines whether an improvement has occurred in getting the care plan on the chart in 10 hours.
C. Methods of monitoring nursing care.
1. Nursing audit: examination of the client's records, either retrospectively (after discharge) or concurrently (while client is receiving care).
2. Peer review: practicing nurses evaluate peer performance based on standards and criteria.
3. Benchmarking: nurse quality indicator results are compared against the results of similar institutions locally and nationally.
4. Client satisfaction: questionnaire is given to clients to determine satisfaction regarding perceptions of the care they received.

## Interprofessional Communication

A. Assertive communication.
1. Has clearly defined goals and expectations.
2. Includes verbal and nonverbal messages that are congruent.
3. Is critical to the directing aspect of management.

**TEST ALERT:** Nurse leaders promote motivation and employee collaboration and communication through positive feedback, respect, and seeking input. Effective leaders use assertive communication. Focus of test item responses is about demonstrating these behaviors.

B. Conflict management.
1. Causes of conflict.
   a. Role conflict—when two people have same or related responsibilities with ambiguous boundaries
   b. Communication conflict—failing to discuss differences with one another can lead to problems with communication.
   c. Goal conflict—when one nurse places his or her personal achievement and advancement above everyone else's, conflict can occur.
   d. Personality conflict—interpersonal conflict among staff, clients, etc., in which they do not get along because of attitudes, values, personal characteristics, etc.
   e. Ethical or values conflict—different types of nurses have different value systems.
2. Ways to resolve conflict.
   a. Win/Lose: Example—competition; based on power; is aggressive and uncooperative.
   b. Lose/Lose: Example—avoidance; escapes and withdraws from the situation; tries to remain neutral.
   c. Lose/Win: Example—accommodation; tries to make peace; maintains harmony; dreads conflict.
   d. Modified Win/Lose or a No Lose/No Win: Example—compromise; takes a middle-of-the-road position; give and take by both parties.
   e. Win/Win: Example—collaboration; assertive and cooperative; objectively views situation; often leads to creativity and satisfaction.

**TEST ALERT:** The effective nurse leader and manager uses collaboration or compromise to resolve conflict.

## Interprofessional Practice

A. Involves health care professionals across disciplines working together to provide client care.
B. Nursing roles: care provider, educator, advocate, leader, change agent, manager, delegator, researcher, and collaborator.
C. Roles and responsibilities of health care team members. (Table 5-2)

## Interprofessional Collaboration

A. Communicating effectively using technology.
1. Don't misuse or overuse email, text messages, or fax machines.
2. When you leave someone a voicemail message, speak slowly and distinctly.
3. With a teleconference, make sure each party is introduced to each other; know how to turn on and off the "mute" setting to reduce background noise.
4. Do not send emotional outbursts in emails.
5. Carefully proofread emails before sending and include your name and a subject line.
6. Learn to use basic computer software.

B. Telephone and other verbal orders (Box 5-4).
1. Write down the telephone order or enter telephone order into the electronic health care record and read it back; receive confirmation from the prescriber that the order is correct.
2. Do not take verbal orders with the physician present when it is not an urgent situation.
3. Orders left on voicemail are not acceptable; the nurse must call the health care provider to obtain the order directly.
4. Verbal orders left with unlicensed assistive personnel (UAP), health unit coordinators, clients, or family members are not acceptable; the nurse must call the health care provider and obtain the order directly.
5. Obtain needed signature promptly.

C. Changes in client's condition.

**TEST ALERT:** Follow up on unresolved issues regarding client care. Evaluate and revise plan of care as needed (change in client condition).

1. Notify appropriate individuals: supervisor, physician, health care provider.
2. Challenge failure to provide appropriate care after notification of significant change in client condition.
3. Document changes and events surrounding the change in the client's status.
4. The nurse is responsible for assessing and evaluating client care and for taking action, obtaining assistance, or notifying appropriate individuals of the change in client condition.
5. Follow up on assessments of client problems and what nursing action was taken to resolve the problem. For example, the nurse may carefully document the events surrounding a client's fall, but it is also critical to follow up on what was done to provide care and to protect the client after the fall.
6. Have all information necessary when you contact the physician regarding a client problem. Follow good communication guidelines for telephone communications (Boxes 5-5 and 5-6).
7. Use an interactive communication method understandable for all interdisciplinary teams—I-SBAR-R (Figure 5-5):
   *I*dentification—Identify yourself and your client (two identifiers to be used).
   *S*ituation—What is happening at the present time?
   *B*ackground—What are the circumstances leading up to this situation?
   *A*ssessment—What do I think the problem is?

### Table 5-2 INTERPROFESSIONAL HEALTH CARE TEAM ROLES

| Team Member | Description of Role |
|---|---|
| Advanced practice registered nurse (APRN) | Has advanced education in pathophysiology, pharmacology, and physical assessment and certification and expertise in a specialized area of practice; conducts physical examinations, diagnoses and treats illnesses, and counsels on preventive health care in collaboration four core roles for the APRN: clinical nurse specialist (CNS), certified nurse practitioner (CNP), certified nurse midwife (CNM), and certified RN anesthetist (CRNA). |
| Dietitian | Provides general nutrition services, including dietary consultation regarding health promotion or specialized diets to manage disease. |
| Occupational therapist (OT) | May assist clients with disabilities, illness, or injury by helping them regain skills of activities of daily living, improve cognitive–perceptual skills, and assist with the construction or use of assistive or adaptive equipment. |
| Pastoral care | Offer spiritual support and guidance to clients and caregivers. |
| Pharmacist | Dispense medications and infusion products. |
| Physical therapist (PT) | Works with clients on improving strength and endurance, gait training, transfer training, and developing a client education program to restore function. |
| Physician assistant (PA) | Works under the direction of a physician to diagnose and treat clients, conducts physical examinations, performs diagnostic procedures and treatments, orders prescriptions. |
| Physician (medical doctor [MD], doctor of osteopathy [DO]) | Diagnoses and treat illness and injury by prescribing medication; ordering, performing, and interpreting diagnostic tests and evaluations, performing surgery; and providing other medical services and advice. |
| Respiratory therapist | Delivers specialized respiratory treatments to improve the client's ventilation and oxygenation status. |
| Social worker (MSW) | Assists clients in obtaining tangible services (financial, housing, etc.), performs counseling and psychotherapy, makes referrals to home and social services and agencies. |
| Speech and language pathologist (speech therapist) | Assesses, diagnoses, treats, and helps to prevent communication and swallowing disorders in clients. |
| Unlicensed assistive personnel (UAP): nursing assistant (NA), patient care associate (PCA), nursing technician, clinical assistants, orderlies, health aides, nurse's aide, nurse extender | Is an unlicensed health care worker trained to function in an assistive role to the RN by performing delegated client-care activities. |

Sources: US Department of Labor Bureau of Labor Statistics. (2017). *Occupational outlook handbook*. Retrieved from https://www.bls.gov/ooh/; and Lewis, S. L., et al. (2016). *Medical-surgical nursing: Assessment and management of clinical problems* (10 ed.). St. Louis, MO: Elsevier.

---

### Box 5-4    STEPS IN TRANSCRIBING ORDERS

1. Read all of the order(s).
2. Determine whether all request forms (laboratory, medication, diagnostic test) and/or contacts have been initiated.
3. Review notes for order entries.
4. Follow institution policy for rechecking orders and signing off.

From Rangel, J. (2018). Building nursing management skills. In J. Zerwekh & A. Garneau (Eds.), *Nursing today: Transitions and trends* (9th ed.). St. Louis, MO: Elsevier Saunders.

*R*ecommendation or Request—What should we do to correct the problem?

*R*eadback or Response—Receiver acknowledges information given: What is his or her response?

8. The oncoming nurse is responsible for the nursing care required on his or her shift.
   a. Status of IVs and amount of fluid to count.

### Box 5-5    TIPS FOR COMMUNICATING WITH PHYSICIANS ON THE TELEPHONE

- Use the I-SBAR-R technique.
- Say who you are right away and what unit you are calling from.
- Do not apologize for phoning.
- State your business briefly but completely.
- Ask for specific orders when appropriate.
- If you want the physician to assess the client, say so.
- If the physician is coming, ask when to expect him or her.
- If you get disconnected, call back.
- Document attempts to reach the physician. If you cannot reach a physician or health care provider or get what you need, notify your chain of command.

From Rangel, J. (2018). Building nursing management skills. In J. Zerwekh & A. Garneau (Eds.), *Nursing today: Transitions and trends* (9th ed.). St. Louis, MO: Elsevier Saunders.

## Box 5-6 SAFETY STEPS FOR VERBAL AND PHONE ORDERS

Step 1: Order is communicated verbally.
Step 2: Order is documented verbatim.
Step 3: Documented order is read directly back to the person who gave it for confirmation that it is accurate and understood correctly.

From Rangel, J. (2018). Building nursing management skills. In J. Zerwekh & A. Garneau (Eds.), *Nursing today: Transitions and trends* (9th ed.). St. Louis, MO: Elsevier Saunders.

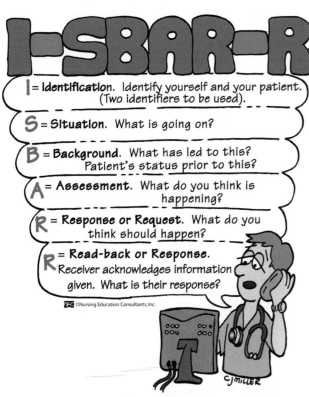

**FIGURE 5-5 I-SBAR-R.** (From Zerwekh, J., Garneau, A., & Miller, C. J. [2017]. *Digital collection of the memory notebooks of nursing* [4th ed.]. Chandler, AZ: Nursing Education Consultants, Inc.)

b. Any abnormal conditions (vital signs, pain, special treatments).
c. Status of client with regard to diagnosis (e.g., cardiac client—presence or absence of chest pain and dysrhythmias; surgical client—voiding, incision status; orthopedic client—circulation distal to cast or traction).
d. Psychosocial status of the client.

**TEST ALERT:** Provide and receive report on assigned clients.

D. Do not resuscitate (DNR) orders.
   1. Written by the physician based on the client's written medical directives or surrogate decision maker's request in consultation with the physician.
   2. Nurses are obligated to respect and observe the DNR order.
   3. Health care personnel should be advised of the DNR order.

## MANAGEMENT CONCEPTS

### Time Management

A. Get organized before the change-of-shift report.
   1. Develop a flow sheet to write down information you need to coordinate care for your clients.
B. Prioritize your care.
   1. Remember Maslow's hierarchy of needs.
C. Organize your work by client.
   1. Multitask to accomplish several objectives in one visit to the client's room.
D. Managing others
   1. Use assertive communication techniques.
   2. Delegate tasks to other assistive personnel.

### Criteria for Providing Constructive Feedback

A. Sandwich the constructive feedback between layers of recognition and positive reinforcement.
B. Keep in mind that when providing constructive feedback, you are simply providing your evaluation of an individual's performance, not his or her character.
C. When providing constructive feedback:
   1. Actively listen to the individual's perception of the situation.
   2. Focus on the facts.
   3. Provide an opportunity for the individual to self-reflect.
   4. Support the individual.

### Client Care Assignments and Delegation

A. The RN is responsible for delegating client care and for supervision of the implementation of care (Figure 5-6).

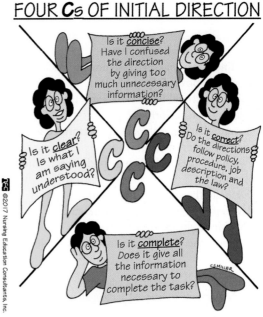

**FIGURE 5-6 Four Cs of Initial Direction.** (From Zerwekh, J., Garneau, A., & Miller, C. J. [2017]. *Digital collection of the memory notebooks of nursing* [4th ed.]. Chandler, AZ: Nursing Education Consultants, Inc.)

**Delegation:** "ANA and NCSBN both defined delegation as the process for a nurse to direct another person to perform nursing tasks and activities. NCSBN describes this as the nurse transferring authority while ANA calls this a transfer of responsibility. Both mean that a registered nurse (RN) can direct another individual to do something that that person would not normally be allowed to do. Both papers stress that the nurse retains accountability for the delegation." (NCSBN, p. 1)

**Supervision:** "to be the provision of guidance and oversight of a delegated nursing task. ANA refers to on-site supervision that is the active process of directing, guiding, and influencing the outcome of an individual's performance of a task and NCSBN refers to direct supervision, as the provision of guidance or direction, oversight, evaluation and follow-up by the licensed nurse for the accomplishment of a delegated nursing task by assistive personnel. Both have to do with the physical presence and immediate availability of the supervising nurse. The ANA refers to off-site supervision, and NCSBN refers to direct supervision. Both have to do with availability of the supervising nurse through various means of written and verbal communication." (NCSBN, p. 1)

**Accountability:** "Being answerable for what one has done, and standing behind that decision and/or action." (Hansten & Jackson)

**Assignment:** "as the distribution of work that each staff member is responsible for during a given work period. The NCSBN uses the verb "assign" to describe those situations when a nurse directs an individual to do something the individual is already authorized to do (e.g., when an RN directs another RN to assess a patient, the second RN is already authorized to assess patients in the RN scope of practice)." (NCSBN, p. 1)

Hansten, R., & Jackson, M. (2009). *Clinical delegation skills: A handbook for professional practice* (4th ed., p. 79). Sudbury, MA: Jones & Bartlett.
National Council of State Boards of Nursing (NCSBN). (2006). Joint statement on delegation. American Nurses Association (ANA) and the National Council of State Boards of Nursing (NCSBN). Retrieved from https://www.ncsbn.org/Delegation_joint_statement_NCSBN-ANA.pdf

B. Guidelines for making assignments, delegation, and supervision (Boxes 5-7 and 5-8).
   1. Give directions with clear expectations of how the task is to be performed.
   2. Ensure that the task is being performed according to standards of practice.
   3. Monitor the task being performed; intervene if necessary.
   4. Evaluate the status of the client.
   5. Evaluate the performance of the task.
   6. Provide feedback as necessary.
   7. Reassess the plan of care; modify as needed.

> **TEST ALERT:** Ensure appropriate education skills and experience of personnel performing assigned or delegated tasks.

C. Assignments are based on the RN determining the client needs, the availability of qualified staff, the scope of

**Right Task**
One that is delegable for a specific patient

**Right Circumstances**
Appropriate patient setting, available resources, and other relevant factors considered

**Right Person**
Delegating the right task to the right person to be performed on the right person

**Right Direction/Communication**
Clear, concise description of the task, including its objective, limits, and expectations

**Right Supervision**
Appropriate monitoring, evaluation, intervention (as needed), and feedback

Modified from National Council of State Boards of Nursing. (1995). *Delegation: Concepts and decision-making process.* Chicago: National Council of State Boards of Nursing.

practice of the available staff (RN, LVN, UAP), and the job descriptions of the institution.
   1. UAP (client care assistant, nurse's aide, certified nursing assistant) delegate activities that have specific guidelines (e.g., bed making, bathing, feeding, ambulating, general activities of daily living).
   2. LPN or LVN performs nursing actions (e.g., suctioning, catheterization) requiring knowledge of sterile technique, administers medication, gathers data regarding client progress, and provides information to RN.
   3. RN implements the nursing process, develops nursing care plan, implements teaching plan, and plans for client discharge.

> **NURSING PRIORITY:** Initial client assessment, provision of care to unstable clients requiring nursing judgment, discharge planning, and planning for client education are responsibilities of the RN.

   a. Performs the nursing assessment and analyzes data for client plan of care.
   b. Determines appropriate nursing diagnoses and nursing actions.
   c. Assigns most ill or unstable clients to RNs.
   d. Responsible for making decisions regarding client care; uses nursing judgment to determine care required of unstable clients.
   4. The nurse who delegates tasks and activities to a UAP and makes assignments to other nursing personal is responsible for supervision or periodic inspection to determine whether the task has been accomplished.
   5. Nurse practice acts of each state may dictate the specific activities of LPNs and RNs.
D. Considerations for assigning client rooms.
   1. Clients who need frequent nursing assessment or intervention should be assigned rooms near the nurses' station.

2. Group client assignments geographically together to assist in the organization of the work schedule of the nurse.
3. Consider the client's diagnosis in planning assignments of care and client room assignments. Refer to the Centers for Disease Control and Prevention website (https://www.cdc.gov/) for additional guidelines for client placement.
   a. Consider the needs of immunosuppressed clients; do not put them at increased risk for developing opportunistic infections.
   b. Do not put clients at increased risk. A client with human immunodeficiency virus (HIV) infection should not share a room with a client with an upper respiratory tract infection; a client with wound infection should not share a room with a client who has an open lesion caused by poor circulation.
   c. Be aware of clients who will require additional levels of isolation precautions and private rooms.
      Example: Children with rotavirus or respiratory syncytial virus; clients with methicillin-resistant *Staphylococcus aureus* (MRSA) infections.
   d. When a group of clients is assigned to one nurse, consider the potential for cross-infections.
      Example: A client who is immunosuppressed and a client with an MRSA infection should not be assigned to the same nurse.

**TEST ALERT:** Make client room assignments.

E. Prioritizing client care assignments.
   1. Identify the most ill or unstable client on your assignment; assess and care for that client first.
      a. Determine which of the client's needs is most urgent.
      b. Determine which of the client's conditions is most unstable.
   2. Guidelines for prioritization of client needs:
      a. Physiologic needs are a priority (Maslow; see Figure 3-1). Of the physiologic needs, airway, breathing, and circulation (ABCs) are the priority. Education, communication, and psychosocial needs can wait until physiologic needs have been met.
         (1) Client needs that are life threatening (e.g., dysrhythmias, airway obstruction) are the first priority.
         (2) Clients who have changing needs and are likely to experience harm if their needs are not met immediately (e.g., an older adult client who is vomiting; a client with difficulty breathing, incisional evisceration, or chest pain).
      b. Nursing process: assessment is the first step; adequate assessment must be done before nursing intervention can be determined.
      c. Considering time and resources, what can be done to benefit the client in the most expedient manner? For example:
         (1) Client with difficulty breathing—sit client up, clear the airway, begin administering oxygen.
         (2) Client with evisceration—put client in supine position with knees bent, cover the incision with sterile dressing soaked in normal saline solution, notify physician.

**TEST ALERT:** Assess and triage a group of clients to prioritize the order of care to be delivered.

# Study Questions
# Nursing Management

More questions on
evolve

1. The physician asks the nurse to give a client a medication that the nurse knows the client has reported an allergy to. When the nurse tries to point this out to the physician, the physician threatens to tell the nurse's supervisor. What is the best response?
   1. Tell the physician to give the medication himself.
   2. Walk away and ignore him.
   3. Agree to give the medication but do not initial the dose.
   4. Suggest a meeting involving the nurse, supervisor, and physician.

2. The nurse receives a hand-off communication report for the change of shift. Which client should the nurse see first?
   1. A 50-year-old woman who is scheduled for a breast biopsy this morning and is crying.
   2. An 85-year-old man admitted during the night because of increasing confusion and who remains disoriented this morning.
   3. A 65-year-old woman who had a thoracotomy the previous day and has two midline chest tubes.
   4. A 40-year-old man who is complaining of chills and painful urination and is scheduled for a colon resection in 2 hours.

3. The charge nurse is planning assignments for the nursing staff. One of the staff nurses is pregnant. Which client would *not* be appropriate to assign to this nurse?
   1. Child with a brain tumor being treated with radiation.
   2. Infant with respiratory syncytial virus receiving ribavirin.
   3. Toddler who is HIV-positive and has an opportunistic respiratory tract infection
   4. Child with leukemia who is receiving vincristine and allopurinol.

4. A nurse manager has been notified to obtain a bed for a client. Of the following clients, which one would the nurse anticipate being able to discharge?
   1. A client who had a myocardial infarction (MI) 2 days ago. She has the following vital signs: blood pressure (BP) 150/94 mmHg, pulse 84 beats/min and irregular, respiration 28 breaths/min, minimal chest pain.
   2. A client who underwent an abdominal aortic aneurysm resection 3 days ago. He has the following vital signs: BP 130/88 mmHg, pulse 88 beats/min, respiration 22 breaths/min, and oral temperature 101°F (38.3°C). He is beginning oral intake without problems.
   3. A client who has a subdural hematoma. He is lethargic; his pulse is 60 beats/min, BP is 150/90 mmHg, respiration is 28 breaths/min, and temperature is 99°F (37.2°C).
   4. A client who had abdominal exploratory surgery for a bowel obstruction 4 days ago. He has bowel sounds, is taking fluids orally, has an abdominal Penrose drain, and is continuing to experience abdominal pain.

5. Which of the following clients would the emergency room (ER) nurse see first?
   1. A client with a fractured left femur.
   2. A client with closed head injury.
   3. A client with third-degree burns to the face.
   4. A client with severe diarrhea and vomiting.

6. After morning report, the nurse prioritizes care of the following assigned clients. Which client would the nurse see first?
   1. A client with a leaky colostomy bag.
   2. A client who will be undergoing lumbar puncture at noon.
   3. A client receiving packed red blood cells and the bag is half empty.
   4. A child in sickle cell crisis with an infiltrated intravenous (IV) line.

7. The nurse and an unlicensed nursing assistant are caring for an older adult client with a diagnosis of emphysema. Which nursing task could be delegated to the nursing assistant to improve oxygenation? Select all that apply.
   1. Elevating the head of the bed.
   2. Obtaining oxygen tubing from the supply closet.
   3. Adjusting the flow of oxygen and turning it on.
   4. Teaching pursed lip breathing.
   5. Providing rest periods when assisting the client to ambulate.
   6. Assisting the client with morning care.

8. The nurse is preparing to delegate care for a client with neutropenia. Which nursing measures should be delegated to the LPN/LVN? Select all that apply.
   1. Instruct visitors about hand hygiene.
   2. Check skin, oral mucosa, and perineal area for signs of infection.
   3. Screen visitors for communicable diseases.
   4. Monitor for signs and symptoms of infection.
   5. Obtain vital signs.
   6. Assess client for subtle signs of infection.

9. The nurse received a report on the assigned clients for the shift. Which client should the nurse see first?
   1. A client who underwent thoracotomy 3 days ago; his vital signs are as follows: temperature of 101°F (38.3°C), pulse of 100 beats/min, and respiration of 28 breaths/min; he is complaining of chest pain when he coughs.
   2. An 85-year-old client who has a fractured hip and is in traction; she is complaining of pain and she is scheduled for surgery in 4 hours.
   3. An adult male client admitted 3 hours ago for dehydration; the vital signs are temperature of 99°F (37.2°C), irregular pulse of 100 beats/min, respiration of 24 breaths/min, and BP of 118/80 mmHg.
   4. A cardiac client whose cardiac monitor is beginning to show multifocal, trigeminal premature ventricular contractions (PVCs).

10. The nurse is planning assignments for the care of a group of clients. Which client would be a good assignment for an LPN/LVN?
    1. A client who is newly admitted with possible thrombophlebitis and is receiving IV heparin.
    2. A client with liver cirrhosis, severe ascites, and orthopnea.
    3. A client scheduled for repair of a fractured hip who has been placed in Buck's traction.
    4. A client with a suspected MI who is having shortness of breath.

# Answers to Study Questions

**1.** *4*

Suggesting that the physician meet with the nursing supervisor would be the most appropriate approach, giving the physician enough time to rethink his position. Giving the medication would place the nurse in a position of liability, and not signing for it would increase the legal liability. Arguing with the physician would only escalate the issue. (Zerwekh & Garneau, 9 ed., pp. 221, 474)

**2.** *4*

The client is scheduled for surgery and is beginning to exhibit symptoms of a urinary tract infection. The client needs to be assessed immediately for an infection, and the doctor must be notified. If an infection is present, the surgery may be postponed or canceled. The other clients are not unstable, and their needs do not have to be addressed immediately. (Zerwekh & Garneau, 9 ed., p. 245)

**3.** *2*

A child with RSV may involve contact with ribavirin, a teratogenic medication that is classified as Pregnancy Risk Category X. The nurse who is pregnant should not come in contact with this medication. The other clients do not pose any particular risk to the pregnant nurse. (Hockenberry & Wilson, 10 ed., p. 1190)

**4.** *4*

The client with the abdominal exploratory surgery represents the most stable client who could be discharged. The clients with an MI and subdural hematoma are showing signs of being unstable with their diagnoses. The client with the abdominal aortic aneurysm is stable, but because of the extensiveness of his surgery and because he had surgery only 3 days ago, he is a less likely candidate to move than the client with the exploratory abdominal surgery. (Zerwekh & Garneau, 9 ed., p. 245)

**5.** *3*

A client with third-degree burns to the face would have a high probability of an inhalation burn injury, which would swell the epiglottis closed. Airway issues take first priority. The next client to be seen by the ER nurse would be the one with the closed head injury, followed by the client with the fractured left femur, because of the neurovascular compromise. The client with severe diarrhea and vomiting would be seen last. There is no evidence of dysrhythmias in the client with diarrhea and vomiting. (Zerwekh & Garneau, 9 ed., p. 245)

**6.** *4*

The priority client is the child with sickle cell crisis. Treatment for sickle cell crisis is hydration to prevent clumping. Maintaining an IV line is important in maintaining this client's hydration status and provides a means of administering pain medication. The other clients do not have issues related to oxygenation. (Zerwekh & Garneau, 9 ed., p. 245)

**7.** *1, 2, 5, 6*

The nursing assistant may assist the nurse with care of the client that may include elevating the head of the bed, retrieving medical supplies, ambulating, and assisting with activities of daily living, such as morning care. The nursing assistant may not administer medications, which include oxygen, or provide teaching, because these actions are professional nursing functions. (Zerwekh & Garneau, 9 ed., pp. 306–309)

**8.** *2, 4*

The LPN/LVN can check skin, oral mucosa, and the perineal area for signs of infection and monitor for signs and symptoms of infection, which would be reported to the RN. Any type of teaching, such as instructing visitors about hand hygiene, screening visitors for communicable diseases, and performing assessments on clients, is the scope and practice of the RN. (Zerwekh & Garneau, 9 ed., pp. 306–309)

**9.** *4*

The client with cardiac disease is the most unstable and is beginning to exhibit symptoms that could be warning signs of increasing cardiac irritation. The client needs to be assessed immediately, and the nurse should anticipate administration of IV medication. The client who had a thoracotomy may be developing hypostatic pneumonia, but the situation does not require immediate attention. The client with a fractured hip is also not in an unstable situation, even though she is uncomfortable. The client with dehydration is exhibiting symptoms of his dehydration but is not unstable at this time. (Zerwekh & Garneau, 9 ed., p. 245)

**10.** *3*

The nurse should assign the client who is the most stable and requires the least complicated nursing care to an LPN/LVN. The client with a repair of a fractured hip is the most stable and would not require as much assessment and nursing judgment. The client with thrombophlebitis is at risk for a pulmonary embolism. The client with cirrhosis is experiencing respiratory difficulty. The client with a suspected MI is not stable and may be experiencing cardiac problems. (Zerwekh & Garneau, 8 ed., p. 309)

# 6 Ethical and Legal Concepts

Ethics, Health Care Law

## LEGAL ASPECTS

### Types of Law

A. Nurses need to understand how laws affect nursing practice.

B. Sources of law that directly or indirectly have an impact on the practice of nursing. (Box 6-1)

### Nursing Practice Regulations

A. Elements of a nurse practice act.
   1. Establishes and authorizes a regulatory agency; each state has a regulatory agency.
   2. Defines nursing practice within the jurisdiction.
   3. Mission: to protect the public by ensuring that any individual holding a license is competent to practice entry-level nursing safely.
   4. Provides the method and the requirements of licensure.
      a. Examination: successful completion of the National Council Licensure Examination for Registered Nurses (NCLEX-RN).
      b. Endorsement: applying for a license in a state or jurisdiction when already licensed in another state.
      c. Nurse licensure compact (NLC) states: As of January 2018, 25 states have adopted a nurse licensure compact agreement (24 of those states have adopted the enhanced nurse licensure compact eNLC) in which the state recognizes the nurse's license from another compact state. The license to practice must be issued from the state of primary residence (i.e., where you hold a driver's license, are registered to vote, and/or file federal income tax). (Visit https://www.ncsbn.org/nlc.htm for specific state information.)
      d. Requirements for foreign graduates.
         (1) Information on the federal screening process may be obtained from the Commission on Graduates of Foreign Nursing Schools (CGFNS, http://www.cgfns.org/).
         (2) Individual states may require completion of the CGFNS test *before* a candidate can take the NCLEX-RN.
         (3) Complete state requirements for NCLEX-RN.

B. How to protect your license. (Box 6-2)
   1. Unsafe practice.
      a. Repeatedly and carelessly failing to perform nursing in conformity with generally acceptable levels of nursing practice.
      b. Improper management of client records.
      c. Inappropriate delegation when result can reasonably be expected to result in unsafe care.
      d. Inability to practice safely.
   2. Misconduct.
      a. Falsifying reports, client documentation, or other documents.
      b. Causing or permitting physical, emotional, or verbal abuse or injury or neglect to the client or the public or failing to report same to employer, appropriate legal authority, or licensing board.
      c. Violating professional boundaries of the nurse–client relationship.
      d. Engaging in sexual conduct with a client, touching a client in a sexual manner, or using language or behavior suggestive of the same.
      e. Misappropriation in connection with the practice of nursing.
      f. Threatening or violent behavior in the workplace.
      g. Drug diversion.
      h. Failure to repay federal student loans or pay court-ordered child support.
      i. Patient abandonment.

C. Good Samaritan laws: enacted by individual states with the purpose of protecting health care providers who assist at accidents and emergencies.
   1. Care provided in good faith.
   2. Care must be gratuitous; no compensation is received for the care rendered.
   3. Care provided should be within the normal standard of care.
   4. Once aid is provided, the nurse must remain with the victim until stable or until another provider with equivalent or higher training provides relief.

D. Standard of care.
   1. The American Nurses Association's "Standards of Nursing Practice" and "Code for Nurses," the American Hospital Association's "A Patient's Bill of Rights," and individual states' nurse practice acts provide the guidelines for safe, ethical nursing practice.
   2. Determining standard of care involves the legal concept of a functional, reasonable, prudent individual of the same education and profession against which another professional's performance is judged.
   3. The guidelines are used to determine whether the nurse provided care in a reasonable, prudent manner.

**Statutory law**—most common type of law affecting nurses
- Nurse Practice Acts are examples of state statutory laws.

**Administrative law**—law made by administrative agencies that have been given authority to pass rules and regulations and render opinions of state statutes on a particular subject area
- Administrative agency is the State Board of Nursing.
- Nursing advisory opinions are examples of administrative law.

**Constitutional law**—refers to rights, privileges, and responsibilities as set forth by the U.S. Constitution, including the Bill of Rights

**Criminal law**—decisions made by judges in court cases; involves prosecution and punishment for conduct deemed a crime; *misdemeanor* is a less serious offense; *felony* is a more serious offense

**Case law**—also referred to as common law is composed of decisions rendered in court cases by appeals courts

**Tort law**—a civil wrong is committed against a person, which allows the injured person to file a law suit and seek damages against the party who caused the injury

From Austin, N. (2018). Legal issues. In J. Zerwekh & A. Garneau (Eds.), *Nursing today: Transitions and trends* (9th ed.). St. Louis, MO: Elsevier Saunders.

- Periodically check to make sure that you are in good standing at the Board of Nursing (BON) because of issues related to identity theft.
- Be sure that the BON knows whenever you change your address, whether you move across the street or across the nation.
- Practice nursing according to the scope and standards of practice in your state.
- Know the Nurse Practice Act in your state.
- Meet all renewal requirements on time.
- Always respond to correspondence from your state board of nursing.
- Know the self-reporting laws and self-report when required.

From Austin, N. (2018). Legal issues. In J. Zerwekh & A. Garneau (Eds.), *Nursing today: Transitions and trends* (9th ed.). St. Louis, MO: Elsevier Saunders.

4. Expert nurse witnesses may be used to establish whether a nurse's performance met or was below the standard of care.

E. External forces regulating nursing practice.
   1. The Joint Commission (TJC): one of several voluntary programs that evaluates and accredits health care organizations.
      a. Purpose is to improve the safety and quality of care provided by health care organizations.
      b. Sets standards for health care organization licensure and accreditation. These standards are frequently used to determine the standard of care for nurses working in the facility.

2. Occupational Safety and Health Administration (OSHA): goal is to ensure a safe and healthy workplace and to prevent injury to employees in the United States.
3. Health Insurance Portability and Accountability Act of 1996 (HIPAA): provides protection for the privacy and security of client's health information.
4. Centers for Medicare & Medicaid Services (CMS): branch of the U.S. Health & Human Services that administers the Medicare program; monitors the state Medicaid programs along with the State Children's Health Insurance Program (S-CHIP) and health insurance portability standards.

## Client Rights

A. Patient Bill of Rights – a previous listing of client's rights and hospital responsibilities that has been replaced by the American Hospital Association (AHA) with the Patient Care Partnership. (Box 6-3)
B. The Joint Commission – Speak Up™ program is about a patient's rights and role regarding treatment and care, which are summarized in the following acronym. (Box 6-4)

**S**peak up if you have questions or concerns.
**P**ay attention to the care you get.
**E**ducate yourself about your illness.
**A**sk a trusted family member or friend to be your advocate (advisor or supporter).
**K**now what medicines you take and why you take them.
**U**se a health care organization that has been carefully checked out.
**P**articipate in all decisions about your treatment.

## Liability for Actions

A. Individual liability: each person is liable for his or her own conduct; liability may be shared by another person or group (e.g., the doctor, another nurse, or the hospital), but it cannot be removed by the statements or actions of another.

- High-quality hospital care.
- A clean and safe environment.
- Involvement in your care.
  - Discussing your medical condition and information about medically appropriate treatment choices.
  - Discussing your treatment plan.
  - Getting information from you.
  - Understanding your health care goals and values (e.g., advance directives, end-of-life care).
  - Understanding who should make decisions when you cannot.
- Protection of your privacy.
- Help when leaving the hospital.
- Help with your bill and filing insurance claims.

Source: American Hospital Association. (2003). *The patient care partnership.* Retrieved from http://www.aha.org/content/00-10/pcp_english_030730.pdf

- You have the right to be informed about the care you will receive.
- You have the right to get important information about your care in your preferred language.
- You have the right to get information in a manner that meets your needs, if you have vision, speech, hearing or mental impairments.
- You have the right to make decisions about your care.
- You have the right to refuse care.
- You have the right to know the names of the caregivers who treat you.
- You have the right to safe care.
- You have a right to have your pain addressed.
- You have the right to care that is free from discrimination.
- You have the right to know when something goes wrong with your care.
- You have the right to get a list of all your current medicines.
- You have the right to be listened to.
- You have the right to be treated with courtesy and respect.
- You have the right to have a personal representative, also called an advocate, with you during your care. Your advocate is a family member or friend of your choice.

From The Joint Commission. (2002). Speak Up™. Retrieved from https://www.jointcommission.org/assets/1/6/Know_Your_Rights_brochure.pdf

B. Vicarious liability: liability is shared, but individual liability is not lessened.
   1. Respondent superior: employer can be held liable for the actions of an employee.
   2. Supervisory negligence—supervisors can share liability if:
      a. Assignments are not within the capabilities of the health caregiver (registered nurse [RN], licensed practical nurse [LPN]/licensed vocational nurse [LVN], unlicensed assistive personnel [UAP]).
      b. Assignments are not appropriate for educational level of health caregiver (RN, LPN/LVN, UAP).
      c. Assignments are not within legal limitations of nursing practice.
      d. Supervision of the activities assigned does not reflect actual limits and abilities of that individual.
   3. Physician may share liability but *cannot* alter an individual nurse's personal liability by a statement of *agreement to assume liability*.

## Civil Torts

A. Torts: intentional or unintentional civil wrongs against individuals or groups. Compensation may be awarded to the victim.
B. Negligence: unintentional harm to a client that occurs through failure to act in a reasonable and prudent manner.
C. Malpractice: professional practice that injures a client through failure to meet the proper standard of care.
   1. Elements of a malpractice suit.
      a. A nurse–client relationship must exist; the nurse must owe a duty to the client.
         (1) Assignment to specific nursing team or client.

         (2) Nursing care given to client regardless of formal assignment.
      b. A professional must breach the duty by not conforming to the established standards of care.
      c. Harm must occur to client.
      d. Direct cause-and-effect relationship must exist between the breach (nurse's action) and the harm (injury to the client), which may be financial or emotional.
      e. Foreseeability: a professional could reasonably expect injury to occur as a result of the breach of duty.
   2. It is the responsibility of the client's (plaintiff's) attorney to prove that each element occurred.
D. Invasion of privacy: protection of the constitutional right to be free from undesired publicity and exposure to public view.

**TEST ALERT:** Provide care within legal scope of practice. Client confidentiality is a nursing legal and ethical responsibility.

1. Medical records.
   a. Records should be released only with written client consent.
   b. Release for medical "need to know" limited to health care providers only.
   c. Client has right to inspect and receive a copy of records.
   d. Electronic medical records are password protected; never give another individual access to your password.
2. Belongings must be protected and may not be searched without specific authorization. The nurse should document the client's belongings. The list of belongings should be reviewed by the client and/or family, signed, and placed in the client's chart.
3. Confidentiality.
   a. Conversations are confidential; care should be taken to prevent conversations from being overheard.
   b. Photographs and viewing of procedures require consent of client.
   c. Control visitor access to client and client information: includes family and/or friends as designated by the client.
   d. Client information may not be released without client consent to family member, press, or friend.
   e. Protect the medical record from being read by unauthorized individuals. Do not leave charts or computer screens open where visitors can read them.
   f. Health professionals are obligated to maintain confidentiality of client's health information in accordance with the HIPAA regulations.

4. Physical privacy.
   a. Properly cover the body during procedures or examination.
   b. Close curtains or doors when procedures are performed.
   c. Individuals may not observe a procedure without permission from the client.
5. Exceptions to privacy requirements: some information is required by law to be reported.
   a. Certain communicable diseases.
   b. Injuries that are, or could be, caused by physical violence (gunshot and knife wounds).
   c. Child or adult abuse.
   d. Deaths occurring under suspicious circumstances.
   e. Animal bites.
   f. Deaths while in restraints.
   g. Others defined by individual state statute.
6. Confidentiality rights may be waived by the client. Obtain written consent to photograph client or to have others present during discussions regarding care, treatment, or procedure.

E. Defamation of character: written or oral communication to other persons concerning matters that may injure an individual's reputation.
   1. Slanderous or libelous statements made about client, staff, and/or coworkers.
   2. Defenses to defamation action.
      a. Truth: the communication is true, but be aware that truth may be a matter of perspective.
      b. Privilege: statements that are legally protected from a defamation action (e.g., lawyer/client information).
F. False imprisonment: unlawfully restraining personal liberty; unlawful detention.
   1. Actual: use of physical force to prevent departure of client; inappropriate use of restraints.
   2. Implied: use of words, threats, or gestures to restrain client.
      a. Refusing to allow client to leave hospital, with or without signing against medical advice (AMA) form.
      b. Refusing to release newborn.
   3. Exceptions depend on state laws.
      a. Refusing to allow departure of individual with communicable disease.
      b. Refusing to allow departure of incompetent or mentally ill client if there is imminent threat of serious injury to self or other as determined by a physician.

G. Assault and battery: nonconsensual threat (assault) or actual touching (battery).
   1. For a client seeking health care, touching is usually expected. However, the client in the hospital does not surrender his or her rights to refuse treatment or to refuse to be touched.
   2. The nurse cannot threaten the client with bodily harm to coerce him or her into a procedure or activity.

## Protective Procedures

A. Documentation: written record of events surrounding client's hospital stay.
   1. Protects client by promoting good communication among health care providers.
   2. Provides evidence in court of care given.
      a. Courts will not assume care is given unless it is recorded.
      b. Demonstrates meeting standard of care.
      c. Demonstrates decision making of nurse.
B. Effective documentation. (Box 6-5)
   1. Documentation, either on paper chart or electronically, should follow the format required by the agency.
   2. Electronic documentation.
      a. Do not give your access code or password to anyone. Any documentation entered will have your entry code on it.
      b. Do not print pages or share pages from the chart; this could be interpreted as a breach of confidentiality or privacy.
      c. Follow the institution guidelines for making corrections in charting and policies for correct documentation.
   3. Use descriptive, objective information based on what is seen, heard, felt, and smelled.
   4. Complete an honest record of events.
      a. Record all events, even unusual events, factually.
      b. Give all appropriate information about each documentation note (e.g., intravenous [IV] site, location, color, temperature, size [swelling, etc.], dressing, and condition).
      c. Do not include any reference to "incident report" filed.
      d. Do not alter record at any time.
      e. Explain omissions in care.
      f. Enter exception documentation as necessary to provide accurate picture of client's situation.
   5. Do not skip lines; do not leave any blank spaces on the paper chart for additional information to be entered.
   6. Correct errors properly.
      a. On paper charting, draw a straight line through error; date and initial.

## Box 6-5   GUIDELINES FOR EFFECTIVE DOCUMENTATION

- All entries should be accurate. Avoid stating your personal opinion. Report only the facts.
- Make corrections appropriately and according to agency or hospital policies. Do not obliterate any information that is written on the paper chart.
- If there is information that should have been charted and was not, make a "late entry," indicating the time the charting actually occurred and the specific time the charting reflects. *Example:* 10/13/16. 10:00 a.m. late entry, charting to reflect 10/12/16.
- All identified client problems, nursing actions taken, and client responses should be noted. Do not describe a client problem and leave it without including nursing actions taken and the client's response.
- It is often as important to document why you did not do something that you would routinely do, as why you did something. For instance: "Pt. refused to ambulate because of . . ."
- Be as objective as possible in charting. Rather than charting "The client tolerated the procedure well," chart the specific parameters checked to determine that conclusion. A chart entry worded "ambulated, tolerated well" would be more effective if charted "ambulated complete length of hall, no shortness of breath noted, pulse rate at 98, respirations at 22."
- Each page of the paper chart or each computer entry should contain the current date and time. Each time you enter information, make sure it reflects the current time of charting.
- Each page of the paper chart or each computer entry should include the full name and professional designation of the person making the entry.
- Document who saw the client and what measures were initiated. Particularly note when the physician visited; if you had to call a physician or health care provider because of a problem, record their response. If orders were received, be sure they are signed according to policy. This is especially important if you had to make several calls to health care provider.
- Make sure your notes on the paper chart are legible and clearly reflect the information you intended. It is a good idea to read over your nurse's notes from the previous day to see whether they still make sense and accurately portray the status of the client. If the notes do not make sense to you the next day, imagine how difficult it would be to decipher the information at a later date.
- Charting by exception may be available on electronic and paper charts. In this case the nurse may be required to document only significant findings or exceptions. It is important that exception notes are entered and provide a clear picture of the client's care or status.

Modified from Austin, N. (2018). Legal issues. In J. Zerwekh & A. Garneau (Eds.), *Nursing today: Transitions and trends* (9th ed.). St. Louis, MO: Elsevier Saunders.

b. Add omitted information by means of an "addendum" or "late entry": give date and time of original note *and* date and time of addendum.
7. Use meaningful, specific language. Do not use words you do not understand or unaccepted abbreviations. Avoid texting language.
8. Use standardized abbreviations as defined by the institution and by The Joint Commission (TJC).

9. Avoid texting results via personal telephone or pager not permitted by the institution.

> **TEST ALERT:** Use documents to record and communicate client information (medical record, referral and transfer form). Enter computer documentation accurately, completely, and in a timely manner.

C. Incident reports. (Box 6-6)
   1. Only the person directly involved in the incident should document the facts in the report.
   2. Do not complete an incident report for someone else.
   3. Document the facts.
      a. *Do not* draw conclusions or speculate on who caused or who was responsible for the incident.
      b. *Do not* state opinions or make judgments.
   4. Report does not replace the documentation of the incident in the chart.
   5. Do not document any reference to the incident report in the chart; the same factual information filed on the incident report should be included on the chart.
   6. Failure to complete an incident report could be considered a cover-up.
   7. Follow the line of authority within the institution for reporting an incident.
D. Know your limits.

> **TEST ALERT:** Recognize task/assignments you are not prepared to perform and seek assistance.

   1. Physical–emotional: be aware of fatigue and exhaustion because they can lead to increased risk of errors.
   2. Practice competency.
      a. Do not perform procedures without adequate preparation, knowledge, and experience. Request supervision if you are unsure of your skills.
      b. Report unsafe practices and misconduct to your supervisor.
      c. Report evidence of any fraudulent activity.
      d. Do not allow anyone to talk you into doing something you are not sure of by letting him or her agree to take the liability or telling you that you should do it.

## Box 6-6   INCIDENTS THAT NEED TO BE REPORTED

- Administration of wrong medication or vaccine.
- Exposure incidents to the skin, eye, mucous membranes with blood or a potentially infectious material occurs (e.g., needlestick injuries).
- Property damage or missing articles of client's belongings.
- Client falls.
- Visitor, client, or employee falls or any other injuries or accidents occurring on health care premises.
- Procedure-related or equipment-related accidents or injuries.
- Visitor exhibiting signs and symptoms of a communicable disease.

3. Floating.
   a. Floating (assigning nurses to work in areas outside their primary area of practice) is common in hospitals to reduce staffing costs and to enhance efficiency.
   b. When floating to another area, the nurse should be oriented and competencies evaluated to avoid a task or render a service for which he or she lacks the skill or knowledge to perform competently.
   c. Ask the supervisor for assignment of a "backup resource" nurse to be available for assistance.
   d. The nurse's right to refuse a floating assignment has not been supported in all situations. The best solution is to negotiate with the supervisor for an acceptable compromise while ensuring client safety.

## Responsibility for Professional Practice

A. To maintain the standards of nursing care and to protect the client, the nurse should report anyone in the health care setting who engages in illegal, unethical, or incompetent practices.
B. Examples of frequently occurring issues confronting nurses include:
   1. Medication errors that are made and not reported/corrected.
   2. Physical and verbal abuse of client.
   3. Providing care while grossly fatigued or under the influence of alcohol or drugs.
   4. Breach of client confidentiality and privacy. (Box 6-7)
   5. Jeopardizing a client's well-being by withholding treatment.
   6. Lack of informed consent.
   7. Potential differences between nurse and client belief systems involving abortion, euthanasia, organ procurement, and donation.

C. Challenge inappropriate orders.
   1. Identify the problem; obtain current, accurate information; and contact the health care provider.
   2. Follow institution's policy and chain of command if provider is not available or if there is not an appropriate resolution to the situation.
   3. Document the nursing action taken regarding the order.

## Box 6-7 HIPAA PRIVACY RULE

**Who Must Follow the Law?**
- **Health Plans**, including health insurance companies, health maintenance organizations (HMOs), company health plans, and certain government programs that pay for health care, such as Medicare and Medicaid
- **Most Health Care Providers (HCP)**—those that conduct certain business electronically, such as electronically billing your health insurance—including most doctors, clinics, hospitals, psychologists, chiropractors, nursing homes, pharmacies, and dentists
- **Health Care Clearinghouses**—entities that process nonstandard health information they receive from another entity into a standard (i.e., standard electronic format or data content), or vice versa

**What Information Is Protected?**
- Information doctors, nurses, and other health care providers put in a patient's medical record
- Conversations physicians or health care providers have about care or treatment with nurses and others
- Information about the patient's health insurer's computer system
- Billing information about the patient
- Most other health information about the patient held by those who must follow these laws

**How Is This Information Protected?**
- Safeguards must be in place to protect a patient's health information.
- HCP must reasonably limit uses and disclosures to the minimum necessary to accomplish their intended purpose.
- There must be contracts in place with their contractors and others ensuring that they use and disclose a patient's health information properly and safeguard it appropriately.
- There must be procedures in place to limit who can view and access a patient's health information, as well as groups who must follow the law; need to implement training programs for employees about how to protect a patient's health information.

**What Rights Does the Privacy Rule Give Patients Over Their Health Information?**
Health insurers and providers must comply with the patient's right to:
- Ask to see and get a copy of health records
- Have corrections added to health information
- Receive a notice that tells the patient how your health information may be used and shared

**Who Can Look at and Receive Patient Health Information?**
The privacy rule sets rules and limits on who can look at and receive patient health information.

Reference: Understanding HIPAA Privacy (n.d.). U.S. Department of Health & Human Services. Retrieved from http://www.hhs.gov/ocr/privacy/hipaa/understanding/index.html
*The HIPAA Privacy Rule provides federal protections for personal health information held by covered entities and gives patients an array of rights with respect to that information.*

D. Provide safe environment.
   1. Restraints may be physical or chemical and are used only to protect the physical safety of the client and others.
      a. Should be adequate and appropriate for the purpose.
      b. Use of a restraint on a client requires a physician's order that includes:
         (1) Type and location of restraint.
         (2) Type of behavior for which restraint is to be used.
         (3) Time frame that the order for the restraint covers.
      c. In an emergency situation, physical restraints may be used without a doctor's order for a limited period of time.
      d. Safe nursing practice for the care of a client in restraints includes:
         (1) Check restrained client every 30 minutes and provide for physiologic needs.
         (2) Remove restraints and provide range of motion every 2 hours.
         (3) Document the time of each check and the neurovascular status of client's extremities.
         (4) Remove restraints as soon as possible.
         (5) Secure restraints to the bed frame, not to the side rails.
         (6) Discuss with family the rationale for and purpose of restraints.
         (7) Investigate all alternatives to restraints: family involvement, methods to increase client orientation, scheduled toileting activities.

**TEST ALERT:** Apply and maintain prescribed restraints, bed alarms, or safety devices according to facility policy. Monitor client response to restraints. Evaluate appropriateness of the type of restraint used.

   2. Prevention of falls.
      a. Educate the staff on fall reduction protocol.
      b. Perform appropriate assessment of client at increased risk.
      c. Orient client to call light and bathroom; give instructions about calling for assistance.
      d. Keep all personal items within client reach.
      e. Keep bed in low position.
      f. Advise all personnel of clients at high risk for falling.
      g. Use side rails appropriately.
      h. Obtain adequate assistance for ambulation.
      i. Ensure appropriate lighting.
      j. Remove all obstacles or dangers on floor or in path.
      k. Check and use locks on wheelchairs, beds, stretchers.
      l. Establish toileting schedule.

## Specific Situations of Risk

**TEST ALERT:** Ensure proper identification of client when providing care.

A. Client identification—The Joint Commission (TJC) requirements:
   1. Two identifiers are required (e.g., the date of birth and the client's name on the armband or other person-specific identifier).
   2. Many institutions use barcoded technology to identify clients.
      a. A bar-coded label is placed on the identification band, specimen, or other patient items for identification.
      b. Barcode technology is often used for proper client identification with medication administration, specimen collection, and nutrition.
   3. The methods of identification should be appropriate to the care setting and individuals served.
      a. The room number is not considered an identifier.
      b. In newborn nurseries or neonatal units, another identifier may be required because multiple newborns have the same dates of birth.
   4. If client does not have an armband, then the individual's stated name would be one identifier; the client's date of birth, social security number, address, or phone number could serve as the second identifier.
   5. Client's current photograph or visual recognition may be used as one identifier in long-term care facilities, home care settings, or behavioral care facilities. For short-term clients, facilities with unstable staffing, and/or high-risk medications, the two-identifier requirement is necessary.
   6. The client does not have to state his or her name as an identifier.

**NURSING PRIORITY:** Always check client identification according to The Joint Commission (TJC) guidelines.

B. Medication errors.

## Legal Documents

A. Client's medical record or chart.
B. Advance medical directive: a written document regarding a client's desires for provision of medical care if that person is unable to make his or her own choices or decisions; examples include living wills and medical powers of attorney.
   1. Patient Self-Determination Act (1990): ensures that clients know about advance directives (ADs); requires facilities receiving Medicare or Medicaid funds to ask adult clients whether they have ADs and to advise clients of their rights.
      a. Living will (natural death act): a written document describing the client's wishes and special instructions regarding life support measures in the event that the client is incapacitated.
      b. Medical power of attorney for health care.
         (1) Identifies the person designated by the client to ensure that previously agreed ADs are carried out according to the client's direction.

## Box 6-8 INFORMED CONSENT

Informed consent is the process whereby the client is informed of the risks, benefits, and alternatives of certain procedures and gives consent for a procedure to be done.

### What It Includes
- The nature of the proposed care, treatment, services, medications, interventions, or procedures
- The potential benefits, risks, or side effects, including potential problems related to recuperation
- The likelihood of achieving care, treatment, and service goals
- Reasonable alternatives and their respective risks and benefits, including the alternative of refusing all interventions

### Nursing Considerations
- Nurses witness signatures to determine client competency, validate the signature, and ensure that the consent is voluntary.
- Witnessed signature: Do not witness unless you know the client has all information needed to make informed decision.
- The procedure is specified in terms the client can understand.
- Client appreciates the benefits and consequences of the procedure.
- Client understands alternatives to the procedure.
- Client is informed of the health care provider performing the procedure.
- The consent form is signed while the client is free from mind-altering drugs or conditions.
- Consents are legal documents.

### Withdrawal of Consent
- Can be written or verbal
- Can occur at any time, even after the procedure has begun

### Exceptions
- Life-threatening emergencies or urgent situations
- Minors: For clients up to age 18, a parent's signature is generally required for consent.
- Emancipated minor: Definition may vary, but usually this is a minor who is self-supporting and living away from home.
- Mentally incapacitated individual: Consent is required of legal guardian or person specified in medical power of attorney.

### Treatments Needing Informed Consent
- Most surgeries, even when they are not done in the hospital
- Advanced or complex medical tests and invasive procedures, such as an endoscopy and needle biopsy of the liver
- Radiation or chemotherapy to treat cancer
- Most vaccines
- Some blood tests, such as HIV testing (need for written consent varies by state)

**TEST ALERT:** Ensure that client has given informed consent for treatment. Participate in obtaining informed consent. Describe components of informed consent.

---

(2) Identifies the person designated to make health care decisions for the client if the client is incapacitated.

2. ADs may be changed or revoked by the client at any time.

**TEST ALERT:** Inform client of his or her rights (e.g., advance directives, confidentiality, etc.)

C. Consent forms.
   1. Informed consent. (Box 6-8)
   2. A minor may not give consent; consent must be obtained from the parent or legal guardian.
   3. Minors giving birth or emancipated minors may give consent based on individual state laws.

## ETHICAL CONCERNS

A. Resources.
   1. International Council of Nurses Code for Nurses (2012) states that nurses have four fundamental responsibilities: to promote health, to prevent illness, to restore health, and to alleviate suffering. The need for nursing is universal.
   2. American Nurses Association Code of Ethics (2015) provides direction for ethical decisions and behavior emphasizing the obligations and responsibilities of the nurse–client relationship.
B. Ethical principles. (Figure 6-1)

C. Ethical decision making.
   1. Determine the facts of the situation; legal versus ethical along with identification of emotional dynamics involved.
   2. Identify the ethical issues of the situation and the understanding of those involved.
   3. The Patient Care Partnership from the American Hospital Association and Speak Up™ from The Joint Commission provide clear guidelines as to how health care providers ensure a health care ethic that respects the role of the client in decision making about treatment choices and other aspects of their care.
   4. Determine the possible courses of action and the potential outcomes, best done by way of consensus for all those involved.
   5. After a course of action has been implemented, evaluate the perception of the outcome by those involved.
D. Interdisciplinary ethics committee: usually consists of physicians, clergy, social workers, attorneys, and nurses. Any member of the health care team should have access to the committee. The committee offers unbiased opinions, clarifies issues, offers support, and suggests a course of action.
E. Advocacy: the nurse serves as an advocate for the client by respecting the client's rights and facilitating communication between the client and the health care team.

**TEST ALERT:** Intervene to promote ethical practice; inform client, family, significant others, and health care team members of ethical issues regarding client care. Ethical issues often involve strong emotions. It is important to identify those emotions as a component of the concern.

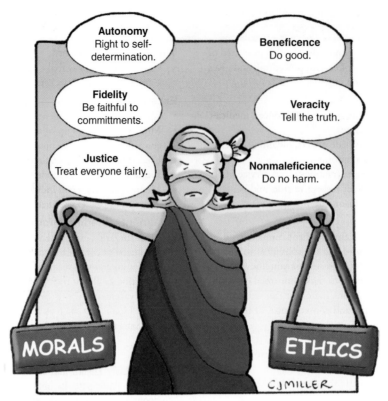

**FIGURE 6-1  Ethical Principles.** From Melonovich, P. (2018). Ethical issues. In J. Zerwekh & A. Garneau (Eds.), *Nursing today: Transitions and trends* (9th ed.). St. Louis, MO: Elsevier Saunders.

## Study Questions
## Ethical and Legal Concepts

More questions on

1. The nurse enters data on a paper chart and then discovers the entry was written on the wrong chart. How is this error best corrected?
   1. White-out the wrong information and write over it.
   2. Recopy the page with the error so that the chart will be neat.
   3. Draw a straight line through the error, initial, and date.
   4. Obliterate the error so that it will not be confusing.

2. Most states have reporting laws that require health care workers to report certain situations and behavior to authorities. Which is *not* usually a reportable matter?
   1. Child abuse
   2. Communicable disease
   3. Gunshot wounds
   4. Attempted suicide

3. What would *not* be considered a violation of HIPAA?
   1. Providing client information to an individual who claims to be a family member
   2. Allowing a student nurse, who is taking care of the client, to make copies of laboratory results
   3. Discussing the client's condition on the telephone with a family member who has provided the client information code
   4. Reviewing the client's chart with the CEO of the hospital, who is the client's brother-in-law

4. Which would the nurse identify as an indication that the client understands the informed consent document?
   1. The client states that the physician has explained the procedure to him.
   2. The nurse finds the informed consent form already signed.
   3. The client can give a return verbal explanation of the informed consent document.
   4. The client states that his wife read it and said it was okay.

5. While caring for an 8-year-old child with a broken wrist, the nurse notices red, raised streaks on the child's back. The child's father enters the room and the child becomes quiet and distant, leaning away from the father as he approaches. What is the best nursing action?
   1. Chart that the child was probably beaten by the father.
   2. Notify the supervisor to report possible child abuse.
   3. Disregard suspicions and care for the immediate needs of the child.
   4. No action is required; there is no actual proof of abuse to the child.

6. What is the nurse's best approach to avoid claims of negligence?
   1. A strong and binding contract for services
   2. Adherence to all hospital policies
   3. Competent practice of nursing
   4. Keeping a current license

7. The nurse is involved in a legal case against the hospital. Which judgment error by the nurse would be considered most damaging?
   1. Making illegal changes in the chart
   2. Arguing with the plaintiff over the case
   3. Withholding information from the hospital attorney
   4. Being argumentative while on the witness stand

8. The nurse stopped on the highway at a multiple-fatality accident to provide assistance. Immediately after the incident, the family members were appreciative of the help the nurse provided. They offered to replace the nurse's soiled clothes. If the nurse accepts, which rights were in violation?
   1. ANA Code of Ethics
   2. HIPAA
   3. Patient Self-Determination Act
   4. Good Samaritan Act

9. The physician asks the nurse to give a client a medication to which the nurse knows the client has reported an allergy. When the nurse tries to point this out to the physician, the physician threatens to tell the nurse's supervisor. What is the best response?
   1. Tell the physician to give the medication himself.
   2. Walk away and ignore him.
   3. Agree to give the medication but do not initial the dose.
   4. Suggest a meeting involving the nurse, supervisor, and physician.

10. Which of the following most clearly represents a situation of assault?
    1. In the emergency department, a client is intoxicated and verbally abusive; the nurse tells him she will put him in restraints if he does not quit talking.
    2. A client is in labor and has not received any medication for pain; she tells the nurse she does not want anything for pain; the nurse administers the pain medication ordered.
    3. The client advises the nurse that he is leaving; the nurse tells the client he cannot leave and threatens to restrain him if necessary.
    4. A pastor calls regarding a client's condition; the nurse provides the pastor with detailed information regarding the client's condition.

## Answers to Study Questions

**1.** *3*

Drawing a straight line through the error and initialing and dating it is the recommended procedure for correcting an error. Errors in charting on a paper chart should never be obliterated, recopied, or covered with correction fluid. When the erroneous information is not legible, it raises questions as to what the person was trying to cover up. (Zerwekh & Garneau, 9 ed., pp. 464–466)

**2.** *4*

Legal reporting laws include exceptions for the invasion of privacy (including suicide attempts). Communicable diseases, gunshot and knife wounds, and child abuse must be reported. (Zerwekh & Garneau, 9 ed., p. 470)

**3.** *3*

Many institutions provide a specific code word to identify individuals who are allowed to have access to the client care information based on the client providing permission for the access. The nurse should not assume that any individual is truly a family member—this must be verified. Copies of client's charts or records should not be made by anyone. The chart should not be reviewed by anyone who does not have a need to know to provide care. The CEO does not provide care. (Zerwekh & Garneau, 9 ed., p. 451)

**4.** *3*

The client needs to show an understanding of the informed consent document by giving an explanation in his own words. He should also be able to tell you what he expects to happen regarding the procedure and the possible complications. It is the physician's responsibility to provide the client with this information. It is not the wife's responsibility to have read it and to agree to it because it is the client giving the informed consent. (Zerwekh & Garneau, 9 ed., p. 471)

**5.** *2*

The physical characteristics and the child's emotional response to the father are suspicious. Further assessment and documentation need to occur. Any suspected child abuse situation should be reported to the nursing supervisor, who is obligated to report it through the facilities channels to the appropriate agencies. (Zerwekh & Garneau, 9 ed., p. 470)

**6.** *3*

The nurse needs to keep skills and nursing knowledge current to deliver competent, safe care. A contract and current license are not protection against negligence. It is important to follow hospital policy, but if the nurse feels the hospital policy is inadequate and/or incomplete, the established competencies for nursing practice should be followed. (Zerwekh & Garneau, 8 ed., p. 474)

**7.** *1*

The chart is considered a legal document. Any illegal alterations can be considered fraud. Arguing and withholding information are not wise and will certainly not benefit the case, but making illegal changes in the chart would be the most damaging error because this is a clear violation of the law. (Zerwekh, Garneau, & Garneau, 9 ed., pp. 464–466)

**8.** *4*

The nurse was in violation of the Good Samaritan Act. Allowing the family to replace the soiled clothes was a form of compensation, which is in direct violation of the Good Samaritan Act. None of the other choices is applicable to the situation. The ANA Code of Ethics provides principles to facilitate ethical problem solving. HIPAA is a law providing confidentiality for the client to protect written and verbal communication about the client. The Patient Self-Determination Act requires that hospitalized patients indicate whether they have an advance directive. (Zerwekh & Garneau, 9 ed., p. 457)

**9. *4***

Suggesting that the physician meet with the nursing supervisor would be the most appropriate approach, giving the physician enough time to rethink his position. Giving the medication would place the nurse in a position of liability, and not signing for it would increase the legal liability. Arguing with the physician would only escalate the issue. (Zerwekh & Garneau, 9 ed., p. 476)

**10. *1***

The nurse in the emergency department has threatened the client with physical restraint if he does not quit being verbally abusive; the threat is considered an assault. When the nurse gives a medication the client does not want, it is a situation of battery or abuse, as well as nonconsensual touching. The nurse is committing false imprisonment when she threatens the client with physical restraint to prevent him from leaving. When the nurse does not check to see whether the pastor had permission from the client to receive this information, it describes a breach of confidentiality and invasion of privacy. (Zerwekh & Garneau, 9 ed., p. 450)

# CHAPTER SEVEN

# Emergency and Disaster Preparedness and Bioterrorism

**7**

Health Care Organizations, Health Policy

## DEFINITIONS

A. Emergency preparedness, as it relates to the nurse, can be divided into two major categories:
   1. Clinical preparedness.
      a. Focus on agent identification, education, and clinical response for the various threats.
      b. Inclusive of early client symptom recognition and efficacious diagnosis and treatment.
   2. Community-based approaches.
      a. Administrative and regulatory efforts to increase preparedness and epidemiologic clues that may indicate a public health event has occurred.
      b. Inclusive of identification of public and private stakeholders necessary to execute an effective public health response.
B. Disaster nursing integrates a wide range of nursing-specific knowledge and practices that facilitate the promotion of health while minimizing health hazards and peripheral life-damaging factors.
   1. Types of disasters (Box 7-1).
   2. Natural disasters: The Centers for Disease Control and Prevention (CDC) has identified more than 10 types of natural disasters (https://www.cdc.gov/disasters/index.html); the five most frequent are:
      a. Hurricane.
      b. Flu pandemic.
      c. Earthquake.
      d. Flooding.
      e. Tornado.
   3. Although each disaster has specific response capacities inherent to that disaster, there are some commonalities to all of these natural disasters. The clinical nurse must be cognizant of each of the following when preparing and responding to natural disasters:
      a. Acute illness (increased presentations of infections from vaccine-preventable diseases (diphtheria, tetanus, hepatitis A).
      b. Carbon monoxide exposures.
      c. Unsanitary food and water.
      d. Animal bites and vector (insect) issues.
      e. Cleanup and associated physical injuries.
      f. General environmental concerns (urban sanitation/trash).
      g. Mold.
      h. Power outages.
      i. Mental health issues (specifically in longer-duration events).
   4. Disaster or emergency management cycle—four stages.
      a. Prevention or mitigation: heightened inspections; improved surveillance and security, testing, immunizations, isolation, or quarantine; and halting chemical, biologic, radiologic, nuclear, and explosive (CBRNE) threats
      b. Preparedness.
         (1) Personal: availability of emergency supplies; plans for family, pets, and own needs; disaster kits.
         (2) Professional: understanding and competence at using personal protection equipment (PPE), involvement in National Disaster Medical System (NDMS), Disaster Medical Assistance Team (DMAT), and other opportunities with American Red Cross, Community Emergency Response Team (CERT), etc.
         (3) What nurses need to know and do to be prepared for a disaster (Box 7-2).
         (4) Community preparedness (discussed later in the chapter).
      c. Response: mobilization at local level of responders, then assessment of scope of disaster.
      d. Recovery: returning to a "new normal" for the community.
   5. Three levels of disaster nursing.
      a. Level I Disaster—in these small-scale disasters (e.g., car accident, house fire), the nurse works in cooperation with local emergency medical systems and the community to provide medical support.
      b. Level II Disaster—these larger disasters (e.g., airplane crash, building collapse, tornado) require the nurse to respond in a greater capacity using larger casualty practices in coordination with regional response agencies, such as state health and emergency management agencies.
      c. Level III Disaster—these large-scale disasters (e.g., earthquakes, pandemics, hurricanes) consume local, state, and federal resources to the fullest extent and require an extended response time of the nurse that can last weeks and even months.

**Natural Disasters**
- Weather-related (blizzards, avalanches, droughts, hailstorms, hurricanes, tornadoes, cyclones, typhoons, floods, heat waves)
- Communicable disease epidemics
- Earthquakes, tsunamis
- Volcanic eruptions
- Wildfires

**Manmade Disasters**
- Terrorism (chemical and biological)
- Toxic or hazardous spills
- Food and/or water contamination
- Transportation accidents
- Riots, bombings, explosions
- Buildings, bridges, and other structural collapses
- Arson/fires
- Wars

- Specific type of disasters that can threaten their community
- Types of injuries to expect from different disaster situations
- Evacuation routes for agency and community
- Locations of shelters
- Understanding and recognition about warning systems (radio, television, emergency apps on phone for weather, etc.)
- Information to educate others about disasters and how to prepare for and respond to them.
- Maintain competency in lifesaving measures (e.g., basic first aid, cardiopulmonary resuscitation [CPR], and use of automated external defibrillators)

**TEST ALERT:** The nurse needs to understand the process of implementing emergency response plans in both an internal (hospital/agency) or external disaster (hurricane, bioterrorism event) and how to participate in an agency's security plan (e.g., bomb threats, newborn nursery security) and in disaster planning activities and drills.

C. Bioterrorism.
1. Weapons of mass destruction—weapon is designed or intended to cause death or serious bodily injury.
   a. Any weapon through release, dissemination, or impact of *toxic or poisonous chemicals*, or their precursors (ricin, tetrodotoxin, mycotoxins).
   b. Any weapon involving a *disease organism.*
      (1) High-priority agents are anthrax, botulism, plague, smallpox, tularemia, and viral hemorrhagic fevers (Ebola virus, Marburg, or Lassa).
      (2) Second-highest priority agents are brucellosis, *Clostridium perfringens,* or food threats by infections with *Salmonella, Escherichia coli* O157:H7, or *Shigella.*

# CLINICAL PREPAREDNESS

A. Biologic agents. (Table 7-1)
B. Chemical agents.
   1. Nerve agents: sarin, soman, tabun, VX gas.
      a. Symptoms: constricted pupils, runny nose, shortness of breath, diaphoresis, vomiting, seizures, cessation of respiration.
      b. Onset: seconds to minutes.
      c. Treatment: MARK-1 kit, diazepam (Valium).
      d. Infection control: gross decontamination before client admission; bleach/water for skin decontamination; standard PPE precautions.
   2. Cyanide.
      a. Symptoms: loss of consciousness, convulsions, temporary cessation of respiration, metabolic acidosis.
      b. Onset: seconds.
      c. Treatment: amyl nitrate, hydroxocobalamin, diazepam, and sodium bicarbonate.
      d. Infection control: gross decontamination before client admission; no decontamination usually needed for skin; standard PPE precautions.
   3. Blister agents: mustard gas, lewisite.
      a. Symptoms: redness of the skin, blisters, eye irritation, cough, shortness of breath.
      b. Onset: hours.
      c. Treatment: none; supportive therapy only.
      d. Infection control: gross decontamination before client admission; standard PPE precautions.
   4. Pulmonary agents: chlorine, phosgene, ammonia.
      a. Symptoms: coughing, shortness of breath.
      b. Onset: hours.
      c. Treatment: none.
      d. Infection control: gross decontamination before client admission; standard PPE precautions.
   5. Riot control agents: BZ (3-quinuclidinyl benzilate), fentanyl, and other opioids.
      a. Symptoms: burning, stinging of eyes, nose, airways, skin.
      b. Onset: seconds.
      c. Treatment: none.
      d. Infection control: gross decontamination before client admission; water for skin decontamination; standard PPE precautions.
C. Radiologic weapons. Any weapon designed to release *radiation or radioactivity* at a level dangerous to human life.
   1. Myriad isotopes exist to be considered for potential weaponized use, but the most common expected isotopes are tritium (H-3), cesium-137, cobalt-60, strontium-90, phosphorus-32, and radium-226. The health effects for each of these isotopes are similar.
      a. Acute radiation syndrome (radiation sickness): an acute illness caused by irradiation of the entire body (or most of the body) by a high dose of penetrating radiation in a short period of time (usually a matter of minutes), resulting in a depletion

**Table 7-1 BIOLOGIC AGENTS**

| Agent | Etiology | Signs and Symptoms | Transmission | Isolation/Prevention/Treatment |
|---|---|---|---|---|
| Anthrax | *Bacillus anthracis* | *Pulmonary:* Flulike Respiratory failure Hemodynamic collapse Usually fatal *Integumentary:* Local skin—head, forearms, hands<br><br>Localized itching followed by a papular lesion that turns vesicular and develops a black eschar in 2–6 days; edema, lymph node enlargement Responds well to antibiotics<br><br>*Gastrointestinal:* Abdominal pain, ascites, nausea, vomiting, fever Bloody diarrhea, emesis Usually fatal | Anthrax is a durable spore that lives in the soil; transmission by inhalation of the spore, contact with the spore, and the ingestion of contaminated food | • Vaccine is available. (This vaccine is recommended for high-risk groups and not traditionally given to health care workers.)<br>• Standard isolation precautions are used, but once the client is sick, there is no person-to-person transmission.<br>• Antibiotics – ciprofloxacin or doxycycline. |
| Botulism | *Clostridium botulinum*— produces a neurotoxin | "Dozen D's for clinical progression: **d**ry mouth, **d**iplopia, **d**ilated pupils, **d**roopy eyes, **d**roopy face, **d**iminished gag reflex, **d**ysphagia, **d**ysarthria, **d**ysphonia, **d**ifficulty in lifting head, **d**escending paralysis, and **d**iaphragmatic paralysis | Ingestion of toxin-contaminated food; the toxin can be made into an aerosol and inhaled (manmade) | • Antitoxin therapy with trivalent A-B-E antitoxin given as soon as possible.<br>• Supportive care only is provided.<br>• No isolation precautions are implemented. |
| Plague | *Yersinia pestis* | Fever, cough, chest pain Hemoptysis Sputum can be thick and very purulent or watery with gram-negative rods Bronchopneumonia | In a bioterrorist event, most likely to be aerosolized; can be transmitted with direct contact of infected person or ingestion of contaminated food | • There is no proven vaccine for the pneumonic plague, which is the most likely version in a bioterrorist event.<br>• Droplet isolation precautions are used.<br>• IV antibiotics: gentamicin or streptomycin.<br>• Oral antibiotics (if client stable): tetracycline or doxycycline. |
| Smallpox | *Variola major virus* | Prodrome of fever, myalgia Vesicles on the distal limbs (hands, feet) as opposed to truncated vesicles with chickenpox | Transmitted via direct contact from person to person Spread by airborne droplets and direct contact with contaminated objects | • Vaccine available for exposure; vaccinia immune globulin (VIG). Routine vaccination ceased with eradication of smallpox in 1979.<br>• Airborne precautions are used in the hospital setting (N-95 mask recommended, especially if pocks develop inside the buccal cavity). |

*Continued*

**Table 7-1    BIOLOGIC AGENTS—cont'd**

| Agent | Etiology | Signs and Symptoms | Transmission | Isolation/Prevention/Treatment |
|---|---|---|---|---|
| Tularemia | *Francisella tularensis* | Sudden onset of high fever, sore throat, headache, swollen lymph nodes<br>Skin ulcer from tick bites<br>Progresses to pneumonia, pleural effusion with weight loss | Incubation period 1–21 days<br>No person-to-person spread<br>Spread by rabbits and ticks<br>Ingestion of contaminated water, aerosols, or agricultural dusts | • Standard precautions.<br>• Gentamicin treatment of choice.<br>• Vaccine under development.<br>• Mortality 35% without treatment. |
| Viral hemorrhagic fevers<br>Marburg virus<br>Ebola virus<br>Lassa fever | Carried by rodents and mosquitos<br>Virus can be aerosolized | Fever, conjunctivitis, headache, malaise, prostration, nausea, vomiting<br>Hemorrhage of tissues and organs<br>Hypotension<br>Organ failure | Marburg: 5–10 day incubation<br>Ebola: 2–21 day incubation<br>Lassa fever: 1–3 weeks incubation | • No vaccine or drug therapy available; however, ribavirin effective in some cases.<br>• Isolation for containment - use Standard, Contact, and Droplet Precautions, including PPE.<br>• Supportive treatment and care. |

*PPE*, personal protection equipment.
From Zerwekh, T., & Zerwekh, J. (2018). Emergency preparedness. In J. Zerwekh & A. Garneau (Eds.), *Nursing today: Transition and trends* (9th ed.). St. Louis: Elsevier/Saunders.

of immature parenchymal stem cells in specific tissues.
  b. Radioactive contamination: Radioactive contamination occurs when radioactive material is deposited on or in an object or a person. Radioactive materials released into the environment can cause air, water, surfaces, soil, plants, buildings, people, or animals to become contaminated. A contaminated person has radioactive materials on or inside his or her body.
    (1) Internal contamination: Internal contamination occurs when people swallow or breathe in radioactive materials or when radioactive materials enter the body through an open wound or are absorbed through the skin. Some types of radioactive materials stay in the body and are deposited in different body organs. Other types are eliminated from the body in blood, sweat, urine, and feces.
    (2) External contamination: External contamination occurs when radioactive material, in the form of dust, powder, or liquid, comes in contact with a person's skin, hair, or clothing. In other words, the contact is external to a person's body. People who are externally contaminated can become internally contaminated if radioactive material gets in their bodies.
  2. The remaining information regarding clinical care, handling, and diagnosis of clients with acute radiation exposure can be found in Table 7-2.
D. Natural disasters: The CDC has identified more than 10 types of natural disasters; the five most frequent are highlighted here:
  1. Hurricane.
  2. Flu pandemic.
  3. Earthquake.
  4. Flooding.
  5. Tornado.

Although each disaster has specific response capacities inherent to that disaster, there are some commonalities to all of these natural disasters. The clinical nurse must be cognizant of each of the following when preparing and responding to natural disasters:
  1. Acute illness (increased presentations of infections from vaccine-preventable diseases such as diphtheria, tetanus, hepatitis A).
  2. Carbon monoxide exposure.
  3. Unsanitary food and water.
  4. Animal bites and vector (insect) issues.
  5. Cleanup and associated physical injuries.
  6. General environmental concerns (urban sanitation/trash).
  7. Mold.
  8. Power outages.
  9. Mental health issues (specifically in longer duration events).
E. "Active shooter" events
  1. An active shooter is an individual actively engaged in killing or attempting to kill people in a populated area, and recent active shooter incidents have underscored the need for a coordinated response by public health, medical, clinical, and law enforcement professionals to save lives.
  2. Since 2000, more than 282 active shooter events have occurred in schools, hospitals, public buildings, movie theaters, and churches, among other venues.
  3. Wounds and/or trauma to the patient, gunpowder particles on the clothing, or other unique presentations can have considerable investigative value as evidence and should not be modified.
  4. Doffing of patient clothing should be done in a manner that will minimize the loss of physical evidence. If

## Table 7-2 ACUTE RADIATION SYNDROMES

| Syndrome | Dose* | Prodromal Stage | Latent Stage | Manifest Illness Stage | Recovery |
|---|---|---|---|---|---|
| Hematopoietic (bone marrow) | Above 0.7 Gy (above 70 rads) *(Mild symptoms may occur as low as 0.3 Gy or 30 rads.)* | • Symptoms are anorexia, nausea, and vomiting.<br>• Onset occurs 1 hour to 2 days after exposure.<br>• Stage lasts for minutes to days. | • Stem cells in bone marrow are dying, although client may appear and feel well.<br>• Stage lasts 1–6 weeks. | • Symptoms are anorexia, fever, and malaise.<br>• Drop in all blood cell counts occurs for several weeks.<br>• Primary cause of death is infection and hemorrhage.<br>• Survival decreases with increasing dose.<br>• Most deaths occur within a few months after exposure. | • In most cases, bone marrow cells will begin to repopulate the marrow.<br>• Full recovery is probable for a large percentage of individuals; recovery process may last from a few weeks up to 2 years after exposure.<br>• Death may occur in some individuals at 1.2 Gy (120 rads).<br>• The $LD_{50}/60^\dagger$ is about 2.5–5 Gy (250–500 rads). |
| Gastrointestinal (GI) | Above 10 Gy (above 1000 rads) *(Some symptoms may occur as low as 6 Gy or 600 rads.)* | • Symptoms are anorexia, severe nausea, vomiting, cramps, and diarrhea.<br>• Onset occurs within a few hours after exposure.<br>• Stage lasts about 2 days. | • Stem cells in bone marrow and cells lining GI tract are dying, although client may appear and feel well.<br>• Stage lasts less than 1 week. | • Symptoms are malaise, anorexia, severe diarrhea, fever, dehydration, and electrolyte imbalance.<br>• Death is due to infection, dehydration, and electrolyte imbalance.<br>• Death occurs within 2 weeks of exposure. | • The $LD_{100}^\ddagger$ is about 10 Gy (1000 rads). |
| Cardiovascular (CV)/central nervous system (CNS) | Above 50 Gy (5000 rads) *(Some symptoms may occur as low as 20 Gy or 2000 rads.)* | • Symptoms are extreme nervousness and confusion; severe nausea, vomiting, and watery diarrhea; loss of consciousness; and burning sensations of the skin.<br>• Onset occurs within minutes of exposure.<br>• Stage lasts for minutes to hours. | • Client may return to partial functionality.<br>• Stage may last for hours but often is less. | • Symptoms are return of watery diarrhea, convulsions, and coma.<br>• Onset occurs 5–6 hours after exposure.<br>• Death occurs within 3 days of exposure. | • No recovery is expected. |

*The absorbed doses quoted here are "gamma equivalent" values. Neutrons or protons generally produce the same effects as gamma, beta, or x-rays but at lower doses. If the client has been exposed to neutrons or protons, consult radiation experts on how to interpret the dose.
†The $LD_{50}/60$ is the dose necessary to kill 50% of the exposed population in 60 days.
‡The $LD_{100}$ is the dose necessary to kill 100% of the exposed population.
From Zerwekh, T., & Zerwekh, J. (2018). Emergency preparedness. In J. Zerwekh & A. Garneau (Eds.), *Nursing today: Transition and trends* (9th ed.). St. Louis: Elsevier/Saunders.

the clothing is bloody, do not allow blood and debris from one area or garment to contaminate another area or garment.

5. Do not roll garments up in a ball. Never put wet or bloody garments in plastic bags. Carefully place garments in paper bags (one item per bag), seal, date, and initial.

6. Pertinent items that could be considered evidence but need to stay with the patient, such as health aids, should be documented by the nurse and then notification submitted to law enforcement.

7. The clinical and community health nurse must be aware of the risk present in active shooter events,

which further underscores the need for appropriate and repeated training within the ICS and Triage systems described previously

## Triage

Triage is a standardized system of sorting clients according to medical need when resources are unavailable for all persons to be treated.

A. The overall goal of triage is to determine whether a client is appropriate for a given level of care and to ensure that hospital resources are used effectively.

B. Triage scoring (color) levels used during a mass casualty incident (MCI) (Figure 7-1).

1. **Green (minimal):** Also referred to as "the walking wounded," these clients require medical attention *after* higher prioritized clients have been tended to. They usually do not require monitoring or stabilization (e.g., broken arm, cut on leg requiring stitches).

2. **Yellow (delayed):** Casualty requires medical attention, but treatment can wait until after red clients have been tended to; commonly this includes those who can withstand medical attention for a maximum

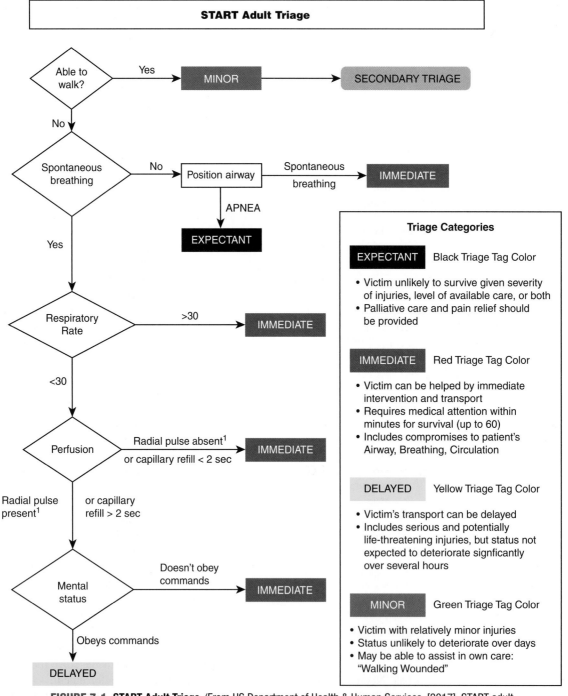

**FIGURE 7-1  START Adult Triage.** (From US Department of Health & Human Services. [2017]. START adult triage algorithm. Retrieved from https://chemm.nlm.nih.gov/StartAdultTriageAlgorithm.pdf)

of 6 hours (e.g., open thoracic wound, penetrating abdominal wound).

3. **Red (immediate):** Casualty requires immediate—usually within 1 hour—medical attention and will not survive without it. Any compromise to the casualty's respiration, hemorrhage control, or shock control could be fatal (e.g., cannot walk, airway passage obstructed, unconscious, acute myocardial infarction).

4. **Black (expectant or morgue):** The victim is not likely to survive because of the severity of injuries, level of care, or both. Palliative care and pain relief should be administered (e.g., cardiac arrest, severe head or chest trauma, large area burns across body) (see Figure 7-1, Box 7-3).

C. Triage scoring used in emergency room is the Five-Level Emergency Severity Index. After an emergency assessment, the nurse conducts a primary and secondary survey to further assess and evaluate the extent of injuries in the trauma patient.

1. Primary survey: Think ABCs (airway, breathing, circulation) and disability.
   a. Clients with head and neck injuries, foreign objects occluding the airway, or who are aspirating take priority during the primary survey because the potential for airway occlusion/obstruction is high.
   b. Clients with breathing difficulty from impaired gas exchange problems such as pulmonary emboli or a pneumothorax need to be assessed and evaluated.
   c. Clients with circulatory problems are also triaged immediately during the primary survey (cardiovascular, neurovascular, and peripheral vascular); examples include myocardial ischemia/infarction, hemorrhage, hypovolemic shock.
   d. Assess and evaluate for disabilities by conducting a focused neurologic examination (e.g., Glasgow Coma Scale). Stroke and unconscious clients fall under the disability category.

2. Secondary survey: Immediately follows the primary survey.
   a. After all life-threatening injuries are treated and stabilized, a focused assessment is undertaken to assess for additional injuries.
   b. A body-systems approach is used (client history, HEENT, integumentary, pulmonary, GI/GU, musculoskeletal).

---

### Box 7-3 THINK OF THE HELPFUL MNEMONIC IDME FOR USING THE START TRIAGE SYSTEM

**I**mmediate—red
**D**elayed—yellow
**M**inimal—green
**E**xpectant—black

For mass casualty incidents (MCI), clients are sorted into groups—remember the mnemonic **MASS:**
**M**ove
**A**ssess
**S**ort
**S**end

---

3. Intervention and evaluation: Ongoing monitoring and evaluation of interventions aimed at managing the trauma client.

> **TEST ALERT:** Airway and breathing always take priority in determining which client you will assess first.

## COMMUNITY NURSING PREPAREDNESS

A. Administrative concepts.
1. Health Resources and Services Administration (HRSA)/Assistant Secretary for Preparedness and Response (ASPR).
   a. Nurses who work in health care facilities receiving HRSA/ASPR funding have been subjected to increasing federal and state standards and regulations to prepare and respond to public health emergency events.
   b. These hospitals and nurses must comply with the application of the National Incident Management System (NIMS).
   c. Hospital Incident Command System (HICS) training, which is a standardized approach to hospital emergency response.
2. The Joint Commission.
   a. Hospitals and health care facilities were required by The Joint Commission to be NIMS compliant by the end of 2007, to confirm successful training of hospital staff under NIMS, and to implement the HICS emergency response command structure during hospital emergency responses (Figure 7-2).
   b. EC 4.10, 4.20, IC 6.10, and IM 2.30 are all Joint Commission standards regarding hospital emergency preparedness and response that are measured and graded during Joint Commission inspections (see Figure 7-2).

B. Community health nursing concepts.
1. Epidemiology of emergencies.
   a. Nurses (and specifically infection control nurses) must know how to perform acute identification and recognition of epidemiologic clues that could signal a public health event. Early recognition of these clues can be achieved through surveillance (passive and active) and monitoring of clients presenting to health care facilities and clinics.
   b. *Syndromic surveillance* applies health-related data such as trends in client symptomatology or disease presentation that precedes clinical diagnosis and can indicate a substantial probability of an outbreak that would warrant further investigation and a public health response (Box 7-4).
2. Strategic National Stockpile (SNS).
   a. National inventory (delivered within 12 hours of request) of antibiotics, chemical antidotes, antitoxins, airway maintenance supplies, and other medical equipment that supports and refreshes existing community resources being implemented during a public health emergency.

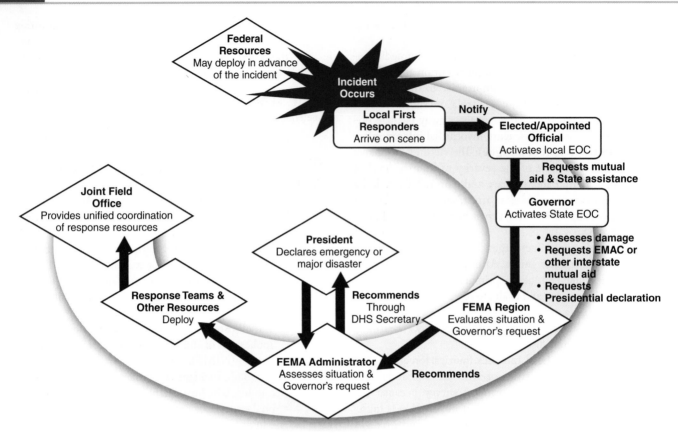

**FIGURE 7-2** Overview of the Stafford Act support to states, tribal, and local governments that are affected by a major disaster or emergency. *DHS,* Department of Homeland Security; *EMAC,* Emergency Management Assistance Compact; *EOC,* Emergency Operation Centers; *FEMA,* Federal Emergency Management Agency. (From US Department of Homeland Security. National response framework. Retrieved from https://www.fema.gov/pdf/emergency/nrf/nrf-stafford.pdf)

---

**Box 7-4   EPIDEMIOLOGIC CLUES THAT COULD SIGNAL A BIOLOGIC EVENT**

- Large numbers of ill persons with a similar clinical presentation, disease, or syndrome
- An increase in unexplained diseases or deaths
- Unusual illness in a population
- Higher morbidity and mortality in association with a common disease or syndrome or failure of such clients to respond to regular therapy
- Single case of disease caused by an uncommon agent, such as smallpox, Machupo hemorrhagic fever, pulmonary anthrax, glanders
- Several unusual or unexplained diseases coexisting in the same client without any other explanation
- Disease with an unusual geographic, temporal, or seasonal distribution—for instance, influenza in the summer or Ebola hemorrhagic fever in United States

- Similar disease among persons who attended the same public event or gathering
- Illness that is unusual or atypical for a given population or age group
- Unusual or atypical disease presentation
- Unusual, atypical, unidentifiable, or antiquated strain of an agent
- Unusual antibiotic resistance pattern
- Endemic disease with a sudden, unexplained increase in incidence
- Atypical disease transmission through aerosols, food, or water, which suggests deliberate sabotage
- Many ill persons who seek treatment at about the same time

From Zerwekh, T., & Zerwekh, J. (2018). Emergency preparedness. In J. Zerwekh & A. Garneau (Eds.), *Nursing today: Transition and trends* (9th ed.). St. Louis: Elsevier/Saunders.

---

b. The Cities Readiness Initiative (CRI) of CDC's SNS was established in 2004 and focuses on enhancing preparedness in the nation's largest cities and metropolitan statistical areas (MSA), where more than 50% of the US population resides. Through CRI, state and large metropolitan public health departments have developed plans to respond to a large-scale bioterrorist event by dispensing antibiotics to the entire population of an identified MSA within 48 hours.

3. CHEMPACK.
   a. Federal forward deployment program to supplement the medical response in the event of a chemical nerve agent release.

b. Caches contain such chemical antidotes as MARK-1 kits (intramuscular auto-injectors of atropine and pralidoxime [2-PAM]), atropine injectors, PAM kits, diazepam, and sterile water.

c. The public health nurse must be aware of the possibility of administering such medications during a chemical weapon event and must be refreshed on the proper dosage and clinical practice applications.

4. Emergency System for Advance Registration of Volunteer Health Professionals (ESAR-VHP).

a. Federally funded program through HRSA/ASPR that maintains a database of credentialed health professional volunteers that can be used in emergencies.

b. Each state's ESAR-VHP system is built to standards that will allow quick and easy exchange of health professionals with other states, thereby maximizing the size of the population able to receive services during public health emergencies.

5. Disaster Medical Assistance Team (DMAT).

a. DMAT consists of 35 deployable units divided by geographic region that can be deployed federally on request.

b. The responsibilities of DMAT teams include triage of victims at a disaster site, medical care at the site, and staging of locations outside the disaster site for transportation of clients to alternative health care facilities.

c. DMAT teams also serve as care centers for evacuation areas, where they can set up mobile medical care facilities for injured and trauma persons evacuating a declared disaster area.

6. Medical Reserve Corps (MRC).

a. MRC volunteers supplement existing emergency and public health resources by including medical and public health professionals such as physicians, nurses, pharmacists, dentists, veterinarians, and epidemiologists.

b. Primary objectives of MRC units are to improve health literacy, increase disease prevention, eliminate health disparities, and, most important, to improve public health preparedness.

7. Community/Individual Preparedness.

a. The community health nurse has a responsibility in delivering primary prevention methodologies related to disaster and emergencies preparedness, which includes mental health preparedness, family/individual preparedness, and business preparedness.

b. The website https://www.ready.gov is an excellent and preferred resource to ascertain specific information about family and individual preparedness items, checklists, kits, evacuation plans, etc. (Box 7-5).

---

**Box 7-5 RECOMMENDED DISASTER PREPAREDNESS KIT**

**Recommended Items to Include in a Basic Emergency Supply Kit**
- Water
- One gallon of water per person per day, for drinking and sanitation
- Children, nursing mothers, and sick people may need more water
- If you live in a warm-weather climate, more water may be necessary
- Store water tightly in clean plastic containers such as soft drink bottles
- Keep *at least* a 3-day supply of water per person
- Food—*at least* a 3-day supply of nonperishable food
- Battery-powered or hand-crank radio and an NOAA (National Oceanic and Atmospheric Administration) weather radio with tone alert and extra batteries for both
- Flashlight and extra batteries
- First aid kit
- Whistle to signal for help
- Dust mask, to help filter contaminated air, and plastic sheeting and duct tape to shelter-in-place
- Moist towelettes, garbage bags, and plastic ties for personal sanitation
- Wrench or pliers to turn off utilities
- Can opener for food (if kit contains canned food)
- Local maps

**Additional Items to Consider Adding to an Emergency Supply Kit**
- Prescription medications and glasses
- Infant formula and diapers
- Pet food and extra water for your pet
- Important family documents such as copies of insurance policies, identification, and bank account records in a waterproof, portable container
- Cash or traveler's checks and change
- Emergency reference material such as a first aid book or information from https://www.ready.gov/
- Sleeping bag or warm blanket for each person; consider additional bedding if you live in a cold-weather climate
- Complete change of clothing including a long-sleeved shirt, long pants, and sturdy shoes; consider additional clothing if you live in a cold-weather climate
- Household chlorine bleach and medicine dropper (A solution of 9 parts water to 1 part bleach can be used as a disinfectant. Or in an emergency, you can treat water by adding 16 drops of household liquid bleach per gallon of water. Do not use scented or "color-safe" bleaches or bleaches with added cleaners.)
- Fire extinguisher
- Matches in a waterproof container
- Feminine supplies and personal hygiene items
- Mess kits, paper cups, paper plates, plastic utensils, paper towels
- Paper and pencil
- Books, games, puzzles, or other activities for children

From Zerwekh, T., & Zerwekh, J. (2018). Emergency preparedness. In J. Zerwekh & A. Garneau (Eds.), *Nursing today: Transition and trends* (9th ed.). St. Louis: Elsevier/Saunders. Courtesy Department of Homeland Security (www.ready.gov).

8. Disaster-related mental health.
   a. The community health nurse must focus and be aware of the development of psychological reactions that persist from days to months to years after the public health event.
   b. The first practice a community nurse should implement is the cognizance and awareness of onset of psychological reactions in persons suffering from disaster-related mental health symptomatology.
   c. Assist in helping the client address the associated symptom progression.
   d. Identification of clients whose symptomatology could progress to long-term mental afflictions.
C. Funding and Sustainment of Emergency Preparedness Initiatives.
   a. Since 2002, the Public Health Emergency Preparedness cooperative agreement has provided more than $11 billion to public health departments across the nation.
   b. Aids health departments and health care facilities to build and strengthen their abilities in responding to a range of public health threats, including infectious diseases, natural disasters, and biological, chemical, nuclear, and radiologic events.
   c. Presidential administration can have a significant impact on funding allocations. As of FY18, an estimated $136.3 million has been recommended for reductions in funding, which further elucidates the need for constant vigilance and cognizance of emergency preparedness/response principles and practices when the clinical and community health nurse is faced with an emergent health event.

## Study Questions
## Emergency and Disaster Preparedness and Bioterrorism

More questions on

1. Which of the following is a Centers for Disease Control and Prevention (CDC) Category A biologic agent?
   1. Smallpox
   2. Sarin
   3. West Nile Virus
   4. Tritium

2. What is the most likely source of exposure in a biologic weapon attack?
   1. Absorption
   2. Adsorption
   3. Inhalational
   4. Dermal

3. Which of the following is an example of a Level I disaster?
   1. Category 5 hurricane in a major metropolitan city
   2. Three-car automobile accident with injuries
   3. F-4 tornado destruction through three cities
   4. 8.0 scale earthquake in a coastal city

4. Which of the following is an example of a Level II disaster?
   1. Train derailment that spills hazardous chemicals into a small city
   2. A tsunami that strikes a major metropolitan area
   3. A three-alarm house fire
   4. A novel virus pandemic

5. Which of the following events is an example of a Level III disaster?
   1. A small building collapse that traps 115 workers
   2. A bus accident carrying 13 passengers
   3. An 8.0 scale earthquake in a major city
   4. F-4 tornado destruction through three cities

6. Which of the following conditions satisfies a "green" triage tag in an emergency triage scenario?
   1. A broken thumb from falling debris
   2. Burns over 98% of body from a chemical fire
   3. A 3-inch laceration on the forearm from window glass in a building explosion
   4. Tension pneumothorax

7. Hospitals and health care facilities were required by The Joint Commission to be compliant with this program by the end of calendar 2007. This program is called:
   1. Emergency System for the Advance Registration of Volunteer Health Professionals (ESAR-VHP)
   2. Medical Reserve Corps (MRC)
   3. CHEMPACK
   4. National Incident Management System (NIMS)

8. The National Preparedness Goal has now focused efforts in preparing for, responding to, and recovering from:
   1. Bioterrorism events
   2. Chemical terrorism events
   3. Natural disaster events
   4. All-hazard events

9. Which of the following is a comprehensive incident management system intended for use in both emergent and nonemergent situations for hospitals and health care agencies?
   1. NIMS: National Incident Management System
   2. HICS: Hospital Incident Command System
   3. START: Simple Triage and Rapid Treatment
   4. DIME: Delayed, Immediate, Minor, Expectant

10. Which of the following is not considered a component of the medical assets stored in a Strategic National Stockpile?
   1. Antibiotics
   2. Ventilators
   3. Chemical antidotes
   4. Personal protective equipment

11. Which of the following potential bioterrorism agents has three routes of exposure to humans?
    1. Smallpox
    2. Anthrax
    3. Botulism
    4. Tularemia

12. The nurse understands that there are no isolation precautions for clients with:
    1. Tuberculosis (TB)
    2. Plague
    3. Smallpox
    4. Botulism

13. Which of the following biologic agents are disseminated by airborne release?
    1. Botulism and anthrax
    2. Anthrax and plague
    3. Plague and smallpox
    4. Botulism and smallpox

14. Which term describes the sorting of clients according to medical need when resources are unavailable for all persons to be treated?
    1. Tasking
    2. Delegating
    3. Triage
    4. Prioritize

15. Which of the following are agents listed by the CDC as agents most likely to be involved in bioterrorism? **Select all that apply.**
    1. Influenza
    2. West Nile virus
    3. Cryptosporidiosis
    4. Anthrax
    5. Plague
    6. Smallpox

## Answers to Study Questions

**1. *1***
Smallpox is considered a Category A biologic agent. Sarin is a chemical nerve agent weapon. West Nile virus is a CDC Category 3 biologic agent. Tritium is a radiologic weapon. (Zerwekh & Garneau, 9 ed., p. 598)

**2. *3***
Inhalational exposure provides the most effective way of disseminating a biologic weapon. Absorption exposure route is the uptake of substances through tissues and is not an effective delivery method of biologic weapons. Adsorption is the process of a gas or liquid adhering to a solid and is an ineffective mechanism for biologic weapon exposure. Dermal exposure is possible with a biologic weapon, but the effectiveness of weapon delivery is minor compared with inhalational exposure. (Zerwekh & Garneau, 9 ed., pp. 598–602)

**3. *2***
Level I disasters include local emergency medical systems and the community to provide medical support. A Category 5 hurricane is a Level III disaster that consumes local, state, and federal resources to the fullest extent and requires an extended response time of the nurse. An F-4 tornado is a Level II disaster that requires the nurse to respond in a greater capacity using larger casualty practices in coordination with regional response agencies. An 8.0 scale earthquake is a Level III disaster that consumes local, state, and federal resources to the fullest extent and requires an extended response time of the nurse. (Zerwekh & Garneau, 9 ed., p. 608)

**4. *1***
Level II disasters require the nurse to respond in a greater capacity using larger casualty practices in coordination with regional response agencies, which include local emergency medical systems and the community, to provide medical support, as would be needed with a train derailment with a hazardous spill. A tsunami that strikes a major metropolitan area is a Level III disaster that consumes local, state, and federal resources to the fullest extent and requires an extended response time of the nurse. A three-alarm house fire is a Level I disaster in which the nurse works in cooperation with local emergency medical systems and the

community to provide medical support. A novel virus pandemic is a Level III disaster that consumes local, state, and federal resources to the fullest extent and requires an extended response time of the nurse. (Zerwekh & Garneau, 9 ed., p. 608)

**5. *3***
Level III disasters consume local, state, and federal resources to the fullest extent and require an extended response time of the nurse, which would be an 8.0-scale earthquake in a major city. A small building collapse is a Level II disaster that requires the nurse to respond in a greater capacity using larger casualty practices in coordination with regional response agencies. A bus accident is a Level I disaster that includes local emergency medical systems and the community to provide medical support. An F-4 tornado is a Level II disaster that requires the nurse to respond in a greater capacity using larger casualty practices in coordination with regional response agencies. (Zerwekh & Garneau, 9 ed., p. 608)

**6. *1***
A "green" triage tag, also referred to as the "walking wounded," would be a broken thumb from falling debris. Burns over 98% of the body are declared "black" because the injured person is not breathing and is beyond the scope of available medical assistance. A 3-inch laceration on the arm is labeled "yellow" because such injured persons can be assisted after "immediate (red)" clients, such as the person with a tension pneumothorax, are medically cared for first. (Zerwekh & Garneau, 9 ed., p. 609)

**7. *4***
Hospitals and health care facilities were required by The Joint Commission to be compliant with The National Incident Management System (NIMS) criteria by the end 2007, to confirm successful training of hospital staff under NIMS, and to implement the Hospital Incident Command System (HICS) emergency response command structure during hospital emergency responses. ESAR-VHP is a federally funded program through HRSA that forms a national system that allows efficient utilization of health professional volunteers in emergencies. MRC is a program administered through the office of the US Surgeon General that uses mostly nonclinical

community members to serve as volunteers to health response agencies during emergencies. CHEMPACK is a CDC program that forward-deploys antidotes and medical assets in the event of a chemical weapon release. (Zerwekh & Garneau, 9 ed., p. 610)

**8.** *4*
The National Preparedness Goal is now focused on all-hazard events. Bioterrorism, chemical, and natural disasters are all specific types of events that warrant a collaborative emergency response. The goal shifted in 2005 after Hurricane Katrina in which a greater emphasis was focused on all events and not necessarily just bioterrorism. (Zerwekh, Garneau, 9 ed., p. 610)

**9.** *2*
The Hospital Incident Command System (HICS) is the comprehensive system intended for use in both emergent and nonemergent situations in hospitals and health care agencies. National Incident Management System (NIMS) is the overarching federal initiative that requires health care emergency responders to be trained in HICS. START is a type of triage methodology employed in hospitals and in the field. DIME is a type of triage mnemonic used to remember the immediate prioritization of clients in an emergency. (Zerwekh & Garneau, 9 ed., pp. 608–611)

**10.** *3*
Chemical antidotes are stored in CHEMPACK containers used in the forward deployment for response to a chemical terrorist event. Antibiotics, ventilators, and personal protective equipment are all components of a Strategic National Stockpile push pack. (Zerwekh & Garneau, 9 ed., p. 612)

**11.** *2*
Infection with *Bacillus anthracis,* the cause of anthrax, can occur via three routes of exposure: cutaneous, gastrointestinal, and inhalation. Botulism can be transmitted via ingestion of toxin-contaminated food. The toxin can be aerosolized and inhaled (manmade). Tularemia is not known to be spread from person to person and is caused by the bacterium *Francisella tularensis,* which is found in animals (especially rodents, rabbits, and hares). (Zerwekh, Garneau, 9 ed., p. 600)

**12.** *4*
Botulism is transmitted by ingestion of toxin-contaminated food. It can be aerosolized and inhaled. The client needs supportive care only; no isolation precautions are necessary. Tuberculosis (TB), smallpox, and plague require droplet precautions. (Zerwekh & Garneau, 9 ed., p. 600)

**13.** *1*
Both anthrax and botulism can be aerosolized and inhaled and disseminated by airborne release. Plague and smallpox are spread person to person. (Zerwekh & Garneau, 9 ed., p. 600)

**14.** *3*
Triage can be used by lightly trained emergency department (ED) personnel and is not to supersede or instruct medical techniques. A common triage system used is known as START (simple triage and rapid treatment). Triage is used during natural disasters and mass casualty events. Delegation, assigning tasks, and prioritizing care are daily functions of the nurse manager. (Zerwekh & Garneau, 9 ed., p. 608)

**15.** *4, 5, 6*
Anthrax, smallpox, and plague are all bioterrorism agents that may be spread through the air and cause significant morbidity and mortality. Influenza is a viral respiratory infection. West Nile virus is a vector-borne disease. Cryptosporidiosis is a waterborne diarrheal disease. (Zerwekh & Garneau, 9 ed., p. 600)

CHAPTER EIGHT

# Pharmacology and Medication Administration

**8**

## PRIORITY CONCEPTS

Clinical Judgement, Safety

## GENERAL CONCEPTS

No medication has a single action; all medications have the potential to alter more than one body function.

> **NURSING PRIORITY:** Many medications have several desirable actions. Carefully evaluate the question as to what the desired response of the medication is for the specific client situation. Example: Acetylsalicylic acid (ASA) is used to prevent platelet aggregation to prevent strokes and cardiac disease, but it is also used as an antipyretic and for pain control in arthritis.

A. Drug names: The Drug Amendments Act of 1962 made it mandatory that each medication have one official name.
   1. Generic name (nonproprietary): the official designated name under which the medication is listed in official publications (e.g., acetaminophen).
   2. Chemical name: designates the specific chemical composition of the medication; usually quite long and complicated to pronounce and spell (e.g., *N*-acetyl-*para*-aminophenol).
   3. Trade name (proprietary, brand name): the name designated and registered by a specific manufacturer (e.g., Tylenol).

> **NURSING PRIORITY:** The medications on the NCLEX-RN examination will be identified by generic names—for example, diazepam, the generic name for Valium, will be used on the NCLEX-RN examination. You may still encounter trade names in the clinical setting.

B. Abuse potential: The Controlled Substances Act of 1970 defines rules for the manufacture and distribution of drugs that are considered to have a potential for abuse.
   1. Defines drugs in five categories—Schedules I, II, III, IV, V: potential for abuse becomes lower with each subsequent category; thus, the higher the schedule number, the lower the potential for abuse.
   2. Schedule I drugs are highly addictive (e.g., heroin) and are not used for medicinal purposes in the United States. Schedule V drugs (e.g., diphenoxylate hydrochloride [Lomotil]) pose the lowest risk for abuse and represent the lowest level of pharmacokinetics.

C. Pharmacokinetic process: consists of four phases acting together to determine the concentration of a drug at its site of action. Use the acronym **ADME** to remember these processes.
   1. **A**bsorption: movement of the drug from site of administration to the systemic circulation.
      a. Drug action may be increased or decreased by alterations in the gastric emptying time, presence of food, changes in gastric or plasma pH, or the drug form (e.g., tablets or capsules).
      b. Method of administration affects absorption (e.g., intravenous [IV] versus oral).
   2. **D**istribution: movement of the drug by the systemic circulation throughout the body.
      a. Based on blood flow of drug to tissue, ability of the drug to leave the vascular system, and ability of the drug to enter the tissue cells.
      b. Degree of binding to plasma proteins or other substances in the body. Albumin (protein) always remains in the bloodstream; drugs that are protein-bound restrict the drug distribution.
   3. **M**etabolism: the enzymatic alteration of the drug structure; most drug metabolism occurs in the liver.
      a. Most important action of drug metabolism is promoting the renal excretion of the drug.
      b. Converts drugs to inactive compounds; also increases or decreases toxicity.
      c. Rates can be influenced by genetic factor, aging, drug interactions, and coexisting pathologies (chronic liver disease).
   4. **E**xcretion: the removal of drugs from the body.
      a. Kidney is the most important organ for excretion of a drug; in renal failure, the duration and the intensity of drug action may increase.
      b. Kidney of a newborn is not fully developed; infants have a limited ability to excrete drugs.
      c. Aging can affect drug excretion (e.g., at the age of 80, renal clearance rate typically decreases half of what it was at age 30).
      d. Drugs are also excreted in breast milk, bile, and the lungs.

D. Pharmacogenomics: Genetically determined responses to drugs can be identified through family health histories.

E. Pharmacovigilance: The process of detecting, assessing, and attempting to prevent adverse drug effects or other related problems.

**117**

⚠ **OLDER ADULT PRIORITY:** Creatinine clearance should be monitored to evaluate renal function, not serum creatinine levels. The source of serum creatinine (lean muscle mass) decreases with the decline in renal function, which may reveal normal serum creatinine levels even though renal function is decreased.

## Drug Actions

A. **Desired action**: the desired, predictable response for which the medication is administered.
   1. Therapeutic range: the range of plasma drug levels that produces a therapeutic response and that which results in toxicity.
B. **Adverse drug reactions (ADR):** any noxious, unintended, and undesired effect that occurs with normal drug doses.

⚠ **OLDER ADULT PRIORITY:** ADRs are seven times more common in older adults than in young adults.

   1. **Side effects:** undesirable drug effects ranging from mild untoward effects to severe responses that occur at normal drug dosages.
   2. **Toxicity:** drug reactions that primarily occur because of receiving an excessive dose (e.g., medication error, poisoning). However, toxicity also may result in severe reactions (anaphylaxis) that occur regardless of the dose.
   3. **Allergic reactions:** drug reactions that occur as a result of prior sensitization and result in an immune response. Intensity can range from very mild to very severe.
   4. **Idiosyncratic effect:** an uncommon drug response.

**TEST ALERT:** Assess client for actual or potential side effects and adverse effects of medications; identify symptoms/evidence of allergic reactions to medications; implement procedures to counteract adverse effects of medications; evaluate and document client response to actions taken to counteract side effects and adverse effects of medications.

C. Factors influencing dose-response relationships.
   1. Age: young infants and older adult clients are generally more sensitive to medications.
   2. Medication history: a new medication may produce an interaction with one of the prescription medications, dietary supplements, or over-the-counter (OTC) medications the client is currently taking.
   3. Drug half-life: the time required for the amount of the drug in the body to be decreased by 50%.
      a. Some drugs have short half-lives; they leave the body quickly. Drugs with long half-lives leave the body more slowly. For example, morphine has a short half-life (approximately 3 hours), whereas levothyroxine has a half-life of 7 days.
      b. The half-life of the drug determines the dosing intervals.

   4. Presence of disease process, specifically kidney (excretion) and liver (metabolism) problems.
   5. Method of administration.
   6. Adequate cardiac output.
   7. Emotional factors: clients are more likely to respond to a medication in a positive manner if they have confidence in the physician and anticipate therapeutic effects.
   8. Pregnancy: always ask a woman of childbearing age if she is pregnant.
   9. Breastfeeding: advise women who are lactating to always advise their health care provider; medications may be excreted in breast milk.
D. Tolerance: increased dose required to maintain expected drug response (e.g., when a client with chronic pain requires higher doses of a strong opioid agonist [morphine sulfate] to achieve pain relief).
E. Dependence: an expected response to repeated use of a drug, resulting in physical signs and symptoms of withdrawal when the serum drug level decreases suddenly (e.g., when a client abruptly stops taking a strong opioid agonist [methadone] and develops irritability, nausea, vomiting, muscle spasm, and musculoskeletal pain).
F. Addiction: the continued use of a psychoactive substance regardless of physical, psychological, or social harm.

## Drug Interactions

A. Synergistic or potentiation effect: If two or more drugs are given together and this increases the therapeutic effects, it is beneficial; if it increases adverse effects, it may be detrimental.
   *Example: A desirable potentiation effect occurs when a diuretic and a beta-blocker are given for hypertension. An undesirable effect can occur when warfarin and aspirin (both anticoagulants) are given together, because this increases the risk for spontaneous bleeding.*
B. Antagonistic or inhibitory effect: if two or more drugs are given together, one may inhibit the effect of the other; this may be beneficial or detrimental.
   *Example: When you administer an adrenergic beta-blocker propranolol with an adrenergic beta stimulant isoproterenol, the action of each drug is canceled. However, the use of naloxone to suppress the effects of morphine results in a desirable inhibitory effect.*
C. Unique response effect: this occurs when two drugs are given together and the effect creates a new response not seen when each drug is used alone.
   *Example: When you administer disulfiram and the client has ingested alcohol or is using products containing alcohol, the effects are undesirable.*
D. Drug incompatibility: a chemical or physical reaction that occurs when two or more drugs are combined in vitro (outside the body).
   1. Do not combine two or more drugs in the same container unless it has been established that an interaction will not occur.
   2. When intravenous (IV) drugs are combined, they may form a precipitate. Do not give an IV solution in which a precipitate has formed after mixing drugs.

E. Drug–food interactions.
1. Food can bind with drugs and delay drug absorption.
   *Example: Tetracyclines bind with dairy products, leading to a decrease in the plasma tetracycline level.*
2. Food increases the absorption of nitrofurantoin, an antiinfective; metoprolol, a beta-blocker; and lovastatin, an antilipemic.
   *Example: Grapefruit juice can raise drug levels of calcium-channel blockers because it decreases metabolism of the drug by inhibiting an intestinal isoenzyme, CYP3A4, which is needed for drug metabolism in the intestines.*
3. Foods can have a direct effect on drug action.
   *Example: Monoamine oxidase inhibitors (e.g., isocarboxazid): these antidepressants, when taken with tyramine-rich foods (e.g., cheese, wine, organ meats, beer, yogurt), may lead to a hypertensive crisis; or foods rich in vitamin K can inhibit the therapeutic effect of warfarin, decreasing its effect.*
F. Drug–laboratory value interactions.
1. Abnormal plasma levels can affect drugs. Many drugs bind with protein (plasma albumin).
   a. The amount of drug molecules to plasma albumin is determined by the strength of attachment and the individual's plasma albumin level.
   b. Additionally, because the number of binding sites on each protein molecule is limited, drugs will compete with one another for binding. Only drug molecules that are not bound (free) can leave the vascular system and reach their site for action, metabolism, or excretion.
   *Example: The attraction between albumin and warfarin is extremely strong (99% bound to albumin), whereas gentamicin and albumin have a weak attraction (only 10% is bound, leaving 90% free).*
2. Abnormal serum electrolyte levels can affect drugs.
   *Example: Digitalis toxicity can occur when a client's serum potassium and magnesium levels are decreased and the serum calcium level is increased.*

G. Adverse drug events.
1. Unintentional medication poisoning is twice as common with children under 5 years as with other children. Primary root cause is accidental consumption due to nonsupervision.
2. Adverse drug reactions in older adults are commonly related to warfarin, insulin, phenytoin, digoxin, and other cardiac medications.
3. Antibiotics are one of the highest drug classifications resulting in adverse drug events, usually due to allergic reactions.

## Drug Therapy Considerations Across the Life Span

A. Pediatric implications (Table 8-1).
1. Younger clients are more sensitive to drugs than adult clients due to organ system immaturity.
2. Although pharmacokinetically similar to adults by age 1, children differ in one important way: they metabolize drugs faster than adults.
B. Older adult implications (Table 8-2).
1. Avoiding adverse drug reactions.
   a. Obtain a complete drug history that includes OTC drugs, herbs, and other supplements.
   b. Monitor client responses and drug levels.

| Table 8-1 PEDIATRIC PHARMACOLOGY AND NURSING IMPLICATIONS | |
|---|---|
| **Pharmacokinetics** | ***Body Effects and Possible Drug Responses*** |
| **Absorption** | Gastric emptying time is prolonged and irregular until about 6 months; delayed gastric emptying enhances drug absorption. Drugs administered intramuscularly to newborns may be poorly absorbed; by early infancy, drugs are absorbed more rapidly. Topical drugs may be absorbed more quickly than in adults because infants have a proportionally greater body surface area; infant's skin is thin and drugs pass through more readily. |
| **Distribution** | Protein-binding capacity does not reach adult values for 10–12 months; dosages for protein-bound medications may need to be reduced in infants. Blood–brain barrier is not fully developed in infants; therefore it is easier for drugs and chemicals to enter the central nervous system. Infants and children have lower blood pressure. The liver and brain are proportionally larger and receive more blood flow. |
| **Metabolism** | Drug metabolizing is decreased in the infant because of an immature liver. Liver does not develop to full capacity until about 1 year. |
| **Excretion** | Blood flow volume through the kidneys is less than in adults, and glomerular filtration rate is significantly lower. At birth there is a significant decrease in drug excretion by the kidney. Adult level of renal excretion occurs around 1 year. |

### Table 8-2 OLDER ADULT PHARMACOLOGY AND NURSING IMPLICATIONS

| Pharmacokinetics | Body Effects and Possible Drug Responses |
| --- | --- |
| **Absorption** | Slowed because of decreased gastric motility and blood flow; drug responses may be delayed; absorption is slowed but not decreased.<br>Decreased peristalsis with delayed gastric and intestinal emptying time.<br>Gastric acidity is reduced and may alter the absorption of some drugs. |
| **Distribution** | Decreased serum protein and albumin; drugs with a high affinity for protein compete for protein-binding sites with other drugs.<br>Drug interactions result because of a lack of protein sites and an increase in free drugs, intensifying drug effects. |
| **Metabolism** | Decreased hepatic blood flow, enzyme function, and total liver function result in reduction in drug metabolism.<br>With a reduction in metabolic rate, the half-life of drugs increases and drug accumulation can result. Drug toxicity may occur when the half-life is prolonged. |
| **Excretion** | Renal function is decreased; therefore, a decrease in drug excretion and drug accumulation results. Continual assessment for drug toxicity is needed while the client is taking the drug. |

> **⚠ NURSING PRIORITY:** An adverse drug reaction secondary to a decrease in renal function is the primary cause of adverse drug reactions in the older client.

c. Keep dosing regimen as simple as possible; use daily dosing when possible rather than twice a day.

d. Emphasize to clients the importance of disposing of medications they are no longer taking.

2. Promoting compliance: intentional under dosing (by clients) is the most common reason for nonadherence to drug regimen.

   a. Provide written instructions to clients regarding medication administration and why they are taking the medication.

   b. Ask the pharmacist to label drug containers with large type.

   c. Provide drug containers that can be opened easily.

   d. Encourage clients to use a system to record or track their drug doses (calendar, pill organizer).

   e. Determine whether clients can afford their medications.

C. Food and Drug Administration (FDA) pregnancy risk categories (Table 8-3).

### Table 8-3 FOOD AND DRUG ADMINISTRATION PREGNANCY RISK CATEGORIES

| Category | Description |
| --- | --- |
| A | *Remote Risk of Fetal Harm:* Controlled studies in women have been done and have failed to demonstrate a risk of fetal harm during the first trimester, and there is no evidence of risk in later trimesters. |
| B | *Slightly More Risk Than A*: Animal studies have revealed no evidence of harm to the fetus, but there are no adequate and well-controlled studies in pregnant women.<br>*Or*<br>Animal studies do show a risk of fetal harm, but controlled studies in women have failed to demonstrate a risk during the first trimester, and there is no evidence of risk in later trimesters. |
| C | *Greater Risk Than B:* Animal studies show a risk of fetal harm, but no controlled studies have been done in women.<br>*Or*<br>No animal studies or studies in pregnant women have been conducted. |
| D | *Proven Risk of Fetal Harm:* Studies in women show proof of fetal damage, but the potential benefits of use during pregnancy may be acceptable despite the risks (e.g., treatment of life-threatening disease for which safer drugs are ineffective). A statement on risk will appear in the "WARNINGS" section of drug labeling. |
| X | *Proven Risk of Fetal Harm:* Studies in women or animals show definite risk of fetal abnormality.<br>*Or*<br>Adverse reaction reports indicate evidence of fetal risk. The risks clearly outweigh any possible benefit. A statement on risk will appear in the "CONTRAINDICATIONS" section of drug labeling. |

Burchum, J.R., & Rosenthal, L.D. (2016). *Lehne's pharmacology for nursing care* (9th ed.). St. Louis: Elsevier.

## Herbal Supplements

A. Biologically based therapies.
1. Dietary supplements – vitamins, minerals, herbs, and other botanical products.
2. Herbal medicines – use of herbs to treat illness.
   a. Herbal medicine can be defined as the use of plant-derived products to promote health and relieve symptoms of disease.
   b. Herbal medicine is the most common form of alternative medicine, which can be defined as treatment practices that are not widely accepted or practiced by mainstream clinicians in a given culture.
   c. The word natural is not synonymous with safe! Remember, poison ivy and tobacco are natural too. (Box 8-1)
   d. All herbal products must be labeled as "dietary supplements."
   e. The product label must state that it is not intended to diagnose, treat, cure, or prevent any disease and that it has not been evaluated by the FDA.
3. Probiotics – live microorganisms (e.g., "good" bacteria) ingested that have similar function to beneficial organisms.

> ❗ **NURSING PRIORITY:** Clients need to be advised that herbal therapy may need to be discontinued 2–3 weeks before surgery.

B. Some commonly used medicinal herbs are identified in Table 8-4.

> ❗ **NURSING PRIORITY:** Unlike conventional drugs, herbal and other dietary supplements can be marketed without any proof of safety or efficacy. Dietary supplements are not regulated by the FDA.

---

### Box 8-1  HARMFUL SUPPLEMENTS TO AVOID

**Comfrey**
- Can cause hepatic venoocclusive disease leading to severe liver damage
- FDA advised manufacturers to remove from market; still widely available

**Kava**
- Can cause hepatotoxicity

**Ma Huang (Ephedra)**
- Elevates blood pressure leading to stroke, MI, and death with high doses
- Stimulates the heart and CNS
- FDA banned ephedra as a dietary supplement, but the ban does not apply to ephedra in Asian medicines

*CNS,* Central nervous system; *FDA,* Food and Drug Administration; *MI,* myocardial infarction.

---

### Table 8-4  COMMONLY USED MEDICINAL HERBS

| Medicinal Herb | Drug Interactions |
| --- | --- |
| **Aloe** is used for topical skin ailments with little or no topical side effects. Oral aloe is used for constipation and can cause severe diarrhea. Fresh aloe is more effective than stored product. | None noted with topical therapy. |
| **Black cohosh** is a popular treatment for acute symptoms of menopause and premenstrual syndrome. Minor side effect of upset stomach may occur. | May potentiate hypotensive effects of antihypertensive drugs, as well as hypoglycemic action of insulin and oral hypoglycemics. |
| **Dehydroepiandrosterone** (DHEA) may increase levels of testosterone and estrogen; has antiaging effects and antidepressant effects. | Carries a risk, especially because it can raise male and female hormone levels. |
| **Echinacea** is used orally to stimulate the immune functions and suppress inflammation; has antiviral properties. Side effects include unpleasant taste, fever, nausea, and vomiting. | May oppose effects of immunosuppressant drugs. |
| **Feverfew** is used for treatment of migraine and fever; it stimulates menstruation and suppresses inflammation. | May suppress platelet aggregation and increase risk for bleeding in clients on anticoagulant medications (aspirin, warfarin, heparin). |
| **Flaxseed** treats constipation and dyslipidemias. | May reduce the absorption of conventional medications. |
| **Garlic** reduces levels of triglycerides and LDLs and raises HDLs. | Suppresses platelet aggregation and can increase the risk for bleeding. |
| **Ginger root** is used for nausea and vomiting caused by motion sickness and perhaps nausea caused by chemotherapy. | Suppresses platelet aggregation and can increase risk of bleeding; lowers blood glucose. |
| **Ginkgo biloba** is used for increased circulation (peripheral vasodilator effects), memory, clear thinking, and impotence. It may cause stomach upset and dose-related headache. | May suppress coagulation and may promote seizures. |

*Continued*

**Table 8-4   COMMONLY USED MEDICINAL HERBS—cont'd**

| Medicinal Herb | Drug Interactions |
|---|---|
| • **Goldenseal** is used for bacterial, fungal, and protozoal infections of mucous membranes in the respiratory, gastrointestinal, and genitourinary tracts. It is also used to treat inflammation of the gall bladder. It is generally well tolerated but can be toxic in high doses. | Contraindicated in pregnancy. |
| • **Glucosamine** is used to treat osteoarthritis symptoms. | May increase the risk of bleeding. |
| • **Melatonin** regulates sleep; treats insomnia and "jet lag." | Large doses can cause hangover, headache, nightmares. |
| • **Milk thistle** has antiinflammatory and antioxidant effects; treats liver and gall bladder disorders. | May mimic the effects of estrogen. |
| • **St. John's wort** is used for depression. Potential interactions with other drugs are possible. | May interfere with oral contraceptives; reduced anticoagulation in clients taking warfarin; decreased effectiveness of cyclosporine; caution in use with antidepressants. |
| • **Saw palmetto** is used to relieve urinary symptoms related to BPH and is well tolerated. May cause a false-negative result on PSA test. | Should not use with finasteride (Proscar) in treatment of BPH; has antiplatelet effect. |
| • **Valerian** is a sedative to promote sleep and reduce restlessness. | Can potentiate the actions of other drugs with CNS-depressant actions; may cause daytime drowsiness. With high doses and long-term use, headache, nervousness, or cardiac abnormalities can occur. |

*BPH,* Benign prostatic hypertrophy; *CNS,* central nervous system, *MAO,* monoamine oxidase; *PMS,* premenstrual syndrome; *PSA,* prostate-specific antigen.

## MEDICATION ADMINISTRATION

**! NURSING PRIORITY:** The nurse's responsibility in administering medication is influenced by three primary factors: nursing guidelines for safe medication administration, pharmacologic implications of the medication, and the legal aspects of medication administration.

### Nursing Responsibilities in Medication Administration

A. Follow the Six Rights of Medication Administration (Figure 8-1).

**TEST ALERT:** Administer medications according to the Six Rights of Medication Administration. Refer to Chapter 6 for responsibilities and legal implications.

B. A nurse should administer *only* those medications that he or she has prepared.
C. Be familiar with medication.
   1. General purpose for which the client is receiving the medication.
   2. Common side effects.
   3. Average dose or range of safe dosage.
   4. Any specific safety precautions that apply before administration (e.g., digoxin: check apical pulse; heparin: check clotting times).
D. Check the medication against the health care provider's orders and document according to policy.

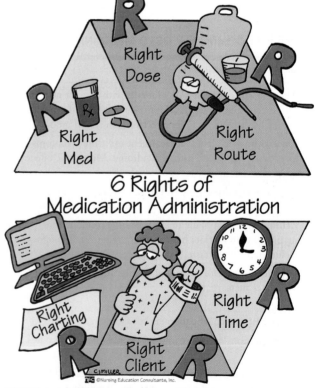

**FIGURE 8-1 6 Rights of Medication Administration.** (From Zerwekh, J., Garneau, A., & Miller, C.J. [2017]. *Digital collection of the memory notebooks of nursing images* [4th ed]. Chandler, AZ: Nursing Education Consultants, Inc.)

E. Evaluate client's overall condition and assess for changes that may indicate the medication is contraindicated (e.g., morphine would be contraindicated in a client who has increased intracranial pressure).

F. Evaluate compatibility with other medications the client is receiving.

G. Use appropriate aseptic technique when preparing and administering medication.

H. Do not leave medications at the client's bedside without a doctor's order to do so.

I. If client is to administer his or her own medication, review the correct method of administration (e.g., eyedrops) with the client.

J. Before procedures, label medications that are not labeled, e.g. medications in syringes, cups, or basins, and do the labeling in the area where medications and supplies are set up.

**TEST ALERT:** Evaluate appropriateness and accuracy of medication order; review pertinent data before medication administration; identify potential and actual incompatibilities of prescribed client medications.

## Nurse's Legal Responsibilities in Administration of Medication

A. The nurse administers a medication only by order of a physician or health care provider and according to provisions of the specific institution.

B. The nurse should not automatically carry out an order if the dosage is outside the normal range or if the route of administration is not appropriate; he or she should consult the physician.

C. The nurse is legally responsible for the medication he or she administers, even when the medication is administered according to a physician's order.

D. The nurse is responsible for evaluating the client before and after the administration of an as-needed (PRN) medication.

E. The medication should be charted as soon as possible after administration.

F. When taking oral orders on the phone, the nurse should carefully repeat all the orders (read-back) to verify they are correct (see Chapter 5, Box 5-5 for additional tips).

Example of a read-back:
*Doctor: "Give 25 mg diphenhydramine IV push."*
*Nurse: "Give 25 mg diphenhydramine IV push."*
*Doctor: "That's correct."*

G. Medication errors (Figure 8-2).
   1. If an error is found in a drug order, it is the nurse's responsibility to question the order.
   2. Always report medication errors to the appropriate health care provider immediately.
   3. It is the nurse's responsibility to carefully assess the client for effects of the erroneous medication.
   4. Medication errors should be documented in an incident report (event report) and on the client's chart.

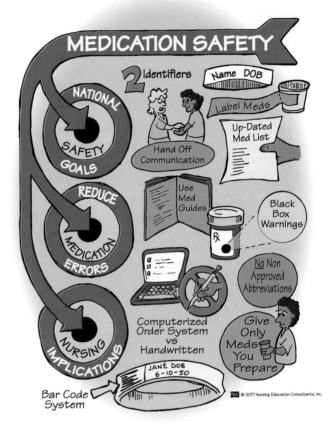

**FIGURE 8-2 Medication Safety.** (From Zerwekh, J., Garneau, A., & Miller, C.J. [2017]. *Digital collection of the memory notebooks of nursing images* [4th ed]. Chandler, AZ: Nursing Education Consultants, Inc.)

   5. The U.S. Pharmacopeia (USP) and the Institute for Safe Medical Practices (ISMP) have developed a nationwide medication error-reporting program called Medication Errors Reporting (MER) Program. Reporting is confidential and can be done via Internet, phone, or fax.

**TEST ALERT:** Identify situations in which the reporting of an incident/event/irregular occurrence/variance is appropriate; report the incident/error/event/occurrence per protocol.

H. High-Alert Medications: Medications that have the highest risk of causing injury and includes insulin, opiates, and narcotics.
   1. The Joint Commission (TJC) and the ISMP have identified specific medications for which errors could have devastating effects on clients.
   2. These medications are identified within the medication tables throughout this book.
   3. TJC requires:
      a. Institution or facility to develop processes to manage High-Alert Medications.
      b. A specific process of communication among health care workers to reconcile medications across the

▲ Box 8-2   NURSING IMPLICATIONS FOR HIGH-ALERT MEDICATIONS

- Maintain good communication and locate easily found information regarding the administration of pain medications to prevent overdose. You may use a visual pain scale. Limit the number of opiates and narcotics that are housed as floor stock. Store narcotics in individual client areas rather than as floor stock.
- Do not store together medications that have the same type of measurements. For example, heparin and insulin are both administered in units.
- Use only accepted abbreviations (see Appendices 8-2 and 8-3).
- Establish a *check* system where one nurse prepares the medication and another nurse reviews it.
- Infusion pump rates and concentrations must have an independent check system.
- Identify and exercise caution with medications that have similar names. For example, hydromorphone and morphine; potassium phosphate and potassium chloride; methyldopa with levodopa or L-dopa.
- Increase the use of standardized concentrations and pre-mixed solutions (potassium chloride, sodium chloride or normal saline) on the nursing unit; decrease the premixing and calculation of medications on the nursing unit.
- Do not store vials or containers of saline in concentrations greater than 0.9% on the nursing unit.
- Use single-dose vials when possible.
- Initiate patient controlled analgesia (PCA) protocols that require double-checks of the drug, the dosage, and pump setting.

continuum of care that includes a process for reconciling the list of medications during transfer, at discharge, and after major procedures.

    4. ▲Nursing Implications for High-Alert Medications (Box 8-2).

## Methods of Medication Administration

**Note:** This section on medications should not be used as a procedure guideline. The purpose is to point out specific characteristics of each method. All medications should be administered according to previously discussed nursing responsibilities in medication administration.

**TEST ALERT:** Administer and document medications given by common routes (e.g., oral, topical), administer and document medications given by parenteral routes (intravenous, intramuscular, subcutaneous), and determine the need for administration of PRN medications.

A. Oral medication.
    1. Assess level of consciousness and ability to follow directions.
      a. Tablets.
        (1) Evaluate swallow reflex.
        (2) Offer water or juice if not contraindicated.

      b. Sublingual.
        (1) Assess the patient's mucous membranes.
        (2) Have client place under tongue and allow to dissolve.
        (3) Caution client not to swallow the tablet.
      c. Buccal.
        (1) Assess the patient's mucous membranes.
        (2) Have client place against the mucous membranes of the cheek until it dissolves.
        (3) Caution client to avoid liquids until after the medication has dissolved.
B. Drugs administered by enteral feeding tubes.
    1. Physical and/or chemical interactions can occur if medications are directly added to enteral feeding formulas.
      a. Stop the feeding and flush the tube with 15 mL of water (use sterile water in immunocompromised or critically ill patients) before and after administering any medication into an enteral feeding tube.
      b. Never mix medications before administering. If multiple medications are to be administered, flush the enteral feeding tube with 15 mL of water after administering each medication.
      c. Always use liquid forms of medications if available and dilute liquid medication to decrease the viscosity of any added thickeners.
C. Topical medications, such as gels, creams, ointments, and aerosol sprays. (Absorption is through the epidermal barrier into underlying tissue with uptake to the system circulation.)
    1. Skin application: Evaluate condition, temperature, and hydration of the skin in the area that the medication is to be applied; if appropriate, rotate sites to prevent irritation.
      a. Presence of rashes, excoriations, fever, or applying an occlusive dressing over the topical medication can increase absorption.
    2. Sublingual: Allow medication to dissolve under the tongue; client should not chew or swallow.
    3. Nasal: Position client to allow nose drops or spray to enter nares directly without contaminating the eyes; the position should foster the movement of the medication to the affected area.
    4. Eyes: Medication must be specifically indicated for ophthalmic use.
      a. Instill one or two drops in the middle of the lower conjunctival sac.
      b. Do not allow tip of applicator to come in contact with the eye.
      c. Do not drop medication directly on the cornea.
      d. Direct client to close his or her eyes gently to distribute the medication.
      e. Make sure you administer the correct medication in the correct eye.
    5. Ears: Medication is instilled into the auditory canal.
      a. Position client with affected ear upward.
      b. Children under 3 years: Pull pinna down and backward.

c. Older children and adults: Pull pinna up and backward.

d. Administer solution at room temperature.

e. Keep client in the same position for appropriate time to prevent medication from coming out.

6. Suppositories.

a. Rectal: absorption of medication from rectal mucosa is slower and less predictable than that of medications administered systemically.

(1) Frequently given for constipation or for nausea and vomiting.

(2) May be preferred route for infant.

b. Vaginal: absorption across vaginal mucous membranes.

(1) Insert suppository about 3 to 4 inches into vagina; client maintains supine position after insertion.

(2) Client should not douche unless advised to do so; maintain good perineal hygiene.

D. Transdermal medication: Medication is stored in a patch or is measured on a dose-determined applicator placed on the skin; absorption occurs through the skin.

1. Provides more consistent blood levels and avoids gastrointestinal problems.

2. Patch sites should be rotated. Old patch should be removed and area should be cleansed after use.

3. Patch should *not* be applied over inflamed areas.

4. Do not allow transdermal medications to come in contact with your skin because medication could be absorbed.

5. Patch must come in contact with skin; excessive body hair may need to be removed. Do not shave the area; use scissors to clip hair from area.

E. Inhalation medication: Medication is in an aerosol or powder form and is inhaled and absorbed throughout the respiratory tract (see Chapter 17).

1. Place client in semi-Fowler's position. (Figure 8-3)

2. Check instructions for use of inhaler and make sure client understands.

a. Shake the metered dose inhaler (MDI) vigorously (3–5 seconds) to mix the medication.

b. Insert the MDI mouthpiece into the spacer and place into the mouth.

c. Press down once while inhaling slowly through the mouth.

d. Hold breath for 10 seconds.

e. Remove the inhaler from the mouth and exhale slowly through pursed lips.

f. Repeat if ordered. (Wait 1 minute between inhalation of bronchodilators to allow medication to take effect.)

g. Rinse mouth with water and spit it out. (Removes remaining medication and reduces risk of infection and irritation.)

F. Parenteral medications: administration of medications by some method of injection.

1. Injection routes (Figure 8-4).

2. Selection of a syringe (Figure 8-5): Select a syringe and type of needle that are appropriate for the type of parenteral medication to be administered.

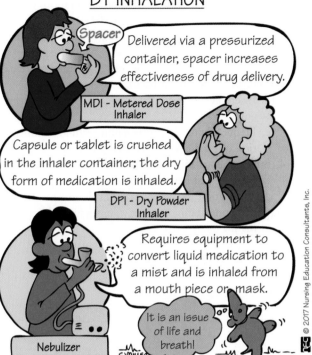

**FIGURE 8-3 Administration of Medications by Inhalation.** (From Zerwekh, J., Garneau, A., Miller, C.J. [2017]. *Digital collection of the memory notebooks of nursing images* [4th ed]. Chandler, AZ: Nursing Education Consultants, Inc.)

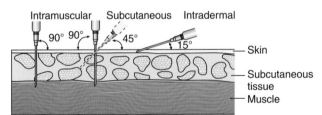

**FIGURE 8-4 Injection Routes.** Needle insertion angles for intramuscular, subcutaneous, and intradermal injections. (From Lilley, L., Collins, S., & Snyder, J. [2017]. *Pharmacology and the nursing process* [8th ed.]. St. Louis, MO: Elsevier.)

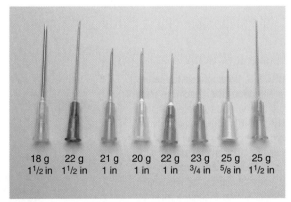

**FIGURE 8-5 Needle Gauges and Lengths.** (From Lilley, L., Collins, S., & Snyder, J. [2017]. *Pharmacology and the nursing process* [8th ed.]. St. Louis, MO: Elsevier.)

3. Intradermal injection: administered just below the skin surface.
   a. Use a syringe with appropriate calibrations because amount is small in volume (0.01–0.1 mL).
   b. Use a tuberculin or 1-mL syringe with a small-gauge (25- or 27-gauge) needle, ⅜ to ⅝ inch long.
   c. Select area where skin is thin (e.g., inner surface of forearm, middle of back).
   d. Insert needle bevel edge up at a 5- to 15-degree angle.
   e. Frequently used for tuberculin testing, administration of local anesthetic, allergy testing.
4. Subcutaneous injection: Medication is injected into fatty tissue just below the dermis.
   a. Medication should be small in volume (0.5–1.5 mL) and nonirritating; smaller volumes for children up to 0.5 mL.
   b. Areas on outer surface of upper arm, anterior surface of the thigh, and the abdomen are frequent sites.
   c. Use a 25-gauge needle that is ⅝ inches long and insert at a 45-degree angle or a 25-gauge needle that is ½ inch long and insert at a 90-degree angle.
5. Intramuscular (IM) injection: injection of medication into the muscle.
   a. The amount of medication is usually 0.5 to 3 mL.
   b. Appropriate sites.
      (1) Deltoid (Figure 8-6).
      (2) Ventrogluteal (Figure 8-7) and vastus lateralis muscles (Figure 8-8).
   c. Use a 1-inch to 1½-inch needle; gauge of needle depends on viscosity of medication; insert needle at 90-degree angle.
      (1) For oil-based or viscous medications, use an 18- to 22-gauge needle.

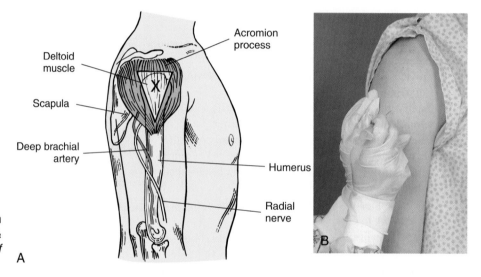

**FIGURE 8-6 Deltoid Muscle Injection Site in the Upper Arm.** (From Potter, P., & Perry, A., et al. [2017]. *Fundamentals of nursing* [9th ed.]. St. Louis, MO: Elsevier.)

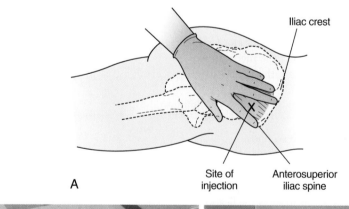

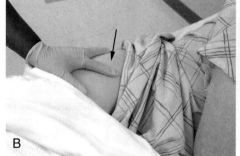
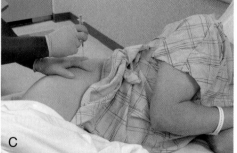

**FIGURE 8-7 Ventrogluteal Intramuscular Injection Site.** Place the palm of your hand over the greater trochanter, with your middle finger pointed toward the iliac crest, your index finger toward the anterosuperior iliac spine, and your thumb toward the client's groin. Administer the injection in the center of the triangle formed by your fingers. (From Lilley, L., Collins, S., & Snyder, J. [2017]. *Pharmacology and the nursing process* [8th ed.]. St. Louis, MO: Elsevier.)

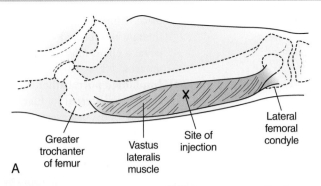

Greater trochanter of femur
Vastus lateralis muscle
Site of injection
Lateral femoral condyle

A

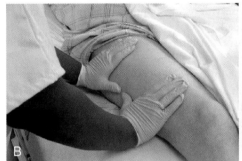

B

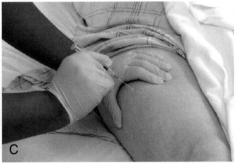

C

**FIGURE 8-8 Vastus Lateralis Intramuscular Injection Site on the Right Thigh.** Place one hand above the knee and the other hand below the greater trochanter. Locate the midline of both the anterior thigh and the lateral side of the thigh. Give the injection within the rectangular area. (From Lilley, L., Collins, S., & Snyder, J. [2017]. *Pharmacology and the nursing process* [8th ed.]. St. Louis, MO: Elsevier.)

(2) For less viscous medications, use a 20- to 22-gauge needle.
d. Aspirate when needle is in place; if no blood returns, administer medication at a rate of 1 mL every 10 seconds.
e. Z-track technique is used to prevent medication from leaking back through the needle track and irritating or staining subcutaneous tissue.
  (1) After medication is drawn up, change the needle.
  (2) Pull skin over to one side at the injection site.
  (3) Inject medication into taut skin at site selected.
  (4) Remove the needle and release the skin. As the stretched skin returns to its original position, the needle track is sealed.

(5) The preferable site is the ventrogluteal area.
f. Intramuscular injections in children.
  (1) Vastus lateralis muscle is common site in infants.
  (2) Ventrogluteal site is the preferred site in children.
  (3) A 22-gauge, 1-inch needle is appropriate for an IM injection in most children.
  (4) See **Calculation of Medication Dosages** section for pediatric calculations.
6. Intravenous (IV) administration: injection of medication into the blood (Table 8-5).
  a. Administration of large volumes of liquid by infusion.

**Table 8-5 INTRAVENOUS MEDICATION ADMINISTRATION**

| Method | Injection Rate | Nursing Implications |
|---|---|---|
| IV push or bolus | Rate of administration is determined by the amount of medication that can be given each minute based on each drug's protocol. | 1. Drug is not diluted and is injected directly into the client's venous system. <br> 2. Access is most often through an existing IV infusion. Use the access port closest to the client. <br> 3. It has a rapid effect on the CNS and cardiopulmonary systems. <br> 4. IV push or bolus is the most dangerous delivery method. Extreme care should be taken in following the drug protocol. If in doubt, do not deliver the bolus. |
| Intermittent infusion or piggyback (IVPB) | Medication is diluted in 25–100 mL and infused over 15–60 minutes. | 1. Drug is diluted to decrease toxicity and hypertonicity of the solution. <br> 2. It is the method of choice for multiple daily doses, especially antibiotics. <br> 3. Concentrated medications require higher dilution and longer infusion time. |
| Constant and variable-rate infusion | Pump is set to deliver constant rate of infusion based on dose of medication and dilution of medication. | 1. This method is used for medications that need to be highly diluted (chemotherapeutic drugs). <br> 2. It provides for continuous medication infusion. |

*CNS,* Central nervous system; *IV,* intravenous.

b. Administration of irritating medications by piggyback method.
   (1) Dilute medication according to directions, usually 25 to 250 mL of a compatible intravenous fluid like normal saline (NS).
   (2) Assess patency of primary infusion.
   (3) Connect medication and adjust flow rate for the time designated, usually 30 to 45 minutes.
   (4) Administration of medications through IV piggyback method enhances the action of the medication.
c. Administration of a specific medication into an already present IV infusion by IV push or bolus method.
   (1) Clamp tubing of primary IV line, inject the medication slowly, and observe the client's response.
   (2) Be aware of the institution's policy regarding guidelines for IV push medications.

> **TEST ALERT:** Access venous access devices, including tunneled, implanted, and central lines; monitor infusions and maintain sites (e.g., central, peripherally inserted central catheter [PICC], epidural, and venous access.)

d. **Vascular access device (VAD) or central IV therapy:** placed in a central bold vessel such as the superior vena cava (SVC). Multiple types are available, depending on the purpose, the duration of the therapy being administered, and the availability of insertion sites.
   (1) **Peripherally inserted central catheter (PICC):** inserted through a vein of the antecubital fossa with the distal tip residing in the SVC where blood flow will dilute administered medication quickly. Teach client to avoid excessive physical activity requiring muscle contraction in the arm to avoid catheter dislodgment and lumen occlusion.
   (2) **Nontunneled percutaneous central catheter:** inserted through the subclavian or jugular vein with the distal tip residing in the SVC. Usually used for short-term therapy and not recommended for home care. (After insertion, validate with chest x-ray and monitor client for complications related to pneumothorax.)
   (3) **Tunneled central catheter** has a portion of the catheter "tunneled" through the subcutaneous tissue. Catheter is composed of a rough materials cuff to which the client's tissue granulates; this provides a mechanical barrier to microorganisms and anchors the catheter in

place. Tunneled catheter is used when infusion therapy is expected to be long term, such as when a client requires parenteral nutrition for months.
   (4) **Implanted port:** catheter inserted in the subclavian or internal jugular vein attached to a "portal body or reservoir" that is surgically inserted into a subcutaneous pocket. Once healed, there is no external catheter that requires dressing changes. The nurse administers the infusion therapy by accessing the reservoir using a noncoring needle (Huber needle).
e. **Epidural catheter:** inserted in the epidural space allowing for the administration of bolus or continuous infusion. Analgesia administered into the epidural space can reach the systemic circulation in significant amounts, which could cause respiratory depression.

## Forms of Medication Preparations

A. Solids.
   1. Capsule: Medication is placed in cylindrical gelatin container.
   2. Pills, tablets: Medication is pressed into solid form in various shapes and colors.
      a. Enteric-coated: prevents medication from being released in stomach; dissolves in intestine. Do not crush enteric-coated, extended-release (ER), or sustained-release (SR) tablets.
      b. Lozenge: flavored tablet is held in the mouth for slow release of medication.
   3. Suppositories: generally keep these in cool area; will melt at body temperature; may produce local or systemic effects.
      a. Rectal.
      b. Vaginal.
   4. Ointments: used for external application.
   5. Powders: finely ground medications that are stable only in dry form; frequently mixed with solution before administration.
B. Solutions.
   1. Syrups: medication prepared in an aqueous sugar solution.
   2. Elixirs: solutions containing alcohol, sugar, and water.
   3. Suspensions: finely ground particles of medication dispersed in a liquid; shake all suspensions well before preparing dose (antacids).
   4. Emulsions: medication is dispersed in an oil or fat solution; shake all emulsions well before preparing dose.
   5. Liniments, lotions: medication dispersed in a mixture of oil, soap, alcohol, or water; used for external application.

## Calculation of Medication Dosages

Occasionally, the physician or health care provider orders medications in amounts not supplied by the pharmacy. In these situations, the nurse must calculate the correct dosage. Another important area of calculation is in the administration of IV solutions. Thus it is essential that the nurse have a good working knowledge of the fundamental principles of mathematics to calculate medication dosages correctly.

### Oral Medication Calculations

Dose desired ÷ Dose on hand = Amount to give

*Example: Order reads to give cephalexin 500 mg.* Dose on hand is 250 mg capsules.

500 ÷ 250 = 2 capsules
Dose desired ÷ Dose on hand × Quantity =
Amount to give

*Example: Order reads to give ampicillin 350 mg.* Dose on hand is 250 mg in 5 mL.

350 ÷ 250 × 5 = x
350 ÷ 250 = 14
14 × 5 mL = 7 mL

The problem also can be set up as an algebraic proportion:

350/x = 250/5 mL
250x = 1750
x = 7 mL

### Parenteral Medication Calculations

Dose desired ÷ Dose on hand × Quantity of
solution = Amount to give

*Example: Order reads gentamicin 60 mg IM.* Dose on hand is 80 mg in 1 mL.

60 mg ÷ 80 mg × 1 mL = x
60 ÷ 80 = 0.75
0.75 × 1 mL = 3/4 mL or 0.75 mL

Set up as an algebraic proportion, the equation reads:

60 mg/x = 80 mg/1 mL
80x = 60
x = 0.75 mL or 3/4 mL

### Intravenous Medication Calculation

- To determine how long an infusion will run, divide the total number of milliliters to infuse by the hourly infusion rate.

Amount to infuse ÷ Hourly rate = Number of
hours

*Example: Order reads 1000 mL at 125 mL per hour. How long will it take the 1000 mL to infuse?*

1000 ÷ 125 = x
1000 ÷ 125 = 8 hours

- To determine the rate in milliliters per hour at which an infusion will run, divide the total number of milliliters to infuse by the infusion time.

Amount to infuse ÷ Total infusion time =
Rate (mL/hr)

*Example: Order reads 1000 mL to run every 8 hours. At what rate in milliliters per hour will the medication be infused?*

1000 mL ÷ 8 hours = 125 mL/hr

- Calculating drop factors: Check the IV equipment to determine how many drops are delivered in 1 mL. For example purposes, a drop factor of 10 gtt per 1 mL is used. The following are two formulas with which to calculate this factor.

Total mL/Time in min = mL per min ×
Drop factor = gtt per min

*Example: 1000 mL is ordered to infuse in 8 hours. Set drop factor is 10 gtt/mL.*

1000 mL ÷ 480 min = 2.08 mL/min
2.08 × 10 = 20.8 or 21 gtt/min

*Example: 500 mL is ordered to infuse in 2 hours. Set calibration is 10 gtt/mL.*

500 mL ÷ 120 min = 4.16 × 10 =
41.6 or 42 gtt/min

- Determine the number of milliliters per hour and divide by 60 (60 minutes in 1 hour). This equals the number of milliliters per minute. Multiply by set calibration of number of drops per milliliter.

Number of milliliters per hour ÷ 60 = mL/min
Rate (mL/min) × Set calibration = gtt/min

*Example: 500 mL is ordered to infuse in 2 hours. Set calibration is 10 gtt/mL (250 mL/hr to infuse).*

250 mL ÷ 60 = 4.16 mL/min
4.16 mL × 10 = 41.6 or 42 gtt/min

**Note:** There may be a difference of 2 to 4 gtt when different formulas are used.

### Determining Safe Pediatric Dosages

Calculations for pediatric dosage should be considered as an approximation of the safe dose range. These calculations can be used as a guide when evaluating the appropriateness of a medication dose order.

Safe dose/kg × Child's weight in kg = Approximation of safe dose

*Example: Order reads to give cefaclor 50 mg qid.* The child weighs 9.1 kg. Is this a safe dose?
Safe dose range is 20 to 40 mg/kg/day in divided doses.

20 mg × 9.1 kg = 182 mg

40 mg × 9.1 kg = 364 mg/day is the approximate upper limits for maximum safe dose.

The child is receiving 50 mg × 4 doses daily (qid) = 200 mg/day. This dose is within the approximate safe range for a pediatric client.

The safest formula for evaluating drug dosages in children is to calculate the proportional amount of the body surface area (BSA) to the body weight. This requires the use of the West Nomogram (Figure 8-9) for estimation of body surface area.

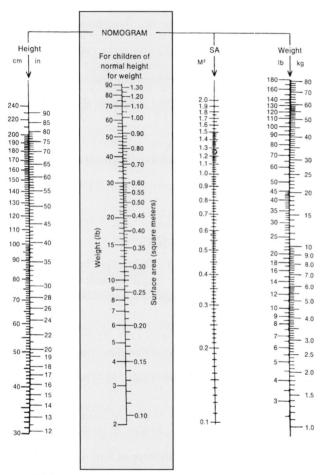

**FIGURE 8-9 West Nomogram for Estimation of Body Surface Area.** Surface area is indicated where a straight line connecting height and weight intersects surface area (SA) column or, if client is approximately of normal proportion, from weight alone *(yellow area)*. (Nomogram modified from data of E. Boyd by C. D. West: From Kliegman, R. M., Stanton, B., St. Geme, J., & Schor, N. F. [Eds.]. [2016]. *Nelson textbook of pediatrics* [20th ed.]. Philadelphia: Elsevier).

### Appendix 8-1 CONVERSIONS

| *Celsius and Fahrenheit* | *Pounds and Grams* |
|---|---|
| Fahrenheit reading = 9/5 × Celsius reading + 32 | 1 pound = 454 gm |
| Example: Temperature is 50°C | To convert pounds to grams, multiply the number of pounds by 454. |
| Fahrenheit = 9/5 × 50 + 32 90 + 32 = 122°F | 7.5 × 454 = 3405 gm |
| | To convert grams to pounds, divide the number of grams by 454. |
| | Example: An infant weighs 3405 gm |
| | 3405/454 = 7.5 lb, or 7 lb 8 oz |

### Appendix 8-2 COMMON ABBREVIATIONS AND SYMBOLS

| | |
|---|---|
| ac | before meals |
| ad lib | as desired |
| bid | twice daily |
| c̄ | with |
| Ca | calcium |
| CBC | complete blood count |
| Cl | chloride |
| gm | gram |
| gtt | drops |
| $H_2O$ | water |
| $H_2O_2$ | hydrogen peroxide |
| K | potassium |
| L | liter |
| Mg | magnesium |
| mL | milliliter |
| mcg | micrograms |
| N | nitrogen |
| Na | sodium |
| NPO | nothing by mouth |
| OOB | out of bed |
| pc | after meals |
| po | by mouth |
| PRN | as needed |
| q2h | every 2 hours |
| q3h | every 3 hours |
| qid | four times a day |
| s̄ | without |
| Stat | immediately |
| tab | tablet |
| tid | three times a day |

## Appendix 8-3 LIST OF "DO NOT USE" ABBREVIATIONS, ACRONYMS, AND SYMBOLS APPROVED BY THE JOINT COMMISSION (TJC)

| Abbreviation | Potential Problem | Preferred Term |
|---|---|---|
| U (unit) | Mistaken for "0" (zero), the number "4" (four) or "cc" | Write "unit" |
| IU (International Unit) | Mistaken for IV (intravenous) or the number 10 (ten) | Write "International Unit" |
| Q.D., QD, q.d., qd (daily) | Mistaken for each other | Write "daily" |
| Q.O.D., QOD, q.o.d, qod (every other day) | Period after the Q mistaken for "I" and the "O" mistaken for "I" | Write "every other day" |
| Trailing zero (x.0 mg)[a] | Decimal point is missed | Write X mg |
| Lack of leading zero (.x mg) | Decimal point is missed | Write 0.x mg |
| MS | Can mean morphine sulfate or magnesium sulfate | Write "morphine sulfate" |
| $MSO_4$ and $MgSO_4$ | Confused for one another | Write "magnesium sulfate" |

From Joint Commission on Accreditation of Healthcare Organizations: *The Official "Do Not Use" List Updated—June 2017*. Retrieved from https://www.jointcommission.org/facts_about_do_not_use_list/
© The Joint Commission, 2017.
[a]**Exception:** A trailing zero may be used only where required to demonstrate the level of precision of the value being reported, such as for laboratory results, imaging studies that report size of lesions, or catheter/tube sizes. It may not be used in medication orders or other medication-related documentation.

## Appendix 8-4 UNDERSTANDING MEDICAL TERMINOLOGY: PREFIXES AND SUFFIXES

**Prefixes**

| | |
|---|---|
| cef- | antibiotic (cephalosporin) |
| ceph- | antibiotic (cephalosporin) |
| nitr- | vasodilator |
| sulf- | antibiotic (sulfonamide) |

**Suffixes**

| | |
|---|---|
| -actone | potassium-sparing diuretic |
| -ane | general anesthetics |
| -ase | thrombolytic |
| -azine | antiemetic |
| -azole | antifungal |
| -azosin | alpha blocker |
| -barbital | barbiturate (sedative-hypnotics) |
| -caine | local anesthetic |
| -cillin | antibiotic (penicillin) |
| -coxib | COX-2 inhibitors |
| -cycline | antibiotic (tetracycline) |
| -dipine | calcium-channel blocker |
| -done | opioid analgesics |
| -dronate | bisphosphonates |
| -floxacin | antibiotic (fluoroquinolones) |
| -gliptin | oral hypoglycemic (DPP-4 inhibitors) |
| -glitazone | oral hypoglycemic (glitazones) |
| -ide | oral hypoglycemic and loop diuretic |
| -kinase | thrombolytic |
| -lam | antianxiety agent; benzodiazepines |
| -mide | diuretics |
| -mycin (micin) | antibiotic (aminoglycosides, macrolides) |
| -nium | neuromuscular blocking agents |
| -olol | beta-blockers |
| -oxin | cardiac glycoside |
| -pam | antianxiety agent |
| -parin | anticoagulant |
| -phylline | bronchodilator |
| -prazole | proton pump inhibitor (PPI) |
| -pril | angiotensin-converting enzyme (ACE) inhibitor |
| -profen | NSAID |
| -ridone | atypical antipsychotic |
| -sartan | angiotensin II blocker |
| -sone | steroid |
| -statin | antihyperlipidemic; HMG-CoA reductase inhibitor |
| -stigmine | cholinergic |
| -stine | antineoplastic |
| -tidine | H2 receptor antagonist (antiulcer) |
| -triptan | antimigraine |
| -vir | antiviral (protease inhibitors) |
| -zepam, -zolam | benzodiazepine |
| -zide | thiazide diuretic |
| -zine | phenothiazines |
| -zole | antifungal (azoles) |
| -zone | oral hypoglycemic (glitazones) |

Use these helpful prefixes and suffixes to assist in identifying medication generic names.

# Study Questions
# Pharmacology and Medication Administration

More questions on

evolve

1. The nurse is preparing to administer an intramuscular injection to an infant who is 8 months old. Which muscle would be the most appropriate injection site?
   1. Deltoid
   2. Dorsogluteal
   3. Vastus lateralis
   4. Ventrogluteal

2. The doctor has indicated that ampicillin and gentamicin are to be given piggyback in the same hour, every 6 hours (12-6-12-6). How would the nurse administer these drugs?
   1. Combine the drugs into 100 mL NS and administer.
   2. Give each drug separately, flushing between drugs.
   3. Retrograde both drugs into the tubing.
   4. Give one drug every 4 hours and the other every 6 hours.

3. At the shift hand-off report, a nurse is told that one of her clients is becoming tolerant to his pain medication. What nursing observation would be in agreement with this conclusion?
   1. The current medication order, which has previously been effective, is no longer providing adequate pain relief.
   2. The client becomes irritable and confused before the next scheduled dose of medication.
   3. Pain medication is being administered every 3 to 4 hours around the clock for adequate pain relief.
   4. The client is sleeping and arouses with physical and verbal stimulation but is very lethargic.

4. What should the nurse take into consideration when giving medication to an older adult client?
   1. The serum albumin level of an older adult is lower, thus decreasing drug metabolism.
   2. The older adult client metabolizes and excretes at a decreased rate.
   3. Medication affects the older adult client during the early hours of the morning.
   4. Medication has an increased effect on the respiratory system of the older adult client.

5. What is the first step the nurse should take to ensure that the right medication is being given to a client?
   1. Check the client's ID band.
   2. Read the information insert for directions as to correct administration.
   3. Check the order with the medication administration sheet.
   4. Check the expiration date on the medication.

6. The nurse prepares a liquid medication and then finds that the client no longer needs the medication. What is the most appropriate nursing action?
   1. To keep the count correct, record that the dose was taken.
   2. Charge for the dose because it must be paid for.
   3. Record the medication as "not taken" and discard the poured dose.
   4. Pour the medication back into the container.

7. The nurse is working in the pediatric unit and receives a phone order from the doctor for a 10-year-old client who weighs 40 kg. The order is for ceftazidime 1.5 gm every 8 hours IV. The therapeutic dosage range is 90 to 150 mg/kg/24 hr. What would be the best nursing action?
   1. Administer the medication because it is within the therapeutic dosage range.
   2. Call the doctor to clarify the order because it is outside the therapeutic dosage range.
   3. Call the hospital pharmacist and ask him or her to calculate the dosage.
   4. Notify the nursing supervisor and request assistance.

8. The nurse is caring for a client who had a stroke (brain attack) 3 months ago and is taking warfarin 5 mg by mouth (PO). The client tells the nurse she has started taking some herbal and vitamin supplements. She gives the nurse a list of the supplements she is taking. What supplements would cause concern for the client who is on warfarin? **Select all that apply.**
   1. Garlic
   2. Cyanocobalamin (vitamin B12)
   3. St. John's wort
   4. Vitamin E (alpha tocopherol)
   5. Saw palmetto
   6. Ginkgo biloba

9. The nurse is preparing medications for a client. The medication order is for cefaclor 0.1 gm PO. The dose available in the unit is 125 mg/5 mL. How many milliliters will the nurse need to give?
   Answer: _____ mL

10. A client is receiving IV antibiotic therapy. The order is for methicillin 750 mg IV. The nurse has a vial on hand that contains 1 gm. The instructions for reconstitution say to add 1.5 mL sterile water. Reconstituted solution will contain 500 mg methicillin per milliliter. How much will the nurse give?
    Answer: _____ mL

11. The nurse is verifying whether to give a medication to a client. What would be the first nursing action?
    1. Check the client's name and hospital number.
    2. Validate the expiration date of the drug.
    3. Determine the appropriate route of delivery.
    4. Review the orders on the medication administration record.

12. A client is scheduled for a total hip replacement, and he has a history of using several herbal and vitamin products. What would the nurse advise the client to discontinue at least 2 weeks before surgery? **Select all that apply.**
    1. Garlic
    2. Vitamin C
    3. Ginger root
    4. St. John's wort
    5. Ma huang
    6. Black cohosh

13. A client asks the nurse about an alternative remedy for hot flashes. Which dietary supplement is the client asking the nurse about?
    1. Ginseng.
    2. Valerian.
    3. Feverfew.
    4. Black cohosh.

14. A client who is being seen at the urgent care clinic with complaints of abdominal pain tells the nurse he has been taking kava. Which nursing intervention would be a priority at this time?
    1. Obtain the electrocardiogram (ECG) results.
    2. Assess breath sounds and respiratory effort.
    3. Review liver function studies.
    4. Review complete blood count results.

15. The physician orders an IV piggyback of cefotetan 1 gm in 100 mL D₅W to run over 30 minutes. The drop factor for the tubing is 10 gtt/mL. At what rate in drops per minute would you run the IV?
    1. 33 gtt/min
    2. 25 gtt/min
    3. 12 gtt/min
    4. 50 gtt/min

16. The physician calls the unit and leaves an order for a client. The order is for cefaclor 0.1 gm PO. The dose available in the unit is 125 mg/5 mL. How many milliliters will the nurse give?
    Answer: _____ mL

17. A client is receiving IV antibiotic therapy. The order is for methicillin 750 mg IV. The nurse has a vial on hand that contains 1 g. The instructions for reconstitution say to add 1.5 mL sterile water. Reconstituted solution will contain 500 mg methicillin per milliliter. How much will the nurse give?
    Answer: _____ mL

## Answers to Study Questions

1. *3*
The vastus lateralis is the preferred site for an infant because the muscle is not located near any vital nerves or blood vessels. It is the best choice for IM injections for children younger than 3 years of age. The deltoid muscle has too little muscle mass in a young infant or toddler and is unable to hold large injected volumes of medication. (Hockenberry & Wilson, 10 ed., p. 917)

2. *2*
Only one antibiotic should be administered at a time; therefore if the medications are given during the same hour, the IV tubing will need to be flushed between administrations. Both drugs should be administered at the time ordered. (Potter & Perry, 9 ed., pp. 667–670)

3. *1*
Tolerance occurs when there is a decrease in the response to a drug after repeated drug administration. More of the analgesic is needed to maintain the same level of pain control. Requiring pain medication around the clock for adequate pain relief is not tolerance because the client is obtaining proper pain relief. Irritability and confusion before the next dose may be an adverse reaction to the medication, or another problem may be occurring. Sleepiness and lethargy may indicate that the client is overmedicated. (Burchum & Rosenthal, 9 ed., pp. 74–75)

4. *2*
The ability to metabolize and excrete medication decreases with the aging process. For example, at the age of 80 years, the ability to metabolize medications decreases approximately 50% compared with a 30-year-old. Medications do not have an increased effect in the morning, nor do they specifically affect the respiratory system of the older adult. (Burchum & Rosenthal, 9 ed., pp. 92–93)

5. *3*
The first step in drug delivery to a client is to check the order with the medication administration sheet for possible discontinuance or a change in dose, route, or time. The question asks for steps to ensure the right medication is being given, not for client identification. (Potter & Perry, 9 ed., p. 635)

6. *3*
The dose should be recorded as "not taken," and the poured dose should be discarded. If the dose is a controlled substance, the discarded dose must be witnessed. Checking the medication administration record or the medication order for changes before preparing the medication helps eliminate waste and/or mistakes. (Burchum & Rosenthal, 9 ed., p. 69)

7. *1*
Administer the medication ceftazidime as ordered. The therapeutic dosage is 90 to 150 mg/kg/day.
    Ordered: 1.5 gm every 8 hours = 1.5 gm × 3 doses = 4.5 gm per day
    Minimum therapeutic dose: 90 mg × 40 kg = 3600 mg or 3.6 gm per day
    Highest safe dose: 150 mg × 40 kg = 6000 mg or 6 gm per day
    (Potter & Perry, 9 ed., p. 620)

8. *1, 4, 6*
Garlic, ginkgo biloba, and vitamin E may interfere with platelet aggregation and increase the risk for bleeding in clients who are taking warfarin. (Burchum & Rosenthal, 9 ed., pp. 1321–1324)

9. *4 mL*

$$1 \text{ gm} = 1000 \text{ mg; therefore, } 0.1 \text{ gm} = 100 \text{ mg}$$
$$125 \text{ mg} : 5 \text{ mL} :: 100 \text{ mg} : x \text{ mL}$$

Formula: 125 × x = 125x (Note: Multiply the two outside numbers of the ratio equation together, then the two inside numbers; solve for x by dividing the total of the inside numbers with the outside numbers.)

$$5 \times 100 = 500$$
$$x = 500/125 = 4 \text{ mL}$$

(Potter & Perry, 9 ed., pp. 618–620)

10. *1.5 mL*

$$500 \text{ mg} : 1 \text{ mL} :: 750 \text{ mg} : x$$

$$\text{Formula: } 500 \times x = 500x$$
$$1 \times 750 = 750$$
$$x = 750/500 = 1.5$$

The dosage calculation cannot be made from the amount of solution added to the vial. The ratio of mg per mL after reconstitution is 500 mg/mL. (Potter & Perry, 9 ed., pp. 618–620)

11. *4*

The medication administration record should be reviewed for current physician's orders. Medication administration records are routinely reviewed to determine the currency of medication orders. The client's name and hospital number are checked to validate client identification before administration of the medication. The nurse should check the medication for the expiration date when she prepares the medication, and the physician will order the route of administration. (Potter & Perry, 9 ed., p. 626.)

12. *1, 3, 5*

Garlic and ginger root can prolong bleeding time by suppressing platelet aggregation. Ma huang is ephedra and affects the blood pressure. St. John's wort, vitamin C, and black cohosh are safe to continue before surgery. (Burchum & Rosenthal, 9 ed., pp. 1321–1328)

13. *4*

Black cohosh is an herbal supplement used for treating symptoms of menopause, including hot flashes, vaginal dryness, palpitations, depression, irritability, and sleep disturbance. The nurse should determine whether the client's symptoms are caused by tamoxifen and other selective estrogen receptor modulators, if this is the situation, then black cohosh should not be used. Ginseng improves mood, boosts endurance, and may lower blood glucose. Feverfew is taken for migraine prophylaxis. Valerian has sedative properties that promote sleep and reduce anxiety. Burchum & Rosenthal, 9 ed., pp. 1321–1328)

14. *3*

Kava is an herbal supplement that is used to relieve anxiety, promote sleep, and relax muscles and is known to be hepatotoxic. Monitoring liver function studies would be an appropriate action. Ma huang (ephedra) is an herbal supplement that can cause hypertension and stimulates the central nervous system. (Burchum & Rosenthal, 9 ed., pp. 1328–1329)

15. *1*

The calculation would be 100 mL/30 min × 10 gtt/mL = 33.3 or 33 gtt/min. (Potter & Perry, 9 ed., pp. 618–620)

16. *4 mL*

$$\text{Rationale: } 1 \text{ gm} = 1000 \text{ mg;}$$
$$\text{therefore, } 0.1 \text{ gm} = 100 \text{ mg}$$
$$125 \text{ mg} : 5 \text{ mL} :: 100 \text{ mg} : x \text{ mL}$$

Formula: 125 × = 125x (Note: multiply the two outside numbers of the ratio equation together, then the two inside numbers; solve for x by dividing the total of the inside numbers with the outside numbers.)

$$5 \times 100 = 500$$
$$x = 500/125 = 4 \text{ mL}$$

(Potter & Perry, 9 ed., pp. 618–620)

17. *1.5 mL*

$$\text{Rationale: } 500 \text{ mg} : 1 \text{ mL} :: 750 \text{ mg} : x$$
$$\text{Formula: } 500 \times x = 500x$$
$$1 \times 750 = 750$$
$$x = 750/500 = 1.5$$

The dosage calculation cannot be made from the amount of solution added to the vial; the ratio of mg per mL after reconstitution is 500 mg per mL. (Potter & Perry, 9 ed., pp. 618–620)

# CHAPTER NINE

# Homeostasis Concepts

**9**

Acid–Base Balance, Fluid & Electrolyte Balance, Infection, Inflammation

## FLUID AND ELECTROLYTES

### Physiology

A. Basic concepts of body fluid.
  1. Water is the primary component of body fluid. It is used to transport nutrients, electrolytes, and oxygen to the cells and to remove waste products.
  2. Intracellular fluid: provides the cell with internal fluid necessary for cellular function.
     a. Approximately 40% to 50% of body weight (two-thirds of total body water).
     b. Electrolytes: potassium (primary), magnesium, phosphate.
  3. Extracellular (intravascular and interstitial) fluids: transport system for cellular waste, oxygen, electrolytes, and nutrients; help regulate body temperature; lubricate and cushion joints.
     a. Approximately 20% to 30% of body weight (one-third of total body water).
     b. An infant maintains a larger percentage of extracellular fluids than does an older child or adult.
     c. Vascular: circulating plasma volume.
     d. Interstitial: fluid surrounding tissue cells.
     e. Electrolytes: sodium (primary), chloride, bicarbonate.
B. Dynamic transport of fluid and electrolytes.
  1. Osmosis: movement of water between two compartments separated by a semipermeable membrane, from an area of low-solute concentration to an area of high-solute concentration.
     a. Oncotic pressure: the osmotic pressure created by plasma proteins; proteins pull fluid from the tissue space to the vascular space.
     b. Osmotic pressure is the amount of pressure required to stop the flow of water. It is determined by the concentration of solutes in solution.
  2. Hydrostatic pressure: the pressure created by the fluid volume in the vascular bed.
C. Fluid movement in capillaries.
  1. Filtration occurs in the arterial end of the capillaries because the hydrostatic pressure is higher than the oncotic pressure. Fluid then moves out of the vascular bed into the tissue.

  2. Capillary hydrostatic pressure and interstitial oncotic pressure move water out of the capillaries. At the venous end of the capillaries, the oncotic pressure is greater, and the fluid moves back into the vascular volume.
  3. Osmolality refers to the concentration of the dissolved particles in a solution; osmolality controls the movement of fluid in each of the compartments.
     a. Hyper-osmolar (hypertonic): fluids in which the concentration of solutes is higher than in the cells.
     b. Hypo-osmolar (hypotonic): fluids in which the concentration of solutes is less than in the cells.
     c. Iso-osmolar (isotonic): fluids with the same osmolality as the cell normal distribution of solutes and water in body fluid.
D. Fluid shifts.
  1. Plasma to interstitial fluid shift (edema).
     a. Edema: accumulation of fluid in interstitial spaces.
        (1) Venous hydrostatic pressure increases (client with fluid overload in heart failure).
        (2) Decrease in oncotic pressure, as in a client with excessive protein loss (renal disease).
        (3) Increased interstitial oncotic pressure, as in trauma and burns where the capillary wall has been damaged and plasma protein moves to the interstitial space.
     b. Hypovolemia may occur as a result of excessive fluid shift into the interstitial spaces, resulting in circulatory collapse (client with burns).
  2. Interstitial to plasma fluid shift: movement of fluid back into the circulatory volume, as in a client with mobilization of burn edema or in the case of excessive administration of hypertonic solution, causing the interstitial water to be returned to the plasma; client may demonstrate symptoms of circulatory overload.
  3. Fluid spacing.
     a. First spacing: normal distribution of fluids.
     b. Second spacing: abnormal accumulation of interstitial fluid—edema.
     c. Third spacing: fluid that is trapped and cannot easily move back into extracellular fluid (ECF) (e.g., edema associated with burns and ascites).
E. Homeostatic mechanisms.
  1. Endocrine system.
     a. Hypothalamus secretes antidiuretic hormone, which regulates the water reabsorption by the kidneys.
     b. Adrenal cortex secretes aldosterone, which promotes sodium retention and potassium excretion, thereby causing an increase in plasma volume.

2. Lymphatic system: assists in the return of excessive protein and fluid, which escapes into the tissue, to the plasma volume.
3. Cardiovascular system maintains blood pressure to ensure adequate renal perfusion.
4. Kidneys maintain fluid volume and concentration of urine via the glomerular filtration rate and by the renin angiotensin aldosterone system.

> **TEST ALERT:** Understand general principles of pathophysiology.

## Fluid Imbalances

A. Fluid deficit: extracellular fluid volume deficit hypovolemia results from vascular fluid volume loss.
   1. Sensible fluid loss: fluid loss of which an individual is aware, as in urine.
   2. Insensible fluid loss: fluid loss of which an individual is not aware (approximately 600 to 900 mL of fluid is lost every 24 hours through the skin and lungs in a healthy adult).
   3. Causes of fluid deficit (all result from loss of both water and sodium).
      a. Decreased fluid intake.
      b. Loss of fluid through the gastrointestinal tract, as in vomiting, nasogastric suctioning, diarrhea.
      c. Excessive excretion due to renal disease; inappropriate antidiuretic hormone secretion.
      d. Iatrogenic loss due to overuse of diuretics or inadequate replacement of fluid loss.
      e. Increased insensible fluid loss through skin and lungs due to febrile state, increased respiratory rates.
      f. Loss of fluid through impaired integrity of the skin as in burns, wounds, and hemorrhages.

> **⚠ NURSING PRIORITY:** Sodium is the major electrolyte that affects fluid balance. "Where sodium goes so goes the water."

   4. Clinical manifestations (Figure 9-1).
      a. Restlessness, lethargy, confusion.
      b. Dry skin and thirst (dry mucous membranes).
      c. Poor skin turgor.
         (1) Assess skin turgor on the abdomen or the inner thigh in children (unless abdominal distention is present).
         (2) Assess skin turgor on the sternum or below the clavicle in older adult clients.
         (3) Assess skin turgor on the back of hand and anterior forearm in adults.
      d. Weight loss.
      e. Oliguria (less than 400 mL/24 hours), concentrated urine.
      f. Postural hypotension.
      g. Increased respiratory and cardiac rate.
      h. Decreased central venous pressure (CVP).
      i. Infants and children: poor perfusion, poor capillary refill resulting in mottled skin color changes.

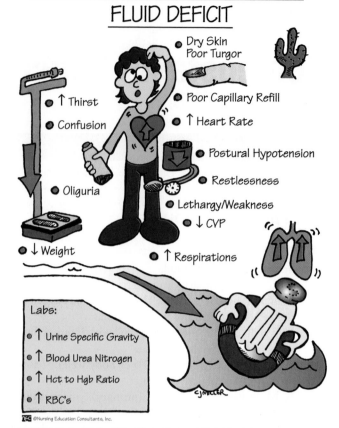

## CLINICAL MANIFESTATIONS OF FLUID DEFICIT

- Dry Skin Poor Turgor
- ↑ Thirst
- Confusion
- Poor Capillary Refill
- ↑ Heart Rate
- Postural Hypotension
- Restlessness
- Oliguria
- Lethargy/Weakness
- ↓ CVP
- ↓ Weight
- ↑ Respirations

Labs:
- ↑ Urine Specific Gravity
- ↑ Blood Urea Nitrogen
- ↑ Hct to Hgb Ratio
- ↑ RBC's

©Nursing Education Consultants, Inc.

**FIGURE 9-1 Clinical Manifestations of Fluid Deficit.** (Zerwekh, J., & Garneau, A., J., Miller, C. J. [2017]. *Digital collection of the memory notebooks of nursing* [4th ed.]. Chandler, AZ: Nursing Education Consultants, Inc.).

      j. Weakness, confusion, speech difficulty in the older adult client.
   5. Laboratory findings.
      a. Increased urine specific gravity and osmolarity.
      b. Increased blood urea nitrogen (greater than 25 mg/dL (8.92 mmol/L) without increase in creatinine.
      c. Increased hematocrit (the normal ratio of hematocrit to hemoglobin is 3:1 (e.g., 12 g hemoglobin to 36% hematocrit) (120 g/L to 0.36 proportion of 1).
      d. Increased electrolyte levels from hemoconcentration.

> **TEST ALERT:** Identify signs and symptoms for client with fluid and/or electrolyte imbalances.

B. Extracellular fluid volume excess (circulatory overload): the retention of sodium and water in the intravascular and interstitial spaces.
   1. Causes of fluid excess.
      a. Excessive oral fluid intake.
      b. Failure to excrete fluids, as in renal disease, cardiac failure, and hormone imbalance.
      c. Iatrogenic: fluid increase due to excessive infusion of hypotonic or isotonic fluids.

2. Clinical manifestations.
  a. Pitting edema, sacral edema.
  b. Dyspnea, crackles, possible pulmonary edema.
  c. Bounding pulse, weight gain.
  d. Lethargy, dizziness, headache, confusion.
  e. Increased central venous pressure (CVP), jugular vein distention.
  f. Increased blood pressure.
3. Laboratory findings: based on the area of the body in which the shift occurs.
  a. Decreased specific gravity of urine (less than 1.010).
  b. Decreased hematocrit.
  c. Decreased serum sodium secondary to dilution.
  d. Large fluid shifts occur in severe injuries, burns, intestinal perforations and obstruction, and lymphatic obstruction.

**TEST ALERT:** Implement interventions to restore client fluid and/or electrolyte balance.

C. Nursing management of client with fluid imbalances.
1. Assessment.
  a. Evaluate client's history and predisposing factors contributing to the problem.
  b. Assess for direction of fluid problem: fluid excess or deficit.
  c. Evaluate appropriate laboratory data.
  d. Evaluate client's ability to tolerate and correct the problem.
  e. Older adult clients are more likely to develop extracellular fluid volume excess because of chronic diseases (renal, cardiac).
2. Nursing intervention.
  a. Maintain accurate intake and output records.
  b. Obtain accurate daily weight.

**! NURSING PRIORITY:** Daily weight is the most reliable indicator of fluid loss or gain in all clients, regardless of age. Accurate daily weight: same time each day (preferably before breakfast), same scales, same clothing. *NOTE: 1 L of fluid equals 2.2 lb. or 1 kg.*

  c. Evaluate for presence of edema.
  d. Maintain intravenous (IV) replacement fluids at prescribed flow rate.
  e. Monitor cardiovascular changes.
   (1) CVP, status of jugular vein.
   (2) Changes in blood pressure. (Blood pressure is not a reliable indicator of early problems of fluid balance in infants and children.)
  f. Monitor for changes in respiratory status.
  g. Maintain good skin care: practice good oral hygiene, elevate edematous extremities, avoid soap, use measures to prevent skin breakdown.
  h. Assess laboratory data for changes in the problem.
  i. Carefully monitor older adult and pediatric clients and clients with cardiac disease for tolerance of fluid replacement.

**! NURSING PRIORITY:** Increased urine specific gravity, dark urine, decreased urine output, and postural hypotension are objective clues to intravascular volume deficit.

3. See Appendix 9-1 for more on electrolyte imbalances and replacement.

## INTRAVENOUS FLUID REPLACEMENT THERAPY

### Isotonic Solutions
A. Used to expand ECF volume and for intravascular dehydration.
B. Solutions.
  1. $D_5W$: 5% dextrose in water (physiologically hypotonic).
  2. 0.9% NaCl (normal saline solution).
  3. Lactated Ringer's solution.
C. May be used to dilute medications or to keep the vein open.

**! NURSING PRIORITY:** In $D_5W$ the dextrose is metabolized rapidly, leaving free water to be absorbed. It does not replenish electrolytes; it is contraindicated for clients with head injuries and should be used with caution in children because of the potential for increase in intracranial pressure.

### Hypotonic Solutions
A. Solutions containing more water and less basic electrolytes.
B. 0.45% or half-strength NaCl (normal saline solution).
C. May be used to replenish cellular fluid.
D. Monitor closely for intravascular fluid loss, hypotension, changes in level of consciousness, and edema.

### Hypertonic Solutions
A. Administered slowly; can cause intravascular volume overload; carefully monitor serum sodium, lung sounds, and blood pressure.
B. Solutions.
  1. Dextrose 5% in 0.45% or half-strength NaCl (normal saline).
  2. Dextrose 5% in 0.9% NaCl (normal saline).
  3. Dextrose 5% in lactated Ringer's.
C. Used to treat situations of hyponatremia and hypovolemia.

### Nursing Implications in Administration of Intravenous Fluid

**TEST ALERT:** Apply knowledge of nursing procedures and motor skills when caring for a client receiving intravenous and parenteral therapy.

#### Selection of Site and Equipment
A. Vein selection (Figure 9-2).
  1. Distal veins of the upper extremities should be used first. Subsequent venipuncture should be proximal to or higher than the previous site.

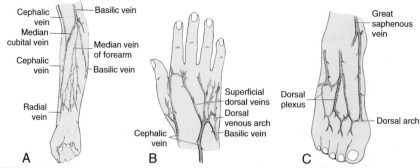

**FIGURE 9-2  Common IV Sites.** (A) Inner arm. (B) Dorsal surface of hand. (C) Dorsal surface of foot (infants and children). (From Potter, P. A., & Perry, A. G. [2017]. *Fundamentals of nursing* [9th ed.]. St. Louis, MO: Mosby.)

2. Veins above or below an area of flexion.
3. Try to select a site on the client's nondominant extremity.
4. Select a vein large enough to accommodate the catheter.
B. Infants: scalp veins are frequently used because of easy access and less movement in the area; it is also easier to stabilize the insertion site.
C. Children: veins on the dorsal surface of the foot are frequently used. (These should *not* be used as an access site in *adults* because of the risk for developing thrombophlebitis.)

**TEST ALERT:** Know which veins should be accessed for various therapies.

D. IV sites to avoid.
  1. Areas of flexion, especially the antecubital area.
  2. Veins previously injured by infiltration or phlebitis.
  3. Veins of an affected extremity: mastectomy, dialysis access.
  4. Veins of an extremity affected by stroke or neurologic trauma.
  5. Veins in the lower extremities and sclerosed or irritated veins.
  6. Avoid previous venipuncture sites, areas of inflammation or bruising.
E. Venous access devices (Figure 9-3).
  1. Butterfly needle: has wings for stabilization of needle; used for blood draws or a short-term infusion.
  2. Plastic cannula/catheter: tubing threaded over a needle; used for infusions over several days and often with IV antibiotics.
  3. Needle: used for short-term infusions.
  4. Select the smallest gauge needle or cannula for the type of fluid infused. The larger the gauge of the needle or cannula, the *smaller* the needle or cannula.
    a. A 22-gauge needle or catheter is most common for IV fluids.
    b. An 18- or 20-gauge needle or catheter for blood or rapid administration of fluids.
    c. May convert a cannula into a saline lock if continuous fluids are not infusing.
  5. Central line (see Appendix 9-4).
  6. Implantable or tunneled ports (see Appendix 9-4).

**TEST ALERT:** Access implanted venous access devices.

7. Saline lock: may be an IV cannula or a butterfly needle.
  a. Used for intermittent access.
  b. May be flushed with a saline flush solution at regular intervals to maintain patency and prevent clot formation of line.
8. Site may be converted to fluid infusion if necessary.

**NURSING PRIORITY:** If the institution is using heparin for flushing locks and tubing, make sure the heparin flush solution (hep-lock)—1 mL per 100 units—is used. It is easy to mistake heparin 1 to 10,000 units as a flush solution.

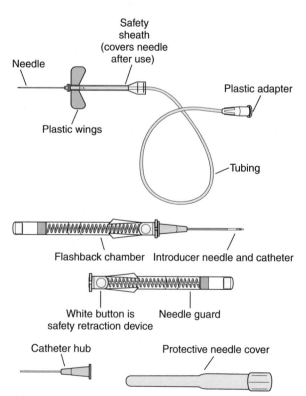

**FIGURE 9-3 IV Access Options.** (From Potter, P. A., & Perry, A. G., Stockert, P. [2017]. *Fundamentals of nursing* [9th ed.]. St. Louis, MO: Mosby.)

*Starting an Intravenous Infusion*

A. Cleanse site thoroughly; recleanse the site if area was palpated before insertion.
B. Wear gloves during insertion of the needle and as long as there is possibility of skin contact with the client's blood.
C. Apply the tourniquet 4 to 6 inches above the site and insert the needle with the bevel up at a 15- to 30-degree angle.
D. After the needle has advanced into the vein and there is good blood return, release the tourniquet.
E. If the stylet has been removed (IV catheter or cannula), do not attempt to reinsert the stylet into the catheter shaft.
F. Always obtain a new catheter or needle if the insertion attempt was unsuccessful.
G. Cover the insertion site (transparent dressing or sterile gauze); do not place tape directly over the insertion site.
H. Label the site with time, date, catheter/needle size, and initials of nurse.
I. Label the infusion container with:
   1. Time container was hung; rate of infusion.
   2. Any medications that were added.
J. Do not encircle the arm with tape; this can restrict circulation to the extremity.

*Maintenance of Intravenous Infusions*

A. Factors influencing rate of fluid administration.
   1. Type of fluid, age of client, and client's response to fluids.
   2. Cardiac and renal status.
   3. Size of the vein and gauge of catheter or needle.
B. Maintain accurate intake and output records.
C. Average maintenance fluid rate is 2000 to 3000 mL over 24 hours, depending on body weight and client's condition.
D. Peripheral IV infusion sites are commonly changed every 72 to 96 hours (3 to 4 days, depending on institution policy) unless complications (inflammation, irritation, or fluid extravasation) occur at the site.
E. Carefully monitor the infusion rate: control with either a roller clamp or an infusion pump.

 F. Pediatric considerations.
   1. Children are very susceptible to rapid fluid shifts; cerebral edema may occur with infusion of $D_5W$. Most common IV solutions are a combination of saline (0.9%) and 5% dextrose to decrease the possibility of an untoward fluid shift.
   2. Volume chambers holding no more than a 3- to 4-hour supply of fluid or controlled infusion devices (pumps) should be used for children to prevent the inadvertent rapid infusion of too much fluid.
   3. Always make sure infants and young children are voiding before beginning IV infusion of fluids containing added potassium.

*Indications for Use of Infusion Pumps*

A. To deliver a medication that requires a precise rate of administration (vasopressor agents, patient-controlled analgesia).
B. To deliver fluids that would precipitate adverse effects if administered too rapidly (total parenteral nutrition).
C. To deliver fluids in controlled amounts to clients very sensitive to volume administered (infants, children younger than 10 years of age, older adult clients, clients with pulmonary edema, cardiac problems, hypertension, and with decreased renal function).

### Complications of Peripheral Intravenous Therapy
(Figure 9-4)

*Infiltration*

A. Common causes: dislodging of the needle/catheter by client movement or obstruction of fluid flow.
B. Signs and symptoms: edema, *blanching of skin*, discomfort at site, fluid that is flowing slowly or has stopped, *cooler skin temperature.*
C. Preventive nursing management: use the smallest gauge of catheter possible; use an arm board to stabilize catheter, especially for restless, confused clients or those with catheters placed in the antecubital fossa area; check frequently for coolness of skin around site; avoid looping tubing below bed level; check IV flow rate at least every 1 to 2 hours.
D. Nursing interventions.
   1. Discontinue IV solution and remove catheter.
   2. Apply warm, moist heat for 20 minutes to increase fluid absorption (if not contraindicated); may reapply warm, moist heat 3 to 4 times throughout the day; raise affected extremity to increase venous return and reduce swelling.
   3. If infiltrated solution contains an irritating medication (chemotherapy, vasoconstrictive fluids), call the health care provider for orders to counteract effects of medication in the subcutaneous tissue.

## COMPLICATIONS OF PERIPHERAL IV THERAPY

**FIGURE 9-4 Complications of Peripheral IV Therapy.** (From Zerwekh, J., Claborn, J., & Gaglione, T. [2010]. *Mosby's fluids and electrolytes memory notecards: Visual, mnemonic, and memory aids for nurses* [2nd ed.]. St. Louis, MO: Mosby.)

### Phlebitis

A. Common causes: overuse of a vein; irritating infusion solutions or medications; catheter left in vein for too long; use of large-gauge catheters.
B. Signs and symptoms: tenderness, pain along the course of the vein, edema, *redness at insertion site*, red streak along course of vein, *extremity with IV feels warmer than other extremity.*
C. Preventive nursing management.
   1. Change IV site every 72 to 96 hours or per policy.
   2. Use large veins to administer irritating solutions.
   3. Stabilize cannula.
   4. Dilute medications adequately and infuse at prescribed rates.
   5. Choose the smallest-gauge catheter possible to administer solutions.
D. Nursing interventions: apply warm, moist compresses to stimulate circulation and promote absorption.

**TEST ALERT:** Evaluate client response to parenteral fluid therapy.

E. Prevention of infections related to IV therapy (Box 9-1).

**TEST ALERT:** Delegate and assign appropriate task based on client's needs to personnel with competency to perform task.

F. Delegation of IV therapy

- Use a >0.5% chlorhexidine skin preparation with alcohol for antisepsis.
- Avoid routine replacement of central venous catheters.
- Select catheters on the bases of intended duration of use, known infectious and non-infectious complications and experience of individual catheter operators.
- Use a midline catheter or peripherally inserted central catheter instead of a short peripheral catheter when the duration of IV therapy will likely exceed six days.
- Remove peripheral venous catheters if the patient develops signs of phlebitis, infection, or a malfunctioning catheter.
- When adherence to aseptic technique cannot be ensured, replace the catheter as soon as possible.
- Perform hand hygiene by washing hands with conventional soap and water or with alcohol-based hand rubs. Hand hygiene should be performed before and after palpating, inserting, replacing, accessing, repairing or dressing an intravascular catheter site.
- Use either sterile gauze or sterile, transparent, semipermeable dressing to cover the catheter site.
- Replace catheter site dressing if the dressing becomes damp, loosened, or visibly soiled.
- Do not use topical antibiotic ointment on insertion sites.
- Replace dressings gauze dressings every 2 days and transparent dressings every 7 days.
- Use a sutureless securement device to reduce the risk of infection for IV catheters.
- Replace tubing used for blood, blood products, or fat emulsions within 24 hours of initiating the infusion.
- Replace tubing used to administer propofol infusions every 6 to 12 hours.

*Recommendation Update 2017: For patients aged 18 years and older, chlorhexidine-impregnated dressings with an FDA-cleared label that specifies a clinical indication for reducing catheter-related bloodstream infection (CRBSI) or catheter-associated bloodstream infection (CABSI) are recommended to protect the insertion site of short-term, non-tunneled central venous catheters. *IV,* Intravenous.
From Centers for Disease Control and Prevention (CDC). *2011 Guidelines for the prevention of intravascular catheter-related infections.* Updated February 15, 2017. Retrieved from https://www.cdc.gov/infectioncontrol/guidelines/BSI/index.html

## ACID–BASE BALANCE

### Basic Concepts of Acid–Base Balance

A. Terms used to describe acid–base balance.
   1. pH: the chemical abbreviation for negative logarithm of hydrogen ion concentration.
   2. $CO_2$: carbon dioxide.
   3. $Paco_2$: pressure of dissolved $CO_2$ gas in the blood.
   4. $O_2$: oxygen.
   5. $PaO_2$: pressure of dissolved $O_2$ gas in the blood.
   6. $HCO_3^-$: bicarbonate.
   7. mmHg: millimeters of mercury.
   8. $H^+$: hydrogen ion concentration.
B. Normal blood gas values (Table 9-1).
C. The hydrogen ion ($H^+$) concentration determines the acidity or alkalinity of a solution (pH); the higher the $H^+$ concentration, the more acidic the solution. An inverse

## Table 9-1 BLOOD GAS VALUES

| Component | Normal Values |
|---|---|
| pH | 7.4 (7.35–7.45) |
| $Pao_2$ | 80–100 mmHg |
| $Paco_2$ | 35–45 mmHg |
| $HCO_3^-$ | 22–26 mEq/L(mmol/L) |

### Acid Base Mnemonic (ROME)

Remember ROME—the acid–base mnemonic to interpret blood gas values.

| R | Respiratory |
|---|---|
| O | Opposite<br>pH ↑ $Pco_2$ ↓ Alkalosis<br>pH ↓ $Pco_2$ ↑ Acidosis |
| M | Metabolic |
| E | Equal<br>pH ↑ $HCO_3^-$ ↑ Alkalosis<br>pH ↓ $HCO_3^-$ ↓ Acidosis |

relationship exists between pH and $H^+$ concentration: Increased pH has fewer $H^+$ ions and is more alkaline; decreased pH has more $H^+$ ions and is more acidic (Figure 9-5).

D. Acid–base ratio is determined by sampling arterial blood. This provides a reliable index of overall body function.

E. The body maintains a normal or neutral state of acid–base balance. The stable concentration of $H^+$ balance is reflected in arterial blood with a relatively constant pH of 7.35 to 7.45.

F. It is necessary for the pH to remain relatively constant for the various enzyme systems of all body organs to function correctly.

G. $O_2$ saturation levels reflected in blood gas readings do not have a direct effect on the acid–base balance but are used to identify status of oxygenation.

H. A state of acid–base decompensation exists when the pH is either below 7.35 or above 7.45.

I. Compensation: The system not primarily affected is responsible for returning the pH to a more normal level.

J. Full compensation: the problem in the system primarily affected is corrected, thereby returning the pH to a more normal level.

K. $Paco_2$ imbalance: the origin or primary system is respiratory or it is compensating for a metabolic problem.

L. $HCO_3^-$ imbalance: the origin or primary system is metabolic or it is compensating for a respiratory problem.

M. The major clinical manifestations of an acid–base imbalance are indicative of central nervous system (CNS) involvement. The severity of the symptoms depends on the length of time the imbalance exists and the severity of the deviation.

1. Acidosis (metabolic or respiratory): symptoms are indicative of depression of the CNS; this is common.
2. Alkalosis (metabolic or respiratory): symptoms are indicative of increased stimulation of the CNS; death is a rare occurrence.

N. The normal ratio of $HCO_3^-$ to $Paco_2$ is 20:1; when this ratio is maintained, the pH is normal.

### Regulation of Acid–Base Balance

A. Buffer system: continuously regulates acid–base balance.
1. A buffer is a chemical that helps maintain a normal pH.
2. The buffer system chemicals are paired. The primary buffer chemicals are sodium bicarbonate ($NaHCO_3^-$) and carbonic acid ($H_2CO_3$). The buffers are capable of absorbing or releasing $H^+$ ions as indicated.
3. The body buffers an acid more effectively than it neutralizes a base.
4. An effective buffer system depends on normal-functioning respiratory and renal systems.

B. Respiratory system: the second most rapid response in regulating the acid–base balance. Carbonic acid is transported to the lungs, where it is converted to $CO_2$ and water, then excreted.
1. The amount of $CO_2$ in the blood is directly related to the carbonic acid concentrations.
2. Increased respirations will decrease $CO_2$ levels, thus decreasing the carbonic acid concentration and resulting in decreased $H^+$ concentration and an increase in the pH.
3. Decreased respirations will cause retention of $CO_2$, increasing the carbonic acid concentrations and resulting in increased $H^+$ concentration and a decrease in the pH.
4. With excessive acid formation, the respiratory center in the medulla is stimulated, which results in an increase in the depth and rate of respirations. This causes a

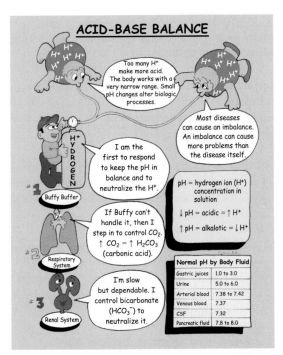

**FIGURE 9-5 Acid–Base Balance.** (From Zerwekh, J., Claborn, J., & Gaglione, T. [2010]. *Mosby's fluids and electrolytes memory notecards: Visual, mnemonic, and memory aids for nurses* [2nd ed.]. St. Louis, MO: Mosby.)

decrease in the $CO_2$ levels and returns the pH to a more normal point.

5. With excessive base formation, the respiratory rate slows to promote retention of $CO_2$ and decrease the alkalotic state. $CO_2$ is considered an acid substance because it combines with water to form carbonic acid. The $Paco_2$ levels are influenced only by respiratory causes.

6. If the respiratory system is the source of the pH alteration, then it loses the ability to correct the problem.

C. Renal system: the slowest, but very effective, mechanism of acid–base regulation.
1. The kidneys reabsorb sodium (Na) and produce and conserve sodium bicarbonate ($NaHCO_3^-$).
2. In acidosis, the $H^+$ concentration is increased; therefore, the $H^+$ ions are excreted before the potassium ($K^+$) ions, thereby precipitating hyperkalemia. When the acidosis is corrected, the potassium moves back into the cell.
3. In alkalosis, the $H^+$ concentration is decreased; there is an augmented renal excretion of $K^+$ ions, thereby precipitating hypokalemia.
4. If the renal system is the source of the pH alteration, it loses the ability to correct the problem.

## Alterations in Acid–Base Balance

**TEST ALERT:** Know laboratory values for arterial blood gases (ABGs), evaluate results of diagnostic testing, and intervene as needed.

A. **Respiratory acidosis:** characterized by excessive retention of $CO_2$ due to hypoventilation; therefore an increased carbonic acid concentration produces an increase in $H^+$ ions and a decrease in the pH (decreases below 7.35).
1. Causes.
   a. Depression of the respiratory center.
      (1) Head injuries.
      (2) Oversedation with sedatives and/or narcotics.
   b. Conditions affecting pulmonary function.
      (1) Obstructive pulmonary diseases.
      (2) Pneumonia.
      (3) Atelectasis.
   c. Conditions that interfere with chest wall excursion.
      (1) Thoracic trauma: flail chest.
      (2) Diseases affecting innervation of thoracic muscle (Guillain–Barré syndrome, myasthenia gravis, polio).
      (3) Mechanical hypoventilation.
2. Clinical manifestations.
   a. Rapid, shallow respirations (hypoventilation).
   b. Disorientation, decreased level of consciousness.
   c. Decreased blood pressure.
   d. Ventricular irritability related to hyperkalemia.
   e. Hypoxemia secondary to respiratory depression.

3. Blood gas values.
   a. pH decreases below 7.35.
   b. $Paco_2$ increases above 45 mmHg.
   c. $HCO_3^-$ remains normal, unless compensating, then increases.
4. Compensation/correction.
   a. Compensation: renal system will compensate by retaining $HCO_3^-$ and excreting increased amounts of $H^+$ ions.
   b. Correction: vigorous pulmonary hygiene to improve ventilation and decrease $Paco_2$ levels; may require mechanical ventilation and administration of sodium bicarbonate in select cases.
5. Nursing management.
   a. Preventive management.
      (1) Have client turn, cough, and deep breathe every 2 hours after surgery.
      (2) Use narcotics judiciously in the immediate postoperative period.
      (3) Maintain adequate hydration.
   b. Use semi-Fowler's position to facilitate deep breathing.
   c. Thoroughly assess client's pulmonary function.
   d. Perform postural drainage and percussion, followed by suction, to remove excessive pulmonary secretions.
   e. Anticipate the need for mechanical ventilation if client does not respond to pulmonary hygiene.
   f. Anticipate use of bronchodilator.
   g. Administer $O_2$ with caution, because it may precipitate $CO_2$ narcosis.
   h. Evaluate for hyperkalemia.
   i. Support renal system to promote adequate compensation.

**TEST ALERT:** Identify changes in respiratory status; provide pulmonary hygiene. The concept of respiratory acidosis may be tested in a variety of situations.

B. **Respiratory alkalosis:** characterized by a low $Paco_2$ due to hyperventilation. An excessive amount of $CO_2$ is exhaled, resulting in a decrease in $H^+$ concentration and an increase in pH (above 7.45).
1. Causes of respiratory alkalosis.
   a. Primary stimulation of CNS: hyperventilation.
      (1) Emotional origin (anxiety, fear, apprehension).
      (2) CNS infection (encephalitis).
      (3) Salicylate poisoning.
   b. Reflex stimulation of CNS.
      (1) Hypoxia stimulates hyperventilation (heart failure, pneumonia, pulmonary emboli).
      (2) Fever.
   c. Mechanical hyperventilation resulting in "overbreathing."
2. Clinical manifestations.
   a. Deep, rapid breathing (hyperventilation).
   b. CNS stimulation, resulting in confusion, lethargy, seizures.

c. Hypokalemia.

d. Hyperreflexia, muscle weakness, tingling of extremities.

3. Blood gas values.

a. pH increases above 7.45.

b. $Paco_2$ decreases below 35 mmHg.

c. $HCO_3^-$ remains normal, unless compensating, then decreases.

4. Compensation/correction.

a. Compensation: renal system will compensate by increasing $HCO_3^-$ excretion and retaining $H^+$ ions, thus returning pH to a more normal level.

b. Correction: prevent loss of $CO_2$ from respiratory systems.

5. Nursing management.

a. Identify and eliminate (if possible) causative factor.

b. Evaluate need for sedation.

c. Use rebreathing mask or techniques (paper bag, cupped hands) to increase $CO_2$ levels.

d. Remain with client to decrease anxiety levels.

C. **Metabolic acidosis:** characterized by a decrease in $HCO_3^-$ level in the serum, leading to an increase in $H^+$ concentration and a decrease in pH (below 7.35).

1. Causes (deficit of a base or an increase in acid).

a. Incomplete oxidation of fatty acids.

(1) Diabetic ketoacidosis.

(2) Starvation.

(3) Shock, resulting in lactic acidosis.

b. Abnormal loss of alkaline substances.

(1) Deep, prolonged vomiting may cause excessive loss of base products.

(2) Severe diarrhea and loss of pancreatic secretions.

c. Renal insufficiency and failure: kidneys lose ability to compensate for acid overload; thus $H^+$ ions are not excreted, nor is $HCO_3^-$ retained in normal amounts.

d. Salicylate poisoning due to accumulation of ketone bodies produced as a result of the increased metabolic rate.

2. Clinical manifestations.

a. Drowsiness, confusion, headache, disorientation.

b. Deep, rapid respirations (Kussmaul) compensatory action by the lungs.

c. GI problems: nausea, vomiting, diarrhea.

d. Dysrhythmias related to hyperkalemia.

e. Decreased blood pressure.

3. Blood gas values.

a. pH decreases below 7.35.

b. $Paco_2$ remains normal.

c. $HCO_3^-$ decreases below 22 mEq/L (mmol/L).

4. Compensation/correction.

a. Compensation: respiratory system compensates by increasing rate and depth of respirations to blow off $CO_2$ and increase the pH.

b. Correction: identification of the underlying problem and promotion of optimal function.

5. Nursing management.

a. Assist in identification of underlying problem.

b. In severe acidosis, $HCO_3^-$ may be given intravenously to neutralize acid and return pH to normal.

c. In clients with diabetes, evaluate for ketoacidosis and administer insulin accordingly.

d. Assess renal function and hydration status.

e. Maintain accurate intake and output records.

f. Evaluate laboratory values for hyperkalemia.

g. Support respiratory system to promote compensation.

D. **Metabolic alkalosis:** characterized by an increase in the $HCO_3^-$ levels in the serum, leading to a decrease in the $H^+$ concentration and an increase in the pH (increase above 7.45).

1. Causes (either an increase in serum $HCO_3^-$ or a decrease in serum $H^+$ concentration).

a. Diuretic therapy: loss of $H^+$, chloride ($Cl^-$), $K^+$ precipitates an increase in the $HCO_3^-$ level in the serum.

b. Excessive loss of $H^+$ ions.

(1) Prolonged nasogastric suctioning without adequate electrolyte replacement.

(2) Excessive vomiting, resulting in loss of hydrochloric acid and $K^+$.

c. Prolonged steroid therapy: loss of $H^+$, $Cl^-$, and $K^+$ ions, leading to an increased retention of $HCO_3^-$ by the kidneys.

d. Excessive intake of bicarbonate (baking soda).

e. Hypokalemia.

2. Clinical manifestations.

f. Nausea, vomiting.

g. Increased irritability, disorientation, restlessness.

h. Muscle cramping, tremors, seizures.

i. Shallow, slow respirations (hypoventilation).

j. Dysrhythmias (tachycardia) related to hypokalemia.

3. Blood gas values.

d. pH increases above 7.45.

e. $Paco_2$ remains normal.

f. $HCO_3^-$ increases above 26 mEq/L (28 mmol/L).

4. Compensation/correction.

a. Compensation: respiratory system will compensate by retaining $CO_2$ (hypoventilation) to compensate for the alkalosis.

b. Correction: replacement of electrolytes and fluids lost due to excessive renal excretion or due to excessive gastric loss of acid.

5. Nursing management.

a. Preventive.

(1) Provide foods high in potassium and chloride for client receiving diuretics.

(2) Administer potassium supplement to client receiving long-term diuretic therapy.

(3) Administer IV solution with replacement electrolytes.

b. Maintain accurate intake and output records.

c. Evaluate the laboratory values for a decrease in serum potassium levels.

# INFLAMMATION

Inflammation is the tissue response to localized injury or trauma. It is an expected response to tissue injury.

## Basic Concepts of Inflammation

A. Acute.
  1. Occurs rapidly.
  2. Neutrophils (white blood cells) arrive first and are usually the predominant cell.
  3. Essential for normal tissue repair.
B. Chronic.
  1. Characterized by pain, redness, and swelling.
  2. Persists longer than 2 weeks; has a damaging course that lasts for weeks, months, or even years.
  3. Examples: rheumatoid arthritis, tuberculosis, chronic glomerulonephritis.
C. Inflammatory response.
  1. Vascular response.
    a. Initial local vasoconstriction caused by tissue injury.
    b. Vasodilatation in area of injury.
    c. Hyperemia and increased capillary permeability lead to changes in osmotic pressure and a leakage of fluid (results in edema).
  2. Systemic response.
    a. Fever.
    b. Leukocytosis (increased numbers of neutrophils in circulation).
    c. Weight loss and nausea.
    d. Increased pulse and respiration.
    e. Increased erythrocyte sedimentation rate (ESR, sed rate).
D. Cardinal signs of inflammation (Table 9-2).
E. Healing process (see Wound Care in Chapter 3).

> ⚠ **NURSING PRIORITY:** Inflammation is necessary for normal healing to occur. A decrease in the normal inflammatory response will result in a decreased ability to heal.

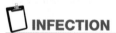

# INFECTION

**Infection is the process by which an organism (pathogen, pathogenic agent) invades the host and establishes a parasitic relationship. Infection may be localized, disseminated, or systemic.**

A. Health care–associated infections (HAIs, nosocomial infections): infections acquired from exposure to pathogens in a hospital setting or health care setting.
B. Development of multiple drug–resistant organisms (MDRO) has further complicated treatment of infections (they are resistant to antibiotics) such as methicillin-resistant *Staphylococcus aureus* (MRSA) and vancomycin-resistant *Enterococcus faecalis* (VRE).

## Chain of Transmission

A. Pathogens.
  1. Incubation period: the period of time from exposure to the pathogen until symptoms of infection occur in the host.
  2. A person can be asymptomatic and still transmit a pathogen that will produce an infection in someone else.
  3. Toxigenicity refers to the destructive potential of the toxin that is released by the pathogen.
B. Reservoir.
  1. Environment within which the organism can live and multiply; provided by some organic substance, human or animal.
  2. A carrier provides an environment in which the pathogen can grow and multiply but shows no symptoms of the infection.
C. Portal of exit.
  1. How the infection leaves the host.
  2. Common ports of exit include skin, mucous membranes, respiratory tract, feces, and body fluids.
  3. Understanding port of exit is necessary to prevent transmission of pathogens.
D. Route of transmission.
  1. Method by which the pathogen moves to another host.
  2. Direct transmission occurs by immediate transfer from one host to another, as in sexually transmitted diseases or by inhalation of contaminated droplets from respiratory tract infections.
  3. Indirect transmission occurs via an intermediate carrier (e.g., health care workers, mosquitoes, contaminated water, contaminated food).
E. Port of entry into susceptible host.
  1. May enter the host by inhalation or ingestion, through the mucous membranes, or percutaneously.
  2. Biologic and personal characteristics of the new host will determine the lines of defense that the host will have against the invading pathogen.
F. Control of transmission.
  1. Transmission of a contagious disease can be broken by interfering with any link of the transmission chain.
  2. Treatment is aimed at breaking the transmission chain at the most vulnerable and cost-effective point.
    a. Barrier precautions: gloves, gowns, condoms.
    b. Proper handling of food and water supplies.
    c. Avoidance of high-risk behavior: unsafe sex, IV drug use.

| Table 9-2 | CARDINAL SIGNS OF INFLAMMATION |
|---|---|
| *Clinical Symptom* | *Pathophysiology* |
| Redness | Hyperemia from vasodilation |
| Heat | Increased metabolism at site and local vasodilation |
| Pain | Pressure from fluid exudate on adjacent nerve endings, which leads to nerve stimulation; change in local pH |
| Edema | Fluid shift and accumulation in interstitial spaces |
| Loss of function | Decreased movement due to swelling and pain |

## Box 9-2 HAND HYGIENE

### Hand Hygiene With Soap and Water
- Handwashing should be done under flow of warm water.
- Using antibacterial soap, lather and wash hands using friction for 15 to 20 seconds, covering all surfaces of the hands and fingers.
- Rinse hands thoroughly under running water.
- Pat dry thoroughly using disposable towels and use towel to turn off the faucet.
- Wash hands with soap and water whenever hands are visibly soiled; otherwise, you can use hand rub (antiseptic cleanser).
- Wash hands before eating and after using a restroom.

### Hand Hygiene With Antiseptic Cleanser
- Rub hands together covering all surfaces of the hands and fingers with cleanser.
- Procedure should take 20 seconds.
- Rub hands together until cleanser is dry.
- Use if hands are not visibly soiled.
- Should not be used if client has *Clostridium difficile*, *Bacillus anthracis*, or *infectious diarrhea during norovirus* infection.

**NURSING PRIORITY:** Hand hygiene is the most important and most basic action to prevent transmission of infections. Hand hygiene must be performed before and after the use of gloves.

Centers for Disease Control and Prevention (CDC). *Hand hygiene in healthcare settings*. Retrieved from: https://www.cdc.gov/HandHygiene/

d. Good hand hygiene technique and good personal hygiene (Box 9-2).
e. Identification of carriers: skin test for tuberculosis, cultures for *Staphylococcus*.
3. Host susceptibility can be greatly reduced through immunizations (see Chapter 2).

## Prevention of Transmission of Infection in the Health Care Setting

A. Maintain standard precautions (see Appendix 9-3), especially good hand hygiene.
B. Consider all blood and body fluids from all clients to be contaminated.
C. Avoid contaminating outside of container when collecting specimens.
D. Do not recap needles and syringes.
E. Cleanse work surface areas with appropriate germicide (household bleach in concentration of 1:10 is effective).
F. Clean up spills of blood and body fluid immediately. Remove as much of the body fluid as possible, then wash the area with a germicide solution.
G. Follow Centers for Disease Control and Prevention (CDC) recommendations for immunization of health care workers (see Table 2-2).

**TEST ALERT:** Apply principles of infection control; understand incubation periods for infectious diseases; evaluate client response to treatment.

### Nursing Interventions
**Goal:** To prevent infection.

A. Hand hygiene is the single most effective mechanism for preventing spread of infection (see Box 9-2).
B. Monitor vital signs: increase in pulse, respiration, and temperature occurring 4 to 5 days after surgery may indicate infectious process.
C. Monitor for *Staphylococcus* and *Pseudomonas* pathogens (produce purulent, draining wounds).
D. Maintain aseptic technique in dressing changes and wound irrigations.
E. Maintain standard precautions (see Appendix 9-3).
F. Administer antibiotic medications (see Appendix 9-2).
G. Identify clients at increased risk for infections.
   1. Older adults (Box 9-3).
   2. Immunocompromised clients.
   3. Clients compromised by chronic health care problems.
   4. Poorly nourished clients.
   5. Client with high-risk lifestyle (IV drug use, unprotected sex).

**Goal:** To promote healing.

A. Encourage high fluid intake when client has a fever: 2000 to 3000 mL daily for adults.
B. Encourage a diet high in protein, carbohydrates, and vitamins—specifically vitamins A, C, and B complex.
C. Immobilize an injured extremity with a cast, splint, or bandage.
D. Administer antipyretic medications (see Appendix 3-2).
E. Identify early signs of infection to facilitate treatment (Box 9-4).

**Goal:** To decrease pain.

A. Cold packs applied after initial trauma may help decrease swelling and pain.
B. Heat may be used later to promote healing and to localize the inflammatory agents.
C. Elevate the injured area to decrease edema and promote venous return.

**TEST ALERT:** Use correct hand hygiene techniques—soap and water or an antimicrobial cleanser.

## Box 9-3 OLDER ADULT CARE FOCUS

### Infections
- Infection may be manifested by changes in behavior: confusion, disorientation.
- Client may not exhibit fever or pain.
- Closely monitor client response to antibiotics, especially with regard to renal function.
- Maintain adequate hydration.
- Monitor gastrointestinal function; diarrhea is common with antibiotics.

Box 9-4   SIGNS OF INFECTION

**Generalized**
- Fever, chills, increased pulse, increased respiratory rate, localized inflammation, joint pain, fatigue, and increased white blood cells

**Gastrointestinal Tract**
- Diarrhea, nausea, and vomiting

**Respiratory Tract**
- Purulent sputum, sore throat, chest pain, and congestion

**Urinary Tract**
- Urgency and frequency, hematuria, purulent discharge, dysuria, and flank pain

**Goal:** To prevent complications.

A. Identify clients with compromised immune response; they are at high risk for opportunistic infection.
B. Increase surveillance for clients with leukopenia or impaired circulation, clients receiving steroids or drugs that depress bone marrow, and clients exposed to a communicable disease.
C. Protect healing wounds from injury that could be caused by pulling or stretching.

**TEST ALERT:** Protect immunocompromised clients.

## Antibiotic-Resistant Infections
A. Common antibiotic-resistant organisms
 1. Methicillin-resistant *Staphylococcus aureus:* wound, skin and soft tissue, pneumonia, and bloodstream infections.
 2. Methicillin-resistant *Staphylococcus epidermidis*: skin and mucosa, common with catheter and implants.
 3. Aminoglycoside-resistant *Enterococcus faecalis and faecium*: oral root canals and urinary tract infections.
 4. Penicillin-resistant *Streptococcus pneumoniae:* pneumonia.
 5. Cephalosporin-resistant *Klebsiella pneumoniae:* pneumonia.
 6. Cephalosporin-resistant *Neisseria gonorrhoeae*: sexually transmitted infections
B. Transmission.
 1. Most common mode of transmission is from person to person, including from health care workers to hospitalized clients.
 2. HAIs.
C. Clients at increased risk.
 1. Treatment with multiple antibiotics.
 2. Multiple hospitalizations.
 3. Older adults with chronic conditions.
 4. Clients with compromised immune function.

*Treatment*
Cultures, followed by administration of antibiotics sensitive to bacteria.

*Nursing Interventions*
**Goal:** To decrease spread of infection.

A. Routine cultures of health care workers.
B. Identification of clients at increased risk.
C. Add contact precautions to the standard precautions.
 1. Private room.
 2. Gown and gloves.
 3. Masks are not necessary unless the client has a respiratory tract infection.
 4. Teach family the importance of gloves and gowns.
D. Notify nurse epidemiologist when client is diagnosed with an antibiotic-resistant infection.
E. A common mode of transmission is via the hands of health care workers; handwashing is critical, even before and after removal of gloves.

## CRITICAL CARE NURSING

## Sepsis
**Sepsis causes a systemic inflammatory response to infection.**

A. Gram-negative and gram-positive bacteria are primary organisms.
B. Increased risk in clients with urinary catheters, respiratory infections, invasive procedures (arterial lines, CVP, any indwelling line).
C. At-risk clients: older adults, clients with chronic health problems, clients with immunosuppression, and clients who are malnourished.
D. Exaggerated body response to an antigen, resulting in release of endotoxins that affect platelets and cause vasodilatation, increased capillary permeability, and development of multiple organ dysfunction syndrome (MODS).
E. Clinical manifestations.
 1. Hypo- or hyperthermia.
 2. Compromised respiratory function.
   a. Initially, hyperventilation occurs as a compensating mechanism.
   b. Hypoventilation and respiratory acidosis occur when compensation fails.
   c. Respiratory failure and development of adult respiratory distress syndrome (ARDS) (see Chapter 17).
 3. Compromised cardiac function.
   a. Tachycardia.
   b. Initially increased cardiac output with decreased systemic vascular resistance (SVR) secondary to hypermetabolic state.
   c. Cardiac decompensation with development of severe hypotension and MODS.
   d. Altered mental status.
   e. Significant edema.
   f. Oliguria.
 4. Development of severe hypotension progressing to septic shock despite adequate fluid resuscitation.
 5. Development of systemic inflammatory response syndrome (SIRS) progressing to MODS.

F. Diagnostics.
1. Leukocytosis or leukopenia.
2. Arterial hypoxemia.
3. Increased creatinine.
4. Coagulation abnormalities.
5. Thrombocytopenia.
6. Hyperglycemia.
7. Hyperlactatemia.
8. Hyperbilirubinemia.

*Treatment*

A. Prevention of infection.
B. Aggressive treatment of infections—administration of broad-spectrum antibiotic as soon as blood cultures are obtained.
C. Aggressive pulmonary support.
D. Fluid resuscitation—aggressive colloid therapy. Albumin if required to maintain hemodynamics.
E. Vasopressor—administration to maintain blood pressure.
F. Inotropic therapy—administration to maintain cardiac output.

*Nursing Interventions*

See care of a client in shock (Chapter 18).

## Systemic Inflammatory Response Syndrome and Multiple Organ Dysfunction Syndrome

**SIRS is a systemic inflammatory response secondary to a major body insult or trauma. MODS is the failure of two or major organ systems and occurs as a result of SIRS.**

A. Characteristics.
1. Risk factors.
a. SIRS occurs as a result of tissue injury.
(1) Tissue trauma: burns, crush injuries, surgery.
(2) Ischemic or necrotic tissue: infarctions (myocardial, intestinal), pancreatitis, vascular disease.
(3) Invasion of pathogens (bacterial, viral, fungal infection).
(4) Endotoxin release from gram-negative and gram-positive bacteria.
b. SIRS is characterized by overwhelming inflammation of organs involved.
c. Transition from SIRS to MODS is not clearly understood.
d. Organ perfusion is compromised secondary to hypertension, decreased perfusion, microemboli, and shunting of blood flow.
B. Clinical manifestations.
1. Precipitating event.
2. Respiratory: increased vascular permeability leads to alveoli collapse and development of ARDS.
3. Cardiac compromise, decreased SVR, and vasodilation lead to severe hypotension and decreased cardiac output.
4. Neurologic problems of confusion, agitation, and lethargy.
5. Acute renal failure secondary to decreased renal perfusion.
6. Gastrointestinal (GI) tract problems are abdominal distention and paralytic ileus.
7. Hypermetabolic response with hyperglycemia and insulin resistance.
8. Failure of the coagulation system leads to development of disseminated intravascular coagulopathy (DIC).
9. Electrolyte imbalances: hypokalemia, hypocalcemia, hypomagnesemia, and hypophosphatemia.

*Treatment*

A. Prevention.
1. Prevent development of HAIs.
2. Surgical removal or debridement of necrotic or damaged tissue.
3. Maintain positive nitrogen balance for wound healing.
B. Aggressive treatment of existing infection.
C. Support of involved organs.

*Nursing Interventions*

**Goal:** Prevention and/or early detection of infection.

A. Identify clients at increased risk for development of SIRS and MODS.
B. Strict asepsis for clients with urinary catheter, IV sites, endotracheal tube, arterial line, and wound care.
C. Aggressive pulmonary hygiene.
D. Strict adherence to standard precautions (see Appendix 9-3).

**Goal:** Maintain tissue oxygenation (see Chapter 17).

A. Monitor for respiratory failure and hypoxia.
B. Decrease oxygen demand and increase oxygen delivery: supplemental oxygen, adequate hemoglobin level, sedation, mechanical ventilation.

**Goal:** Support nutritional needs.

A. Provide protein and calories to support hypermetabolic state.
B. Provide enteral feedings to maintain positive nitrogen balance (see Appendix 20-3).
C. Monitor glucose levels; preferably maintain levels below 150 mg/dL.
D. Close monitoring of fluid balance.

**Appendix 9-1    POTASSIUM, SODIUM, AND CALCIUM IMBALANCES AND CORRECTING MEDICATIONS**

## Electrolyte Imbalances: Potassium

| *Causes* | *Symptoms* | *Nursing Implications* |
|---|---|---|

**Normal Serum Potassium (K) Levels:** 3.5–5.0 mEq/L (mmol/L)

**Hypokalemia:** Serum $K^+$ below 3.5 mEq/L (mmol/L)

| Causes | Symptoms | Nursing Implications |
|---|---|---|
| Decreased intake of K<br>GI loss:<br>   Vomiting<br>   Diarrhea<br>   Fistulas<br>Nasogastric suction without replacement<br>Skin loss: diaphoresis<br>Excessive renal excretion:<br>   Loop diuretics<br>   Increasing aldosterone<br>   Alkalosis<br>Steroid therapy<br>Diabetics: insulin and glucose moves<br>   $K^+$ into cell | Fatigue, muscle weakness, hyporeflexia<br>Decreased muscle tone and reflexes<br>Confusion, drowsiness, fatigue bradycardia,<br>   weak irregular pulse<br>ECG changes: flat T wave, S-T depression,<br>   U waves, PVCs<br>GI: Decreased bowel sounds, develop-<br>   ment of ileus, nausea, vomiting | 1. Identify source of depletion.<br>2. Monitor $K^+$ levels.<br>3. Encourage foods high in $K^+$.<br>4. Replace $K^+$ (oral potassium supplements<br>   and IV).<br>5. Maintain accurate I&O records.<br>6. Evaluate for digitalis toxicity (low serum $K^+$<br>   potentiates digitalis).<br>7. Evaluate for alkalosis.<br>8. Provide client education regarding diuretics. |

**Hyperkalemia:** Serum $K^+$ above 5.0 mEq/L (mmol/L)

| Causes | Symptoms | Nursing Implications |
|---|---|---|
| Decreased urinary excretion:<br>   Renal failure<br>Decreased aldosterone<br>Decreased secretion<br>Potassium-sparing diuretics<br>Massive tissue injury:<br>   Burns<br>   Trauma<br>   Fever, sepsis<br>Excessive administration of IV $K^+$<br>Salt substitutes containing potassium<br>ACE inhibitors<br>Acidosis | Drowsiness<br>Muscle weakness and twitching paresthesia<br>   of hands and feet and around the mouth<br>GI—diarrhea with hyperactive bowel<br>   sounds<br>ECG changes:<br>   Peaked T waves<br>   Prolonged P-R interval<br>   Widened QRS complex<br>Dysrhythmias:<br>   Bradycardia with ventricular ectopic<br>     beats (irregular pulse)<br>   Ventricular fibrillation<br>   Cardiac arrest (Figure 9-6) | 1. Identify origin of increase.<br>2. Monitor $K^+$ levels.<br>3. Administer loop or thiazide diuretics and<br>   fluids, if renal function is adequate.<br>4. Administer insulin to initiate $K^+$ transfer into<br>   cell and hypertonic glucose (dextrose 50%).<br>5. Use exchange resins: sodium polystyrene<br>   sulfonate.<br>6. Place on cardiac monitor. Be prepared for a<br>   cardiac emergency.<br>7. Maintain accurate I&O records.<br>8. Sodium bicarbonate (1 mEq/kg) for acidosis. |

## Medications to Correct Potassium Imbalance

### Potassium Supplements

Oral:
- Potassium chloride (KCl)
- Sustained release:
  - K-Dur, Micro-K, Slow-K
  - Potassium gluconate

IV:
- Potassium chloride
- ▲ High-Alert Medication (Box 8-1)

1. Sustained-release preparations are better tolerated and more convenient.
2. Oral preparations generally have unpleasant taste and are irritating to GI system; they should be administered with a full glass of water or juice.
3. Make sure client is urinating adequately before beginning supplementation. Monitor BUN and creatinine.
4. IV potassium *must* be diluted and administered by slow IV drip. Do not give $K^+$ IM or by IV push; may cause cardiac arrest. Administer no faster than 10 mEq/hr in adults.
5. IV potassium solutions are irritating to the vein and must be diluted (preferably to 40 mEq/L or less). If pain occurs, either slow the infusion rate or dilute solution in larger volume of fluid.
6. Administer with caution to clients with heart disease and those taking digitalis preparations.

### Exchange Resin

Sodium polystyrene sulfonate:
PO or rectal retention enema
(Medication is not absorbed
   systemically.)

1. Laxatives are given to facilitate excretion of the resin.
2. Cleansing enema precedes the sodium polystyrene sulfonate retention enema to enhance effectiveness.
3. Carefully evaluate the client with HF and/or hypertension.
4. Monitor serum electrolytes.
5. Use with caution in clients requiring sodium restriction.

**Appendix 9-1 POTASSIUM, SODIUM, AND CALCIUM IMBALANCES AND CORRECTING MEDICATIONS—cont'd**

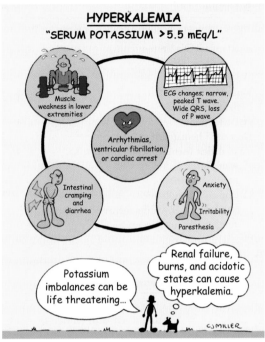

**FIGURE 9-6 Hyperkalemia.** (From Zerwekh, J., Claborn, J., & Gaglione, T. [2010]. *Mosby's fluids and electrolytes memory notecards: Visual, mnemonic, and memory aids for nurses* [2nd ed.]. St. Louis, MO: Mosby.)

## Electrolyte Imbalances: Sodium

| Causes | Symptoms | Nursing Implications |
|---|---|---|

**Normal Serum Sodium (Na⁺) Levels:** 135–145 mEq/L (mmol/L)

**Hyponatremia:** Serum Na⁺ below 135 mEq/L (mmol/L) (loss of sodium or water excess)

| Causes | Symptoms | Nursing Implications |
|---|---|---|
| Inadequate Na⁺ intake (rare)<br>Loss of sodium-rich fluids<br>Cystic fibrosis<br>Fluid gain, overhydration (dilutional)<br>Increased renal excretion:<br>• Thiazide diuretics<br>• Adrenal insufficiency—Addison disease<br>• Increased ADH or SIADH<br>Edema<br>Excessive administration of D₅W<br>GI losses<br>Massive tissue injury:<br>• Burns<br>• Trauma | **Solution deficit (Na⁺ loss):**<br>CNS problems: changes in level of consciousness, confusion, seizures<br>Weakness, restlessness<br>Oliguria<br>Abdominal cramps<br>Postural hypotension<br>Cold and clammy skin<br>*Dilutional hyponatremia (water excess):*<br>CNS problems: confusion, headache, seizures<br>Hypertension<br>Muscle twitching, cramping<br>Increased urine<br>Weight gain | 1. Identify source of depletion.<br>2. Maintain accurate I&O records, and determine weight daily (best measurement of fluid status).<br>3. Irrigate nasogastric tubes with normal saline solution.<br>4. 0.9% NaCl (normal saline) IV or half-strength 0.45% NaCl if client has sodium deficit.<br>5. If seizures are present, may administer IV hypertonic solution containing 3% NaCl.<br>6. Monitor blood pressure.<br>7. Restrict fluid intake if client has fluid excess.<br>8. Occurs in clients who are NPO, taking diuretics, perspiring, vomiting, having diarrhea, and in clients with burns or excessive administration of D₅W.<br>9. Occurs in renal disease, Addison disease, and diabetic acidosis. |

⚠ **NURSING PRIORITY:** Older adult clients and infants are at higher risk because of variations in total body water; carefully monitor clients receiving fluid replacement with D₅W.

*Continued*

**Appendix 9-1   POTASSIUM, SODIUM, AND CALCIUM IMBALANCES AND CORRECTING MEDICATIONS—cont'd**

| Causes | Symptoms | Nursing Implications |
|---|---|---|

**Hypernatremia:** Serum Na+ above 145 mEq/L (mmol/L) (sodium retention or water loss)

| Causes | Symptoms | Nursing Implications |
|---|---|---|
| Decreased fluid intake<br>Excessive salt intake<br>Excessive water loss:<br>• Diarrhea<br>• Febrile state<br>Increased renal retention<br>Cushing syndrome | Fluid excess (Na$^+$ retention):<br>Pitting edema<br>Weight gain<br>Flushed skin<br>Lethargic<br>Hypertension<br>Decreased hematocrit<br>Fluid deficit (hemoconcentration of Na, water loss):<br>Concentrated urine<br>Dry mucous membranes<br>Flushed skin, tachycardia increased temperature, weight loss, decreased CVP | 1. Identify origin of increase.<br>2. Maintain accurate I&O records, and determine weight daily.<br>3. Administer D$_5$W IV if fluid is normal or there is a fluid deficit.<br>4. Administer diuretics to remove excess Na$^+$<br>5. Restrict fluid intake if client has fluid excess.<br>6. Assess for cerebral edema—lethargy, headache, nausea, vomiting, increased BP. |

## Medications to Correct Sodium Imbalance

| Medication | Nursing Implications |
|---|---|
| **Sodium Supplements**<br>Sodium chloride (NaCl, table salt)<br>Saline solutions: 3%, 0.9%, and 0.45% saline solution for infusion<br>▲ High-Alert Medication | 1. Administer with caution to clients with CHF, renal problems, edema, or hypertension.<br>2. Determine weight daily; maintain accurate I&O records to evaluate fluid retention.<br>3. Evaluate serum Na$^+$ levels.<br>4. Do not store containers of sodium chloride above a concentration of 0.9% (normal saline) on the nursing unit. |

## Electrolyte Imbalances:  Calcium

| Causes | Symptoms | Nursing Implications |
|---|---|---|

**Normal  Serum  Calcium  (Ca$^{++}$)  Levels:** 9–11 mg/dL (2.25-2.75 mmol/L) Hypocalcemia: Serum Ca$^{++}$ below 9 mg/dL (2.25 mmol/L) or below 3.0 mg/dL (1.1 mmol/L) in infants

* Note: A reciprocal relationship exists between phosphorus and calcium. (Figure 9-7)

| Causes | Symptoms | Nursing Implications |
|---|---|---|
| Acute pancreatitis<br>Laxative abuse<br>Dietary lack of Ca$^{++}$ and vitamin D<br>Hypoparathyroidism<br>Hyperphosphatemia<br>Excessive blood transfusions<br>Excessive IV fluids<br>Alkalosis | Tetany: $^{++}$Chvostek sign; $^{++}$Trousseau sign (Chapter 15)<br>Neuromuscular irritability<br>Numbness and tingling in extremities or around mouth<br>Laryngeal stridor<br>Seizures<br>Abdominal cramping and distention<br>Hyperreflexia<br>Dysrhythmias | 1. Identify origin of deficiency.<br>2. Keep Ca$^{++}$ replacement medications easily accessible for clients who have had thyroid or parathyroid surgically removed.<br>3. Assess for tetany.<br>4. Reduce environmental stimuli for both adults and infants.<br>5. Institute seizure precautions.<br>6. Provide client education regarding Ca$^{++}$ intake. |
| **Infants:**<br>*Early onset*—decreased activity of parathyroid; infants of diabetic mothers; premature infants; exchange transfusion<br>*Late onset*—decreased dietary intake; infants who are fed evaporated milk formulas containing phosphorus; intestinal malabsorption | *Early onset in infant:* restlessness, edema, apnea, intermittent cyanosis, vomiting, abdominal distention, high-pitched cry<br>*Late onset in infant:* increasing CNS excitability | 1. Teach parents to use infant formulas and/or oral supplements until the child is 1 year old.<br>2. Do not give a child whole cow's milk until 1 year old. |

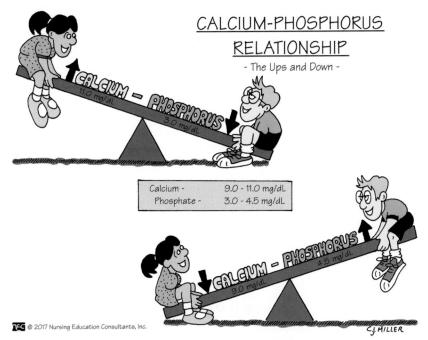

**FIGURE 9-7 Calcium–Phosphorus Relationship.** (Zerwekh, J., & Garneau, A., J., Miller, C. J. [2017]. *Digital collection of the memory notebooks of nursing* [4th ed.]. Chandler, AZ: Nursing Education Consultants, Inc.).

| Causes | Symptoms | Nursing Implications |
|---|---|---|
| **Hypercalcemia:** Serum Ca$^{++}$ above 11 mg/dL (2.75 mmol/L) | | |
| Metastatic malignancy<br>Hyperparathyroidism<br>Thiazide diuretics<br>Prolonged immobilization<br>Vitamin D overdose | Anorexia, nausea, constipation<br>CNS depression<br>Decreasing muscle tone, coordination<br>Pathologic fractures<br>Dysrhythmias—increases sensitivity to digitalis preparations<br>Kidney stones | 1. Identify origin of increase.<br>2. Administer loop diuretics to facilitate removal of serum Ca$^+$, normal saline fluid replacement.<br>3. Increase client's fluid intake 3000–4000 mL/24 hours.<br>4. Decrease Ca$^{++}$ intake.<br>5. Encourage client mobility.<br>6. Provide client education regarding supplemental vitamins.<br>7. Increase fiber intake.<br>8. Assess client taking digitalis for symptoms of toxicity. |

**Medications to Correct Calcium Imbalance**

| Medication | Action | Nursing Implications |
|---|---|---|
| **Calcium Salts** | | |
| Calcium citrate: PO<br>Calcium gluconate: IV, PO<br>Calcium carbonate: PO<br>Loop diuretics may be used to enhance excretion of calcium in treatment of hypercalcemia. | Activator for coagulation enzyme factors<br>Necessary for cardiac muscle function<br>IV infusion for treatment of hypocalcemic tetany<br>Adjunctive therapy to prevent hypocalcemia during exchange transfusion | 1. May be given in conjunction with vitamin D to enhance absorption.<br>2. PO supplements are more effective if taken ½–1 hr after meals.<br>3. Prevent IV infiltration; Ca1$^+$ solutions cause tissue hypoxia and sloughing.<br>4. Do not add Ca$^{++}$ preparations to solutions containing carbonates or phosphates.<br>5. Use with caution for client receiving digitalis.<br>6. Monitor infusion rate carefully; sudden increase in serum Ca$^{++}$ level may precipitate severe cardiac dysrhythmias.<br>7. Corticosteroids decrease Ca$^{++}$ absorption. Administer several hours apart. |

*Continued*

**Appendix 9-1   POTASSIUM, SODIUM, AND CALCIUM IMBALANCES AND CORRECTING MEDICATIONS—cont'd**

## Electrolyte Imbalances: Phosphorus

| Causes | Symptoms | Nursing Implications |
|---|---|---|

### Normal Serum Phosphorus Level (PO₄): 2.4–4.4 mg/dL (0.78–1.42 mmol/L)

### Hypophosphatemia: Serum phosphorus below 2.4 mg/dL (0.78 mmol/L)

*Note: A reciprocal relationship exists between phosphorus and calcium. (Figure 9-7)

| Causes | Symptoms | Nursing Implications |
|---|---|---|
| Malabsorption<br>Chronic diarrhea<br>Malnutrition, vitamin D deficiency<br>Parenteral nutrition<br>Chronic alcoholism<br>Phosphate-binding antacids<br>Diabetic ketoacidosis<br>Hyperparathyroidism<br>Refeeding syndrome<br>Respiratory alkalosis | CNS depression (confusion, coma)<br>Muscle weakness, including respiratory muscle weakness<br>Polyneuropathy, seizures<br>Cardiac problems (dysrhythmias, heart failure)<br>Osteomalacia, rickets<br>Rhabdomyolysis | 1. Identify origin of deficiency.<br>2. Increase oral intake of foods high in phosphate and/or administer a supplement, e.g., dairy.<br>3. Symptomatic clients may require IV administration of sodium phosphate or potassium phosphate.<br>4. Monitor for hypocalcemia, hyperkalemia, hypotension, and dysrhythmias during IV administration. |

### Hyperphosphatemia: Serum Phosphorus above 4.4 mg/dL (1.42 mmol/L)

| Causes | Symptoms | Nursing Implications |
|---|---|---|
| Renal failure<br>• Phosphate enemas (e.g., Fleet enema)<br>Excessive ingestion (e.g., phosphate-containing laxatives)<br>Rhabdomyolysis<br>Tumor lysis syndrome<br>Thyrotoxicosis<br>Hypoparathyroidism<br>Sickle cell anemia, hemolytic anemia<br>Hyperthermia | Hypocalcemia<br>Numbness and tingling in extremities and region around mouth<br>Hyperreflexia, muscle cramps<br>Tetany, seizures<br>Calcium-phosphate precipitates in skin, soft tissue, cornea, viscera, blood vessels | 1. Identify origin of increase and treat underlying cause.<br>2. Administer oral phosphate-binding agents (e.g., calcium carbonate) to facilitate removal of excess.<br>3. Restrict foods high in phosphate (e.g., dairy products).<br>4. Increase client's fluid intake 3000–4000 mL/24 hours.<br>5. Volume expansion and forced diuresis with a loop diuretic may facilitate phosphorus excretion.<br>6. Hemodialysis may be required with severe cases. |

## Medications to Correct Phosphorus Imbalance

| Medication | Action | Nursing Implications |
|---|---|---|
| **Inorganic Phosphates**<br>**Calcium-Based Phosphate Binders**<br>Calcium carbonate: PO<br>Calcium acetate: PO<br>**Calcium-Free Phosphate Binders**<br>Sevelamer carbonate: PO<br>Lanthanum: PO | Both groups of binders have GI effects<br>Calcium-based phosphate binders promote hypercalcemia | 1. Medication taken daily with meals.<br>2. Monitor calcium levels with calcium-based phosphate binders.<br>3. Calcium-free phosphate binders are more expensive but do not promote hypercalcemia or metabolic acidosis. |

## Electrolyte Imbalances: Magnesium

| Causes | Symptoms | Nursing Implications |
|---|---|---|

### Normal Serum Magnesium (Mg⁺) Levels: 1.5–2.5 mg/dL (0.75–1.25 mmol/L)

### Hypomagnesemia: Serum Mg⁺ below 1.5 mg/dL (0.75 mmol/L)

| Causes | Symptoms | Nursing Implications |
|---|---|---|
| GI tract fluid losses (e.g., diarrhea, NG suction)<br>Chronic alcoholism<br>Malabsorption syndromes<br>Prolonged malnutrition<br>↑ Urine output<br>Hyperglycemia<br>Proton pump inhibitor therapy | * Symptoms similar to hypocalcemia<br>Confusion<br>Muscle cramps<br>Tremors, seizures<br>Vertigo<br>Hyperactive deep tendon reflexes<br>Chvostek's and Trousseau's signs<br>↑ Pulse, ↑ BP, dysrhythmias<br>Associated with digitalis toxicity | 1. Identify origin of deficiency.<br>2. Administer oral magnesium supplements and encourage foods high in magnesium (e.g., dark chocolate, avocados, nuts, legumes, tofu, leafy greens).<br>3. Assess for tetany.<br>4. Reduce environmental stimuli for both adults and infants.<br>5. Institute seizure precautions.<br>6. If hypomagnesemia is severe or if hypocalcemia is present, IV magnesium (e.g., magnesium sulfate) is administered.<br>7. Assess client taking digitalis for symptoms of toxicity. |

| Appendix 9-1 | POTASSIUM, SODIUM, AND CALCIUM IMBALANCES AND CORRECTING MEDICATIONS—cont'd |
|---|---|

| Causes | Symptoms | Nursing Implications |
|---|---|---|

**Hypermagnesemia:** Serum Mg⁺ above 2.5 mg/dL (1.25 mmol/L)

| Renal failure<br>IV administration of<br>  magnesium, especially<br>  for treatment of<br>  eclampsia<br>Tumor lysis syndrome<br>Hypothyroidism<br>Metastatic bone disease<br>Adrenal insufficiency<br>Antacids, laxatives | Lethargy, drowsiness<br>Muscle weakness<br>Urinary retention<br>Nausea, vomiting<br>Diminished deep tendon reflexes<br>Flushed, warm skin, especially facial<br>↓ Pulse, ↓ BP | 1. Identify origin of increase.<br>2. Limit dietary intake of foods high in magnesium (e.g., dark chocolate, avocados, nuts, legumes, tofu, leafy greens).<br>3. Administer diuretics if client's renal function is adequate to promote urinary excretion of magnesium.<br>4. Increase client's fluid intake 3000–4000 mL/24 hours.<br>5. Administer IV calcium gluconate, if client is symptomatic to oppose the effect of the high level of Mg on cardiac muscle. |

### Medications to Correct Magnesium Imbalance

| Medication | Action | Nursing Implications |
|---|---|---|
| Magnesium oxide: PO<br>Magnesium sulfate: IV | Excessive levels of magnesium cause neuromuscular blockade – leads to respiratory depression<br>Excessive oral doses may cause diarrhea | 1. IV administration preferred treatment for severe deficiency.<br>2. Calcium gluconate can reverse excess effects.<br>3. See Appendix 26-2 for obstetrical implications of magnesium administration. |

*ADH*, Antidiuretic hormone; *BP*, blood pressure; *CNS*, central nervous system; *CVP*, central venous pressure; *D₅W*, 5% dextrose in water; *ECG*, electrocardiogram; *GI*, gastrointestinal; *HF*, heart failure; *I&O*, intake and output; *IM*, intramuscularly; *IV*, intravenous; *NPO*, nothing by mouth; *PO*, by mouth (orally); *PVCs*, premature ventricular contractions; *SIADH*, syndrome of inappropriate antidiuretic hormone secretion.

| Appendix 9-2 | MEDICATIONS: ANTIINFLAMMATORY AND ANTIBIOTIC |
|---|---|

### Antiinflammatory Medications General Nursing Implications

- Give oral medications with or after meals to decrease GI irritation and side effects.
- After therapy, withdrawal from steroids *must be done* gradually.
- For clients on long-term therapy, increased amounts of corticosteroids will be required during periods of stress such as surgery.
- Decreases client's ability to respond to and fight infection.
- Closely evaluate the client on digitalis preparations and thiazide diuretics for the development of hypokalemia.
- Use with nonsteroidal antiinflammatories (NSAIDs) increases risk for intestinal irritation and perforation (see Appendix 3-2).
- Uses: inflammatory conditions—respiratory, gastrointestinal, joint inflammation, and skin conditions. Adrenocortical hormone replacement is necessary if adrenal glands are insufficient or have been removed. Suppress rejection of transplanted organs.

| Medications | Side Effects | Nursing Implications |
|---|---|---|

**Adrenocortical Hormones (Corticosteroids, Glucocorticoids) Antiinflammatory Action:** Inhibit synthesis of chemical mediators (histamine, prostaglandins), thereby suppressing inflammatory response. Suppress infiltration of area by phagocytes and suppress production of lymphocytes, further reducing the immune response and inflammation. During stress, an increased release of corticosteroids occurs to maintain blood pressure and plasma levels of glucose. Used as immunosuppressant for delaying organ rejection. Long-term use will suppress the function of the adrenal glands.

| Hydrocortisone base: PO<br>Hydrocortisone sodium<br>  succinate: IV, IM<br>Dexamethasone: PO, IV, IM,<br>  topical<br>Prednisone: PO<br>Methylprednisolone: PO, IM,<br>  IV<br>Methylprednisolone sodium<br>  succinate: IV | Increased susceptibility to infections (bodywide)<br>GI upset, gastric irritation<br>Osteoporosis<br>Psychological disturbances (depression, euphoria)<br>Hypokalemia<br>Hyperglycemia<br>Hypertension (caused by sodium and water retention)<br>Cushing syndrome: moon face, buffalo hump, distended abdomen, thin arms and legs, excessive hair growth<br>Cataracts | 1. Administer medication before 9:00 a.m. to decrease adrenal cortical suppression.<br>2. Monitor for psychological changes.<br>3. Decrease salt intake in diet; encourage high-protein and high-potassium diet.<br>4. Determine weight daily; evaluate weight gain and blood pressure.<br>5. Topical steroids usually do not provoke physical evidence of absorption. |

*Continued*

**Appendix 9-2  MEDICATIONS: ANTIINFLAMMATORY AND ANTIBIOTIC—cont'd**

| *Medications* | *Side Effects* | *Nursing Implications* |
|---|---|---|

| | | *Teaching:* Take medication in the morning with food. |

| | 🛑 **NURSING PRIORITY:** It is critical that clients on corticosteroids do not stop taking the medications abruptly. This can result in a significant drop in blood pressure and hypoglycemia. Clients should advise all their health care providers if they are on steroids. | Diet should include adequate $K^+$ intake and decreased $Na^+$ intake. <br> Do not stop taking the medication or change the dosing without a doctor's order. <br> Report to health care provider: any early signs of infection; or a weight gain of 5 lb or more in a week. <br> Do not take a live virus vaccine (MMR, varicella). <br> Do not take with aspirin products. |

## Antibiotic Medications: General nursing implications

- Always assess for antibiotic allergies, especially for penicillin and sulfa, before administration.
- If cultures are ordered, they should be obtained before the administration of the first dose.
- Teach the client to finish the entire prescribed course of medication even though he or she may feel well.
- Schedule PO, IM, and IV administration at evenly spaced intervals around the clock.
- Give most oral antibiotic drugs on an empty stomach (1 hour before or 2 hours after meals) at evenly spaced intervals around the clock.
- Take medications with a full glass of water.
- Observe for *hypersensitivity:*
  - Anaphylaxis—hypotension, respiratory distress, urticaria, angioedema, vomiting, diarrhea
- Serum sickness—fever, vasculitis, generalized lymphadenopathy, edema of joints, bronchospasm
- Observe for *superinfection:*
  - Stomatitis—sore mouth, white patches on oral mucosa, black furry tongue
  - Pseudomembranous colitis—diarrhea, abdominal pain, and cramping
  - Monilial vaginitis—rash in perineal area, itching, vaginal discharge
  - New localized signs and symptoms—redness, heat, edema, pain, drainage, cough
  - Recurrence of systemic signs and symptoms—elevated WBCs, fever, malaise

## Penicillin: Bactericidal: Interferes with the formation of the bacterial cell wall

| **Natural penicillins** | Parenteral injection—more hazardous than oral administration | 1. Observe for allergic reactions and have emergency equipment available. |
|---|---|---|
| Penicillin G: IM | Diarrhea, especially in children | 2. Amoxicillin can be scheduled without regard to meals. |
| Penicillin V: PO, IV | Allergic reactions: skin rashes, joint pain, dermatitis, kidney damage | 3. Observe client for 30 minutes after IM or IV administration for symptoms of allergic reactions. |
| **Aminopenicillins** | Anaphylactic reaction (hypersensitivity): decreased BP, increased pulse, respiratory distress, diaphoresis | 4. Clients with beta-hemolytic strep infections should receive penicillin for a minimum of 10 days to prevent development of rheumatic fever or glomerulonephritis. |
| Amoxicillin: PO | Ticarcillin—hypernatremia | 5. Discard liquid forms of penicillin after 7 days at room temperature and 14 days when refrigerated. |
| Amoxicillin with clavulanic acid: PO | | 6. For IV administration, dilute reconstituted penicillin in 50–100 mL of 5% dextrose or 0.9% sodium chloride injection and infuse over 30–60 minutes. |
| Ampicillin: PO, IM, IV | | |
| **Penicillinase-Resistant Penicillins** | | |
| Cloxacillin: PO | | |
| Dicloxacillin: PO | | |
| Nafcillin: IV | | |
| Oxacillin: IM, IV | | |
| **Extended-Spectrum Penicillin** | | |
| Carbenicillin: PO | | |
| Piperacillin: IV, IM | | |
| Piperacillin/Tazobactam: IV | | |
| Ticarcillin disodium: IM, IV | | |

## Aminoglycoside: Bactericidal: Interferes with protein synthesis

| Gentamicin: IM, IV | Ototoxicity—hearing loss is irreversible | 1. Monitor serum peak and trough levels to determine toxic levels. |
|---|---|---|
| Amikacin: IM, IV | Nephrotoxicity—albuminuria, casts, oliguria, elevated BUN and serum creatinine | 2. Neurotoxicity may be increased if given soon after surgery. |
| Streptomycin: IM | Skin rash, headache, hypotension, pain, and tenderness at injection site | 3. Assess for ototoxicity (change in hearing, ringing in the ears, dizziness, or unsteady gait) and nephrotoxicity (monitor BUN and creatinine). |
| Tobramycin: IM, IV | Oral neomycin is not absorbed systemically | 4. Not commonly used for long-term therapy. |
| Neomycin sulfate: PO, PR, topical, ophthalmic | | 5. Encourage PO fluids of 2000–3000 mL of fluid daily. |
| | | 6. For IV piggyback medications, administer over 60 minutes. |
| | | 7. Neomycin PO may be used to suppress intestinal flora before surgery and to suppress ammonia formation in clients with cirrhosis. |

**Appendix 9-2    MEDICATIONS: ANTIINFLAMMATORY AND ANTIBIOTIC—cont'd**

| Medications | Side Effects | Nursing Implications |
|---|---|---|

### Cephalosporins: Bactericidal: Broad-spectrum; interfere with the formation of the bacterial cell wall

| Medications | Side Effects | Nursing Implications |
|---|---|---|
| **First Generation**<br>Cefadroxil: PO<br>Cephalexin: PO<br>Cefazolin: IM, IV<br>Cephradine: IV, PO<br>**Second Generation**<br>Cefaclor: PO<br>Cefuroxime: PO, IM, IV<br>Axetil: PO<br>Cefprozil: PO<br>Cefoxitin: IM, IV<br>Cefotetan: IV<br>**Third Generation**<br>Cefpodoxime: PO<br>Ceftibuten: PO<br>Cefdinir: PO<br>Cefotaxime: IV<br>Ceftizoxime: IV<br>Ceftazidime: IM, IV<br>Ceftriaxone: IM, IV<br>**Fourth Generation**<br>Cefepime: IM, IV<br>**Fifth Generation**<br>Ceftaroline: IV | Hypersensitivity—rash, superinfection<br>GI upset, neutropenia (decreased WBCs), pain at injection site, renal damage, seizures | 1. Give oral cephalosporins with food or milk.<br>2. Administer IM medications deep into the muscle.<br>3. Use caution when given to clients with a known allergy to penicillin.<br>4. Decrease phlebitis at IV site by diluting solution and administering it slowly.<br>5. Antibacterial activity increases from first generation to fourth generation: treatment usually begins with first generation to prevent development of increased resistance. |

### Carbapenems: Bactericidal and inhibit cell wall synthesis

| Medications | Side Effects | Nursing Implications |
|---|---|---|
| Imipenem/cilastatin: IM, IV<br>Meropenem<br>Ertapenem<br>Doripenem | Seizures<br>GI upset: diarrhea, nausea, vomiting<br>Thrombocytopenia, elevation of liver enzymes<br>Meropenem can cross blood–brain barrier and is used for bacterial meningitis | 1. Broadest antibacterial action of any antibiotics to date.<br>2. Effective against many gram-positive organisms.<br>3. Risk of cross-allergenicity with penicillin allergy—do not deliver for those with anaphylactic-type reaction to penicillins. |

### Tetracyclines: Bacteriostatic: Broad-spectrum; interfere with protein synthesis of infectious organism and thus diminish its growth and reproduction

| Medications | Side Effects | Nursing Implications |
|---|---|---|
| Tetracycline: PO, IV, IM<br>Doxycycline: PO, IV<br>Demeclocycline: PO<br>Minocycline: PO, IV<br>Oxytetracycline: PO<br>Tigecycline: IV | PO may cause GI irritation (loose stools, diarrhea), sore throat, photosensitivity<br>Diarrhea may indicate severe superinfection (pseudomembranous colitis) in bowel<br>Discoloration of teeth in children up to 8 years old<br>Can cause staining of developing teeth in the fetus if taken after fourth month of gestation and in children before permanent teeth have come in<br>Photosensitivity | 1. Administer on empty stomach; withhold antacids, dairy foods, and foods high in calcium at least 2 hours after PO administration; do not administer with milk.<br>2. Can give doxycycline and minocycline with food.<br>3. Do not give at the same time as iron preparations. Give them as far apart as possible (e.g., 2–3 hours).<br>4. Advise client to avoid direct or artificial sunlight.<br>5. If diarrhea occurs, important to determine cause.<br>6. Observe for development of superinfections. |

### Monobactams: Bactericidal: Synthetic beta-lactam

| Medications | Side Effects | Nursing Implications |
|---|---|---|
| Aztreonam: IM, IV | Rash, nausea, vomiting, and diarrhea | 1. Often combined with other antibiotics for treatment of intraabdominal and gynecologic infections. |

*Continued*

**Appendix 9-2  MEDICATIONS: ANTIINFLAMMATORY AND ANTIBIOTIC—cont'd**

Ⓡ

| Medications | Side Effects | Nursing Implications |
|---|---|---|
| **Sulfonamides:** Bacteriostatic: Suppress bacterial growth by inhibiting synthesis of folic acid | | |
| Sulfisoxazole: PO, IV, IM Trimethoprim sulfamethoxazole (also referred to as TMP-SMZ): PO, IV | Blood dyscrasias—hemolytic anemia Hypersensitivity—rash, "drug fever," photosensitivity Renal dysfunction—crystalluria (irritation and obstruction) (Stevens–Johnson syndrome) | 1. Encourage 8–10 glasses of water per day to prevent crystalluria. 2. Contraindicated during pregnancy and for nursing mothers and infants under 2 months of age. 3. Avoid prolonged exposure to sun. |
| **Macrolides:** Bacteriostatic: Inhibit protein synthesis | | |
| Erythromycin base: PO Azithromycin: PO, IV Clarithromycin: PO | Nausea, vomiting, abdominal distress, diarrhea Cholestatic hepatitis: abnormal liver function studies, jaundice, fever | 1. Administer with a full glass of water. |
| **Quinolones:** Bactericidal: Inhibit bacterial DNA | | |
| Ciprofloxacin: PO, IV Levofloxacin: PO, IV Norfloxacin: PO Moxifloxacin: PO, IV Gemifloxacin: PO | GI: Nausea, vomiting, abdominal distress, diarrhea CNS: dizziness, headache, confusion Superinfections, hypersensitivity Tendon rupture with Cipro | 1. Absorption is reduced by milk products, antacids. 2. Administer IV infusions over 60 minutes. 3. Instruct client to report joint pain promptly. |
| **Other Antibiotics** | | |
| Metronidazole: PO, IV | Nausea, dry mouth, headache Disulfiram reaction when taken with alcohol: nausea, copious vomiting, flushing, palpitations, headache; may last 30 minutes to an hour | 1. Classified as an antiprotozoal antibiotic; is effective against anaerobic microorganisms. 2. Avoid concurrent use with alcohol or products containing alcohol. Will cause a disulfiram (Antabuse) reaction. |
| Clindamycin: PO, IV, topical | Mild nausea, vomiting, or stomach pain, and joint pain. Vaginal itching or discharge Monitor for diarrhea—risk of pseudomembranous colitis. | 1. Bactericidal or bacteriostatic, depends on the concentration of drug. 2. Contraindicated in those with ulcerative colitis or enteritis. 3. High risk for pseudomembranous colitis development. |
| Vancomycin: PO, IV | Ototoxicity, thrombophlebitis at site Red man syndrome: flushing, rash, pruritus, tachycardia, and hypotension | 1. Acts by inhibiting cell wall synthesis; used only for serious infections. 2. IV infusions over at least 60 minutes to prevent adverse effects. 3. Serum peak and trough levels are monitored. 4. Used to treat MRSA. |
| Linezolid: PO, IV | GI: diarrhea, nausea Myelosuppression—anemia, leukopenia, thrombocytopenia | 1. New class of antibiotics—oxazolidinones. 2. Monitor for blood dyscrasias. 3. Reserved for treatment of infections from MDROs especially VRE. |
| **Antifungal** | | |
| Nystatin: PO, topical Amphotericin B: IV Fluconazole: PO, IV | GI: diarrhea, nausea, stomach pain, vomiting Amphotericin B: hypokalemia, cardiac dysrhythmias, neurotoxicity, renal toxicity and infusion-related fever, chills, headaches, malaise, hypotension, anemia. | 1. Used for treatment of candidiasis (mouth, esophagus, vagina). 2. Oral treatment: Encourage client to hold medication in their mouth and "swish" around to provide good contact with all affected areas. |

*BUN,* Blood urea nitrogen; *CBC,* complete blood count; *CNS,* central nervous system; *GI,* gastrointestinal; *IM,* intramuscular; *IV,* intravenous; *MDRO,* multiple drug–resistant organisms; *MRSA,* methicillin-resistant *Staphylococcus aureus;* PO, by mouth; VRE, vancomycin-resistant *Enterococcus faecalis.*

## General Information

- Many clients with disease-specific isolation precautions require only standard precautions.
- The specific substances covered by standard precautions include blood and all other body fluids, body secretions, and body excretions, even if blood is not visible. Moisture from perspiration (sweat) is an exception.
- Transmission-based precautions are followed, in addition to standard precautions, whenever a client is known or suspected to be infected with contagious pathogens.

## Standard Precautions

1. Wash hands before and after client care and after removing gloves. Wash hands immediately with soap and water if visibly contaminated with blood or body fluids.
2. Wear gloves if there is a possibility you might come in contact with any body fluid or contaminated surfaces or objects.
3. Change gloves between tasks and procedures on the same client if moving from a contaminated body area (perineal area) to a clean body area. Do not wash gloves for reuse.
4. Wear gloves, gown, eye protection (goggles, glasses) or face shield and a mask during procedures likely to generate droplets of blood or body fluids.
5. Wear a gown when there is risk clothing will come in contact with body fluids. Perform hand hygiene after removing the gown. Do not reuse gowns, even if they are not soiled.
6. Have used client care equipment properly cleaned; discard any single-use items after use.
7. Ensure that hospital procedures for routine care, cleaning, and disinfection of environmental surfaces, beds, bedrails, and bedside equipment are followed.
8. Place contaminated linens in a leak-proof bag; handle contaminated linens in a manner that prevents contamination and transfer of microorganisms.
9. Discard all sharps in puncture-resistant container. Do not bend, break, reinsert them into their original sheaths, or handle them unnecessarily. Discard them intact immediately after use.
10. Place clients who pose a risk for transmission to others in a private room. This includes clients who cannot contain secretions/excretions or wound drainage and infants with respiratory or intestinal infections.
11. Practice good hand hygiene.

## Respiratory Hygiene and Cough Etiquette

1. Educate health care personnel regarding measures to contain their own respiratory secretions.
2. Post signs in strategic places regarding covering the mouth and nose with a tissue when coughing or sneezing; provide no-touch receptacles for disposal of tissue.
3. Teach client importance of hand hygiene.

## Safe Injection Practices

1. Use single-dose vials for parenteral administration when possible.
2. If multidose vials must be used, the needle or cannula and the syringe used to access the vial must be sterile.
3. Do not use the same syringe to administer medications to multiple clients, even if the needle is changed.
4. Do not keep multidose vials in the immediate client treatment area.

## Airborne Precautions (droplets smaller than 5 micrometers)

1. Place client in airborne isolation infection (negative pressure airflow) room (AIIR) as soon as possible.
2. Personal protection equipment (PPE):
   - Wear respiratory protection (N95 respirator mask approved by the National Institute for Occupational Safety and Health [NIOSH]) when entering the room).
   - Wear gloves and gown when entering the room; remove before leaving room.
3. Limit client transport and client movement out of the room. Health care personnel who are not immune are restricted from entering the client's room.
4. Conditions requiring use of airborne precautions include pulmonary or laryngeal tuberculosis, varicella, rubella, and smallpox.

## Droplet Precautions (droplets larger than 5 micrometers)

1. Applicable to clients known to be, or suspected of being, infected with pathogens that are transmitted via respiratory droplets (sneezing, coughing, talking).
2. Place the client in a private room whenever possible; may place two clients in the same room if they are infected with the same pathogen.
3. PPE:
   - Wear a mask when entering the client room or examination area.
   - No recommendation regarding routine use of eye protection.
4. Place a mask on the client if transporting in the health care setting.
5. Instruct client and family regarding respiratory hygiene/cough etiquette.
6. Limit movement of the client from the room; if the client must leave the room, have him or her wear a surgical mask.

## Contact Precautions

1. Applicable to clients with diseases easily transmitted by direct contact such as gastrointestinal, respiratory tract, skin, or wound infections and clients colonized with multidrug-resistant bacteria.
2. Place the client in a private room if condition (e.g., uncontrolled drainage, incontinence) may facilitate transmission. Two clients infected with same pathogen may be placed in the same room.
3. PPE:
   - Wear a gown when entering the client's room; remove gown before leaving the room.
   - Wear gloves when entering the client's room. Always change gloves after contact with infected material. Remove gloves before leaving the client's room and perform hand hygiene; do not touch anything in the room as you are leaving.
   - Wear gloves when touching the client's intact skin and surfaces and articles in close proximity to the client.
4. Dedicate use of noncritical client care equipment to the single client; if common equipment use is unavoidable, the equipment must be disinfected before use on another client.
5. Limit the transport or movement of the client outside the room; if it is necessary to move the client, ensure that infected or colonized areas of the client's body are contained and covered.

*Continued*

6. Evidence shows that multiple drug–resistant organisms (MDROs) can be carried from one person to another via the hands of health care personnel.

## Protective Environment Precautions

1. Precautions may be used for clients who are severely immuno-suppressed—clients with stem cell transplants, clients with organ transplant, AIDS clients.
2. Place the client in a private room that has positive-pressure air flow and high-efficiency particulate air (HEPA) filtration for incoming air.

3. Wear respiratory protection (N95 respirator mask), gloves, and gown when entering the room.
4. Limit client transport and client movement out of the room.
5. No fresh flowers, fresh fruits/vegetables, or potted plants are allowed in room.

> **TEST ALERT:** Use critical thinking to ensure standard transmission-based precautions are implemented; prevent environmental spread of infectious diseases.

Centers for Disease Control and Prevention: *2007 Guideline for isolation precautions: preventing transmission of infectious agents in healthcare settings.* Retrieved from https://www.cdc.gov/hicpac/pdf/isolation/isolation2007.pdf

---

**Central Line:** A single or multilumen catheter inserted into the venous system and progressed into the thoracic cavity with the end of the line in the superior vena cava or the right atrium

### Nursing Implications for Central Line
- Most common insertion is percutaneous into the subclavian or internal jugular vein.
  - A central line is necessary for a central venous pressure (CVP) reading and for total parenteral nutrition solutions.
  - Obtain a chest x-ray to evaluate for a possible pneumothorax after insertion of catheter into subclavian vein.
- When changing the tubing on central lines, position the client flat (if tolerated), clamp the tubing, and have client hold his or her breath and bear down when the line is opened (Valsalva maneuver). Immediately connect the new line and have the client breathe normally. Because the catheter goes into the thoracic cavity, it is subjected to changes in pressure, which increase the risk for air embolus.
- Maintain sterile technique when changing the dressing on the puncture site and sterility of the connections when changing tubing.

> **TEST ALERT:** Assist with invasive procedures (e.g., central line placement). Obtain blood specimens peripherally or through a central line.

**Vascular Access Devices:** Long-term vascular lines for clients receiving intravenous (IV) therapy for 3 months or longer.

- **Implanted ports (MediPort, Port-A-Cath):** MediPort vascular access line port is implanted under the skin; activities are not restricted (Figure 9-8).
- **Tunneled ports (Hickman, Broviac, Groshong):** Requires surgical placement; has an external port. The distal tip lies in the superior vena cava just above the right atrium. It is not used to obtain CVP readings.
- **PICC:** A peripherally inserted central catheter (PICC) line is inserted into a large peripheral vein of the upper arm and threaded into the subclavian vein and has an external port; the area requires a sterile occlusive dressing; it may be used to obtain blood samples.
- **Triple- or double-lumen lines:** A venous catheter that contains two or three separate ports and lines that are encased and

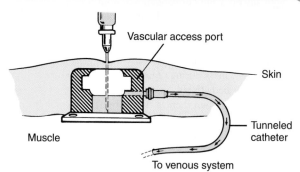

**FIGURE 9-8 Implantable Vascular Access Port and Huber-point Needles.** (From Lewis, S., et.al. (2017). *Medical-surgical nursing: Assessment and management of clinical problems* [10th ed.]. St. Louis, MO: Mosby.)

inserted as one line; may be part of the vascular access device (VAD). Because each line is separate, the infusing solutions do not mix.

### Nursing Implications for Vascular Access Devices
- **Flushing:** Routine flushing may be required unless there is a continuous IV infusion. This may be done with normal saline solution, heparin, or fibrinolytics. Type of solution, frequency, and volume depend on IV therapy and whether blood was drawn from the line, as well as institution policy. Excessive force should never be used to irrigate the line. Syringes smaller than 10 mL should not be used because the smaller the syringe, the greater the pressure exerted. The push-pause technique is a flushing method used to possibly remove debris from ports or catheter lumens.

> **⚠ NURSING PRIORITY:** Do not flush a central catheter if there is resistance or if catheter is occluded; increased pressure may cause catheter to rupture and/or produce a catheter emboli or dislodgment of a clot.

- **Accessing:** Gloves are worn and appropriate skin preparation is performed for implanted ports; external injection ports and connectors are cleansed before accessing.
- **Dressing changes:** Implanted sites require cleansing after exit but do not require a dressing. External sites (PICCs and ports)

require dressings, either gauze or transparent. Gauze dressings are changed if they are contaminated or if observation of the site is required; dressing is routinely changed every 48 hours. Transparent dressings with antimicrobial discs may not be changed for 5 to 7 days.

- **Changing lines:** Clamping may be necessary during a tubing change to prevent air emboli; always use a flat or padded clamp to prevent damaging the line. If the line cannot be clamped, have the client hold his or her breath and bear down (Valsalva maneuver) during the line change.

### Arterial Lines: Used to obtain arterial blood sample for ABGs and for blood pressure monitoring.

- **Measurements:** Arterial lines are used to evaluate blood pressure measurements. Measurement should be obtained at the end of respiration to avoid effect of respiratory cycle on arterial pressure.
- **Arterial blood sample:** Blood is withdrawn to evaluate ABGs.

**Nursing Implications for Arterial Line**
- **Complications:** hemorrhage, infection, thrombus formation, neurologic damage.
- Maintain Leur Lock connections to prevent problem with accidental disconnection and bleeding from site.
- Prevent thrombus formation and maintain line patency by maintaining pressure on line at 300 mmHg to provide continuous flush at 3 to 6 mL/hr.
- Perform Allen's test (see Arterial Blood Gas Studies in Appendix 17-1) to determine adequate circulation to hand before placing line in radial artery.
- Assess for infection at insertion site; if present, remove catheter and change all tubing and equipment for new site.
- Prevent infection by changing pressure tubing, fluid bag, and transducer every 96 hours.
- Assess vascular status distal to arterial line by checking capillary refill and color of extremity.
- Assess neurologic status distal to arterial line by checking for presence of tingling, pain, or paresthesia.

## Study Questions
## Homeostasis Concepts

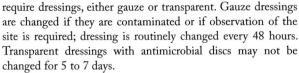

More questions on

1. The nurse is caring for a client with an acute onset of shortness of breath and a respiratory rate of 28 breaths per minute. Arterial blood gasses are pH 7.20; $Paco_2$ 47, $HCO_3^-$ 24. What is the priority plan of care?
   1. Slow the respiratory rate with relaxation and sedation.
   2. Improve the pH by administering sodium bicarbonate.
   3. Determine a cause of the shortness of breath with further assessment.
   4. Intubation to maintain respiratory effort.

2. The nurse is caring for an older adult client with edema, tachycardia, hypertension, and jugular venous distention. Which nursing action should the nurse prioritize to evaluate the client's fluid status?
   1. Measure the intake and output (I&O).
   2. Check for thirst and skin turgor.
   3. Evaluate changes in daily weight.
   4. Evaluate vital signs every 4 hours.

3. The nurse is admitting a client from the post anesthesia care unit. Postoperative prescriptions include $D_5$ ½ NS with 40 mEq/L of KCl @ 100 mL/hr. The current liter of lactated Ringer's solution has 450 mL left in the bag. What should the nurse's next action be?
   1. Finish the current liter of fluid at 100mL/hr.
   2. Assess urine output.
   3. Change the solution to D5 ½ NS with 40 mEq/L KCl at 100 mL/hr.
   4. Assess the IV site.

4. The nurse is reviewing the health care provider's prescriptions for a new client returning from the post anesthesia care unit. The client is NPO, with a nasogastric tube and stable vital signs. Which prescription should the nurse question?
   1. 20 mEq potassium IV push.
   2. 1000 mL D5 ½ NaCl to infuse at 125 mL/hr.
   3. Assist client to dangle at bedside in morning.
   4. Mefoxin 1 gm IV in 50 mL D5W over 30 minutes.

5. The nurse is assisting a client to ambulate. Upon standing at the bedside, the client becomes weak, says "I feel dizzy," and sits back down on the bed. What should be the nurses next action?
   1. Lay the client down in bed.
   2. Obtain a blood pressure.
   3. Ask the client to try again.
   4. Find additional help for ambulation.

6. The nurse is planning to educate colleagues on best practices in decreasing central line infections. What practices should be included in staff education? **Select all that apply.**
   1. Follow agency policy for dressing and tubing changes.
   2. Use clean technique when changing caps and dressings.
   3. Report sites that are reddened.
   4. Change dressings that have moisture.
   5. Gauze dressings need changing less frequently

7. A client in the emergency department has been hydrated with normal saline over the last hour for hypovolemia. Assessment changes now include a rapid bounding pulse and shortness of breath. What additional information would the nurse want to gather? Select all that apply.
   1. Blood pressure
   2. Level of consciousness
   3. Urinary output
   4. Hemoglobin level
   5. Oxygen saturation

8. The nurse is admitting a 5-month-old infant. The health care provider has ordered an IV solution of normal saline. There is also an order for potassium chloride (KCl) to be added to the solution. The infant's temperature is 101°F (38.8°C) rectally, and the pulse is 120 beats/min; the infant is irritable and has not voided. What is the priority nursing action?
   1. Wait for 1 hour from admission time and then begin the infusion of normal saline with the KCl.
   2. Feed the infant before adding the KCl to the infusing solution.
   3. Consider the order a stat order and begin the infusion immediately.
   4. Start the normal saline infusion and hold the KCl until adequate urinary output has been documented.

9. The nurse is caring for a client with excess fluid volume. Which action will best evaluate a change in the client's condition?
   1. Obtaining the client's daily weight before breakfast each day
   2. Measuring fluid intake and output and comparing with values from the previous day
   3. Assessing the blood pressure and comparing it with previous readings
   4. Auscultating the lungs for the presence of adventitious breath sounds

10. An older adult client has a prescription for continuous fluid replacement at 75 mL/hr. The nurse is preparing to start the IV. Which option would be best?
    1. A 22-gauge butterfly needle, right arm antecubital area.
    2. An 18-gauge, 3-inch IV cannula, inserted in the left hand.
    3. An 18-gauge, 1-inch IV cannula, in the antecubital area of left arm.
    4. A 22-gauge, 1-inch IV cannula, top of the left hand.

11. A client has just received 250 mL of packed cells and is now receiving 1000 mL of D$_5$W at 150 mL/hr. The client tells the nurse that he feels dizzy and has a headache. The nurse observes the distended jugular veins with the client in a semi-Fowler's position. What should be the nurse's initial response?
    1. Notify the health care provider of the client's symptoms.
    2. Check vital signs.
    3. Reduce the D5W infusion to keep vein open rate.
    4. Lay the client flat.

12. The nurse is performing a dressing change on a client who has a *Staphylococcus* infection in an abdominal incision. Which infection-control precautions will the nurse implement? **Select all that apply.**
    1. Wear clean gloves to remove the old dressing.
    2. Put on a gown when entering the room.
    3. Wear a face shield.
    4. Dispose of the gown and mask in container outside the client's door.
    5. Leave all extra dressing supplies in the room.
    6. Carefully cleanse the stethoscope and scissors before taking them out of the room.

13. The client is receiving an IV of 0.9% NaCl at 125 mL/hr. The client had a colon resection this morning. He has a nasogastric tube to suction and an ileostomy, and he is becoming increasingly restless. The nurse reviews the serum laboratory values. Which value should the nurse consider a priority?
    1. Blood urea nitrogen 28 mg/dL (10 mmol/L).
    2. Serum glucose 155 mg/dL (8.6 mmol/L).
    3. Hemoglobin 13.5 mmol/L, hematocrit 41% (0.41).
    4. Sodium 155 mEq/L (mmol/L).

14. A client has returned to the room from the postoperative recovery area. He is lethargic but responsive. He has O$_2$ via nasal cannula at 4 L/min and an IV infusing at 125 mL/hr. On the initial nursing assessment, the nurse notes that the O$_2$ saturation is 82%. What is the priority nursing action?
    1. Perform a complete neurologic check.
    2. Increase the O2 flow and recheck the pulse oximetry.
    3. Suction the client and recheck the vital signs.
    4. Stimulate the client to cough and deep breathe.

15. The nurse is admitting a client with type 1 diabetes. What values on the arterial blood gases would indicate the client is developing a complication because of his poorly controlled diabetes?
    1. Paco$_2$ 48 mmHg, pH 7.34, Pao2 98 mmHg, HCO3$^-$ 24 mEq/L (mmol/L).
    2. Paco$_2$ 33 mmHg, pH 7.48, Pao2 88 mmHg, HCO3$^-$ 26 mEq/L (mmol/L).
    3. Paco$_2$ 40 mmHg, pH 7.45, HCO3$^-$ 32 mEq/L (mmol/L), O2 saturation 90%.
    4. Paco$_2$ 38 mmHg, pH 7.31, HCO3$^-$ 20 mEq/L (mmol/L), base excess −2.

16. A client has pain at the peripheral IV site. The nurse determines the IV is not infusing; assesses the site; and finds the area swollen, pale, and cool to touch. What is the best nursing action?
    1. Discontinue the IV and apply warm, moist packs to the involved area.
    2. Slow the IV infusion and see whether the swollen area decreases.
    3. Notify the health care provider regarding the status of the IV.
    4. Discontinue the IV and start another IV in the same vein, distal to the current site.

17. A client is being seen in the emergency department after an accident. He has no obvious physical injuries, and his blood pressure is 158/90 mmHg. He is crying loudly, wringing his hands, and pacing the floor. His respiratory rate is 32 breaths/min, and he says he feels lightheaded. What is the best nursing response?
    1. Have him lie down and begin O$_2$ per nasal cannula at 4 L/min.
    2. Put him on a stretcher and begin a head-to-toe assessment.
    3. Perform a quick neurologic examination to determine his level of orientation.
    4. Have him sit down and help him breathe into a paper sack.

18. The nurse is documenting information regarding an IV insertion. What information is important to include? **Select all that apply.**
    1. Time and date of insertion.
    2. Type of catheter and size.
    3. Name of vein used.
    4. Status of fluid infusing.
    5. Protective measures used.
    6. Who ordered the IV and at what time.

19. The nurse is assessing an IV site after the client has verbalized an increase of tenderness. The site is inflamed, streaks of inflammation are progressing up the inside of the client's arm, and the fluid is continuing to infuse at the prescribed rate. What is the best nursing action?
    1. Remove the catheter and place warm packs on the area.
    2. Lower the IV bag below the site to determine whether there is blood return in the line.
    3. Determine what medications the client is receiving that may have caused the irritation.
    4. Decrease the rate of the infusion to decrease the discomfort.

## Answers to Study Questions

1. *3*

Sudden shortness of breath with tachypnea is always a concern and a priority problem. The ABGs show that the client is in a respiratory acidosis that is uncompensated (from the sudden onset of symptoms). Further assessment should include a pulse oximetry reading, blood pressure, heart rate, auscultation of lungs, and assessment for tracheal shift and bilateral lung expansion. Anxiety level is another important assessment and should be addressed. Sedation would be contraindicated, since it would slow the respirator rate causing further retention of $Paco_2$. Sodium bicarbonate is more commonly used in metabolic acidosis, and intubation is not warranted unless the client lacks a breathing response or more severe respiratory acidosis. (Lewis et al., 10 ed., pp. 288, 1616)

2. *3*

The assessment findings demonstrate fluid volume excess. The priority assessment for a client with fluid problems is to obtain the daily weight. Weight gain and loss are the most accurate measurements of fluid gain and loss. Checking tissue turgor on an older adult is not accurate because many older adults have poor turgor. Thirst is too nonspecific and would be a proper assessment for dehydration rather than fluid volume excess. The I&O is important, but it is not as accurate in evaluating the amount of fluid retained as is the daily weight. (Lewis et al., 10 ed., p. 277)

3. *4*

Although the cost-effective decision is to finish the current liter of fluid, at the prescribed rate it will take 4 hours to infuse. Because there is a loss of potassium from urinary and GI loss with surgery, it is important to begin potassium replacement upon arrival to the unit. The initial assessment of the IV site should take place prior to the infusion of potassium. Determination of kidney function and urine output is also important to establish prior to the infusion of potassium, but IV assessment is a higher priority, since it can cause injury to the client if an infiltration is present. (Lewis, et al., 10 ed., p. 282)

4. *1*

Potassium should never be administered by IV push. It is extremely irritating and painful at the catheter site, as well as lethal to the client when administered by IV push. It should be diluted in an IV solution and run over the time of the total infusion (1000 mL $D_5W$ with 40 mEq potassium over 8 hours), or small amounts should be given in less solution (potassium 10 mEq in 250 mL $D_5W$ to run over 3 hours). The other orders listed are all within acceptable limits for a postoperative client. (Lewis et al., 10 ed., p. 282)

5. *1*

With dehydration or fluid deficit, orthostatic hypotension may occur. After the client is safely back in bed, the nurse should assess for other symptoms of fluid volume deficit: decreased blood pressure, weight loss, imbalance of urine output and fluid intake, and dry skin and mucous membranes. Ambulation should be avoided until the symptoms have subsided. (Lewis et al., 10 ed., p. 282)

6. *1, 3, 4*

Central lines have a high rate of infection in hospitalized clients. The Centers for Disease Control and Prevention offers guidelines for prevention of intravascular catheter-related infections. The nurse should follow the agency policy for dressing and tubing changes, which will guide the nurse when in practice. Sterile technique should be used, not clean technique, and gauze dressings need to be changed more frequently, since they are porous. Moisture increases the risk of infection. All signs of infection should be reported, including temperature, increased white blood cells, and redness. (Lewis et al., 10 ed., p. 217)

7. *1, 2, 3, 5*

The client who had been hypovolemic is not demonstrating assessment changes of fluid volume excess. Appropriate assessments include vital signs such as pulse oximetry, weight, urine output, and changes in level of consciousness. Hemoglobin would not be affected by fluid status. (Lewis et al., 10 ed., p. 277)

8. *4*

In infants (and adults), validation of renal function must be established before the delivery of IV KCl. This is necessary to prevent hyperkalemia and possible death. The key point in the question is that the infant has not voided, so the prudent nurse should hold the KCl until adequate urine output is documented. (Lewis et al., 10 ed., p. 277)

9. *1*

Daily weights are an accurate indicator of fluid retained or lost. One liter of fluid is equal to 2.2 pounds (1 kg). Measuring the intake and output does not take into consideration insensible fluid loss and is not as accurate an evaluation as is the daily weight. Changes in vital signs are less reliable because they do not reflect subtle changes in retention of fluid. Although adventitious sounds may be present if the client is overhydrated, the daily weights would have increased before the pulmonary changes occurred. (Lewis et al., 10 ed., p. 277.)

**10.** *4*

With a continuous flow at 75 mL/hour, a small-gauge IV cannula (22 G), 1 inch (2.5 cm) is appropriate. Butterfly needles are used for short-term infusions and drawing blood. IVs should be started in the lowest vein possible and progress upward. The antecubital area is not a preferred area. (Potter & Perry, 9 ed., p. 958)

**11.** *3*

Headache and dizziness in a client receiving IV fluid are frequently signs of fluid overload from the increase in circulating volume, which increases cerebral vascular pressure. After decreasing the IV rate, the nurse should continue with the assessment of the vital signs. If other assessment findings (increased blood pressure, lethargy, bounding pulse, weight gain, adventitious breath sounds) confirm the problem, the physician needs to be notified. If the increase in circulating volume continues, it can cause pulmonary edema. (Lewis et al., 10 ed., p. 709)

**12.** *1, 2, 5*

Contact precautions would require the nurse to wear clean gloves to remove the old dressing, put on a gown when entering the room, and leave all extra dressing supplies in the room. A face shield is not necessary unless splattering of fluids is anticipated. The gown and mask should be disposed of in the client's room; they should not be worn outside the room and should be disposed according to hospital policy. The stethoscope and scissors should not be taken out of the client's room. (Potter & Perry, 9 ed., p. 458)

**13.** *4*

The client is losing fluids, but the replacement fluid only contains sodium. The laboratory value of 155 mEq/L (mmol/L) of sodium indicates that the client has hypernatremia. This increases retention of fluids and subsequently increases the cardiac workload. The glucose level is elevated, but that is not unusual in clients in the immediate postoperative period. The hemoglobin and hematocrit values are within the normal ranges. The blood urea nitrogen (BUN) level is elevated, and this needs to be investigated and correlated with the serum creatinine level. However, it is not alarmingly high and could be an indication of decreased fluids, and it is not the priority concern. (Lewis et al., 10 ed., p. 292)

**14.** *4*

The client is lethargic from the anesthetic and needs to be stimulated to deep breathe to facilitate ventilation. The client is at increased risk for development of respiratory acidosis and hypoxemia. Stimulation should be done before suctioning to determine whether it relieves the problem. Increasing the oxygen flow does not address the problem of hypoventilation. Neurologic checks can be done but are not a priority at this time. (Lewis et al., 10 ed., p. 288)

**15.** *4*

This series of values ($Paco_2$ 38 mmHg, pH 7.31, $HCO_3^-$ 20 mEq/L [mmol/L], base excess $-2$) best represents metabolic acidosis, a complication of type 1 diabetes, which is the correct answer. This series of values ($Paco_2$ 48 mmHg, pH 7.34, $Pao_2$ 98 mmHg, $HCO_3^-$ 24 mEq/L [mmol/L]) reflects respiratory acidosis; notice the elevated $Paco_2$ and decreased pH. This series of values ($Paco_2$ 33 mmHg, pH 7.48, $Pao_2$ 88 mmHg, $HCO_3^-$ 26 mEq/L [mmol/L]) reflects respiratory alkalosis; notice the decreased $Paco_2$ and increased pH. This series of values ($Paco_2$ 40 mmHg, pH 7.45, $HCO_3^-$ 32 mEq/L [mmol/L], $O_2$ saturation 90%) reflects metabolic alkalosis; notice the elevated bicarbonate and pH. (Lewis et al., 10 ed., p. 289)

**16.** *1*

The IV is infiltrated and should be discontinued. A warm, moist pack can be applied for client comfort. The IV should be discontinued but not restarted distal to the previous site; it should be started proximal to or above the current infiltrated site or in the other extremity. (Potter & Perry, 9 ed., p. 961)

**17.** *4*

The client is experiencing acute respiratory alkalosis from hyperventilation caused by anxiety. Rebreathing in a paper sack will help reestablish normal $Paco_2$ levels. The other options do not address the origin of the problem and may further increase his anxiety. (Potter, 9 ed., p. 944)

**18.** *1, 2, 4*

The specific name of the vein is not necessary, but the general location of the site is important. Standard precautions are used for everyone, and it is not necessary to chart that they were used. The order and time for the IV should be on the client's chart; it is not necessary to repeat it in the documentation. The question did not ask for all the information that could be charted. (Potter & Perry, 9 ed., p. 958)

**19.** *1*

Phlebitis has developed at the site, and the catheter should be removed. If continued administration of fluids is necessary, the catheter should be restarted at another site. It does not make any difference whether the catheter is still in the vein. The catheter must be removed because of the inflammation. Assessment of medications causing the problem can be done at a later time after the current problem is resolved. The rate of infusion should remain the same. (Potter & Perry, 9 ed., p. 962)

# CHAPTER TEN

# Immune: Care of Adult, Maternity, and Pediatric Clients

**10**

Immunity, Infection

## PHYSIOLOGY OF THE IMMUNE SYSTEM

A. Functions of the immune system.
1. Defense – protect against invading microorganisms.
2. Homeostasis – removal of damaged cellular substances.
3. Surveillance – recognition of foreign cells and destruction of them.
B. Body recognizes foreign proteins, called *antigens,* which will elicit a response from the immune system—the production of antibodies, which attack and destroy the invading antigens.
1. Antigens are foreign to the body and are frequently associated with bacteria, viruses, or other pathogens; antigens react with antibodies or antigen receptors on B and T cells.
2. Allergens are antigens that produce an allergic response.
C. Inflammatory response—an innate resistance or natural barrier that responds to the site of tissue injury; examples include infection, mechanical injury, ischemia, temperature extremes.
1. Redness, heat, swelling, and pain occur secondary to vasodilation, increased vascular permeability, and white blood cell migration to site of injury.
2. Complement system consists of plasma proteins that directly destroy pathogens, activated by the formation of an antigen–antibody complex (immune complex).
3. Complement cells are found in the innate and the acquired immune response.

### Immunologic Responses

A. Humoral response.
1. Antibodies produced by the plasma cells circulate through the blood and bind to and inactivate antigens or infectious agents.
2. B lymphocytes (plasma cells) recognize the antigen and become activated, differentiated plasma cells, which produce immunoglobulins (e.g., IgM, IgG, IgA, IgE, IgD).
B. Cell-mediated response—stem cells originate in the bone marrow and travel to the thymus, where they mature into functional T cells.
1. A response is initiated through recognition of antigens by T cells (T lymphocytes, macrophages, and natural killer cells).

2. Differentiation of the T cells into specific cells that react directly with the antigen (e.g., CD8, CD4, and NK cells).
3. Provides cellular immunity, delayed hypersensitivity reactions; recognizes tumor cells and inhibits tumor growth; rejects foreign tissue (organ transplants) and produces autoimmune disorders.
C. Humoral and cellular responses are not independent—but *inter*dependent—and an effective immune response is based on the interactions of both responses.
D. Properties of the immunologic response. (Figure 10-1)
1. *Specificity:* the formation of a specific antibody for each antigen; antibodies produced against one pathogen will not protect the body from other pathogens.
2. *Memory:* both responses are capable of "remembering" the antigen and responding more rapidly if exposed to same antigen again.
3. *Self-recognition:* the immune system has the ability to distinguish self or self-antigens from nonself or foreign antigens; the self-antigens do not illicit the immune response.
E. Inflammatory response.
1. Early inflammatory response is self-limiting. It destroys injurious agents and removes them from the site. It also confines agents to the area, stimulates the immune response, and promotes healing.
2. Chronic inflammation lasts 2 weeks or longer and is frequently preceded by an unsuccessful acute response. Infiltration of lymphocytes and macrophages occur in an attempt to protect the body; the area may be walled off to form a granuloma (e.g., the granuloma associated with tuberculosis).
F. Types of specific immunity.
1. Innate immunity: present at birth; is not antigen specific and involves a nonspecific response; first line of defense.
2. Acquired immunity: develops either actively or passively (Table 10-1).
G. Effects of aging on immune response.
1. Infants are protected at birth by maternal antibodies that cross the placenta; an infant's antibody system begins to function around 6 months of age.
2. With aging there is a diminished response of cell-mediated immunity. A decline in efficiency of humoral immunity also occurs because of a decrease in antibody production in response to antigens; lymphocyte production is decreased.

# IMMUNE SYSTEM RESPONSE

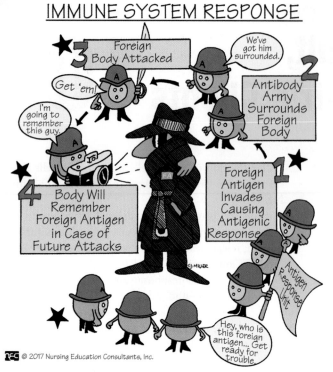

**FIGURE 10-1 Immune System Response.** (From Zerwekh, J., Garneau, A., & Miller, C. J. [2017]. *Digital collection of the memory notebooks of nursing* [4th ed.]. Chandler, AZ: Nursing Education Consultants, Inc.)

3. Older clients are at increased risk for impaired inflammation and wound healing secondary to chronic diseases (cardiovascular, diabetes) and medications that impair the inflammatory response (steroids).

> **⚠ NURSING PRIORITY:** Clients who have a compromised immune system, from either disease or medications, should not take any immunizations until they have checked with their doctor.

# DISORDERS OF THE IMMUNE SYSTEM

### 📋 *Hypersensitivity*

A. Type I (IgE-mediated reaction; IgE antibodies involved).
   1. Occurs when a person has been previously sensitized to a specific antigen.
   2. When same antigen reappears, it interacts with the IgE; this activates the release of chemical mediators, primarily histamine.
   3. Histamine: major chemical mediator.
      a. Smooth muscle contraction (spasms of bronchial muscles and airway obstruction).
      b. Capillary vasodilation and increased capillary permeability leading to vascular collapse (decreased blood pressure).
      c. Increased nasal stuffiness and bronchial secretions.
      d. Reaction usually begins within minutes after exposure.
   4. Conditions associated with type I.
      a. Anaphylaxis (most severe).
      b. Latex allergy (occurs within minutes).
      c. Atopic reactions (most common).
         (1) Allergic rhinitis (hay fever).
         (2) Atopic dermatitis.
         (3) Urticaria (hives).
         (4) Angioedema.
B. Type II (cytotoxic; direct binding of IgG and IgM antibodies to an antigen).
   1. Antibodies destroy cell on which antigen is bound, causing tissue injury.
   2. The normal process of phagocytosis is accelerated and begins to damage healthy body tissue.
   3. Conditions associated with type II.
      a. Hemolytic disease of the newborn (Rh factor).
      b. Leukopenia and thrombocytopenia.
      c. ABO blood incompatibility (hemolytic reaction).
      d. Goodpasture syndrome (an antibody-mediated reaction involving the lungs and kidneys).

### Table 10-1 ACQUIRED IMMUNITY

| Type | Characteristics | Examples |
|---|---|---|
| *Active:* Antibodies synthesized by body in response to antigen stimulation | *Natural:* Contact with an antigen through exposure develops slowly but often provides lifetime protection. | Recovery from childhood diseases (e.g., chicken pox, measles, mumps) |
| | *Artificial:* Immunization with an antigen (like a vaccine) develops slowly; it may provide protection for several years, but "boosters" may be required. | Immunization with live or attenuated vaccines (varicella, IPV, MMR) Toxoid immunization (tetanus toxoid, diphtheria toxoid) |
| *Passive:* Antibodies produced in one individual and transferred to another | *Natural:* Immunity from placenta and colostrum is transferred from mother to child and provides immediate temporary protection. | Maternal immunoglobulin in the neonate |
| | *Artificial:* Injection of serum from immune human or animal offers short-lived but immediate immunity. | Gamma globulin; injection of animal hyperimmune serum (diphtheria antitoxin, tetanus antitoxin) |

*IPV,* Inactivated polio vaccine; *MMR,* measles–mumps–rubella vaccine.

C. Type III (immune complex; IgG and IgM antibodies involved).
   1. Circulating immune complexes (antibody–antigen complex) are too small to be effectively removed and are deposited in the body tissue.
   2. When the immune complex is deposited in the body tissue (kidneys, skin, joints, blood vessels, and lungs), local tissue inflammation and cell wall damage occur.
   3. Symptoms depend on the number of complexes present and the area of the body involved (autoimmune conditions).
      a. Persistent infections (streptococcal infections) combined with a poor antibody response may lead to the formation of immune complexes that are eventually deposited in an affected organ.
         (1) Endocarditis (see Chapter 19).
         (2) Acute glomerulonephritis (see Chapter 25).
      b. Rheumatoid arthritis (see Chapter 23).
      c. Systemic lupus erythematosus (SLE).
D. Type IV (cell-mediated; delayed hypersensitivity).
   1. The T cells are sensitized to an antigen from a previous exposure; occurs 24 to 48 hours after exposure, may take 72 hours to reach maximum intensity.
   2. The sensitized T cells initiate the inflammatory response, leading to cellular damage and damage to the surrounding tissue.
   3. Conditions associated with type IV.
      a. Tuberculosis, skin testing.
      b. Contact dermatitis (poison ivy).
      c. Transplant rejection.
      d. Latex allergy (result of chemicals used in manufacturing latex gloves; contact dermatitis occurs within 6–48 hours) (Box 10-1).

---

**Box 10-1   GUIDELINES FOR PREVENTING ALLERGIC LATEX REACTIONS[a]**

- Be aware of latex-containing products—gloves, blood pressure cuffs, stethoscopes, tourniquets, IV tubing, syringes, electrode pads, oxygen masks, tracheal tubes, colostomy and ileostomy tubes, urinary catheters, anesthetic masks, and adhesive tape.
- Use latex-free gloves and powder-free gloves.
- Do not use oil-based hand creams or lotions when wearing gloves.
- Always wash hands after removing gloves.
- Frequently clean areas and equipment contaminated with latex-containing dust.
- Recognize symptoms of latex allergy—skin rash; hives; flushing; itching; nasal, eye, and sinus symptoms; asthma; (rarely) anaphylaxis.
- Always ask client if they have a latex allergy before using any possible latex-containing product.
- Wear a medic alert bracelet if latex sensitive and carry an epinephrine pen.

Source: National Institute for Occupational Safety and Health (NIOSH): *Latex Allergy a Prevention Guide.* Retrieved from http://www.cdc.gov/niosh/docs/98-113

[a]*Note: The more frequent and prolonged the exposure to latex, the greater the likelihood of developing latex allergy.*

## Anaphylactic Reaction

**Type I occurs in clients who are highly sensitized to a specific allergen—medications, blood products, insect stings. The antigen–antibody response precipitates the release of histamine, causing vasodilation and increased capillary permeability (Figure 10-2).**

### Assessment

A. Risk factors.
   1. History of exposure to allergen.
      a. Amount of allergen.
      b. Absorption of ingested allergen.
      c. Antibody levels from previous exposure.
      d. Occupational, social, and environmental factors.
   2. The more rapid the onset of symptoms after exposure, the more severe the reaction.
B. Clinical manifestations—depend on the level of prior sensitivity and the amount of allergen.
   1. Mild to moderate: peripheral tingling/itching (pruritus, urticaria), sensation of warmth, edema of the lips and tongue, nasal congestion, flushing, anxiety.
   2. May rapidly progress to acute anxiety, difficulty breathing (bronchospasm, laryngeal edema), gastrointestinal (GI) cramping, cyanosis, and hypotension; can be fatal.

### Diagnostics

According to symptoms and exposure to allergen.

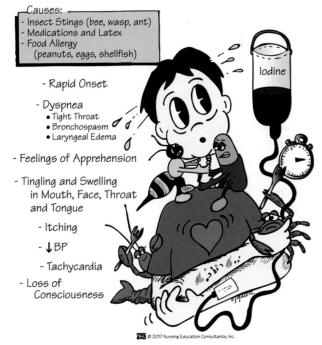

**FIGURE 10-2  Anaphylaxis.** (From Zerwekh, J., Garneau, A., & Miller, C. J. [2017]. *Digital collection of the memory notebooks of nursing* [4th ed.]. Chandler, AZ: Nursing Education Consultants, Inc.)

*Treatment*

A. Mild to moderate reactions—antihistamines (SQ or IV) and/or epinephrine (1:1000 solution), 0.3–0.5mg IM or IV, can repeat every 5 to 15 minutes; lower dose for mild to moderate reactions (Appendix 10-1).

> ⚠ **NURSING PRIORITY:** When administering epinephrine, make sure you have the correct concentration of solution. It is administered in concentrations of 0.1% or 1:1000 subcutaneously or IM, and 0.01% or 1:10,000 IV or intracardiac. Intravenous solutions are more dilute because of potential fatal reactions.

B. Severe reactions—epinephrine (1:1000 solution), 0.3–0.5mg IM or IV, can repeat every 5 to 15 minutes; higher dose administered for severe reactions.
C. Oxygen in high concentrations.
D. IV fluids (lactated Ringer's solution or 0.9% saline), vasopressor agents, and volume expanders to maintain circulatory status.
E. Maintain patent airway—intubation or tracheostomy may be necessary.
F. Corticosteroids to reduce inflammatory response (see Appendix 9-2).

> ⚠ **TEST ALERT:** Manage a medical emergency. Anaphylaxis is an immediate response, and symptoms progress rapidly. Emergency treatment should be initiated immediately if anaphylaxis is suspected. Death from an anaphylactic reaction is most often caused by bronchospasm and edema of the airway.

*Nursing Interventions*

**Goal:** To identify clients with a predisposition to hypersensitivity reactions.

> ⚠ **TEST ALERT:** Assess for client allergies.

A. Evaluate client history regarding reactions to:
   1. Medications, especially penicillin.
   2. Foods (e.g., seafood or iodine, eggs, peanuts).
   3. Insect bites.
   4. Vaccines, especially egg-cultured types.
   5. Blood products (transfusion reaction).
   6. Diagnostic agents (e.g., iodine-based contrast media).
B. If hypersensitivity is suspected, a localized skin test may be done before the administration of substance.
C. Prevention is the priority.

**Goal:** To maintain adequate ventilation.

> ⚠ **NURSING PRIORITY:** Airway positioning and mouth-to-mouth resuscitation will not provide adequate ventilation when client has airway edema. An emergency tracheotomy or intubation may be indicated.

A. Maintain bed rest; place client in low Fowler's position with the legs elevated.

B. High oxygen concentrations if airway is compromised.
C. Anticipate use of airway adjuncts (tracheostomy, endotracheal intubation).
D. Administration of medications to reverse bronchospasm (albuterol, corticosteroid, epinephrine).

**Goal:** To restore adequate circulation.

A. Administer IV fluids (normal saline or lactated Ringer's solution) to correct loss of fluid to third-space shifts and vasodilation.
B. Carefully titrate fluid replacement with vital signs.

> ⚠ **NURSING PRIORITY:** Monitor the client's fluid status closely; as fluid begins to shift back into the vascular compartment, it is easy to cause fluid overload.

C. Vasopressors and volume expanders may be used to increase blood pressure if fluid replacement is not effective.

**Goal:** Client will verbalize actions to prevent recurrence.

A. Once causative agent is identified, instruct client accordingly.
B. Advise client to wear identification tag or medic-alert bracelet.
C. Explain to client that if he or she had any level of allergic reaction previously, the next exposure could be worse (penicillin, insect stings, etc.).

## Autoimmune Conditions

A. Conditions in which body tolerance has been disrupted and the body tissue or cells cannot recognize their own cells (self-recognition). A critical aspect of the immune response is the ability of the body to recognize normal tissue and to not invade or destroy it.
B. An autoimmune condition occurs when the immune system can no longer recognize the normal tissue; it reacts against self-antigens and begins to destroy the host tissue.
C. Autoimmune response and disease occurrence.
   1. The direct action of the autoantibody on the cell surface. This causes destruction of the cell (cytotoxic); may activate the inflammatory response.
   2. An alteration of both B cells and/or T cells can produce auto-sensitized T cells and cause tissue damage.
D. Autoimmune response may be systemic or organ specific. *Note: diseases are discussed in various chapters.*
   1. Systemic diseases (rheumatic disorders: autoimmune and inflammatory).
      a. Chronic pain and progressive immobility involving the joints are characteristics.
      b. Connective tissue disorders: SLE.
      c. Rheumatic disorders: rheumatoid arthritis.
      d. Scleroderma.
   2. Organ-specific diseases.
      a. Myasthenia gravis, multiple sclerosis, Guillain-Barré syndrome.

b. Hyperthyroid (Graves' disease), celiac disease.

c. Addison disease, glomerulonephritis.

d. Type 1 diabetes mellitus, pernicious anemia.

## Systemic Lupus Erythematosus (SLE)

**SLE is a multisystem inflammatory autoimmune disorder; the disease affects multiple organs. SLE is characterized by a diffuse production of autoantibodies that attack and cause damage to body organs and tissue.**

A. Tissue injury in SLE results from deposition of the immune complexes throughout the body (kidneys, heart, skin, brain, and joints); this activates the inflammatory response.

B. The severity of symptoms varies greatly throughout the course of the disease; periods of exacerbation and remission occur.

### Assessment

A. Risk factors.

1. More common in women 20 to 40 years of age.

2. Familial tendencies.

3. More prevalent in African Americans, Asian Americans, Hispanics, and Native Americans than in Caucasians.

4. May be triggered by environmental stimulus, infections, and medications; sun exposure most common.

B. Clinical manifestations (Figure 10-3).

1. Initially may be nonspecific: weight loss, fatigue, and fever.

2. Integumentary: characteristic "butterfly" rash over face in 55% to 85% of clients; erythematous rash on areas of the body exposed to sunlight (photosensitivity); ulcerations involving oral mucosa, alopecia, dry scaly scalp, palmer erythema.

3. Musculoskeletal: arthritis, diffuse swelling with joint and muscle pain.

4. Renal system involvement: lupus nephritis, proteinuria, and glomerulonephritis.

5. Cardiovascular system hypertension, dysrhythmias.

a. Raynaud's phenomenon: caused by peripheral vasospasm.

b. Pericarditis: may progress to endocarditis.

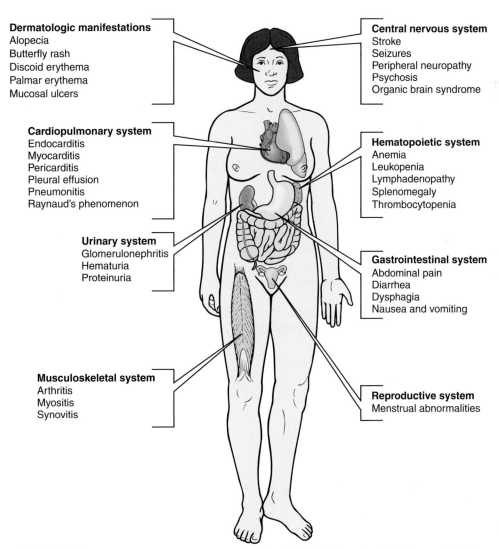

**FIGURE 10-3 Systemic Lupus Erythematosus.** (From Lewis, S. L., Dirksen, S. R., Heitkemper, M. M., & Bucher, L. [2017]. *Medical-surgical nursing: Assessment and management of clinical problems* [10th ed.]. St. Louis, MO: Mosby.)

c. Vascular inflammation of the small vessels; most commonly affects the small vessels of the fingers and the gastrointestinal tract.

6. Neurologic disorders: seizures, cognitive dysfunction.

7. Hematologic disorders: anemia, leukopenia, thrombocytopenia.

8. Emotional lability: severe depression and anxiety.

9. Respiratory system: dyspnea and pleurisy.

10. Gastrointestinal system: ulcers in the oral mucosa or nasopharyngeal membranes.

### Diagnostics

A. No specific test is diagnostic; assess configuration of symptoms.

B. Presence of antinuclear antibody (ANA), high levels of anti-DNA, and presence of anti-Smith (Sm) are most suggestive of a diagnosis of SLE.

C. C-reactive protein (CRP), erythrocyte sedimentation rate (ESR)—monitor progress of inflammation and therapy effectiveness.

### Treatment

SLE has no known cure.

A. Nonsteroidal antiinflammatory drugs (NSAIDs) (see Appendix 3-3).

B. Corticosteroids for exacerbations polyarthritis (see Appendix 9-2).

C. Immunosuppressants (see Appendix 25-2).

D. Antimalarial agents (e.g., hydroxychloroquine).

E. Steroid-sparing drugs (e.g., methotrexate).

### Nursing Interventions

**Goal:** To prevent exacerbations.

A. Maintain good nutritional status; eat a low-cholesterol diet.

B. Avoid exposure to infections.

C. Teach client about skin problems: discoid lesions, loss of hair, dry scaly scalp.

D. Teach client personal hygiene to prevent urinary tract infections.

E. Make sure client understands how to take medications.

F. Avoid exposure to sunlight; use a sunscreen with a minimum SPF 30 when exposure is unavoidable.

G. Contact physician before participating in any immunization procedures.

H. Counsel regarding pregnancy.

**Goal:** To maintain adequate tissue perfusion.

A. Assess for indications of impaired peripheral perfusion—numbness, tingling, and weakness of hands and feet.

B. Prevent injury to extremities, especially fingers.

C. Carefully evaluate fluid status with regard to cardiac status, fluid retention, and weight gain.

**Goal:** To promote effective pain control.

A. Establish schedule to conserve energy, but still maintain physical activity.

B. NSAIDs to control arthritic pain.

C. Nonpharmacologic therapies to supplement analgesics (see Chapter 3).

D. Evaluate response of pain to decreased inflammation from corticosteroids.

**Goal:** To maintain renal function.

A. Monitor for peripheral edema, hypertension, hematuria, and decreased output.

B. Monitor blood urea nitrogen and creatinine levels.

C. Monitor for urinary tract infections (glomerulonephritis).

D. Assess for peripheral edema and excess fluid volume.

**Goal:** To assist client to maintain psychological equilibrium.

A. Observe for behavioral changes that may indicate central nervous system involvement: headaches, inappropriate speech, difficulty concentrating.

B. Encourage client to participate in support groups and to seek counseling to deal with stress.

## Human Immunodeficiency Virus Infection

A. **Human immunodeficiency virus (HIV) infection is caused by a retrovirus that causes immunosuppression.**

B. **The person infected with HIV is more susceptible to infection due to the diminished response of the immune system.**

### Transmission of Human Immunodeficiency Virus

A. Blood transmission.

1. Needlesticks that occur when the client has a high viral load carry a higher risk than those that occur when client is at a low viral load.

2. Exposure to an infected client's blood via open wounds or mucous membranes carries a lower risk than does a needlestick.

3. Transmission via blood transfusions has been greatly reduced with the screening of donated blood.

a. A risk remains when the blood is donated within the first few months of infection and the screening blood test does not identify the donor as being HIV positive.

B. Sexual transmission—most common mode of transmission.

1. Sexual practices, not preferences, place people at increased risk.

2. Risk for infection is greater for the partner who receives the semen during oral, vaginal, or anal sex.

3. Any sexual activity that involves direct contact with vaginal secretions and semen may transmit HIV.

C. Perinatal transmission.

1. Exposure can occur during pregnancy, at the time of delivery, or during the postpartum period through breast milk.

2. Twenty-five percent of infants born to untreated HIV-positive mothers are infected.

3. Prophylactic antiretroviral medications (zidovudine, AZT) during pregnancy can reduce rate of transmission to less than 2%.

4. Decreased incidence occurs with cesarean delivery of HIV-positive mothers.

D. HIV *cannot* be transmitted by:
1. Hugging, kissing, holding hands, or other nonsexual contact.
2. Inanimate objects (money, doorknobs, bathtubs, toilet seats, etc.).
3. Dishes, silverware, or food handled by an infected person.
4. Animals or insects.
E. CD4$^+$ T helper cells are the regulating cells in the immune system; the level of CD4$^+$ T cells is used to monitor the stages and progression of the virus; normal CD4$^+$ T-cell count is at least 800 cells/μL (0.80 × 10$^9$/L) of blood.
F. The viral load in the semen, blood, vaginal secretions, or breast milk is an important variable in the transmission. The higher the viral load, the greater the risk of transmission.

> **■ NURSING PRIORITY:** As a nurse, it is essential for you to know the modes of transmission of HIV; activities that do *not* transmit the virus; and the nursing care to protect yourself, your clients with AIDS, and other clients you are caring for.

*Clinical Manifestations*
A. Acute HIV infection.
1. Intense viral replication and dissemination of HIV throughout the body.
2. Symptoms are mild, ranging from no symptoms to flulike symptoms (fever, swollen lymph glands, muscle and joint pain, diarrhea, sore throat, headache).
3. Window of seroconversion: period from when the person is infected with the virus until HIV antibodies can be detected.
4. Average time for seroconversion to occur is 1 to 3 weeks.
5. A client may have vague, nonspecific symptoms for years.
6. During this period, there is a high viral load, and the CD4$^+$ T-cell count falls but only temporarily.
B. Chronic HIV infection.
1. Asymptomatic infection—CD4$^+$ T-cell count greater than 500 cells/μL (0.50 × 10$^9$/L) and low viral load.
   a. Viral replication has reached a steady state.
   b. Considered asymptomatic phase, but chronic vague symptoms persist (fatigue, fever, headache, night sweats).
   c. Persistent generalized lymphadenopathy.
2. Symptomatic infection—CD4$^+$ T-cell count between 200 and 500 cells/μL (0.02 and 0.50 × 10$^9$/L) and increased viral load.
   a. Exacerbation of symptoms.
   b. Client begins to experience localized infections, increased lymphadenopathy, and neurologic manifestations.

c. *Candida* is a common problem—persistent oropharyngeal or vulvovaginal candidiasis.
d. Hairy oral leukoplakia, which may also be indication of progression of disease.
e. Shingles, oral or genital herpes lesions.
f. Kaposi sarcoma.
   (1) A cutaneous skin lesion that looks like a bruise; later will turn dark violet or black.
   (2) Invades body organs, extremities, skin, and torso.
   (3) May become painful.
3. Acquired immunodeficiency syndrome (AIDS)—CD4$^+$ T-cell count less than 200 cells/μL (0.20 × 10$^9$/L) and viral load increases. A diagnosis of AIDS is made when the HIV-positive client develops at least one of the following disease processes.
   a. CD4$^+$ T-cell count below 200 cells/μL (0.20 × 10$^9$/L).
   b. AIDS dementia complex.
   c. Wasting syndrome caused by HIV.
   d. At least one opportunistic cancer—invasive cervical cancer, Kaposi sarcoma, Burkitt's lymphoma, immunoblastic lymphoma, primary lymphoma of the brain.
   e. At least one opportunistic infection—viral (cytomegalovirus), fungal (*Pneumocystis jiroveci* pneumonia, coccidioidomycosis), bacterial, or protozoal infection.

*Opportunistic Diseases*
A. Diseases and infections that occur in clients with AIDS are called opportunistic because they take advantage of the suppressed immune system.
1. The type of infection and its extent varies with each client, depending on the extent of immunosuppression.
2. Single opportunistic infections are rare; a client usually has multiple infections.
B. Infections may be delayed or prevented by antiretroviral therapy, vaccines (hepatitis B, influenza, and pneumococcal), and disease-specific prevention.
C. *Coccidioides jiroveci* pneumonia, *Pneumocystis jiroveci* pneumonia (previously called *Pneumocystis carinii* and abbreviated as PJP or PCP).
1. May be caused by a pathogen in the body that is dormant.
2. Is not common in healthy individuals; immune system must be compromised for the infection to occur.
3. Symptoms: fever, night sweats, nonproductive cough, progressive dyspnea.
D. Tuberculosis (see Chapter 17).
E. Fungal infections: histoplasmosis (pneumonia, meningitis), coccidioidomycosis (pneumonia).
F. Kaposi's sarcoma: a bruised, dry-appearing skin lesion; may be present internally as well.
G. Candidiasis of the esophagus, mouth, vagina.
H. Viral infections: cytomegalovirus (CMV), CMV retinitis, herpes simplex with chronic ulcers or bronchitis, esophagitis, or pneumonitis.

## Diagnostics

> **⚠ NURSING PRIORITY:** A positive test result means the person has HIV—it does not predict the course of the disease. A negative test result means that HIV antibodies were not detected, but this can occur during the window period of seroconversion.

A. HIV antibody/antigen testing (fourth-generation testing): highly sensitive test that detects antibodies and antigens associated with HIV.
   1. Fourth-generation testing algorithm includes confirmatory testing with HIV viral load testing for any indeterminate results.
   2. If the client has a negative fourth-generation test but reports risky behavior, encourage retesting in 4 to 6 weeks.
   3. If results are positive, assist in finding follow-up HIV primary care.
B. Rapid HIV tests—ready within 20 minutes but results are preliminary and must be confirmed.
   1. Client needs to return for a standard HIV assay if the results are positive.
   2. In-home testing kits available that use an oral fluid sample (saliva).
C. CD4$^+$ T cell (receptor cell on the T4 helper cell) count: below 200 cells/μL ($0.20 \times 10^9$/L) in an HIV-positive client indicates progression to acute HIV infection (T4, T4 helper, and CD4$^+$ are synonymous terms).
D. Serum monitoring after diagnosis.
   1. CD4$^+$ T-cell counts and plasma assays (HIV RNA viral load).
   2. Evaluation for drug resistance.

## Treatment

A. Medications: antiretroviral therapy (ART) (see Appendix 10-1).
   1. Prescribed according to the viral load and the CD4$^+$ T-cell counts.
   2. Combination of at least three or more ART drugs.
   3. Women should begin ART even if they are pregnant, except for Sustiva, which can cause fetal anomalies.
   4. Combination drug therapy attacks virus at different stages of replication.
   5. Over-the-counter drugs and herbal therapies, especially St. John's wort, may cause reactions or interfere with ART drugs.
B. Medications do not cure the client but decrease the viral replication and slow disease process.
C. Adherence to drug schedules is critical; nonadherence to drug regimen can lead to mutations of the virus and increased virus resistance.

> **⚠ NURSING PRIORITY:** Frequently, the treatment for the client with AIDS causes problems in other areas: the high-dose antibiotics may increase the level of leukopenia, and the chemotherapy medications will further decrease the bone marrow functions. The client with AIDS receiving chemotherapy will be even further immunosuppressed.

## Nursing Interventions

See Nursing Interventions for immunocompromised clients.

**Goal:** To provide and promote client and public education regarding transmission of HIV.

Public and client teaching regarding the transmission of the HIV is vital in the control of this disease. The period from when the client is infected until the condition is diagnosed is when the majority of new infections are transmitted.

A. Safe sex.
   1. Maintain monogamous relationships.
   2. Sex with female or male prostitutes is a high-risk activity.
   3. Avoid all direct contact with a partner's mouth, penis, vagina, or rectum if the HIV status of the partner is not known.
   4. Avoid all sexual activities that cause cuts or tears in the vagina, on the penis, or in the rectum.
   5. Males should wear a condom if multiple partners are involved.
   6. If the HIV status of a sexual partner is not known, a condom should always be used during intercourse.
   7. Anyone who has been involved in any high-risk sexual activities or who has injected IV recreational drugs should have a blood test to determine presence of the HIV.
B. Needles should not be recapped or shared. Dispose of them in an impenetrable sealed container.

## Home Care

A. An employee in a health care setting should advise employer of HIV-positive status.
B. Kitchen and bathroom facilities may be shared, provided that normal sanitary practices are observed.
C. Clean up spills of body fluids or waste immediately with a solution of 1 part bleach to 10 parts water. A bleach solution can be used to disinfect kitchen and bathroom floors, showers, sinks, and toilet bowls.
D. Towels and washcloths should not be shared without laundering.
E. Sanitary napkins, tampons, and any bloody dressings should be wrapped in a plastic bag and placed in a trash container.
F. Needles should not be recapped. Dispose of them in an impenetrable sealed container.
G. Do not donate blood or plasma, body organs, or semen.

## ⚕ Pediatric Acquired Immunodeficiency Syndrome

The majority of children with AIDS were infected in the perinatal period. Cases related to blood transfusions are relatively rare.

> **⚠ NURSING PRIORITY:** HIV-positive mothers should not breastfeed their infants.

## Assessment

A. Risk factors.
1. Sexual activity and IV drug use are the major causes of HIV infection in adolescents.
2. Infants born to mothers who are HIV positive account for the majority of children with HIV infection; ART during pregnancy reduces risk for transmission to fetus.
3. Children rarely have Kaposi sarcoma.
4. *P. jiroveci* pneumonia (PJP, PCP) is the most common opportunistic infection.

B. Clinical manifestations.
1. Infants affected during the prenatal period have rapid disease progression.
2. HIV-positive infants usually have symptoms by 18 to 24 months of age.
3. Infants diagnosed within the first year of life have a poor prognosis, as do those who develop *P. jiroveci* pneumonia (PJP, PCP) and progressive encephalopathy.
4. Symptoms include lymphadenopathy, hepatosplenomegaly, oral candidiasis, chronic diarrhea, failure to thrive, developmental delay, and parotitis.
5. Severe symptoms in adolescents include the AIDS-defining illnesses such as PCP or PJP, wasting syndrome, HIV encephalopathy, *Candida* esophagitis, and cryptosporidiosis.
6. Immune categories are based on CD4$^+$ T-cell counts; these are age adjusted.

## Diagnostics

A. Enzyme-linked immunoassay (ELISA), also known as enzyme immunoassay (EIA), and Western blot (WB) for children 18 months or older.
B. Newborn: polymerase chain reaction (PCR); p24 antigen detection; majority of infants who are HIV positive can be identified by 3 months of age.
C. Maternal antibodies to HIV may persist for up to 18 months; then the infant may seroconvert to a negative status.
D. Positive results on two separate occasions and from separate blood specimens for p24 antigen detection, PCR, and virus culture are required to confirm diagnosis of HIV infection.

## Treatment

Treatment for children is essentially the same as that for an adult.

## Nursing Interventions Specific to Children

**Goal:** To maintain homeostasis.

A. Infants and children should receive the standard immunizations against childhood diseases. Measles–mumps–rubella (MMR) and varicella (chickenpox) vaccines may be given if the child is not severely immunocompromised or HIV$^+$.
B. Pneumococcal and influenza vaccines are recommended.
C. Nutritional support; high-calorie, high-protein diet.
D. Antifungal medications to prevent fungal infections.
E. Educate adolescents regarding safe sex.

## Home Care

A. Teach parent(s) how to care for the child.
1. How to administer medications and importance of administering medications as scheduled.
2. Symptoms of complications: *P. jiroveci* pneumonia (PJP, PCP), *Candida,* failure to thrive.
3. Teach parents standard precautions, including proper handling of diapers and avoidance of contact with blood and body fluids.
4. Prevent biting behaviors in young children.
5. Help parents deal with child's pain—multiple procedures, infections (abscessed tooth, otitis media).
   a. Aggressive management of pain with NSAIDs, opioids, muscle relaxants.
   b. Ongoing assessment of pain in nonverbal children— irritability, lack of interaction, lack of play.

B. Teach parents how to prevent transmission of disease.
C. Course of disease in infants and children is unpredictable.
D. Work with school personnel to maintain privacy/confidentiality.
E. Promote normal growth and development.

## Nursing Interventions for Immunocompromised Clients

**Goal:** To monitor for and/or prevent opportunistic infections

A. The type, location, and severity of the infection depend on the disease progress and the client's immunosuppressive state.
B. Antimicrobial medications are given in high doses for an extended period. Medications may cause neutropenia.
C. Protect from iatrogenic infections or hospital-associated infections.
D. Observe hospitalized client and/or teach client symptoms of opportunistic infections.
1. Persistent unexplained fever, night sweats.
2. Thrush (white spots in the mouth).
3. Persistent diarrhea and weight loss.

**Goal:** To maintain ventilation and prevent pulmonary involvement.

A. PCP prophylaxis may be maintained with trimethoprim-sulfamethoxazole.
B. Rifabutin is used for *Mycobacterium avium* prophylaxis.
C. Frequent assessments for pulmonary changes and hypoxemia.
D. Activities may be unlimited, or bed rest may be prescribed.
E. Supplemental oxygen.
F. Coughing and deep-breathing exercises.
G. Carefully evaluate respiratory function if narcotic analgesics are used.
H. Assess activity tolerance.

**Goal:** To minimize the effects of neurologic changes.

A. Frequent assessment of neurologic status.
B. Assess for visual changes.
C. Observe for neurologic infections, specifically meningitis.
D. If client is confused, provide care directed to reorientation.

E. Provide a safe and supportive environment, according to the neurologic deficits.

**Goal:** To maintain adequate nutritional intake.

A. Teach client regarding nutrition and caloric intake (high-calorie, high-protein diet; nutrition to correct deficiencies).
B. Encourage high-calorie snacks throughout the day.
C. Encourage client to eat several small meals throughout the day.
D. May need to include dietary supplements.
E. Assess client for lactose intolerance.
F. Avoid foods or beverages that may cause oral, esophageal, or gastric irritation.
G. Tube feedings or parenteral nutrition may be necessary.

**Goal:** To maintain fluid and electrolyte status.

A. Evaluate weight gain and loss.
B. Assess for chronic diarrhea.
C. Encourage fluids that assist in maintaining electrolyte balance.

**Goal:** To prevent formation of pressure ulcers and excoriation of the skin.

A. Wash perineal and anal areas; allow areas to dry thoroughly.
B. Observe bony prominence for adequacy of circulation and development of a pressure ulcer.
C. Do not massage or put any lotions on reddened areas or open lesions.
D. Teach client the importance of frequent changes in position.

E. Use gel pads, foam mattress pads, and other pressure-relieving devices to prevent skin breakdown in pressure prone areas (heels and sacrum).

**Goal:** To assist client to maintain psychological equilibrium.

A. Encourage client to express feelings and concerns.
B. Assess for altered self-esteem, family stress, and economic pressures; provide referrals and assistance.
C. Encourage client to maintain as much independence as possible.
D. Help client take advantage of community services available.
E. Do not be judgmental regarding client's lifestyle.
F. Maintain frequent contact with the client.

### Home Care for the Immunocompromised Client

A. Maintain personal hygiene and practice standard precautions; wash hands frequently.
B. Do not share personal items such as toothbrushes, razors, and enema equipment.
C. Teach client how to prevent infection.
   1. Cook all vegetables and meats and peel fruit before eating; this eliminates many sources of microorganisms.
   2. Avoid contact with animal waste (e.g., litter boxes, bird cages, or fish); this further decreases contact with microorganisms.
   3. Avoid crowds and people with respiratory tract infections.
D. Do not get pregnant.

---

## Appendix 10-1 MEDICATIONS

### Antiretroviral Therapy (ART)

#### General Nursing Implications
- Highly active antiretroviral therapy (ART) is used for treatment of clients with HIV infection and AIDS.
- Report any sore throat, white patches on tongue or throat, fever, or other signs of infection to the health care provider.
- It is important to administer the medication at the same time each day to maintain consistent blood levels and to decrease drug resistance.
- No vaccines or immunity-conferring agents should be administered while client is immunosuppressed.
- Maintain standard precautions; use contact, droplet, and airborne precautions as indicated.
- Medications do not cure AIDS or reduce the risk for transmission.

| Medications | Side Effects | Nursing Implications |
|---|---|---|
| **Nonnucleoside Reverse Transcriptase Inhibitors (NNRTIs):** All bind directly to the HIV transcriptase and inhibit the enzyme. | | |
| Efavirenz: PO | CNS symptoms, rash, hepatotoxic, teratogenic | Efavirenz: Monitor LFTs; avoid getting pregnant; avoid taking with St. John's wort. |
| Nevirapine: PO | Rash (may be severe—blistering, joint pain, oral lesions), hepatotoxic, hepatitis | Nevirapine: Monitor LFTs; rash may be so severe that drug is discontinued; resistance may occur if drug is used alone; therefore administer concurrently with another antiretroviral drug. |
| Delavirdine: PO | Rash (may be severe), hepatotoxic, GI symptoms | Delavirdine: Monitor LFTs; rash may be so severe that drug is discontinued. |

### Nucleoside/Nucleotide Reverse Transcriptase Inhibitors (NRTIs): All NTRIs suppress the synthesis of viral DNA by reverse transcriptase. Medications are given with other antiretroviral agents; they are not used alone because of rapid development of resistance.

**Appendix 10-1 MEDICATIONS—cont'd**

R

| Medications | Side Effects | Nursing Implications |
|---|---|---|
| **Adverse Effects of All NRTIs:** Potentially fatal lactic acidosis with hepatic steatosis can occur. Avoid NRTIs during pregnancy because of increased risk of lactic acidosis and hepatic steatosis. | | |
| Zidovudine: PO, IV | Bone marrow suppression, anemia, neutropenia | Maintain upright position to decrease esophageal irritation; monitor levels of anemia and neutropenia. |
| Didanosine: PO | Nausea, diarrhea, peripheral neuropathy, liver damage, pancreatitis | Food decreases absorption; give on empty stomach 30 min before eating or 2 h after. |
| Stavudine: PO | Pancreatitis, lactic acidosis, diarrhea, peripheral neuropathy | Report peripheral neuropathy. Monitor serum amylase and triglyceride levels. |
| Lamivudine: PO | Headache, nausea, malaise/fatigue, diarrhea | St. John's wort may decrease concentration. |
| Abacavir: PO | Hypersensitivity, pulmonary problems | ETOH increases risk for hypersensitivity reactions; report respiratory changes. |

**Protease Inhibitors (PIs):** Bind to the active site of the HIV and render the virus immature and noninfectious; PIs are not given alone because of the development of increased resistance; often given in combination with NRTIs.

**Adverse Effects of all PIs:** Fat maldistribution, hyperlipidemia, hyperglycemia, bone loss, hepatotoxicity, increased bleeding.

**Shared Interactions:** St. John's wort, decreases the effectiveness of PIs.

| Medications | Side Effects | Nursing Implications |
|---|---|---|
| Saquinavir: PO | GI effects | Do not give with grapefruit juice; take with food; check for drug interactions. |
| Ritonavir: PO | Nausea, diarrhea, altered taste, perioral paresthesia | Food increases levels; take with food for tolerance. |
| Indinavir: PO | GI discomfort, renal stones | Take 1 h before or 2 h after meals. |
| Nelfinavir: PO | Diarrhea, rash | Take with food. |
| Amprenavir: PO | N/V, diarrhea, rash | Contraindicated in pregnancy, renal or hepatic failure; high-fat meals decrease absorption. |
| Lopinavir/ritonavir: PO | N/V, diarrhea, increased fatigue | Moderate fat meal increases absorption; take with food; avoid alcohol. |

**Integrase Inhibitor:** Inhibits the enzyme integrase needed for HIV replication.

| Medications | Side Effects | Nursing Implications |
|---|---|---|
| Raltegravir: PO | Insomnia, headache, itching, skin reactions | Women should not breastfeed. *Rifampin can lower levels of the drug.* |
| Dolutegravir: PO | Allergic reactions (may be life threatening), rash | Do not take dolutegravir with dofetilide, which is an antiarrhythmic. |

**HIV Fusion Inhibitor:** Blocks entry of HIV into CD4 T cells.

| Medications | Side Effects | Nursing Implications |
|---|---|---|
| Enfuvirtide: subQ | Injection site reaction, bacterial pneumonia, hypersensitivity reactions | Use small-gauge needle to decrease skin reaction; requires twice-daily subcutaneous injections; monitor respiratory status. |

**CCR5 Antagonist:** Binds CCR5 that HIV must bind within order to enter CD4 cells.

| Medications | Side Effects | Nursing Implications |
|---|---|---|
| Maraviroc: PO | Cough, dizziness, fever, rash, abdominal pain, jaundice; liver injury precipitated by an allergic reaction | Use with caution in clients with cardiovascular risk factors. Inform client of possible signs associated with liver injury (rash, jaundice, pruritis). |

## Medications for Allergic Reactions

**Antihistamines:** Selectively block histamine receptor sites.

*Continued*

---

**Appendix 10-1   MEDICATIONS—cont'd**

| Medications | Side Effects | Nursing Implications |
|---|---|---|
| **H1 Antagonist—First Generation** | | |
| Diphenhydramine: PO, IM, IV<br>Clemastine: PO<br>Promethazine: PO, IV, IM | Dry mouth, dizziness, blurred vision, urinary retention, constipation, and sedation<br>Children: paradoxical reactions; promethazine is contraindicated | 1. Advise client not to engage in activity that requires mental alertness for safety.<br>2. Should not take medication with alcohol.<br>3. Should not be used in clients with asthma.<br>4. Older adults are especially sensitive to CNS and anticholinergic effects. |
| **H1 Antagonist—Second Generation (nonsedating)** | | |
| Cetirizine: PO<br>Fexofenadine: PO<br>Loratadine: PO | Dry mouth and throat<br>Paradoxical reaction in children | 1. Second generation is nonsedating.<br>2. Do not have anticholinergic properties of first generation.<br>3. Should not be taken with alcohol.<br>4. Are much more expensive than first generation. |
| **Intranasal Glucocorticoids** | | |
| Fluticasone<br>Triamcinolone | Nasopharyngeal irritation, sore throat, epistaxis, headache | 1. Teach client to clear nasal passages before using nasal spray.<br>2. Hold spray bottle upright and insert tip into nostril.<br>3. Used to treat allergic rhinitis. |

**Adrenergic Agonist:** Stimulates alpha$_1$, alpha$_2$, beta$_1$, and beta$_2$ adrenergic receptors.

**Action:** Relaxes smooth muscle of bronchial tree (decreases respiratory distress), cardiac stimulant (increases cardiac rate), produces vasoconstriction (increases blood pressure), drug of choice for anaphylactic reactions.

| | | |
|---|---|---|
| Epinephrine, epinephrine auto-injector: subQ, IV<br>1%—1:100—oral inhalation<br>0.1%—1:1000—subQ, IM, IV<br>0.01%—1:10,000—IV, intracardiac | Hypertension, dysrhythmias, angina pectoris, hyperglycemia<br>Necrosis at IV site if extravasation occurs | 1. Clients at risk for anaphylaxis should carry emergency auto-injector epinephrine.<br>2. Auto-injector epinephrine is sensitive to extreme heat and light; discard if it is brown in color, has a precipitate, or has passed its expiration date.<br>3. Advise clients to obtain medical assistance immediately if epinephrine is used.<br>4. Drug of choice for severe anaphylactic reactions.<br>5. Closely monitor pulse rate and blood pressure. |

*AIDS,* Acquired immunodeficiency syndrome; *CNS,* central nervous system; *DNA,* deoxyribonucleic acid; *ETOH,* ethanol; *GI,* gastrointestinal; *HIV,* human immunodeficiency virus; *IV,* intravenous; *LFTs,* liver function tests; *N/V,* nausea/vomiting; *PO,* by mouth (orally); *subQ,* subcutaneous.

---

# Study Questions
# Immune: Care of Adult, Maternity, and Pediatric Clients

More questions on

1. To evaluate the progress of the client's systemic lupus erythematosus (SLE), the nurse evaluates which data?
   1. Increased serum complement fixation, which correlates with reduction of "butterfly" rash
   2. Increasing levels of C-reactive protein (CRP) and erythrocyte sedimentation rate (ESR)
   3. Overall bone marrow proliferation, which correlates with symptoms of inflammation
   4. Presence of antinuclear antibodies (ANA), which correlates with a diminishing immune process

2. The mother of a 15-month-old child who is immunosuppressed asks about continuation of the childhood vaccines. Which immunizations are not recommended to be given to the child during immunosuppression?
   1. Diphtheria, tetanus, and pertussis (DTaP); hepatitis B
   2. *Haemophilus influenzae* B
   3. Varicella; measles–mumps–rubella (MMR)
   4. Inactivated polio; diphtheria, tetanus, and pertussis (DTaP)

3. A client returns to the clinic to receive evaluation of his routine purified protein derivative (PPD) test for tuberculosis screening. The test result is positive. What is the best nursing interpretation of this information?
   1. This is a serious type II reaction and could indicate that he has active tuberculosis; he will need further evaluation immediately.
   2. The positive results indicate the client has been exposed to the tuberculosis bacilli and has had a delayed type IV response.
   3. The client's immune system has been compromised, which allows the immune system to build up antibodies against the pathogen.
   4. An autoimmune response has occurred, and the client will need further evaluation to determine appropriate treatment.

4. A nurse is caring for a client who received a penicillin injection about 15 minutes earlier. The client complains of itching around the mouth, and this rapidly progresses to severe dyspnea and respiratory distress. What are the priority nursing actions?
   1. Anticipate need for possibility of endotracheal intubation, begin oxygen, call for assistance, and obtain emergency cart.
   2. Place the client in supine position and assess for patent airway and presence of breath sounds.
   3. Start oxygen at 6 L/min via nasal cannula; review chart for history of a penicillin allergy.
   4. Place the client in semi-Fowler's position, perform a chin lift to open the airway, and assess for air movement.

5. The nurse is administering medications to a client who has no allergy band on his arm. The nurse tells the client she has his penicillin medication. The client states that the last time he had penicillin, it made his mouth tingle and his hands itch. What would the best nursing action be?
   1. Administer the medication because there is no indication that the client is allergic to penicillin.
   2. Hold the medication and contact the physician regarding the client's statement about his previous experience with penicillin.
   3. Hold the medication and review the client's chart to determine whether there is a penicillin allergy noted.
   4. Notify the nursing supervisor regarding the client's statement and request further evaluation of the client.

6. A client has systemic lupus erythematosus (SLE). What statement best describes this client's immune response?
   1. A delayed hypersensitivity that is cell mediated
   2. An immediate reaction to prior exposure
   3. An immune complex that forms with antibody production
   4. An immune response that no longer recognizes normal body tissue

7. A client is diagnosed with an immunodeficiency disease. The nurse would understand what is characteristic of this condition?
   1. Occurs when a client's body is unable to defend itself from an invading microorganism
   2. Creates a severe, sudden problem that is characterized by increased vascular permeability
   3. Is precipitated by the destruction of the normal lymphocytes in the attempt to reduce the serum level of the antigen
   4. Is a condition in which the normal immune response is interrupted and the body cells do not recognize healthy tissue

8. An infant has an active acquired immunity. Which statement best explains this type of immunity?
   1. The infant has received immunizations.
   2. Immunity was transferred from the mother to the infant.
   3. The infant is recovering from a childhood disease that conferred immunity.
   4. The infant has received gamma globulin after exposure to hepatitis.

9. The nurse is preparing discharge teaching for a woman newly diagnosed with SLE. What will be important for the nurse to include in the teaching plan? **Select all that apply.**
   1. Wear sunscreen and protective clothing when in direct sunlight.
   2. Avoid nonsteroidal antiinflammatory drugs to prevent bleeding episodes.
   3. Plan activities that encourage range of motion in extremities.
   4. Advise the client that pregnancy is contraindicated.
   5. Observe fingertips for changes in circulation.
   6. Help the client prioritize self-care activity.

10. Which of the following statements are correct about latex allergy? **Select all that apply.**
    1. Typical reactions include skin redness, urticaria, and rhinitis.
    2. Latex allergy involves only type I allergic reactions.
    3. The more frequent the exposure to the latex, the more likely a person will develop an allergy.
    4. Hand lotions should be applied before putting on gloves to reduce exposure.
    5. Wash hands with mild soap after removing gloves.
    6. Persons should wear a medic alert bracelet and carry an epinephrine pen.

11. A client with a diagnosis of AIDS has developed *P. jiroveci* pneumonia (PJP, PCP). What will be important for the nurse to include in the nursing care plan?
    1. Put a mask on the client whenever he has visitors in his room.
    2. Explain to the client why he cannot go outside his room.
    3. Wear a mask and gown when providing direct care to the client.
    4. Wear a gown and gloves when assisting the client with personal hygiene.

12. A client is worried he may have been exposed to AIDS. What will be important for the nurse to explain to this client?
    1. Symptoms of AIDS will develop immediately in sexually active individuals.
    2. Clients may remain asymptomatic for an indefinite period of time.
    3. Symptoms of AIDS are usually seen before the client is found to be HIV-positive.
    4. After exposure to the virus, symptoms may develop within 6 to 12 weeks or as late as 6 months.

13. The nurse is caring for a client who is categorized as HIV positive, acute infection. What would the nurse anticipate finding on the nursing assessment?
    1. Fever, swollen lymph glands, nausea
    2. Confusion, wasting syndrome, localized infections
    3. Dyspnea, dementia, persistent fever
    4. Night sweats, low-grade fever, generalized lymphadenopathy

14. A woman explains to the nurse that she thinks she has been exposed to HIV. However, she had a test 1 week after the exposure, and the result was negative. What is most important for the nurse to explain to this client?
    1. Make sure she understands the importance of safe sex practices, especially the use of condoms and contraceptive practices to prevent pregnancy.
    2. Even though the client tested negative, she needs to have a series of follow-up blood tests because of the possibility of seroconversion.
    3. It is important that she obtain counseling regarding the transmission of the virus and how she may protect herself and her partner.
    4. The client should abstain from sexual activity for the next 3 months until the blood test confirms that she is negative for HIV.

15. A client is experiencing difficulty breathing, periorbital swelling, flushing, and itching. He had a diagnostic test in which an iodine-based dye was used about an hour earlier. What medication will the nurse anticipate administering immediately?
    1. A bronchodilator such as aminophylline
    2. A corticosteroid such as dexamethasone
    3. An antihistamine such as diphenhydramine
    4. An adrenergic agonist such as epinephrine

16. The nurse is reviewing with a certified nursing assistant (CNA) the care for a child who is diagnosed with acquired immunodeficiency syndrome (AIDS) and has developed *P. jiroveci* pneumonia (PJP, PCP). Which of the following precautions would the nurse review with the CNA?
    1. Strict handwashing
    2. Airborne precautions
    3. Contact precautions
    4. Standard precautions

17. The nurse is assisting a client with his antiretroviral therapy. What can the nurse do to help the client take his medications as prescribed?
    1. Assess the client's activities of daily living and his lifestyle routine to determine when he can most easily remember to take his medications.
    2. Provide the client with brochures that explain the side effects of the medications and why it is so important for him to adhere to his medication schedule.
    3. Plan for him to visit with other clients who use the same antiretroviral therapy and have them explain to the client how they handle their medications.
    4. Emphasize to the client how important it is to take the medications on the schedule prescribed so that the virus will not get stronger.

18. The nurse is caring for a client who is experiencing a severe anaphylactic reaction caused by an allergy to peanuts. After administering subcutaneous epinephrine and beginning oxygen administration, what would be the next most important nursing action?
    1. Administer analgesics to relieve the pain.
    2. Start an IV for fluid administration.
    3. Insert a catheter to determine urinary output.
    4. Obtain a history of possible reactions to penicillin.

19. A client with AIDS has several cutaneous lesions identified as Kaposi sarcoma. How will the nurse care for these areas?
    1. Gently cleanse the areas, keeping them dry and free of abrasions.
    2. Place sterile, saline-soaked gauze over the areas.
    3. Apply a topical corticosteroid cream.
    4. Decrease infection by applying an antibiotic ointment.

20. What is an allergic reaction that can quickly deteriorate into shock and death?
    1. Anaphylaxis
    2. Graft-versus-host disease
    3. Type III, immune complex formation
    4. Delayed sensitivity

# Answers to Study Questions

1. *2*
The ESR and the CRP are indicators of inflammation in the body. Neither is diagnostic of SLE, but the level of inflammation is an index to the progress of the condition. Presence of ANA is characteristic of SLE, but it does not indicate progression. Complement fixation does not indicate progression, nor does absence or presence of the butterfly rash. (Lewis et al., 10 ed., p. 1540)

2. *3*
Live viruses are usually not administered when a client is immunosuppressed. Frequently, measles–mumps–rubella (MMR) vaccine and varicella vaccine are not given to the immunocompromised client; they may be administered when the client has a more competent immune system. Childhood vaccinations are encouraged when the client is not immunocompromised (in remission or not on immunosuppressant medications). (Hockenberry & Wilson, 9 ed., p. 1455)

3. *2*
Type IV (cell-mediated, delayed hypersensitivity) reaction is a delayed response that occurs 24 to 72 hours after exposure to the allergen (e.g., PPD). The client has been sensitized to tuberculosis. There is no indication of active TB, and it is not a type II reaction. The client's immune system has not been compromised; rather, it has responded normally with the production of antibodies after exposure to the allergen. This does not represent an autoimmune response. (Lewis et al., 10 ed., pp. 199–200)

4. *1*
This situation best describes an anaphylactic reaction to the penicillin injection. This is a rapidly occurring response that may result in a life-threatening occlusion of the airway (laryngeal edema, bronchospasm). The client may require an emergency tracheotomy or endotracheal intubation. Time should not be wasted on checking the chart or further assessment. The client is obviously in distress,

and the presence of breath sounds will not be significant in determining the nursing actions. The chin lift is not an effective method for opening an airway that is occluded from edema or bronchospasm. Epinephrine is the drug of choice for a serious anaphylactic reaction. (Lewis et al., 10 ed., p. 201)

**5.** *2*

Even though there is no allergy band, if the client provides information that may indicate a previous reaction to a medication (especially penicillin), hold the medication. With each exposure to an allergen, the reaction could become worse (type I reaction). Notifying the supervisor is not necessary; there is enough information for the nurse to make this decision. (Lewis, 10 ed., pp. 201–202)

**6.** *4*

SLE is characterized as an autoimmune disorder in which the body begins to invade and destroy normal tissue. A delayed hypersensitivity is a type IV response that is characteristic of a transplant rejection or reaction to tuberculin skin testing. An immediate reaction describes a type I reaction characterized by a prior exposure to antigen. This occurs with atopic reactions and anaphylaxis. An immune complex that forms with antibody production is a type III response, which occurs with acute glomerulonephritis. (Lewis et al., 10 ed., pp. 197–200)

**7.** *1*

Immunodeficiency is the condition when the immune system is depressed, weak, or compromised and is unable to defend the body from invading microorganisms. Immunodeficiency may be primary if it is caused by an absence of immune cells or by poorly developed immune cells. It is secondary if it is caused by illnesses or treatment. A severe, sudden problem characterized by increased vascular permeability describes an anaphylactic reaction. The destruction of normal lymphocytes in the attempt to reduce the serum level of the antigen reflects phagocytosis as the white cells destroy the foreign protein. When the normal immune response is interrupted and body cells do not recognize healthy tissue, this is characteristic of an autoimmune condition. (Lewis et al., 10 ed., pp. 205–206)

**8.** *1*

Active acquired immunity occurs when a client (infant, child, or adult) receives an immunization against a specific disease. Natural active immunity occurs when the client has had the disease. Natural passive immunity occurs with transfer of antibodies from the mother to the infant at birth or through breast milk. Passive artificial immunity occurs with injection of gamma globulins; the response is immediate but short term. (Lewis et al., 10 ed., p. 192)

**9.** *1, 3, 5, 6*

The client with SLE is photosensitive and needs protection from sunlight. The client needs to keep joints mobilized because of the invasion of the lupus erythematosus cells into the joints. This condition also affects the circulation in the fingertips, and Raynaud's phenomenon is characteristic of the disease. Fatigue is a problem, and the client needs to prioritize activities of daily living. NSAIDs are frequently used to reduce the musculoskeletal discomforts. Although individual disease progression and course of therapy need to be considered in consultation with health care providers, there is no specific contraindication to pregnancy. The woman should be advised regarding individual risk, but she can carry and deliver a healthy infant. (Lewis et al., 10 ed., pp. 1538–1542)

**10.** *1, 3, 5, 6*

It is important for the nurse to recognize symptoms of latex allergy—skin rash, hives, flushing, and itching; nasal, eye, and sinus symptoms; asthma and (rarely) anaphylaxis. The nurse should also be aware of latex-containing products—gloves, blood pressure cuffs, stethoscopes, tourniquets, IV tubing, syringes, electrode pads, oxygen masks, tracheal tubes, colostomy and ileostomy tubes, urinary catheters, anesthetic masks, and adhesive tape. The use of nonlatex gloves and powder-free gloves, along with the elimination of oil-based hand creams or lotions when wearing gloves, can reduce exposure. Always wash hands after removing gloves. Individuals with latex allergy should wear a medic alert bracelet if latex sensitive. The more frequent and prolonged the exposure to latex, the greater the likelihood of developing latex allergy. There are two types of latex allergy: type IV allergic contact dermatitis (delayed reaction) and type I allergy reaction (immediate response). (Lewis et al., 10 ed., pp. 203–204)

**11.** *4*

*P. jiroveci* pneumonia (PJP, PCP) is not easily transmitted from an infected person to a healthy person. The pathogen is frequently dormant in the body and is reactivated when the client's immune system is significantly depressed. There is no need for airborne or droplet precautions, but standard precautions must be strictly adhered to with this client. (Lewis et al,. 10 ed., p. 222)

**12.** *4*

Clients usually have symptoms within 6 to 12 weeks of exposure, but symptoms may not develop until 6 months after exposure. This is the period of seroconversion. The symptoms do not develop immediately in sexually active individuals. The client may remain asymptomatic for an undetermined period of time. The client may be HIV positive for years before he is diagnosed as having AIDS. (Lewis et al., 10 ed., p. 220)

**13.** *1*

An acute infection occurs when the primary condition is identified or the client has recently been infected. The client may be asymptomatic at this time or they may have flulike symptoms and early nonspecific changes characterized by fatigue, sore throat, fever, diarrhea, muscle and joint pain, diffuse rash, and swollen lymph glands. The other items are symptoms noted with chronic HIV infection. Chronic HIV infection can be either *asymptomatic* (fatigue, headache, low-grade fever, night sweats, persistent generalized lymphadenopathy), *symptomatic* (symptoms become worse, leading to persistent fever, frequent drenching night sweats, chronic diarrhea, recurrent headaches, and fatigue severe enough to interrupt normal routines with localized infections, lymphadenopathy, and nervous system problems), or *AIDS* (development of opportunistic infections, wasting syndrome, dementia). The symptoms noted in the remaining options are seen with chronic disease. (Lewis et al., 10 ed., pp. 220–221)

**14.** *2*

After initial infection, there is a window of seroconversion in which the virus begins to replicate and produce antibodies. The client may have a negative test result early in the window. When the body begins to produce antibodies against the virus, the test result will convert to a positive. She should not get pregnant, but contraceptives (oral birth control) do not protect her against human immunodeficiency virus (HIV). Abstaining from sexual activity is frequently unrealistic, and counseling would be beneficial, but it is not the priority. Although emphasizing the importance of safe sex practices is correct, it is not the best response. The priority in this situation is the necessity for follow-up blood tests because of the initial negative test result. (Lewis et al., 10 ed., pp. 220–221; 225–226.)

**15.** *4*

Epinephrine, given subcutaneously or intravenously, is the drug of choice for anaphylactic reactions. The reaction described is a mild to moderate anaphylactic reaction. The other medications listed may be used in treatment of the reaction, but epinephrine is the immediate drug of choice. (Lewis et al., 10 ed., pp. 202–203.)

**16.** *4*

The CDC recommends standard precautions for all clients; this is particularly important for the client with AIDS. Although strict handwashing is not an incorrect response, this should be performed when caring for all clients and is a part of standard precautions. Airborne precautions are not indicated for clients with opportunistic infections such as *P. jiroveci* pneumonia (PJP, PCP). Protective isolation is indicated for clients who are severely immunocompromised (e.g., clients who have undergone transplants). (Lewis et al., 10 ed., p. 218)

**17.** *1*

It is important to identify the client's routines and discuss how he can adapt those routines to take his medications as prescribed. Discussing with the client the importance of taking the medications does not assist him to identify ways in which he can incorporate the medications into his daily routines. Talking to and working with another client is positive, but it still does not incorporate the medication routine into his own daily living routines. (Lewis et al., 10 ed., pp. 228–229)

**18.** *2*

Shock is a common problem in anaphylactic reactions; therefore it is important to establish an IV for fluid and medication administration. There should be no pain, and there is no reason the client cannot void on his or her own. A history can be taken at a later time. (Lewis et al., 10 ed., p. 202)

**19.** *1*

There is no specific nursing care required for Kaposi sarcoma lesions. Gently cleansing the area and protecting it from abrasive trauma, which could open the lesions, would be appropriate. Dressings, steroid cream, and antibiotic ointment are not indicated. Standard precautions should be followed when caring for the lesions. (Lewis et al., 10 ed., pp. 222–223)

**20.** *1*

Anaphylaxis is a massive antigen–antibody response, causing a physiologic system shutdown and possible death. Graft-versus-host disease (GVHD) occurs when antibodies in the transplanted organ attack the host's antigens. An immune complex formation occurs when antigen–antibody complex is deposited in body tissue. A delayed sensitivity is a reaction that occurs after cells are sensitized to an antigen, as seen in the tuberculosis skin testing. (Lewis et al., 10 ed., pp. 197–199)

# CHAPTER ELEVEN

# Cancer Concepts

## PRIORITY CONCEPTS

Cellular Regulation, Palliation, Safety

## CHARACTERISTICS OF CANCER

Cancer must be regarded as a group of disease entities with different causes, manifestations, treatments, and prognoses. The basic disease process begins when normal cells undergo change and begin to proliferate in an abnormal manner.

### Major Dysfunction in the Cell

A. Cellular proliferation: Cancer cells divide in an indiscriminate, unregulated manner and exhibit significant variations in structure and size.

B. Loss of contact inhibition: Cancer cells have no regard for cellular boundaries; normal cells respect boundaries and do not invade adjacent areas or organs.

C. Cancer can arise from any cell in the body that can evade the normal regulatory controls of proliferation or growth and cellular differentiation.

D. Cell biology.
1. Predetermined means that the stem cell of specific tissue will differentiate and mature for only that tissue.
2. A state of equilibrium is constantly being maintained between cellular proliferation and cellular degeneration.
3. Cancer cells divide indiscriminately.

E. Tumors (neoplasms) (Table 11-1).
1. Benign: encapsulated neoplasm that remains localized in the tissue of origin and is typically not harmful.
   a. Exerts pressure on surrounding organs.
   b. Will decrease blood supply to the normal tissue.
2. Malignant: nonencapsulated neoplasm that invades surrounding tissue. Depends on the stage of the neoplasm as to whether metastasis (spreading to distant body parts) occurs. The neoplasm spreads by means of four primary mechanisms:
   a. Vascular system: Cancer cells penetrate vessels and circulate until trapped. The cancer cells may penetrate the vessel wall and invade adjacent organs and tissues.
   b. Lymphatic system: Cancer cells penetrate the lymphatic system and are distributed along lymphatic channels.
   c. Implantation: Cancer cells implant into a body organ. Certain cells have an affinity for particular organs and body areas.
   d. Seeding: A primary tumor sloughs off tumor cells into a body cavity, such as the peritoneal cavity.
3. Common sites for metastasis: brain, liver, lungs, adrenals, spinal cord, and bone (Figure 11-1).

### Etiology

A. Viruses: incorporate into the genetic structure of the cell, causing mutations (e.g., Kaposi sarcoma from HIV, hepatitis B virus and hepatocellular cancer, human papilloma virus and cervical cancer).

B. Radiation: exposure to sunlight and radiation (e.g., bone cancer in radiologists, UV radiation and melanoma).

C. Chemical agents: produce toxic effects by altering DNA structure in body cells (e.g., dyes, asbestos, tars, tobacco use, chronic irritation, or inflammation); there may be an extended latency period from time of exposure to development of the cancer.

D. Genetic and familial factors: DNA damage occurs in cells where chromosomal patterns are abnormal, which increases the individual's susceptibility to cancer.

E. Hormonal agents: Tumor growth is promoted by disturbances in hormonal balance of the body's own (endogenous) hormones or administration of exogenous hormones (e.g., prolonged estrogen replacement, oral contraceptives).

F. Idiopathic: Many cancers—breast, colon, rectal, lymphatic, bone marrow, and pancreatic cancers—arise spontaneously from unknown causes.

### Prevention

A. Cancer prevention.
1. Eat a balanced diet that includes fresh fruits and vegetables, adequate amount of fiber and whole grains, and decreased fats and preservatives; avoid smoked and salt-cured foods containing increased nitrates (see Figure 2-4).
2. Avoid exposure to known carcinogens (e.g., cigarette smoking, tanning beds, and sun exposure).
3. Keep weight in normal range; obesity is associated with cancer of uterus, gallbladder, breast, and colon.
4. Get enough rest and sleep—at least 6 to 8 hours per night.
5. Decrease stress, or perception of stress, and improve ability to effectively manage stress.
6. Engage in at least 30 minutes of moderate to vigorous exercise 5 days a week.
7. Limit alcohol use.

**Table 11-1   COMPARISON OF BENIGN AND MALIGNANT TUMORS**

| Characteristic | Benign | Malignant |
|---|---|---|
| Cell division | Continuous or inappropriate | Rapid and continuous |
| Appearance | Specific morphologic features | Anaplastic |
| Cell characteristics | Fairly normal; similar to parent cells | Cells abnormal; become more unlike parent cells |
| Encapsulated | Usually | Rarely |
| Differentiated functions | Many | Some or none |
| Metastasis or migration of cells | Absent | Yes |
| Recurrence | Rare | Possible |
| Vascularity | Slight | Moderate to marked |
| Mode of growth | Expansive | Infiltrative, invasive, and expansive |

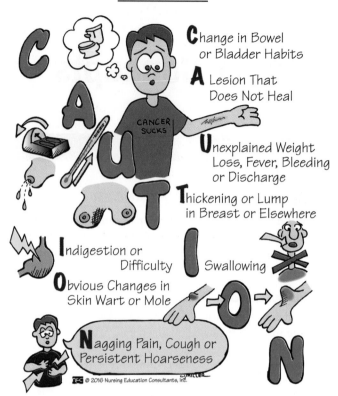

**FIGURE 11-2 Caution.** (From Zerwekh, J., Garneau, A., & Miller, C. J. [2017]. *Digital collection of the memory notebooks of nursing* [4th ed.]. Chandler, AZ: Nursing Education Consultants, Inc.)

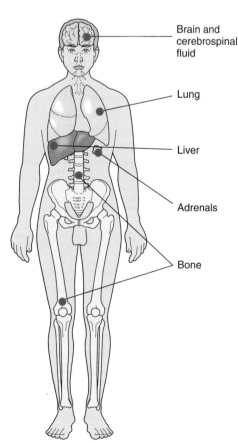

**FIGURE 11-1 Main Sites of Metastasis.** (From McCance, K., & Huether, S. [2014] *Pathophysiology: The biologic basis for disease in adults and children* [7th ed.]. St. Louis, MO: Elsevier.)

B. Screening guidelines—early detection is important. Know the seven warning signs of cancer and encourage early reporting of any change in an individual's normal body function. (Figure 11-2) (See the U.S. Preventive Services Task Force information at http://www.uspreventiveservicestaskforce.org/Page/Name/tools-and-resources-for-better-preventive-care)

1. Cervical: Screening should begin at age 21; between ages 21 and 29 should have a Pap test every 3 years; between ages 30 and 65 should have a Pap test plus an HPV test every 5 years; if vaccinated against HPV, should still follow the screening recommendations.

2. Prostate: The pros and cons of prostate cancer screening should be discussed with men beginning at age 50. Testing could include a digital rectal examination (DRE) or prostate-specific antigen blood test. African American men and those men with strong family history should have this talk beginning at age 45.

3. Colorectal: For ages 50 to 75, all clients should have one of the following: a flexible sigmoidoscopy every 5 years, a colonoscopy every 10 years, a double contrast barium enema every 5 years, a computed tomography (CT) colonography (virtual colonoscopy) every 5 years, a yearly highly sensitive fecal occult blood test (FOBT), or a yearly fecal immunochemical test (FIT). Screening selection will be determined on the basis of the client's history and what schedule works best for the client.

4. Breast: Women should undergo annual screening mammography from ages 45 to 54. At 55 years, women may transition to biennial screening. Screening mammography should continue as long as life expectancy is 10 years or longer.
5. Testicular self-examination: monthly from ages 20 to 40 (see Chapter 24).
6. Endometrium: At menopause, all women should be informed about the risks and symptoms of endometrial cancer. Women should report unexpected bleeding or spotting.

## Classification of Malignant Tumors

A. Cellular origin or anatomic classification: tumor is identified by the tissue of origin.
   1. Epithelial tissue *(-carcinoma):* surface epithelium—carcinoma; glandular epithelium—adenocarcinoma.
   2. Connective tissue *(-sarcoma):* cartilage—chondrosarcoma; striated muscle bone—rhabdomyosarcoma; fibrous tissue—fibrosarcoma; bone—osteosarcoma.
   3. Nervous system tissue *(-oma):* meninges—meningeal sarcoma; nerve cells—neuroblastoma.
   4. Hematopoietic tissue *(-oma):* lymphoid tumors—Hodgkin's lymphoma, non-Hodgkin's lymphoma; plasma cells—multiple myeloma; bone marrow—lymphocytic and myelogenous leukemia.
B. TNM classification (staging) (Box 11-1).

---

### Box 11-1  TNM STAGING CLASSIFICATION

T: Tumor size
N: Degree of involvement of lymph nodes
M: Absence or presence of metastasis

**T: Primary Tumor**
TX: Tumor cannot be evaluated
T0: No evidence of primary tumor
Tis: Cancer is in situ (tumor has not started growing into the surrounding structures)
T1–T4: Describe the size and/or level of invasion into nearby structures—the higher the T number, the larger the tumor and/or the further it may have grown into nearby structures

**N: Regional Lymph Nodes**
NX: Nearby lymph nodes cannot be evaluated
N0: No regional lymph node involvement (no cancer in the lymph nodes)
N1–N3: Describe the size, location, and/or the number of lymph nodes involved—the higher the N number, the more lymph nodes are involved

**M: Distant Metastasis**
M0: No distant metastases
M1: Distant metastases present
   *Example:* Tis, NX, MO—cancer in situ; unable to clinically assess distant lymph nodes; no evidence of distant metastasis

Adapted from American Joint Committee on Cancer: *What is cancer staging?* Retrieved from http://www.cancerstaging.org/references-tools/Pages/What-is-Cancer-Staging.aspx

---

# TREATMENT OF CANCER

## Diagnostics

A. Common cancer diagnostic studies.
   1. X-ray.
   2. Tissue biopsy.
   3. Radiographic studies: mammography, ultrasonography, CT scans, or magnetic resonance imaging (MRI).
   4. Radioisotopic scans: bone, liver, lung, brain.
   5. Cytology studies (bone marrow aspiration, urine and cerebrospinal fluid analysis, cell washings, Pap smears, and bronchial washings).
   6. Position emission tomography (PET) scan.
   7. Tumor markers; genetic markers.
   8. Endoscopic examinations: upper GI, sigmoidoscopy, or colonoscopy examinations—including stool for occult blood.
   9. Complete blood count (CBC), chemistry profile, liver function tests.
   10. Bone marrow examination (if hematolymphoid malignancy is suspected).
   11. Molecular receptor status (estrogen and progesterone receptors).

> **TEST ALERT:** Assist client in maintaining an optimum level of health; evaluate incorporation of healthy behaviors into lifestyle (screening, immunizations); instruct client on ways to promote health.

B. Biopsy.
   1. Used for definitive diagnosis.
   2. Needle: Tissue samples are obtained by a small-gauge aspiration needle (fine-needle aspiration) or with a large-bore needle (large-core biopsy).
   3. Incisional: Scalpel or dermal punch is used to obtain a tissue sample.
   4. Excisional: involves removal of the entire tumor.
   5. Endoscopic biopsy: direct biopsy through an endoscopy of the area (gastrointestinal, respiratory, genitourinary tracts).

## Goals of Cancer Therapy

A. Prophylaxis: to provide treatment when no tumor is detectable but when client is known to be at risk for tumor development, spread, or recurrence.
B. Cure: Client will be disease-free and live to normal life expectancy.
C. Control: Client's cancer is not cured but controlled by therapy over long periods of time.
D. Palliation: to maintain as high a quality of life for the client as possible when cure and control are not possible.

## Personalized Cancer Care

A. Cancer treatments chosen for the individual are based on the client's specific genetic information rather than just their disease and stage.

B. Can lead to better outcomes for the client, since the treatment is specific to the client.

## Modalities of Cancer Treatment

> ⚠ **NURSING PRIORITY:** Therapy generally involves using two or more modalities of treatment.

A. Surgery.
   1. Diagnostic surgery: obtains tissue samples (biopsies) for diagnostic purposes and to determine methods of treatment.
   2. Clinical staging surgery: determines the extent of the cancer; presence and location of metastatic lesions.
   3. Curative and/or control surgery: removal of cancers that are localized to the area of origin; extent of resection determined by the type and spread of tumor.
   4. Palliative surgery: does not impair the growth or spread of the cancer but improves the client's quality of life; may be done to relieve pain, decrease obstruction, relieve pressure, and/or to prevent hemorrhage.
   5. Supportive care: surgeries to support cancer treatment (e.g., suprapubic cystostomy for prostate cancer, feeding tubes).
   6. Reconstructive surgery: restoration of the client's form, function, and appearance after radical surgery for cancer.
   7. Preventive surgery: For clients who are in a high-risk category, certain surgical procedures may prevent the future development of cancer (e.g., prophylactic mastectomy).
B. Chemotherapy: Overall goal of chemotherapy is to destroy the cancer cells without excessive damage to normal cells (see Appendix 11-1).

> ⚠ **NURSING PRIORITY:** The therapeutic ratio is the guiding principle of chemotherapy. The aim is to administer an antineoplastic agent dose large enough to eradicate cancer cells but small enough to limit adverse effects to safe and tolerable levels.

   1. Medications are highly toxic and destroy healthy cells as well as cancer cells.
   2. Combination chemotherapy is more effective than single-dose therapy.
   3. Adjuvant therapy: after the initial therapy (surgical or radiation), medications are used to eliminate or slow replication of any remaining cancer cells. For example, tamoxifen may be given in the early stages of breast cancer to block the effects of estrogen, thereby helping prevent the development of cancer in the other breast.
   4. Myelosuppressive effects usually peak in 7 to 10 days after chemotherapy, causing low platelet counts and critically low white blood cell counts (leukopenia/neutropenia). The period of time when a client is at the lowest level of neutrophil count is called the nadir; this represents the point at which the client is at the highest risk for infection.

> **TEST ALERT:** Follow procedures for handling biohazardous materials (e.g., chemotherapeutic agents, radiation sources).

   5. Vascular access methods of administration (see Appendix 9-4).
      a. Peripherally inserted central catheters (PICC): external access central lines.
      b. Tunneled venous access port: catheter is tunneled from exit site to the venous insertion site (Hickman catheter or Groshong catheter).
      c. Implanted infusion venous access port: a single or double subcutaneous injection port is connected to a central venous catheter. The catheter is placed in a vein, and the other end is connected to a port that is sutured or implanted into the chest wall (Port-A-Cath).
C. Regional chemotherapy.
   1. Intrathecal or intraventricular: delivery of chemotherapy into the cerebrospinal fluid; often administered via a surgically implanted device positioned under the scalp (Ommaya reservoir).
   2. Intraperitoneal: delivery of chemotherapy into the peritoneal cavity.
   3. Intraarterial: catheter placed into an artery and then connected to an infusion pump.
   4. Intravesical bladder chemotherapy: delivery of chemotherapy into the bladder using a urinary catheter.
D. Nursing interventions in chemotherapy (Table 11-2).
   1. Assess client for symptoms of bone marrow suppression (increased bruising and bleeding, sore throat, fever, increased fatigue).
   2. Prevent exposure of client to people with communicable diseases or infections.
   3. Before therapy, establish a baseline regarding intake and output, bowel habits, oral hygiene, mental health status, and family relationships.
   4. Monitor intake and output; maintain adequate hydration to prevent urinary complications.
   5. Inform client that alopecia, if it occurs, is usually transient.
   6. Some chemotherapeutic medications are highly irritating (vesicant) and must be administered intravenously into an area of high blood flow (central venous access devices [CVADs]) to provide rapid dilution and prevent extravasation.
E. Radiation therapy: radiation destroys the cell's ability to reproduce by damaging the cellular DNA. Cells that are rapidly reproducing are vulnerable to the effects of

**Table 11-2   NURSING IMPLICATIONS AND CHEMOTHERAPY**

| Problem | Nursing Implications |
|---|---|
| Bone marrow suppression <br> • Thrombocytopenia (decreased platelets) | 1. Initiate bleeding precautions (e.g., decrease invasive procedures; minimize injections). <br> 2. Observe for bleeding tendency (bruising, hematuria, bleeding gums, etc.). <br> 3. Monitor platelet counts. |
| • Anemia (decreased hemoglobin) | 1. Fatigue is normal with chemotherapy; client should report any significant increase in fatigue. <br> 2. Encourage diet high in protein, calories, and iron; administer iron supplements and erythropoietin. <br> 3. Monitor hemoglobin level. |
| • Leukopenia (decreased white cells) | 1. Advise health care provider regarding any unexplained temperature elevation greater than 100°F or other signs of infection. <br> 2. Protect client from exposure to infections (e.g., frequent hand hygiene, location of room, screen visitors, etc.). <br> 3. Monitor WBC count, especially neutrophil levels. <br> 4. Administer WBC growth factors. |
| Pneumonitis (pulmonary toxicity) | 1. Monitor for persistent nonproductive cough, fever, exertional dyspnea, and tachypnea. <br> 2. Most cases are cumulative dose–related and can be fatal. |
| Hyperuricemia (increased serum levels of uric acid) | 1. Encourage fluid intake up to 3000 mL daily, if allowed. <br> 2. Assess for involvement of the kidney, ureters, and bladder. <br> 3. Allopurinol may be used as prevention or as treatment. |
| Alopecia | 1. Encourage client to wear something to cover the scalp (e.g., wig, scarf, turban, hat). <br> 2. Avoid exposure of scalp to sunlight. <br> 3. Do not rub scalp; do not use hair rollers, hair dryers, curlers, or curling irons. <br> 4. Avoid excessive shampooing, brushing, or combing of hair. <br> 5. Hair usually grows back in 3–4 weeks after chemotherapy; it is usually a different texture and color. |
| Stomatitis (mucositis) | 1. Encourage good oral hygiene and frequent oral checks. <br>    a. Encourage frequent mouth rinses of saline or salt and soda solution to keep mucous membranes moist. <br>    b. Brush teeth with a small, soft toothbrush after every meal and at bedtime. <br>    c. Remove dentures to prevent further irritation. <br> 2. Avoid alcohol and spicy or hot foods; a mechanical soft, bland diet may be ordered. <br> 3. Rinse mouth with topical anesthetics, such as viscous lidocaine, for pain control. |
| GI: anorexia, nausea and vomiting, diarrhea, and constipation | 1. Assist client to maintain good nutrition. <br>    a. Discuss food preferences with client and dietitian; encourage small, frequent meals. <br>    b. Correlate meals with antiemetic medications. <br>    c. Encourage family to provide client with favorite foods. <br>    d. Increase calories, protein, and iron; encourage supplemental vitamins. Nutritional supplements may be indicated. <br> 2. Monitor weight, hydration status, and electrolyte imbalances. <br> 3. Evaluate skin around anal area in the client with diarrhea; prevent excoriation. <br> 4. If prone to constipation, maintain high fluid and high fiber intake; use stool softeners as needed. <br> 5. If experiencing diarrhea, encourage fluids, low-fiber, low-residue diet. |
| Tissue irritation, necrosis, ulceration from infusion therapy | 1. Vesicant medications should be administered via a central line to promote dilution of medication. Monitor site for infection. <br> 2. If multiple drugs are administered, flush between each administration. |

> **⚠ NURSING PRIORITY:** Observe client for side effects of a chemotherapeutic agent. If extravasation occurs with a vesicant medication in a peripheral site:
> 1. Stop the infusion: Remove any remaining drug in the tubing or needle.
> 2. Contact physician and consult hospital policy and precautions for specific medication.
> 3. Antidote medication may be instilled directly into the infiltrated area.
> 4. Ice or heat may be applied to site, depending on the medication; the extremity may be elevated for the first 24–48 hours after extravasation.

*GI*, Gastrointestinal; *IV*, intravenous; *WBC*, white blood cell.

radiation. Radiation treats select regions of the body to achieve a focused control of the disease.

1. Types of radiation therapy.
   a. External beam therapy (teletherapy): radiation source is outside the body and directed toward the area of the tumor.
      (1) Decreases the incidence of skin surface damage.
      (2) Client should not wash off the markers for the radiation sites.

> **⚠ NURSING PRIORITY:** Clients who receive radiation therapy should not be bathed with soap over the radiation site and should avoid use of lotions and powders.

   b. Internal radiation (brachytherapy, close therapy, sealed source therapy): the sealed source of radiation is implanted directly in the tumor or in a body cavity around a tumor.
      (1) *Brachy* means "short distance"—radiation given very close to the tumor, where it can be focused precisely on abnormal cells.
      (2) May be used to treat gynecologic malignancies and lung or head and neck malignancies.
      (3) Sealed sources of radiation are temporarily implanted in the tumor area (see Box 11-2).
   c. Unsealed source (radiopharmaceutical or isotope): radioisotopes may be given intravenously or orally. Body fluids become contaminated.
2. Adverse effects of radiation therapy.

> **⚠ NURSING PRIORITY:** Adverse effects are related to radiation dose delivered within a specified time, method of delivery, and client's overall health status.

   a. Skin reactions.
      (1) Skin erythema, followed by dry desquamation of the skin in the treatment field.
      (2) Wet desquamation, particularly in areas of skinfolds (breast, perineum, axillary); skin may be blistered.
      (3) Loss of hair on the skin in the treatment field.
      (4) Skin hyperpigmentation and discoloration.
   b. GI disturbances are more pronounced when radiation is delivered to the area closely associated with the GI tract.
   c. Cystitis when radiation source is near the urinary tract.
   d. Radiation pneumonitis develops 2 to 3 months after start of treatment.
   e. Pericarditis may occur when chest wall receives radiation.
3. Safety precautions to prevent excessive exposure for health care providers (Figure 11-3; also see Box 11-2).
   a. Time: coordinate client care to minimize caregiver's exposure to the client.
   b. Distance: maintain the maximum distance possible to provide client care. Attempt to maintain distance of 6 feet from the source of radiation.

---

### Box 11-2 RADIATION SAFETY PRECAUTIONS AND NURSING IMPLICATIONS

**Internal Implant (Sealed Source)**
- Provide private room and bath.
- Plan care so minimal time is spent in the room.
- When prolonged care is required, use a lead shield or wear a lead apron.
- Wear a film badge to measure exposure; do not share badges.
- Mark on the room and in the Kardex that pregnant women, infants, and young children should not come in contact with the client during treatment.
- Check all linens and materials removed from the bed for presence of foreign bodies that could be a source of radioactivity.
- Keep long-handled forceps and lead container in the room of a client with an implant in place.
- Post notice on client's door—visits should be limited to 30 minutes per day and advise them to stay about 6 feet from the client.

**External Radiation**
- Do not wash off marks placed on client's body for purpose of identifying area for external radiation.
- Skin reactions after radiation therapy may not develop for 10–14 days and may not subside until 2–4 weeks after treatment.
- Gently cleanse skin with a mild soap; do not remove skin markings.
- Avoid tight-fitting clothing; encourage loose-fitting cotton clothes.
- Avoid direct sunlight on radiation area.
- Avoid exposure of treatment area to all heat and/or cold sources (hot baths, hot water bottles, ice packs)
- Do not apply any perfumed or medicated lotions or creams.
- Advise client to avoid swimming during treatment period; chemicals can irritate the skin.
- Do not use tape, adhesive bandages, cosmetics, lotions, perfumes, powders, or deodorants on the skin in the treatment field.
- Closely monitor skin condition on area where x-ray treatment is directed.

   c. Shielding: in practice, lead shielding is difficult to work with and is generally not necessary if time and distance principles are observed.
   d. Film badge: always wear a film badge (dosimeter) when providing care.

> **TEST ALERT:** Follow procedures when handling biohazardous materials (e.g., radiation therapy implants, chemotherapeutic agents). Time, distance, and shielding are critical concepts (cardinal principles) in caring for a client with a radiation implant.

4. Nursing implications for client receiving internal (sealed source) and external radiation. (see Box 11-2)
5. Nursing implications for the client receiving systemic radiation therapy.
   a. Systemically administered radionuclides—radioisotopes (e.g., $I^{131}$ for thyroid cancer)—will initially cause radioactive body secretions.

## RADIATION SAFETY

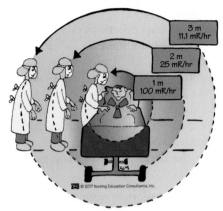

- Time, distance, and shielding are important safety precautions to prevent excessive exposure to health care providers.
- The closer you are to the patient the more exposure to radioactivity, so minimize time spent at a close distance.
- Try to maintain a minimum distance of 6 feet or 2 meters from the source of radiation.

**FIGURE 11-3 Radiation Safety.** (From Zerwekh, J., Garneau, A., & Miller, C. J. [2017]. *Digital collection of the memory notebooks of nursing* [4th ed.]. Chandler, AZ: Nursing Education Consultants, Inc.)

b. Keep linens, dressings, and trash in client's room until radiation safety office determines how and when they can be removed.

c. Be aware of the type of radiation administered and the half-life of the isotope; this will determine how long the body secretions are radioactive.

F. Immunotherapy: agents modify the relationship between the host and the tumor by altering the biologic response of the host to the tumor cells. Immunotherapy can (1) have direct antitumor effects or (2) boost or manipulate the immune system so that cancer cells are unable to grow.

G. Targeted therapy: interferes with cancer growth by targeting cellular receptors and pathways important in tumor growth. Targeted therapies are able to kill cancer cells with less damage to normal cells compared with chemotherapy.

H. Hematopoietic stem cell transplantation: allows for very high doses of chemotherapy and/or radiation therapy to be given, which clears the bone marrow to allow the transplanted healthy stem cells to engraft.

I. Hematopoietic growth factors: support cancer patients as they are treated for their disease.

J. Pediatrics: long-term effects of treatment on the child.
1. Impaired growth and development, especially from radiation to growth centers of the bone during early childhood and adolescence.
2. Damage to the central nervous system.
3. Gonadal aberrations, including reproductive, hormonal, genetic, and teratogenic effects.
4. Disturbances to other organs, including pneumonitis, pericarditis, pleurisy, hypothyroidism, and cystitis.

## Oncologic Emergencies

A. Life-threatening problems arising from tumor progression, response to chemotherapy or radiation therapy, extensive surgical resection.

B. Obstructive emergencies: caused by tumor growth and obstruction of an organ or blood vessel.
1. Superior vena cava syndrome (SVCS): may be associated with non-Hodgkin's lymphoma, metastatic breast cancer, or lung cancer.
    a. Symptoms: periorbital and facial edema; distention of the veins in the head, neck, and chest; headache and possible seizures.
    b. Treatment: radiation or chemotherapy.
2. Tracheobronchial compromise: may occur in the upper or lower airway; most commonly occurs secondary to a lung tumor.
    a. Symptoms: stridor and hypoxia.
    b. Treatment: bronchodilators, steroids, and possible intubation.
3. Spinal cord compression: caused by tumor growth into the epidural space of the spinal cord.
    a. Symptoms: intense, severe back pain; motor weakness and dysfunction; sensory paresthesia; changes in bowel and bladder.
    b. Treatment: radiation and corticosteroids.
4. Intestinal obstruction from tumor growth (see Chapter 20).

C. Third-space syndrome: fluid shifts from the vascular space to the interstitial space; may be associated with extensive surgical resection.
1. Symptoms: hypovolemia with hypotension, tachycardia, low central venous pressure (CVP), decreased urine output.
2. Treatment: fluid, electrolyte, and plasma protein replacement, but hypervolemia easily can occur.

D. Metabolic emergencies.
1. Syndrome of inappropriate antidiuretic hormone (SIADH): results from production of antidiuretic hormone (ADH) by the cancer cells or by stimulation of ADH production by the chemotherapy.
    a. Symptoms: sustained production of ADH, leading to water retention, hyponatremia (dilutional), weight gain, weakness, GI disturbances.
    b. Treatment: correct sodium–water imbalance; treat underlying malignancy.
2. Hypercalcemia: results from metastatic disease of the bone or secretion of parathyroid-like hormone by the cancer cells (see Chapter 9). Immobility and dehydration also contribute to development of hypercalcemia.
    a. Symptoms: apathy, fatigue, muscle weakness, polyuria, GI disturbances, electrocardiogram changes.
    b. Treatment: long-term treatment aimed at primary malignancy; hydration, diuretics, and bisphosphonates.
3. Tumor lysis syndrome (TLS): often triggered by chemotherapy when a large number of cancer cells die

and a host of intracellular components are released into the blood.

   a. Symptoms: four hallmark signs—hyperuricemia, hyperphosphatemia, hyperkalemia, and hypocalcemia—may occur within the first 24 to 48 hours after initiation of treatment.
   b. Treatment: increase fluids to support renal function, correct electrolyte imbalances, ensure adequate hydration to decrease uric acid concentrations.

E. Infiltrative emergencies.
   1. Cardiac tamponade (see Chapter 19).
   2. Carotid artery rupture: associated with head and neck cancer and neck radiation therapy; treatment involves ligation of the carotid artery.

### Nursing Interventions

**Goal:** To maintain client at optimum psychosocial level.

A. Encourage verbalization.
B. Assist client to understand disease process and therapeutic regimen.
C. Include family in the care.
D. Assist client to cope with changes in body image caused by alopecia (see Table 11-2).
E. Assess client's coping skills and support systems. Encourage communication and be an active listener.
F. Recognize client's emotional outbursts and anger as part of the coping process.
G. Encourage measures to maintain client's ego.
   1. Allow client to participate in his or her own care and make decisions.
   2. Maintain active listening.
   3. Encourage personal lifestyle choices (clothing, makeup, hobbies, etc.).
   4. Discuss body image issues.

**Goal:** To maintain nutrition (see Table 11-2).

A. Diet: appropriate to age level.
B. Total parenteral nutrition (see Chapter 20) to maintain adequate intake.
C. Prevent and/or decrease complications associated with nutrition.

**Goal:** To maintain healthy, intact skin.

A. Teach client about radiation-induced skin reactions and provide nursing care for these skin reactions.
   1. Moisturize skin three to four times a day with non-perfumed, nonmedicated cream or lotion.
   2. If moist desquamation occurs, cleanse gently with normal saline solution; area should be gently patted dry or air-dried; expose areas to air for 10 to 15 minutes three times a day.
   3. Avoid use of perfumes, deodorants, powders, and cosmetics to affected area.
   4. Wear loose-fitting cotton clothing; avoid swimming.
   5. If dry desquamation is present, apply lotion that is not perfumed, not medicated, and does not contain alcohol.
B. Monitor skin integrity and report any signs of skin infection.

**Goal:** To maintain normal elimination pattern (see Table 11-2).

A. Prevent and/or decrease complications of diarrhea.
B. Prevent constipation.
C. Prevent urinary tract infections, primarily cystitis.
   1. Maintain adequate fluid intake (at least 3000 mL per day).
   2. Frequently assess for symptoms of cystitis (see Chapter 25).
   3. Avoid bladder catheterization if possible.
   4. Check urine for presence of hematuria.
   5. Encourage frequent voiding.
D. Assess for the development of vesicovaginal or rectovaginal fistulas.

**Goal:** To prevent and/or decrease infectious process (see Table 11-2).

A. Monitor white cell counts; be aware of onset and point of nadir.
B. Monitor temperature routinely.
C. Meticulous personal hygiene including frequent handwashing.
D. Child should be isolated from others with communicable diseases.
E. Frequently assess for potential infectious processes.
F. Fresh fruits and vegetables should be eaten only after they have been cooked, peeled, or washed thoroughly.
G. See goals for self-care.

**Goal:** To decrease hematologic complications.

A. Evaluate for decreasing platelet levels and thrombocytopenia.

> **⚠ NURSING PRIORITY:** Institute bleeding precautions if platelet count is less than 50,000/mm³.

B. Administer platelets as indicated.
C. Evaluate areas of potential bleeding.
   1. Mucous membranes, nosebleed (epistaxis).
   2. Urinary tract (hematuria).
   3. GI bleeding (hematemesis), stool (melena).
   4. Implement bleeding precautions (see Box 16-1).

> **⚠ NURSING PRIORITY:** Advise client to use electric razor and a soft-bristle toothbrush.

D. Anemia (see Table 11-2).
   1. Maintain adequate rest; encourage client to pace activities to avoid fatigue.
   2. Maintain adequate oxygenation.
   3. Assess for problems with erythropoiesis.
   4. Evaluate respiratory and cardiac systems for mechanisms of compensation.
   5. Administer red blood cell transfusions as indicated.

**Goal:** To relieve pain (see Chapter 3).

A. Evaluate client and family responses to pain.
B. Evaluate characteristics of pain: determine whether pain control is to be palliative.

C. Administer medications for pain relief.

D. Utilize nonpharmacologic approaches to pain relief (positioning, imagery, hypnosis, etc.).

**Goal:** To recognize complications specific to radiation and chemotherapy.

A. Alopecia.

B. Hemorrhagic problems.

C. Gastrointestinal distress (anorexia, ulcerations, nausea, vomiting).

D. Bone marrow depression (myelosuppression).
   1. Thrombocytopenia.
   2. Anemia.
   3. Neutropenia.

E. Skin reactions.

F. Decreased immune response.

> ∎ **NURSING PRIORITY:** It is important for the nurse to be able to differentiate between toxic effects of medication or radiation therapy and the progression of the disease process.

 **Home Care**

**Goal:** To effectively manage pain to provide client optimal rest and pain relief.

A. Assess quality, intensity, timing, and location of pain to establish baseline.

B. Identify provoking and alleviating factors and adjust environment accordingly.

C. Assess other psychological factors affecting pain tolerance (fear, anxiety, agitation, and past experiences with pain).

D. Discuss questions regarding addiction to opioid analgesics.

E. Assist client with nonpharmacologic pain therapies (Chapter 3).

F. Layer pain management strategies as needed; medicate with opioids, nonsteroidal antiinflammatories (NSAIDs), and adjuvant pain medications as necessary.

G. Assess effectiveness of therapies and medications and modify as necessary.

H. Provide a calm, healthy environment with appropriate lighting and personal belongings as warranted by disease progression.

I. When appropriate, suggest hospice care, which can provide compassion, concern, and support for the terminally ill client.

**Goal:** To decrease or limit exposure to infection.

A. Limit number of people having direct contact with the client.

B. Good oral hygiene: regular flossing if there is no bleeding problem and no tissue irritation; soft toothbrush; avoid irritating foods.

C. Client should avoid coming in direct contact with animal excreta (cat litter boxes, bird cages, etc.).

D. Teach client to take his or her temperature daily and report temperature over 100.4°F (38°C).

E. Use antipyretics cautiously because they tend to mask infection.

F. Teach client that peak of neutropenia (nadir), or highest risk for infection, occurs within 7 to 10 days after the administration of chemotherapy.

G. Teach client importance of frequent handwashing.

**Goal:** To maintain optimum psychosocial function.

A. Assess coping mechanisms.

B. Assess family/significant other resources.

C. Provide opportunities for client to express feelings, concerns, and fears.

D. Encourage activity; one of the best activities is walking for about 30 minutes at a rate that is comfortable.

---

## Appendix 11-1   CANCER CHEMOTHERAPY

### General Nursing Implications

- Observe for adverse effects (see Table 11-2).
- Dosage is usually based on client's body weight and height using the body surface area calculation.
- Monitor client and laboratory values for evidence of bone marrow suppression: infection from loss of neutrophils, bleeding from loss of thrombocytes, and anemia from loss of erythrocytes.
- Avoid contact with skin when preparing chemotherapy medications that are vesicants.
- Do not administer a vesicant through a hand or wrist intravenous site; most are administered via a CVAD.
- General side effects of antineoplastic agents are nausea, vomiting, diarrhea, anorexia, alopecia, hyperuricemia, nephrotoxicity, and bone marrow suppression.
- Monitor renal and hepatic function to evaluate ability of client to break down and excrete chemotherapeutic agents.

| Medication | Side Effects | Nursing Implications |
|---|---|---|
| **TEST ALERT:** Follow procedure for handling biohazardous materials (e.g., chemotherapeutic agents). | | |

**Alkylating Agents:** Kill cells by alkylation of the DNA; all are dose limiting by bone marrow suppression.

| | | |
|---|---|---|
| Cyclophosphamide | Renal, hepatotoxic | 1. Monitor for hemorrhagic cystitis; encourage high fluid intake. |
| Mechlorethamine (nitrogen mustard) | Blood dyscrasias | 1. Strong vesicant; prevent extravasation and direct contact with the skin. |

*Continued*

**Appendix 11-1   CANCER CHEMOTHERAPY—cont'd**                                                                                           ℞

| Medication | Side Effects | Nursing Implications |
|---|---|---|
| Chlorambucil | Pulmonary infiltrates and pulmonary fibrosis, hepatotoxic | 1. Monitor respiratory status and maintain good respiratory hygiene. |
| Busulfan | Pulmonary infiltrates and pulmonary fibrosis, sterility | 1. Monitor respiratory status and maintain good respiratory hygiene. |
| Ifosfamide | Hemorrhagic cystitis | 1. High risk for cystitis; urinalysis done before each dose. |
| Carmustine | Crosses the blood–brain barrier<br>May have delayed bone marrow suppression | 1. Nadir occurs at 4–6 weeks after beginning treatment.<br>2. May have severe nausea and vomiting. |

**Platinum Compounds:** Have a similar action as the alkylating agents and are cell-cycle nonspecific.

| | | |
|---|---|---|
| Cisplatin<br>Carboplatin | Neurotoxicity, ototoxicity<br>Dose limited by bone marrow suppression<br>Renal damage is dose-limiting factor | 1. Produces nausea and vomiting within an hour of administration.<br>2. Assess for tinnitus and hearing loss.<br>3. Encourage high fluid intake; may be coupled with diuretics. |

**Antimetabolites:** Disrupt critical cellular metabolism; cell-cycle specific; dose limited by bone marrow suppression.

**Folic Acid Analogs:** Interfere with the conversion of folic acid to its active form

| | | |
|---|---|---|
| Methotrexate sodium | Pulmonary infiltrates and fibrosis; oral and GI ulceration<br>High doses can damage kidney<br>Teratogenic | 1. Leucovorin may be administered to increase uptake; it can be potentially dangerous, especially if the *right dose* is not administered at the *right time*, in which case it could be fatal.<br>2. Monitor GI status; potential of intestinal perforation; nausea and vomiting occur early.<br>3. Encourage high fluid intake to promote drug excretion.<br>4. Avoid pregnancy for at least 6 months.<br>5. Do not take folic acid. |
| Pemetrexed | Teratogenic<br>GI toxicity—stomatitis and diarrhea may be dose limiting | 1. Vitamin $B_{12}$ and folic acid to decrease bone marrow and GI toxicity.<br>2. Avoid in pregnancy. |

**Pyrimidine Analogs:** Disrupt nucleic acid function; inhibit biosynthesis of DNA and RNA.

| | | |
|---|---|---|
| Cytarabine | High doses may cause pulmonary edema and cerebellar toxicity | 1. Nausea and vomiting after bolus administration.<br>2. Monitor pulmonary status and fluid balance. |
| 5-Fluorouracil | Stomatitis, GI ulceration | 1. Monitor and report early GI symptoms; may be discontinued. |

**Purine Analogs:** Disrupt nucleic acid function and multiple biochemical processes of the cell.

| | | |
|---|---|---|
| Mercaptopurine | Hepatotoxicity common, GI ulceration<br>Mutagenic—avoid in pregnancy | 1. Monitor for jaundice.<br>2. Allopurinol increases risk for toxicity. |
| Thioguanine | Hepatic dysfunction; GI ulceration | 1. Monitor for jaundice. |

**Antitumor Antibiotics:** Interfere with DNA synthesis; are not used to treat infections; poor GI absorption, given IV.

**Anthracyclines:** Cause bone marrow suppression and cardiac damage

| | | |
|---|---|---|
| Doxorubicin<br>Daunorubicin | Acute dysrhythmias, delayed cardiotoxicity; heart failure | 1. Dysrhythmias may occur minutes after administration.<br>2. Monitor cardiac status and rhythm.<br>3. Encourage follow-up after therapy to evaluate cardiac status. |

## Appendix 11-1 CANCER CHEMOTHERAPY—cont'd

| Medication | Side Effects | Nursing Implications |
|---|---|---|
| **Nonanthracyclines: Do not injure the heart but do have serious toxicities.** | | |
| Dactinomycin | Bone marrow suppression and GI mucositis are dose limiting | 1. Strong vesicant.<br>2. Monitor mouth for ulcerations. |
| Bleomycin | Pulmonary injury (pneumonitis) is dose limiting | 1. Monitor pulmonary functions and report any adverse changes. |
| Mitomycin | Bone marrow suppression is dose limiting | 1. Nadir occurs in about 4–6 weeks.<br>2. Monitor for anemia and renal damage. |
| **Mitotic Inhibitors: Prevent cell division** | | |
| **Vinca Alkaloids: Derived from the periwinkle plant.** | | |
| Vincristine | Peripheral neuropathy is dose limiting<br>Autonomic nerve system damage | 1. Assess reflexes, weakness, paresthesias, sensory loss.<br>2. Autonomic nervous system: constipation and urinary hesitancy.<br>3. Severe vesicant. |
| Vinblastine | Dose limiting by bone marrow suppression | 1. Severe vesicant.<br>2. Neurotoxicity can occur but is less severe than what occurs with vincristine. |
| **Taxanes: Severe hypersensitivity reactions.** | | |
| Paclitaxel | Severe hypersensitivity reactions (hypotension, dyspnea, urticaria), dose limiting by bone marrow suppression, peripheral neuropathy, and cardiac problems | 1. Administered by 24-hour infusion.<br>2. Assess for bradycardia, heart block, and hypersensitivity.<br>3. Assess reflexes, weakness, paresthesias, sensory loss. |
| Docetaxel | Neutropenia, hypersensitivity, fluid retention, especially with abnormal liver function | 1. Monitor liver function studies.<br>2. Assess for hypotension, bronchospasm, rash. |
| **Hormonal Agents: Mimic or block the action of hormones.** | | |
| **Androgen Antagonist: Used to treat prostate cancer** | | |
| Leuprolide | Hot flashes, impotence, increased risk for fractures | 1. Encourage activity to minimize bone loss; increase intake of calcium and vitamin D; increase weight-bearing activities. |
| Flutamide | Gynecomastia, nausea, vomiting | 1. Monitor liver function studies. |
| **Antiestrogens: Used to treat breast cancer.** | | |
| Tamoxifen | Increases incidence of endometrial cancer and thromboembolic problems | 1. Dosage for prevention of breast cancer continues for 5 years.<br>2. Teach activities to prevent venous stasis. |
| Raloxifene<br>Fulvestrant | Does not increase incidence of endometrial cancer<br>Increases risk for osteoporosis | 1. Used to treat breast cancer in postmenopausal women.<br>2. Encourage activity to minimize bone loss: increase intake of calcium and vitamin D; increase weight-bearing activities. |
| **Aromatase Inhibitors: Used to treat estrogen receptor (ER) positive breast cancer in postmenopause.** | | |
| Anastrozole | Joint and musculoskeletal pain<br>Increased risk for osteoporosis | 1. NSAIDs for joint pain.<br>2. Encourage activity to minimize bone loss: increase intake of calcium and vitamin D; increase weight-bearing activities. |

*Continued*

## Appendix 11-1   CANCER CHEMOTHERAPY—cont'd

| Medication | Side Effects | Nursing Implications |
|---|---|---|
| **Immunostimulants:** Biologic response modifiers that alter the host response to cancer cells. | | |
| Interferon Alfa-2a Interferon Alfa-2b | Flulike symptoms (fever, chills, fatigue, myalgia); profound fatigue may be dose limiting | 1. Symptoms tend to diminish with continued therapy. |
| Aldesleukin | Flulike symptoms (fever, chills, fatigue), nausea, vomiting, diarrhea Hypotension, anemia Hepatotoxicity, nephrotoxicity Capillary leak syndrome (CLS): hypotension, reduced organ perfusion, pulmonary edema | 1. Toxicity is common in most clients; may be administered in an intensive-care setting; toxicity occurs soon after administration. 2. CLS: observe for adequate renal perfusion, hypotension. 3. Monitor urine output and liver and renal function studies. |
| **Targeted Drugs:** Bind with specific molecules that drive tumor growth. | | |
| Trastuzumab | Cardiotoxicity, hypersensitivity reactions, pulmonary problems | 1. Used for metastatic and aggressive breast cancer with tumors that overexpress human epidermal growth factor receptor 2 (HER2). |
| EGFR-Tyrosine Kinase Inhibitors Cetuximab | Severe infusion reactions, severe acne-like rash | 1. Monitor IV administration. 2. Assess skin (face, upper torso) for rash. 3. Limit sunlight exposure; wear sunblock. |
| BCR-ABL Tyrosine Kinase Inhibitors Imatinib | Nausea, vomiting, diarrhea, fluid retention; avoid use during pregnancy | 1. Monitor for fluid retention, pulmonary edema, and ascites. |
| CD20-Directed Antibodies Rituximab | Severe infusion-related hypersensitivity, TLS, Stevens–Johnson syndrome | 1. Monitor for TLS, infusion hypersensitivity. |
| Angiogenesis Inhibitors Bevacizumab | Block growth of new blood vessels Hypertension, GI perforation, impaired wound healing, thromboembolism | 1. Watch for impaired wound healing; monitor blood pressure. |
| **Hematopoietic Growth Factors:** Used to support cancer client. | | |
| Erythropoietin | Hypertension, cardiovascular events | 1. Monitor hemoglobin and hematocrit—not to exceed 12 g/dL. 2. Assess for cardiovascular problems—stroke, heart failure, thromboembolism. |
| Filgrastim | Bone pain, leukocytosis | 1. Monitor WBC counts. |
| Oprelvekin | Fluid retention, cardiac dysrhythmias, severe allergic reactions (anaphylaxis) | 1. Assess for peripheral edema and expansion of fluid volume—dyspnea. 2. Monitor pulse for tachycardia. |

*BP*, Blood pressure; *CVAD*, central venous access device; *ECG*, electrocardiogram; *GI*, gastrointestinal; *IV*, intravenous; *TLS*, tumor lysis syndrome; *WBC*, white blood cell.

# Study Questions
# Cancer Concepts

More questions on

1. The nurse receives report on assigned clients. One client is reported to be at the nadir for his cancer chemotherapy. How will this affect the nursing care plan?
   1. Implement bleeding precautions.
   2. Reinforce measures and teaching regarding preventing infections.
   3. Anticipate nutritional problems caused by nausea and vomiting.
   4. Assess for problems with fluid balance.

2. The nurse is assessing a client after beginning external radiation. What is a nursing observation that confirms the presence of early side effects of the radiation?
   1. A gradual weight loss and GI disturbances
   2. Skin erythema followed by dry desquamation
   3. Vertigo when sitting up quickly
   4. Excoriation and blisters on the affected skin

3. What are the nursing interventions regarding care of a client with a vaginal radium implant?
   1. Clamp and drain the urinary retention catheter.
   2. Provide a high-residue diet.
   3. Place the client in a semiprivate room.
   4. Raise the head of the bed no more than 20 degrees.

4. What is an important aspect of client teaching regarding external radiation therapy?
   1. Remain isolated after treatments.
   2. Fast before the treatment.
   3. Schedule treatments monthly.
   4. Leave skin markings between treatments.

5. A client is receiving chemotherapy with several antineoplastic agents. Which nursing observation is considered a common side effect of chemotherapy?
   1. Slow, slurred speech
   2. Increased leukocytes on complete blood count
   3. Stomatitis and oral ulcers
   4. Sinus dysrhythmias with bradycardia

6. A client is going to begin external radiation therapy for his lung cancer. Which comment by the client would indicate to the nurse the need for additional teaching?
   1. "I will shower with a mild soap and check my skin for areas of redness."
   2. "I am looking forward to swimming laps again for my exercise."
   3. "I am going to eat small meals and increase the protein and fiber in my diet."
   4. "I will use only unscented emollient creams to the dry skin areas on my chest."

7. The nurse is evaluating a central venous line before administering the client's chemotherapy. What observation would cause the nurse the most concern?
   1. Nurse is unable to withdraw blood into line.
   2. Dressing was changed 24 hours ago.
   3. Inflammation and exudate are present at the insertion site.
   4. Fluid infusing is D5W and 0.45% normal saline.

8. The nurse understands that the following are general adverse effects of antineoplastic drugs. **Select all that apply.**
   1. Urinary retention
   2. Infertility
   3. Stomatitis
   4. Bone marrow depression
   5. Extravasation
   6. Nausea

9. The nurse is updating a teaching plan for a client who has cancer and has been taking doxorubicin for the past several months. What is important to review with the client?
   1. Report symptoms of hematuria.
   2. Increase intake of oral fluids.
   3. Avoid folic acid intake.
   4. Report symptoms of dyspnea.

10. A client is receiving busulfan. The nurse would notify the physician regarding which assessment finding?
    1. Persistent, nonproductive, dry cough
    2. Hemoglobin 13 g/dL (130 g/L), hematocrit 38% (0.38 proportion of 1)
    3. Nausea and vomiting
    4. Low serum uric acid

11. A client asks the nurse why he has to take several chemotherapy agents at the same time. The nurse's response would be based on which principle?
    1. The more medications that can be given together, the shorter the treatment period.
    2. The cost is decreased because the medications are administered at the same time.
    3. Multiple medications given together will attack the cancer cells at different levels.
    4. One medication will interact with another to reduce incidence of side effects.

12. A client has developed stomatitis while receiving chemotherapy. What would be an appropriate intervention to suggest for the pain associated with the stomatitis?
    1. Use lemon-flavored glycerin swabs.
    2. Apply antacid coating solutions and viscous lidocaine.
    3. Brush oral plaques off with a soft toothbrush.
    4. Have client swish mouth with a weak hydrogen peroxide solution.

13. What is a common side effect of radiation therapy that is not associated with the effect of radiation in the treatment field?
    1. Reddened skin
    2. Bone marrow suppression
    3. Fatigue
    4. GI disturbances

14. The nurse understands what major difference between benign and malignant tumors? Malignant tumors:
    1. Are encapsulated and immovable
    2. Grow at a faster rate than benign tumors do
    3. Invade adjacent tissue and metastasize
    4. Cause death, whereas benign tumors do not

15. A client is being referred to the hospice nurse for care. The nurse explains to the client and the family that the primary goal of hospice differs from the goal of traditional care in what way? Hospice care:
    1. Provides support to the family and to the client with a terminal illness
    2. Is delivered only at home, so that no extraordinary means are initiated to prolong life
    3. Provides a Medicare-supported pain regimen so pain medications are affordable
    4. More readily recognizes advance directives related to the "right to die"

16. The nurse is caring for a client who is being treated with chemotherapy for his lung cancer. The client has had two treatments in the last 2 days, and the nurse notes hyperkalemia and hyperuricemia on the latest serum laboratory values. The nurse understands that these are symptoms of:
    1. Third-space syndrome
    2. Syndrome of inappropriate antidiuretic hormone
    3. Tumor lysis syndrome
    4. Parathyroid deficiency

17. Combined therapy of radiation and chemotherapy can have a significant therapeutic impact on the survival of an individual with cancer. The nursing priority for these clients includes measures to:
    1. Monitor for acute renal tubular necrosis
    2. Control nausea and vomiting
    3. Prevent infection
    4. Maintain hydration and nutrition

18. The nurse recognizes which of the following conditions as an oncologic emergency? **Select all that apply.**
    1. Cardiac tamponade
    2. Leukopenia
    3. Syndrome of inappropriate antidiuretic hormone
    4. Hypercalcemia
    5. Hypophosphatemia
    6. Tumor lysis syndrome

19. The nurse is reviewing the chart of a client who recently had a cervical biopsy. The test results indicate Tis, N0, M0. How will the nurse interpret this information?
    1. The cancer is in situ, which means it is localized and not invasive at this time.
    2. The origin of the cancer is probably in the uterus, and further testing will be necessary.
    3. The lymph nodes are involved, and the presence of distant metastasis cannot be determined.
    4. There is no cancer present; the tissue was normal.

## Answers to Study Questions

1. *2*
The nadir refers to the point in the chemotherapy when the leukocytes or neutrophils are at the lowest level. The client's ability to resist infections is at the lowest point, and the client is at the highest risk for developing an infection. Bleeding precautions are implemented with thrombocytopenia or decreased platelets. Nutritional problems are common throughout chemotherapy, and there is no increased risk for development of problems with fluid balance. (Lewis et al., 10 ed., pp. 250–254)

2. *2*
Abnormal skin pigmentation, erythema, and dry desquamation may develop within a few days of beginning the radiation treatment. Wet desquamation may occur with progression of the radiation treatment, but the skin does not have blisters. Vertigo may be a sign of orthostatic hypotension associated with hypovolemia. The weight loss occurs, but it is not due to the radiation; it is most often due to the malignancy. (Lewis et al., 10 ed., pp. 250–256)

3. *4*
Once the implant is in place, keeping it in the exact measured position without disruption is a primary goal of care. Strict bed rest is maintained. The head of the bed should be raised only slightly to accomplish this. A urinary retention catheter is placed for gravity drainage. The client should be in a private room. Constipation should be avoided, but a high-residue diet will increase the bulk of the stool and possibly dislodge the implant. (Lewis et al., 10 ed., p. 250)

4. *4*
Skin markings are used by the radiotherapist to delineate the exact area of the body to be irradiated. Treatments are completed in a series, depending on the location of the malignancy and the level of radiation being administered. The treatments do not require isolation, fasting, or any form of activity restriction. (Lewis et al., 10 ed., pp. 249–250)

5. *3*
A common side effect of chemotherapy is stomatitis. It may be manifested as inflammation of the gums and ulcerations in the mouth. There is a decrease in leukocytes, making the client less resistive to infection. Dysrhythmias are not common in cancer therapy; they may occur with electrolyte imbalances secondary to chemotherapy. The slowed speech may occur with hypercalcemia as a complication involving the parathyroid gland. (Lewis et al., 10 ed., pp. 250–256)

6. *2*
The client should avoid swimming during the treatment period because of the irritating chemicals in swimming pools. The other options—showering with a mild soap, eating small nutritious meals, and using an emollient cream—are correct for external radiation. (Lewis et al., 10 ed., p. 255)

7. *3*
Irritation at the insertion site is a problem in a client who is immunocompromised. Checking the IV site and surrounding area for signs of infection is a priority nursing action. Frequently, central lines are long and narrow, and withdrawing blood may not occur. Transparent dressings are changed on an as-needed basis. Opaque (gauze) dressings are usually changed every 48 hours. (Lewis et al., 10 ed., pp. 295–297)

8. *3, 4, 6*
Adverse effects of antineoplastic drugs can be classified as acute, delayed, or chronic. Acute toxicity includes nausea, vomiting, arrhythmias, and allergic reactions. Delayed side effects include stomatitis, alopecia, and bone marrow depression. Chronic toxicity involves organ damage. Common urinary problems include cystitis and nephrotoxicity. Extravasation is not an adverse effect but a complication of an infiltrated IV running a chemotherapy medication that is a vesicant. (Lewis et al, 10 ed., pp. 250–256)

**9.** *4*

One of the most common and most severe toxicities of doxorubicin is cardiotoxicity. After months of treatment, this can manifest as heart failure (dyspnea, tachycardia, peripheral edema). Early side effects include dysrhythmias and electrocardiogram (ECG) changes. These can occur within hours of receiving the medication. (Lewis et al., 10 ed., p. 256)

**10.** *1*

Pulmonary toxicity (dry nonproductive cough, crackles, dyspnea, tachypnea) is an adverse effect of busulfan. It can lead to pulmonary fibrosis. Hemoglobin is within normal limits. The nausea and vomiting may be a side effect of the chemotherapy, and the client would be treated for this. Problems occur with a high (not low) serum acid level. (Lehne, 9 ed., p. 1226)

**11.** *3*

Combination drug therapy is important because different drugs inhibit cancer cell growth at various phases of cellular replication. This makes each of the medications more effective. Medications are given together because this is a more effective method of treatment, not because of cost or to reduce the side effects. (Lewis et al., 10 ed., p. 248)

**12.** *2*

Ulcerations in the mouth (stomatitis) can occur when a client is receiving chemotherapy medication. Alleviation of the pain can be achieved by administering systemic or local analgesics and coating agents such as antacids. Frequent saline rinses are encouraged. Lemon–glycerin swabs may irritate the mucosa and lead to further pain, as would trying to remove oral plaques. (Lewis et al., 10 ed., pp. 251–254)

**13.** *3*

A general body or system effect is fatigue because it occurs as a result of changes in cell cycle patterns and toxic effects from cell destruction. The other problems (reddened skin, bone marrow suppression, GI disturbance) occur when radiation is directed at specific parts of the body. (Lewis et al., 10 ed., pp. 250–256)

**14.** *3*

The primary difference between benign and malignant tumors is the ability of the malignant tumor to invade adjacent tissues and metastasize. Benign tumors tend to be encapsulated, and both types of tumors can lead to death. As benign tumors expand, they can adversely affect organ function. The growth of malignant and nonmalignant tumors varies, depending on the characteristics and location of the tumor. (Lewis et al., 10 ed., p. 240)

**15.** *1*

Hospice care provides compassion, concern, and support for the dying client and family. It may or may not be delivered in the home. Pain control is an issue for the hospice client and for any client with cancer. Advance directives are recognized in all health care settings. (Potter & Perry, 9 ed., pp. 761–762)

**16.** *3*

These two findings, hyperuricemia and hyperkalemia, are hallmark symptoms of tumor lysis syndrome, which often occurs at the onset of chemotherapy when a large number of tumor cells are destroyed. This process yields fatal biochemical changes of hyperkalemia, hyperuricemia, hypocalcemia, and hyperphosphatemia if not averted with adequate fluids. (Lewis et al., 10 ed., p. 263)

**17.** *3*

The statistics indicate that infection is the most common cause of morbidity in clients with cancer. Good handwashing, monitoring white blood cell counts, checking temperatures (watching for elevations), and providing protective isolation when needed (when clients are severely immunosuppressed) are the primary measures to prevent infection. (Lewis et al., 10 ed., p. 262)

**18.** *1, 3, 4, 6*

Metabolic emergencies, including SIADH, hypercalcemia, and TLS; infiltrative emergencies, including cardiac tamponade; and obstructive emergencies are life-threatening complications of cancer or cancer therapy. Leukopenia is an expected side effect. Hypophosphatemia is not common. (Lewis et al., 10 ed., p. 263)

**19.** *1*

The cancer is in situ (Tis), which means the cancer is localized to the cervix; there is no evidence of either lymph node involvement (N0) or of invasive activity (M0). Because it is not invasive at this time, there is no immediate need for treatment. The client's history and risk factors will influence the decisions for further diagnostic testing or treatment. (Lewis et al., 10 ed., p. 241)

# 12 Psychosocial Nursing Care

Addiction, Anxiety, Coping, Interpersonal Violence, Mood and Affect, Psychosis, Safety, Stress

## SELF-CONCEPT

A. *Self-concept:* all beliefs, convictions, and ideas that constitute an individual's knowledge of himself or herself and influence the individual's relationships with others.
B. *Self-esteem:* an individual's personal judgment of his or her own worth obtained by analyzing how well his or her behavior conforms to his or her self-ideal.

> **! NURSING PRIORITY:** A healthy self-concept, (i.e., positive self-esteem) is essential to psychological well-being; it is universal.

## Assessment

A. Factors affecting self-esteem.
   1. Parental rejection in early childhood experiences.
   2. Lack of recognition and appreciation by parents as child grows older.
   3. Overpossessiveness, overpermissiveness, and control by one or both parents.
   4. Unrealistic self-ideals or goals.

> **! OLDER ADULT PRIORITY:** The use of wheelchairs, canes, walkers, hearing aids, adaptive devices, or any combination of these will affect the self-esteem of the older client.

B. Behaviors associated with low self-esteem.
   1. Self-derision and criticism: describes self as stupid, no good, or a loser.
   2. Self-diminution: minimizes one's ability.
   3. Guilt and worrying.
   4. Postponing decisions and denying pleasure.
   5. Disturbed interpersonal relationships.
   6. Self-destructiveness and boredom.
   7. Conflicted view of life.

> **TEST ALERT:** Promoting a positive self-concept is basic to all psychotherapeutic interventions. Look for options that focus on this concept; acknowledging the client as a person is an example.

## Nursing Interventions

A. Expand self-awareness.
   1. Promote an open, trusting therapeutic relationship.

   2. Maximize the client's participation in the therapeutic relationship.
B. Self-exploration.
   1. Encourage the client to accept his or her own feelings and thoughts.
   2. Help the client clarify his or her concept of self and relationship with others through appropriate self-disclosure.
   3. Explore with the client false assumptions such as:
      a. Catastrophizing: thinking that the worst will happen.
      b. Minimizing and maximizing: tendency to minimize the positive and maximize the negative.
      c. All-or-nothing thinking: tendency to look at situations in extremes; no middle ground.
      d. Overgeneralization: thinking that if something happens once, it will happen again.
      e. Filtering: selectively taking certain details out of context while neglecting to look at more positive facts.
   4. Communicate empathically, not sympathetically, and remind the client that he or she has the power to change himself or herself.
C. Self-evaluation.
   1. Encourage client to define and identify problem.
   2. Identify irrational beliefs such as:
      a. "I must be loved by everyone."
      b. "I must be competent and never make mistakes."
      c. "My whole life is a disaster if it doesn't turn out exactly as planned."
   3. Identify areas of strength by exploring, for example, the client's hobbies, skills, work, school, character traits, personal abilities.

> **! PEDIATRIC PRIORITY:** If parents help children identify and accomplish goals that are important to them, children begin to develop a sense of personal competence and independence.

   4. Explore client's adaptive and maladaptive coping responses.
      a. Determine "pay-offs" for maintaining self-defeating behaviors such as:
         (1) Procrastination.
         (2) Avoiding risks and commitments.
         (3) Retreating from the present situation.
         (4) Not accepting responsibility for one's actions.
      b. Identify the disadvantages of the maladaptive coping responses.

# BODY IMAGE

## Evaluation of Body Image Alteration

A. Types of body image disturbances.
1. Changes in body size, shape, or appearance (rapid weight gain or loss, plastic surgery, pregnancy, burns, hair loss, hirsutism).
2. Pathologic processes causing changes in structure or function of one's body (e.g., Parkinson disease, cancer, heart disease).
3. Failure of a body part to function properly (paraplegia or stroke).
4. Physical changes associated with normal growth and development (puberty, aging process).
5. Threatening medical or nursing procedures (fecal or urinary diversion, radiation therapy, organ transplantation).

B. Principles.
1. Body characteristics that have been present from birth or acquired early in life seem to have less emotional significance than those arising later.
2. Body image changes, handicaps, or changes in body function that occur abruptly are far more traumatic than ones that develop gradually.
3. The location of a disease or injury greatly affects the emotional response to it; internal diseases are generally less threatening than external diseases (trauma, disfigurement).
4. Changes in genitals or breasts are perceived as a great threat and reawaken fears about sexuality and virility.

# SPECIFIC SITUATIONS OF ALTERED BODY IMAGE AND NURSING INTERVENTIONS

**TEST ALERT:** Facilitate client's adjustment to changes in body image.

## Obesity

### Assessment

A. Body weight exceeds 20% above the normal range for age, sex, and height.
B. Feeding behavior is gauged according to external environmental cues (i.e., odors, stress, availability of food) rather than hunger (increased gastrointestinal motility).
C. Increased incidence of diabetes, cardiovascular disease, cancer, and delayed wound healing.
D. Obese client often has symptoms of depression, fatigue, dyspnea, tachycardia, and hypertension.

### Nursing Interventions

A. Encourage behavior modification programs.
B. Promote activities and interests not related to food or eating.
C. Identify client's need to eat and relate the need to preceding events or situations.
D. Decrease guilt and anxiety related to being obese.
E. Provide long-range nutritional counseling.
F. Encourage an exercise program.
G. Assess for complications (hypertension, cardiovascular disease).

## Stroke

### Assessment

A. Change of body function due to loss of bowel and bladder control, speech, and cognitive skills.
B. Disordered orientations in relationship to body and position sense in space; body image boundaries disrupted.

### Nursing Interventions

A. Decrease frustration related to speech problems by encouraging speech effort, speaking slowly, and clarifying statements.
B. Promote reintegration of altered body image caused by paralyzed body part by means of tactile stimulation and verbal reminders of the existing body part.

## Amputation

### Assessment

A. Feelings of loss, lowered self-esteem, guilt, helplessness.
B. Depression, passivity, and increased emotional vulnerability.
C. Phantom limb pain occurs in most clients: increased experience if amputation occurs after 4 years of age; almost universal experience after 8 years of age.

### Nursing Interventions

A. Anticipatory guidance and therapeutic preparation of a client who is to undergo amputation.
B. Discussion of phantom limb phenomenon and exploration of client's fears regarding amputation.
C. Assist family members to work through their feelings and to accept client as a whole person.
D. Acknowledge phantom limb pain; reassure client that this is a normal process.
E. Provide pain medication as needed.
F. Educate client and family members on proper fitting of prosthesis (if applicable).

## Pregnancy

### Assessment

A. Produces marked changes in a woman's body, resulting in major alterations in body configuration within a short period.
B. Second trimester: woman becomes aware that her body is widening and requires more space.
C. Third trimester: woman is very much aware of increased size; may feel ambivalent about the changes in her body.
D. Woman perceives her body as vulnerable yet also as a protective space for the unborn.
E. Significant other experiences change body image and sympathetic symptoms during a woman's pregnancy.

### Nursing Interventions

A. Explain and offer reassurance about the normal physiologic changes that are occurring.

B. Provide discussions of alterations in body image for both mates.

C. Encourage verbalization of feelings relating to changed body image.

## Cancer

### Assessment

A. Clients with cancer may experience many changes in body image.

B. Side effects of chemotherapy, radiation, and surgery may affect body image.

C. Removal of sex organs (breasts, uterus) has a significant effect on a client's perception of sexuality.

D. Disfiguring head-and-neck surgery has a devastating effect on body image because the face is one of the primary means by which people communicate.

E. Symptoms of depersonalization, loss of self-esteem, and depression may occur.

### Nursing Interventions

A. Assess client for depression.

B. Provide anticipatory guidance to help client cope with crisis of changed body image.

C. Set long-term goals to help client with cancer adjust to physiologic and psychological changes.

## Enterostomal Surgery

### Assessment

A. Client is often shocked at initial sight of ostomy.

B. Client may experience lowered self-esteem, fear of fecal or urine spillage, alteration in sexual functioning, and feelings of disfigurement and rejection.

### Nursing Interventions

A. Preoperative explanation by use of drawings, models, or pictures of how stoma will appear.

B. Reassurance that reddish appearance of stoma and large size will diminish in time.

C. Encourage discussion and recognize importance of client talking with a "successful ostomate."

D. Educate client on performing ostomy care (pouching ostomy, emptying drainage bag/reservoir, observing peristomal skin).

## HUMAN SEXUALITY

### Key Nursing Concepts

A. Growth and development.
1. Observable differences in male and female behavior are seen as early as infancy.
2. Core gender identity develops in the healthy child at about 3 or 4 years of age.
3. Sexual problems seen in childhood are as follows: sexual misconception, gender identity disturbances (gender dysphoria), and home settings that cause sexual confusion.
4. Rapid biologic changes seen in adolescence result in anxiety about maturation.

5. Sexual problems seen in adolescents include: guilty feelings regarding masturbation, integration of transient homosexual experiences into heterosexual relationship, resolution of conflicts related to premarital intercourse, and obtaining sex-related health services (e.g., birth control). Adolescents and adults with gender dysphoria may verbalize a desire to be the other sex and be treated as if they were the other sex.
6. The young adult faces the task of establishing a pattern of heterosexual intimacy.
7. The middle-age adult faces the task of adjusting to physiologic changes in sexual function and the responsibilities of parenting.
8. The older adult faces the task of reflecting back on life experiences and examining whether life goals have been accomplished.

B. Sexual activity and interest may continue into old age.

C. Principles.
1. Sexual role identity may be altered during the illness process.
2. Cultural variables influence one's expression of sexuality.
3. Sexual problems are addressed through short-term, behavior-oriented treatment; the goal is to decrease fear of performance and to facilitate communication.
4. Nursing plays a key role in sex-health education; nurses need to be aware of their own attitudes toward sex to respond helpfully to clients.

### Changes in Sexuality

A. Effect of illness and injury on sexuality.
1. Depressive episodes often precipitate a decrease in libido.
2. Sexual preoccupations and overtones may be experienced by the client with psychosis.
3. Certain medications contribute to sexual dysfunction, failure to reach orgasm in women, and impotence or failure to ejaculate in men (e.g., antipsychotic agents, reserpine, phenothiazine, and estrogen use in men decreases libido; androgen use in women increases libido).
4. Clients with spinal cord injuries may lose sexual functioning.
5. Trauma and disfigurement may precipitate an alteration in sexuality.

B. Effect of the aging process on sexuality.
1. Physiologic changes in women are frequently caused by decreasing estrogen supply, which results in decreased vaginal lubrication, shrinkage and loss of elasticity in vaginal canal, and decrease in breast size.
2. Physiologic changes in men include a decrease in testosterone, decrease in spermatogenesis, and a longer length of time to achieve erection along with a decrease in the firmness of erection.
3. Prolonged abstinence from sexual activity can lead to disuse syndrome, in which the physiologic changes are experienced to a greater degree.

# CONCEPT OF LOSS

A. Definition
1. Includes both biologic and physiologic aspects; loss of function.
2. Components of loss include death, dying, grief, and mourning.
    a. Grief: the sequence of subjective states that follow loss and accompany mourning.
    b. Anticipatory grief: grief that occurs before the actual loss (e.g., diagnosis of a terminal illness, client receiving hospice care).
    c. Maladaptive grief: loss that is not associated with normal grieving (e.g., disenfranchised grief, chronic grief, delayed grief, exaggerated grief, masked grief).
B. Nursing care of the dying client (see Chapter 3).

## Coping and Reactions to Death Throughout the Life Cycle

 A. Infant-toddler (ages 1–3).
1. Reactions to death and dying.
    a. No specific concept of death: thinks only in terms of living.
    b. Reacts more to pain and discomfort of illness and immobilization, separation anxiety, intrusive procedures, change in ritualistic routine.
2. Nursing interventions.
    a. Assist parents to deal with their feelings.
    b. Encourage parents' participation in child's care.
    c. Promote decreased separation anxiety by providing arrangements for parents to stay with child.

**NURSING PRIORITY:** Parents of a dying child may have feelings of guilt and may need to talk out these feelings before being able to help each other and their child.

B. Preschooler (ages 3–5).
1. Reactions to death and dying.
    a. Death is viewed as a departure, a kind of sleep.
    b. No real understanding of the universality and inevitability of death.
    c. Life and death can change places with one another.
    d. Death is viewed as gradual or temporary; the person is still alive but under a different set of conditions.
    e. Often views illness and death as a punishment for his or her own thoughts or actions.
    f. If a pet dies, may request a funeral, burial, or some other type of ceremony to symbolize the loss.
2. Nursing interventions.
    a. Use play therapy for expression of thoughts and feelings regarding death and dying.
    b. Provide a clear explanation of what death is; that is, death is not sleep—it is final.

c. Permit a choice of attending a funeral; if child decides to attend, explain what will take place.

 **NURSING PRIORITY:** A young child's fear of death is often a fear of aloneness, of being away from the parents. It is important for parents to interact with the nurse in the child's presence so that the nurse can be identified as a trustworthy substitute caretaker.

C. School-age child (ages 5–12).
1. Reactions to death and dying.
    a. Death is personified; fantasies of a separate person or distinct personality (e.g., skeleton-man, devil, ghost, or death-man).
    b. Fantasies about the unknown are often frightening.
    c. Fear of mutilation and punishment is often associated with death; anxiety is released by nightmares and superstitions.
2. Nursing interventions.
    a. Respond to questions regarding funerals, burials, and memorial services.
    b. Accept regressive or protest behavior.
    c. Encourage verbalization of feelings and emotional reactions.
D. Adolescent (ages 12–18).
1. Reactions to death and dying.
    a. Has a mature understanding of death.
    b. Concerned more with the here and now (i.e., the present).
    c. May have strong emotions about death (anger, frustration, despair); silent, withdrawn.
    d. Often worries about physical changes in relationship to terminal illness.
    e. May ask difficult, open questions regarding death.
2. Nursing interventions.
    a. Support maturational crises relating to identity.
    b. Encourage verbalization of feelings.
    c. Promote peer and parental emotional support.
    d. Respect need for privacy and personal expressions of anger, sadness, or fear.
    e. Model appropriate grieving behavior.
E. Adult.
1. Concerned about death as a disruption in lifestyle and its effect on significant others.
2. Adults tend to think about loss in terms of unmet goals and/or an impediment to future plans; often experience delayed grief and threat to emotional integrity.
F. Older adult.
1. Aware of death as inevitable; life is over.
2. Emphasis on religious belief for comfort; a time of reflection, rest, and peace.

## CULTURAL DIVERSITY

> **TEST ALERT:** Include client's cultural beliefs and practices in planning and providing nursing care.

> **! NURSING PRIORITY:** Certain psychopathologic conditions may change a diagnostic category entirely in different cultures. Misinterpretation and misunderstanding of clients' presenting symptoms can lead to problems in the nurse–client relationship. For example, a Vietnamese mother coining (vigorously rubbing a coin across the body) her child in an attempt to restore hot–cold balance and alleviate illness might be viewed by health care providers as child abuse.

### Assessment of Cultural Aspects

A. Communication styles.
  1. Does the client speak English fluently? If not, what language is preferred?
  2. Is a medical interpreter needed?

> **! NURSING PRIORITY:** Use a medical interpreter from the health care facility and avoid using family members.

B. Ethnic or religious group.
  1. With what particular group does the client identify?
  2. How closely does the client adhere to the traditional beliefs of the group?
C. Nutrition.
  1. Are there certain ethnic or religious preferences about the selection or preparation of foods?
  2. Are there foods to be encouraged (or avoided) when a person is ill?
D. Family relationships.
  1. Is the family matriarchal or patriarchal?
  2. What role in the family does the client hold?
E. Health beliefs.
  1. Does the client rely on folk medicine practices or complementary and alternative therapies?
  2. Has the client been recently treated by a *curandero*, shaman, voodoo doctor, medicine man, or Chinese herbalist?
  3. Does the client take any herbal supplements or over-the-counter medications?

## PSYCHOSOCIAL ASSESSMENT

> **! NURSING PRIORITY:** Strong evidence suggests that factors such as genetics, environment, diet, and cultural beliefs are responsible for ethnic variations in psychotropic drug use (e.g., poor metabolism of certain psychotropic drugs because of genetic factors has been found to be responsible for drug effects in some ethnic groups).

Complete assessment includes descriptions of the intellectual functions, behavioral reactions, emotional reactions, and dynamic issues of the client relative to adaptive functioning and response to present situations.

> **TEST ALERT:** Assess client's response to illness, identify coping mechanisms of client and family, and assess the family's emotional reaction to client's illness.

## Psychiatric History

Purpose: A psychiatric history is used to obtain data from multiple sources (e.g., client, family, friends, police, mental health personnel) as a means of identifying patterns of functioning that are healthy and patterns that create problems in the client's everyday life.

> **! OLDER ADULT PRIORITY:** Allow ample time to gather psychosocial data from older clients.

A. General history of client.
  1. Demographic information, such as address, age, religious affiliation, occupation, and insurance company.
  2. Pertinent personal history, such as birth, growth and development, illness, and marital history.
  3. Previous mental health hospitalizations or treatment.
B. Components of psychiatric history.
  1. Chief complaint: main reason client is seeking psychiatric help.
    a. Use client's own words as to why he or she is hospitalized or seeking help.
    b. Check for recent difficulties or alterations in relationships, level of functioning, behavior, perceptions, or cognitive abilities.
  2. Presenting symptoms: onset and development of symptoms or problems.
    a. Check for increased feelings of depression, anxiety, hopelessness, suspiciousness, confusion, fear.
    b. Assess for changes in bowel habits, insomnia, lethargy, weight loss or gain, anorexia, palpitations, pruritus, headaches.
  3. Family history.
    a. Have any of client's family members sought psychiatric treatment?
    b. Who was important to client in childhood? In adolescence?
    c. Was there physical, emotional, or sexual abuse?
    d. Did parents drink or use drugs?
  4. Personality profile.
    a. Assess client's interests, feelings, mood, and usual leisure activities or hobbies.
    b. How does client cope with stress?
    c. Inquire about sexual patterns: sexually active? sexual orientation? sexual difficulties?
    d. Have client describe social relationships: Who are client's friends? Who is important to client? What is a usual day like?

## Mental Status Exam

The mental status exam differs from the psychiatric history in that it is used to identify an individual's present mental status.

*Aspects of the Examination*

A. Mini-Mental State Examination (MMSE): developed by Folstein, Folstein, and McHugh (1975).
   1. Widely used common mental status assessment for cognitive function. A score of 23 or less may indicate cognitive impairment.
   2. Quickly administered—questions related to orientation (person, place, and time), registration (repeating items, give client three common words and ask him to repeat the words), naming (point to a chair or object and ask client to name it), and reading (ask client to read and follow directions from a simple sentence).
   3. Excludes assessment of mood, abnormal psychological experiences (hallucinations, delusions, illusions), and content and process of thinking.
B. General appearance, attitude, and behavior.
   1. Descriptors: posture, gait, activity, facial expression, mannerisms.
   2. Disturbances include deviations of activity, distortions in mobility (waxy flexibility or dyskinesia), uncooperativeness, and changes in personal hygiene.
C. Characteristics of talk and stream of thought.
   1. Descriptors: emphasis on *form*, rather than content, of client's verbal communication; loudness, flow, speed, quality, logic, level of coherence.
   2. Disturbances include these patterns:
      a. Perseveration: pattern of repeating same words or movements.
      b. Flight of ideas: rapid speech, loosely connected thoughts.
      c. Blocking: sudden silence, often associated with intrusion of delusional thoughts or hallucinations.
      d. Echolalia: repeating of words, sentences, or phrases.
      e. Neologism: coining of new words.
      f. Word salad: jumbling several words together that make no sense.
D. Emotional state.
   1. Descriptors: client's report of subjective feelings (mood or affect) and examiner's observation of client's pervasive or dominant emotional state.
   2. Disturbances include deviations such as elation, depression, apathy, incongruence, and disassociation.
E. Content of thought.
   1. Descriptors: What is central theme? How does client view himself or herself (self-concept)? Is suicidal or homicidal ideation present? If so, what is potential lethality?
   2. Disturbances include special preoccupations and experiences such as hallucinations, delusions, illusions, depersonalization, obsessions or compulsions, phobias, fantasies, and daydreams.
F. Sensorium and intellect.
   1. Determine the degree of client's awareness and level of intellectual functioning, general ability to grasp information and calculate, abstract thinking, memory (recall of remote past experiences or recent past experiences, retention and recall of immediate impressions), reasoning, and judgment.
   2. Disturbances of orientation in terms of time, place, person, and self; memory, retention, attention, information, and judgment are assessed through use of standardized tests and questions.

G. Insight evaluation: determine whether the client can understand and appreciate the nature of his or her condition and the need for treatment.

## STRESS AND ADAPTATION

**Stress is a state produced by a change in the environment that is perceived as challenging, threatening, or damaging to the individual's equilibrium.**

**Adaptation is a constant, ongoing process that occurs along the time continuum, beginning with birth and ending with death.**

### Stressors

A. Physiologic stressors.
   1. Chemical agents: drugs, poisons, alcohol.
   2. Physical agents: heat, cold, radiation, electrical shock, trauma.
   3. Infectious agents: viruses, bacteria, fungi.
   4. Environment: noise and air pollution.
   5. Faulty immune mechanisms.
   6. Genetic disorders.
   7. Nutritional imbalance.
   8. Hypoxia.
B. Psychosocial stressors.
   1. Accidents and the survivors (e.g., airplane crash, hurricane, and earthquake survivors).
   2. Death of a close friend; neighbor being robbed and/or beaten.
   3. Horrors of history: Auschwitz, Hiroshima, Chernobyl, etc.
   4. Fear of aggression, mutilation, and destruction.
   5. Events of history brought into our living rooms through various media.
   6. Life crises: situational, developmental, role.
   7. Inherent conflicts in all social relations.

## Stress Response

> **!! NURSING PRIORITY:** Understanding of the stress response is basic to many nursing interventions.

A. Sympathetic: adrenal medullary response; fight-or-flight response (Box 12-1, Figure 12-1).
  1. Increased pulse, blood glucose level, and coagulability of blood.
  2. Pupils dilated.

---

### Box 12-1 SELYE'S GENERAL ADAPTATION SYNDROME (GAS)

**Stage I: Alarm Stage (or Acute Stress)**
Mobilization of the body's defensive forces (antiinflammatory) and activation of the fight-or-flight mechanism.

**Stage II: Stage of Resistance (Adaptation Stage)**
Optimal adaptation to stress within a person's capabilities.

**Stage III: Stage of Exhaustion**
Loss of the ability to resist stress because of depletion of body resources; failure to adapt leads to death.

---

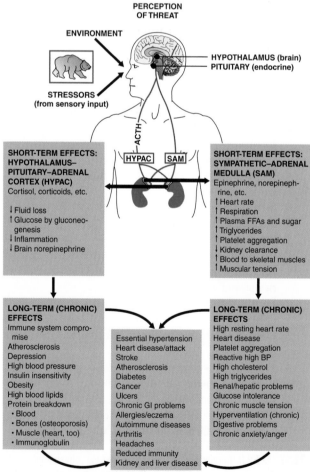

**FIGURE 12-1 The Stress Response.** (From Halter, M. [2014]. *Varcarolis' foundations of psychiatric mental health nursing: A clinical approach* [7th ed.] St. Louis, MO: Elsevier.)

  3. Mental activity enhanced.
  4. Cold, clammy skin.
  5. Respirations rapid and shallow.
B. Pituitary–adrenal cortical response.
  1. Increased production of adrenocorticotropic hormone (ACTH) and mineralocorticoids (aldosterone); increased release of glucagon and decreased fluid loss.
  2. Includes the fight-or-flight response and takes minutes to hours to produce a desired effect.

### Stress Reduction Methods

A. Proper nutrition, regular exercise, physical activity, and recreation; meditation, breathing exercises, guided imagery, mindfulness.
B. Biofeedback, progressive muscle relaxation, journaling.
C. Relaxation response.
  1. Quiet environment.
  2. Passive attitude.
  3. Comfortable position.
  4. A mental device or object, such as a word, sound, or phrase, to occupy the mind and keep out thoughts.
D. Group process and social support.
E. Thought-stopping, self-hypnosis, refuting irrational self-talk, cognitive reframing.

## 📋 CONCEPT OF ANXIETY

**Anxiety is an emotion, a subjective experience; a feeling state that is experienced as vague uneasiness, tension, or apprehension; it occurs when the ego is threatened, is provoked by the unknown, and precedes all new experiences.**

A. Assessment (Table 12-1).
B. Nursing management (Table 12-2).

> **TEST ALERT:** Plan measures to help a client cope with anxiety.

### Defense Mechanisms

**Defense mechanisms are specific defense or coping processes used by individuals to relieve or decrease anxieties caused by uncomfortable situations that threaten self-esteem.**

A. Related principles.
  1. Primary functions are to decrease emotional conflicts, provide relief from stress, protect from feelings of inadequacy and worthlessness, prevent awareness of anxiety, and maintain an individual's self-esteem.
  2. Everyone uses defense mechanisms to a certain extent. If used to an extreme degree, defense mechanisms distort reality, interfere with interpersonal relationships, limit one's ability to work productively, and may lead to pathologic symptoms.
B. Common defense mechanisms (see Appendix 12-1).
C. Nursing management.
  1. Accept defense mechanisms.
  2. Discuss alternative coping mechanisms and problem-solving techniques.
  3. Assist the client in learning new or alternative coping patterns for a healthier adaptation.
  4. Use techniques to decrease anxiety.

## Table 12-1    ASSESSMENT OF ANXIETY

| Physiologic | Psychological |
|---|---|
| **Sympathetic Responses** | **Behavioral Responses** |
| Tachycardia | Restlessness |
| Elevated blood pressure | Agitation |
| Increased perspiration | Tremors (fine to gross shaking of the body) |
| Dilated pupils | Startle reaction |
| Hyperventilation with difficulty breathing | Rapid speech |
| Cold, clammy skin | Lack of coordination |
| Dry mouth | Withdrawal |
| Constipation | |
| **Parasympathetic Responses** | **Cognitive Responses** |
| Urinary frequency | Impaired attention |
| Diarrhea | Poor concentration |
| | Forgetfulness |
| | Blocking of thought |
| | Decreased perceptual field |
| | Decreased productivity |
| | Confusion |
| **Related Responses** | **Affective Responses** |
| Headaches | Tension |
| Nausea or vomiting | Jittery feeling |
| Sleep disturbances | Worried |
| Muscular tension | Apprehension, nervousness |
| | Irritability |
| | Dread |
| | Fear |
| | Panic |
| | Fear of impending doom |

# THERAPEUTIC NURSING PROCESS

Therapeutic interpersonal relationship is the interaction between two persons: The nurse promotes goal-directed activities that help alleviate the discomfort of the client by promoting growth and satisfying interpersonal relationships.

## Characteristics

A. Goal-directed.
B. Empathetic understanding.
C. Honest, open communication.
D. Concreteness; avoids vagueness and ambiguity.
E. Acceptance; nonjudgmental attitude.
F. Involves nurse's understanding of self and personal motives and needs.

## Interview Process

A. Establish rapport with the client.
B. Focus on client needs.
C. Obtain pertinent client data.
D. Initiate client assessment.
E. Make practical arrangements for treatment.

## Phases

A. Preorientation phase: Goal is to *obtain* relevant client data.
   1. During this phase, the nurse obtains relevant information from another caregiver regarding the client's care.
   2. The nurse locates a comfortable setting for interviewing the client.
B. Orientation phase: Goal is to *build trust*.
   1. Explore the client's perceptions, thoughts, feelings, and actions.

## Table 12-2    NURSING MANAGEMENT OF ANXIETY

| Level of Anxiety | Assessment | Goal | Nursing Management |
|---|---|---|---|
| Mild | Increased alertness, motivation, and attentiveness | To assist client to tolerate some anxiety | 1. Help the client identify and describe feelings. 2. Help the client develop the capacity to tolerate mild anxiety and use it consciously and constructively. |
| Moderate | Perception narrowed, selective inattention, poor concentration, physical discomforts | To reduce anxiety; directed toward helping client understand cause of anxiety and new ways of controlling it | 1. Provide an outlet for tension, such as walking, crying, or working at simple, concrete tasks. |
| Severe | Behavior becomes automatic; connections between details are not seen; senses are drastically reduced | To assist in channeling anxiety | 1. Recognize own level of anxiety. 2. Link the client's behavior with feelings. 3. Protect defenses and coping mechanisms. 4. Identify and modify anxiety-provoking situations. |
| Panic | Overwhelmed; inability to function or communicate; potential for bodily harm to self and others; loss of rational thought; hallucinations or delusions may be present | To be supportive and protective | 1. Provide a nonstimulating, structured environment. 2. Avoid touching. 3. Stay with the client. 4. Medicate the client with tranquilizers if necessary. |

2. Identify the purpose of the meeting and the client's problem.
3. Assess levels of anxiety of self and client.
4. Mutually define specific goals to pursue.
5. Establish stated or written contract.

C. Working phase: Goal is *behavioral change.*
1. Encourage client participation.
2. Focus on problem-solving techniques; choose between alternate courses of action and practice skills.
3. Explore thoughts, feelings, and emotions.
4. Develop constructive coping mechanisms.
5. Increase independence and self-responsibility.

D. Termination phase: Goal is to *evaluate goals* set forth and terminate relationship.
1. Plan for termination early in formation of relationship (in orientation phase).
2. Discuss client's feelings about termination.
3. Evaluate client's progress and goal attainment.

> **！NURSING PRIORITY:** To effectively interview a client, be sure to start with a broad, empathetic statement; explore normal behaviors before discussing maladaptive behaviors; phrase inquiries or questions sensitively to decrease the client's anxiety; ask the client to clarify vague statements; refocus on pressing problems when the client begins to ramble; interrupt nonstop talking by the client as tactfully as possible; express empathy toward the client while he or she is expressing feelings.

## Communication Theory

A. Levels of communication.
1. Verbal communication: occurs through the medium of words—spoken or written.
2. Nonverbal communication: includes everything that does not involve the spoken or written word; it involves the five senses.
   a. Vocal cues: tone of voice, quality of voice, nervous coughing, sounds of hesitation.
   b. Action cues: body movement, posture, facial expressions, gestures, mannerisms.
   c. Object cues: dress, appearance to convey a certain "look" or message.
   d. Space: distance between two people; intimate, personal, public space.
   e. Touch: universal and basic to all nurse–client relationships; response to touch is influenced by the setting, cultural background (of client and of nurse), type of relationship, sex of communicators, and expectations.

B. Therapeutic nurse–client communication techniques.
1. Planning and goals.
   a. Demonstrate active listening; use face-to-face contact.
   b. Demonstrate unconditional positive regard, interest, congruence, respect.
   c. Develop trusting relationship; accept client's behavior and display nonjudgmental, objective attitude.
   d. Be supportive, honest, authentic, genuine.
   e. Focus on emotional needs and emotionally charged area.

f. Focus on here-and-now behavior and expression of feelings.
g. Attempt to understand the client's point of view.
h. Develop an awareness of the client's likes and dislikes.
i. Encourage expression of both positive and negative feelings.
j. Use broad openings and ask open-ended questions; avoid questions that can be answered by "yes" or "no."
k. Use reflections of feelings, attitudes, and words.
l. Explore alternatives rather than answers or solutions.
m. Focus feedback on *what* is said rather than *why* it is said.
n. Paraphrase to assist in clarifying client's statements.
o. Promote sharing of feelings, information, and ideas instead of giving advice.
2. Examples of therapeutic communication responses (Table 12-3).
3. Examples of nontherapeutic communication responses (Table 12-4).

### Table 12-3　THERAPEUTIC COMMUNICATION

| Response | Example |
|---|---|
| 1. Exploring | "What seems to be the problem?"<br>"Tell me more about . . ." |
| 2. Reflecting | Client: "I am really mad at my mother for grounding me."<br>Nurse: "You sound angry." |
| 3. Focusing | "Give an example of what you mean."<br>"Let's look at this more closely." |
| 4. Clarifying | "I'm not sure that I understand what you're saying."<br>"Do you mean . . . ?" |
| 5. Using general leads | "Go on . . ."<br>"Talk more about . . ." |
| 6. Broad opening leads | "Where would you like to begin?"<br>"Talk more about . . ." |
| 7. Validating | "Did I understand you to say . . . ?" |
| 8. Informing | "The time is . . ."<br>"My name is . . ." |
| 9. Accepting | "Yes."<br>"Okay."<br>Nodding, "Uh hmm." |
| 10. Sharing observations | "You appear anxious. I noticed that you haven't been coming to lunch with the group." |
| 11. Presenting reality | "I do not hear a noise or see the lights blinking."<br>"I am not Cleopatra; I am your nurse." |
| 12. Summarizing | "During the past hour we talked about . . ." |
| 13. Using silence | Nurse remains silent to allow time for client to gather thoughts and begin speaking. |

## Table 12-4   NONTHERAPEUTIC COMMUNICATION

| Response | Example |
|---|---|
| 1. False reassurance | "Don't worry; you will be better in a few weeks." "Don't worry. I had an operation just like it; it was a snap." |
| 2. Giving advice | "What you should do is . . ." "If I were you, I would do . . ." |
| 3. Rejecting | "I don't like it when you . . ." "Please, don't ever talk about . . ." |
| 4. Belittling | "Everybody feels that way." "Why, you shouldn't feel that way." |
| 5. Probing | "Tell me more about your relationships with other men." |
| 6. Excessive questioning | "Hi, I am JoAnn, your student nurse. How old are you? What brought you to the hospital? How many children do you have? Do you want to fill out your menu right now?" |
| 7. Asking "why" questions | "Why are you crying?" |
| 8. Clichés | "Gee, the weather is beautiful outside." "Did you watch that new TV show last night? Everybody's talking about it." |

**TEST ALERT:** Listen to the client's concerns and use therapeutic interventions to increase client's understanding of his or her behavior.

## INTERVENTION MODALITIES

### Crisis Intervention

**A crisis is a self-limiting situation in which usual problem-solving or decision-making methods are not adequate.**

A. Crisis types.
   1. Maturational (birth of child, leaving home to go to college).
   2. Situational (divorce, death of spouse, debilitating physical or mental illness).
   3. Adventitious (mass-casualty incident; earthquake, terrorist attack, war, and rape).
B. Crisis intervention strategy views people as capable of personal growth and able to control their own lives.
C. Types of crisis intervention strategies.
   1. Individual crisis counseling.
   2. Crisis groups.
   3. Telephone counseling.
D. Crisis intervention requires support, protection, and enhancement of the client's self-image.
E. Goals of crisis intervention are to promote client safety and reduce client's anxiety by providing anxiety reduction techniques.

**TEST ALERT:** Identify the client in crisis; provide opportunity for the client to express feelings about the crisis.

### Group Therapy

**Group therapy is a structured or semistructured process in which individuals (7–12 members is an ideal size) are interrelated and interdependent and may share common purposes and norms.**

A. Emphasis on clear communication to promote effective interaction.
B. Disturbed perceptions can be corrected through consensual validation.
C. Socially ineffective behaviors can be modified through peer pressure.
D. See Table 12-6: Group Modalities for Older Adult Clients.

**⚠ NURSING PRIORITY:** Determining a client's perception of reality is an important consideration when selecting the client to be a member of a group. For instance, a person who is psychotic would not be a good selection as a group member.

### Family Therapy

**TEST ALERT:** Provide emotional support to family, assess dynamics of family interactions, assess family's understanding of illness and emotional reaction, and help family adjust to role changes.

Family therapy is a treatment modality designed to bring about a change in communication and interactive patterns between and among family members.

A. A family can be viewed as a system that is dynamic. A change or movement in any part of the family system affects all other parts of the system.
B. A family seeks to maintain a balance or "homeostasis" among various forces that operate within and on it.
C. Emotional symptoms or problems of an individual may be an expression of the emotional symptoms or problems in the family.
D. Therapeutic approaches involve helping family members look at themselves in the here and now and recognize the influence of past models on their behavior and expectations.

### Milieu

**TEST ALERT:** Maintain a therapeutic milieu/environment.

**Milieu is a scientifically planned, purposeful manipulation in the environment aimed at causing changes in the behavior and personality of the client.**

A. Nurse is viewed as a facilitator and a helper to clients rather than as a therapist.
B. The *therapeutic community* is a special kind of milieu therapy in which the total social structure of the treatment unit is involved as part of the helping process.
C. Emphasis is placed on open communication both within and between staff and client groups.

## Complementary and Alternative Medicine (CAM) Therapies

These alternative therapies are different from traditional Western medicine and are often influenced by traditional Chinese medicine, which focuses on maintaining unity with nature and balancing our energy systems.

A. Energy therapies.
   1. Healing touch—use of gentle touch on or close to the body to bring balance and healing.
   2. Therapeutic touch: the practitioner directs their balanced energy through the use of the practitioner's hands and directs it toward the client to enhance healing.
   3. Reiki therapy—hands are placed on or above the body and a transfer or "universal life energy" flows from practitioner to client.
B. Body-based or manipulative therapies.
   1. Acupressure—digital pressure is applied to an area of the body to reduce pain or regulate body function.
   2. Chiropractic medicine—movement and manipulation of the spine column and neck; includes physiotherapy and nutritional therapy.
   3. Massage—use of touch that unblocks energy flow and connects client with practitioner; stroking, rubbing, or kneading soft tissue to improve circulation, muscle tone, and promote relaxation.
C. Mind–body therapies.
   1. Biofeedback—electronic monitoring of a normally automatic bodily function (e.g., blood pressure, pulse, etc.) is used to train client to acquire voluntary control of that function.
   2. Guided imagery—change reality by creating a different mental picture.
   3. Music therapy—use of music as an intervention to improve the client's psychosocial, emotional, and cognitive needs by creating, singing, moving to, and/or listening to music.
   4. Transcendental meditation—quiet meditation focusing on getting beyond the self and becoming one with the universal energy source.
   5. Tai chi—slow, rhythmic, meditative movements designed to help the client find peace and calm.
   6. Yoga—involves breath control, simple meditation, and the adoption of specific bodily postures to promote health, relaxation, flexibility.
   7. Pilates—a type of movement therapy using specialized equipment to improve physical strength, flexibility, posture, and improve mental awareness.
D. Whole medical systems.
   1. Ayurvedic medicine—health and wellness depend on a delicate balance between the mind, body, and spirit; main goal is to promote good health, not fight disease, via dietary and lifestyle changes, herbal remedies and purgatives, massage, meditation, and exercise.
   2. Homeopathic medicine—certain diseases can be cured by giving small, highly diluted doses of substances made from naturally occurring plant, animal, or mineral substances that would in larger amounts produce in healthy persons symptoms similar to those of the disease; goal is to stimulate the vital force of the body to heal itself.
   3. Naturopathic medicine—belief that diseases can be successfully treated or prevented without the use of drugs, through techniques such as diet changes, exercise, and massage; goal is to treat the whole person rather than the disease.
   4. Traditional Chinese medicine (TCM)—focus on balancing the yin and yang energies; includes acupuncture, which is the movement of energy through meridians of the body to restore energy balance (Qi), herbal medicines, massage, acupressure, moxibustion (use of heat from burning herbs), Qi gong (balancing energy flow through body movement), tai chi, cupping, and massage.

**TEST ALERT:** Assess client's use of alternative/complementary practices; evaluate client's response to alternative therapy.

## Somatic Therapies

A. Restraints.
   1. Must consider client's civil liberties.
   2. Mechanical restraints include camisoles, wrist and ankle restraints, and sheet restraints.

**! NURSING PRIORITY:** Legally, the nurse must have a physician's order for applying restraints and to provide for clients' biologic needs, (e.g., hygiene, elimination, nutrition, and ability to communicate).

## Other Therapies

A. Activities therapy: a number of vital programs belong in this category, such as pet therapy, music therapy, occupational therapy, art therapy, recreational therapy, ropes course therapy, dance or movement therapy, etc.

## COMMON BEHAVIORAL PATTERNS

**TEST ALERT:** Identify inappropriate behavior, use client behavior modification techniques, and use therapeutic interventions to increase client's understanding of his or her behavior.

### Interpersonal Withdrawal

Interpersonal withdrawal is behavior characterized by avoidance of interpersonal contact and a sense of unreality.

A. Physical withdrawal: client sits or stands apart from others; may hide, assume a catatonic posture, or (in extreme form) attempt suicide.
B. Verbal withdrawal: avoidance through silence or (in extreme form) mutism; silence may indicate resistance, a pensive moment, or the indication that nothing more is to be said.

*Nursing Interventions*

A. Avoid punishment of client.
B. Decrease isolation.
C. Invite the client to speak.
D. State the amount of time you are willing to stay with the client, whether he or she chooses to speak or not.
E. Change the context of the contact (e.g., go for a walk together).
F. Encourage the client to share responsibility for the continuance of the relationship.

## Regression

**Regression is a selective, defensive operation in which the individual resorts to earlier, childish, or less complex patterns of behavior that once brought the client attention or pleasure.**

*Nursing Interventions*

A. Avoid fostering dependency and childlike attitudes.
B. Be patient and understanding.
C. Confront client directly about his or her plan.
D. Compliment client when he or she does something unusually well or assumes more responsibility.
E. Promote problem solving, reality orientation, and involvement in social activities.
F. Avoid punishment after periods of regression; instead, explore the meaning of the regressive behavior.
G. Remember that regression is a normal occurrence in young children who are hospitalized.

## Anger

**Anger is an unconscious process used to obtain relief from anxiety that is produced by a sense of danger; it involves a sense of powerlessness.**
   **Fear of expressing anger is related to fear of rejection.**

*Nursing Interventions*

A. Have client acknowledge or name feelings.
B. Explore source of personal fear or perceived threat (e.g., illness, disability, disfigurement, or emotional crisis).
C. Encourage verbalization of anxiety.
D. Explore appropriate external expression of feelings.
E. Avoid arguing with client.
F. Acting-out behavior is often an indirect expression of anger; it attracts attention and often represents the feelings the person is experiencing.

> **! NURSING PRIORITY:** Nontherapeutic responses to a client's anger include defensiveness, retaliation, condescension, and avoidance.

## Hostility/Aggressiveness

**Hostility is an antagonistic feeling; the client wishes to hurt or humiliate others; the result may be a feeling of inadequacy or self-rejection due to a loss of self-esteem.**

*Nursing Interventions*

> **TEST ALERT:** Plan interventions to assist the client in controlling aggressive behavior.

A. Prevent aggressive contact by early recognition of increased anxiety.
B. Maintain client contact rather than avoiding it.
C. Encourage verbalization of feelings associated with a threat of frustration (helplessness, inadequacy, anger).
D. Reduce environmental stimuli.
E. Avoid reinforcement behavior (e.g., joking, laughing, teasing, and competitive games).
F. Use distraction or remove the client from the immediate environment to reestablish self-control.
G. Set limits on unacceptable behavior.
H. Protect other clients.

> **! NURSING PRIORITY:** When two clients are arguing, engage the dominant client first by using distraction or removing the client from the setting to allow time for deescalation and processing of the situation.

## Violence

**Violence is behavior that is physically assaultive and risks injury to the self, others, and the environment.**

*Nursing Interventions*

> **! NURSING PRIORITY:** Immediate intervention should focus on control and safety followed by discussion to alleviate guilt and identify alternative behaviors to help prevent future episodes of violence.

A. Establish eye contact.
   1. Conveys attention and concern.
   2. Elicits more information.
   3. Ask the person to look at you.

> **! OLDER ADULT PRIORITY:** Expect some older clients to have vision problems; they may not know who you are. Hearing problems occur often with older adults; don't shout or talk rapidly.

B. Avoid asking, "Why?" Instead ask, "What's bothering you?"
   1. *Why* questions are threatening and decrease self-esteem.
   2. Open-ended questions seek to identify the problem, convey concern, and elicit more information.
C. Speak to the client softly, slowly, and with assurance.
D. Give directions clearly and concisely. Tell the client what you want him or her to do.
E. Encourage client to verbalize feelings.
   1. Give the client an outlet for the physical tension: "Walk with me. Tell me what happened."
   2. Keep the conversation slow; pace yourself: "Wait, I can't follow that. Tell me what you said."

3. Listen more than talk.
4. Let the client walk or move around or provide something for the client to safely "pound" on to release the tension before you talk.
F. Position yourself near the door.
1. Don't block the door.
2. Don't box the client into a corner.
G. Self-protection and protection of other clients are primary concerns.
1. Never remain alone with a potentially violent client; call security or other personnel.
2. Keep a comfortable distance from client; don't intrude on his or her personal space.
  a. With a client experiencing mild or moderate anxiety: sit near, about 2 feet away.
  b. With a client experiencing severe anxiety or panic: stay 4 to 6 feet away (or farther).
3. Be prepared to move quickly; violent clients act quickly and unpredictably.
4. Determine that the client has no weapons before approaching him or her.
5. Be supportive and intervene to increase client's self-esteem.
6. Be honest; tell the client you are concerned that he or she is out of control, but you are not going to let anyone get hurt.
7. Stay with the client but don't touch him or her until you've asked permission and it has been given to you.
H. Once the client is in control of his or her behavior, review and process the situation to alleviate the client's guilt and to discuss alternatives in case the client becomes anxious or angry in the future.

# ABUSE

*Abuse* is difficult to define because the term has been politicized and is not a clinical or scientific term.

**TEST ALERT:** Report client abuse to authorities, initiate a consultation/referral (e.g., support groups, community programs, social service, etc.), and protect the client from injury.

## Types of Abuse

A. **Physical abuse:** nonaccidental, intentional physical injury inflicted on another person.
B. **Physical neglect:** willing deprivation of essential care needed to sustain basic human needs and to promote growth and development.
C. **Emotional abuse:** use of threats, verbal insults, or other acts of degradation that are intended to be injurious or damaging to another's self-esteem.
D. **Emotional neglect:** absence of a warm, interpersonal atmosphere that is necessary for psychosocial growth, development, and the promotion of positive feelings of self-worth and self-esteem.
E. **Economic abuse:** failing to provide financial support to an individual, even though funds are available (e.g., not

paying utility bills and water/electricity being shut off to home).
F. **Sexual abuse:** lack of comprehension and consent on the part of the individual involved in sexual activities that are either exploitative or physically intimate in nature (e.g., rape, fondling, oral or genital contact, masturbation, unclothing, etc.).
G. **Incest:** sexual activity performed between members of a family group.

## Family Violence

**Patterns of dysfunctional, violent families can frequently be traced back for several generations. Adult behavior and role models for parenting are influenced by the childhood experiences within the family system.**

**TEST ALERT:** Assess dynamics of family interactions; identify risk factors; plan interventions to assist the client and family to cope.

A. The incorporation of violence within the family teaches children that the use of violence is appropriate. When the children grow up and form their own families, they tend to recreate the same parent–child, husband–wife relationships experienced in their original family.
B. Frequently, the abuser has inappropriate expectations of family members; the abuser may expect perfection and may be obsessed with discipline and control.
C. Family members are confused regarding their roles in the family; parents may be unable to assume adult roles in the family. Adult family members who feel inadequate in their roles may use violence in an attempt to prove themselves and to maintain superiority.
D. Family is usually isolated both physically and emotionally. The family tends to have few friends and is frequently isolated from the extended family. Family members are ashamed of what is occurring and tend to withdraw from social contacts in fear that the family activities might become known to others.
E. The *hostage response* is when victims assume responsibility for the violence inflicted on them.

## Characteristics of Abuse: The Perpetrator

A. The person who abuses—the perpetrator.
1. Perpetrator has an inability to control impulses; explosive temper; low tolerance for frustration.
2. Possesses greater physical strength than the victim.
3. Has low self-esteem and depression; feels he or she is a victim.
4. Tends to project shortcomings and inadequacies onto others.
5. Emotional immaturity; decreased capacity to delay satisfaction.
6. Suspicious of everyone; fear of being exposed; tends to isolate self from family.
7. High incidence of drug and alcohol abuse.
8. Often has experienced abuse as a child; has a greater tendency to demonstrate violence in his or her adult relationships.

B. Similarities between person who abuses and victim.
1. Poor self-concept and feelings of insecurity.
2. Feelings of helplessness, powerlessness, and dependence.
3. Difficulty in handling or inability to handle anger.

## Child Abuse

A. Child neglect: the failure to provide a child with the basic necessities; this may be classified as physical or emotional neglect.
1. Failure to thrive: Infant or child is below the normal ranges on the growth chart.
2. Infant or child does not appear to be physically cared for. Inappropriate diapering, diaper rash, or a strong urine smell to the body may be seen in infants who have been neglected.
3. Evidence of malnutrition.
4. Lack of adequate supervision; child is allowed to engage in dangerous play activities and sustains frequent injuries.
5. Language development may be delayed.
6. Withdrawal; inappropriate fearfulness.
7. Parents may be apathetic and unresponsive to the child's needs. The nurse is most often able to observe the parent–child interaction in school situations, in a doctor's office, or in the emergency department.
B. Physical child abuse.
1. Symptoms.
   a. Bruises and welts from being beaten with a belt, strap, stick, or coat hanger or from being slapped repeatedly in the face.
   b. Rope burns from being tied up or beaten with a rope.
   c. Human bite marks.
   d. Burns.
      (1) Burns on the buttocks from being immersed in hot water.
      (2) Pattern of burns: round, small burns from cigarettes; patterns that suggest an object was used.
      (3) Burns are frequently on the buttocks, in genital area, or on the soles of the feet.
   e. Evidence of various fractures in different stages of healing.
   f. Internal injuries from being hit repeatedly in the abdomen.
   g. Head injuries: skull, facial fractures.
2. Behavior symptoms.
   a. Withdrawal from physical contact with adults.
   b. Inappropriate response to pain or injury; failure to cry or seek comfort from parents.
   c. Infant may stiffen when held; child may stiffen when approached by adult or parent.
   d. Little eye contact with adults.
   e. Child may try to protect abusing parent for fear of punishment if abuse is discovered.
3. Parents or caretakers.
   a. Conflicting stories regarding accident or injury.
   b. Explanation of accident is inconsistent with injuries sustained (fractured skull and broken leg from "falling out of bed").

c. Initial complaint is not associated with child's injury (child is brought to the emergency department with complaints of the "flu," and there is evidence of a skull fracture).
d. Exaggerated concern or lack of concern related to level of child's injury.
e. Refusal to allow further tests or additional medical care.
f. Lack of nurturing response to injured or ill child; no cuddling, touching, or comforting child in distress.
g. Repeated visits to various medical emergency facilities.
h. Unrealistic expectations of the child; lack of understanding about stages of growth and development (e.g., severely spanking or beating a 1-year-old for lack of response to toilet training).

### Nursing Interventions

**Goal:** To establish a safe environment.

A. It is important for the nurse to be knowledgeable of the legal responsibilities in regard to state practice acts and child abuse laws (Box 12-2).

---

**Box 12-2 DOCUMENTATION FOR SUSPECTED ABUSE**

**Procedure**
1. Obtain the client's or parent's permission before photographing the victim.
2. Do not make assumptions about the identity of the perpetrator.
3. Chart the exact words used by the client/child to describe the abuser.
4. Record information very objectively; do not record your feelings, assumptions, or opinions of the incident or how it occurred.

**History**
1. Specify the time, date, and location as described by the client.
2. Report the sequence of events before the abuse/attack.
3. Identify and explain the period of time between the abuse/attack and initiation of medical attention.
4. List other people/children in the immediate vicinity of the abuse/attack.
5. Include quotations from the client.
6. Use objective, specific documentation when recording observations of the client and the person who brought the client to the emergency department.
7. Observe and record the interaction of the child and the parents.
8. Do conduct the interview in private.

**Physical Examination**
1. Be very specific in describing the location, size, and shape of bruises and lacerations. If possible, photograph the client to demonstrate the extent of the injuries.
2. If possible, describe the location and extent of injuries on an anatomic diagram.
3. Identify the presence of other injuries.
4. Describe the victim's reaction to pain, level of pain, and location of pain.

B. All 50 states have a designated agency that is available on a 24-hour basis for reporting child abuse.

C. All states have mechanisms for removing the child from the immediate abusive environment.

**Goal:** To educate the parents and help them identify assistance for long-term supportive care.

A. Educate parents in regard to normal growth and development of children, the role of discipline, and the necessity for having realistic expectations.

B. Become familiar with available community resources such as crisis centers, crisis hotlines, parent effectiveness training groups, Parents Anonymous groups, etc.

## Incest

A. Assessment

1. Victim is usually female; the perpetrator of abuse is primarily male, usually between ages 30 and 50, and often the victim's father or other member of the immediate family.

2. Incest is a symptom of severe dysfunction in an individual and within the family.

3. Perpetrators of sexual exploitation.
   a. Emotionally dependent men.
   b. Feelings of inferiority and low self-esteem.
   c. Perpetrators frequently seduce their victims by being endearing and "good" to the child.
   d. Often, these men are pillars of the community and are involved in many youth activities.
   e. Frequently, the mother is unaware of the problem. If she suspects it, she may feel guilty for having such ideas.

4. Sexually exploited child.
   a. Child may fear retaliation if anyone finds out; she may fear that she will not be believed if she tells anyone.
   b. Child may feel guilty for participating in the sexual activity and afraid of disruption of the family if it is revealed.
   c. Violence rarely accompanies the incest relationship.
   d. The child may be emotionally and physically dependent on the abusing parent.

### Nursing Interventions

**Goal:** To educate children that their bodies belong to themselves and are private.

A. Instruct children to report any type of touching, fondling, or caressing that makes them feel uncomfortable.

B. Provide educational material to help parents talk about sexual assault and inappropriate fondling with their children.

**Goal:** To support the parents and the child and to help them identify assistance for long-term supportive care.

A. Provide support and the opportunity for the child and family members to discuss their feelings.

B. Assist the family to identify community resources; strongly encourage involvement in family counseling.

## Older Adult Abuse

A. Types of older adult abuse (Box 12-3).

B. Typical victim.
   1. Woman of advanced age with few social contacts.
   2. At least one physical or mental impairment that limits the person's ability to perform activities of daily living.

C. Assessment of older adult abuse.
   1. Symptoms: contusions, abrasions, sprains, burns, bruising, human bite marks, sexual molestation, untreated or previously treated conditions, erratic hair loss from hair pulling, fractures, dislocations, head and face injuries (especially orbital fractures, black eyes, and broken teeth).
   2. Behavior: clinging to the abuser, extreme guardedness in the presence of the abuser, wariness of strangers, expression of ambivalence toward family/caregivers, depression, social or physical isolation, denial of abuse for fear of retaliation.

### Nursing Interventions

**To assess for older adult abuse.**

A. Use a private, separate setting for interviewing victim and perpetrator.

B. The interview must be unbiased, accurate, and appropriately documented.

C. Avoid signs of disapproval that might evoke shame or anger in the older client; be nonjudgmental.

**Goal:** To establish a safe environment.

A. It is important for the nurse to be knowledgeable of the legal responsibilities in regard to state practice acts and reporting of abuse (see Box 12-2).

---

### Box 12-3  OLDER ADULT CARE FOCUS

**Older Adult Abuse**
*Types of Older Adult Abuse*
- Physical: willful infliction of injury
- Neglect: withholding goods or services (such as food or attention) to the detriment of the older adult's physical or mental health
- Emotional: withholding affection or imposing social isolation
- Exploitation: dishonest or inappropriate use of the older person's property, money, or other resources

*Neglect Indicators*
- Poor hygiene, nutrition, and skin integrity
- Contractures
- Urine burns/excoriation
- Pressure ulcers
- Dehydration
- Bruises in various stages of healing
- Outdated medications
- No access to assistive devices if used by older adult (i.e., cane, wheelchair, hearing aid)

B. Client and family teaching in the areas of nutrition, general physical care, etc.

## Spousal or Intimate Partner Abuse (Figure 12-2)

A. Most often the spouse abused is the wife; frequently, the violence is a pattern in the woman's life. The violence in the family is frequently associated with alcohol; often there is a history of the woman's parents having a violent relationship.
B. It is not uncommon for the husband or abuser to have been exposed to violent family dynamics during childhood.
C. After the violent attack, the husband is frequently remorseful, kind, and loving. He may promise that he will never do it again.
D. Women tend to stay in abuse situations. Retaliation, loss of home and children, and additional abuse are just a few of the consequences they fear if they try to escape the situation. Abuse may increase if they express a desire to become more independent.

### Physical Assessment

A. Traumatic injury to the upper body, especially the face and breasts.
B. Signs of fear and an expression of helplessness.
C. May avoid friends and family for fear they will find out.
D. May exhibit feelings of shame, guilt, and embarrassment that she must seek treatment for her injuries.

### Nursing Interventions

**Goal:** Primary prevention—education of the community regarding the risks of abuse.
**Goal:** Secondary prevention—screening activities that occur within the community to identify victims of abuse early on and intervene to stop the abuse.
**Goal:** Tertiary prevention—emergency treatment, counseling, and work that goes on in shelters toward rehabilitating and providing long-term support to victims of abuse.

> **! NURSING PRIORITY:** When working with an abused victim, avoid anything that sounds like blaming the individual for his or her situation.

## RAPE

A. Legal definition of rape (varies from state to state): forced, violent sexual attack on an individual without his or her consent. Includes sex acts other than forced intercourse as rape; some states do not recognize rape by the husband.
B. Sexual assault is not a means of sexual gratification; it is a violent physical and emotional attack. Men attack women in an attempt to demonstrate their power and dominance; it is an attempt to control, terrify, and degrade the woman.
C. Majority of rapes are not sudden and impulsive; they are well planned.

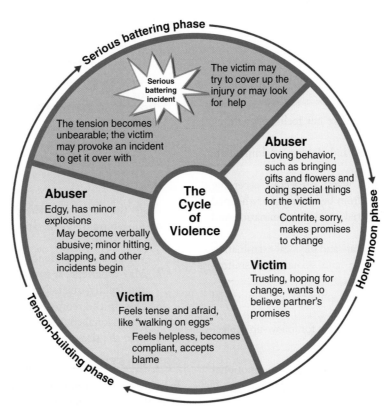

**FIGURE 12-2 The Cycle of Violence.** (From Halter, M. [2014]. *Varcarolis' foundations of psychiatric mental health nursing: A clinical approach* [7th ed]. St. Louis, MO: Elsevier.)

D. Most women know the rapist; most rape assaults occur between people of the same race.

E. Rape-trauma syndrome: variant of posttraumatic stress disorder; has two phases, an acute phase and a long-term reorganization phase.

> ⚠ **NURSING PRIORITY:** Five components are essential in treating the rape victim: treat and document injuries, treat and evaluate for sexually transmitted diseases, evaluate and prevent pregnancy risk, arrange for follow-up counseling, and collect evidence according to protocols.

### Assessment

A. Acute phase: may last a couple of weeks.
1. Woman may experience a wide range of emotional responses: fear, shock, disbelief, anger, denial, guilt, embarrassment, etc. (there is no "normal response" to rape).
2. Somatic reaction: physical trauma, skeletal muscle tension, gastrointestinal and genitourinary symptoms/discomfort.

B. Long-term reorganization phase: occurs 2 weeks or more after rape.
1. Intrusive thoughts (flashbacks, violent dreams, insomnia), fears, phobias.
2. Increased motor activity (moving, taking trips, changing phone numbers) and emotional lability.

C. Advise the woman to not "clean up" after a rape, because the physical evidence may be destroyed; advise the woman to come immediately to the emergency department (ED).

D. Complete physical assessment (Box 12-4).

### Nursing Interventions

**Goal:** To assist the client through the acute phase after the rape experience.

A. Encourage the client to verbalize her feelings regarding the attack.

B. Assist her to set priorities and determine immediate needs.

C. Respond to the client in a warm, respectful, accepting manner; protect the client from becoming overwhelmed and distressed from the initial physical examination and questioning.

D. Discuss need for follow-up care and physical examination regarding possible pregnancy and sexually transmitted disease.

E. Provide information regarding physical and emotional responses to rape.

F. Provide referral information and plan for follow-up contact within the next week.

**Goal:** To assist the client to work through the emotional phases that commonly occur after the initial trauma.

A. Encourage mental health counseling during the first few days after the assault.

---

### Box 12-4 CHECKLIST OF NURSING MANAGEMENT FOR THE RAPE VICTIM

**Medical–Legal**
- Valid written consent for examination, photographs, laboratory tests, release of information, and laboratory samples
- Appropriate "chain of evidence" documentation: follow agency protocol
- Protect legal rights

**Assist With Physical Examination**
- Vital signs and general appearance
- Examine for extragenital trauma: mouth, breasts, neck
- Examine for cuts, bruises, scratches; photograph

**Implement Medical Treatment**
- Care for injuries and emotional trauma
- Antibiotic prophylaxis for STDs
- Emergency contraception prophylactic dose of LO/OVRAL

**Document History**
- Age, marital status, and parity
- Menstrual and contraceptive history
- Time of last coitus before assault
- Change of clothes, bath, douche?
- Use of drugs or alcohol
- Who, what, when, where?
- Penetration, ejaculation, condom, extragenital acts

**Obtain Laboratory Samples**
- Use appropriate *evidence collection kits* and label carefully
- Vaginal smears: Pap smear and gram stain
- Oral or rectal swabs and smears
- Blood tests for serology, blood type, alcohol level
- Cultures: cervix plus other areas, if indicated
- Urine: pregnancy test, drugs
- Hair: comb and clip; obtain fingernail scrapings; comb pubic hairs; clip client's pubic hair or any matted hairs

**Follow-Up and Referral**
- Recommend continued follow-up and services of rape crisis center
- Repeat serology testing for gonorrhea, chlamydia, and HIV at a later date

*HIV,* Human immunodeficiency virus; *STDs,* sexually transmitted diseases.

---

B. Assist the client to understand and recognize the period of long-term reorganization that frequently follows a sexual attack.
1. Victim may experience sexual problems.
2. May experience a strong urge to discuss the incident and feelings related to the attack.
3. During the reorganization phase, client should have professional counseling to assist her to positively cope with the situation.

## PSYCHIATRIC DISORDERS

**It is important to note that emotional disturbances must be evaluated within the context and framework of normal growth and development, because behavior that is acceptable at one age may be a symptom of disease at another age.**

# CHILD-RELATED DISORDERS

## Intellectual Developmental Disorder

**A child who has an intellectual disability has deficits in three areas: intellectual functioning, social functioning, and practical aspects of daily living.** *This was previously called mental retardation.*

### Assessment

A. Causes.
   1. Down syndrome, fragile X syndrome, phenylketonuria, rubella.
   2. Kernicterus (elevated bilirubin level), anoxia, fetal alcohol syndrome.
   3. Lead poisoning, meningitis, encephalitis.
   4. Neoplasms, Tay-Sachs disease.
B. Additional characteristics.
   1. Irritability, temper tantrums, stereotyped movements.
   2. Multiple neurologic abnormalities: dysfunction in vision or hearing or seizure activity.

### Nursing Interventions

**Goal:** To promote optimum development within a family and community setting.

A. Promote feelings of self-esteem, worth, and security.
B. Educate the parents about developmental stages and tasks; deal with child's developmental, *not* chronologic, age.

**Goal:** To promote independence by setting realistic goals.

A. Teach basic skills in simple terms, with steps outlined.
B. Use behavior modification as a method for behavior control.
C. Use the principles of *repetition, reinforcement,* and *routine* when providing information for understanding and learning.

## Down Syndrome

**Down syndrome is a common chromosomal abnormality characterized by an extra chromosome 21 (trisomy 21); incidence increases with maternal age.**

### Assessment

A. Physical characteristics criteria.
   1. Head: small in size; face has flat profile, sparse hair.
   2. Eyes: inner epicanthal folds; short and sparse eyelashes.
   3. Nose: small and depressed nasal bridge (saddle nose).
   4. Ears: small and sometimes low-set.
   5. Mouth: protruding tongue; high arched palate.
   6. Neck: short and broad.
   7. Abdomen: protruding; umbilical hernia.
   8. Genitalia: small penis, cryptorchidism.
   9. Hands: short, stubby fingers; simian crease (transverse palmar crease).
   10. Muscles: hypotonic.
B. Mental characteristics.
   1. Cognitive impairment.
   2. Developmental delay.

### Nursing Interventions

**Goal:** To promote optimal development

A. Involve child and parents in early stimulation program.
B. Promote self-care skills.
C. Help parents identify realistic goals for child.
D. Encourage parents to enroll child in special daycare programs and education classes.
E. Emphasize to parents that child has same needs of play, discipline, and social interaction as all children.

**Goal:** To encourage early identification of Down syndrome.

It is common for pregnant women at risk (older than 35 years, family history of Down syndrome, or previous birth of a child with Down syndrome) to have an amniocentesis before the sixteenth week to rule out Down syndrome.

## Home Care

A. Prevent respiratory tract infections by teaching parents about postural drainage and percussion.
B. Encourage use of cool mist vaporizer.
C. Stress importance of changing infant's position frequently; swaddle infant to prevent heat loss.
D. Explain to parents about feeding difficulties and the need for direct supervision; encourage small, frequent feedings; feed solid food by pushing food back inside of mouth; provide foods that will form bulk to prevent constipation.
E. Discuss alternative options to home care with parents.
F. Individuals with Down syndrome develop a clinical syndrome of dementia that has almost identical clinical and neuropathologic characteristics of Alzheimer disease as described in individuals without Down syndrome.
   1. The main difference is the age of onset of Alzheimer disease in individuals with Down syndrome.
   2. These clients present with clinical symptoms in their late 40s or early 50s.

## Attention-Deficit/Hyperactivity Disorder (ADHD)

**Attention-deficit/hyperactivity disorder is a developmental disorder characterized by inappropriate inattention and impulsivity, which usually appear between 3 and 7 years of age. Names previously used include hyperkinetic syndrome, minimal brain damage, minimal brain dysfunction.**

### Assessment

A. Diagnostic criteria.
   1. Inattention.
      a. Fails to finish things he or she starts.
      b. Often does not seem to listen when spoken to.
      c. Is easily distracted.

d. Has difficulty concentrating.

e. Has difficulty sticking to play activity.

2. Impulsivity.

a. Often acts before thinking.

b. Shifts excessively from one activity to another.

c. Has difficulty organizing work.

d. Needs frequent supervision.

e. Frequently calls out in class.

f. Has difficulty waiting turn in games or group activities.

3. Hyperactivity.

a. Runs about or climbs on things.

b. Has difficulty sitting still; fidgets.

c. Has difficulty staying seated.

d. Moves about excessively during sleep.

e. Is always "on the go."

4. Onset before 7 years of age

5. Duration of at least 6 months.

## Nursing Interventions

**Goal:** To keep child from harming self or others.

A. Assist child to recognize when he or she feels angry.

B. Help child accept his or her feelings of anger.

C. Teach child appropriate expression of angry feelings.

D. Redirect violent behavior with physical outlets for child's anxiety (e.g., use of punching bag, jogging).

E. Confront child; withdraw attention when interactions with others are manipulative or exploitative.

F. Use time out, isolation room, and restraints only when other interventions are unsuccessful. *Note: The nurse should review and be aware of the agency's policies related to the use of chemical and physical restraints.*

**Goal:** To encourage age-appropriate, socially acceptable coping skills.

A. If child is hyperactive, make environment safe for continuous large muscle movement.

B. Provide large motor skill activities for child to participate in.

C. Provide frequent, nutritious snacks for child to "eat on the run."

**Goal:** To decrease anxiety and increase self-esteem.

A. Encourage child to seek out staff to discuss true feelings.

B. Offer support during times of increased anxiety; ensure physical and psychological safety.

**Goal:** To administer prescribed medication.

A. Methylphenidate hydrochloride or dextroamphetamine sulfate may be used; not recommended for children younger than 6 years of age.

B. Prolonged administration may produce a temporary suppression of normal weight gain. Administer in morning (to prevent insomnia) and 30 to 45 minutes before meals.

## Autism Spectrum Disorders (Autism)

**Infantile autism is characterized by a lack of responsiveness to other people, a lack of involvement with others, a lack of verbal communication, a preoccupation with inanimate objects, and ritualistic behavior.**

## Assessment

A. Diagnostic criteria.

1. Onset before 3 years of age.

2. Impairment in social interactions—lack of responsiveness and involvement with others; difficulty maintaining eye contact.

3. Impairment in communication and imaginative activity.

a. Gross deficits in language development: speech is characterized by echolalia, parrot speech (i.e., automatic repetition of words).

b. Pronominal reversal (tendency to use *you* for *I*).

c. Lack of spontaneous make-believe play.

4. Markedly restricted, stereotypical patterns of behavior, interest, and activities.

a. Rigid adherence to routines and rituals.

b. Repetitive motor mannerisms—hand flapping, clapping, rocking, or rhythmic body movements.

5. *Absence* of delusions, hallucinations, and associative looseness, which are characteristics of childhood schizophrenia.

## Nursing Interventions

**Goal:** To increase social awareness.

A. Encourage a significant one-to-one relationship with an adult.

B. Promote and engage in peer interaction.

C. Develop play and self-care skills.

D. Do not force interactions. Begin with positive reinforcement for eye contact. Gradually introduce touch, smiling, and hugging.

**Goal:** To teach verbal (oral) communication.

A. Respond to verbalization by telling the child what you do not understand.

B. Respond to nonverbal cues with verbal (oral) interpretation.

C. Observe and record context in which lack of clarity of spoken word occurred.

D. Use *en face* approach (face-to-face, eye-to-eye) to convey correct nonverbal expressions by example.

**Goal:** To decrease unacceptable behavior.

A. Encourage child to recognize and respond to own physiologic needs and urges.

B. Encourage verbalization of body needs but do not make an issue of it.

C. Offer fluids and encourage exercise to prevent constipation.

D. Offer the bathroom at appropriate intervals throughout the day.

E. Prevent the child from hurting self or others by setting firm limits and recognizing feelings of anger, fear, and frustration.

## Separation Anxiety Disorder

**Child demonstrates persistent and excessive anxiety on separation from parent or familiar surroundings.**

### Assessment

A. Diagnostic criteria.
  1. Excessive distress when separated from home or parents.
  2. Unrealistic worry about harm occurring.
  3. Refusal to sleep unless near parent.
  4. Refusal to attend school or other activities without parent.
  5. Physical symptoms as a response to anxiety (e.g., upset stomach, vomiting, headache, etc.).
B. Additional characteristics.
  1. Depressed mood.
  2. Excessive conformity; often demonstrates need for constant attention; may be demanding.
  3. Usual age of onset any time between preschool years and 11 or 12 years.

### Nursing Interventions

**Goal:** To reduce the level of anxiety in anxiety-provoking situations.

A. Identify factors that produce anxiety.
B. Turn on nightlights to allay night fears.
C. Offer calm reassurance.

**Goal:** To differentiate between normal separation anxiety, which is seen in early childhood, and excessive anxiety, which is seen in separation anxiety disorders.

## Specific Disorders With Physical Symptoms

### Assessment

A. Dysfluency (stuttering).
  1. Frequent repetitions or prolongations of sounds, syllables, or words.
  2. Unusual hesitations and pauses that disrupt the flow of speech.
  3. Speech may be rapid or slow.
  4. Stuttering is often absent during singing or talking to inanimate objects.
B. Enuresis (bed-wetting).
  1. Repeated involuntary voiding during the day or night.
  2. The involuntary voiding occurs after the age at which it is expected and is not due to any physical disorder.
C. Encopresis (fecal incontinence).
  1. Repeated voluntary or involuntary passage of feces of normal consistency in inappropriate places.
  2. Smearing feces, which should be differentiated from the smearing that takes place involuntarily and in the younger child (1 or 2 years of age).

### Nursing Interventions

**Goal:** To assess and medically evaluate for any physiologic cause related to stuttering, enuresis, or encopresis.

**Goal:** To promote a positive self-concept by helping the child overcome feelings of shame and guilt associated with the disorder.
**Goal:** To identify various approaches to controlling enuresis.

A. Administer imipramine.
B. Restrict fluids before going to bed.
C. Encourage behavioral intervention therapies (a buzzer that wakes child when he or she starts to urinate; bladder training programs).

**Goal:** To identify various approaches to controlling fecal incontinence.

A. If child is retaining feces, initiate a bowel-cleaning regimen.
B. If child has loose stools, he or she needs a daily bulk laxative.
C. If soiling is deliberate, help child express feelings through other means.
D. Educate child about bodily signals (rectal pressure).
E. Teach child to sit on toilet for 10 to 15 minutes after eating to establish regular elimination pattern.

**TEST ALERT:** Initiate a toileting schedule.

## Specific Developmental Disorders

### Assessment

A. Developmental reading disorder.
  1. Impairment in the development of reading skills.
  2. Often referred to as *dyslexia.*
  3. Slow reading speed and reduced comprehension.
B. Developmental arithmetic disorder: impairment in the development of arithmetic skills.
C. Developmental language disorder.
  1. Three major types.
    a. Failure to acquire any language.
    b. Acquired language disability.
    c. Delayed language acquisition.
  2. Often the result of trauma or a neurologic disorder.

### Nursing Interventions

**Goal:** To identify specific developmental disorders in relationship to chronologic age in preschool testing.
**Goal:** To refer child to appropriate developmental program in school.

## Eating Disorders

**This group of disorders is characterized by gross disturbances in eating behavior; it includes anorexia nervosa and bulimia nervosa.**

### Assessment

A. Anorexia nervosa.
  1. Intense fear of gaining weight and/or becoming obese.
  2. Need for control and perfectionism.
  3. Disturbance of body image.
  4. Occurs more often in females than males.
  5. Body weight less than 85% of that expected.
  6. No known physical illness.

7. A life-threatening emergency: Up to 15% of clients with anorexia die of malnutrition, and many are prone to suicide.

B. Bulimia nervosa.
1. Recurrent episodes of binge eating.
2. Awareness that eating pattern is abnormal.
3. Secretive binge eating and purging behaviors (diuretics, laxatives, excessive exercise).
   a. Russell's sign—bruises or calluses on the thumb or hand caused by trauma from self-induced vomiting.
   b. Erosion of tooth enamel, pharyngitis from vomiting.
4. Fear of not being able to stop eating voluntarily.
5. Depressed mood and self-induced vomiting after the eating binges.

### Nursing Interventions

**Goal:** To exhibit no signs or symptoms of malnutrition.

A. If client is unable or unwilling to maintain adequate oral intake, a liquid diet may be administered through a nasogastric tube.
B. Consult with dietitian; determine number of calories required to provide adequate nutrition and realistic weight gain.
C. Explain details of behavior modification program to client.
D. Sit with client during mealtimes for support and to observe amount ingested. A limit (usually 30 minutes) should be imposed on time allotted for meals.
E. Observe client for at least 1 hour after meals.
F. Accompany client to bathroom if self-induced vomiting is suspected.
G. Carefully document intake and output.
H. Weigh client immediately after he or she arises and after first voiding, usually once or twice each week, but not more often to avoid focusing on weight. Always use same scale, if possible, with client's back facing scale.
I. Do not discuss food or eating with client once protocol has been established. Do, however, offer support and positive reinforcement for obvious improvements in eating behaviors.
J. Offer support and use nonjudgmental approach with the client.
K. Administer antidepressants as ordered.

**Goal:** To increase self-esteem, as manifested by verbalizing positive aspects of self and exhibiting less preoccupation with own appearance, by discharge.

A. Assist client to reexamine negative perceptions of self and to recognize positive attributes.
B. Offer positive reinforcement for independently made decisions influencing client's life.
C. Offer positive reinforcement when honest feelings related to autonomy/dependence issues remain separated from maladaptive eating behaviors.
D. Help client develop a realistic perception of body image and relationship with food.

E. Promote feelings of control within the environment through participation and independent decision making.
F. Allow client to make decisions when appropriate and realistic.
G. Help client realize that perfection is unrealistic and explore this need with the client.
H. Help client claim ownership of angry feelings and recognize that expressing them is acceptable if it is done in an appropriate manner. Be an effective role model.

**Goal:** To identify an eating disorder and rule out a physiologic cause
**Goal:** To recognize complications.

A. Anorexia nervosa—refeeding syndrome can result if system is replenished too quickly, leading to cardiovascular collapse.
B. Bulimia nervosa—if syrup of ipecac is used to induce vomiting, and vomiting does not occur, the absorption of the ipecac can lead to cardiotoxicity and heart failure. Watch for edema and check breath sounds.

## NEUROCOGNITIVE DISORDERS

Neurocognitive disorders manifest deficits in memory, problem solving, perception, reasoning, and judgment. Delirium and dementia are common neurocognitive disorders.

### Delirium

**Delirium is a neurocognitive disorder that is always secondary to another physiologic process. Clinical manifestations usually develop over a short period of time. The constellation of symptoms typically fluctuates and is often reversible and temporary once the underlying physiologic cause is treated.**

### Assessment

A. Diagnostic criteria.
1. A clouded sensorium or state of consciousness.
2. Memory loss for both recent and remote events; disorientation.
3. Signs and symptoms develop over a short period and tend to fluctuate during the day.
4. Confusion, hallucinations, and delusions.
5. Sleep disturbances.
6. Motor activity may be increased or decreased.
7. Speech may be incoherent.
8. Confusion Assessment Method (CAM) is a standardized diagnostic tool for detecting and diagnosing delirium.

B. Additional characteristics.
1. Emotional disturbances: anxiety, fear, depression, anger.
2. Age at onset: common in older adult clients.
C. Etiologic factors.
1. Systemic infection: meningitis, encephalitis, respiratory and urinary infection.
2. Metabolic disorders: fluid or electrolyte imbalance.
   a. Hypoglycemia.
   b. Dehydration, vomiting.
   c. Hypoxia.

3. Hepatic or renal disease; thiamine deficiency.
4. Drug intoxication and withdrawal.
5. Pain and sleep deprivation.
6. Circulatory problems associated with hypertension.
7. Head trauma: seizure activity.
8. Change in caregiver or location.

### Nursing Interventions

**Goal:** To diminish effect of causative agent such as drugs, infectious organisms, physiologic or psychosocial stressors, or a circulatory–metabolic disorder.

A. Administer medications: antipyretics, antibiotics, or sedatives.
B. Assess for contributing factors/agents and eliminate when possible.
C. Prevent further damage by assessing for possible complications.

**Goal:** To provide adequate nutrition.

A. Encourage diet high in calories, protein, and vitamins, especially thiamine (vitamin $B_1$).
B. Encourage adequate intake and output.

**Goal:** To prevent complications and provide a safe environment.

A. Provide a quiet, nonstimulating environment to prevent hallucinations.
B. Ensure that safety needs are met (may fall out of bed).
C. Remove potentially harmful articles from a client's room: cigarettes, matches, lighters, sharp objects.
D. Pad side rails and headboard of bed for client with a seizure disorder.

### Dementia

**Dementia is a neurocognitive disorder characterized by loss of intellectual abilities to such an extent that social and occupational functioning are negatively affected; it involves memory, judgment, abstract thought, and changes in personality. Often the disorders are progressive and follow an irreversible course in which the damage remains permanent(Box 12-5).**

A. Diagnostic criteria.
1. Loss of intellectual abilities that interfere with social and occupational functioning.
2. Memory impairment and confusion.
3. Impairment in judgment, comprehension, abstract thinking, and language (Figure 12-3).
4. Personality change demonstrated by exaggeration of previous personality traits.
5. Mini-Mental State Examination shows disorientation and lack of recall.
6. Brain atrophy present on computed tomography (CT) and positron emission tomography (PET) scans
B. Additional characteristics.
1. Anxiety or depression may be apparent.
2. Behavior may demonstrate excessive orderliness, social withdrawal, or the tendency to relate an event in excessive detail.
3. Age at onset: found predominantly in older adults.

---

### Box 12-5 KEY POINTS: COGNITIVE DISORDERS

- Clients have varying degrees of awareness of the changes that are occurring, which is emotionally painful to them.
- Often depression is mistaken for the early onset of dementia.
- Dementia disrupts the older adult couple's final stage of family development (generativity, retirement, etc.).
- Dementia interferes with family intergenerational development when adult offspring are unable to rectify past injustices, conflicts, and disappointments with parents.
- Caregiver coping is highly stressful and can be handled with a more positive approach when there is a focus on problem solving and education.
- Clients with Alzheimer disease have loss of memory, intellectual functioning, orientation, affective regulation, motor coordination, and personality, with eventual loss of bowel and bladder control to the point of total incapacitation.

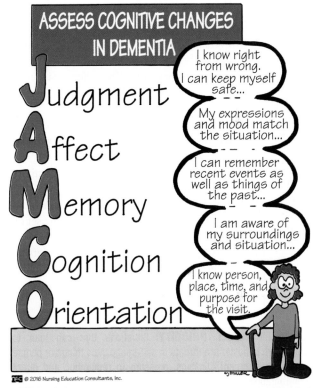

**FIGURE 12-3 JAMCO.** (From Zerwekh, J., & Garneau, A., J., Miller, C. J. [2017]. *Digital collection of the memory notebooks of nursing* [4th ed.]. Chandler, AZ: Nursing Education Consultants, Inc.)

C. Etiologic factors.
1. Neurologic diseases: Huntington disease, multiple sclerosis, Parkinson disease.
2. Cardiovascular disorders causing anoxia and brain damage: cerebral arteriosclerosis, cerebral vascular accident (stroke).
3. Central nervous system (CNS) infections: tertiary neurosyphilis, tuberculosis, fungal meningitis, viral encephalitis.

4. Brain trauma: chronic subdural hematoma.
5. Alcohol-related disorder: Korsakoff syndrome (thiamine deficiency)
6. Toxic effects: metabolic disturbance.
   a. Pernicious anemia, hypothyroidism.
   b. Folic acid deficiency.
7. Loss of brain tissue and function in presenile conditions.

> ⚠ **OLDER ADULT PRIORITY:** The cardinal rule: do not push too fast in getting information, assisting with activities of daily living, or insisting that the person socialize. Continued pressure and insistence on a task may result in combative behavior. Watch for reasons for confusion; it could be due to depression, infection, dehydration, and electrolyte imbalance.

a. Alzheimer disease (most common form of dementia) (Table 12-5).
   (1) More commonly seen in older adult clients.
   (2) Five As—anomia, apraxia, agnosia, amnesia, aphasia (Figure 12-4).
   (3) Irreversible—cerebral atrophy and neuritic plaques.
   (4) Recent memory loss. The client can recall events and activities of 10 years ago but not 10 minutes ago.
   (5) Sundowner syndrome—confused, disoriented behavior that becomes noticeable after the sun goes down and during the night.
   (6) Wandering behavior, restlessness, activity-seeking behavior.
   (7) Disorientation and inability to sustain intentions; the person forgets what he or she set out to do.
   (8) Catastrophic reactions: heightened anxiety occurring during interviewing or questioning, when a person cannot answer or perform.
   (9) Combative behavior.

> ⚠ **OLDER ADULT PRIORITY:** Situations that can lead to combative behavior are threats to self-image, new things or people in the environment, illusions, pressure to remember, and direct confrontation.

> ⚠ **NURSING PRIORITY:** The three Rs—routine, reinforcement, and repetition—are key aspects of care not only for the intellectually disabled but also for the older adult client with dementia.

### Nursing Interventions

**Goal:** To administer medication to slow the dementia disease process (see Appendix 10-2).
**Goal:** To provide a quiet, structured environment to increase consistency and promote feelings of security.

A. Avoid dependency.
B. Establish routine for activities of daily living.
C. Meet client's physical needs.

D. Do not isolate client from others in the unit.
E. Provide handrails, walkers, and wheelchairs.
F. Do not change schedules suddenly: *routine, reinforcement,* and *repetition* are the key aspects of care.
G. Check for hazards in the environment (e.g., rugs on floor); make sure environment is well lighted.
H. Prevent client from wandering away from care area.

> **TEST ALERT:** Orient the client to reality and monitor activities of the confused client. (Knowledge about providing care for the older client, especially the client with Alzheimer disease, is often tested.)

**Goal:** To promote contact with reality.

A. Make brief and frequent contact.
B. Give feedback.
C. Supply stimulation to motivate client to engage in activities.
D. Use concrete ideas in communication.
E. Maintain reality orientation by encouraging client to reminisce (Table 12-6).

> ⚠ **NURSING PRIORITY:** Reminiscence and life review help the client resume progression through the grief process associated with disappointing life events and increase self-esteem as successes are reviewed.

F. Orient client frequently to reality and surroundings.
   1. Allow client to have familiar objects around him or her.
   2. Use other items such as clocks, calendars, and daily schedules.
G. Use simple explanations and face-to-face interaction.
H. Do not shout message into client's ear.
I. Allow sufficient time for client to complete projects.
J. Reinforce reality-oriented comments and orientation to time, place, and date.

> ⚠ **NURSING PRIORITY:** Speaking slowly and in a face-to-face position is most effective when communicating with an older adult experiencing a hearing loss. Visual cues facilitate understanding. Shouting causes distortion of high-pitched sounds, and in some instances creates a feeling of discomfort for the client.

**Goal:** To provide diversion activities that enhance self-esteem.

A. Name sign and picture on door identifying client's room.
B. Identifying sign on outside of dining room door.
C. Large clock, with oversized numbers and hands, appropriately placed.
D. Large calendar, indicating one day at a time, with month, day, and year identified in bold print.

> ⚠ **NURSING PRIORITY:** The three Ps for clients with dementia: protecting dignity, preserving function, and promoting quality of life.

### Table 12-5  STAGES OF ALZHEIMER DISEASE

| Stage | Hallmarks |
|---|---|
| No impairment | No memory problems |
| **Stage 2**<br>Very mild cognitive decline (may be age-related or due to dementia) | Aware of memory lapses<br>Forgetting familiar words or the location of everyday objects<br>No symptoms of dementia can be detected during a medical examination or by friends, family, or coworkers |
| **Stage 3**<br>Mild cognitive decline (early-stage Alzheimer can be diagnosed in some, but not all, individuals with these symptoms) | Others begin to notice difficulties<br>Noticeable problems coming up with the right word or name<br>Trouble remembering names when introduced to new people<br>Noticeable difficulty performing tasks in social or work settings<br>Forgetting material that one has just read<br>Losing or misplacing a valuable object<br>Increasing trouble with planning or organizing |
| **Stage 4**<br>Moderate cognitive decline (mild or early-stage Alzheimer disease) | Forgetfulness of recent events<br>Impaired ability to perform challenging mental arithmetic<br>Difficulty performing complex tasks, such as planning dinner for guests, paying bills, or managing finances<br>Becoming moody or withdrawn, especially in socially or mentally challenging situations |
| **Stage 5**<br>Moderately severe cognitive decline (moderate or midstage Alzheimer disease) | Gaps in memory and thinking are noticeable, and individuals begin to need help with day-to-day activities. At this stage, individuals may:<br>Be unable to recall their own addresses or telephone numbers or the high schools or colleges from which they graduated<br>Become confused about where they are or what day it is<br>Have trouble with less challenging mental arithmetic<br>Need help choosing proper clothing for the season or the occasion<br>Still remember significant details about themselves and their families<br>Still require no assistance with eating or using the toilet |
| **Stage 6**<br>Severe cognitive decline (moderately severe or midstage Alzheimer disease) | Personality changes may take place, and sufferers may need extensive help with daily activities<br>At this stage, individuals may:<br>Lose awareness of recent experiences as well as of their surroundings<br>Remember their own names but have difficulty with their personal histories<br>Distinguish familiar and unfamiliar faces but have trouble remembering the name of a spouse or caregiver<br>Need help dressing properly and may, without supervision, make mistakes such as putting pajamas over daytime clothes or shoes on the wrong feet<br>Experience major changes in sleep patterns (sleeping during the day, becoming restless at night)<br>Need help handling details of toileting<br>Have increasingly frequent trouble controlling their bladder or bowels<br>Experience major behavioral changes, including suspiciousness and delusions or compulsive, repetitive behavior<br>Tend to wander or become lost |
| **Stage 7**<br>Very severe cognitive decline (severe or late-stage Alzheimer disease) | In the final stage of this disease, individuals lose the ability to respond to their environment, to carry on a conversation, and, eventually, to control movement<br>May still say words or phrases<br>At this stage, individuals need help with much of their daily personal care, including eating and using the toilet<br>May also lose the ability to smile, sit without support, and hold their heads up<br>Reflexes become abnormal<br>Muscles grow rigid<br>Swallowing is impaired |

Used with permission and adapted from Alzheimer's Association. (2013). *Seven stages of Alzheimer's*. Retrieved from http://www.alz.org/alzheimers_disease_stages_of_alzheimers.asp

## Anxiety Disorders

Anxiety can be a predominant disturbance (panic and generalized anxiety), or anxiety can be experienced as a person attempts to confront a dreaded situation (phobic disorder) or resist the obsessions and compulsions of an obsessive–compulsive disorder. In general, these are common responses to emotional problems that are seldom treated in a psychiatric setting because the person does not have a great defect in reality testing and does not demonstrate severe antisocial behavior. Pressures of decision making and decisions that are made in the early adult years seem to act as precipitating events in the development of anxiety disorders (Table 12-7).

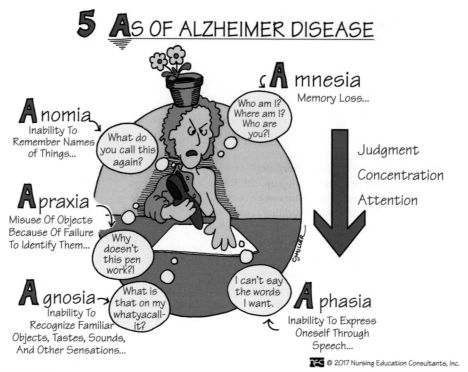

**FIGURE 12-4 Five As of Alzheimer Disease.** (From Zerwekh, J., & Garneau, A., J., Miller, C. J. [2017]. *Digital collection of the memory notebooks of nursing* [4th ed.]. Chandler, AZ: Nursing Education Consultants, Inc.)

### Table 12-6 GROUP MODALITIES FOR OLDER ADULT CLIENTS

| *Remotivation Therapy* | *Reminiscing Therapy* | *Psychotherapy* |
|---|---|---|
| **Purpose of Group** | | |
| Resocialize regressed and apathetic older adult clients | Share memories<br>Increase socialization<br>Enhance self-esteem | Alleviation of presenting psychiatric problems<br>Promote ability to interact with others in a group<br>Increase ability to make decisions and function more independently |
| **Format** | | |
| 10–15 clients in a group<br>Meet 1–2 times per week<br>Meetings highly structured in a classroom setting<br>Each session has a specific topic | 6–8 clients in a group<br>Meet 1–2 times per week<br>Topics include holidays, travel | 6–12 group members<br>Members share problems and problem-solving strategies with each other<br>Group meets at regularly scheduled times |
| **Desired Outcomes** | | |
| Increases group members' sense of reality<br>Encourages a more objective self-image | Assists in alleviating depression<br>Use of process of reorganization and reintegration provides an avenue for older adults to achieve a sense of identity and positive self-concept | Decreases sense of isolation<br>Promotes new roles and reestablishes old roles<br>Provides group support for increasing self-esteem |

From Matteson, M. A., & McConnell, E. S. (Eds.). (1988). *Gerontological nursing: Concepts and practice* (p. 80). Philadelphia: Saunders. As cited in M. J. Halter, *Varcarolis' foundations of psychiatric mental health nursing* (p. 580).

**TEST ALERT:** Identify effects of environmental stressors on client; plan measures to deal with client's anxiety; encourage client to use problem-solving skills; teach stress-reduction techniques; and provide support to client who is upset or distraught.

### Nursing Interventions

**Goal:** To promote techniques to reduce anxiety.

A. Systematic desensitization/exposure therapy: Client is exposed serially to a specific list of anxiety-provoking situations; through techniques of progressive relaxation, the client becomes desensitized to each stimulus.

B. Reciprocal inhibition: The anxiety-provoking stimulus is paired with another stimulus that is associated

## Table 12-7  SELECTED ANXIETY DISORDERS

| Problem | Description | Nursing Intervention |
|---|---|---|
| **Panic disorder** (with or without agoraphobia): an extreme level of anxiety | Agoraphobia (fear of being in places or situations; crowds, traveling) May experience shortness of breath, dizziness, diaphoresis, palpitations, feeling of impending doom; misinterprets reality (may exhibit hallucinations or delusions) | **Goal:** To reduce panic level anxiety feelings by reinterpreting the feelings correctly (see Table 10-2). 1. Stay with client; maintain calm manner and use simple, direct statements. 2. Reduce environmental stimuli (lights, noise alarms). |
| **Phobia:** an intense, irrational fear of a specific object, activity, or situation | Fear of being alone or in public places Claustrophobia (fear of enclosed spaces) Acrophobia (fear of heights) Social phobia (fear of circumstances that may be humiliating, e.g., speaking in public, being called on in a classroom) | **Goal:** To reduce phobic behavior. 1. Do not force client to come in contact with the feared object or source of anxiety. 2. Have client focus on awareness of self. 3. Distract client's attention from phobia. |
| **Obsessive–compulsive disorder:** unconscious control of anxiety by the use of rituals, thoughts, obsessions, or compulsions | **Obsessions:** recurrent, persistent ideas, thoughts, or impulses that are not voluntarily produced *Most common obsessions include thoughts of violence, need for order, contamination, and doubt.* **Compulsions:** repetitive, ritualistic behaviors that are performed in a certain fashion to relieve an unbearable amount of tension *Most common compulsions include handwashing, counting, checking.* | **Goal:** To assist in coping with the compulsive behavior. 1. Accept rituals and avoid punishment or criticism; do not interrupt ritual, because this will increase anxiety. 2. Plan for extra time because of slowness and client's need for perfection. 3. Prevent physical deterioration or harm, and set limits only to prevent harmful acts (such as handwashing so excessively that it removes the skin from the hand surface). **Goal:** To encourage client to develop different ways of handling anxiety. 1. Reduce demands on the individual. 2. Convey acceptance of the client, regardless of behavior. 3. Encourage alternative activity. |
| **Posttraumatic stress disorder:** involves the development of characteristic symptoms after a traumatic psychological event in which the individual is unable to adapt or adjust (e.g., rape, military combat, airplane crashes, torture, or abuse) | Client reexperiences the traumatic event (e.g., flashbacks). Client withdraws, becomes isolated, and restricts emotional response. Experiences hyperalertness, insomnia, nightmares, depression, and anxiety | **Goal:** To determine precipitating stress factor in client's reaction. 1. Reduce and prevent chronic disability. 2. Encourage verbalization of the traumatic event. **Goal:** To maintain personal integrity. 1. Provide physical, social, or occupational rehabilitation. 2. Administer SSRI (selective serotonin reuptake inhibitor); first-line treatment. |
| **Generalized anxiety disorder:** unrealistic or excessive anxiety and worry about life's circumstances; differs from panic disorder in that it never remits and onset is at early age | Physical symptoms associated with disorder are restlessness, apprehension, tension, irritability, "free-floating" anxiety. | **Goal:** To reduce level of anxiety. 1. Administer benzodiazepines for immediate relief of symptoms. 2. Teach anxiety-reducing techniques. 3. Reduce pressure and anxiety-provoking situations around client. 4. Divert attention from symptoms. |

with an opposite feeling to diminish the effect of the anxiety.

C. Cognitive therapy: internal dialogue or self-talk on feelings, emotions, and behavior.

D. Regular daily exercise.

E. Other therapy: hypnosis, meditation, imagery, yoga, biofeedback training.

 ## Somatic Symptom Disorders

**Somatic symptom disorders are disorders in which the person has physical symptoms suggesting a physiologic etiology, but after in-depth assessment and diagnostic testing, no organic disease or physiologic abnormalities are found.**

### Assessment

A. Conversion disorder is a loss of, or alteration in, voluntary and/or sensory functioning that suggests a neurologic disorder but is related to expression of a psychological conflict or need; person appears calm while experiencing symptoms.
   1. Development of one or more voluntary and/or sensory impairments (e.g., blindness, deafness, loss of sensation), suggesting a neurologic disorder.
   2. Symptoms are not under voluntary control.
   3. *La belle indifference:* an attitude toward the symptoms in which there is a lack of concern.
   4. "Classic conversion symptoms" usually suggest neurologic disease: paralysis, aphonia, blindness, and paresthesias.
B. Illness anxiety disorder, previously referred to as hypochondriasis, is a distorted interpretation of existing physical signs or bodily sensations occurring for at least 6 months that leads the client to an unrealistic belief and preoccupation with the fear or belief of having a serious, debilitating disease.
   1. Preoccupied with bodily functioning: focusing on heartbeat, breathing, digestion, or a minor aliment, such as a small scratch or a cough.
   2. Physical evaluation does not support the diagnosis of any physical problem.
   3. Fear or belief of having medical illness despite medical reassurance.
C. Body dysmorphic disorder is a preoccupation with an imagined flaw in appearance in a normal-appearing person.
   1. Excessive concern and focus on facial defect; less commonly on other parts of the body; preoccupies and dominates client's life.
   2. Social isolation and depression leading to suicidal threats and repeated hospitalizations.
   3. May seek plastic surgery.

### Nursing Interventions

**Goal:** To divert attention from preoccupation with self and symptomatology.

A. Encourage purposeful activity that promotes interest and success.
B. Promote attitude that acknowledges personal integrity and self-worth.
C. Provide for client's physical needs as necessary.
D. Correct any misinformation and give correct information.
E. Encourage client to develop new interests and gain satisfaction from them.
F. Promote a good sense of humor.

**Goal:** To identify primary or secondary gain.

A. Primary gain: symptom has symbolic meaning to client; keeps client unaware of internal conflict and anxiety.
B. Secondary gain: a gain of attention and sympathy along with reinforcement of maladjusted behavior.

**Goal:** To avoid secondary gains as a source of reward and reinforcement for the disorder.

A. Focus on the individual and his or her feelings, *not* on the symptoms.

B. A calm, warm, supportive approach promotes understanding and acceptance.

**Goal:** To avoid reinforcing the client's symptoms.

A. Focus on feelings, *not* on symptoms.
B. Reduce pressure and anxiety-provoking situations around client.
C. Divert attention from symptoms.
D. Provide recreational activity.
E. Avoid pity and sympathetic approach to client's "illnesses" or "symptoms."

**Goal:** To be aware of personal response to the client.

A. Recognize and understand the client's self-perception as unable to cope.
B. Promote a nonjudgmental, understanding attitude.

**Goal:** To provide a supportive approach that does not focus on physical condition.

A. Help client understand how he or she uses illness to avoid dealing with life's problems.
B. Offer empathy without sympathy.

**Goal:** To support alternative therapy.

A. Behavior modification.
B. Insight-oriented psychotherapy.
C. Hypnosis.
D. Acupuncture.

### Dissociative Disorders

**Dissociative disorders involve five primary symptoms: amnesia (memory loss), derealization (objects in external environment take on a quality of unreality and estrangement), depersonalization (alteration in the perception or experience of self), identity confusion (sense of conflict, puzzlement, or uncertainty in relation to one's identity), and identity alteration (organized shift in personality that occurs without the individual's awareness); not caused by substance abuse, physiologic, or psychological disorders.**

### Assessment

A. Dissociative amnesia.
   1. A sudden inability to recall important personal information.
   2. Usually begins suddenly after severe psychosocial stress.
   3. Most often observed in the adolescent and young adult female, rarely in older adults.
B. Dissociative fugue.
   1. Sudden, unexpected travel away from home with the assumption of a new identity.
   2. An inability to recall one's previous identity or past.
   3. No recollection of events that took place during the fugue state.
   4. May be present in clients with posttraumatic stress disorder (PTSD).
C. Dissociative identity disorder (DID).
   1. The existence of two or more distinct personalities, each of which determines the nature of his or her

behavior and attitudes while uppermost in the person's consciousness.
2. Transition from one personality to another is sudden and often stressful.
3. Best-known examples found in literature: *Sybil* and *The Three Faces of Eve*.
D. Depersonalization disorder.
1. An alteration in the perception of the self so that the usual sense of one's own reality is temporarily lost or changed.
2. Sensations of unreality (e.g., feelings that one's extremities have changed size).
3. Onset is rapid; disappearance is gradual.

### Nursing Interventions

**Goal:** To assist in ruling out a physical or organic disease as the cause of the dissociative disorder.

A. Many behaviors resemble postconcussion amnesia and temporal lobe epilepsy.
B. Accurate observation and description of character, duration, and frequency of the symptoms are important.

**Goal:** To minimize anxiety.

A. Redirect client's attention away from self.
B. Increase socialization activities.
C. Include family members in learning new ways to deal with client's behavior.

**Goal:** To provide insight into past traumatic experiences and learn new coping methods.

A. Long-term therapy is aimed at insight into pain of past experiences and conflicts that have been repressed.
B. Encourage awareness that dissociative behaviors are reactivated by current situations that arouse emotional pain.

## PERSONALITY DISORDERS

**Personality disorders create disruptive lifestyles and are characterized by inflexible and maladapted behaviors. Those with personality disorders clash with society and with cultural norms and are often placed in correctional systems, mental hospitals, and child placement facilities.**

### Common Characteristics

A. Problems are expressed through behavior rather than as physical symptoms of stress.
B. Disruptive lifestyle is deeply ingrained and quite difficult to change; usually related to some form of abnormal behavior or the development of a particular pattern or trait.
C. Often comes in conflict with others.
D. Pleasure principle is dominant with inadequate superego control; has difficulty with problem solving.
E. Unable to develop meaningful relationships with others and communicate effectively.
F. Rarely acknowledges that there is a problem.

### Assessment
See Table 12-8 on personality disorder types.

**NURSING PRIORITY:** Personality disorders occur when traits become rigid and manipulative.

### Nursing Interventions

**Goal:** To promote communication and socialization in the paranoid personality.

A. Decrease social isolation.
B. Verbal and nonverbal messages should be clear and consistent.
C. To decrease anxiety, plan several brief contacts rather than one prolonged contact.
D. Promote trust by following through on commitments.
E. Be open and honest to avoid misinterpretation.

**Goal:** To convey to the schizoid or schizotypal client the idea that you do not perceive reality the same way as he or she does but are willing to listen, learn, and offer feedback about his or her experiences.

**Goal:** To promote a positive, therapeutic, interpersonal relationship.

A. Set realistic expectations.
B. Provide a model of mature behavior.
C. Use problem-solving techniques to encourage a client to make changes.
D. Anticipate and deal with depression in a client who gradually acquires enough insight to realize and accept responsibility for his or her behavior.
E. Common sources of frustration for nurses.
1. Client's immature behavior.
2. Poor communication skills.

**Goal:** To minimize manipulation and "acting-out" behaviors and encourage verbal communication.

A. Set firm, consistent limits without being punitive.
B. Be aware of how client may manipulate other staff members (e.g., playing one against the other or splitting).
C. Promote expression of feelings versus acting out.
D. Promote client's acceptance of responsibility for his or her own actions and a social responsibility to others.

**NURSING PRIORITY:** A client with borderline personality disorder has a tendency to cling to one staff member, if allowed, transferring his or her maladaptive dependency to that individual. This dependency can be avoided if the client is able to establish therapeutic relationships with two or more staff members who encourage independent self-care activities.

**Goal:** To assist client to manage anxiety.

A. Anticipate client's needs before he or she demands attention.
B. Teach client to express his or her ideas and feelings assertively.
C. Watch for signs of defensiveness, because a client is unlikely to recognize this as a mechanism of anxiety.

**Goal:** To set realistic limits.

## Table 12-8 PERSONALITY DISORDERS

| Paranoid Personality | Antisocial Personality | Avoidant Personality |
|---|---|---|
| Suspicious and mistrustful of people<br>Secretive<br>Questions loyalty of others<br>Jealous<br>Overly concerned with hidden motives and special meanings<br>Hypersensitive and alert<br>Exaggerates<br>Unable to relax<br>Takes offense quickly<br>Impaired affect<br>Unemotional and cold<br>No sense of humor<br>Absence of soft, tender, sentimental feelings<br>Distorts reality<br>Uses projection | Violates rights of others<br>Lacks responsibility<br>Manipulative<br>Unable to sustain a job; frequent job changes and lengthy periods of unemployment<br>Financial dependency<br>Common behaviors observed—lying, stealing, truancy<br>Excessive drinking and drug use<br>Criminality<br>Vagrancy<br>Lack of remorse | Fear of criticism or disapproval<br>Hypersensitive to potential rejection<br>Views self as socially inept, personally unappealing, and inferior to others<br>Inhibited in interpersonal relationships<br>Reluctant to take personal risks<br>Unwilling to get involved with people unless certain of being liked |
| **Schizoid Personality** | **Borderline Personality** | **Dependent Personality** |
| Unable to form social relationships<br>Cold and aloof; flat affect<br>Indifferent to praise or criticism<br>Has little or no desire for social involvement<br>Appears reserved, withdrawn, and seclusive; emotionally detached from others | Unstable interpersonal relationships and moods; splitting behavior (admires then devalues a person)<br>Impulsiveness and unpredictability that may be self-damaging (e.g., spending, sex, reckless driving, drug use)<br>Identity disturbance<br>Recurrent suicidal behavior, gestures, or threats<br>Self-mutilating behavior<br>Inappropriate, intense anger; lack of anger control; shifts in mood<br>Chronic feelings of emptiness | Submissive; clinging behavior<br>Fear of separation<br>Difficulty making everyday decisions<br>Needs others to assume responsibility<br>Wants others to take care and nurture<br>Feels uncomfortable or helpless when left alone<br>Difficulty initiating projects independently |
| **Schizotypal Personality** | **Histrionic Personality** | **Obsessive-Compulsive Personality** |
| Magical thinking (e.g., telepathy, superstition)<br>Ideas of reference<br>Social isolation<br>Recurrent illusion<br>Oddities of thought, perception, speech, and behavior<br>Inappropriate affect<br>Excessive social anxiety | Excessive emotionality and attention-seeking behavior<br>Uncomfortable when not center of attention<br>Uses physical appearance to draw attention to self<br>Self-dramatization, theatrical, and exaggerated expression of emotion<br>Easily suggestible | Preoccupation with rules, lists, organization, schedules<br>Perfectionistic<br>Excessive devotion to work<br>Overly conscientious and inflexible<br>Reluctant to delegate tasks<br>Hoards money; frugal<br>Rigid and stubborn in thoughts |
| | **Narcissistic Personality** | |
| | Grandiose self-importance<br>Preoccupation with fantasies of success<br>Belief that he or she is "special or unique"<br>Need for excessive amount of admiration<br>Unrealistic sense of entitlement<br>Interpersonal exploitation<br>Lack of empathy<br>Arrogant and haughty<br>Fears rejection by others | |

A. Break the health-attention-avoidance cycle that usually exists in relating to this type of client.

B. Support the client who is gradually making more decisions on his or her own.

C. Offer assistance only when needed.

# SUBSTANCE USE DISORDERS

**Substance use disorders are characterized by behavior changes, regular use of a substance (alcohol or another drug) that affects the CNS, and withdrawal symptoms when the substance is not taken. The term "addiction" is defined as a chronic disease of brain reward, motivation, memory, and related brain circuitry.**

**Polydrug dependence involves the regular use of three or more psychoactive substances over a period of at least 6 months.**

> **TEST ALERT:** Identify signs and symptoms of substance abuse/chemical dependency.

A. Substance abuse.
  1. A pattern of pathologic use.
     a. Intoxication during the day.
     b. Inability to cut down or stop drinking.
     c. Daily need of the substance to function.
     d. Blackouts and medical complications from use.
  2. Impairment of social or occupational functioning.
     a. Failure to meet important obligations to friends, family, and employer.
     b. Inappropriate display of erratic and impulsive behavior.
     c. Inappropriate expression of aggressive feelings.
  3. Minimum duration of at least 1 month of substance use.
  4. Tolerance.
     a. Increased amounts of the substance are required to achieve the desired effect.
     b. Markedly diminished effect with regular use of the same dose.
  5. Withdrawal: a specific syndrome of symptoms that develops when the person abruptly stops ingesting the substance.
B. Psychological dependence.
  1. Habituation: the need to take the substance.
  2. Physiologic dependence is not necessary.
  3. No physiologic symptoms on withdrawal.
C. Common health problems.
  1. Acute problems.
     a. Poor nutritional status, loss of appetite, nausea, vomiting, and diarrhea.
     b. CNS dysfunction and irritability, seizures, tremors, motor restlessness, sensitivity to light, auditory or visual disturbances, insomnia.
     c. Susceptibility to recurrent respiratory tract infections.
  2. Chronic problems.
     a. Liver dysfunction, cirrhosis, pancreatitis, hypertension.

b. Chronic brain damage and mental deterioration, poor hygiene, dermatologic changes.
     c. Human immunodeficiency virus (HIV) seropositivity.
D. Dysfunctional behavior patterns.
  1. Manipulation.
     Examples: Legal difficulties, crime, physical assault, taking advantage of generosity.
  2. Impulsiveness.
     Examples: Inconsistent work patterns, overdose, recklessness.
  3. Dysfunctional anger.
  4. Grandiosity.
     Example: Belief that nobody has done worse things or has lost as much or taken drugs or drunk as much.
  5. Denial.
  6. Codependency: extreme emotional, social, or physical focus on another person, place, or thing.
E. Treatment modalities.
  1. Detoxification: controlled withdrawal from alcohol or drugs by means of a medical protocol.
  2. Drug treatment and rehabilitation: comprehensive program based on client outcomes; may include detoxification, family education, group counseling, and 12-step programs.
  3. 12-step self-help groups: recovery built on abstinence as a daily process; requires peer support and acknowledgment that client has addiction.
  4. Drug-free residential communities: therapeutic community based on a hierarchical community structure and governance, peer support, and a disciplined lifestyle.
  5. Pharmacologic therapy: use of methadone for opiate abuse to eliminate craving for drug.
  6. Psychotherapy: may be individual, group, family, or a combination of all three; facilitates behavioral and lifestyle changes by dealing with personality issues and psychological conflicts.

## Alcohol Dependence (Alcoholism)
**A chronic pattern of pathologic alcohol use is characterized by impairment in social or occupational functioning along with tolerance or withdrawal symptoms.**

### General Concepts
A. Incidence.
  1. Alcohol abuse is more common in men than women.
  2. Only 25% of individuals with alcohol dependence seek treatment.
B. Effects of use.
  1. CNS depressant drug.
  2. Requires no digestion; 20% is absorbed unchanged from the stomach; 80% is absorbed from the small intestine.
  3. Absorbed slowly in a full stomach.
  4. Measured in the bloodstream by the blood alcohol level (BAL).
  5. Can be measured within 15 to 20 minutes after ingestion; reaches a peak in 60 to 90 minutes; is completely metabolized by 12 to 24 hours after the last drink.

6. Decreases inhibitions and enhances mood; slows motor reactions and subsequently prolongs reaction time.
7. In low doses, tends to increase sexual arousal; in high doses, tends to decrease it.
8. Affects critical thinking, judgment, and memory.
9. A BAL of 8% to 10% (0.08 mg to 0.10 mg) or more is considered the legal level of intoxication in most states.

### Assessment

A. Risk factors.
   1. History of alcoholism in family.
   2. History of total abstinence.
   3. Broken or disrupted home.
   4. Last or near-last child in a large family.
   5. Heavy smoking.
   6. Cultural groups: Irish, Eskimo, Scandinavian, Native American.
B. Diagnostics.
   1. BAL.
      a. BAL is determined by how much alcohol is consumed, how fast it is consumed, and body weight.
      b. The larger the person, the more alcohol he or she can tolerate.
   2. Breathalyzer.
      a. About 5% (0.05 mg) to 10% (0.10 mg) of the alcohol is excreted through breathing.
      b. Used for monitoring the use of alcohol and to identify persons who are driving while intoxicated (DWI) or driving under the influence (DUI).
C. General personality characteristics of alcoholics.
   1. Dependent behavior along with resentment of authority.
   2. Demanding and domineering with a low tolerance for frustration.
   3. Dissatisfied with life; tendency toward self-destructive acts, including suicide.
   4. Low self-esteem and poor self-concept.
D. Signs and symptoms of possible alcohol abuse.
   1. Sprains, bruises, and injuries of questionable origin.
   2. Diarrhea and early morning vomiting.
   3. Chronic cough, palpitations, and infections.
   4. Frequent Monday morning illnesses; blackouts (inability to recall events or actions while intoxicated).
E. Alcohol withdrawal syndrome. The withdrawal syndrome develops in heavy drinkers who have increased, decreased, or interrupted the intake of alcohol.
   1. Alcohol withdrawal.
      a. Anorexia, irritability, nausea, and tremulousness.
      b. Insomnia, nightmares, irritability, hyperalertness.
      c. Tachycardia, increased blood pressure, and diaphoresis.
      d. Onset within several hours after cessation of drinking (usually 48–72 hours); clears up within 5 to 7 days.
   2. Alcohol withdrawal delirium (Figure 12-5).
      a. Autonomic hyperactivity: tachycardia, sweating, increased blood pressure.

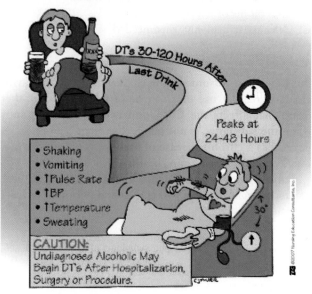

### Alcohol Withdrawal Delirium 'Delirium Tremens (DTs)'

**FIGURE 12-5 Alcohol Withdrawal Delirium.** (From Zerwekh, J., & Garneau, A., J., Miller, C. J. [2017]. *Digital collection of the memory notebooks of nursing* [4th ed.]. Chandler, AZ: Nursing Education Consultants, Inc.)

   b. Vivid hallucinations, delusions, confusion.
   c. Coarse, irregular tremor is almost always seen; fever may occur.
   d. Onset within 24 to 72 hours after the last ingestion of alcohol; usually lasts 2 to 3 days.
   e. Convulsions/seizures may occur.
F. Wernicke encephalopathy.
   1. An acute, reversible neurologic disorder.
   2. Triad of symptoms: global confusion, ataxia, and eye movement abnormality (nystagmus).
   3. Occurs primarily in clients with chronic alcoholism; may develop in illnesses that interfere with thiamine (vitamin $B_1$) absorption (e.g., gastric cancer, malabsorption syndrome, regional enteritis).
   4. Treatment: high doses of thiamine; 100 mg, given intramuscularly, usually reverses nystagmus within 2 to 3 hours of treatment.
G. Korsakoff syndrome (alcohol amnesiac disorder).
   1. A chronic, *irreversible* disorder, often following Wernicke encephalopathy.
   2. Triad of symptoms: memory loss, learning deficit, confabulation (filling in of memory gaps with plausible stories).
H. Other disorders associated with chronic alcoholism: pneumonitis, esophageal varices, cirrhosis, pancreatitis, diabetes (these are covered in the appropriate chapter discussing the system).

### Nursing Interventions

**Goal:** To assess for alcoholism in a client through careful questioning.

A. Frequently used acronym—*CAGE-AID*—suggests asking the following questions. An answer of "yes" to any question can indicate a problem.
   1. Have you ever felt the need to:
      **C**ut down on your drinking?
   2. Have you ever felt:
      **A**nnoyed by criticism of your drinking?
   3. Have you had:
      **G**uilty feelings about drinking?
   4. Do you ever take a morning:
      **E**ye-opener?
   5. **AID**—**A**dapt questions to **I**nclude **D**rugs.
B. Identify the alcoholic client in the preoperative period.
   1. Often, alcoholics are undiagnosed at the time of surgery and may go into withdrawal or alcohol withdrawal delirium after the NPO (nothing by mouth) period.
   2. Preoperative medication doses need to be adjusted; usually, if tolerant of alcohol, clients are also tolerant of other medications, including anesthetics.
   3. Client usually takes longer to be fully responsive during postoperative period; client is susceptible to severe respiratory complications; client has more difficulty with healing because of poor nutritional state.

**Goal:** To assist in the medical treatment of alcohol withdrawal.

A. Benzodiazepines for agitation (see Appendix 12-2).
B. Thiamine (vitamin $B_1$) to prevent Wernicke encephalopathy.
C. Magnesium sulfate is used to increase effectiveness of vitamin $B_1$ because it helps reduce postwithdrawal seizures.
D. Anticonvulsant (phenytoin or carbamazepine), if necessary, for seizure control.
E. Encourage use of multivitamins, especially folic acid, $B_{12}$, and vitamin C.
F. Antipsychotic agents (chlorpromazine or haloperidol) for alcohol withdrawal delirium
G. Beta-adrenergic blockers (atenolol, propranolol) to improve vital signs; encourage intake of fluids but do not force.

**Goal:** To provide for the basic needs of rest, comfort, safety, and nutrition.

A. Safety measures, such as bed rest and use of bed rails, may be necessary.
B. If client is experiencing delirium tremens, stay with him or her.
C. Have room adequately lit to help reduce confusion and avoid shadows and unclear objects.
D. Monitor vital signs every 1 to 4 hours.
E. Encourage a high-carbohydrate, soft diet.

**Goal:** To recognize complications of alcohol use.

A. Obstetric implications.
   1. Two ounces (60 mL) of alcohol per day may produce a BAL in the pregnant woman, leading to fetal alcohol syndrome.
   2. Chronic alcoholism can lead to maternal malnutrition, especially folic acid deficiency, bone marrow suppression, infections, and liver disease.
   3. Alcohol withdrawal syndrome may occur in the intrapartal period as early as 12 to 48 hours after the last drink.
   4. Alcohol withdrawal delirium may occur in the postpartum period.
B. Neonatal implications (fetal alcohol syndrome).
   1. Teratogenic effects may be seen along with growth and developmental delay.
   2. Increased risk for anomalies of the heart, head, face, and extremities.
   3. Withdrawal symptoms can occur shortly after birth and are characterized by tremors, agitation, sweating, and seizure activity.
   4. Maintain seizure precautions.
C. Medical complications of alcohol abuse.
   1. Trauma related to falls, burns, hematomas.
   2. Liver disease: cirrhosis, esophageal varices, hepatic coma.
   3. Gastrointestinal disease: gastritis, bleeding ulcers, pancreatitis.
   4. Nutritional disease: malnutrition, anemia caused by iron or vitamin $B_{12}$ deficiency, thiamine deficiency.
   5. Infections, especially pneumonia.
   6. Neurologic disease: polyneuropathy and dementia.

**Goal:** To assist in the long-term rehabilitation of the client.

A. Avoid sympathy, because clients tend to rationalize and use dependent, manipulative behavior to seek privileges.
B. Maintain a nonjudgmental attitude.
C. Set behavior limits in a firm but kind manner.
D. Place responsibility for sobriety on client; do not give advice or punish or reprimand client for failures.
E. Provide opportunities to decrease social isolation by encouraging participation in social groups and activities.
F. Encourage client to develop coping mechanisms other than alcohol to deal with stress.
G. Refer clients and family to available community resources.
   1. Alcoholics Anonymous (AA): a self-help group focusing on education, guidance, and the sharing of problems and experiences unique to the individual.
   2. Al-Anon: a self-help support group for the spouses and significant others of the alcoholic.
   3. Alateen: the support group for teenagers with an alcoholic parent.
   4. Adult Children of Alcoholics (ACOA): support group for adult children of alcoholics and dysfunctional individuals.
   5. Families Anonymous: support group for the families whose lives have been affected by the addicted client's behavior.
   6. Codependents Anonymous: support group for codependents who may be alcoholics or drug addicts and for persons who are close to an addict.

H. Promote adherence to prescribed therapeutic regimens.
  1. Disulfiram: a drug that produces intense side effects after ingestion of alcohol (severe nausea, vomiting, flushed face, hypotension, and blurred vision).
  2. Naltrexone: opioid antagonist that decreases the craving for alcohol.
  3. Acamprosate: a drug that helps clients abstain from alcohol.

## Polydrug Dependence

**Polydrug dependence is the regular use of three or more psychoactive substances over a period of at least 6 months.**

### General Concepts

A. Effects of use.
  1. Relieves anxiety.
  2. Overdose can occur.
  3. Factors affecting the degree of dependence.
    a. Physiologic and psychological makeup of the abuser.
    b. Drug's pharmacologic action.
    c. External social and cultural factors.
B. General personality characteristics.
  1. Inability to cope with stress, frustration, or anxiety.
  2. Rebellious, immature, desire for immediate gratification.
  3. Passivity and low self-esteem.
  4. Difficulty forming warm, personal relationships.
  5. Uses defense mechanisms: denial, rationalization, intellectualization.

### Assessment

A. General assessment.
  1. Determine the pattern of drug use.
    a. Which drugs are being used by the client?
    b. When was the last use?
    c. How much does client use and how often?
    d. How long has client been using drugs?
    e. What combination of drugs is being used?
  2. Determine whether there are any physical changes present (e.g., needle tracks, swollen nasal mucous membranes, reddened conjunctivae).
B. Narcotic dependence.
  Examples of narcotics: opium, heroin, morphine, codeine, fentanyl, methadone, oxycodone.
  1. Street names: horse, junk, smack (heroin); black poppy (opium); M (morphine); dollies (methadone); terp (terpin hydrate or cough syrup with codeine).
  2. Administration.
    a. Heroin: sniffed, smoked, injected intravenously (mainlining), injected subcutaneously (skin popping).
    b. Other narcotics are usually taken orally or by injection.
  3. Symptoms of use.
    a. Drowsiness and decreased blood pressure, pulse, and respiratory rate.
    b. Pinpoint pupils, needle tracks, scarring.
    c. Overdose effects: slow, shallow breathing, clammy skin, convulsions, coma, pulmonary edema, possible death.

  4. Withdrawal symptoms.
    a. Onset of symptoms approximately 8 to 12 hours after the last dose.
    b. Lacrimation, sweating, sneezing, yawning.
    c. Gooseflesh (piloerection), tremor, irritability, anorexia.
    d. Dilated pupils, abdominal cramps, vomiting, involuntary muscle spasms.
    e. Symptoms generally subside within 7 to 10 days.
C. Sedative-hypnotic dependence.
  Examples of sedative-hypnotics: barbiturates (pentobarbital, secobarbital) and the benzodiazepines (chlordiazepoxide, diazepam).
  1. Street names: green and whites, roaches (*chlordiazepoxide);* red birds, red devils (secobarbital); blue birds (amobarbital capsules); yellow birds (*pentobarbital);* downers, rainbow, 7145 (barbiturates; tranquilizers).
  2. Administration: oral or injected.
  3. Symptoms of use.
    a. Alterations in mood, thought, behavior.
    b. Impairment in coordination, judgment.
    c. Signs of intoxication: slurred speech, unsteady gait, decreased attention span or memory.
    d. Barbiturate use: often violent, disruptive, irresponsible behavior.
  4. Withdrawal symptoms.
    a. Insomnia, anxiety, profuse sweating, weakness.
    b. Severe reactions of delirium, grand mal seizures, cardiovascular collapse.

> **! NURSING PRIORITY:** Abrupt withdrawal of CNS depressants may lead to death. Client must be tapered off drug slowly.

D. Cocaine abuse.
  1. Street names: coke, toot, nose candy, snow, C, powder, lady.
  2. Administration: intranasal ("snorting") or by intravenous or subcutaneous injection; also smoked in a pipe (free-basing).
  3. Symptoms of use.
    a. Euphoria, grandiosity, and a sense of well-being.
    b. Amphetamine-like or stimulant-like effects such as increased blood pressure, racing of the heart, paranoia, anxiety.
    c. Used regularly, cocaine may disrupt eating and sleeping habits, leading to irritability and decreased concentration.

> **! NURSING PRIORITY:** Crack (rock) has been labeled the most addictive drug. It is a potent form of cocaine hydrochloride mixed with baking soda and water, heated (cooked), allowed to harden, and then broken or "cracked" into little pieces and smoked in cigarettes or glass water pipes. Cardiac dysrhythmias, respiratory paralysis, and seizures are some of the dangers associated with crack use.

4. Withdrawal symptoms.
   a. Severe craving.
   b. Coming down from a "high" often leads to a severe "letdown," depressed feeling.
   c. Psychological dependence often leads to cocaine becoming a total obsession.
E. Methamphetamine dependence.
   Example: dextroamphetamine.
   1. Street names: meth, crystal, crank, bennies, wake-ups, uppers, speed (amphetamines).
   2. Administration: inhalation, oral or injected.
   3. Symptoms of use.
      a. Elation, agitation, hyperactivity, irritability, visual and auditory hallucinations, paranoia, and profound dental caries ("meth mouth").
      b. Increased pulse, respiration, and blood pressure.
      c. Fine tremor, muscle twitching, and mydriasis (pupillary dilation).
      d. Large doses: convulsions, cardiovascular collapse, respiratory depression, coma, death.
   4. Withdrawal symptoms.
      a. Appear within 2 to 4 days after the last dose.
      b. Depression, overwhelming fatigue, suicide attempts.
F. PCP (phencyclidine hydrochloride) abuse.
   1. Street names: peace pill, hog, super pill, elephant tranquilizer, angel dust, rocket fuel, primo.
   2. Administration: snorted, smoked, or orally ingested; usually smoked along with marijuana.
   3. Symptoms of use.
      a. Euphoria, feeling of numbness, mood changes.
      b. Diaphoresis, eye movement changes (nystagmus), hypertension, catatonic-like stupor with eyes open.
      c. Seizures, shivering, decerebrate posturing, possible death.
      d. Synesthesia: experiencing one sense when another is actually being stimulated (e.g., seeing colors when a loud sound occurs).
   4. Overdose symptoms ("bad trip"): psychosis, possible death.
      a. User may become violent, destructive, and confused.
      b. Users have been known to go berserk; users may harm themselves and others.
      c. Intoxicating symptoms lighten and worsen over a period of 48 hours.
G. Hallucinogen abuse.
   Example: LSD (lysergic acid diethylamide), psilocybin ("magic mushroom"), mescaline (peyote), DMT, MDA.
   1. Street name: acid.
   2. Administration: usually oral, but LSD and mescaline can be injected.
   3. Symptoms of use.
      a. Pupillary dilation, tachycardia, sweating.
      b. Visual hallucinations, depersonalization, impaired judgment and mood.
      c. Flashbacks and "bad trips."
      d. Usually no signs of withdrawal symptoms after use has been discontinued.

H. Marijuana dependence.
   Example: marijuana, hashish, tetrahydrocannabinol (THC).
   1. Street names: joints, reefers, pot, grass, shit, Mary Jane (marijuana), hash (hashish).
   2. Administration: oral, sniffed, and smoked.
   3. Symptoms of use.
      a. Euphoria, relaxation, tachycardia, and conjunctival congestion.
      b. Paranoid ideation; impaired judgment.
      c. Rarely, panic reactions and psychoses.
      d. Heavy use leads to apathy and general deterioration in all aspects of living.
      e. Overdose effects: flashbacks, bronchitis, personality changes.
   4. Withdrawal symptoms.
      a. Anxiety, sleeplessness, sweating.
      b. Lack of appetite, nausea, general malaise.
I. Designer drugs.
   1. Street names: ecstasy, Adam (MDMA [methylenedioxymethamphetamine]), China white (MTPT).
   2. Called *analog drugs* because they retain the properties of controlled drugs (e.g., MTPT is an analog of meperidine).
   3. Symptoms of use and side effects are similar to those associated with the controlled substance from which they are derived.
J. Bath salts (synthetic marijuana).
   1. Symptoms are similar to those of stimulants and include euphoria, an elevated mood, and an intense "rush."
   2. Hypertension, chest pain, hallucinations, bizarre behavior may also be present.
   3. Although the bath salts are illegal in the United States, sellers of the drug have gotten around this by modifying the chemical components found in the drug.

### Nursing Interventions

**Goal:** To assess the drug use pattern.
**Goal:** To assist in medical treatment during detoxification or withdrawal.

A. Narcotics.
   1. Narcotic antagonists, such as naloxone, nalorphine, or levallorphan, are administered intravenously for narcotic overdose.
   2. Withdrawal is managed with methadone tapering and naltrexone chloride. Substitution therapy with buprenorphine may be instituted to decrease withdrawal symptoms for longer effects.
B. Opiates.
   1. Substitution therapy with methadone hydrochloride may be instituted to decrease withdrawal symptoms.
   2. Some physicians prescribe buprenorphine as needed for objective symptoms, gradually decreasing the dosage until the drug is discontinued.
C. Stimulants.
   1. Treatment of overdose is geared toward stabilization of vital signs.

2. IV antihypertensives may be used, along with IV diazepam, to control seizures.
3. Chlordiazepoxide may be administered orally for the first few days while client is "crashing."
4. Withdrawal symptoms are managed with tricyclic antidepressants such as desipramine and dopamine agonists such as bromocriptine.
D. Hallucinogens and marijuana.
   1. Medications are normally not prescribed for withdrawal from these substances.
   2. In the event of overdose, diazepam or chlordiazepoxide may be given as needed to decrease agitation.
E. Be aware that gradual withdrawal, detoxification, or dechemicalization is necessary for the client addicted to barbiturates, narcotics, and tranquilizers.
F. Abrupt withdrawal, or quitting "cold turkey," is often dangerous and can be fatal.
G. Maintain a patent airway; have oxygen available.
H. Provide a safe, quiet environment (i.e., remove harmful objects, place bed in low position).

**Goal:** To decrease problem behaviors of manipulation and "acting out."

A. Set firm, consistent limits.
B. Confront client with manipulative behaviors.

**Goal:** To promote alternative coping methods.

A. Encourage responsibility for own behavior.
B. Encourage the use of hobbies, exercise, or alternative therapies as a means to deal with frustration and anxiety.

**Goal:** To recognize complications of substance abuse.

A. Obstetric implications.
   1. Narcotic addiction.
      a. Increased risk for pregnancy-induced hypertension, malpresentation, and third-trimester bleeding.
      b. Provide methadone maintenance therapy for the duration of the pregnancy—withdrawal is not advisable because of the risk to the fetus.
   2. Use of other drugs causes increased risk to mother and fetus.
B. Neonatal complications.
   1. Withdrawal symptoms depend on type of drug mother used.
   2. Restlessness, jitteriness, hyperactive reflexes, high-pitched shrill cry, feeds poorly.
   3. Maintain seizure precautions.
   4. Administer antiepileptics to treat withdrawal and prevent seizures.
   5. Swaddle infant in snug-fitting blanket.
   6. Increased risk for congenital malformations and prematurity.
C. Medical implications.
   1. Increased risk for hepatitis, malnutrition, and infections in general.

**Goal:** To assist in the long-term process of drug rehabilitation.

A. Refer client to drug rehabilitation programs.
B. Promote self-help residential programs that foster self-support systems and use ex-addicts as rehabilitation counselors.
C. Methadone maintenance programs.
   1. Must be 18 years old and addicted for more than 2 years, with a history of detoxification treatments.
   2. Methadone is a synthetic narcotic that appeases desire for opiates.
      a. Controlled substance; given only under urinary surveillance.
      b. Administered orally; prevents opiate withdrawal symptoms.
D. 12-step self-help groups.
   1. Narcotics Anonymous: support group for clients who are addicted to narcotics and other drugs.
   2. Nar-Anon: support group for relatives and friends of narcotic addicts.
   3. Families Anonymous.

## MOOD DISORDERS

**The major mood disorders are characterized by disturbances of mood.**

### General Concepts

A. Incidence.
   1. More prevalent among family members when there is a positive family history.
   2. Major depression is seen more often in women.
   3. More common in higher socioeconomic groups.
B. Causes.
   1. A variety of theories may explain affective disorders.
   2. Depressive: loss of significant others or objects; changes in levels of serotonin and norepinephrine (decrease) and steroids (increase); loss of self-esteem leading to hopelessness, helplessness, and pessimism toward self and others.
   3. Manic: unresolved diffuse anger and hostility; denial of depression; may develop from early childhood as a result of high parental expectations.
C. Personality characteristics associated with affective disorders.
   1. Depressive: lacking in confidence, introverted, unassertive, dependent, pessimistic, feelings of inadequacy.
   2. Manic: extroverted, confident, manipulative, and obsessive.

### Psychodynamics

A. Manic.
   1. During infancy, needs and narcissistic goals are not met, which leads to impairment in the development of self-esteem.
   2. Low self-esteem and helplessness lead to need for excessive attention, affection, warmth, and appreciation.
   3. Usually a massive denial of depression.
   4. The air of happiness and self-confidence is a defense against dependency feelings.

B. Depressive.
1. Loss, either real or perceived, of a loved person or object.
2. Turning aggressive feelings inward and displacing them onto the self; accompanied by feelings of guilt.
3. Ambivalent feelings toward the valued/lost object.
4. Repressive guilt, which leads to feelings of helplessness and hopelessness.

*Assessment*

A. Bipolar disorder (Figure 12-6). There are currently three types of bipolar disorder, ranging from mild to severe forms. They include bipolar I disorder (most severe), bipolar II disorder (low-level severity), and cyclothymic disorder (low-level severity; more common in children).
- Bipolar I disorder exhibits features of mania for at least 1 week with psychotic features (hallucinations, delusions).
- Bipolar II disorder exhibits features of low-level mania (hypomania) followed by profound depression.
- Cyclothymic disorder resembles similar manifestations of bipolar II disorder but is typically seen more frequently in children.
1. Mania.
a. Onset before the age of 30 years.
b. Mood: elevated, expansive, or irritable.
c. Speech: loud, rapid, difficult to interpret, punning, rhyming, and clanging (using words that sound like the meaning rather than the actual word).
d. Cognitive skills: flight of ideas, grandiose delusions, easily distracted.
e. Psychomotor activity: hyperactive, decreased need for sleep, exhibitionistic, vulgar, profane, may make inappropriate sexual advances and be obscene.
f. Course of manic episode: begins suddenly, rapidly escalates over a few days, and ends more abruptly than major depressive episodes.

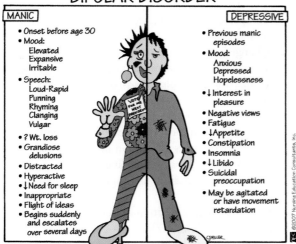

## BIPOLAR DISORDER

**MANIC**
- Onset before age 30
- Mood:
  Elevated
  Expansive
  Irritable
- Speech:
  Loud-Rapid
  Punning
  Rhyming
  Clanging
  Vulgar
- ? Wt. loss
- Grandiose delusions
- Distracted
- Hyperactive
- ↓Need for sleep
- Inappropriate
- Flight of ideas
- Begins suddenly and escalates over several days

**DEPRESSIVE**
- Previous manic episodes
- Mood:
  Anxious
  Depressed
  Hopelessness
- ↓Interest in pleasure
- Negative views
- Fatigue
- ↓Appetite
- Constipation
- Insomnia
- ↓Libido
- Suicidal preoccupation
- May be agitated or have movement retardation

**FIGURE 12-6 Bipolar Disorder.** (From Zerwekh, J., Garneau, A., & Miller, C. J. [2017]. *Digital collection of the memory notebooks of nursing* [4th ed.]. Chandler, AZ: Nursing Education Consultants, Inc.")

2. Hypomania (depressive).
a. Has had one or more manic episodes.
b. Mood: dysphoric, depressive, despairing, loss of interest or pleasure in most usual activities.
c. Cognitive process: negative view of self, world, and of the future; poverty of ideas; crying; and suicidal preoccupation.
d. Psychomotor: may have either agitation or retardation in movements, feelings of fatigue, lack of appetite, constipation, sleeping disturbances (insomnia or early morning wakefulness), and a decrease in libido.

B. Major depressive disorder.
1. May occur at any age.
2. Differentiated as either a single episode or a recurring type.
3. Severity and type of depression vary with the ability to test reality.
a. Psychotic: feels worse in the morning and better as the day goes on.
b. Neurotic: wakes up feeling optimistic; mood worsens as the day passes. Diagnosis is made when five or more of the following symptoms identified are present nearly every day over a 2-week period:
(1) Depressed mood most of day.
(2) Anhedonia.
(3) Insomnia or hypersomnia.
(4) Weight loss or weight gain.
(5) Increased or decreased psychomotor activity.
(6) Suicidal thoughts or plan to harm self.
(7) Anergia (loss of energy).
(8) Feelings of worthlessness or guilt.
(9) Poor concentration; unable to make decisions.
c. Delusional thoughts or hallucinations present with psychotic major depression.

C. Other disorders (not considered part of the major affective type classification).
1. Persistent depressive disorder.
a. Depressed mood with loss of interest in most usual daily activities for at least 2 years.
b. No delusions or hallucinations.
c. Common disorder in adolescence and early adulthood; chronic course.
2. Premenstrual dysphoric disorder.
a. Symptoms similar to major depression occur in female 1 week before onset of menses.
b. Once client has menstrual period, symptoms subside.

*Nursing Interventions (Manic Episode)*

**Goal:** To provide for basic human needs of safety and rest/activity.

A. Reduce outside stimuli and provide a nonstimulating environment.
B. Monitor food intake: provide a high-calorie, high-vitamin, high-fiber diet with finger foods to be eaten as the client moves about.

❗ **NURSING PRIORITY:** Physiologic needs are the first priority in providing client care.

C. Encourage noncompetitive solitary activities such as walking, swimming, or painting.
D. Assist with personal hygiene.

❗ **NURSING PRIORITY:** During the manic phase, the client's physical safety is at risk because the hyperactivity may lead to exhaustion and ultimately cardiac failure.

**Goal:** To establish a therapeutic nurse–client relationship.

A. Use firm, consistent, honest approach.
B. Assess client's abilities and involve client in his or her own care planning.
C. Promote problem-solving abilities; recognize that a false sense of independence is often demonstrated by loud, boisterous behavior.
D. Do not focus on or discuss grandiose ideas.

**Goal:** To set limits on behavior.

A. Instructions should be clear and concise.
B. Initiate regularly scheduled contacts to demonstrate acceptance.
C. Maintain some distance between self and client to allow freedom of movement and to prevent feelings of being overpowered.
D. Maintain neutrality and objectivity: realize that client can be easily provoked by harmless remarks and may demonstrate a furious reaction but calm down quickly.
E. Use measures to prevent overt aggression (e.g., distraction, recognition of behaviors of increased excitement).

**Goal:** To promote adaptive coping with constructive use of energy.

A. Do not hurry client; this leads to anxiety and hostile behavior.

❗ **NURSING PRIORITY:** In a hyperactive state, the client is extremely distractible, and responses to even the slightest stimuli are exaggerated.

B. Provide activities and constructive tasks that channel the agitated behavior (e.g., cleaning game room, going for a walk, gardening, playing catch).

**Goal:** To assist in the medical treatment.

A. Administer lithium carbonate.
B. Teach client about lithium medication instructions (see Appendix 12-2).
C. Divalproex or valproic acid is used to treat lithium nonresponders.
D. Carbamazepine can be used with lithium or an antipsychotic for treatment-resistant bipolar disorder.
E. Antipsychotic drugs such as olanzapine and quetiapine may be better tolerated than lithium.

F. Risperidone is a first-line treatment for severe mania.
G. Lamotrigine is a first-line treatment for acute manic episodes and maintenance therapy.
   1. Clients taking lamotrigine need to be instructed to seek immediate medical attention if a skin rash appears, because this drug can cause a severe potentially life-threatening rash.

*Nursing Interventions (Depressive Episode)*

❗ **NURSING PRIORITY:** Depression and suicidal behaviors may be viewed as anger turned inward on the self. If this anger can be verbalized in a nonthreatening environment, the client may be able to resolve these feelings, regardless of the discomfort involved.

**Goal:** To assess for suicide potential.

A. Recognition of suicidal intent.
   1. Self-destructive behaviors are viewed as attempts to escape unbearable life situations.
   2. Anxiety and hostility are overwhelmingly present.
   3. There is the presence of ambivalence; living versus self-destructive impulses.
   4. Depression, low self-esteem, and feelings of hopelessness are critical to evaluate because suicide attempts are often made when the client feels like giving up.
   5. Assess for *indirect* self-destructive behavior: any activity that is detrimental to the physical well-being of the client in which the potential outcome is death.
      a. Eating disorders: anorexia nervosa, bulimia, obesity, and overeating.
      b. Noncompliance with medical treatment (e.g., diabetic who does not take insulin).
      c. Cigarette smoking, gambling, criminal and/or socially deviant activities.
      d. Alcohol and drug abuse.
      e. Participation in high-risk sports (e.g., automobile racing; skydiving).
B. Suicide danger signs (Box 12-6).
   1. The presence of a suicide plan: specifics relating to method, its lethality, and likelihood for rescue.
   2. Change in established patterns in routines (e.g., giving away personal items, making a will, saying goodbye).
   3. Anticipation of failure: loss of a job, preoccupation with physical disease, actual or anticipated loss of a significant other.
   4. Change in behavior, presence of panic, agitation, or calmness; often, as depression lifts, client has enough energy to act on suicidal feelings.
   5. Hopelessness: feelings of impending doom, futility, and entrapment.
   6. Withdrawal and rejection of help.
C. Clients at risk (Box 12-7).
   1. Adolescents and older adults; males more likely to complete the suicide act.
   2. Clients experiencing recent stress of a maturational or situational crisis.

## Box 12-6 SAD PERSONS SCALE

One of the most popular and easy-to-use tools available to help assess suicide risk. The more areas checked, the higher the risk.

___ **S**ex (males are more likely to successfully commit suicide)
___ **A**ge (younger than 19 or older than 45 years of age)
___ **D**epression
___ **P**revious suicide attempt
___ **E**thanol (alcohol) abuse
___ **R**ational thinking (impaired)
___ **S**ocial support lacking (including recent loss of loved one)
___ **O**rganized plan
___ **N**o spouse
___ **S**ickness (especially chronic)

Total score ranges from 0 (lowest risk) to 10 (highest risk). Scores of 3–4 require psychiatric consultation (psychiatric history and comprehensive assessment). This scale should be used as a guideline only; use your judgment and don't neglect unspecified factors.

## Box 12-7 ADOLESCENT SUICIDE

### Characteristics
- History of suicide ideation
- Previous suicide attempt
- Long-term use of drugs
- Acting-out behaviors: delinquency, stealing, vandalism, academic failure, promiscuity, loss of boyfriend/girlfriend

### Family Characteristics
- Unproductive, conflictual communication
- Impaired problem-solving ability
- Inconsistent positive reinforcements, plus a greater number of negative reinforcements
- Unstable home environment

3. Clients with chronic or painful illnesses.
4. Clients with previous suicide attempts or suicidal behavior.
5. Withdrawn, depressed, or hallucinating clients.
6. Clients with sexual identity conflicts and those who abuse alcohol and drugs.

**Goal:** To provide for basic human needs of safety and protection from self-destruction.

A. Remove all potentially harmful objects (e.g., belts, sharp objects, matches, lighters, strings, etc.).
B. Maintain a one-to-one relationship and close observation.

> **! NURSING PRIORITY:** Be aware of special times when client might be suicidal (e.g., when suddenly cheerful, when there are fewer staff members available, on arising in the morning, or during a busy routine day). When drug therapy is started, the client may feel better emotionally and act on suicidal ideations.

C. Have client make a written contract agreeing not to harm himself or herself; provide an alternative plan of coping.
D. Administer lamotrigine, if ordered.

**Goal:** To provide for physical needs of nutrition and rest/activity.

A. Assess for changes in weight (weight loss may indicate deepening depression).
B. Encourage increased bulk and roughage in diet along with sufficient fluids if client is constipated.

> **! NURSING PRIORITY:** Depressed clients are particularly vulnerable to constipation as a result of psychomotor retardation.

C. Provide for adequate amount of exercise and rest; encourage client not to sleep during the day.
D. Assist with hygiene and personal appearance.

**Goal:** To promote expression of feelings.

A. Encourage expression of angry, guilty, or depressed feelings.
B. Convey a kind, pleasant, interested approach to promote a sense of dignity and self-worth in the client.
C. Support the client's expression of feelings by allowing the client to respond in his or her own time.
D. Seek out the client; initiate frequent contact.
E. Assist with decision making when depression is severe.

**Goal:** To provide for meaningful socialization activities.

> **! NURSING PRIORITY:** The depressed client often has impaired decision-making/problem-solving ability and needs structure in his or her life. The nurse must devise a plan of therapeutic activities and provide the client with a written time schedule. **REMEMBER:** The client who is moderately depressed feels best early in the day, whereas later in the day is a better time for the severely depressed individual to participate in activities.

A. Encourage participation in activities (e.g., plan a work assignment with client to do simple tasks: straightening game room, picking up magazines).
B. Assess hobbies, sports, or activities client enjoys; encourage client's participation.
C. Encourage client to participate in small-group conversation or activity and to practice social skills through role-playing and psychodrama.
D. Encourage activities that promote a sense of accomplishment and enhance self-esteem.

**Goal:** To assist in medical treatment.

A. Administer antidepressant medication (see Appendix 12-2).
B. Assist in electroconvulsive therapy (ECT) (Box 12-8).

## Box 12-8    ELECTROCONVULSIVE THERAPY (ECT)

ECT is an electric shock delivered to the brain through electrodes that are applied to both temples. The shock artificially induces a grand mal seizure.

### Indications
1. Severely depressed clients who do not respond to medication
2. High risk for suicide/starvation
3. Major depression with delusions or hallucinations
4. Number of treatments: usually given in a series that varies according to the client's presenting problem and response to therapy; 2–3 treatments per week for a total of 6–12 treatments

### Nursing Intervention
- To prepare client for ECT
  1. Assess client's record for routine pretreatment checklist for information
  2. Teach client about procedure: what to expect before, during, and after
  3. NPO (nothing by mouth) status for 6 hours before treatment
  4. Remove dentures
- To provide support and care immediately after treatment
  1. Provide orientation to time
  2. Temporary memory loss is usually confusing; explain that this is a common occurrence
  3. Assess vital signs for 30 minutes to 1 hour after treatment
  4. Deemphasize preoccupation with ECT; promote involvement in regularly scheduled activities
- Long-term goal: to promote and develop a positive self-concept and realistic perception of self
  1. Encourage problem solving in social relationships; identify problem areas in relationships with others
  2. Acknowledge and encourage statements that reflect positive attributes and/or skills
  3. Reinforce new, alternative coping methods, especially if client uses a new method to handle sad situations and painful feelings

## SCHIZOPHRENIC DISORDERS

**! NURSING PRIORITY:** Schizophrenia constitutes the largest group of psychotic disorders in society (approximately 1% of the U.S. population).

### Schizophrenia and Schizophrenia Spectrum Disorders

**Schizophrenia is a brain disorder characterized by a number of common behaviors involving disorders of thought content, mood, feeling, perception, communication, and interpersonal relationships. Onset of symptoms usually occurs in early adulthood (ages 19–21 years) with a duration of symptoms of at least 6 months.**

### General Concepts
A. Loss of ego boundaries.
B. May result from many possible factors.
  1. Organic or physiologic: genetic, biochemical (overactivity of dopamine, an insufficiency of norepinephrine, or an imbalance of both; decreased monoamine oxidase activity), immunologic imbalance, a structural deviation of brain tissue, or enlarged brain ventricles.
  2. Psychosocial: individual adaptive patterns to stress, double-bind communication pattern, poor family relationships, past traumatic experiences, lack of ego strength, or a deficit in cognitive development caused by perinatal, nutritional, and maturational factors.
C. Primary defense mechanisms are repression, regression, projection, and denial.
D. Failure or inability to trust self or others.
E. Security and identity are threatened, prompting the client to withdraw from reality.

### Prepsychotic Personality Characteristics
A. Aloof and indifferent.
B. Social withdrawal; peculiar behavior.
C. Relatives and friends note a change in personality.
D. Unusual perceptual experiences and disturbed communication patterns.
E. Lack of personal grooming.

### Psychodynamics of Maladaptive Disturbances
A. Disturbed thought processes.
  1. Confused, chaotic, and disorganized thinking.
  2. Communicates in symbolic language in which all symbols have special meaning.
  3. Belief that one's thoughts or wishes can control other people (i.e., magical thinking).
  4. Retreats to a fantasy world, rejecting the real world of painful experience while responding to reality in a bizarre or autistic manner.
B. Disturbed affect.
  1. Difficulty expressing emotions.
  2. Absent, flat, blunted, or inappropriate affect.
  3. Inappropriate affect makes it difficult to form close relationships.
C. Disturbance in psychomotor behavior.
  1. Display of disorganized, purposeless activity.
  2. Behavior may be uninhibited and bizarre; abnormal posturing (agitated or retardation catatonia); waxy flexibility.
  3. Often appears aloof, disinterested, apathetic, and lacking motivation.
D. Disturbance in perception.
  1. Hallucinations and delusions; auditory forms are most common.
  2. Abnormal bodily sensations and hypersensitivity to sound, sight, and smell.
E. Disturbance in interpersonal relationships.
  1. Establishment of interpersonal relationships is difficult because of inability to communicate clearly and react appropriately.
  2. Difficulty relating to others.
    a. Unable to form close relationships.

b. Has difficulty trusting others and experiences ambivalence, fear, and dependency.

c. "Need-fear dilemma": withdraws to protect self from further hurt and consequently experiences lack of warmth, trust, and intimacy.

d. "As if" phenomenon: feels rejected by others, which leads to increased isolation, perpetuating further feelings of rejection.

### Symptoms of Schizophrenia

A. Positive symptoms—the presence of something that is not normally present.
   1. Hallucinations and delusions (Figure 12-7).
   2. Regressive and bizarre behavior.
   3. Disorganized, incoherent speech, "word salad," associative looseness.
B. Negative symptoms—the absence of something that should be present.
   1. Anhedonia, blunted affect, loss of motivation "avolition."
   2. Rigidity and mutism.
   3. Poverty of thought "alogia."
C. Cognitive symptoms—symptoms associated with cognition, thinking.
   1. Difficulty concentrating.
   2. Problems with decision making.
   3. Impaired judgment.
   4. Memory impairment.
D. Affective symptoms—symptoms that involve emotions and expression of emotion.
   1. Suicidal ideation.
   2. Hopelessness.
   3. Dysphoria.

### Assessment

A. Four As: Eugen Bleuler's classic symptoms.
   1. Associative looseness: lack of logical thought progression, resulting in disorganized and chaotic thinking.
   2. Affect: emotion or feeling tone is one of indifference or is flat, blunted, exaggerated, or socially inappropriate.
   3. Ambivalence: conflicting, strong feelings (e.g., love and hate) that neutralize each other, leading to psychic immobilization and difficulty in expressing other emotions.
   4. Autism: extreme retreat from reality characterized by fantasies, preoccupation with daydreams, and psychotic thought processes of delusion and hallucination.
      a. Hallucinations: false sensory perceptions with no basis in reality; may be auditory, olfactory, tactile, visual, gustatory.
      b. Delusions: fixed, false beliefs not corrected by logic; develop as a defense against intolerable feelings or ideas that cause anxiety.
         (1) Delusions of grandeur: related to feelings of power, fame, splendor, magnificence.
         (2) Delusions of persecution: belief that others are out to harm, injure, or destroy.
      c. Ideas of reference: belief that actions and speech of others have reference to oneself; ideas symbolize feelings of guilt, insecurity, and alienation.
      d. Depersonalization: feeling alienated from oneself; difficulty distinguishing self from others; loss of boundaries between self and environment.
B. Additional characteristics.
   1. Regression: extreme withdrawal and social isolation.
   2. Negativism: doing the opposite of what is asked; typical behavior is to speak to no one and answer no one; used to cover feelings of unworthiness and inadequacy.
   3. Religiosity: excessive religious preoccupation.
   4. Impulsivity: unable to resist impulses.
   5. Motor retardation: slowed movement.
   6. Motor agitation: pacing or running; constantly on the move.

### Nursing Interventions

**Goal:** To build trust.

> **TEST ALERT:** Building trust is the primary goal when working with the client with schizophrenia. Maintain a therapeutic milieu; stay with client to promote safety; reducing fear and assisting client to communicate effectively are important nursing care measures.

A. Encourage free expression of feelings (either negative or positive) without fear of rejection, ridicule, or retaliation.
B. Use nonverbal level of communication to demonstrate warmth, concern, and empathy, because client often distrusts words.

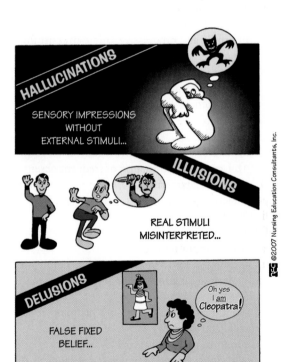

**FIGURE 12-7 Hallucinations, Illusions, and Delusions.** (From Zerwekh, J., Garneau, A., & Miller, C. J. [2017]. *Digital collection of the memory notebooks of nursing* [4th ed.]. Chandler, AZ: Nursing Education Consultants, Inc.")

C. Consistency, reliability, acceptance, and persistence build trust.

D. Allow client to set pace; proceed slowly in planning social contacts.

**Goal:** To provide a safe and secure environment.

A. Maintain familiar routines. Make sure persons who come in contact with the client are recognizable to the client.

B. Avoid stressful situations or increasing anxiety.

**Goal:** To clarify and reinforce reality.

A. Involve client in reality-oriented activities.

B. Help client find satisfaction in the external environment and ways of relating to others.

C. Focus on clear communication and the immediate situation.

**Goal:** To promote and build self-esteem.

A. Encourage simple activities with limited concentration and *no* competition.

B. Provide successful experiences with short-range goals that are realistic for client's level of functioning.

C. Relieve client of decision making until he or she is ready.

D. Avoid making demands.

**Goal:** To encourage independent behavior.

A. Anticipate and accept negativism.

B. Avoid fostering dependency.

C. Encourage client to make his or her own decisions, using positive reinforcement.

**Goal:** To provide care to meet basic human needs.

A. Determine client's ability to meet responsibilities of daily living.

B. Attend to nutrition, elimination, exercise, hygiene, and signs of physical illness.

**Goal:** To assist in medical treatment. Administer antipsychotic medications (see Appendix 12-2).

**NURSING PRIORITY:** As the client's symptoms lessen, he or she will often discontinue therapy and medication, which can lead to recurrence of symptoms.

**Goal:** To deal effectively with withdrawn behavior.

A. Establish a therapeutic one-to-one relationship.
   1. Initiate interaction by seeking out client at every opportunity.
   2. Maintain a nonjudgmental, accepting manner in what is said and done.
   3. Attempt to draw client into a conversation without demanding a response.

B. Promote social skills by helping client feel more secure with other people.
   1. Accept one-sided conversations.
   2. Accept client's negativism without comments.

C. Attend to physical needs of client as necessary.

D. Have client focus on reality.

E. Protect and restrain client from potential destructiveness to self and others.

**Goal** To deal effectively with hallucinations.

A. Clarify and reinforce reality.
   1. Help client recognize hallucination as a manifestation of anxiety.
   2. Provide a safe, secure environment.
   3. Avoid denying or arguing with client when he or she is experiencing hallucinations.
   4. Acknowledge client's experience but point out that *you* do not share the same experience.
   5. Do not give attention to content of hallucinations.
   6. Direct client's attention to real situations, such as singing along with music.
   7. Protect client from injury to self or others when he or she is prompted by "voices" or "visions."

B. Encourage social interaction to help client find satisfactory ways of relating with others.
   1. Increase interaction gradually.
   2. Respond verbally to anything real that client talks about.

## Disorders of Impulse Control

**In disorders of impulse control, there is failure to resist an impulse, drive, or temptation to perform some act that may be harmful to others; failure to resist is usually preceded by an increasing amount of tension before the act is committed but is followed by an outcome of pleasure or gratification.**

*Assessment*

A. Pathologic gambling.
   1. Diagnostic criteria.
      a. A chronic and progressive failure to resist impulses to gamble.
      b. Disrupts, damages, or compromises family, personal, and vocational pursuits.
         (1) Evidence of forgery, fraud, embezzlement.
         (2) Unable to pay debts or meet other financial obligations.
         (3) Borrows money either legally or illegally.
         (4) Loss of work because of frequent absenteeism.
   2. Additional characteristics.
      a. Overconfident, energetic, "big spender."
      b. Often begins in adolescence.

B. Kleptomania (shoplifting).
   1. Recurrent impulse to steal objects.
   2. Characterized by increasing tension before stealing and a feeling of pressure or release after the act is committed.
   3. Usually done without long-term planning.

C. Pyromania (setting fires).
   1. Recurrent impulse to set fires.
   2. Usually characterized by increased amount of tension before the fire is set, with subsequent release after the act is committed.

D. Explosive disorder.
   1. A loss of control of aggressive impulses, resulting in assault or destruction of property.

2. Behavior is usually out of proportion to the precipitating stressor.
3. Individual usually describes "spells" or "attacks"; usually regrets the display of aggression.

*Nursing Interventions*

**Goal:** To encourage client to develop alternative ways of dealing with stress.

A. Refer client to self-help groups: Gamblers Anonymous (GAM-ANON).
B. Assist client in determining when anxiety and tension are increasing and provide a plan of action to prevent acts of stealing, setting fires, or destroying property.

---

**Appendix 12-1   UNDERSTANDING DEFENSE MECHANISMS**

| *Name of Defense Mechanism* | *Definition* | *Example* |
|---|---|---|
| Compensation | Attempting to make up for or offset deficiencies, either real or imagined, by concentrating on or developing other abilities | An adolescent who perceives herself as unattractive focuses her energies on cultivating her intellectual abilities and is on the honor roll at school. |
| Conversion | Symbolic expression of intrapsychic conflict expressed in physical symptoms | A man develops blindness after watching his friend get seriously injured in a racecar accident. |
| Denial | Blocking out or disowning painful thoughts or feelings | A young mother with a newborn who has a cleft palate tells her friends everything is okay with her baby. |
| Displacement | Feelings are transferred, redirected, or discharged from the appropriate person or object to a less threatening person or object | A man gets reprimanded by his boss. Later, he yells at his wife when dinner is not ready. |
| Dissociation | Separating and detaching an idea, situation, or relationship from its emotional significance; helps the individual put aside painful feelings and often leads to a temporary alteration of consciousness or identity | A young adolescent who was the lone survivor of an airplane crash now experiences amnesia. |
| Identification | Attempting to pattern or resemble the personality of an admired, idealized person | A young man chooses to become a professional football player like his father. |
| Intellectualization | Attempt to avoid emotional conflict by focusing on concrete, logical events | A man is given a diagnosis of prostate cancer and focuses on medical management and survival rates of his cancer rather than addressing his feelings about having cancer. |
| Introjection | Acceptance of another's values and opinions as one's own | A young woman takes on the values and opinions of her peer group. |
| Projection | Attributing one's own unacceptable feelings and thoughts to others | A student who feels like a failure after getting an F on an important examination says, "It's the teacher's fault. He doesn't know how to write a test." |
| Rationalization | Attempting to justify or modify unacceptable needs and feelings to the ego in an effort to maintain self-respect and prevent guilt feelings | A man drinks several alcoholic beverages each evening, saying, "I work hard, so I need to relax when I get home." |
| Reaction formation | Assuming attitudes and behaviors that one consciously rejects | A man is extremely polite and courteous to his mother-in-law, whom he dislikes intensely. |
| Regression | Retreating to an earlier, more comfortable level of adjustment | A young preschool child begins to suck his thumb and wet the bed shortly after the birth of a sibling. |
| Repression | An involuntary, automatic submerging of painful, unpleasant thoughts and feelings into the *unconscious* | A woman is unable to remember being sexually abused as a child. |
| Splitting | Unable to integrate positive and negative attributes of one's self or others into a cohesive image (all-or-nothing thinking) | Belief that all Republicans are conservative and Democrats are liberal. |
| Sublimation | Diversion of unacceptable instinctual drives into personally and socially acceptable areas to help channel forbidden impulses into constructive activities | A man who has strong competitive or aggressive drives channels his energy into building a successful business. |

*Continued*

## Appendix 12-1 UNDERSTANDING DEFENSE MECHANISMS—cont'd

| Name of Defense Mechanism | Definition | Example |
|---|---|---|
| Suppression | Intentional exclusion of forbidden ideas and anxiety-producing situations from the *conscious* level; a voluntary forgetting and postponing mechanism | A young man is thinking so much about his date that it is interfering with his work. He decides to put it out of his mind until he leaves the office. |
| Undoing | Actually or symbolically attempting to erase a previous consciously intolerable experience or action; an attempt to repair feelings and actions that have created guilt and anxiety | A mother who has unjustly punished her child decides to bake the child's favorite cookies. |

> **! NURSING PRIORITY:** Recognize client's use of defense mechanisms.

## Appendix 12-2 MEDICATIONS: ALZHEIMER, ANTIANXIETY, ANTIMANIC, ANTIDEPRESSANT, AND ANTIPSYCHOTIC

## Alzheimer Medications

### General Nursing Implications

- Two types: (1) *cholinesterase inhibitors,* which prevent the breakdown of acetylcholine, thus making it available at the cholinergic synapses and resulting in enhanced transmission of nerve impulses and (2) *NMDA receptor antagonist*—which blocks calcium influx and modulates the effects of glutamate (major excitatory transmitter in CNS). Glutamate causes neurodegeneration in excessive amounts.
- Drugs do not cure and do not stop disease progression, but they may slow down the progression by a few months.

| Medications | Side Effects | Nursing Implications |
|---|---|---|
| **Cholinesterase Inhibitors** Donepezil: PO Galantamine: PO Rivastigmine: PO, transdermal | GI symptoms: nausea, vomiting, dyspepsia, diarrhea Dizziness and headache Bradycardia, syncope | 1. Abrupt withdrawal of medication can lead to a rapid progression of symptoms. 2. Monitor for side effects because the drug is typically given in high doses to produce the greatest benefit. 3. Donepezil is better tolerated. |
| **NMDA Receptor Antagonist** Memantine: PO | Dizziness, headache, confusion, constipation | 1. Used for moderate to severe cases. 2. Better tolerated than cholinesterase inhibitors. 3. Monitor renal function; contraindicated in patients with severe renal impairment. |

## Antianxiety Agents

### General Nursing Implications

- Withhold or omit one or more doses if excessive drowsiness occurs.
- Assess for symptoms associated with a withdrawal syndrome in hospitalized clients: anxiety, insomnia, vomiting, tremors, palpitations, confusion, and hallucinations.
- When discontinuing, the drug dosage should be gradually decreased over a period of months, depending on the dose and length of time the client has been taking the medication.
- Schedule IV drug requires documentation.
- Promote safety with the use of side rails and assistance with ambulation as necessary.
- Teach the client and family that the client should not to drink alcohol while taking an antianxiety agent and not to stop taking the medication abruptly.

**Appendix 12-2  MEDICATIONS: ALZHEIMER, ANTIANXIETY, ANTIMANIC, ANTIDEPRESSANT, AND ANTIPSYCHOTIC—cont'd**

| Medications | Side Effects | Nursing Implications |
|---|---|---|

**Benzodiazepines:** Reduce anxiety by enhancing the action of the inhibitory neurotransmitter GABA on its receptor; also promote anticonvulsant activity and skeletal muscle relaxation.

Alprazolam: PO
Chlordiazepoxide: PO, IM, IV
Diazepam: PO, IM, IV
Clonazepam: PO
Clorazepate: PO
Lorazepam: PO, IV
Midazolam: IM, IV

CNS depression, drowsiness (decreases with use), ataxia, dizziness, headaches, dry mouth

*Adverse effects:* tolerance commonly develops, physical dependency

1. May cause paradoxical effects and should not be taken by mothers who are breastfeeding.
2. Assess for symptoms of leukopenia, such as sore throat, fever, and weakness.
3. Encourage the client to rise slowly from a supine position and to dangle feet before standing.
4. Chlordiazepoxide: Do not inject or add IV chlordiazepoxide to an existing IV infusion; inject directly into a large vein over a 1-minute period.
5. Do not mix chlordiazepoxide or diazepam with any other drug in a syringe or add to existing IV fluids.
6. Versed is commonly used for induction of anesthesia and sedation before diagnostic tests and endoscopic examinations.
7. Flumazenil is approved for the treatment of benzodiazepine overdose; it has an adverse effect of precipitating convulsions, especially in clients with a history of epilepsy.
   *Uses:* anxiety and tension, muscle spasm, preoperative medication, acute alcohol withdrawal, and to induce sleep

**Nonbenzodiazepine Agents:** Interact with serotonin and dopamine receptors in the brain to decrease anxiety; lack muscle-relaxant and anticonvulsant effects; do not cause sedation or physical or psychological dependence; do not increase CNS depression caused by alcohol or other drugs.

Buspirone: PO

Dizziness, drowsiness, headache, nausea, fatigue, insomnia

1. Not a controlled substance
2. Some improvement can be noted in 7–10 days; however, it usually takes 3–4 weeks to achieve effectiveness.
3. Better tolerated than benzodiazepines.
   *Uses:* short-term relief of anxiety and anxiety disorders

## Antimanic Medications

**Lithium Carbonate:** Believed to alter glutamate uptake and release; blocks binding of serotonin to its receptors. *Uses:* bipolar affective disorder (manic episode).

Lithium: PO

*High incidence:* increased thirst, increased urination (polyuria)
*Frequent:* 1.5 mEq/L (1.5 mmol/L) levels or less: nausea, vomiting, slurred speech, dry mouth, lethargy, fatigue, muscle weakness, headache, GI disturbances, fine hand tremors
*Adverse effects:* 1.5–2.0 mEq/L (1.5–2.0 mmol/L) may produce confusion, persistent GI disturbances, ECG changes, drowsiness, incoordination, coarse hand tremors, muscle twitching 2.0–2.5 mEq/L (2.0–2.5 mmol/L) may result in ataxia, tinnitus, seizures, clonic movements, high output of dilute urine, blurred vision, severe hypotension
*Acute toxicity greater than 2.5 mEq/L (2.5 mmol/L):* generalized convulsions, oliguria, coma, death

1. Monitor lithium blood levels: blood samples are obtained 12 hours after dose was given.
2. Teach client the following:
3. Symptoms of lithium toxicity.
4. Importance of frequent blood tests (every 2–3 days) to check lithium levels at the beginning of treatment (maintenance blood levels done every 1–3 months).
5. Importance of taking dose at same time each day, preferably with meals or milk to reduce GI symptoms.
6. Encourage a diet containing normal amounts of salt and a fluid intake of 3 L per day; avoid caffeine because of its diuretic effect.
7. Report polyuria, prolonged vomiting, diarrhea, or fever to physician (may need to temporarily reduce dosage or discontinue use).
8. Do not crush, chew, or break the extended-release or film-coated tablets.
9. Assess clients at high risk for developing toxicity: postoperative, dehydrated, hyperthyroidism, those with renal disease, or those taking diuretics.
10. Blood levels:
    • Extremely narrow therapeutic range: 0.5–1.5 mEq/L (0.5–1.5 mmol/L)
    • Toxic serum lithium level: greater than 2 mEq/L (2 mmol/L)
    • Acute mania: 0.8–1.4 mEq/L (0.8–1.4 mmol/L)
    • Long-term maintenance levels: 0.4–1 mEq/L (0.4–1.0 mmol/L)
11. Management of lithium toxicity: possible hemodialysis.
12. Long-term use may cause goiter; may be associated with hypothyroidism.

*Continued*

| Medications | Side Effects | Nursing Implications |
|---|---|---|
| **Other Agents:** Both of the following medications were originally developed and used for seizure disorders. Both have mood-stabilizing effects. | | |
| Carbamazepine: PO | Drowsiness, dizziness, visual problems (spots before eyes, difficulty focusing, blurred vision), dry mouth<br>*Toxic reactions:* blood dyscrasias | 1. Used primarily for clients who have not responded to lithium or who cannot tolerate the side effects.<br>2. Avoid tasks that require alertness and motor skills until response to drug is established.<br>3. Monitor CBC frequently during initiation of therapy and at monthly intervals thereafter. |
| Valproic acid: PO | Nausea, GI upsets, drowsiness, may cause pancreatitis, hepatotoxicity | 1. Monitor liver function studies.<br>2. Administer with food to avoid GI upset. |

## Antidepressant Medications

### General Nursing Implications
- Selective serotonin reuptake inhibitors (SSRIs) are overtaking tricyclic antidepressants (TCAs) as drugs of choice for depression.
- Because of the potential interactions with other drugs and certain foods, monoamine oxidase inhibitors (MAOIs) are used as second-line drugs for the treatment of depression.
- The therapeutic effect has a delayed onset of 7 to 21 days, but SSRIs may take as long as 4 to 6 weeks to become effective.
- These drugs can potentially produce cardiotoxicity, sedation, seizures, and anticholinergic effects and may induce mania in clients with bipolar disorder (SSRIs are less likely to cause these problems).
- Drugs are usually discontinued before surgery (10 days for MAOIs; 2–3 days for TCAs) because of adverse interactions with anesthetic agents.

**Tricyclic Antidepressants (TCAs):** Prevent the reuptake of norepinephrine or serotonin, which results in increased concentrations of these neurotransmitters.

| | | |
|---|---|---|
| Imipramine hydrochloride: PO, IM<br>Nortriptyline hydrochloride: PO<br>Doxepin hydrochloride: PO<br>Amitriptyline hydrochloride: PO, IM | Drowsiness, dry mouth, blurred vision, constipation, weight gain, and orthostatic hypotension<br>*Adverse reactions:* cardiac dysrhythmias, nystagmus, tremor, hypotension, restlessness | 1. TCAs should not be given at the same time as an MAOI; a time lag of 14 days is necessary when changing from one drug group to the other.<br>2. Because of marked sedation, client should avoid activities requiring mental alertness (driving or operating machinery).<br>3. Instruct client to move gradually from lying to sitting and standing positions to prevent postural hypotension.<br>4. Doxepin is better tolerated by older adults and has less effect on cardiac status; dilute the concentrate with orange juice.<br>5. TCAs are contraindicated in clients with epilepsy, glaucoma, and cardiovascular disease.<br>6. TCAs are usually given once daily at bedtime.<br>7. *Uses:* depression; imipramine is also used to treat enuresis in children. |

**Selective Serotonin Reuptake Inhibitors (SSRIs):** Cause selective inhibition of serotonin uptake and produce CNS excitation rather than sedation; have no effect on dopamine or norepinephrine.

| | | |
|---|---|---|
| Fluoxetine: PO<br>Sertraline: PO<br>Paroxetine: PO<br>Citalopram: PO<br>Escitalopram: PO<br>Fluvoxamine: PO | Nausea, headache, anxiety, nervousness, insomnia, weight gain, skin rash, sexual dysfunction<br>*Adverse reactions (serotonin syndrome):* tachycardia, delirium, restlessness, fever, seizures | Medication is usually given once a day.<br>*Uses:* depression, obsessive–compulsive disorder, bulimia<br>Interacts with St. John's wort and MAOI; may cause serotonin syndrome.<br>Discontinue SSRI 5 weeks before starting MAOI. |

| Appendix 12-2 | MEDICATIONS: ALZHEIMER, ANTIANXIETY, ANTIMANIC, ANTIDEPRESSANT, AND ANTIPSYCHOTIC—cont'd |
|---|---|

| Medications | Side Effects | Nursing Implications |
|---|---|---|

**Monoamine Oxidase Inhibitors (MAOIs):** Inhibit the enzyme monoamine oxidase, which breaks down norepinephrine and serotonin, increasing the concentration of these neurotransmitters.

| Medications | Side Effects | Nursing Implications |
|---|---|---|
| Isocarboxazid: PO<br>Phenelzine sulfate: PO<br>Tranylcypromine: PO | Drowsiness, insomnia, dry mouth, urinary retention, hypotension<br>*Adverse reactions:* Serotonin syndrome, tachycardia, tachypnea, agitation, tremors, seizures, heart block, hypotension | 1. Potentiate many drug actions: narcotics, barbiturates, sedatives, and atropine-like medications.<br>2. Have a long duration of action; therefore 2–3 weeks must go by before another drug is administered while a client is taking an MAOI.<br>3. MAOIs interact with specific foods and drugs (ones containing tyramine or sympathomimetic drugs); and may cause a severe hypertensive crisis characterized by marked elevation of blood pressure, increased temperature, tremors, and tachycardia. Foods and drugs to avoid: coffee, tea, cola beverages, aged cheeses, beer and wine, pickled foods, avocados, and figs and many over-the-counter cold preparations, hay fever medications, and nasal decongestants.<br>4. Monitor for bladder distention by checking urinary output.<br>5. Parnate: most likely to cause hypertensive crisis; onset of action is more rapid.<br>*Uses:* primarily psychotic depression and depressive episode of bipolar affective disorder. |

**Miscellaneous Antidepressants**

| Medications | Side Effects | Nursing Implications |
|---|---|---|
| Trazodone: PO | Sedation, orthostatic hypotension, nausea, vomiting, can cause priapism (prolonged, painful erection of the penis) | See General Nursing Implications. |
| Bupropion: PO | Weight loss, dry mouth, dizziness | See General Nursing Implications. |

**Antipsychotic (Neuroleptic) Medications**

*General Nursing Implications*
- Use cautiously in older adults.
- These drugs should make the client feel better and experience fewer psychotic episodes.
- Maintain a regular schedule; usually take daily dose 1 to 2 hours before bedtime.
- Explain to client and family the importance of compliance with medication regimen.
- Medications are not addictive.
- Discuss side effects and importance of notifying primary care provider if client experiences undesired or side effects.
- When mixing for parenteral use, do not mix with other drugs.
- Inject deep IM; client should stay in reclined position 30 to 60 minutes after dose administration.

*Continued*

| Medications | Side Effects | Nursing Implications |
|---|---|---|
| **Phenothiazines:** Block dopamine receptors and thought to depress various portions of the reticular activating system; have peripherally exerting anticholinergic properties (atropine-like symptoms: dryness of mouth, stuffy nose, constipation, blurring of vision). Classified by chemical type (aliphatic, piperazine, piperidine types) and potency. | | |
| *Aliphatic type:*<br>Conventional/first generation:<br>  Chlorpromazine hydrochloride **(low potency):** PO, IM, IV suppository<br>*Piperazine type:*<br>Conventional/first generation:<br>  Fluphenazine hydrochloride **(high potency):** PO, IM<br>Conventional/first generation:<br>  Trifluoperazine (high potency): PO, IM<br>*Piperidine type:*<br>Conventional/first generation:<br>  Thioridazine **(low potency):** PO | **Extrapyramidal effects (movement disorder):** occur early in therapy and are usually managed with other drugs<br>*Acute dystonia*—painful spasm of muscles of tongue, face, neck, or back; oculogyric crisis (upward deviation of the eyes); opisthotonus (spasm of the back muscles causing trunk to arch forward and limbs to move backward)<br>*Parkinsonism*—muscle tremors, rigidity, spasms, shuffling gait, stooped posture, cogwheel rigidity<br>*Akathisia*—motor restlessness, pacing<br>**Tardive dyskinesia:** occurs late in therapy; symptoms are often irreversible—earliest symptom is slow, wormlike movements of the tongue; later symptoms include fine twisting, writhing movements of the tongue and face, grimacing; lip smacking; involuntary movements of the limbs, toes, fingers, and trunk<br>**Neuroleptic malignant syndrome:** rare problem, fever (41°C, 105°F), "lead pipe" muscle rigidity, agitation, confusion, delirium, respiratory and acute renal failure<br>*Endocrine*—amenorrhea, increased libido in women, decreased libido in men, delayed ejaculation, increased appetite, weight gain, hypoglycemia, and edema<br>*Dermatologic:* photosensitivity<br>*Hypersensitivity reaction:* jaundice, agranulocytosis | 1. Check blood pressure before administration; to avoid postural hypotension, encourage client to rise slowly from sitting or lying position.<br>2. Be aware of the antiemetic effect of the phenothiazines; may mask other pathology such as drug overdose, brain lesions, or intestinal obstruction.<br>3. Client teaching: protect skin from sunlight—wear long-sleeved shirts, hats, and sunscreen lotion when out in the sunlight.<br>4. Explain importance of reporting any signs of sore throat, fever, or symptoms of infection.<br>5. Encourage periodic liver function studies to be done.<br>6. Teach that drug may turn urine pink or reddish brown.<br>7. Extrapyramidal symptoms treated with anticholinergics (e.g., benztropine).<br>8. Long-term use of phenothiazines requires assessment of involuntary movement screening (AIMS).<br>9. *Uses:* severe psychoses, schizophrenia, manic phase of bipolar affective disorder, personality disorders, and severe agitation and anxiety. |
| **Other Antipsychotic Drugs**<br>First generation/Conventional:<br>  Haloperidol: PO, IM | High potency antipsychotic agent<br>Significant extrapyramidal effects; low incidence of sedation, orthostatic hypotension; does not elicit photosensitivity reaction | 1. May reduce prothrombin time.<br>2. Often used as the initial drug for treatment of psychotic disorders. |
| Second generation/Atypical:<br>  Risperidone: PO | Anxiety, somnolence, extrapyramidal symptoms, dizziness, constipation, GI upset, rhinitis | 1. *Uses:* tics, vocal disturbances, and psychotic schizophrenia.<br>2. Risperidone is the most frequently prescribed antipsychotic because of less serious side effects. |
| Second generation/atypical:<br>  Clozapine: PO | Blood dyscrasias (agranulocytosis), sedation, weight gain, orthostatic hypotension, seizures, diabetes | 1. Used with caution in clients with diabetes and those with history of seizures.<br>2. Treatment is started slowly and gradually increased; it is important that the client not stop taking medication. |
| Third generation (dopamine system stabilizer):<br>  Aripiprazole: PO | Very low extrapyramidal effects and tardive dyskinesia, headache, nervousness, insomnia, dizziness | 1. Only medication in this category. |

*CBC,* Complete blood count; *CNS,* central nervous system; *GABA,* gamma-aminobutyric acid; *GI,* gastrointestinal; *IM,* intramuscularly; *IV,* intravenously; *PO,* by mouth (orally).

# Study Questions
## Psychosocial Nursing Care

More questions on

1. A nurse case worker suspects older adult neglect. Which assessment findings during a home visit would confirm this? (Select all that apply.)
   1. Confusion and disorientation
   2. Recent hip fracture
   3. Poor nutrition and hygiene
   4. Dirty dishes in the sink
   5. Outdated prescription bottles
   6. Missing hearing aids

2. The nurse is about to conduct an admission assessment on an 85-year-old female client who is admitted after falling down in her home. When determining the amount of time to set aside for the interview, the nurse will consider which of the following?
   1. Allow ample time to gather psychosocial data from the client.
   2. Skip the psychosocial assessment; it is not important for the client with a physiologic problem.
   3. Interview the client's daughter and son about the client's psychosocial background.
   4. Ask the client whether she has any pressing or major issues she wants to talk about.

3. The nurse notes that a client is quite suspicious during an assessment interview and believes that her family is under investigation by the CIA. What would be appropriate nursing interventions with this client? **Select all that apply:**
   1. Use active listening skills to seek information from the client.
   2. Encourage the client to describe the problem as she sees it.
   3. Ask the client to tell you exactly what she thinks is happening.
   4. Tell the client that she is delusional and you can help her.
   5. Explain to the client that most people are not investigated by the CIA or FBI.
   6. Reassure the client that you are not with the CIA.

4. Which of the following nursing interventions should be instituted for a client experiencing a manic episode?
   1. Place the client in a quiet area, separate from others.
   2. Encourage the client to engage in some physical activity.
   3. Establish firm, set limits on behavior.
   4. Include the client in the group's activities.

5. A client experiencing severe depression is admitted to the inpatient psychiatric unit. During the initial assessment, she says, "I feel like killing myself, but I wouldn't do that because of my kids." The nurse's priority action would be to:
   1. Explore the reasons that the client might want to take her life.
   2. Determine the severity of her suicidal risk.
   3. Prevent the client from harming herself.
   4. Guide her to consider alternative ways of coping.

6. Which of the following signs and symptoms would the nurse assess for in a client with possible lithium toxicity?
   1. Hypotension, bradycardia, polyuria
   2. Tachycardia, hypertension, convulsions
   3. Diarrhea, ataxia, seizures, lethargy
   4. Urinary frequency, vomiting, fever

7. When caring for a client admitted for medically monitored detoxification from alcohol, the nurse would assess for which of the following signs and symptoms of withdrawal?
   1. Anorexia, irritability, nausea, and tremulousness
   2. Bradycardia, hypotension, diaphoresis, and fever
   3. Vivid hallucinations, coarse irregular tremor
   4. Severe craving, euphoria, profuse sweating, and paranoid ideation

8. A client is admitted to the inpatient psychiatric unit for medically monitored detoxification from alcohol. Which of the following actions would be included in the client's plan of care?
   1. Encourage increased fluid intake.
   2. Order a high-protein, high-fat diet.
   3. Provide a high-sodium, low-carbohydrate diet.
   4. Encourage ambulation and deep breathing.

9. A client with a diagnosis of schizophrenia repeatedly states, "There are flies eating my brain and making me feel weird." The client is most likely experiencing which of the following?
   1. Ideas of reference
   2. Grandiose delusions
   3. Somatic delusions
   4. Persecutory delusions

10. When preparing a client for electroconvulsive therapy (ECT), the nurse would include which of the following actions?
    1. Provide orientation to time.
    2. Assess vital signs for 30 minutes to 1 hour.
    3. Remove dentures and maintain NPO status.
    4. Encourage problem solving in social settings.

11. A client is experiencing a lack of logical thought progression, resulting in disorganized and chaotic thinking. The nurse understands this to be:
    1. Delusions of grandeur
    2. Ideas of reference
    3. Depersonalization
    4. Associative looseness

# Answers to **Study Questions**

**1.** *3, 5, 6*
Lack of assistive devices, medication mismanagement, and access to basic physiologic needs such as hygienic care, food, and water are characteristics of neglect in the older adult. A hip fracture is typically caused by osteoporosis in older adults, not neglect. Confusion and disorientation are signs of dementia. Dirty dishes in the sink is not a sign of neglect. (Halter, 7 ed., p. 540)

**2.** *1*
Because older adult clients may be starved for someone to listen to them, the nurse must allow ample time to gather psychosocial data. It would not be good nursing judgment to skip the psychosocial assessment. The nurse should interview the client and, if additional information is required, then the client's family can be interviewed. Although asking the client about pressing or major issues is a good answer, it does not address the importance of allowing sufficient time to actually discuss the pressing or major issues that the client may want to describe. (Potter & Perry, 8 ed., pp. 318–319)

**3.** *1, 2, 3*
The client is demonstrating paranoid behavior, which necessitates a matter-of-fact approach that is nonjudgmental and accepting of the client's statements and shows the nurse's willingness to listen attentively to the issue. Telling the client that she is delusional, explaining that most people are not investigated by the CIA or FBI, reassuring the client that you are not with the CIA do not help the paranoid client gain trust to talk with the nurse. (Halter, 7 ed., p. 465)

**4.** *1*
For the client's protection, he should be moved to a quiet environment away from others. This will help him regain some control and will not produce unneeded stimuli. Setting firm limits would be appropriate for manipulative behavior. Until the manic behavior is under control, including a client in group activities (physical or otherwise) would not be therapeutic for him and would more than likely be disruptive to others. (Halter, 7 ed., p. 237)

**5.** *2*
The priority nursing action is to determine the suicidal lethality. Ask clients whether they plan to hurt themselves, what the method would be, and what factors might interfere with the rescue. The more detailed the plan, the more lethal and accessible the method. The more effort that is exerted to block rescue, the greater the likelihood will be of the suicidal effort being successful. Although the other three options are definitely plausible, they are not the priority. (Halter, 7 ed., pp. 485–486)

**6.** *3*
Lithium toxicity is a serious problem for clients with bipolar disorder. Symptoms include diarrhea, confusion, ataxia, slurred speech, hypotension, seizures, oliguria, coma, and death. (Halter, 7 ed., p. 240)

**7.** *1*
Detoxification or controlled withdrawal from alcohol via a medical protocol includes regular assessment for withdrawal signs and symptoms and administration of prescribed medications. Signs and symptoms of alcohol withdrawal include anorexia, irritability, nausea, tremulousness, insomnia, nightmares, hyperalertness, tachycardia, increased blood pressure, diaphoresis, and anxiety. (Halter, 7 ed., p. 421)

**8.** *1*
When assisting in the medical treatment of alcohol withdrawal, the nurse should encourage intake of fluids. Alcohol depletes the body of fluid, and detoxification is usually smoother if the client takes fluids readily. A high-protein and high-carbohydrate diet would be encouraged, because alcoholic clients often have poor nutrition and become debilitated. (Halter, 7 ed., p. 421)

**9.** *3*
Bizarre ideas that focus on the body being incapacitated are known as somatic delusions and are sometimes observed in schizophrenia. Grandiose delusions are beliefs of being important. Ideas of reference or delusions of reference occur when a person believes or perceives that irrelevant, unrelated, or innocuous things in the world are referring to them directly or have special personal significance. Persecutory delusions are when a person believes (wrongly) that they are being picked on or threatened by someone/something else. (Halter, 7 ed., p. 206)

**10.** *3*
To prepare a client for ECT, the nurse must do the following: check the client's record for routine preoperative information; institute and maintain NPO status for 6 hours before the treatment because the client will be receiving a general anesthetic agent—short-acting barbiturate (methohexital) and muscle paralyzing agent (succinylcholine); have the client remove dentures; and administer preoperative medication. (Halter, 7 ed., p. 271)

**11.** *4*
According to Eugen Bleuler's classic symptoms of schizophrenia, associative looseness is a lack of logical thought progression resulting in disorganized and chaotic thinking. Grandiose delusions are beliefs of being important. Ideas of reference or delusions of reference occur when a person believes or perceives that irrelevant, unrelated, or innocuous things in the world are referring to him or her directly or have special personal significance. Depersonalization is characterized by a change in how an affected individual perceives or experiences his or her sense of self. The usual sense of one's own reality is temporarily lost or changed. A feeling of detachment from, or being an outside observer of, one's mental processes or body occurs such as the sensation of being in a dream. (Halter, 7 ed., p. 213)

# CHAPTER THIRTEEN

# Integumentary: Care of Adult and Pediatric Clients

# 13

## PRIORITY CONCEPTS

Infection, Inflammation, Tissue Integrity

## PHYSIOLOGY OF THE INTEGUMENTARY SYSTEM

A. Structure.
  1. Epidermis—outermost layer; contains the melanocytes and keratinocytes.
  2. Dermis—connective tissue below epidermis. Ridges in this layer form the fingerprints and footprints. Assists in body temperature and blood pressure regulation. Highly vascular.
  3. Hypodermis (subcutaneous)—located below dermis; anchors the muscles and bones to the skin; provides insulation, cushioning, temperature regulation.
  4. Nails.
  5. Hair.
  6. Glands.
     a. Sebaceous glands: produce sebum, an oily secretion that is deposited into the hair shaft.
     b. Apocrine glands: secrete an odorless fluid from the hair shaft, which, on contact with bacteria, produces a distinctive body odor.
     c. Eccrine glands: sweat glands that are stimulated by elevated temperature and emotional stress.
B. Functions of the skin.
  1. Protection: barrier from the external environment is the primary function.
  2. Sensory: major receptor for general sensation such as touch, pain, hot, cold.
  3. Water balance.
     a. Water—600 to 900 mL—is lost daily through insensible perspiration.
     b. Prevents loss of water and electrolytes from the internal environment.
  4. Regulates body temperature in response to external temperature.
  5. Involved in the activation of vitamin D.
  6. Delivery system for drugs.

## System Assessment

A. Health history.
  1. History of rashes/lesions, hair loss, or changes in nails.
  2. Is there any itching, burning, or discomfort associated with the problem?
  3. Contact with irritants, ultraviolet (UV) exposure, cold, unhygienic conditions, insect bites/stings.

  4. Current medications.
  5. Allergies to food, medications, insect stings, etc.
B. Physical assessment (Box 13-1).
  1. Inspection.
     a. Assess skin color.
        (1) Jaundice, cyanosis, erythema.
        (2) Vitiligo: loss of melanin, resulting in white, hypopigmented area.
        (3) Best areas to assess include the sclera, conjunctiva, nail beds, lips, and buccal mucosa.
     b. Assess vascularity.
        (1) Bruising, purpura, or petechiae.
        (2) Presence or absence of blanching with direct pressure.
     c. Assess lesions for:
        (1) Type, shape, color, size, distribution, grouping, and location.
        (2) Use metric rulers to measure the size of the lesion.
        (3) Use appropriate specific terminology to describe and report type of lesion (Table 13-1).
     d. Assess for unusual odors, especially around lesions or in the intertriginous areas (axilla, overhanging abdominal folds, and groin).
     e. Assess for chronic UV exposure and photoaging of skin—appearance of actinic (sun) keratoses (precancerous lesions), wrinkling, and telangiectasia.
        (1) UVB—major factor of sunburn and nonmelanoma skin cancer.
        (2) UVA—carcinogenic and causes accelerated aging effects.
     f. Inspect hair (head and body for distribution) and nails (grooves, pitting, ridges, smoothness–thickness, and detachment from nail bed).
  2. Palpation.
     a. Determine temperature (use back of hand), tissue turgor (pinch under clavicle or back of hand), and mobility.
     b. Evaluate moisture and texture.
C. Cultural considerations: assessment of color in dark skin is most easily determined in areas such as lips, mucous membranes, and nail beds.
D. Health Promotion: sun exposure—use SPF 30 or higher if a history of skin cancer.
E. Diagnostics (see Appendix 13-1).

**TEST ALERT:** Perform a risk assessment—evaluation of skin integrity.

**Differences in Skin Assessment**

*Skin*

- Increased wrinkling and sagging, redundant flesh around eyes, slowness of skin to flatten when pinched together (tenting)
- Dry, flaking skin: excoriation from scratching
- Thinning of skin
- Decreased rate of wound healing
- Increased incidence of bruising/skin tears
- Decreased sensation to touch, temperature, and pain
- Decreased subcutaneous fat, elastic fibers, and collagen stiffening

*Hair*

- Graying; dry, scaly scalp
- Thinning, baldness

*Nails*

- Thick, brittle, hardened, nails; ridging/yellowing
- Prolonged return of blood with blanching
- Increased incidence of fungal infections

### Table 13-1    COMMON DERMATOLOGIC LESIONS

| Primary Lesions | Secondary Lesions |
|---|---|
| **Macule:** Flat, circumscribed area of color change in the skin without surface elevation; less than 1 cm in diameter (freckle, measles) | **Fissure:** Linear crack; may be dry or moist (athlete's foot, crack in corner of mouth) |
| **Papule:** Solid, elevated lesion, less than 1 cm in diameter (wart, elevated mole) | **Scale:** Excess epidermal cells caused by shedding (flaking of the skin) |
| **Plaque:** Circumscribed, solid lesion, greater than 1 cm in diameter (psoriasis, seborrheic keratosis) | **Scar:** Abnormal connective tissue that replaces normal skin (healed surgical incision) |
| **Nodule:** Raised, solid lesion that is larger and deeper than a papule | **Ulcer:** Loss of epidermis and dermis; crater-like; irregular shape (pressure ulcer, chancre) |
| **Vesicle:** Small elevation, usually filled with serous fluid or blood. Bulla: larger than a vesicle. Pustule: vesicle or bulla filled with pus (chickenpox, burn, herpes zoster-shingles) | **Atrophy:** Depression in skin resulting from thinning of the layers (aged skin, striae) |
| **Wheal:** Elevation of the skin caused by edema of the dermis (insect bite, urticaria, allergic reaction) | **Excoriation:** Area where epidermis is missing, exposing the dermis (scabies, abrasion, scratch) |
| **Cyst:** Mass of fluid-filled tissue that extends to the subcutaneous tissue or dermis | **Petechiae:** Small red to purple spots on the skin caused by tiny hemorrhages in the dermal or submucosal layers |
| | **Ecchymosis:** A blue to purple discoloration of the skin caused by leakage of blood into the subcutaneous tissue; usually as a result of tissue trauma |

# BENIGN AND INFLAMMATORY DISORDERS
(Figure 13-1)

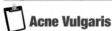

## Acne Vulgaris

**Acne is an inflammatory disorder of the sebaceous glands and their hair follicles.**

### Assessment

A. Risk factors/etiology.
   1. More common in teenagers; may persist into adulthood.
   2. Under hormonal influence during puberty; affected by presence of androgen, which stimulates the sebaceous glands to secrete sebum.
B. Clinical manifestations.
   1. Inflammatory papules or pustules; noninflammatory lesions such as open comedones (blackheads) and closed comedones (whiteheads).
   2. Cysts: deep nodules that may produce scarring.

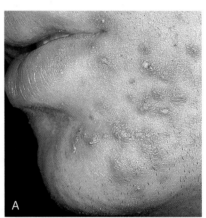

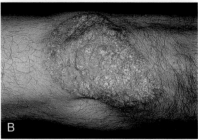

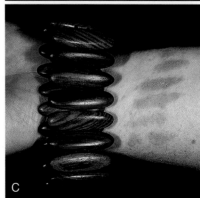

**FIGURE 13-1 Benign and Inflammatory Disorders. (A)** inflammatory acne with pustules and cysts; **(B)** plaque psoriasis; **(C)** allergic contact dermatitis to lacquer on bracelet. (From Habif, T., et al. [2011]. *Skin disease: Diagnosis & treatment* [3rd ed.]. St. Louis, MO: Elsevier.)

## Treatment

A. Medical: topical or systemic therapy.
   1. Antibacterial and peeling agents: benzoyl peroxide and glycolic acid.
   2. Long-term oral antibiotic therapy.
   3. Combination therapy (both oral and topical is common).
   4. Isotretinoin—derivative of vitamin A, may cause serious side effects; may be teratogenic; contraindicated during pregnancy. Client will require two forms of birth control during course of therapy and monitoring (e.g., liver, triglycerides, symptoms of depression).

### Home Care

A. Instruct client to cleanse face twice daily but to avoid overcleansing.
B. May use a polyester sponge pad to cleanse, because it provides a mechanical removal of the epidermal layer.
C. Instruct client to keep hands away from face and to avoid any friction or trauma to the area; avoid propping hands against face, rubbing face, etc. Make sure client recognizes that picking and squeezing lesions will worsen condition.
D. Emphasize the importance of a nutritious diet; encourage adequate food intake and use of vitamin A.
E. Avoid the use of cosmetics, shaving creams, and lotion because they may exacerbate acne; if cosmetics are to be used, water-based makeup is preferable.
F. Instruct the client to administer medication appropriately: topical application; avoid sunlight while using medications, etc.

## Psoriasis

**Psoriasis is a chronic inflammatory autoimmune disorder characterized by rapid turnover of epidermal cells. Can be common in families.**

### Assessment

A. Silvery scaling, plaques on the elbows, scalp, knees, palms, soles, trunk, and outside surface of the limbs.
B. If scales are scraped away, a dark red base of the lesion is seen, which will produce multiple bleeding points.
C. No cure; may improve but then exacerbates throughout life.
D. Bilateral symmetry of symptoms is common.

### Treatment

A. Medical.
   1. Topical therapy.
      a. Coal tar preparation.
      b. Anthralin.
      c. Corticosteroids.
      d. Calcipotriene.
      e. Salicylic acid.
   2. Photo chemotherapy.
      a. (PUVA therapy): **p**soralen, **u**ltraviolet **A** therapy (must wear protective eyewear during treatment and for 24 hours after therapy).
      b. UVB and narrow-band UVB (ultraviolet B radiation).
   3. Systemic therapy: antimetabolites (methotrexate).
   4. Biologic immunotherapy (adalimumab).

### Home Care

A. Encourage verbalization regarding appearance.
B. Instruct client to use a soft brush to remove scales while bathing.
C. Assess client to determine factors that may trigger skin condition (e.g., emotional stress, trauma, seasonal changes).
D. Make sure client understands treatment and implications of care related to PUVA therapy and other treatments.

## Atopic Dermatitis

Atopic dermatitis (also called eczema) is a superficial, chronic inflammatory disorder associated with allergy with a hereditary tendency. The condition commonly occurs during infancy, usually between 2 and 6 months of age and often persists into adulthood.

### Assessment

A. Symptoms are similar with both adults and children: reddened lesions occur on the cheeks, arms, and legs in infants and children and in the antecubital and popliteal space in adults; lesions may have oozing vesicles.
B. Intense itching (worse at night).
C. As the child gets older, the lesions tend to be dry with a thickening of the skin (lichenification).
D. Infants with eczema are more likely to have allergies as children and adults and are at increased risk for developing asthma.

### Treatment

A. Milk, eggs, wheat, and peanuts are the most commonly suspected causes in children; food allergies are not associated with adult atopic dermatitis.
B. Pruritus is treated with oral antihistamines, topical steroids, and immunomodulators.
C. Systemic steroids are prescribed if condition is severe.
D. Antibiotics may be needed if secondary infection occurs.

### Home Care

A. Teach parents about dietary restrictions; provide them with written guidelines.
B. Keep fingernails and toenails cut short.
C. Feed the child when he or she is well rested and is not itching.
D. Assist parents to identify foods that contain eggs and other "hidden" allergenic foods.
E. Avoid overheating; decrease likelihood of perspiration (no nylon clothing).
F. Child should avoid contact with persons who have the chickenpox virus or herpes simplex.
G. Avoid immunizations with live vaccines because of the possibility of severe reactions.

H. Child should wear nonirritating clothing; wool and abrasive fabrics should be avoided.

I. Tepid bath with mild soap or an emulsifying oil followed immediately by application of an emollient; cool compresses decrease itching.

J. Teach adults to avoid things that cause a flare-up of the condition and to treat symptoms with topical medication when they occur.

> **! NURSING PRIORITY:** Apply emollients (medications) to treat dry skin immediately after bathing while skin is slightly moist.

## Contact Dermatitis

Contact dermatitis is an inflammatory skin reaction that results because the skin has come in contact with a specific irritant or allergen. Diaper dermatitis occurs after prolonged contact with urine, feces, ointments, soaps, or friction. Allergic dermatitis is usually a symptom of delayed hypersensitivity.

### Assessment

A. Risk factors/etiology.
  1. Poison ivy and poison oak; fabrics such as wool, polyester.
  2. Cosmetics; household products such as detergents, soap, hair dye.
  3. Industrial substances: paints, dyes, insecticides, rubber compounds, etc.
  4. Prolonged contact with diaper wetness, fecal enzymes, increased skin pH due to urine, and friction/irritation.

B. Clinical manifestations.
  1. Pruritus; hivelike papules, vesicles, and plaques (more chronic).
  2. Sharply circumscribed areas (with occasional vesicle formation) that crust and ooze.

C. Diagnostics.
  1. Skin testing to determine allergen.

### Treatment

A. Medical.
  1. Eliminate allergen.
  2. Topical steroids; oral steroids for severe cases.
  3. Antihistamines, antipruritic agents, and antifungals (diaper dermatitis).
  4. Skin lubrication.

### Home Care

A. Teach importance of washing exposed skin with cool water and soap as soon as possible after exposure (within 15 minutes is best).

B. Provide cool, tepid bath; trim fingernails; and use measures to control itching.

C. Teach about fallacy of blister fluid spreading the disease.

D. Change diaper frequently, keep skin dry, and use protective ointment (zinc oxide or petrolatum).

> **! PEDIATRIC PRIORITY:** Talc powders may keep skin dry, but they are harmful if breathed. Plain cornstarch is safer to use.

## Pressure Injury

A pressure injury (previously called a pressure ulcer; also known as decubitus ulcer, bedsore) is a localized injury to the skin and/or underlying tissue usually over a bony prominence as a result of pressure or pressure in combination with shear and/or friction.

> **TEST ALERT:** Identify potential for skin breakdown: a pressure injury can be and should be prevented. Identify those clients at increased risk for ulcer development and begin preventive care as soon as possible. Do not wait for the reddened area to occur before preventive measures are initiated.

### Assessment

A. Risk factors/etiology.
  1. Immobility/inactivity, shearing/friction/contractures.
  2. Inadequate nutrition.
  3. Fecal/urinary incontinence (maceration/excoriation).
  4. Decreased sensation/pain perception/circulation.
  5. Advancing age (loss of lean body mass; decreased elasticity of the skin; decreased venous and/or arterial blood flow).
  6. Equipment such as casts, restraints, traction devices, etc.
  7. Obesity, diabetes mellitus, low diastolic BP (less than 60 mmHg).

B. Risk assessment instruments.
  1. Braden scale.
    a. Scores six subscales: sensory perception, moisture, activity–mobility, nutrition, friction, and shear.
    b. Total score range is 6 to 23.
      (1) A score of 18 = at risk.
      (2) A score of 12 or less = high risk for development of a pressure ulcer.
    c. Most reliable and most often used assessment scale for pressure ulcer risk.
  2. Pressure Ulcer Scale for Healing (PUSH Tool).
    a. Developed by the National Pressure Ulcer Advisory Panel (NPUAP) as a quick, reliable tool to monitor the change in pressure ulcer status over time.
    b. Ulcers are categorized according to size of the wound, exudate, and degree of tissue involvement.
    c. Monitor scoring over time: 0 = healed; 17 = not healed.

C. Clinical manifestations (Table 13-2).

### Treatment

A. Medical and surgical.
  1. Debridement: initial care is to remove moist, devitalized tissue.
    a. Surgical debridement: use of a scalpel or other instrument; used primarily when there is a large amount of nonviable tissue present.

**Table 13-2 STAGES OF PRESSURE INJURY**

| *Definition* | *Diagram* |
| --- | --- |

### Stage 1: Nonblanchable Erythema of Intact Skin

Intact skin with a localized area of nonblanchable erythema, which may appear differently in darkly pigmented skin. Presence of blanchable erythema or changes in sensation, temperature, or firmness may precede visual changes. Color changes do not include purple or maroon discoloration; these may indicate deep tissue pressure injury.

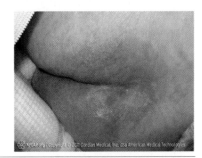

### Stage 2: Partial-Thickness Skin Loss with Exposed Dermis

Partial-thickness loss of skin with exposed dermis. The wound bed is viable, pink or red, moist, and may also present as an intact or ruptured serum-filled blister. Adipose (fat) is not visible and deeper tissues are not visible. Granulation tissue, slough and eschar are not present. These injuries commonly result from adverse microclimate and shear in the skin over the pelvis and shear in the heel. This stage should not be used to describe moisture associated skin damage (MASD) including incontinence associated dermatitis (IAD), intertriginous dermatitis (ITD), medical adhesive related skin injury (MARSI), or traumatic wounds (skin tears, burns, abrasions).

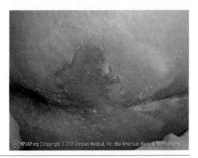

### Stage 3: Full-Thickness Skin Loss

Full-thickness loss of skin, in which adipose (fat) is visible in the ulcer and granulation tissue and epibole (rolled wound edges) are often present. Slough and/or eschar may be visible. The depth of tissue damage varies by anatomic location; areas of significant adiposity can develop deep wounds. Undermining and tunneling may occur. Fascia, muscle, tendon, ligament, cartilage and/or bone are not exposed. If slough or eschar obscures the extent of tissue loss this is an Unstageable Pressure Injury.

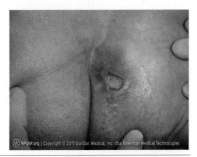

### Stage 4: Full-Thickness Skin and Tissue Loss

Full-thickness skin and tissue loss with exposed or directly palpable fascia, muscle, tendon, ligament, cartilage or bone in the ulcer. Slough and/or eschar may be visible. Epibole (rolled edges), undermining and/or tunneling often occur. Depth varies by anatomic location. If slough or eschar obscures the extent of tissue loss this is an Unstageable Pressure Injury.

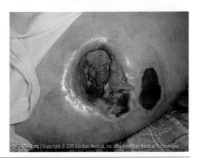

### Unstageable: Obscured Full-Thickness Skin and Tissue Loss

Full-thickness skin and tissue loss in which the extent of tissue damage within the ulcer cannot be confirmed because it is obscured by slough or eschar. If slough or eschar is removed, a stage 3 or stage 4 pressure injury will be revealed. Stable eschar (i.e. dry, adherent, intact without erythema or fluctuance) on the heel or ischemic limb should not be softened or removed.

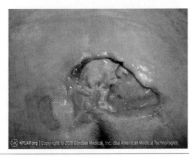

*Continued*

**Table 13-2 STAGES OF PRESSURE INJURY—cont'd**

| *Definition* | *Diagram* |
|---|---|

**Deep Tissue Pressure Injury: Persistent Nonblanchable Deep Red, Maroon, or Purple Discoloration**

Intact or nonintact skin with localized area of persistent nonblanchable deep red, maroon, or purple discoloration or epidermal separation revealing a dark wound bed or blood-filled blister. Pain and temperature change often precede skin color changes. Discoloration may appear differently in darkly pigmented skin. This injury results from intense and/or prolonged pressure and shear forces at the bone-muscle interface. The wound may evolve rapidly to reveal the actual extent of tissue injury, or may resolve without tissue loss. If necrotic tissue, subcutaneous tissue, granulation tissue, fascia, muscle, or other underlying structures are visible, this indicates a full-thickness pressure injury (Unstageable, stage 3, or stage 4). Do not use DTPI to describe vascular, traumatic, neuropathic, or dermatologic conditions.

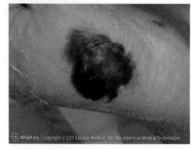

Reprinted with permission from National Pressure Ulcer Advisory Panel: *Updated staging system, 2016.* Available at http://www.npuap.org/resources/educational-and-clinical-resources/pressure-injury-staging-illustrations/

    b. Mechanical debridement: wet-to-dry dressings, hydrotherapy, wound irrigation, and dextranomers (small beads poured over secreting wounds to absorb exudate).

    c. Enzymatic and autolytic debridement: use of enzymes or synthetic dressings that cover wound and self-digest devitalized tissue by the action of enzymes that are present in wound fluids.

  2. Wound cleansing: use normal saline solution for most cases.

    a. Use minimal mechanical force when cleansing to avoid trauma to the wound bed.

    b. Avoid the use of antiseptics (e.g., Dakin's solution, iodine, hydrogen peroxide).

  3. Dressings: (should protect wound, be biocompatible, and hydrate).

    a. Moistened gauze.

    b. Film (transparent).

    c. Hydrocolloid (moisture and oxygen retaining).

    d. Alginate (absorbs exudate).

    e. Impregnated silver dressing (antimicrobial).

    f. Medicinal honey (lowers pH levels in wound, assists in autolytic debridement).

  4. Alternate therapies:

    a. Vacuum-assisted closure (VAC)—uses a wound covering and vacuum device to remove fluids or infectious materials from the wound to enhance healing and promote the growth of granulation tissue.

    b. Electrical stimulation—uses a low-voltage current to stimulate blood supply and promote granulation formation.

    c. Hyperbaric oxygen therapy (HBO)—uses oxygen delivery at high pressure to force concentrated oxygen into the tissue to maximize tissue healing.

    d. Skin substitutes—use of laboratory engineered products. Used as a covering for the wound that is healing or awaiting grafting.

    e. Topical growth factors—facilitate wound healing by stimulating cell development and growth.

> **! NURSING PRIORITY:** Keep the pressure injury tissue moist and the surrounding intact skin dry.

B. Dietary.

  1. Increased carbohydrates and protein.

  2. Increased vitamin C and zinc.

*Nursing Interventions*

**Goal:** To prevent or relieve pressure, stimulate circulation.

A. Frequent change of position; turning frequency individualized based on risk factors, patient condition, and type of mattress; do not position directly on the trochanter.

B. Pressure-relieving mattresses that provide for a continuous change in pressure across the mattress.

C. Memory foam mattresses or gel pads in chairs.

D. Avoid trauma to skin; use lift sheets and/or transfer devices.

E. Keep head of bed elevated less than 30 degrees when in bed.

F. Keep heels off the bed surface.

**Goal:** To keep skin clean and healthy and prevent the occurrence of a pressure injury.

A. Wash skin with mild soap and blot completely dry with soft towel, especially after toileting.

B. Inspect skin frequently, especially over bony prominences and points of pressure.

C. Use moisturizer on dry skin.

D. Keep client well hydrated.

E. Use of topical skin barrier creams, ointments, and pastes.

F. Avoid wrinkles in sheets or clothing that may serve as a source of irritation to the skin.

> **! NURSING PRIORITY:** Avoid massage over bony prominences. When the side-lying position is used in bed, avoid positioning client directly on the trochanter; use the 30-degree lateral inclined position. Do not use donut-type devices. Maintain the head of the bed at or below 30 degrees or at the lowest degree of elevation. Teach chair-bound persons, who are able, to shift weight every 15 minutes.

**Goal:** To promote healing of pressure injury.

A. Specialized support surfaces such as mattresses and cushions.

B. Nutritional supplements. Ensure adequate fluid intake.

C. Wound care dressings.

D. Keep pressure injury area dry.

   1. Minimize skin exposure to moisture caused by incontinence, perspiration, or wound drainage.

   2. Use only underpads or briefs that are made of materials that absorb moisture and provide a quick-drying surface next to the skin.

   3. Use skin barriers to decrease contamination and increase healing of a noninfected ulcer.

   4. Observe the ulcer for signs of infection. Infected ulcers will have to be debrided if healing is to occur.

# SKIN INFECTIONS AND INFESTATIONS
(Figure 13-2)

## Impetigo

**Impetigo is a bacterial skin infection caused by invasion of the epidermis by pathogenic *Staphylococcus aureus* and/or group A beta-hemolytic streptococci.**

### Assessment

A. Pustule-like lesions with moist honey-colored crusts surrounded by redness.

B. Pruritus; spreads to surrounding areas.

C. May appear anywhere on the body but appears most commonly on the face, especially around the mouth.

### Treatment

A. Medical.

   1. Local: topical treatment.

     a. Warm soaks with water or aluminum acetate solution. Gently wash two to three times a day to remove crusts.

     b. Use topical mupirocin antibiotic cream if only a couple of lesions are found.

   2. Systemic antibiotic therapy is the treatment of choice with extensive lesions.

### Home Care

A. Teach the client and family the importance of good handwashing and assure them that lesions heal without scarring.

B. Encourage adherence to therapeutic regimen, especially taking the full course of antibiotics.

C. Untreated impetigo may result in systemic infection and glomerulonephritis.

D. Empirically treat the nares of *Staphylococcus* carriers with mupirocin to prevent spread/reinfection.

## Cellulitis

**Cellulitis is an inflammation of the subcutaneous tissues often occurring after a break in the skin and**

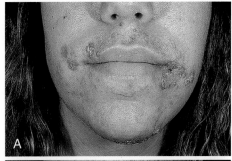

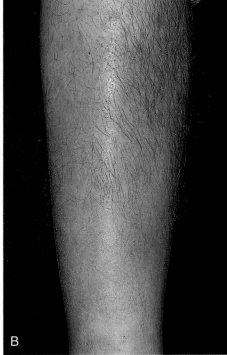

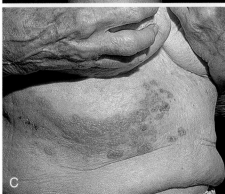

**FIGURE 13-2 Skin Infections. (A)** impetigo; **(B)** cellulitis; **(C)** herpes zoster. (From Habif, T., et al. [2011]. *Skin disease: Diagnosis & treatment* [3rd ed.]. St. Louis, MO: Elsevier.)

**most commonly caused by *Staphylococcus aureus* or *Streptococcus*.**

### Assessment

A. Intense redness, edema with diffuse border, and tenderness; localized warmth.

B. Chills, malaise, and fever.

C. Most common location is the lower legs.

*Treatment*

A. Medical.
1. Moist heat, immobilization, elevation of affected extremity.
2. Systemic antibiotic therapy.

 **Home Care**

A. Teach the client and family the importance of good handwashing.
B. Encourage adherence to therapeutic regimen, especially taking the full course of antibiotics.

 **Fungal (Dermatophyte) Infections**

**The nails, skin, and hair came become infected with fungi because there is a large number of fungi present in the environment.**

*Assessment*

A. Types.
1. Tinea corporis (ringworm): causes a ring-shaped lesion on the skin; temporary hair loss may occur if scalp is affected.
2. Tinea capitis: scaly patches on scalp; areas of alopecia; pruritus.
3. Tinea cruris (jock itch): small, red, scaly patches in the groin area.
4. Tinea pedis (athlete's foot): scaling, maceration, erythema, blistering, and pruritus; usually found between the toes.
5. Tinea unguium (onychomycosis): thickened, crumbling nails (usually toes) with yellowish discoloration.
6. Candidiasis: caused by *Candida albicans*, known as moniliasis or thrush, may affect oral mucosa, vulvovaginal, and rectal areas; causes white plaques in mouth; diffuse red rash with satellite lesions on skin.

*Treatment*

A. Topical antifungal cream (see Appendix 13-2).
B. Oral antifungal medication.
C. Systemic therapy: griseofulvin; used primarily for extensive cases.

 **Home Care**

A. To prevent athlete's foot, client should be instructed to keep feet as dry as possible and wear socks made of absorbent cotton.
1. Talcum powder or antifungal powder may be used; tolnaftate may be applied twice daily.
2. Encourage aeration of shoes to allow them to completely dry out.
B. Client should maintain hygienic measures to prevent the spread of fungal diseases, specifically ringworm of the scalp.
1. Family members should avoid using the same comb or hairbrush.
2. Scarves and hats should be washed thoroughly.
3. Examine family and household pets frequently for symptoms of the disease.

 **Parasite Infestations**

**Parasites are organisms that live off other organisms, or hosts, to survive and obtain their food from or at the expense of the host. Some parasite infections/infestations are easy to treat and others are not.**

A. Pediculosis.
1. Types.
a. *Pediculus humanus capitis:* head lice.
b. *Pediculus humanus corporis:* body lice.
c. *Phthirus pubis:* pubic lice or crabs.
2. Clinical manifestations.
a. Intense pruritus, which may lead to secondary excoriation and infection.
b. Lesions vary by species: head lice (red, noninflammatory papules), body lice (urticarial papule), and pubic lice (gray–blue lesions).
c. Eggs (nits) of both head and body lice are often attached to the hair shafts.
d. Pubic lice are often spread by sexual contact.
B. Scabies: an infestation of the skin by *Sarcoptes scabiei* mites.
1. Intense itching, especially at night.
2. Burrows are seen, especially between fingers, on the surfaces of wrists, and in axillary folds.
3. Redness, swelling, and vesicular formation may be noted.
C. Bedbugs: an infestation caused by the *Cimex lectularius.*
1. Does not live on the human body but survives by feeding on human blood.
2. Bites resemble a mosquito or flea bite, wheal surrounded by a flare, and cause intense itching.

*Treatment*

A. Pediculosis.
1. Permethrin 1% liquid: effective against nits and lice with just one application; shampoo hair first, leave Nix on hair for 10 minutes, rinse off; may repeat in 7 days.
2. Pyrethrin compounds for pubic and head lice.
B. Scabies.
1. Permethrin 5% cream; cream is applied to the skin from head to soles of feet and left on for 8 to 14 hours, then washed off; with a repeat application in 7 days.
C. Bedbugs.
1. Treatment of the bite area is with topical or systemic antihistamines, depending on the extensiveness of the bites.
2. Bedding should be inspected for infestation of the bugs (about the same size, shape, and color of an apple seed).
3. Eradication is by washing clothing and linens in hot water and drying on the hot setting.
4. Bedding and furniture that cannot be washed must be treated by a pest control professional or disposed of.

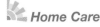 *Home Care*

A. All family members and close contacts need to be treated for parasitic disorders; lice can survive up to 48 hours; nits can hatch in 7 to 10 days when shed in the environment.

B. Bedding and clothing that may have lice or nits should be washed or dry cleaned; furniture and rugs should be vacuumed or treated.

C. Nonwashable items should be sealed in a plastic bag for 14 days if unable to dry clean or vacuum.

D. Nurses should wear gloves when examining scalp to prevent spread to others.

E. When shampooing hair, use a fine-tooth comb or tweezers to remove remaining nits.

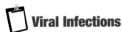 **Viral Infections**

**Viral infections of the skin (similar to body ones) are difficult to treat.**

A. Herpes simplex virus type 1 (HSV-1) (fever blister, cold sore).
   1. Painful local reaction consisting of vesicles with an erythematous base; most often appears around the mouth and/or nose.
   2. Contagious by direct contact; is lifelong and recurrent; there is no immunity.
   3. Chronic disorder that may be exacerbated by stress, trauma, menses, sunlight, fatigue, or systemic infection.
   4. Recurrent episodes are characterized by appearance of lesions in the same place.
   5. Not to be confused with HSV-2, which primarily occurs below the waist (genital herpes).
   6. It is possible for the HSV-1 to cause genital lesions and for HSV-2 to cause oral lesions (see Sexually Transmitted Infections in Chapter 24).

B. Herpes zoster (shingles).
   1. Related to the chickenpox virus: varicella.
   2. Contagious to anyone who has not had chickenpox or who may be immunosuppressed.
   3. Linear patches of vesicles with an erythematous base are located along spinal and cranial nerve tracts, or dermatomes; zosteriform.
   4. Often unilateral and appears on the trunk but may also appear on the face.
   5. Pain, burning, and neuralgia occur at the site before outbreak of vesicles.
   6. Often precipitated by the same factors as herpes simplex infection; incidence increases with age.

*Treatment*

A. Usually symptomatic; application of soothing moist compresses.

B. Analgesics; gabapentin for postherpetic neuralgia; systemic corticosteroids may reduce symptoms.

C. Antiviral agents (see Appendix 13-2).

D. Herpes zoster vaccine is recommended for adults over 60 years regardless of whether they report a prior episode of chickenpox or herpes zoster.

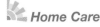 *Home Care*

A. Alleviate pain by administering analgesics.

B. Antihistamines may be administered to control the itching.

C. Usually lesions heal without complications; herpes simplex usually heals without scarring, whereas herpes zoster may cause scarring.

D. If hospitalized, establish contact precautions for herpes zoster.

## NEOPLASMS OF THE INTEGUMENTARY SYSTEM

*Assessment*

A. Risk factors/etiology.
   1. Overexposure to sunlight; indoor tanning.
   2. Fair skin type (blond or red hair and blue or green eyes).
   3. Exposure to chemicals.
   4. Family history of skin cancer.

B. Clinical manifestations.
   1. Actinic keratosis
      a. Most common of all premalignant conditions
      b. Small macules or papules with dry, rough, adherent yellow or brown scales; irregular shape.
      c. Appears on face, neck, back of hand, and forearm.
      d. May slowly progress to squamous cell carcinoma.
   2. Basal cell carcinoma.
      a. Most common type of skin malignancy.
      b. Appears as a small, waxy nodule with a translucent pearly border.
      c. Appears more frequently on the face, usually between the hairline and upper lip.
      d. Rarely metastasize.
   3. Squamous cell carcinoma.
      a. Usually follows excessive sun exposure, irradiation, or trauma causing scarring.
      b. May metastasize.
      c. Appears as an opaque firm nodule (dome-shaped) with an indistinct border, scaling, and ulceration.
      d. Increased risk in immunocompromised and renal transplants.
   4. Malignant melanoma (Figure 13-3).
      a. Some genetic predisposition; also known to be related to UV exposure without protection or overexposure to artificial light (tanning beds).
      b. Highest mortality rate of any form of skin cancer.
      c. Common sites include back and legs in women, and trunk, head, and neck in men.
      d. Characterized by a sudden or progressive change in size, symmetry, color, elevation, or shape of a mole.
      e. Often dark brown or black in color.
      f. Can metastasize to any organ, including brain and heart.

# MALIGNANT MELANOMA
## (SIGNS OF)

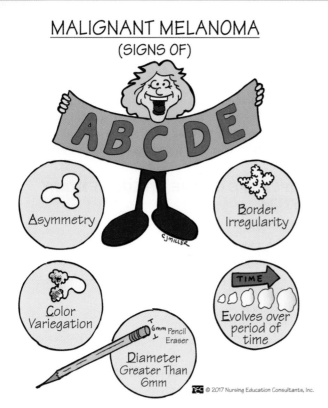

**FIGURE 13-3 Malignant Melanoma.** (From Zerwekh, J., Garneau, A., & Miller, C. J. [2017]. *Digital collection of the memory notebooks of nursing* [4th ed.]. Chandler, AZ: Nursing Education Consultants, Inc.)

## Treatment

A. Medical.
 1. Radiation therapy.
 2. Chemotherapy.
 3. Biological therapy.
B. Surgical.
 1. Excisional surgery/skin grafts.
  a. All suspicious lesions should be biopsied.
  b. Mohs procedure: a specialized form of excision used primarily to treat basal cell and squamous cell cancers; skin grafts may be required because of the extensiveness of the excision.
 2. Laser treatment.
 3. Cryosurgery.

## Nursing Interventions

**Goal:** To assist the client in understanding the disease process, the importance of follow-up treatment, and measures to maintain health.

A. Teach the importance of avoiding unnecessary exposure to sunlight.
B. Apply protective sunscreen when outside (Figure 13-4).
C. Teach the warning signs of cancer.
D. Treat moles found in areas where there is friction or repeated irritation.

**Goal:** To support the client and promote psychological homeostasis.

A. Allow for verbalization of fear and anxiety.

# SUNSCREENS

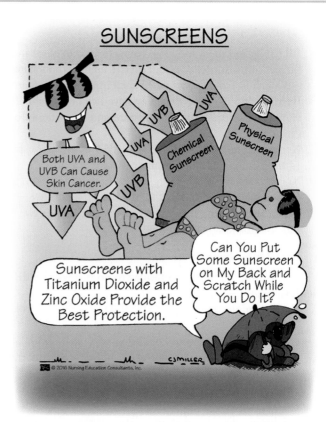

**FIGURE 13-4 Sunscreen.** (From Zerwekh, J., Garneau, A., & Miller, C. J. [2017]. *Digital collection of the memory notebooks of nursing* [4th ed.]. Chandler, AZ: Nursing Education Consultants, Inc.)

B. Encourage verbalization relating to altered body image when large, wide, full-thickness excisions must be made to treat malignant melanoma.
C. Point out client's resources and support effective coping mechanisms.
D. Teach the importance of examining and checking moles and any new lesions (Figure 13-5).

## ELECTIVE COSMETIC/RECONSTRUCTION PROCEDURES

A. Purpose: to improve self-image.
B. Types of elective cosmetic surgery.
 1. Chemical facelift or peel: superficial destruction of the upper layers of skin with a cauterant solution.
 2. Tretinoin and alpha-hydroxy acids: topical application provides reversal of photodamaged skin and normal aging by influencing epithelial cell growth and differentiation.
 3. Microdermabrasion: removal of epidermis to treat acne, scars, wrinkles, etc.
 4. Botulinum toxin injection: neurotoxin that causes temporary interference with neuromuscular transmission, paralyzing the affected muscle.
 5. Facelift (rhytidectomy): lifting and repositioning of facial and neck tissues
 6. Dermal fillers: injection of hyaluronic acid filler to smooth away wrinkles around mouth and nose.

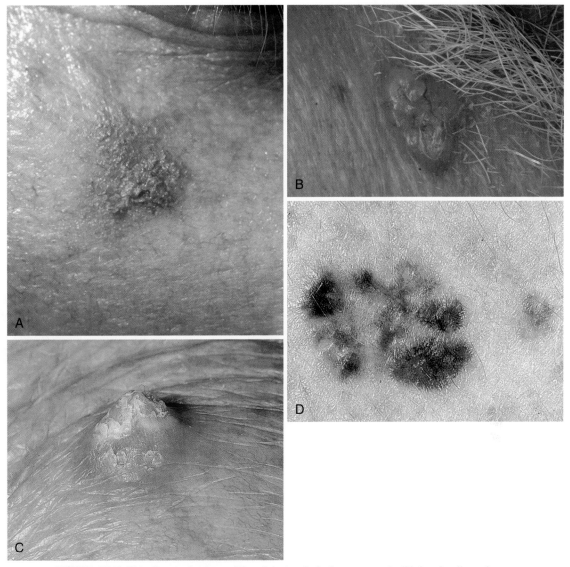

**FIGURE 13-5 Skin Cancer Lesions. (A)** actinic keratosis (precancerous); **(B)** basal cell carcinoma; **(C)** squamous cell carcinoma; **(D)** malignant melanoma (superficial spreading). (From Habif, T., et al. [2011]. *Skin disease: Diagnosis & treatment* [3rd ed.]. St. Louis, MO: Elsevier.)

7. Eyelid lift (blepharoplasty): removal of redundant (excess) eyelid tissue.
8. Liposuction: technique for removing subcutaneous fat from face and body.

*Nursing Interventions*

**Goal:** To provide preoperative care.

A. Reinforce information from informed consent obtained by the physician.
B. Instruct the client to avoid taking vitamin E, nonsteroidal antiinflammatory agents, and aspirin at least 1 week before surgery to prevent bleeding.
C. Explain that wound healing and final results may not be complete until 1 year after procedure.

**Goal:** To provide postoperative care.

A. Administer analgesics for pain management.
B. Observe for bleeding.

C. Teach the client signs and symptoms of infection.
D. Instruct the client to avoid all tobacco products for several weeks after surgery because they constrict blood vessels and delay healing.
E. Teach the client who had a chemical peel to avoid the sun for 6 months to prevent hyperpigmentation, because a reduction of melanin in the skin occurs as a result of the procedure.
F. Teach the client who has liposuction to wear spandex compression garments to reduce the risk of bleeding and to prevent fluid accumulation.

## CRITICAL CARE NURSING

## PRIORITY CONCEPTS

Fluid and Electrolytes, Pain, Tissue Integrity

# BURNS

A. Types of burns.
1. Thermal injury: most common type of burn injury; results from flames, flash (explosion), scald, or direct contact with hot object.
2. Electrical injury: intense heat is generated from electrical current and causes coagulation necrosis as current flows through the body.
3. Chemical injury: results from contact with a corrosive substance.
4. Smoke, inhalation injury, and noxious chemicals.
   a. Inhalation of smoke or superheated air causes swelling and/or occlusion of airway.
   b. Inhalation of carbon monoxide combines with hemoglobin, thereby decreasing availability of oxygen to cells, resulting in hypoxia.

## Assessment

A. Respiratory—determine circumstances surrounding injury: did fire occur in an enclosed space, is there a risk for an inhalation injury?
1. Assess for burns on the face and in the mouth.
2. Examine mouth and sputum for black particles and the nasal septum for edema.
3. Assess for change in respiratory pattern indicating impending respiratory obstruction.
   a. Increased hoarseness
   b. Drooling or difficulty swallowing.
   c. Audible wheezing, crackles, presence of stridor.
4. Assess for development of carbon monoxide poisoning.
   a. Mild: headache, decreased vision.
   b. Moderate: tinnitus, drowsiness, vertigo, altered mental state, decreased blood pressure, "cherry red" color from vasodilation.
B. Evaluate cardiac output and peripheral circulation.
1. Hypovolemic shock may occur early.
2. Sludging (intravascular agglutination) may result from massive fluid shift.
3. Peripheral circulation may be impaired by circumferential burns or edema.
4. Assess these metrics: mean arterial pressure (MAP) greater than 65 mmHg, systolic pressure above 90 mmHg, and pulse less than 120 beats/minute.
C. Determine hydration status.
1. Monitor for acute tubular necrosis.
2. Monitor urine output (should be at least 0.5–1 mL/kg/hr in older children and adults; 1–2 mL/kg/hr in children weighing less than 66 lb [30 kg]).
3. Fluid shift and edema formation occur within first 12 hours post burn and can continue 24 to 36 hours after burn injury.
4. Fluid mobilization and diuresis occur 48 to 72 hours postburn when the capillary integrity is restored.
D. Determine tetanus immunization status.

> **! NURSING PRIORITY:** The client with a burn injury is often awake, mentally alert, and cooperative at first. The level of consciousness may change as respiratory status deteriorates or as the fluid shift occurs, precipitating hypovolemia.

E. Determine the severity of the burn injury (Box 13-2, Figure 13-6).
1. Extent of burn surface (burn surface area)
   a. Rule of nines: generally used for quick estimation in adults and estimation in children.
   b. A more accurate determination uses charts that calculate the total body surface area burned and the depth of the burn based on age of the client (e.g., Lund-Browder chart or Sage Burn Diagram) (Figures 13-7 and 13-8).
2. Area of burn.
   a. Circumferential burns (burns surrounding an entire extremity) may cause severe reduction of circulation to an extremity as a result of edema

---

**Box 13-2    DEPTH OF BURNS**

- *Superficial partial-thickness or first-degree burn:* Area is reddened and blanches with pressure; no edema is present; the area is generally painful to touch.
- *Deep partial-thickness or second-degree burn:* Dermis and epidermis are affected; large, thick-walled blisters form; underlying skin is erythematous; these burns are painful.
- *Full-thickness or third- and fourth-degree burn:* All dermis skin layers are destroyed; subcutaneous tissue and muscle may be damaged; burn usually has a dry appearance, may be white or charred; it will require skin grafting to cover the area; fourth degree involves underlying structures (fascia, tendons, and bones), which are severely damaged, usually blackened.

---

### DEGREE OF BURN BY TISSUE LAYER

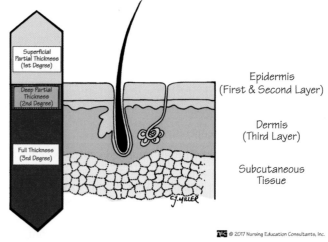

**FIGURE 13-6 Degree of Burn by Tissue Layer.** (From Zerwekh, J., Garneau, A., & Miller, C. J. [2017]. *Digital collection of the memory notebooks of nursing* [4th ed.]. Chandler, AZ: Nursing Education Consultants, Inc.)

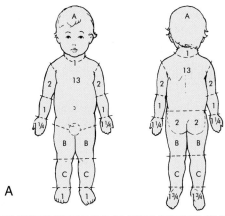

**RELATIVE PERCENTAGES OF AREAS AFFECTED BY GROWTH**

| AREA | BIRTH | AGE 1 YR | AGE 5 YR |
|---|---|---|---|
| A = ½ of head | 9½ | 8½ | 6½ |
| B = ½ of one thigh | 2¾ | 3¼ | 4 |
| C = ½ of one leg | 2½ | 2½ | 2¾ |

A

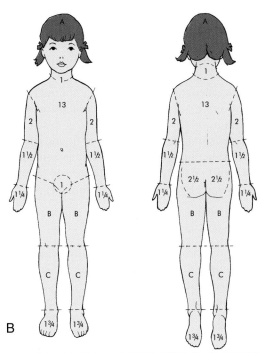

**RELATIVE PERCENTAGES OF AREAS AFFECTED BY GROWTH**

| AREA | AGE 10 YR | AGE 15 YR | ADULT |
|---|---|---|---|
| A = ½ of head | 5½ | 4½ | 3½ |
| B = ½ of one thigh | 4½ | 4½ | 4¾ |
| C = ½ of one leg | 3 | 3¼ | 3½ |

B

**FIGURE 13-7 Estimation of Distribution of Burns in Children.** (A) Children from birth to 5 years. (B) Older children. (From Hockenberry, M. J., & Wilson, D. [2015]. *Wong's essentials of pediatric nursing* [10th ed.]. St. Louis, MO: Elsevier/Mosby.)

formation and lack of elasticity of the eschar, leading to compartmental syndrome.
   b. The location of the burn is related to the severity of the injury:
      (1) Face, neck, chest; respiratory obstruction.
      (2) Hands, feet, joints, and eyes; self-care.
      (3) Ears, nose, genital area; infection.

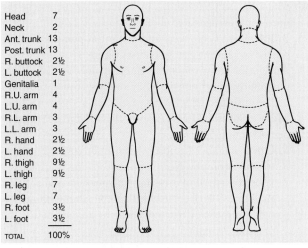

| | |
|---|---|
| Head | 7 |
| Neck | 2 |
| Ant. trunk | 13 |
| Post. trunk | 13 |
| R. buttock | 2½ |
| L. buttock | 2½ |
| Genitalia | 1 |
| R.U. arm | 4 |
| L.U. arm | 4 |
| R.L. arm | 3 |
| L.L. arm | 3 |
| R. hand | 2½ |
| L. hand | 2½ |
| R. thigh | 9½ |
| L. thigh | 9½ |
| R. leg | 7 |
| L. leg | 7 |
| R. foot | 3½ |
| L. foot | 3½ |
| TOTAL | 100% |

**FIGURE 13-8 Lund-Browder Chart.** (From Lewis, S. L., et al. [2017]. *Medical-surgical nursing: Assessment and management of clinical problems* [10th ed.]. St. Louis, MO: Mosby.)

3. Age.
   a. Infants have an immature immune system and poor body defense.
   b. Older adult clients heal more slowly and are more likely to have wound infection problems and pulmonary complications.
4. Presence of other health problems: diabetes and peripheral vascular disease delay wound healing.

*Treatment*

A. Respiratory status takes priority over the treatment of the burn injury. Prophylactic intubation may be performed if inhalation injury is suspected.
B. If the burn area is small (less than approximately 10% body surface area), apply cool compresses or immerse injured area in cool water to decrease heat; ice should not be directly applied to the burn area.
C. Administer tetanus immunization if more than 5 years since last injection.
D. Do not put any ointment or salves on the burn area.
E. If the cause of the burn is chemical, remove all clothing and brush all dry chemicals off the skin before thoroughly flushing the area with large amounts of cool water.
F. Fluid resuscitation.
   1. Used for clients with burns on 15% to 20% or more of body surface area.
   2. Placement of large-bore intravenous catheters.
   3. Fluid replacement: calculation of fluid replacement begins from time of burn, not time of admission to the emergency department.
      a. One-half of first 24-hour fluid replacement amounts given during first 8 hours after burn injury.
      b. One-fourth of remaining amount is given during the second and third 8-hour periods.
      c. Urine output is the most sensitive indicator of fluid status; fluid replacement may be titrated to keep urine output adequate for age of the client.

G. Maintain NPO (nothing by mouth) status; assess the need for a nasogastric tube.

H. Intravenous $H_2$ blockers and/or proton pump inhibitors started to prevent gastric (stress) ulcers.

I. Analgesics are given intravenously; do not give intramuscularly, subcutaneously, or orally because they will not be absorbed effectively.

J. Methods of wound care (area is cleaned and debrided of necrotic burned tissue).

1. Open method (exposure): burn is covered with a topical antibiotic cream and no dressing is applied.
2. Closed method of dressing: fine mesh is used to cover the burned surface; may be impregnated with antibiotic ointment or ointment may be applied before the dressing is applied.
3. Escharotomy: procedure involves excision through the eschar to increase circulation to an extremity with circumferential burns.
4. Enzymatic debriders: collagenase, fibrinolysin, and Accuzyme may be used.
5. Wound grafting: as eschar is debrided and granulation tissue begins to form, grafts are used to protect the wound and to promote healing.

K. Nutritional support.

1. Diet is high in calories and protein.
2. In clients who have large burn surface areas, supplemental gastric tube feedings or hyperalimentation may be used.

### Nursing Interventions

**Goal:** To maintain patent airway and prevent hypoxia.

A. Anticipate respiratory difficulty if there are any indications of inhalation injury.

1. Remain with client; frequent assessment of respiratory status.
2. Supplemental oxygen.
3. Be prepared to intubate client: airway edema can occur rapidly.
4. Assess airway as fluid resuscitation begins; may precipitate more edema.

B. Assess for carbon monoxide poisoning.

C. Anticipate transfer to burn unit if burns cover more than 15% to 20% of body surface area, depending on depth of burn, age of client, and presence of other chronic illnesses.

**Goal:** To evaluate fluid status and determine circulatory status and adequacy of fluid replacement.

A. Obtain client's weight on admission.

B. Assess status and time frame of fluid resuscitation; *calculation of fluid replacement begins at time of burn injury, not on arrival at hospital.*

 C. Evaluate renal status and urine output; adequate output: adults 0.5 to 1 mL/kg/hr, children 1 to 2 mL/kg/hr.

**Goal:** To prevent or decrease infection.

A. Implement infection control procedures to protect the client.

B. After eschar sloughs or is removed, assess wound for infection; infection is difficult to identify before the eschar sloughs.

**Goal:** To maintain nutrition and promote positive nitrogen balance for healing.

A. Work with dietitian to maintain nutritional intake.

B. Provide tube feedings as indicated.

C. Care of total parenteral nutrition as indicated (see Appendix 20-5).

D. Daily weight.

**Goal:** To prevent contractures and scarring.

A. Assist client to attempt mobilization and ambulation as soon as possible.

B. Passive and active range of motion should be initiated from the beginning of burn therapy and throughout therapy.

C. Position client to prevent flexion contractures; position of comfort for the client may increase contracture formation.

D. Use splints and exercises to prevent flexion contractures.

E. Use pressure dressings and garments to contour healing burn area to keep scars flat and prevent elevation and enlargement above the original burn injury area.

**Goal:** To promote acceptance and adaptation to alterations in body image.

A. Employ counselors and resource team members.

B. Maintain open communication and encourage expression of feelings.

C. Anticipate depression as a normal consequence of burn trauma; it should decrease as condition improves.

> **⚠ NURSING PRIORITY:** It is important to recognize that the client's anger is not a direct attack on the care provider; it is an expression of grief and sorrow.

### Home Care

A. Physical therapy.

B. Continue high-calorie, high-protein diet.

C. Wound care management.

D. Avoid exposure of burn area to direct sunlight and irritating agents.

## Appendix 13-1   SKIN DIAGNOSTIC STUDIES

**Skin Testing:** Purpose: to confirm sensitivity to a specific allergen by placing antigen on or directly below skin (intradermal) to check for presence of antibodies.

1. Three methods—allergen applied to arms or back and injected at a 15 degree angle.
   - Cutaneous scratch test (also known as a *tine* or *prick test*): allergen applied to a superficial scratch on skin.
   - Intradermal injection: small amount of the allergen is injected intradermally in rows; more accurate; high risk for severe allergic reaction; used only for those who do not react to cutaneous method.
   - Patch test: used to determine whether client is allergic to testing material (small amount applied on back)—client returns in 48 hours for evaluation.
2. Interpreting results.
   - *Immediate* reaction: appears within minutes after the injection; marked by erythema and a wheal; denotes a positive reaction.
   - *Positive* reaction: indicates an antibody response to previous exposure; local wheal-and-flare response occurs.
   - *Negative* reaction: inconclusive; may indicate that antibodies have not formed yet or that antigen was deposited too deeply in skin (not an intradermal injection); may also indicate immunosuppression.
3. Complications: range from minor itching to anaphylaxis (see Chapter 10).

> **! NURSING PRIORITY:** Never leave the client alone during skin testing, because of the risk for anaphylaxis. If a severe reaction occurs, anticipate antiinflammatory topical cream applied to skin site (scratch test) or a tourniquet applied to the arm (intracutaneous test) and possible oral antihistamines and/or epinephrine injection.

**Wood's Lamp (Black Light):** Purpose: examination of skin with long-wave ultraviolet light that causes specific substances or areas to fluoresce (e.g., *Pseudomonas* species, fungi, patches of vitiligo).

**Biopsy:** Purpose: to determine specific diagnoses and/or malignancy.

Types: punch, excisional, incisional, shave.
1. Verify if informed consent is needed.
2. Apply dressing and give postprocedure instructions—watch for bleeding.

**Skin Culture:** Purpose: identify fungal, bacterial, and viral organisms.

1. Scrap or swab affected area, label specimen, and send to laboratory.

**Microscopic Tests:** Potassium hydroxide (KOH)—identifies fungal infection.

- Tzanck test—diagnoses of herpes infections.
- Mineral oil slides—diagnoses of infestations.
- Immunofluorescence—identifying abnormal antibody proteins (can also be a serum test).

## Appendix 13-2   MEDICATIONS

### Medications Used in Skin Disorders

#### *General Nursing Implications*
- Topical medications are used primarily for local effects when systemic absorption is undesirable.
- For topical application:
  - Apply after shower or bath for best absorption because skin is hydrated.
  - Apply small amount of medication and rub in well.
  - Always wear gloves when applying topical agents

**Antifungal:** Inhibits or damages fungal cell membrane, either altering permeability or disrupting cell mitosis.

| *Medications* | *Side Effects* | *Nursing Implications* |
|---|---|---|
| Clotrimazole: topical and intravaginal<br>Miconazole: intravaginal<br>Nystatin: topical<br>Ketoconazole: PO, topical<br>Griseofulvin: PO<br>Terbinafine: topical | Nausea, vomiting, abdominal pain<br>Hypersensitivity reaction: rash, urticaria, pruritus<br>Hepatotoxicity<br>Gynecomastia (ketoconazole) | 1. Monitor hepatic function (when oral medication is given).<br>2. Avoid alcohol because of potential liver problems.<br>3. Check for local burning, irritation, or itching with topical application.<br>4. Prolonged therapy (weeks or months) is usually necessary, especially with griseofulvin.<br>5. Take griseofulvin with foods high in fat (e.g., milk, ice cream) to decrease GI upset and assist in absorption.<br>6. *Uses:* tinea infections, fungal infections, candidiasis, diaper dermatitis |

*Continued*

## Appendix 13-2 MEDICATIONS—cont'd

| Medications | Side Effects | Nursing Implications |
|---|---|---|
| **Antiviral:** Inhibits viral replication, thereby reducing pain and healing time. | | |
| Acyclovir: topical, PO, IV, topical<br>Valacyclovir: PO<br>Penciclovir: topical<br>Vidarabine: IV, ophthalmic<br>Docosanol: topical<br>Famciclovir: PO | Dizziness, headaches, phlebitis, rash, hives, nausea, vomiting, diarrhea<br>Topical: burning, stinging, pruritus<br>Ophthalmic: burning, itching | 1. Apply topically to affected area six times per day.<br>2. Avoid autoinoculation; wash hands frequently; apply with gloved hand.<br>3. Avoid sexual intercourse while genital lesions are present.<br>4. Maintain adequate fluid intake.<br>5. Treatment should be started at first sign of outbreak (even if in prodromal period).<br>6. Treatment is NOT a cure; it only reduces duration of episodes.<br>7. *Uses:* herpes infections. |
| **Antiinflammatory:** Decreases the inflammatory response. | | |
| Super High Potent<br>Clobetasol propionate .05%<br>Mid-Strength<br>Triamcinolone acetonide 0.1%: topical<br>Low-Potency<br>Hydrocortisone 1% | Skin thinning, superficial dilated blood vessels (telangiectasis), acne-like eruptions, adrenal suppression | 1. Topical steroids come in various strengths and potency. Watch the class and the percent strength. Super high potency is the highest concentration.<br>2. Apply 2–3 times a day.<br>3. Use an occlusive dressing only if ordered.<br>4. Encourage client to use the least amount possible and for the shortest period of time. |
| **Immunosuppressant:** Suppresses T cells and decreases release of inflammatory mediators to decrease severity of atopic dermatitis. | | |
| Pimecrolimus cream: topical<br>Tacrolimus ointment: topical | Increased risk of skin cancer/lymphoma<br>Burning sensation at application site | 1. Teach clients to use sunscreen because medication makes client sensitized to UV light. |
| **Topical Antibiotics:** Prevent and treat infection at the burn site. | | |
| Silver sulfadiazine | Hypersensitivity: rash, itching, or burning sensation in unburned skin | 1. Liberal amounts are spread topically with a sterile, gloved hand or on impregnated gauze rolls over the burned surface.<br>2. If discoloration occurs in the silver sulfadiazine cream, do not use.<br>3. A thin layer of cream is spread evenly over the entire burn surface area; reapplication is done every 12 hours.<br>4. Client should be bathed, "tubbed," or showered daily to aid in debridement.<br>5. Medication does not penetrate eschar.<br>6. For clients with extensive burns, monitor urine output and renal function; a significant amount of sulfa may be absorbed.<br>7. Contraindicated in clients with allergy to sulfonamides. |
| Mafenide acetate | Pain, burning, or stinging at application sites; excessive loss of body water; excoriation of new tissue; may be systemically absorbed and cause metabolic acidosis | 1. Bacteriostatic medication diffuses rapidly through burned skin and eschar and is effective against bacteria under the eschar.<br>2. Dressings are not required but are frequently used. A thin layer of cream is spread evenly over the entire burn surface.<br>3. Monitor renal function and possible acidosis because medication is rapidly absorbed from the burn surface and eliminated via the kidneys.<br>4. Pain occurs on application.<br>5. Watch for hyperventilation, as a compensatory mechanism when acidosis occurs. |

*GI,* Gastrointestinal; *IV,* intravenously; *PO,* by mouth (orally).

More questions on evolve

# Study Questions
## Integumentary: Care of Adult and Pediatric Clients

1. A client has extensive burns with eschar on the anterior trunk. What is the nurse's primary concern regarding eschar formation?
   1. It prevents fluid remobilization in the first 48 hours after burn trauma.
   2. Infection is difficult to assess before the eschar sloughs.
   3. It restricts the ability of the client to move about.
   4. Circulation to the extremities is diminished because of edema formation.

2. A client comes to the outpatient clinic with impetigo on his left arm. What information would the nurse give this client?
   1. Apply antibiotic ointment to the crusted lesions.
   2. Wash the lesions with soap and water and then apply a steroid ointment.
   3. Soak the scabs off the lesions and apply an antibiotic ointment.
   4. Wash the lesions with hydrogen peroxide and apply an antifungal cream.

3. A teacher notifies the school nurse that many of the students in her third-grade class have been scratching their heads and complaining of intense itching of the scalp. The nurse notices tiny white material at the base of a student's hair shaft. What condition does this assessment reflect?
   1. Tinea capitis
   2. Pediculosis capitis
   3. Dandruff
   4. Scabies

4. What is the type of skin cancer that is most difficult to treat?
   1. Dysplastic nevi
   2. Malignant melanoma
   3. Basal cell epithelioma
   4. Squamous cell epithelioma

5. An older adult client has an open wound over the coccyx that extends through the dermis and subcutaneous tissue, exposing the deep fascia. The wound edges are distinct, and the wound bed is a pink–red color. There is no bruising or sloughing. The nurse would correctly document this ulcer as what stage?
   1. Stage I
   2. Stage II
   3. Stage III
   4. Stage IV

6. The nurse understands that scaling around the toes, blistering, and pruritus is characteristic of what condition?
   1. Eczema
   2. Psoriasis
   3. Tinea pedis
   4. Pediculosis corporis

7. What physical characteristics of a client would place the client at highest risk for development of malignant melanoma?
   1. Light to pale skin, blond hair, blue eyes
   2. Olive complexion, oily skin, dark eyes
   3. Dark skin with freckles, dry flaky skin, hazel eyes
   4. Coarse skin, ruddy complexion, brown eyes

8. Herpes zoster has been diagnosed in an older adult client. What will the nursing management include?
   1. Apply antifungal cream to the areas daily.
   2. Maintain client on contact precautions.
   3. Instruct on the need for sexual abstinence.
   4. Closely inspect the perineal area for lesions.

9. Which nursing interventions will assist in reducing pressure points that may lead to pressure ulcers? **Select all that apply:**
   1. Position the client directly on the trochanter when side-lying.
   2. Avoid the use of donut-type devices.
   3. Massage bony prominences.
   4. Elevate the head of the bed no more than 30 degrees when possible.
   5. When the client is side-lying, use the 30-degree lateral inclined position.
   6. Avoid uninterrupted sitting in any chair or wheelchair.

10. The nurse is teaching self-care to an older adult client. What would the nurse encourage the client do for his dry, itchy skin?
    1. Apply a moisturizer on all dry areas daily.
    2. Shower twice a day with a mild soap.
    3. Use a pumice stone and exfoliating sponge on areas to remove dry scaly patches.
    4. Wear protective pads on areas that show the most dryness.

11. What is the priority assessment finding for a client who has sustained burns on the face and neck?
    1. Spreading, large, clear vesicles
    2. Increased hoarseness
    3. Difficulty with vision
    4. Increased thirst

12. A client has sustained a third-degree burn. What would the nurse expect to find during assessment of the burn?
    1. Area reddened, blanches with pressure, no edema
    2. Blackened skin and underlying structures
    3. Thick, clear blisters, underlying skin edematous and erythematous
    4. Dry white, charred appearance, damage to subcutaneous tissues

# Answers to Study Questions

1. *2*
The primary concern would be watching for infection, because the eschar makes it difficult to visually examine the healing skin. Removal of the eschar enhances healing and prevents infection, which occurs because of the moist, enclosed area under the eschar. Eschar formation will not prevent fluid remobilization. It might restrict mobility if the eschar were involving the arm, legs, or joint areas. Circulation to the extremities would not be affected by eschar on the anterior trunk; that would be the case if the eschar were on the extremities. (Lewis et al., 10 ed., p. 443)

2. *3*

Teaching should include the use of warm saline or aluminum acetate soaks followed by soap and water removal of crusts and application of a suitable antibiotic ointment, such as mupirocin (Bactroban). Hydrogen peroxide has little ability to reduce bacteria in wounds and can actually inflame healthy skin cells that surround a lesion, increasing the amount of time the wounds take to heal. Impetigo is caused by group A beta-hemolytic streptococcus or *Staphylococcus* species, which are bacterial and would not be treated by an antifungal cream. If lesions are on the face, a systemic antibiotic also may be given. (Hockenberry & Wilson, 10 ed., p. 226)

3. *2*

Pediculosis capitis (head lice) is characterized by tiny white nits (eggs) that attach to the base of the hair shaft and are highly contagious. Tinea capitis is characterized by a red, scaly, rash with central clearing in the well-defined margins. Dandruff is often mistaken for head lice, but dandruff can be easily removed from the hair shaft. Nits adhere to the hair shaft and are not easy to remove. Scabies form burrows under the skin and cause intense nighttime itching. (Lewis et al., 10 ed., p. 416)

4. *2*

Malignant melanoma is the most difficult to treat; it involves extensive full-thickness skin resections and has the poorest prognosis. Dysplastic nevi are thought to be a precursor of malignant melanoma, although they are not considered malignant in the initial stage. Basal cell epithelioma and squamous cell epithelioma are easier to treat and do not metastasize as does melanoma. (Lewis et al., 10 ed., pp. 411–413)

5. *3*

This is classified as a stage III pressure ulcer because of the full-thickness tissue loss extending to the deep fascia. Subcutaneous fat may be visible, but bone, tendon, or muscle is not exposed. Slough may be present but does not obscure the depth of tissue loss. There may be undermining and tunneling. A stage I pressure ulcer is characterized by intact skin with nonblanchable redness of a localized area usually over a bony prominence. Darkly pigmented skin may not have visible blanching; its color may differ from the surrounding area. A stage II pressure ulcer is characterized by partial-thickness loss of dermis presenting as a shallow, open ulcer with a red–pink wound bed without slough, which also may present as an intact or open/ruptured serum-filled blister. A stage IV pressure ulcer is characterized by full-thickness tissue loss with exposed bone, tendon, or muscle. Slough or eschar may be present on some parts of the wound bed and often includes undermining and tunneling. (Lewis et al 10 ed., p. 173)

6. *3*

Scaling, itching, and redness are common signs of tinea pedis or athlete's foot. Eczema or atopic dermatitis in adults is characterized by reddened lesions in antecubital and popliteal space with pruritus or in children on cheeks, arms, and legs. Psoriasis is a benign condition of the skin where there are silvery scaling plaques on the skin, commonly the elbows, knees, palms, and soles of the feet. Pediculosis corporis is body lice and is a parasitic infection. (Lewis et al., 10 ed., p. 418)

7. *1*

People with light to pale skin and who are excessively exposed to sunlight are most at risk for development of malignant melanoma. Dark-skinned and olive-skinned individuals have more melanin in their skin, which provides a measure of protection from UV exposure. Although those with a ruddy complexion are more prone to development of skin cancers, the coarseness of the skin does provide some protection from the sun's harmful rays. (Lewis et al., 10 ed., p. 411)

8. *2*

Herpes zoster is considered infectious and contact precautions should be used with an older adult client. Antiviral medications would be given instead of antifungal agents. Lesions are usually along the sensory dermatomes (waist, neck, face) and not in the perineal area, which is HSV-2. There is no need for sexual abstinence, although a condom should be worn if contact may occur with the lesions. (Lewis et al., 10 ed., p. 415)

9. *2, 4, 5, 6*

Elevating the head of the bed to 30 degrees or less will decrease the chance of pressure ulcer development from shearing forces. When placing the client in a side-lying position, use the 30 degrees lateral inclined position. Do not place the client directly on the trochanter, which can create pressure over the bony prominence. Avoid the use of donut-shaped cushions because they reduce blood supply to the area, which can lead to extension of the area of ischemia. Bony prominences should not be massaged, because this increases the risk for capillary breakage and injury to underlying tissue leading to pressure ulcer formation. (Ignatavicius & Workman, 8 ed., pp. 436–444)

10. *1*

Dry skin should be moisturized daily and as needed, especially after the client takes a bath. The number of baths and showers should be limited. Exfoliation will remove the dry epidermal layer, but underlying areas also need moisturizing. Protective pads do nothing to provide moisture to dry areas. (Lewis et al., 10 ed., p. 409)

11. *2*

When there is evidence of burns around the face, the airway should be carefully assessed. Increased respiratory rate and hoarseness may be the first sign of respiratory complications. Large, clear vesicles are expected on burns of second degree or worse and are not a sign of a complication. Difficulty with vision may be of concern, but it is not life threatening like respiratory distress. Increased thirst is common in the first few hours after a burn because of fluid shift into the extravascular space. Intubation is often needed within 1 to 2 hours of the injury in burns of the face and neck. (Lewis et al., 10 ed., p. 438)

12. *4*

All of the skin is destroyed in a full-thickness or third-degree burn. Often it has a dry appearance and may be white or charred and usually requires skin grafting to repair. An area reddened that blanches with pressure is indicative of a superficial first-degree burn (partial thickness). Characteristics of a full-thickness fourth-degree burn include blackened skin into underlying muscle and bone structures. Thick, clear blisters, underlying skin edematous and erythematous are characteristics of a deep second-degree burn (partial thickness). (Lewis et al., 10 ed., p. 432)

# Sensory: Care of Adult and Pediatric Clients

# 14

Infection, Safety, Sensory Perception

## THE EYE

## PHYSIOLOGY OF THE EYE

A. Eyes.
  1. External layer.
    a. Sclera: tough, protective covering of the outside of the eye; the "white" of the eye.
    b. Cornea: transparent tissue that covers the front of the eye over the pupil.
    c. Conjunctiva: the thin, transparent mucous membrane that covers the outer surface of the eye and lines the inner surface of the eyelid.
  2. Middle layer.
    a. Choroid: pigmented layer containing large number of blood vessels that nourish the retina.
    b. Ciliary muscle: muscular body that allows the eye to focus through contraction and relaxation.
    c. Ciliary body: produces aqueous humor.
    d. Iris: controls the size of the pupil to regulate the amount of light that enters the eye; gives the eye its characteristic color.
    e. Pupil: the opening in the center of the *iris;* the size of the pupil determines the amount of light that enters the eye.
  3. Inner layer.
    a. Retina: thin innermost lining (or the inside back wall) of the eye; contains millions of light-sensitive nerve cells to coordinate and transmit signals via the optic nerve to the brain; similar to a film in a camera.
    b. Macula: the part of the retina responsible for providing optimum visual focusing.
    c. Aqueous humor: fluid that fills anterior and posterior chambers, circulates through the pupil, and empties into canal of Schlemm.
    d. Trabecula: mesh network through which the aqueous humor fluid drains into the canal of Schlemm.
    e. Vitreous humor: fluid that fills the cavity posterior to the lens.
    f. Crystalline lens: provides for the convergence and refraction of light rays and images onto the retina; enables vision to be focused.

    g. Optic nerve: exits the eye through the retina at the location of the optic disc.
    h. Choroid: blood supply to the retina.
B. Eyelids: protective coverings of the eye.
  1. Conjunctiva: inner lining of the eyelid.
  2. Lacrimal gland: excretes lacrimal fluid (tears) to lubricate, clean, and protect the outer surface of the eye.

### System Assessment

A. External assessment.
  1. Assess position and alignment of the eyes: both eyes should fixate on one visual field simultaneously.
  2. Evaluate for presence of ptosis (drooping eyelids).
  3. Inspect lids and conjunctiva for signs of inflammation such as discharge, erythema, or edema.
  4. Assess eyelids for entropion (turning inward) or ectropion (turning outward).
  5. Assess color of sclera: normally a thin white coating; may yellow with age and with jaundice.
  6. Evaluate size and equality of pupils: both should be equal in size and shape.
  7. Evaluate pupillary reaction to light.
    a. Direct light reflex: constriction of pupil when stimulated with light.
    b. Consensual reflex: constriction of opposite pupil when stimulated with light.
  8. Extraocular muscle function: hold finger or object about 12 inches in front of the eye and ask the client to follow the object with only the movement of the eyes; this helps evaluate for paralysis or weakness in extraocular muscle and cranial nerve function (Figure 14-1).
B. Evaluate visual acuity and check for refractive errors (see Appendix 14-1).
  1. Myopia (nearsightedness): vision for near objects is better than vision for distant objects.
  2. Hyperopia (farsightedness): vision for distant objects is better than vision for near objects.
  3. Assess for any blurred or double vision.
C. Assess for presence of pain and any recent change in vision.

---

**TEST ALERT:** Assist client to cope with sensory impairment (e.g., hearing, sight, etc.).

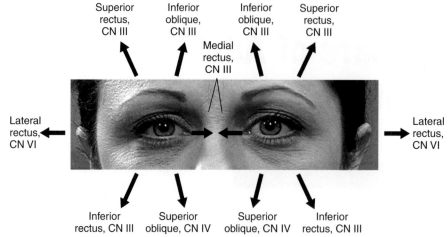

Superior rectus, CN III

Inferior oblique, CN III

Inferior oblique, CN III

Superior rectus, CN III

Medial rectus, CN III

Lateral rectus, CN VI

Lateral rectus, CN VI

Inferior rectus, CN III

Superior oblique, CN IV

Superior oblique, CN IV

Inferior rectus, CN III

**FIGURE 14-1 Extraocular Eye Movements.** (From Ball, J., et al. [2015]. *Seidel's guide to physical examination* [8th ed.]. St. Louis, MO: Elsevier.)

## DISORDERS OF THE EYE

 **Glaucoma**

**Glaucoma is a group of disorders characterized by an increase in intraocular pressure, optic nerve atrophy and progressive loss of peripheral vision. It is an acute or chronic condition and a leading cause of blindness that can be prevented with early detection/treatment.**

### Types

A. Primary open-angle glaucoma (POAG—chronic): most common form.
  1. Flow of aqueous humor is slowed or stopped by obstruction, thus increasing intraocular pressure.
  2. Characterized by a slow onset.
  3. Chronic and progressive peripheral vision loss late in the disease process.
B. Primary angle-closure (PACG—acute) glaucoma.
  1. Rapid increase in intraocular pressure due to a reduction in the outflow of aqueous humor; may also occur in the client with prolonged pupil dilation.
  2. Symptoms occur suddenly, and immediate medical treatment is required because it may cause total blindness within hours to a day.
C. Secondary glaucoma: caused by trauma or optic neoplasm.

### Assessment

A. Risk factors for POAG.
  1. Family history.
  2. Aging—occurs most often in clients more than 40 years of age.
  3. Chronic diseases such as diabetes mellitus.
  4. History of eye injury.
  5. Cataract surgery.
B. Risk factors for PACG.
  1. Anything that causes pupil dilation, such as dark rooms, emotional excitement, or drug-induced mydriasis.

C. Diagnostics: intraocular pressure is greater than 22 mm Hg (see Appendix 14-1).
D. Clinical manifestations of POAG—develop slowly and frequently without symptoms (Figure 14-2).
  1. Gradual loss of peripheral vision (i.e., tunnel vision).
  2. Blindness may occur if untreated.
  3. Central vision is normal, even with loss of peripheral vision.
E. Clinical manifestations of PACG.
  1. Sudden, severe pain in and around the eye.
  2. Nausea and vomiting.
  3. Blurred vision.
  4. Redness of the eye.
  5. Colored halos around lights.

### Treatment

A. Medications (see Appendix 14-2).
  1. Topical (ophthalmic) beta-blockers (can have an additive effect with systemic beta blockers), carbonic anhydrase inhibitors, and alpha adrenergic agonists decrease the amount of aqueous humor produced.
  2. Cholinergics (miotics) and prostaglandin analogs increase the outflow of aqueous humor.
  3. Oral glycerin preparations promote diuresis and lower intraocular pressure.
  4. Medications may be used alone or in combination.
B. Surgical intervention: most often done on outpatient basis with topical anesthetic.
  1. Argon laser trabeculoplasty: microscopic laser burns applied to the trabecula open the fluid channels facilitating outflow of aqueous humor.
  2. Trabeculectomy: creation of an artificial drain to bypass the trabecular meshwork, allowing outflow of aqueous humor.
  3. Laser peripheral iridotomy: may be used for PACG, allowing flow of aqueous humor to occur through a newly created opening in the iris into the normal outflow channels. Permanent change in pupil shape.

# GLAUCOMA
### * Increased Intraocular Pressure & Progressive Vision Loss *

Risk Factors - Familial
- Family History
- Over Age 40
- Diabetes, Hypertension

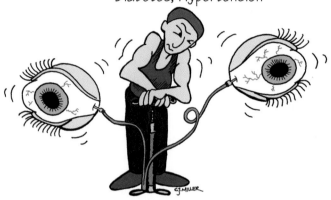

### Primary Open-Angle Glaucoma (POAG)
- Gradual Loss of Peripheral Vision (Tunnel Vision)
- Generally Painless
- Blindness if Untreated
- ↓ Visual Acuity
- ↑ IOP>22mm Hg

© 2017 Nursing Education Consultants, Inc.

**FIGURE 14-2 Glaucoma.** (From Zerwekh, J., Garneau, A., & Miller, C. J. [2017]. *Digital collection of the memory notebooks of nursing* [4th ed.]. Chandler, AZ: Nursing Education Consultants, Inc.)

## Nursing Interventions

**Goal:** To prevent progression of visual impairment.

A. Teaching plan.
1. Explanation of the problem of increased intraocular pressure.
2. Visual damage cannot be corrected, but further damage can be slowed.
3. Correct use of prescribed medications; client must continue to take medication to control disease, otherwise visual problem will progress.
4. Importance of continued follow-up medical care.
5. Advise all health care providers of glaucoma condition.
6. Avoid medications that increase intraocular pressure, such as atropine, antihistamines, and decongestants.
7. Wear medical alert identification.

**Goal:** To decrease intraocular pressure.

A. Avoid straining with defecation, lifting, or stooping.
B. Administer medications to decrease intraocular pressure.

**Goal:** To provide appropriate preoperative nursing measures if surgery is indicated.

A. Surgery and treatments are frequently done on an outpatient basis and with a local anesthetic. Orient the client to the surroundings and sounds that will occur during the procedure.
B. For outpatient surgery, client should wear comfortable clothes and arrange for someone to provide transportation home.
C. Give postoperative instructions to the client or family in writing and verbally clarify any questions the client may have regarding postoperative care.

**Goal:** To prevent client from experiencing postoperative complications (surgery frequently done under local anesthesia).

A. Administer medications: miotics, antibiotics, and steroids.
B. Be sure medication is administered in the eye for which it is ordered; the unaffected eye may be treated with a different medication.
C. Client may eat and ambulate as desired after the initial sedative effect is gone.

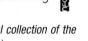 **Home Care**

A. Emphasize the importance of follow-up care.
B. Teach the client not to rub the eyes; wear an eye shield or patch at night to prevent inadvertent rubbing of the eyes.
C. Demonstrate the correct administration of eye medication and have the client return the demonstration.
D. Advise the client to avoid activities that increase intraocular pressure.
E. Teach the client to report pain that is not relieved by prescribed analgesics.

## Cataract

**A cataract is a complete or partial opacity of the lens that compromises the sharpness of images on the retina. It may occur at birth (congenital cataract), but it occurs most commonly in adults past middle age (senile cataracts).**

## Assessment

A. Risk factors.
1. Diabetes mellitus.
2. Corticosteroids: long-term systemic or topical use.

3. Advanced age – due to metabolic changes within the lens.
4. Trauma to the eye.
B. Clinical manifestations.
   1. Painless with gradual decrease in visual acuity, blurry vision.
   2. Pupil appears gray or yellowish brown to milky white.
   3. Red light reflex is distorted on direct ophthalmoscopic examination.
   4. Poor color perception.
   5. Glare due to light scatter on lens; worse at night.
C. Diagnostics (see Appendix 14-1).

### Treatment

A. Nonsurgical: corrective lenses, increased lighting, adaptions in lifestyle.
B. Surgical treatment occurs when palliative measures no longer provide an acceptable level of vision; surgery is usually performed when client begins to experience problems in activities of daily living (Box 14-1). If both eyes require surgical correction, each is treated individually, about 4 to 8 weeks apart.
C. Phacoemulsification (phaco): a small incision is made on the side of the cornea, allowing a tiny probe to be inserted to emit ultrasound, which fragments the lens; cataract is then aspirated.
D. Intraocular lens (IOL) implant is inserted to restore vision.

### Nursing Interventions

**Goal:** To provide appropriate teaching and nursing care.
A. Orient the client to the surroundings and sounds that will occur during the procedure.
B. For outpatient surgery, client should wear comfortable clothes and arrange for someone to provide transportation home.
C. Before surgery, the nurse will instill mydriatic eye drops; frequently, cycloplegic drops also are used; client will be photosensitive; dimming the lighting in the room will help reduce photosensitivity.
D. It is normal for visual acuity to be decreased immediately after surgery.

### Home Care (see Box 14-1)

A. Maintain client's orientation to surroundings.
B. Eye patch may be used for about 24 hours or until the client returns to the physician for a follow-up visit.
C. Client should avoid stooping, lifting, excessive coughing, or straining in the early postoperative period to reduce ocular pressure.
D. Client should avoid sleeping on the affected side.
E. Teach the client to avoid rubbing the affected eye; there should be minimal discomfort, and this is generally relieved by acetaminophen; report any pain that is not easily relieved.
F. Teach client how to administer eye drops (antibiotic and steroid eye drops); have client demonstrate procedure.
G. Provide written instructions; make sure the type is large enough for client to read.

---

**Box 14-1** OLDER ADULT CARE FOCUS

**Promoting Independent Activities of Daily Living for the Client With Diminished Vision**

**Medications**
- When the client is taking several medications, use containers that have different shapes (square, round, triangular).
- Obtain medication boxes with raised letters or numbers on them representing the days of the week.
- Obtain a "talking clock" that states the time or other assistive devices that talk, such as calculator, scales, watches, etc.

**Safety**
- Remove throw rugs.
- Orient the client to his or her environment.
- Increase lighting; avoid glare.
- Use raised buttons on dials of appliances.
- Use unbreakable dishes, cups, and glasses.
- Keep appliance cords short and out of walkways.
- Avoid footstools in favor of a recliner with a built-in footrest.
- Label all cleansers, cleaning fluids, and caustic chemicals with large, raised lettering.
- Have handgrips installed in bathrooms.
- Put nonskid stripping on the surface of the tub floor.
- Encourage use of an electric razor.
- Obtain clearance from a physician before performing hazardous activities such as driving.

**Communication**
- Teach caregivers to always introduce themselves when entering the client's room and before touching the client and let the client know when you leave the room.
- Teach the client to use telephones that have programmable automatic dialing features. Be sure to include emergency phone numbers.
- Recognize that communication is both verbal and nonverbal, therefore frequent clarification of meaning may be required.
- Use printed materials that are high contrast, such as black lettering on white background.
- Leave the client's door open, if appropriate, to facilitate hearing them.

**Daily Living Considerations**
- Provide information on Meals on Wheels for delivery of cooked, ready-to-eat meals.
- Encourage use of a microwave for cooking—it is safer than using a standard stove.
- Encourage the use of large-print books, newspapers, and magazines for reading. Also, many publications are available as audiotapes and CDs at local libraries and vision aid services.
- Avoid rearranging furniture and other belongings.

# Retinal Detachment

Retinal detachment is the separation of the sensory retina and the underlying epithelium, which allows fluid to collect in the space. Untreated symptomatic retinal detachment almost always results in the loss of vision in the eye.

## Assessment

A. Risk factors.
1. Increasing age.
2. Severe myopia (nearsightedness).
3. Trauma, especially to the face or eye.
4. Previous cataract or glaucoma surgery.
5. Family or patient history of retinal detachment.
B. Diagnostics (see Appendix 14-1).
C. Clinical manifestations.
1. Flashes of light, floaters, cobweb, hairnet, or ring in the visual field.
2. Sensation of a curtain, shadow, or ring over a portion of the visual field.
3. Painless loss of peripheral or central vision.

## Treatment

> **⚠ NURSING PRIORITY:** Immediately put the client on bed rest and patch both eyes to prevent further detachment.

A. Surgical repair may be done on an outpatient basis or may require hospitalization.
B. Laser photocoagulation: a laser light beam is used to create inflammation and seal the tear or break.
C. Cryopexy: a "supercooled" probe is directed over the retinal tear to produce inflammation to seal the tear.
D. Scleral buckling: in this extraocular surgery, the sclera is depressed from the outside with the application of a silicone "buckle" to weld the retina in contact with the choroid (Figure 14-3).
E. Intravitreal bubble: injected bubble of gas or oil. Often used in combination with photocoagulation or cryopexy. This treatment requires special positioning of the head postinjection.

## Nursing Interventions

**Goal:** To enable client and significant others to discuss problems associated with detachment of the retina, the rationale for surgery, and anticipated preoperative and postoperative activities.

A. Emotional support, especially in the preoperative period.
B. Discourage client from jerky head movements, stooping, or straining; may have activity restrictions, depending on degree of detachment.
C. Local anesthesia may be used; client may be discharged within hours or may remain in hospital, depending on the degree of detachment and the type of repair.

**Goal:** To prevent postoperative complications.

A. Orient client to surroundings (see Box 14-1).
B. Postoperative pain may require opioid analgesic.
C. Client may experience redness and swelling of the lids.

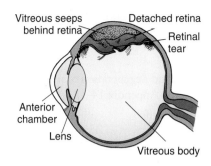

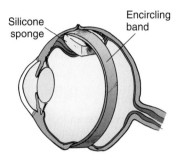

**FIGURE 14-3 Scleral Buckling.** (From Lewis, et al. [2017]. *Medical-surgical nursing: Assessment and management of clinical problems* [10th ed.]. St. Louis, MO: Elsevier Mosby.)

D. Warm or cool compresses may be used to promote comfort.
E. Postoperative medications usually include antibiotic eye drops, ophthalmic steroid drops, and dilating agents.

**Goal:** To help the client understand and perform own eye care.

A. Activities requiring visual acuity may be restricted for several weeks (reading, driving, etc.).
B. Discourage any straining, lifting, vigorous coughing, or stooping during the postoperative recovery period.
C. Make sure client understands symptoms of detachment and importance of seeking immediate attention if it occurs again (increased incidence of reoccurrence).

# Age-Related Macular Degeneration (AMD)

AMD is the most common cause of irreversible central vision loss in clients over 60 years of age; it is related to retinal aging.

## Assessment

A. Risk factors.
1. Familial tendency: gene has been identified.
2. Long-term exposure to UV lights and eye irritants.
3. Cigarette smoking.
B. Clinical manifestations.
1. Blurred, darkened vision.
2. Presence of scotomas (blind spots in visual field).
3. Distortion of vision.
4. Permanent loss of central vision.
5. Wet exudative—more severe form.
   a. Development of abnormal vessels in or near macula.
   b. New vessels begin to leak and form scar tissue.
   c. Rapid onset.

6. Dry nonexudative—less severe form.
   a. More common form.
   b. Accumulation of yellow pigment in retinal epithelium.
   c. Atrophy and degeneration of macular cells.
C. Diagnostics (see Appendix 14-1).

### Treatment

Treatment is directed toward stopping progression; affected vision cannot be restored.
A. Laser treatment (photodynamic therapy) of abnormal vessels, macular photocoagulation of abnormal vessels.
B. Intraocular medications to inhibit growth of endothelial tissue and vessels.

### Nursing Interventions

**Goal:** To promote prevention and/or early identification of problem and care of client with decreased visual acuity.

A. Encourage regular visual checkups.
B. Encourage diet high in dark green leafy vegetables containing lutein (e.g., spinach and kale) and vitamins containing A, C, and E, beta carotene, and zinc.
C. Promote independence in clients with decreased vision (see Box 14-1).
D. Psychosocial support in dealing with issues such as loss of independence (e.g., inability to continue driving as visual impairment progresses).

## Visual Impairment in Children

A. Refractory problems: same as those of an adult (see Appendix 14-1).
B. Amblyopia: reduced visual acuity in one eye; preventable if primary problem is corrected before 6 years of age.
C. Strabismus (misalignment of eyes) may result if amblyopia is not corrected.
D. Retinopathy of prematurity: originally known as *retrolental fibroplasia;* results in vasoconstriction of retina vessels causing retinal damage.

### Nursing Interventions

A. Promote discovery of the problem as early as possible.
   1. Identify children at increased risk because of history (prematurity).
   2. Assess children for behaviors that indicate poor vision.
   3. Encourage screening for visual acuity (schools, clinics).
B. Educate parents regarding importance of therapy and continued medical follow-up.

## Conjunctivitis

**Conjunctivitis is an inflammation of the conjunctiva.**

### Assessment

A. Exposure to bacterial or viral infections, allergens, or chemical irritants.
B. Redness, edema, tearing, and mucopurulent drainage.

### Treatment

A. Antibiotic eye drops for infections: instill after the eye has been cleaned.
B. Antihistamines and corticosteroids for allergic conjunctivitis.
C. Warm, moist compresses are used to remove crust and exudates.

### Nursing Interventions

**Goal:** To prevent the transmission of organisms to the uninfected eye and to others.

A. Always clean eye from inner canthus downward and outward to prevent contamination of the other eye.
B. Highly contagious; spreads easily from one eye to other.
C. Encourage good handwashing and instruct not to share a washcloth with others.

## Eye Trauma

**Eye trauma may include surface injuries (e.g., burns or splash injuries), embedded or impaled objects, or orbital trauma. History is usually congruent with eye injury.**
A. Assessment and treatment are often carried out at the same time.
B. As soon as the eye injury is detected, the client should be seen by a physician (ophthalmologist).

### Assessment

A. Identify eye in which trauma occurred.
B. Determine whether client has a contact lens in the affected eye.
C. Pain, inability to open the eye.
D. Decreased visual acuity: may be unable to distinguish light and images.
E. Ecchymosis, swelling, or visible foreign body.

### Treatment

A. If there is visible trauma but no penetrating object, gently apply dressing soaked with normal saline solution to prevent drying during transport.
B. Any suspected or known corneal abrasion should be examined with fluorescein (see Appendix 14-2), followed by ocular irrigation with normal saline solution (see Appendix 14-3).
C. Nonpenetrating foreign objects may be removed by irrigation with normal saline solution.
D. Penetrating foreign bodies must be removed by a physician (ophthalmologist) as soon as possible. Do not attempt to remove foreign objects from eye but stabilize the object and protect from movement by patching the other eye while seeking emergency care.
E. Do not attempt to stop bleeding from the eye or the eyelid with direct pressure; do not patch the eye until type of injury is determined.
F. For chemical eye burns, before going to emergency department (ED), irrigate the eye with copious amounts of warm tap water to remove chemical. Normal saline irrigation is used in the ED; injury may require short-acting ophthalmic anesthetic drops.

*Nursing Interventions*

**Goal:** To prevent further eye damage

A. Have client "rest" the eyes: provide dimly lit room; use eye patches if necessary.
B. Irrigate eyes with normal saline solution from inner canthus to outer canthus so solution does not flow into unaffected eye.
C. Eye may remain irritated after foreign body is removed and the anesthetic drops wear off; eye patch may be necessary.
D. If penetrating eye injury is present, decrease activities that cause increased ocular pressure, such as any Valsalva maneuver, blowing nose, sneezing, bending at the waist, etc.
E. Keep client immobilized until evaluated by an ophthalmologist.

**Goal:** To care for a client with an enucleation.

A. Immediate: obtain vital signs; monitor for bleeding.
B. Instillation of topical ointments until prosthesis is fitted.
C. A clear "conformer" may be placed in the eye socket to allow the area to heal until a permanent prosthesis can be fitted.
D. Eye prosthesis.
   1. Insertion: notched end of prosthesis should be closest to the client's nose; lift upper eyelid (using nondominant hand) and insert saline solution-rinsed prosthesis into socket area with top edge slipping under upper lid; gently retract lower lid until bottom edge of prosthesis slips behind it.
   2. Removal: retract the lower lid and apply slight pressure just below the eye; this should release the suction holding the prosthesis in place; assess the socket for signs of infection.
   3. The prosthesis is usually cleansed with normal saline.

## THE EAR

## PHYSIOLOGY OF THE EAR

A. External ear (Figure 14-4).
   1. External auditory canal: function is to transmit the collected sound waves to the tympanic membrane; outer half of canal secretes cerumen, or wax, which has a protective function.
   2. Tympanic membrane: a tough membrane separating the external and middle ear; transmits vibrations from external ear to the malleus of the middle ear; normally a pearly gray color.
B. Middle ear.
   1. Middle ear is filled with air at atmospheric pressure by means of the eustachian tubes; the eustachian

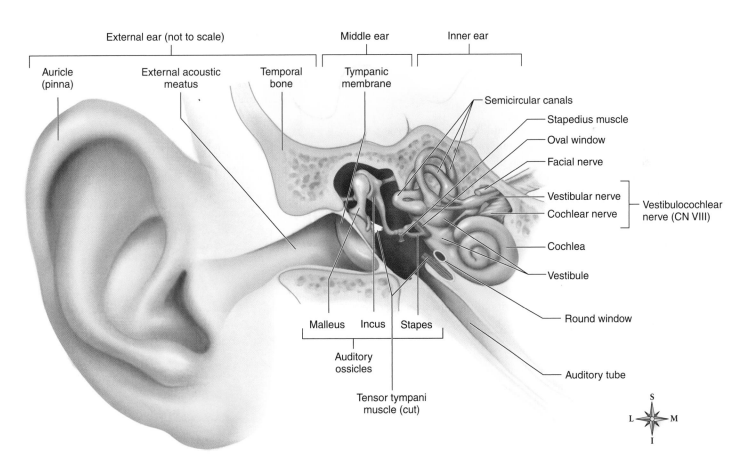

**FIGURE 14-4 Ear Anatomy.** (From Patton, K., & Thibodeau, G. [2013]. *Anatomy & physiology* [10th ed.]. St. Louis, MO: Elsevier.)

tubes of infants and young children are shorter, wider, straighter, and more horizontal than those of adults.
2. The function of the external and middle ear is to transmit and magnify sound waves by air conduction.
3. Problems in the external and middle ear cause conductive hearing loss.
C. Inner ear.
 1. Bony labyrinth.
  a. Vestibule: central area contains oval window and is bathed in fluid.
  b. Semicircular canals: open into the vestibule; related to maintaining equilibrium.
  c. Cochlea: contains organ of Corti, which is the receptive end organ for hearing.
 2. Disease of the inner ear or nerve pathway can result in sensorineural hearing loss.

### System Assessment

A. External assessment of the ear.
 1. Assess placement of the ears: low-set ears may be indicative of congenital anomalies in the newborn.
 2. Movement of the auricle should not elicit pain.
 3. Note presence of any discharge in the external canal.
 4. With an otoscope, examine tympanic membrane for landmarks, color, and intactness.
 5. Note color and consistency of cerumen.
B. Assessment of bone and air conduction (see Appendix 14-1).
C. Assess for vertigo: ask client to close eyes and stand on one foot; have client walk with eyes closed; client may fall to one side or complain of the room spinning.

## DISORDERS OF THE EAR

### Otitis Media

**Otitis media is an infection of the middle ear caused by a viral or bacterial agent. Infants and young children are predisposed to the development of acute otitis media because of the physiologic characteristics of the ear—the eustachian tube is shorter, wider, and straighter in children than in adults.**

#### Assessment

A. Acute otitis media (AOM).
 1. May be purulent (pus filled) or suppurative (capable of producing pus).
 2. Symptoms vary with the severity of the infection.
B. Repeated or persistent acute infections may lead to perforation of the tympanic membrane or more severe complications such as mastoiditis.
C. Chronic otitis media with effusion (OME): a collection of fluid in the middle ear without infection or acute symptoms that result from a blocked eustachian tube; may persist for weeks to months; most common cause of conductive hearing loss.
D. Risk factors.
 1. Age: increased incidence from 6 months to 20 months; decreases with age.

2. Upper respiratory tract infection.
3. Allergies, asthma.
4. Exposure to tobacco smoke.
5. Out-of-home daycare and exposure to siblings or parents with chronic otitis media.
6. Feeding bottle to infant/toddler in the supine position.
7. Pacifier use past 6 months of age.
8. Not receiving immunization with pneumococcal conjugate vaccine (PCV).
E. Clinical manifestations (Figure 14-5).
 1. Otalgia (pain from pressure in the middle ear).
  a. Infants are irritable; may pull at their ears or cry; sucking exacerbates pain.
  b. Young children verbally complain of severe ear pain.
 2. Fever as high as 104°F (40°C) is not uncommon with AOM.
 3. Otoscopic examination.
  a. AOM—tympanic membrane is immobile, bright red, and bulging, with purulent effusion and no light reflex.
  b. OME—tympanic membrane is immobile, dull gray, and may have fluid behind it.
 4. Postauricular and cervical lymph node enlargement.
 5. If tympanic membrane ruptures, purulent drainage or blood may be present in the outer ear; pain will decrease temporarily (AOM and OME).
 6. Conductive hearing loss may occur with recurrent rupture.
 7. Speech and language development may be delayed.

#### Treatment

A. Medications.
 1. Antibiotics, analgesics, antipyretics.

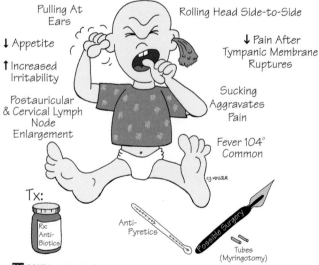

**FIGURE 14-5 Otitis Media.** (From Zerwekh, J., Garneau, A., & Miller, C. J. [2017]. *Digital collection of the memory notebooks of nursing* [4th ed.]. Chandler, AZ: Nursing Education Consultants, Inc.)

2. Ear drops (antibiotic and steroid combination).
3. Decongestants and antihistamines.
4. Corticosteroids for eustachian tube edema as needed.
5. OME does not require antibiotic therapy.
B. Surgical—myringotomy: drainage of the middle ear with insertion of tubes or grommets (or tympanostomy myringotomy) to relieve pressure and promote healing; used for recurrent cases that do not respond to medication; tubes are also known as pressure-equalizing tubes (PE tubes or myringotomy tubes).

> **■ NURSING PRIORITY:** Teach the parents to administer the full course of the antibiotic.

### Nursing Interventions

**Goal:** To enable parents of clients to describe problem, handle medication schedule, and cope with home care.

A. Recurrent infections cause an increased risk for permanent hearing loss or mastoiditis with potential intracranial spread of infection.
B. Antibiotics should be continued until all prescribed medication is taken, even after all symptoms are relieved.
C. Administer acetaminophen or ibuprofen for pain and fever. There should be relief of symptoms within 24 to 72 hours; if not, the health care provider should be contacted.
D. Pain-relieving ear drops (antipyrine, benzocaine, and glycerin) should be used only when there is no tympanostomy tube or rupture of the tympanic membrane.

> **■ NURSING PRIORITY:** Aspirin should not be used for fever or pain in children 18 years of age or younger.

E. Control allergies and upper respiratory congestion, including decreased exposure to those with respiratory infections.
F. The child should be discouraged from forcefully blowing his or her nose or holding his or her nose closed when sneezing.
G. Decrease risk for recurrence by preventing fluids from pooling around eustachian tube.
   1. Hold or elevate infant's head while feeding.
   2. Do not prop bottle or allow infant to fall asleep with a bottle.
   3. Encourage intake of water before sleeping.

**Goal:** Care for child after placement of tympanostomy tubes (myringotomy tubes or grommets).

A. Do not allow any water to get into the child's ears; use of earplugs is currently controversial.
B. Assure parents that if the ear grommet or tube falls out, it is not a significant problem.

### External Otitis

**External otitis is an inflammation or infection of the skin of the auricle of the ear and/or the ear canal.**

### Assessment

A. Risk factors/etiology.
   1. Swimming, especially when the water is contaminated or contains chemicals.
   2. Trauma to the ear, such as piercing.
B. Clinical manifestations.
   1. Ear pain, fever, disturbances of hearing.
   2. Drainage from the ear: blood-tinged or white to green-colored fluid.

### Treatment

A. Antibiotics (typically given as an ear drop; oral preparations for severe cases).

### Nursing Interventions

**Goal:** To prevent and reduce risk factors.

A. Encourage an ear drop drying agent (isopropyl alcohol and glycerin) after swimming, showering, or bathing to dry external ear canal and/or use of earplugs when child goes swimming.
B. Use earplugs if swimming or performing any activities that may precipitate water getting into the ears.
C. Do not use a cotton-tipped applicator to remove water from the ears.

### Acoustic Neuroma

**An acoustic neuroma is a unilateral benign tumor where cranial nerve VIII (acoustic [vestibulocochler]) enters the internal auditory canal.**

### Assessment

A. Clinical manifestations.
   1. Sensorineural hearing loss.
   2. Tinnitus.
   3. Intermittent vertigo.
   4. Impairment of facial movement from tumor compression (CN V, VII).
B. Diagnostics (see Appendix 14-1).
C. Treatment—surgical removal of tumor.

### Nursing Interventions

**Goal:** Promote communication and prepare client for surgery

A. Assist hearing-impaired client with communication (Box 14-2).
B. Determine presence of vertigo and plan for client safety.
C. Preoperative preparation (see Chapter 3).
   1. Assess level of hearing loss and communication skills.
   2. Encourage client to discuss fear regarding loss of hearing on affected side.
   3. Establish communication system for postoperative period.

**Goal:** To provide postoperative craniotomy care (see Chapter 22).

A. Assess for surgical interference with other cranial nerves (V, trigeminal; VII, facial; IX, glossopharyngeal).
   1. Assess for equal movement of face: smile, show teeth.
   2. Evaluate for problem swallowing.
   3. Evaluate speech.

---

**Box 14-2  OLDER ADULT CARE FOCUS**

**Improving Communication With Hearing-Impaired Clients**
- Stand in front of the client at eye level to speak. An adequate light source on your face will help with speech reading (i.e., reading lips).
- Lower the tone of your voice because high-pitched hearing loss is the first to go, so lower tones are easier to hear.
- Get the client's attention by raising your hand or arm.
- Do not walk back and forth in front of the client while speaking.
- Speak clearly and in an even tone; do not shout.
- Do not chew gum, cover your mouth, or smile excessively while talking.
- Because clients rely on visual cues, watch your facial expressions.
- Encourage professional counseling in speech reading and sign language.
- Assist the client in obtaining a hearing aid; if appropriate, promote social interaction.
- Do not avoid conversation with the client; do not depend on family to interpret information.
- Investigate use of TDD (telecommunication device for the deaf).
- Use light-activated devices: doorbell, smoke alarms, telephones.
- Client should avoid noisy environments where it is difficult to interpret sound.
- Provide client instruction in a quiet room with minimal distractions.

---

B. Assess for and teach patient to report any clear, colorless discharge from the nose (cerebral spinal fluid).
C. Evaluate balance and hearing loss regarding activities of daily living and safety.

## Hearing Loss
**Hearing loss results from an impairment of the transmission of sound waves.**
A. Conductive hearing loss results from mechanical dysfunction in transmission of sound from the outer or middle ear or both. Client will be able to benefit from a hearing aid. An example of conductive hearing loss is impacted cerumen, which often occurs in older adults.
B. Sensorineural (perceptive) hearing loss results from a problem in the inner ear (cochlea) or auditory nerve pathway. It often results from injury to cilia that transmit sound. Incoming sound cannot be analyzed correctly. Client may benefit from cochlear implant. An example of sensorineural hearing loss is presbycusis, which occurs in older adults.
C. Otosclerosis: an immobilization of the small bones in the inner ear; it occurs most often in women; an autosomal dominant disease that is usually bilateral.
D. Congenital: rubella or nutritional deficiencies.
E. Toxicity from aminoglycosides or other ototoxic drugs
F. Occupational/environmental/recreational: exposure to loud noises.

**Assessment**
A. Risk factors.
  1. Prolonged exposure to high-intensity sound waves.

> **⚠ NURSING PRIORITY:** Earplugs should be worn when the potential for exposure to loud noise exists.

  2. Repeated, chronic ear infections.
  3. Prenatal problems of rubella and eclampsia.
  4. Ototoxic medications: aminoglycosides, diuretics.
  5. Female with family history of otosclerosis.
B. Diagnostics (see Appendix 14-2).
C. Clinical manifestations.
  1. Speech problems: deterioration of present speech or delayed speech development.
  2. Fails to respond to oral communication or responds inappropriately.
  3. Excessively loud speech.
  4. General indifference to sound.
  5. Tinnitus.
  6. Responds more to facial expressions than to verbal ones.
  7. Inappropriate emotional response.

**Treatment**
A. Speech therapy.
B. Sign language.
C. Stapedectomy for otosclerotic lesions.
D. Cochlear implants for profound sensorineural hearing loss.

**Nursing Interventions**
**Goal:** To promote communication and socialization of the hearing-impaired client (see Box 14-2).

A. Teach client how to care for hearing aid (Box 14-3).

---

**Box 14-3  OLDER ADULT CARE FOCUS**

**Hearing Aid Care**
- Keep the hearing aid dry; do not wear it while bathing or swimming.
- Avoid using hair spray, cosmetics, or oils around the ear.
- Clean hearing aid with soft cloth and recommended cleanser; do not immerse in water.
- At night turn it off and open the battery compartment to prevent draining the battery.
- Avoid exposing it to extreme temperatures (e.g., leaving it on a window ledge in the sunlight).
- When cleaning the hearing aid, use a toothpick or pipe cleaner to remove any debris or cerumen from the hole in the middle part of the device that goes in the ear.
- If the hearing aid does not work, change the battery or check the on/off switch; check the connection between the ear mold and receiver; clean it using the steps described earlier, or take it to an authorized hearing aid service center.
- Keep extra batteries on hand for the hearing aid.

B. Teach client how to remove earwax if impacted cerumen is a problem; may need an ear irrigation (see Appendix 14-3).

**Goal:** To prevent complications after stapedectomy.

A. Assess client for dizziness, nausea, and vomiting.
B. Teach client to avoid sudden movement to prevent dizziness.
C. Maintain safety measures.
D. Instruct client that hearing may not improve until edema subsides in the operative area.

> **TEST ALERT:** Hearing loss is common in older adult clients. Watch for questions about hearing loss to be incorporated into test situations pertaining to other chronic health care problems.

## Balance Disorders

**The vestibular system of the inner ear maintains balance and coordination.**

A. Disorders.
  1. Ménière disease: an inner ear disorder of unknown origin but characterized by excess endolymph in the vestibular and semicircular canals, causing increased fluid pressure in the inner ear; also known as endolymphatic hydrops.
  2. Labyrinthitis: an inflammation of the cochlear and/or vestibular portion of the inner ear.

### Assessment

A. Diagnostics (see Appendix 14-2).
  1. Results of Weber test and auditory testing may indicate hearing loss.
  2. Romberg test (see Chapter 22 for Neurologic System Assessment).
B. Clinical manifestations.
  1. Vertigo: a sense of moving or spinning that is usually stimulated by sudden movement of the head; may occur when lying down.
  2. Sudden, severe paroxysmal episodes of vertigo (Ménière disease).
    a. Severe nausea, vomiting.

b. Nystagmus.
    c. Loss of balance.
    d. No pain or loss of consciousness.
  3. Fluctuating hearing loss and tinnitus (Ménière disease).
  4. Client may have no symptoms between attacks.
  5. Manifestations become less severe with time.
  6. Hearing loss increases with each attack (Ménière disease).

### Treatment

A. Medications (Ménière disease).
  1. During an acute attack, antihistamines (e.g., diphenhydramine), anticholinergics (e.g., atropine), and benzodiazepines (e.g., lorazepam) may be used to decrease abnormal sensations and lessen nausea and vomiting.
  2. Antiemetics (e.g., prochlorperazine), sedatives (e.g., diazepam), and antivertigo medications (e.g., meclizine) for motion sickness, in addition to bed rest.
  3. Diuretics, antihistamines, and calcium channel blockers may be prescribed for use between attacks.
B. Diet: low sodium.

### Nursing Interventions

**Goal:** To provide patient safety, emotional and physical support during an acute attack.

A. Maintain bed rest in a quiet, dimly lit room; avoid flickering lights and television.
B. Secure a position of comfort.
C. Avoid unnecessary nursing procedures.
D. Minimize stimulation and sudden position changes.
E. If client is severely nauseated, administer medications via routes other than oral.
F. Instruct client to always call before getting out of bed.
G. Rise and change positions (especially the head) slowly.

> **NURSING PRIORITY:** As a safety precaution, instruct the client to lie down immediately if an attack feels imminent.

---

### Appendix 14-1 OPHTHALMIC AND HEARING DIAGNOSTICS

#### Ophthalmic Diagnostics

The **Snellen chart** is used in screening for visual acuity problems. Client is placed 20 feet (6 meters) from the chart, and visual acuity is expressed as a ratio (what the client *should* see at 20 feet [6 meters] with normal vision compared with what he or she *can* see at 20 feet [6 meters]). A ratio of 20/50 means that the client can see at 20 feet (6 meters) what he or she should see at 50 feet (15 meters). Normal visual acuity is 20/20. Legal blindness is defined as the best-corrected vision in the better eye of 20/200 or less.

A **noncontact tonometer** is an instrument used to measure intraocular pressure noninvasively. Normal pressure is 12 to 22 mmHg. A puff of air is directed toward the cornea, which causes

indentation and allows measurement of intraocular pressure, a screen for diagnosis of glaucoma.

**Direct ophthalmoscopy** is examination of the fundus or back portion of the interior of the eyeball, which provides for visual evaluation of the retina, vascular patterns, and optic disk.

**Biomicroscopy** (slit-lamp examination) is used to assess the anterior eye for problems of the cornea, iris, and lens and to evaluate the depth of the anterior chamber.

**Refractive error evaluation** determines what refractive errors have occurred because light is not correctly focused on the retina. Conditions that occur in refractive errors are:
• **Myopia** (nearsightedness)—sees near objects clearly; light ray is focused in front of the retina

*Continued*

- **Hyperopia** (farsightedness)—sees distant objects clearly; light ray is focused behind the retina
- **Presbyopia**—a decrease in the elasticity of the lens that causes poor accommodation for near vision (common in older adults)
- **Astigmatism**—an uneven curvature of the cornea; light rays do not focus on the retina at the same time.

## Hearing Diagnostics

**Audiometry** is used to measure a client's hearing by the use of various tones and intensities of sound produced by an audiometer.

The **Rinne test** is conducted by holding a tuning fork on the mastoid bone (bone conduction). When the client indicates that he or she no longer hears sound, the vibrating tuning fork is moved to about 2 inches (5 cm) from the external ear (air conduction). The

client who hears normally will continue to hear the vibrations. This demonstrates that air conduction will last twice as long as bone conduction (2:1 ratio). When the tone is louder through air, the test result is positive and indicates normal hearing. If the bone conduction is louder than air conduction, it is indicative of a conductive loss.

The **Weber test** is conducted by placing a vibrating tuning fork on top of the client's head or in the middle of the forehead; the sound should be heard equally well in each ear. Lateralization of sound indicates pathology. Sound is heard better in impaired ear with conduction deafness, and sound is heard only in normal ear with sensorineural hearing loss.

**Otoscopy** is the examination of the external ear and the tympanic membrane by the use of an otoscope.

Appendix 14-2   OPHTHALMIC MEDICATIONS

### General Nursing Implications

Only use ophthalmic preparations of medications; the container should say for "ophthalmic use only."

- To decrease systemic absorption of ophthalmic topical medications, teach the client to apply gentle pressure (punctal occlusion) to the nasolacrimal duct (tear duct) for 30 to 60 seconds immediately after instillation of drops.
- Instruct the client or family in proper administration of eye drops or ointment (i.e., maintain sterile technique and prevent dropper contamination; clearly mark each container to indicate what eye medication is for, and do not share medication).
- Expect some blurriness from ointments; apply at bedtime, if possible, to avoid safety problems from diminished vision.
- Instruct the client to report changes in vision, blurring, difficulty breathing, or flushing.
- Teach the client to gently close eye and allow medication to distribute evenly over eye.

| Medications | Side Effects | Nursing Implications |
|---|---|---|
| **Glaucoma Medications** | | |
| **Alpha₂ Adrenergic Agonists—Decrease the production of aqueous humor and increase outflow.** | | |
| Brimonidine<br>Dipivefrin | Dry mouth, ocular hyperemia, local burning and stinging<br>Systemic absorption: hypotension<br>Dipivefrin may cause hypertension and tachycardia | 1. Can be absorbed into contact lens, wait 15 minutes after drops are instilled to replace contacts.<br>2. Dipivefrin is contraindicated in clients with narrow-angle glaucoma. |
| **Beta-Blockers**<br>Contraindicated with a history of cardiac problems such as bradycardia, heart block, or hypertension. | | |
| **Nonselective Beta₁ and Beta₂ Blockers—Decrease the production of aqueous humor.** | | |
| Timolol maleate<br>Carteolol | Eye irritation, dry eyes<br>Bradycardia, AV block, bronchospasm | 1. Assess for cardiac and respiratory changes with systemic absorption.<br>2. Contraindicated in patients with COPD or asthma. |
| **Selective Beta₁ Blockers—Decrease the production of aqueous humor.** | | |
| Betaxolol | Bradycardia, AV block | 1. Recommended for use in clients with history of chronic pulmonary disease.<br>2. Contraindicated in clients with bradycardia or overt cardiac failure.<br>3. Assess for systemic absorption. |
| **Prostaglandin Analogs—Increase the outflow of aqueous fluid from the eye.** | | |
| Latanoprost<br>Travoprost<br>Bimatoprost | Increases pigmentation of eyelid and growth of eyelashes; conjunctiva hyperemia | 1. Systemic effects are minimal.<br>2. May cause local brown pigmentation of the iris. |

## Appendix 14-2 OPHTHALMIC MEDICATIONS—cont'd

| Medications | Side Effects | Nursing Implications |
|---|---|---|
| **Cholinergics—Direct Acting:** Contract the ciliary muscle, which causes the iris to be withdrawn, permitting drainage of aqueous humor and decreased pressure within the eye. | | |
| Pilocarpine hydrochloride: 0.25%–10% solutions; 5 mg and 7.5 mg tablets | Conjunctive irritation Provocation of asthma Headache, ciliary spasm | 1. Cholinergics are contraindicated in clients with inflammatory eye conditions. 2. Miotic; causes constriction of pupil. |

> ⚠ **NURSING PRIORITY:** Only use ophthalmic preparations of any clinically indicated medication (drops or ointment) that is instilled into the eye.

| | | |
|---|---|---|
| **Cycloplegic and Mydriatics:** These agents work by blocking the response of the sphincter muscle of the iris to produce dilation of the pupil; they may cause paralysis of accommodation. They are used in eye examination and diagnosis. All are contraindicated in glaucoma because dilated pupils cause an increase in intraocular pressure. | | |
| Atropine sulfate Cyclopentolate HCl Tropicamide | Blurred vision, photophobia, headache, hyperemia; systemic effects: flushing, sweating, dry mouth, dizziness | 1. These are contraindicated in clients with glaucoma. 2. Dark glasses may be worn to decrease discomfort from photophobia. 3. Use only ophthalmic preparations. |

| | | |
|---|---|---|
| **Diagnostics:** Surface of eye absorbs dye, thus enhancing the visualization of corneal abrasions in eye trauma. | | |
| Fluorescein sodium | Stinging, burning sensation | 1. Cornea remains uncolored; abrasions and defects turn green. |

| | | |
|---|---|---|
| **Antiinfectives:** Used for treatment of eye infections. | | |
| Neomycin–polymyxin Erythromycin ophthalmic ointment | Drops and ointment may cause burning or irritation. | 1. Vision may be blurred. 2. Teach correct application of medication. 3. Use only eye preparations of medications. |

*AV,* Atrioventricular; *CNS,* central nervous system; *GI,* gastrointestinal; *IV,* intravenously; *PO,* by mouth (orally).

## Appendix 14-3 NURSING PROCEDURE: EAR AND EYE IRRIGATION

### Ear Irrigations

**Common Solutions**

- Warm tap water or normal saline solution
- Prescribed solution

### ✓ KEY POINT: Irrigation

- Before irrigation, visually inspect the external ear canal with an otoscope to ensure that tympanic membrane is intact and that the auditory canal is not obstructed by a foreign body. Do not irrigate an ear with otitis media present.
- Temperature of irrigating solution should be near body temperature (37°C, approximately 98°F). If the solution is too cold or hot, dizziness and/or nausea may occur.
- Cerumen may be softened by adding a few drops of warm mineral oil or an over-the-counter preparation.
- A rubber bulb syringe or a water pressure device may be used.
- Straighten the ear canal by either pulling the outer ear up and back for adults or down and back for children under 3 years of age.
- Direct water flow toward the top of the ear canal to create a circular motion but never on the eardrum itself.
- Do not forcefully push fluid into the ear canal because this may rupture the eardrum. If severe pain, nausea, vomiting, or dizziness develops, stop the irrigation immediately.
- Position the client to allow drainage of solution from the ear after irrigation.

### Eye Irrigations

**Common Solutions**

- Normal saline

### ✓ KEY POINT: Eye Irrigation

- Place client in position with head turned onto the affected side so that the solution does not run into unaffected eye.
- Small amount of fluid.
- Moderate amount of fluid: use a needleless syringe and direct fluid along conjunctiva and over the eye from inner to outer canthus.
- Large amount of fluid: bags of intravenous solutions may be used to provide constant stream and adequate flushing of chemical from the eye.
- Do not allow tip of irrigating equipment to touch the eye or eyelashes.
- Immersion technique: place entire face in basin of lukewarm water and have client open and close eyes repeatedly.
- Avoid use of contact lenses for a period of time after eye irritation.

## Study Questions
## Sensory: Care of Adult and Pediatric Clients

More questions on<br />evolve

1. The nurse would question which medication order for a client with PACG (primary angle-closure glaucoma)?
   1. Atropine 1 to 2 drops in each eye now
   2. Hydrochlorothiazide 25 mg PO daily
   3. Propranolol 20 mg PO two times a day
   4. Carbamylcholine eye drops, 1 drop two times a day

2. A client who has glaucoma is concerned about her adult children "inheriting" the condition. What is the best nursing response?
   1. "There is no need for concern; glaucoma is not a hereditary disorder."
   2. "Your children should have an ophthalmologic examination with screening for glaucoma around age 40. After that, examinations should be done every 2 to 3 years."
   3. "There may be a genetic factor with glaucoma, and your children over 30 years of age should be screened yearly."
   4. "Are your grandchildren complaining of any eye problems? Glaucoma generally skips a generation."

3. The nurse is evaluating a client recently diagnosed with primary open-angle glaucoma (POAG). What will be an important nursing action(s)? **Select all that apply.**
   1. Review all medications the client is currently taking to determine whether any of them cause an increase in intraocular pressure as a side effect.
   2. Determine whether the client has experienced any sudden loss of vision accompanied by pain.
   3. Discuss with the client the importance of controlling blood pressure to decrease the potential loss of peripheral vision.
   4. Instruct the client to take analgesics as soon as any discomfort occurs in the eye and to notify clinic if pain is not relieved.
   5. Have the client demonstrate the use of eye drops.
   6. Assess the client for chronic diseases such as diabetes.

4. A child is scheduled for a myringotomy with placement of tympanostomy tubes. What is the long-term goal of this procedure that the nurse will discuss with the parents?
   1. To decrease pressure on the tympanic membrane
   2. To irrigate the eustachian tube
   3. To correct a malformation in the inner ear
   4. To prevent recurrent ear infections

5. A client comes to the clinic with decreased hearing. Examination of the ear canal reveals a large amount of cerumen. What is the recommended method for removal of the cerumen?
   1. Curettage with suction and irrigation
   2. Warm sterile solution irrigation
   3. Cool tap water irrigation
   4. Cotton swab applicator

6. The nurse is admitting a postoperative client after removal of an acoustic neuroma. What would be most important to include in the postoperative nursing care for this client?
   1. Determining when the client will begin chemotherapy
   2. Evaluating hearing status
   3. Assessing for clear, colorless nasal discharge
   4. Encouraging the client to discuss problems with hearing loss

7. A client's eye has been anesthetized for an ophthalmology examination. What instructions will be important for the nurse to give the client?
   1. Do not watch television for at least 24 hours.
   2. Do not rub the eye for 15 to 20 minutes.
   3. Irrigate the eye every hour to prevent dryness.
   4. Wear sunglasses when in direct sunlight for the next 6 hours.

8. A teenager is diagnosed with conjunctivitis. Which statement indicates that the teenager understood the nurse's teaching?
   1. "I can let my friends use my sunglasses while we are together."
   2. "It's okay for me to softly rub my eye, as long as I use the back of my hand."
   3. "I can pick the crusty stuff out of my eyelashes with my fingers when I wake up in the morning."
   4. "I will use my own wash cloth and towel for my face while my eyes are sick."

9. An unknown chemical was splashed into a client's eyes. What is most important for the nurse to tell the client to do immediately?
   1. Rinse the eye with a large amount of water or saline solution.
   2. Put a pad soaked in sterile saline solution over the eye.
   3. Go to the closest emergency department.
   4. Have a coworker visually check the eye for a foreign body.

10. Which client is at highest risk for retinal detachment?
    1. A 4-year-old with amblyopia
    2. A 17-year-old who plays physical contact sports
    3. A 33-year-old with severe ptosis and diplopia
    4. A 72-year-old with nystagmus and Bell palsy

11. When teaching a family and a client about the use of a hearing aid, the nurse will base the teaching on what information regarding the hearing aid?
    1. It provides mechanical transmission for the damaged part of the ear.
    2. It stimulates the neural network of the inner ear to amplify sound.
    3. It amplifies sound and directs it into the ear canal.
    4. It will assist the client to interpret the incoming sounds more effectively.

12. A parent and an 8-month-old child come into a public health clinic for a well-child checkup. The parent tells the nurse the child has been crying more than usual. What information obtained during the nursing assessment would cause the nurse the most concern?
    1. Crying when sucking on his bottle
    2. Crying when placed in crib at night
    3. On-and-off crying throughout the day
    4. Crying when left at the child care center

13. The nurse is discharging a client with bilateral cataracts following cataract surgery on one eye. What statement by the client would indicate to the nurse the need for additional teaching?
    1. "I'll call if I have a significant amount of pain."
    2. "I'll remember to wash my hands before changing the eye dressing."
    3. "I'll be okay by myself at home today."
    4. "I will have someone help me with my eye medications."

14. A client is walking down the hall, and he begins to experience vertigo. What is the most important nursing action when this occurs?
    1. Have the client sit in a chair in a brightly lit room.
    2. Administer meclizine PO.
    3. Help the client sit or lie down.
    4. Assess whether the problem is vertigo or dizziness.

15. A 3-year-old child had a myringotomy about a week ago. The mother calls the nurse to report that one of the tubes fell out. She found the tube on the child's pillow. After the nurse makes an appointment for the child to be seen in the clinic, what would be important to tell the mother?
    1. Observe for any purulent or bloody drainage from the ear.
    2. Rinse the tube in soapy water and keep it.
    3. Do not allow any water to get into the child's ears.
    4. Do not allow the child to play outside.

16. The nurse is evaluating a teenager for hearing loss. In reviewing the client's history, the nurse knows that which finding is not associated with a hearing loss?
    1. Listening to loud music on an iPod
    2. Repeated chronic ear infections
    3. Taking penicillin and cephalosporin medication
    4. History of increased ear cerumen

17. A client is being admitted for problems with Ménière disease. What is most important for the nurse to assess to promote the client's safety?
    1. Diet history
    2. Screening hearing tests
    3. Effect on client's activities of daily living (ADLs)
    4. Frequency and severity of attacks

18. The nurse prepares to irrigate the external auditory canal for a client with impacted cerumen. What would be included in the correct technique for irrigation?
    1. Use cool tap water.
    2. Pour solution into ear canal.
    3. Assess for signs of pain and tenderness in the ear.
    4. Use a cotton-tipped applicator to clean near the tympanic membrane.

19. Which of the following are appropriate nursing actions when measuring visual acuity using a Snellen chart? **Select all that apply.**
    1. Position the client 30 feet (9 meters) away from the chart.
    2. Have the client first read the chart with both eyes open.
    3. Record visual acuity as the largest line that the client can read correctly.
    4. Test each eye individually with the opposite eye covered.
    5. Repeat the test with the client wearing corrective lenses.
    6. Use a picture chart if the client is unable to read.

## Answers to Study Questions

1. *1*
Atropine causes mydriasis or pupillary dilation, which can precipitate an attack of acute glaucoma. It should be questioned if it is ordered for a client with glaucoma. The other drugs would be safe for a client with glaucoma. (Lewis et al., 10 ed., p. 379)

2. *2*
Blindness from glaucoma is preventable. A comprehensive eye examination should be done around age 40, then every 2 to 4 years until 64 years, and then every 1 to 2 years after age 65. There is a familial tendency and a significantly higher incidence in African Americans. Therefore African Americans should have ophthalmic examinations more frequently. (Lewis et al., 10 ed., pp. 380, 382)

3. *1, 5, 6*
Medications must be evaluated in terms of their potential for increasing intraocular pressure. Ophthalmic eye drops are often prescribed for the client with glaucoma, and clients should know how to administer them correctly. Diabetes is a risk factor for the development of glaucoma, and management of the diabetes is important in helping to prevent progression of the glaucoma. An increase in intraocular pressure could cause further damage to the eye in the client with glaucoma. The question states the client has already been diagnosed; primary open-angle glaucoma (POAG) is painless and is not correlated with the blood pressure. (Lewis et al., 10 ed., pp. 379–382)

4. *4*
The goal of a myringotomy is to allow draining of the fluid within the ear that will help prevent recurrent ear infections. It will decrease the pressure immediately, but this is not the long-term goal.

It neither corrects a malformation in the inner ear nor provides a way to irrigate the eustachian tube, and you do not want excessive fluid in the middle ear. (Lewis et al., 10 ed., p. 385)

5. *2*
Although the structures of the outer ear are not sterile, sterile drops and solutions are used for irrigations in case the tympanic membrane is ruptured. The addition of nonsterile solutions may result in possible infections of the middle ear. Cool irrigants will be uncomfortable, and tap water is not considered sterile. Curettage with suction and irrigation and use of a cotton swab applicator can damage the tympanic membrane. (Lewis et al., 10 ed., p. 385)

6. *3*
The removal of an acoustic neuroma may result in a cerebrospinal fluid (CSF) leak that would be a significant risk of infection, which would be noted by clear, colorless nasal discharge. This symptom requires immediate assessment and intervention. The tumor is benign; therefore the client will not begin chemotherapy. The nurse will need to evaluate the hearing loss in the affected ear as well as the effect of hearing loss on the client's body image and ability to perform ADLs; however, these are secondary to the assessment of a possible CSF leak. Hearing loss may also occur after this procedure, but this would not be as much a priority as the possible CSF leak. (Lewis et al., 10 ed., p. 387)

7. *2*
The eye has been anesthetized, therefore there is no feeling or sensation in it for 15 to 20 minutes. It would be very easy to rub the eye and cause damage. Not watching television for a day would have no effect on the safety. Irrigating the eye every hour is not

necessary. Because there is no effect on the client's tolerance of direct sunlight, sunglasses would be optional. (Lilley, 8 ed., p. 916)

**8.** *4*

Conjunctivitis is contagious through physical contact. The teenager should be directed not to touch the eye, if possible. Handwashing should be stressed after any contact with the eye, and the teen should not share any items that might be contaminated, such as facial towels. Conjunctivitis may be bacterial or viral, and sharing of possibly contaminated objects may result in the spread of infection. Rubbing or picking at the eyelashes may result in further irritation or contamination of the hands, which would further the risks of infection transmission. (Lewis et al., 10 ed., pp. 371–373)

**9.** *1*

When an unknown solution has been splashed in the eyes, it is most important to remove as much of the solution as possible by rinsing the eyes with large amounts of water or normal saline solution, if available. Placing a pad soaked in sterile saline solution over the eye, going to the closest emergency department, and having a coworker visually check the eye for a foreign body do not address removing the excess solution from the eye to prevent further damage. (Lewis et al., 10 ed., p. 371)

**10.** *2*

Participating in physical contact sports puts this person at the highest risk for retinal detachment because trauma is a leading cause. The other pathologies (amblyopia, ptosis, diplopia, nystagmus, and Bell palsy) will affect eye function but have minimal likelihood of causing retinal detachment. (Lewis et al., 10 ed., p. 376)

**11.** *3*

The hearing aid amplifies sound but does not change the overall ability to interpret incoming sound. Sensorineural hearing loss is the inability of the client to interpret the sounds. A hearing aid is used for clients with conductive hearing loss or a mix of conductive and sensorineural loss. The hearing aid does not stimulate the neural network to amplify sound, such as a cochlear implant. (Lewis et al., 10 ed., p. 391)

**12.** *1*

Pain during feeding may indicate increased inner ear pain during sucking. With effusion in the middle ear space, negative pressure draws mucus into the middle ear in response to a child crying, or sucking on a nipple, resulting in increased pressure and pain. Crying when placed in a crib and on and off during the day is normal in childhood development. Separation anxiety is not an uncommon problem. (Hockenberry & Wilson, 10 ed., pp. 1179–1181)

**13.** *3*

This client may experience visual impairment and difficulty with self-care the day of surgery because the operative eye will be patched and the other eye still has a cataract. This client may need some special assistance at home until the vision improves, especially the first 24 hours while the operative eye is patched. Discomfort after cataract surgery is minimal, thus there should be no significant amount of pain. Proper hygiene is important to prevent wound/eye contamination during dressing changes. Eye drops may be difficult for the client to administer, so assistance is a good idea. (Lewis et al., 10 ed., p. 373)

**14.** *3*

The client experiencing vertigo is severely imbalanced and at high risk of falling, thus client safety is the priority. He should be assisted to sit or lie down immediately or he may fall. The client should be safely sitting or lying down before any treatment or further assessment can continue. Although sitting in a chair is not a bad option, the fact that the rest of the statement includes sitting in a well-lit room would not be prudent. The preferred action during an acute attack would be to have the client lie down in a quiet, darkened room. (Lewis et al., 10 ed., p. 386)

**15.** *3*

There may still be an opening in the eardrum where the tube was placed. It is important to continue to keep all water out of the child's ear to prevent infection. Observing for drainage is important for the mother to do, but not allowing water to get into the ears is more important. The tube is usually thrown away. There is no need to wash it, and the child can play outside if he is comfortable. (Hockenberry & Wilson, 10 ed., pp. 1181–1182)

**16.** *3*

Penicillin and cephalosporin medications are not ototoxic. Aminoglycosides are ototoxic. The other three options—listening to loud music on an iPod, repeated chronic ear infections, and a history of increased ear cerumen—are risk factors for hearing loss. (Lewis et al., 9 ed., p. 391; Lehne, 9 ed., p. 1056.)

**17.** *4*

The nurse must assess the frequency and severity of attacks to plan best for the client's safety. Although hearing tests and diet may be of some significance, they will not protect the client immediately. After the client's immediate safety needs are met, the nurse will want to determine the effect that Ménière's disease has on the client's ADLs. (Lewis et al., 10 ed., p. 386)

**18.** *3*

Before performing the irrigation, the nurse should assess the client for pain and tenderness, which could be caused by a perforated eardrum or impaction of a foreign body, and for dizziness caused by disequilibrium. The temperature of the water or saline solution should be comfortable to the wrist of the client or nurse, and it should be sterile. The nurse uses an ear syringe to inject water onto the superior side of the ear canal. The client should be sitting or lying down to facilitate drainage and to maintain safety in case the client gets dizzy from the irrigation. Cotton-tipped applicators should only be used on the outer (pinna or auricle) ear. (Lewis et al., 10 ed., p. 384)

**19.** *2, 4, 5, 6*

The nurse should position the client 20 feet (6 meters) away from the chart, not 30 feet (9 meters). Record the smallest line that can be correctly read, not the largest. Each eye is tested separately with the opposite eye covered. The eye test is repeated with the client wearing corrective lenses. You may use an "E" chart or a picture chart if the client is unable to read. (Lewis et al., 10 ed., p. 355)

CHAPTER FIFTEEN

# Endocrine: Care of Adult, Maternity, and Pediatric Clients

**15**

## PRIORITY CONCEPTS

Glucose Regulation, Hormonal Regulation, Patient Education

## PHYSIOLOGY OF THE PITUITARY GLAND

The pituitary gland is often referred to as the "master gland" and is located deep in the brain. It secretes hormones that control hormone secretion of other endocrine glands (Figure 15-1). It has two lobes—anterior and posterior pituitary—that secrete hormones promoting growth, water absorption by the kidney, and sexual development and function.

### 🦎 System Assessment

A. Assess for growth imbalance.
   1. Evaluate overall growth pattern of child.
   2. Assess for excessive or retarded growth.
      a. In adults, assess for excessive growth of small bones and soft tissue.
      b. In children, assess for excessive or retarded growth in height.
   3. Evaluate excessive weight gain or loss.
B. Evaluate familial tendencies.
   1. Parents who displayed slower growth patterns.
   2. Compare rate of growth of siblings at age comparable to that of client.
   3. Assess for specific characteristics and/or genetic traits in the adults of the immediate family.
C. Assess for secondary sexual characteristics appropriate to age and gender.
D. Assess for emotional, intellectual, and mental characteristics appropriate to physical development and age.
   1. Intelligence.
   2. Increased excitability.
   3. Mental confusion, apathy.

## DISORDERS OF THE PITUITARY GLAND

### 📋 Hyperpituitary: Acromegaly

**Acromegaly is most often the result of a benign slow-growing tumor (pituitary adenoma) that secretes growth hormones. It occurs after the closure of epiphyses of the long bones.**

#### Assessment

A. Clinical manifestation.
   1. Enlargement of the hands and feet and hypertrophy of the skin.

2. Peripheral neuropathy may also be present.
3. Changes in facial features: protruding jaw, slanting forehead, and an increase in the size of the nose.
4. Severe enlargement of the pituitary gland may cause pressure on the optic nerve, resulting in changes in vision and headaches.

B. Diagnostics (see Appendix 15-1).
C. Complications.
   1. Headache and visual field disturbances.
   2. Diabetes mellitus/glucose intolerance.
   3. Obstructive sleep apnea.

#### Treatment

A. Treatment consists of surgery, radiation therapy, drug therapy, or a combination of these therapies.
B. Surgical intervention includes a hypophysectomy, which may be accomplished by the transsphenoidal approach (Figure 15-2).

#### Nursing Interventions

**Goal:** To provide supportive preoperative care (see Chapter 3).
**Goal:** To decrease the chances of complications after hypophysectomy.

A. Elevate the head of the bed 30 degrees.
B. Assess for signs of cerebrospinal fluid (CSF) leakage (client swallowing frequently or complaints of postnasal drip or headache); monitor gauze pad placed under the nose regularly for drainage. If any clear drainage is present, check for glucose and protein using a urine dipstick.
C. Discourage bending, coughing, sneezing, or Valsalva maneuver to prevent CSF leak.
D. Assess for symptoms of increasing intracranial pressure (see Chapter 22).
E. Evaluate urine for excessive increase in volume (>200 mL/hr for 3 consecutive hours) or specific gravity less than 1.005 (i.e., development of diabetes insipidus). Replace fluids to avoid hypovolemia.
F. Do not brush teeth, and rinse frequently with nonirritating solutions.

**Goal:** To assist client to reestablish hormone balance after hypophysectomy (adrenal insufficiency and hypothyroidism are most common complications).

A. Administer corticosteroids.
B. If output becomes excessive (because of decrease in antidiuretic hormone [ADH]), anticipate administration of ADH-regulating medications (see Appendix 15-2).

277

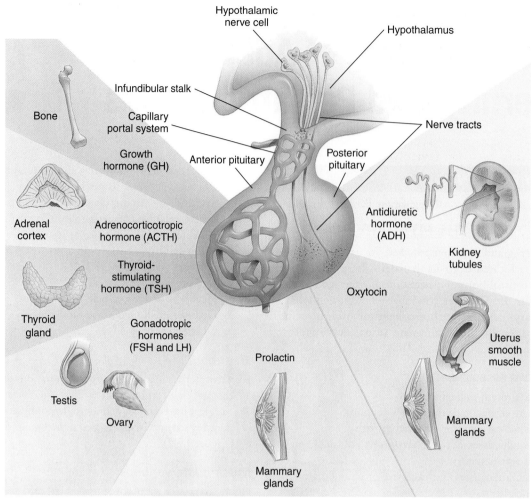

**FIGURE 15-1  Pituitary Hormones and Target Organs.** (From Patton, K. T., & Thibodeau, G. A. [2014]. *The human body in health and disease* [6th ed.]. St. Louis, MO: Elsevier/Mosby.)

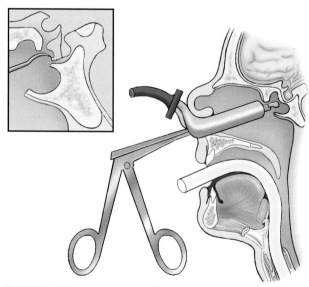

**FIGURE 15-2  Surgery on the Pituitary Gland is Most Commonly Performed with the Transsphenoidal Approach.** An incision is made in the inner aspect of the upper lip and gingival. The sella turcica is entered through the floor of the nose and sphenoid sinuses. (From Lewis, S. L., et al. [2017]. *Medical-surgical nursing: Assessment and management of clinical problems* [10th ed.]. St. Louis, MO: Mosby.)

C. Evaluate serum glucose levels for significant changes.

D. Monitor for problems related to hypothyroidism.

**Goal:** To cope with altered body image.

A. Infertility will frequently be experienced as a result of hormone changes.

B. Skeletal changes before surgery are not reversible.

C. Medication.

1. Cortisone and thyroid hormone replacement throughout lifetime.

2. ADH-regulating medications.

3. Medication to support target organs involved (pancreas, thyroid, gonads).

## DISORDERS OF THE POSTERIOR PITUITARY

### Diabetes Insipidus

Diabetes insipidus (DI) is characterized by a deficiency of ADH or kidney's inability to respond to ADH. When it occurs, it is most often associated with neurologic conditions, surgery, tumors, head injury, or inflammatory problems.

A. When there is a decreased or inadequate amount of ADH (either failure in synthesis of ADH or the inability of the kidneys to respond to ADH), this deficiency results in large volumes of dilute urine (polyuria).

B. The large loss of water leads to dehydration and increased plasma osmolarity, leading to thirst.

### Assessment

A. Risk factors/etiology: problems with the pituitary or hypothalamus gland, hypophysectomy, infections, brain tumor, head injury, medications such as lithium and demeclocycline and other conditions that reduce or interfere with ADH production.

B. Clinical manifestations.
1. Polyuria: excretion of excessive amounts urine (2 to 20 L/day).
2. Polydipsia.
3. Low urine specific gravity (<1.005).
4. Severe dehydration (tachycardia, poor skin turgor, dry mucous membranes, hypotension).
5. Hypernatremia and elevated serum osmolality (>295 mOsm/kg 295 mmol/kg)
6. Hemoconcentration (increased hemoglobin, hematocrit, blood urea nitrogen [BUN]).

C. Diagnosis: water deprivation test; measurement of ADH level.

### Treatment

A. Administration of ADH-regulating medications (desmopressin, vasopressin) (see Appendix 15-2).

### Nursing Interventions

**Goal:** To maintain fluid and electrolyte balances (see Chapter 9).

A. Encourage intake of fluids containing electrolytes.
B. Monitor intake and output carefully. Weigh daily.
C. Evaluate urine specific gravity for changes.
D. Assess hydration status.
E. Correlate hydration status with weight gain or loss.
F. Closely monitor sodium and potassium levels with fluid shifts (hypernatremia).

**Goal:** To understand the implications of the condition.

A. DI caused by other problems is usually self-limiting.

### Syndrome of Inappropriate Antidiuretic Hormone

The syndrome of inappropriate antidiuretic hormone (SIADH) is a condition in which there is continued release or high production of ADH, regardless of the level of plasma osmolarity, which may be normal or low.

A. When the normal feedback mechanism for ADH fails and the level of ADH is sustained, there is excessive water retention in the body.

B. When the serum osmolality is considerably lower than the urine osmolality, this indicates the *inappropriate* excretion of concentrated urine in the presence of dilute serum.

### Assessment

A. Risk factors/etiology: malignancy is the most common cause, especially small cell lung cancer; other causes include head injury, other central nervous system disorders, and some medications.

B. Clinical manifestations.
1. Low urinary output with weight gain and no obvious edema.
2. Decreased (dilutional hyponatremia) serum sodium level (less than 134 mEq/L 134 mmol/L) and hypochloremia.
3. Gastrointestinal (GI) disturbances (anorexia, nausea, abdominal cramps).
4. Cerebral edema: altered mental status, headaches, seizures.
5. High specific gravity (>1.025).
6. Fatigue and muscle aches.

### Treatment

A. Treat underlying cause.
1. Fluid restriction (limit fluids to 800–1000 mL/24 hr).
2. Monitor sodium correction carefully. Correct deficit slowly.

### Nursing Interventions

**Goal:** To maintain fluid and electrolyte balances (see Chapter 9).

A. Restrict fluids.
B. Monitor intake and output carefully. Weigh daily.
C. Evaluate urine specific gravity for changes.
D. Assess hydration status.
E. Correlate hydration status with weight gain or loss.
F. Closely monitor sodium and potassium levels with fluid shifts (hyponatremia).
G. Seizure and fall precautions.

## PHYSIOLOGY OF THE THYROID GLAND

The thyroid gland is located in the anterior portion of the neck below the Adam's apple and in front of the trachea. Primary function of thyroid hormone is to control the level of cellular metabolism by secreting thyroxin ($T_4$) and triiodothyronine ($T_3$).

### System Assessment

A. Assess for changes in metabolism.
1. Significant increase or decrease in weight.
2. Diarrhea or constipation.
3. Increase or decrease in appetite.
4. Changes in vital signs.
5. Changes in skin texture or appearance.

B. Assess for intellectual development and mental changes.
1. Intellectual level appropriate for age.
2. Increased irritability, excitability, nervousness.
3. Mental confusion, lethargy.

## DISORDERS OF THE THYROID GLAND

### Hyperthyroidism

**Hyperthyroidism (also called Graves' disease) or thyrotoxicosis is caused by excessive amounts of thyroid hormones. Thyrotoxicosis can also be related to excessive intake of levothyroxine.**

*Assessment*

A. Risk factors.
 1. More prevalent in women, with the highest frequency in persons 20 to 40 years old.
 2. Probably an autoimmune disorder.
B. Clinical manifestations (Figure 15-3).
 1. Increased rate of body metabolism.
  a. Intolerance to heat.
  b. Significant weight loss, despite increased appetite and food intake.
  c. Tachycardia, increase in systolic blood pressure.
  d. Increased peristalsis, leading to diarrhea.
  e. Hand tremors and hyperactive deep tendon reflexes.
 2. Visual problems.
  a. Exophthalmos (bulging eyeballs).
  b. Changes in vision.
  c. Eyelid retraction (lid lag).
 3. Changes in menstrual cycle.
 4. Enlarged, palpable thyroid gland.
 5. Labile emotional state.
C. Diagnostics (see Appendix 15-1).
 1. Increase in $T_3$, $T_4$, and free $T_4$ serum levels.
 2. Decrease in TSH.
 3. Radioactive iodine uptake test greater than 50%.
 4. Client's physical appearance and symptoms.

*Complications*

A. Acute thyrotoxicosis (also called thyroid storm or crisis) may occur from stressors, after surgery or treatment with radioactive iodine.
 1. Systolic hypertension, tachycardia, heart failure.
 2. Increased temperature (>102°F [38.9°C]); hyperthermia up to 105.3°F (40.7°C).

# HYPERTHYROIDISM

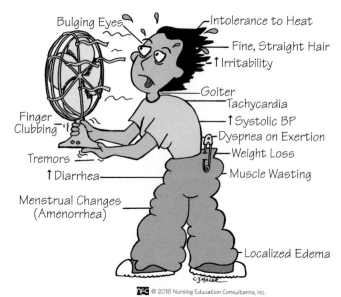

Bulging Eyes
Intolerance to Heat
Fine, Straight Hair
↑Irritability
Goiter
Tachycardia
↑Systolic BP
Dyspnea on Exertion
Weight Loss
Muscle Wasting
Finger Clubbing
Tremors
↑Diarrhea
Menstrual Changes (Amenorrhea)
Localized Edema

© 2016 Nursing Education Consultants, Inc.

**FIGURE 15-3 Hyperthyroidism.** (From Zerwekh, J., Garneau, A., & Miller, C. J. [2017]. *Digital collection of the memory notebooks of nursing* [4th ed.]. Chandler, AZ: Nursing Education Consultants, Inc.)

 3. Increased agitation, seizures, delirium, coma.
B. Calcium deficit may occur as a result of trauma to the parathyroid (see Hypoparathyroidism section later in this chapter).

*Treatment*

A. Surgical: thyroidectomy.
B. Medical.
 1. Destroy or damage thyroid tissue: radioactive iodine therapy, eventually resulting in hypothyroid state.
 2. Decrease thyroid hormone synthesis and release with antithyroid medications (see Appendix 15-2).

*Nursing Interventions*

**Goal:** To decrease effects of excess thyroid hormone.

A. Decrease environmental stress (lights, visitors, noise, etc.).
B. Cool environment.
C. Assess vital signs.
D. Well-balanced meals (high in calories and high in vitamins); small meals served 4 to 6 times per day.

**Goal:** To protect eyes of client experiencing complications caused by eye changes.

A. Artificial tears.
B. Assess for excess tearing, a sign of dry cornea.
C. Eye patches or light taping of eyelids may be necessary at night.
D. Salt restrictions and elevating head of bed to reduce periorbital edema.

**Goal:** To prevent complications of thyroid storm (or crisis) (thyrotoxicosis).

A. Identify risk factors precipitating thyroid crisis.
 1. Inadequate preoperative preparation.
 2. Infection, increased emotional lability.
 3. Surgical removal of thyroid gland.
 4. After treatment with radioactive $I^{131}$ ablation.
B. Assess for increase in hyperthyroid state.
 1. Increase in temperature, dehydration.
 2. Tachycardia.
 3. Pulmonary edema.
 4. Nausea, vomiting, diarrhea.
 5. Increase in agitation.

**Goal:** To maintain homeostasis in client experiencing thyroid storm (or crisis).

A. Decrease body temperature and heart rate.
 1. Keep room cool.
 2. Acetaminophen to decrease fever.
 3. Propranolol or atenolol to treat cardiac issues.
B. Oxygen to meet increased metabolic demands.
C. Intravenous (IV) fluids.
D. Hydrocortisone for shock and adrenal insufficiency.
E. Iodine preparations to decrease $T_4$ output.
F. Assess for cardiac tachydysrhythmias.
G. Propylthiouracil (PTU) or methimazole given to inhibit formation of thyroid hormone.

**Goal:** To provide preoperative nursing measures if surgery is indicated.

A. Demonstrate to client how to provide neck support after surgery.
B. Administer iodine preparations to decrease vascularity of the thyroid gland.
C. Establish baseline data for postoperative comparison.

**Goal:** To maintain homeostasis after thyroidectomy.

A. Maintain semi-Fowler's position to avoid tension on the suture line.
B. Administer analgesics for pain.
C. Administer IV fluids until nausea and swallowing difficulty subside.
D. Check dressings on the side and back of the neck for bleeding.
E. Assess for hematoma around the wound.
F. Evaluate calcium levels and assess for tetany because parathyroid may have been damaged or accidentally removed.
G. Evaluate temperature elevations; temperature increase may be early indication of thyroid storm.

> **NURSING PRIORITY:** Monitor status of client who has undergone surgery (hemorrhage, airway, wound).

**Goal:** To prevent complication of respiratory distress after thyroidectomy.

A. Assess client frequently for noisy breathing and increased restlessness.
B. Evaluate voice changes; increasing hoarseness (some hoarseness is to be expected) may be indicative of laryngeal edema.
C. Keep suction equipment and tracheotomy set readily available.

**Goal:** To decrease radiation side effects in a client being treated with radioactive iodine.

A. Treat throat dryness with sips of water and ice chips.
B. If irritation persists, use a salt water gargle.
C. Monitor client for a transient period of several days to weeks, when the symptoms of hyperthyroidism may actually worsen after radioactive iodine therapy

> **TEST ALERT:** Observe client for side effects of chemotherapy or radiation.

 **Home Care**
A. Thyroid levels checked every 6 to 12 months.
B. Lifelong thyroid replacement.
C. If excessive fatigue or tachycardia and tremors become consistent problems, notify health care provider.

## Hypothyroidism

**Hypothyroidism is characterized by a slow deterioration of thyroid function. It occurs primarily in older adults and five times more frequently in women (ages 30–60)** than in men. **Myxedema coma is a life-threatening form of hypothyroidism. Hashimoto thyroiditis is a chronic autoimmune disorder that may lead to a goiter and hypothyroidism.**

### *Assessment*

A. Risk factors.
   1. More prevalent in women.
   2. Can be associated with using medications such as amiodarone and lithium.
B. Early clinical manifestations (Figure 15-4).
   1. Extreme fatigue, menstrual disturbances.
   2. Hair loss, brittle nails, and dry/coarse skin.
   3. Intolerance to cold.
   4. Constipation, apathy.
C. Late clinical manifestations.
   1. Subnormal temperature.
   2. Cardiac complications (bradycardia, heart failure, hypotension).
   3. Weight gain and edema, thickened skin.
   4. Change or decrease in level of consciousness.
D. Diagnostics.
   1. Decrease in serum $T_3$ and $T_4$ levels.
   2. Increase in serum TSH level.

### *Treatment*

A. Medical management.
   1. Replacement of thyroid hormone.
   2. Low-calorie diet to promote weight loss.
   3. Minimize constipation; increase fiber in diet and fluids.

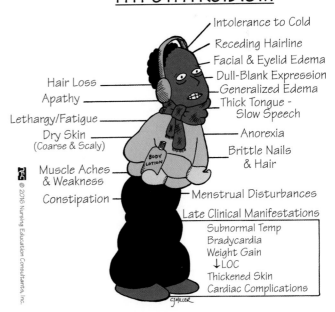

# HYPOTHYROIDISM

Intolerance to Cold
Receding Hairline
Facial & Eyelid Edema
Dull-Blank Expression
Generalized Edema
Thick Tongue - Slow Speech
Hair Loss
Apathy
Lethargy/Fatigue
Dry Skin (Coarse & Scaly)
Anorexia
Brittle Nails & Hair
BODY LOTION
Muscle Aches & Weakness
Menstrual Disturbances
Constipation
Late Clinical Manifestations

Subnormal Temp
Bradycardia
Weight Gain
↓LOC
Thickened Skin
Cardiac Complications

© 2016 Nursing Education Consultants, Inc.

**FIGURE 15-4 Hypothyroidism.** (From Zerwekh, J., Garneau, A., & Miller, C. J. [2017]. *Digital collection of the memory notebooks of nursing* [4th ed.]. Chandler, AZ: Nursing Education Consultants, Inc.)

### Complications

A. Thyroid hormone replacement will increase the workload of the heart and increase myocardial oxygen requirements.
B. Observe the client for the development of cardiac failure.
C. Have the client report tachycardia, chest pain, tremors, weight loss, insomnia.

### Nursing Interventions

**Goal:** To assist the client to return to hormone balance.

A. Begin thyroid replacement and evaluate client's response; advise the client that it will be about 7 days before he or she begins to feel better.
B. Provide a warm environment.

> ⚠ **NURSING PRIORITY:** Administer sedatives and hypnotics with caution because of increased susceptibility. These medications tend to precipitate respiratory depression in the client with hypothyroidism.

C. Prevent and/or treat constipation.
D. Assess progress.
  1. Decrease in body weight.
  2. Intake and output balance.
  3. Decrease in visible edema.
  4. Energy level and mental alertness should increase in 7 to 14 days and continue to rise until normal.
E. Evaluate cardiovascular response to medication.

**Goal:** To assist client to understand implications of disease and requirements for health maintenance.

A. Need for lifelong drug therapy.
B. Client with diabetes needs to evaluate blood glucose levels more frequently; thyroid preparations may alter effects of hypoglycemic agents.
C. Continue to reinforce teaching as client begins to make progress; early in the disease, the client may not comprehend importance of information.

### 🌲 Congenital Hypothyroidism

Congenital hypothyroidism (formerly known as cretinism) is a deficiency of thyroid hormones present at birth. Symptoms depend on the amount of thyroid hormones present at birth.

### Assessment

A. Condition is not generally evident in the newborn because of thyroid hormones received through the maternal circulation; may become evident at 3 to 6 months of age.
B. Early clinical manifestations.
  1. Thick, dry, mottled skin.
  2. Bradycardia, hypotonia, hyporeflexia.
  3. Poor feeding.
  4. Hypotonic abdominal musculature.
    a. Constipation.
    b. Protruding abdomen (umbilical hernia).

C. Diagnostics.
  1. Filter-paper blood-spot thyroxine ($T_4$) test; if result is low, then a TSH test is done.
  2. Mandatory test in all states; should be done within 24 to 48 hours after birth.

### Treatment

Medical management includes replacement of thyroid hormones. (If replacement is accomplished shortly after birth, it is possible that the child will have normal physical growth and intellectual development.)

### Nursing Interventions

**Goal:** To identify neonates experiencing congenital hypothyroidism.
**Goal:** To assist parents to understand the implications of the disease and requirements for continued health maintenance.

A. Child will require lifelong medication.
B. Continue medical care to evaluate changes in thyroid replacement as the child grows.

## PHYSIOLOGY OF THE PARATHYROID

Four small parathyroid glands are located near or embedded in the thyroid gland. The hormone secreted is parathyroid hormone (PTH), also called parathormone, which is primarily involved in the control of serum calcium levels.

### 🩺 System Assessment

A. History of problems of calcium metabolism and/or thyroid surgery.
B. Assess for changes in mental or emotional status.
C. Evaluate reflexes and neuromuscular response to stimuli.
D. Evaluate serum and urine calcium levels.

## DISORDERS OF THE PARATHYROID

### 📋 Hyperparathyroidism

**Hyperparathyroidism is characterized by excessive secretion of PTH, resulting in hypercalcemia.**

A. Normal function of PTH is to maintain serum calcium and phosphate levels.
B. Excessive PTH leads to bone damage, hypercalcemia, and kidney damage.

### Assessment

A. Risk factors: more common in women in their 40s and 50s.
B. Clinical manifestations.
  1. Primary hyperparathyroidism is due to adenomas, hyperplasia, or carcinomas. Bone cysts and pathologic fractures occur because of bone decalcification. Calcium is released into the blood, causing hypercalcemia.
  2. Secondary hyperparathyroidism is frequently due to chronic renal failure.
    a. Renal calculi, azotemia.
    b. Hypertension caused by renal failure.
    c. Repeated urinary tract and renal infections.

3. Central nervous system problems of lethargy, stupor, and psychosis.
4. GI problems.
   a. Anorexia, nausea, and vomiting.
   b. Constipation, development of peptic ulcer.
C. Diagnostics.
   1. Increased level of serum total calcium; decreased level of serum phosphorous; increased PTH.
   2. Computed tomography (CT) scan and/or x-ray film show demineralized cystic areas in bone.
   3. Increased urine calcium and phosphorous levels.

### Treatment

A. Decrease level of circulating calcium.
B. Parathyroidectomy.

### Nursing Interventions

**Goal:** To decrease the level of serum calcium.

A. High fluid intake to dilute serum calcium and urine calcium levels.
B. If IV is necessary, generally administer normal saline solution.
C. Furosemide, a loop diuretic, may be used to increase excretion of calcium.
D. Encourage mobility, because immobility increases demineralization of bones.
E. Limit foods high in calcium.
F. Phosphate replacement.

**Goal:** To assess client's tolerance of and response to increased PTH level.

A. Assess for skeletal involvement.
B. Assess for renal involvement.
   1. Strain urine for stones.
   2. Evaluate for low back pain (renal).
   3. Check for hematuria.
   4. Assess intake and output carefully.
C. Assess for presence of bone pain.
D. Assess cardiac response to increased level of calcium.

**Goal:** To provide appropriate preoperative measures if surgery is indicated (see Chapter 3).

**Goal:** To prevent postoperative complications of parathyroidectomy.

A. Care of client who has undergone parathyroidectomy is same as that for client who has undergone thyroidectomy.
B. Bone pain is relieved shortly after surgery; bone lesions frequently heal; serious renal disease may not be reversible.

### 📋 Hypoparathyroidism

**Hypoparathyroidism is characterized by a decrease in the PTH level, resulting in hypocalcemia and elevated serum phosphate levels. Severe hypocalcemia results in tetany.**

### Assessment

A. Risk factors or precipitating causes.
   1. Adults: inadvertent removal of parathyroid gland during thyroidectomy or radical neck dissection.
   2. Children: primary cause is idiopathic (unknown).
B. Clinical manifestations.
   1. Insidious onset.
      a. Muscle weakness/spasms.
      b. Loss of hair; dry skin.
   2. Overt/acute tetany (potentially fatal).
      a. Bronchospasm, laryngospasm.
      b. Seizures, cardiac dysrhythmias.
      c. Circumoral paresthesia.
      d. Abdominal cramps, nausea, vomiting, diarrhea, anorexia.
      e. Positive Chvostek sign (sign is positive when sharp tapping over the facial nerve elicits mouth, nose, and eye twitching) (Figure 15-5).
      f. Trousseau phenomenon (present when carpopedal spasm is precipitated by occluding blood flow for 3 minutes to the upper portion of the upper extremity with a blood pressure cuff).

   3. Pediatrics.
      a. Carpopedal spasms, muscle cramps, twitching.
      b. Seizures: generalized or absence.
      c. Brittle hair, thin nails.
C. Diagnostics.
   1. Decreased serum calcium levels.
   2. Increased serum phosphate levels.
   3. Low PTH levels.

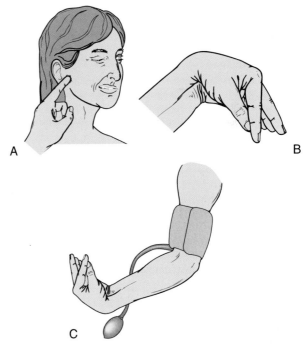

**FIGURE 15-5 Tests for Hypocalcemia. (A)** Chvostek sign is contraction of facial muscles in response to a light tap over the facial nerve in front of the ear. **(B)** Trousseau sign is a carpal spasm induced by inflating a blood pressure cuff above the systolic pressure for a few minutes **(C)**. (From Lewis, S. L., et al. [2017]. *Medical-surgical nursing: Assessment and management of clinical problems* [10th ed.]. St. Louis, MO: Mosby.)

*Treatment*

A. Vitamin D to enhance calcium absorption.
B. Increased calcium in the diet and supplements.

**TEST ALERT:** Adjust food and fluid intake to improve fluid and electrolyte balances.

C. Acute.
  1. Replace calcium through slow IV drip (calcium gluconate, calcium chloride).
  2. Monitor IV calcium administration with electrocardiogram. Potential for serious cardiac dysrhythmias, especially if taking digoxin.
  3. Sedatives, anticonvulsants.

*Nursing Interventions*

**Goal:** To assist client to increase serum calcium levels.

A. Administer calcium preparations.
B. Evaluate for an increase in serum calcium levels and a decrease in serum phosphate levels.
C. Client will require lifelong medical care to maintain homeostasis.

**Goal:** To prevent complications of neuromuscular irritability.

A. Quiet environment.
B. Low lights.
C. Seizure precautions.
D. Have client breathe in and out of a breathing mask or bag (reduces serum pH, thereby increasing total calcium available in its free form.)

**Goal:** To help client avoid complications of respiratory distress.

A. Bronchodilators.
B. Tracheotomy and suction set readily available.
C. Frequent assessment of respiratory status.

**Goal:** To prevent complications of cardiac problems.

A. Assess client for history of cardiac problems.
B. Assess frequently for dysrhythmias.
C. Calcium will potentiate effects of digitalis; use cautiously together.

## PHYSIOLOGY OF THE PANCREAS

The pancreas is located in the upper left aspect of the abdominal cavity and produces the enzymes trypsin, amylase, and lipase, along with insulin and glucagon from the islets of Langerhans.

### System Assessment

A. Evaluate changes in weight, particularly weight gain in an adult and weight loss in a child.
B. Evaluate alterations in fluid balance.
C. Evaluate changes in mental status.
D. Evaluate serum glucose and pancreatic enzyme studies.
E. Evaluate the abdomen for epigastric pain and abdominal discomfort.

## DISORDERS OF THE PANCREAS

### Diabetes Mellitus

Diabetes mellitus (DM) is a complex, multisystem disease characterized by the absence of—or a severe decrease in—the secretion or utilization of insulin.

A. Pathophysiology.
  1. The primary function of insulin is to facilitate the movement of glucose from the blood into the cell, thus decreasing the blood glucose level.
    a. Necessary for the transport of glucose into the cells of the liver, muscles, and other tissues.
    b. Regulates the rate of carbohydrate metabolism and conversion to glucose; normally insulin is decreased during fasting and increased after eating (prandial).
  2. Insulin is secreted by the beta cells in the islets of Langerhans in the pancreas.
  3. Insulin allows the body to use carbohydrates more effectively for conversion of glucose for energy.
    a. Adequate intake of carbohydrates.
    b. Available insulin to facilitate the movement of glucose into cells.
    c. Adequate reserves of glucagon (released by pancreas; converts glycogen to glucose in the liver).
  4. If carbohydrates are not available to be used for energy, cells will begin to oxidize the fats and protein stores.
    a. Breakdown of fat results in the production of ketone bodies.
    b. Protein is wasted during insulin deficiency. Protein is broken down and converted to glucose by the liver, thus contributing to the increase in circulating glucose.
    c. When fats are used as the primary energy source, the serum lipid level rises and contributes to the accelerated development of atherosclerosis.
  5. When circulating glucose cannot be used for energy, the level of serum glucose will increase (hyperglycemia).
    a. Hyperglycemia will cause an increase in the osmotic gradient; water moves out of the cells into the circulating volume to decrease the osmolarity. This results in an increase in urinary output.
    b. The increase in circulating glucose exceeds the renal threshold, and glucose spills into the urine.
  6. Pathophysiologic bases for symptoms.
    a. Polyuria: because of the increased serum osmolarity, there is more circulating volume; water is not reabsorbed from the renal tubules, and there is a significant increase in urine output.
    b. Polydipsia: increased loss of fluids precipitates dehydration, causing thirst.
    c. Polyphagia: tissue breakdown and wasting cause hunger.
    d. Weight loss (with type 1 DM): glucose is not available to the cells; body begins to break down fat and protein stores for energy.
B. Classification.
  1. Type 1: absolute lack of insulin secretion.
    a. Absence of insulin production; client is dependent on insulin to prevent ketoacidosis and maintain life.

b. Generally affects people under 40 years of age but can occur at any age.

c. Previously called juvenile diabetes or insulin-dependent diabetes mellitus.

d. Familial tendencies in transmission.

e. Client will have type 1 diabetes for the rest of his or her life.

2. Type 2: combination of insulin resistance and inadequate insulin secretion to compensate.

a. Insulin deficiency caused by defects in insulin production or by excessive demands for insulin; client is not dependent on insulin.

b. Ketoacidosis is generally not a problem because of limited insulin production.

c. Mostly in adults (peaking in the 50s), but becoming more common in children due to childhood obesity.

d. Previously called adult-onset diabetes mellitus (AODM) or noninsulin-dependent diabetes mellitus (NIDDM).

e. Associated with obesity; overweight people require more insulin.

f. If not associated with obesity, there is usually a strong family history.

g. Blood sugar often controlled by diet and oral hypoglycemics but during episodes of stress may require insulin for control.

3. Prediabetes.

a. Increased risk for developing type 2 diabetes.

b. Defined as impaired glucose tolerance test, impaired fasting glucose, or both.

c. Asymptomatic, although long-term damage may be occurring.

d. Lifestyle changes can reduce the risk of developing overt type 2 diabetes.

4. Pregestational diabetes mellitus.

a. Woman has either type 1 or type 2 diabetes before becoming pregnant.

b. Insulin dependent during pregnancy.

c. Increased risk of intrauterine fetal demise (IUFD), sometimes called *stillbirth*, and congenital malformations (cardiovascular, central nervous system, and skeletal system).

5. Gestational diabetes mellitus (GDM).

a. Develops during pregnancy; usually detected at 24 to 28 weeks' gestation by a screening glucose test; if screen is positive (130–140 mg/dL [7.2–7.8 mmol/L] blood sugar), then an oral glucose tolerance test (OGTT) is ordered.

b. Higher risk for cesarean delivery, and infants have increased risk for perinatal death, birth injury, and neonatal complications.

c. Infant may be large for gestational age and may experience hypoglycemia shortly after birth.

d. Glucose tolerance usually returns to normal soon after delivery.

e. Commonly occurs again in future pregnancies; client is at increased risk for development of glucose intolerance and type 2 diabetes later in life.

## Assessment

A. Clinical manifestations.

1. Types 1 and 2.

a. Three Ps: polyphagia, polydipsia, polyuria.

b. Fatigue, increased frequency of infections.

2. Type 1.

a. Weight loss, excessive thirst.

b. Bed-wetting, blurred vision.

c. Enuresis in children, nocturia in adults.

d. Complaints of abdominal pain.

e. Rapid onset, generally over days to weeks.

3. Type 2 (most clients asymptomatic first 5–10 years).

a. Weight gain (obese), visual disturbances.

b. Slow onset; may occur over months.

c. Fatigue and malaise.

d. Recurrent vaginal yeast or monilial infections—frequently, this is the initial symptom in women.

e. Older adult assessment considerations (Box 15-1).

B. Diagnostics (the criteria for diagnosis is made using one of the following methods) (see Appendix 15-1).

1. $A_{1c}$ (glycosylated hemoglobin) of 6.5% or higher.

2. Fasting blood glucose level: above 126 mg/dL (7 mmol/L) (normal glucose below 100 mg/dL [5.6 mmol/L]) after no caloric intake for at least 8 hours.

3. Two-hour plasma glucose level greater than or equal to 200 mg/dL (11.1mmol/L) during an oral glucose tolerance test, using a glucose load of 75 g.

4. When symptoms of hyperglycemia (polyuria, polydipsia, unexplained weight loss) or hyperglycemic crisis, a random plasma glucose greater than or equal to 200 mg/dL (11.1 mmol/L) is diagnostic.

5. Prediabetes: intermediate stage between normal and diabetes.

a. Impaired glucose tolerance (IGT): 2 hours after a meal, plasma glucose is greater than 140 mg/dL

---

**Box 15-1    OLDER ADULT CARE FOCUS**

**Diabetic Assessment Considerations and Care**

- Determine mental status and manual dexterity to handle injections.
- Determine whether the client can access the injection sites.
- Is the client alert and mentally capable of making judgments on medications?
- Determine whether the client can pay for supplies.
- What is the client's attitude about needles and injections?
- Assess how many other medications the client is taking. Are there problems with "polypharmacy" (too many medications)?
- Discuss the risk of hypoglycemia unawareness (e.g., does not experience early signs of hypoglycemia related to age and use of beta-adrenergic blockers).
- Determine family's or client's ability to accurately perform serum glucose testing.
- What is the client's support system?

(7.8 mmol/L) to 199 mg/dL (11.0 mmol/L) or higher during an oral glucose tolerance test.
b. Impaired fasting glucose (IFG): fasting blood glucose is greater than 100 mg/dL (5.6 mmol/L) but less than 126 mg/dL (7 mmol/L).

> ❗ **NURSING PRIORITY:** The glycosylated hemoglobin A$_{1c}$ level will indicate overall glucose control for approximately the past 120 days. This allows evaluation of control of the blood glucose level, regardless of increases or decreases in the blood glucose level immediately before the sample was obtained.

### Treatment

A. Factors in diabetes management (Figure 15-6).
   1. Regular physical activity.
   2. Diet.
   3. Pharmacologic intervention.
▲ B. Hypoglycemic agents.
   1. Insulin: may be used in both type 1 or 2 diabetes (Table 15-1).
      a. Insulin may be delivered subcutaneous, intravenous, inhaled or via pump.
      b. Only regular insulin can be given intravenously.
      c. Combination premixed insulin therapy eliminates problem of mixing different types (example: NPH/regular 70/30—number refers to percentage of each type of insulin).
      d. Insulin will be used for glucose control during pregnancy.

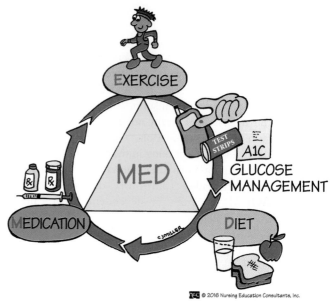

# TRIANGLE OF DIABETIC MANAGEMENT

**FIGURE 15-6  Triangle of Diabetes Management.** (From Zerwekh, J., Garneau, A., & Miller, C. J. [2017]. *Digital collection of the memory notebooks of nursing* [4th ed.]. Chandler, AZ: Nursing Education Consultants, Inc.)

## Table 15-1  PROFILE OF INSULINS

| Insulin | Nursing Implications |
|---|---|
| **Action** — Rapid-acting: lispro, aspart, glulisine — Onset: 15 minutes, Peak: 60-90 minutes, Duration: 3-4 hours (graph from 6 AM, Noon, 6 PM, Midnight, 6 AM) | **Rapid-Acting** Lispro Aspart Glulisine Should be used in combination with intermediate-acting insulin. ❗ **NURSING PRIORITY:** Because of quick onset of action, client must eat immediately. |
| Short-acting: regular — Onset: ½ -1 hour, Peak: 2-3 hours, Duration: 3-6 hours (graph from 6 AM, Noon, 6 PM, Midnight, 6 AM) | **Short-Acting** Regular Usually given 20–30 minutes before meals. May be given alone or in combination with longer-acting insulins. Given for sliding scale coverage. ❗ **NURSING PRIORITY:** When administering injections: • May mix regular insulin with other insulins. • Only regular insulin may be given IV. |

**Table 15-1   PROFILE OF INSULINS—cont'd**

| *Insulin* | *Nursing Implications* |
|---|---|

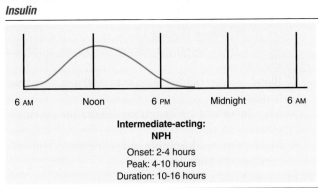

**Intermediate-acting:**
**NPH**
Onset: 2-4 hours
Peak: 4-10 hours
Duration: 10-16 hours

**Intermediate-Acting**
NPH
Hypoglycemia tends to occur in mid to late afternoon.
Never give IV. May only be given subQ.
May be mixed with regular insulin.
May be given at bedtime for nighttime coverage.

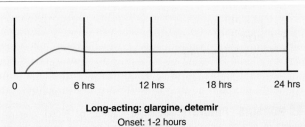

**Long-acting: glargine, detemir**
Onset: 1-2 hours
Peak: no pronounced peak
Duration: 24+ hours

**Long-Acting**
Glargine
Detemir
Degludec
Glargine and detemir CANNOT be diluted or mixed with other insulins.
Usually given once a day at bedtime but can be administered during the day.
Detemir can be given twice daily.
May only be given subQ.

Onset: 12–15 min
Peak: 60 min
Duration: 2.5–3 hr.

**Inhaled Insulin Powder**
Afrezza
1. Not for use with clients who smoke or recently stopped smoking.
2. Can cause bronchospasm.
3. Taken at the beginning of the meal.

> **TEST ALERT:** Assess the client for signs of hypoglycemia/hyperglycemia. Know various insulins and nursing implications for mixing medications from two vials when necessary. Administer insulin according to blood glucose levels.

Figures from Lewis, S. L., et al. (2017). *Medical-surgical nursing: Assessment and management of clinical problems* (10th ed.). St. Louis, MO: Mosby.

2. Oral hypoglycemic agents for type 2 diabetes mellitus (see Appendix 15-2).
3. Insulin requirement increases when:
   a. Client is seriously ill.
   b. An infection develops.
   c. Client experiences physical trauma (surgery or accidents).
   d. Growth spurts occur during adolescence and puberty.
4. Diabetic diet.
   a. Client with type 1 diabetes mellitus should coordinate insulin dosing with eating habits and activity pattern in mind. Food selection is flexible.
   b. Client with type 2 diabetes mellitus should strive for glucose, lipid, and blood pressure goals. Modest weight loss has been associated with improved insulin resistance for those who are overweight or obese.
   c. Meal plan.
      (1) Individualized carbohydrate intake (prefer whole grains, fruits, vegetables, low-fat milk). May include carbohydrate counting.
      (2) Fiber intake goal of 25 to 30 grams/day.
      (3) Less than 200 mg/day of cholesterol and limited trans fats.
      (4) Protein intake for those with normal renal function is the same as the general population.
      (5) Alcohol consumption can cause hypoglycemia in clients on insulin or oral hypoglycemic medications (due to inhibiting of gluconeogenesis) and require close monitoring of glucose levels.
5. Exercise.
   a. Recommended to exercise 150 min/week (30 minutes/5 days/week) in a moderate-intensity aerobic physical activity.
   b. Those with type 2 diabetes should also perform resistance training 3 times/week.

> **TEST ALERT:** Intervene to control symptoms of hypoglycemia or hyperglycemia.

> **! NURSING PRIORITY:** Metabolic effects of exercise:
> 1. Reduces insulin needs by reducing the blood glucose level.
> 2. Contributes to weight loss or maintenance of normal weight.
> 3. Helps the body metabolize cholesterol more efficiently.
> 4. Promotes less extreme fluctuations in blood glucose levels.
> 5. Decreases blood pressure.

### Complications of Insulin Therapy

A. Hypoglycemia (Table 15-2).
B. Allergic reaction.
   1. Localized reactions may occur and often resolve in 1 to 3 months.
   2. Allergic reactions may also be from the preservatives used or the latex or rubber stoppers of the syringe or vial.
C. Lipoatrophy and lipodystrophy.
   1. May result from poor rotation of injection sites.
   2. Use of human insulin greatly decreases the chance of this occurring.
D. Somogyi effect (Figure 15-7).
   1. Physiologic reflex: rebound hyperglycemia from an unrecognized hypoglycemic state.
   2. Most often occurs at night.
   3. May be treated by decreasing the evening insulin dose or by increasing the calories in the bedtime snack.
E. Dawn phenomenon (Figure 15-8).
   1. Results from nighttime release of growth hormone and cortisol.
   2. Blood glucose elevates at 5:00 to 6:00 a.m. (predawn hours).
   3. May be treated by increasing insulin for overnight period.
   4. Most severe in adolescence and young adulthood with peak growth hormone.
F. Hormones that counteract insulin.
   1. Glucagon.
   2. Epinephrine.
   3. Cortisol.
   4. Growth hormone.

> **! NURSING PRIORITY:** Intensive control of blood glucose levels in clients with type 1 diabetes can prevent or ameliorate many of the complications.

### Table 15-2 COMPARISON OF DIABETIC KETOACIDOSIS (DKA), HYPEROSMOLAR HYPERGLYCEMIC SYNDROME (HHS), AND HYPOGLYCEMIA

| | DKA | HHS | Hypoglycemia |
|---|---|---|---|
| Age | All ages, increased incidence in children | Adult (usually seen in older adults with underlying chronic disease) | All ages |
| GI | Abdominal pain, anorexia, nausea, vomiting, diarrhea | Normal | Normal; may be hungry |
| Mental state | Dull, confusion increasing to coma | More severe neurologic symptoms due to increased osmolarity and high blood glucose level | Difficulty concentrating, coordinating; eventually coma |
| Skin temperature | Warm, dry, flushed | Warm, dry, flushed | Cold, clammy |
| Pulse | Tachycardia, weak | Tachycardia | Tachycardia |
| Respirations | Initially deep and rapid; lead to Kussmaul respirations | Tachypnea | Shallow |
| Breath odor | Fruity, acetone | Normal | Normal |
| Urine output | Increased | Increased | Normal |
| **Laboratory Values** | | | |
| Glucose | >250 mg/dL (13.9 mmol/L) | >600 mg/dL (33.3 mmol/L) | Below 70 mg/dL (3.9 mmol/L) |
| Ketones | High/large | Normal | Normal |
| pH | Acidotic (less than 7.3) | Normal | Normal |
| Hematocrit | High due to dehydration | High due to dehydration | Normal |
| **Laboratory Values: Urine** | | | |
| Sugar | High | High | Negative |
| Ketones | High | Negative | Negative |
| Onset | Rapid (less than 24 hr) | Slow (over many days) | Rapid |
| Classification of diabetes | Primarily type 1; type 2 in severe distress | Type 2 | Type 1 and type 2 |

*DKA*, Diabetic ketoacidosis; *GI*, gastrointestinal; *HHS*, hyperosmolar hyperglycemic syndrome.

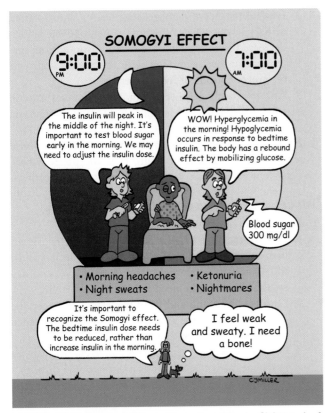

FIGURE 15-7 **Somogyi Effect.** (From Zerwekh, J., Claborn, J., & Gaglione, T. [2011]. *Mosby's pathophysiology memory notecards* [2nd ed.]. St. Louis, MO: Mosby.)

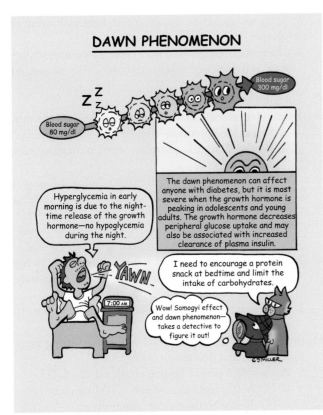

FIGURE 15-8 **Dawn Phenomenon.** (From Zerwekh, J., Claborn, J., & Gaglione, T. [2011]. *Mosby's pathophysiology memory notecards* [2nd ed.]. St. Louis, MO: Mosby.)

## Complications Associated With Poorly Controlled Diabetes

A. Diabetic ketoacidosis.
1. An extreme increase in the hyperglycemic state.
2. An increase in the mobilization of fat and protein as energy sources.
3. Metabolism of fat results in the production of fatty acids, which are converted to ketone bodies.
4. An increase in circulating ketone bodies precipitates the state of acidosis.
5. Occurs predominately in type 1 diabetes.

B. Clinical manifestations of diabetic ketoacidosis (see Table 15-2).
1. Onset.
   a. May be acute or occur over several days.
   b. May result from stress, infection, surgery, or lack of effective insulin control.
   c. Results from poorly controlled diabetes.
2. Severe hyperglycemia (blood glucose levels >250 mg/dL [13.9 mmol/L]).
3. Presence of metabolic acidosis (low pH [6.8–7.3] and serum bicarbonate level less than 16 mEq/L [mmol/L]).
4. Hyperkalemia, hypokalemia, or normal potassium level, depending on amount of water loss.
5. Urine ketone and sugar levels are increased.
6. Excessive weakness, increased thirst.
7. Nausea, vomiting.
8. Fruity (acetone) breath.
9. Kussmaul respirations.
10. Decreased level of consciousness.
11. Dehydration.
12. Increased temperature caused by dehydration.

C. Hyperglycemic–hyperosmolar syndrome.
1. Occurs primarily in older adult clients with type 2 diabetes.
2. Insulin production is adequate to prevent the breakdown of fat for cellular function, but severe hyperglycemia exists.
3. Severe electrolyte imbalance and dehydration exist in the absence of the acidotic state.
4. Characterized by extreme hyperglycemia (values >600 mg/dL [33.3 mmol/L]).
5. Because of the ability of the body to maintain a low level of insulin production, the breakdown of fat and the production of ketone bodies do not occur. This prevents the client from developing acidosis.
6. Osmotic diuresis occurs as a result of the hyperglycemia; the client becomes dehydrated very rapidly.

D. Clinical manifestations of HHS (see Table 15-2).
1. Warm, flushed skin, lethargy.
2. Weakness, thirst, decreased level of consciousness.
3. Increased temperature from dehydration.
4. Tachycardia, decrease in blood pressure.
5. Generally no GI problems.
6. No acetone odor to breath or glycosuria.
7. Severe hyperglycemia (>600 mg/dL [33.3 mmol/L]).
8. Serum pH is normal; urine output is increased.

E. Electrolyte imbalance.
1. As acidosis develops in DKA, potassium ions move out of cells; this leaves cellular potassium levels depleted, but the serum potassium level may be normal because of excessive excretion.
2. As osmotic diuresis occurs from the hyperglycemic/hyperosmolar state, serum potassium is excreted.
3. As the client becomes more dehydrated, the serum potassium becomes concentrated and does not reflect the potassium loss.
4. As the osmolarity and acidosis are corrected, along with the administration of insulin, the potassium will move back into the cells and result in severe hypokalemia. The client must be cardiac monitored for life-threatening arrhythmias.

## Complications of Long-Term Diabetes

A. Angiopathy: premature degenerative changes in the vascular system.
1. May affect the large vessels (macroangiopathy, early onset of atherosclerosis, and arteriosclerotic vascular problems).
2. May affect the small vessels (microangiopathy); problems are specific to diabetes.
B. Peripheral vascular disease: combination of both types of angiopathy.
C. Hypertension.
D. Diabetic gastroparesis: delayed gastric emptying.
E. Cerebrovascular disease.
F. Coronary artery disease.
G. Ocular complications: retinopathy, cataracts, glaucoma.

> **! PEDIATRIC PRIORITY:** An ophthalmologic examination should be obtained once the child is 10 years of age and has had diabetes for 3 to 5 years.

H. Nephropathy.
1. Microangiopathy primarily affects the glomerular capillaries, resulting in thickening and increased permeability of the glomerular basement membrane; will progress to end-stage renal disease.
2. Recurrent pyelonephritis, particularly in women.
3. Diabetic effects on the kidneys are the single most common cause of end-stage renal failure.
I. Neuropathy: inadequate blood supply to the nerve tissue and high blood glucose levels cause metabolic changes within the neurons.
1. Peripheral neuropathy: may be general pain and tingling; may progress to painless neuropathy.

> **! NURSING PRIORITY:** Painless peripheral neuropathy is a very dangerous situation for the client with diabetes. Severe injury to the lower extremities may occur, and the client will not be aware of it. Clients should be taught to visually inspect their feet and legs daily.

2. Autonomic nerve damage: diarrhea or constipation, urinary incontinence or retention, neurogenic bladder, decreased sweating, and orthostatic hypotension; impotence in men. Interferes with the client's ability to recognize episode of hypoglycemia.
3. Approximately 60% of clients with diabetes experience neuropathy; it is the most common chronic complication.
J. Infections: an alteration in immune system response results in impairment of white cells for phagocytosis. Persistent glycosuria potentiates urinary tract infections.

## Clinical Implications of Diabetes in Pregnancy

A. Effects of pregnancy on diabetes.
1. During the first trimester of pregnancy, there is an increase in the fetal need for glucose and amino acids; this lowers the maternal blood glucose level and decreases the maternal need for additional insulin.
2. During the second and third trimesters, the need for insulin will increase as a result of insulin resistance from major hormone changes.
3. Oral hypoglycemic agents are *not used* to control diabetes in the pregnant client who has **pregestational** diabetes.
4. Glyburide is being used more frequently with women who have gestational diabetes (GDM) instead of insulin.
B. Effects of diabetes on pregnancy.
1. Increased tendency toward the development of metabolic acidosis caused by an increase in metabolic rate.
2. Placental antagonist to insulin will decrease the effectiveness of insulin.
3. Fetal antagonists to insulin decrease the utilization of glucose.
4. Hormonal changes lead to decreased tolerance to glucose and increased insulin resistance (begins around 14–16 weeks).
C. Influence of pregnancy on diabetic control.
1. Insulin requirements for **pregestational** diabetic mother.
   a. Weeks 3 to 7 gestation—insulin requirement increased.
   b. Weeks 7 to 15 gestation—insulin requirements decrease.
   c. Increase in insulin requirements during the second and third trimesters of pregnancy may double or quadruple prepregnancy amounts.
   d. At week 35 gestation—insulin requirements plateau and often drop significantly after 38 weeks.
2. Insulin-dependent pregnant women are prone to hypoglycemia during the first trimester of pregnancy; may need to reduce insulin dosage.
3. Tendency to intensify the existing complications of diabetes.
D. Monitoring fetal and maternal well-being during pregnancy, labor, and delivery.
1. Antepartum period for pregestational and GDM.
   a. For both pregestational and GDM mothers.
      (1) Home blood glucose monitoring.
      (2) Diet: well balanced, avoid refined sugar; no skipping meals or snacks.
      (3) Exercise as prescribed.

b. For pregestational diabetic mothers.
   (1) Maternal alpha-fetoprotein measured around 15 to 20 weeks' gestation due to increased risk of neural tube defects.
   (2) Fetal echocardiography performed between 20 and 22 weeks; repeated at 34 weeks.
   (3) Mother should be taught to take daily fetal movement counts beginning at 28 weeks' gestation.
   (4) Biophysical testing once or twice weekly is begun around 28 to 34 weeks' gestation, depending on glucose control and/or presence of hypertension.
   (5) Labor induction at 38 to 40 weeks; fetal lung maturity determined by amniocentesis if delivery is before 38.5 weeks.
2. Intrapartum period.
   a. For GDM, as long as there is evidence of adequate placental function and the infant's response to stress is appropriate, the pregnancy is allowed to progress to term, with an anticipated vaginal delivery.
   b. For pregestational diabetes, blood glucose levels are maintained with IV glucose and regular insulin.
   c. GDM mothers may need rapid-acting insulin IV; IV glucose is avoided.
   d. Fetal monitoring during labor.
3. Postpartum period.
   a. Endocrine and metabolic changes will occur rapidly after delivery.
   b. Insulin requirements for mother will be markedly decreased and will fluctuate over next few weeks.
   c. Pregestational diabetic mother must go through a period of diabetic reregulation.
   d. GDM mother's glucose returns to normal after delivery.
E. Presence of diabetes predisposes the mother to an increased incidence of:
   1. Pregnancy-induced hypertension.
   2. Hemorrhage.
   3. Polyhydramnios (increase in volume of amniotic fluid >2000 mL).
   4. Vaginal and urinary tract infections.
   5. Premature delivery.
   6. Intrauterine death in third trimester.
   7. Compromised newborn.
      a. Respiratory distress syndrome.
      b. Hypoglycemia.
      c. Hyperbilirubinemia.
      d. Congenital anomalies associated with pregestational diabetes.

### Nursing Interventions (All Types)

> ❗ **NURSING PRIORITY:** Evaluating client's control of diabetes:
> 1. Normal fasting blood glucose 110–115 mg/dL (6.1–6.38 mmol/L).
> 2. Two hours after meals or after glucose load, blood glucose is no higher than 140 mg/dL (7.77 mmol/L).
> 3. Client is in good general health and is of normal weight.
> 4. Glycosylated hemoglobin $A_{1c}$ is less than 6.5% (0.07 proportion of total hemoglobin).

> **Box 15-2  IMPLICATIONS IN THE ADMINISTRATION OF INSULIN**
>
> 1. Do not administer cold insulin; it increases pain and causes irritation at injection site.
> 2. An open 10 mL vial of unrefrigerated insulin should be discarded after 30 days, regardless of how much was used.
> 3. Do not allow insulin to freeze, and keep it away from heat and sunlight.
> 4. Insulin pens (NPH and 70/30) should be discarded after 1 week of storage at room temperature. Regular cartridges, which do not contain preservatives, may be left unrefrigerated for up to 1 month.
> 5. Extreme temperatures (less than 36°F [2.2°C] or greater than 86°F [30°C]) should be avoided.
> 6. Roll the vial between the palms of the hands to decrease the risk for inconsistent concentration of insulin.
> 7. The abdomen is the primary site for subcutaneous injections of insulin. Rotate injection sites within one particular anatomic location; injection sites should be 1 inch apart.
> 8. Abdomen area provides most rapid insulin absorption.
> 9. Use only insulin syringes to administer insulin.
> 10. Check expiration date on the insulin bottle.
> 11. When drawing up regular insulin with a long-acting insulin, draw up the regular (clear) insulin before the longer-acting (cloudy) insulin.
> 12. Regular insulin is used for administration by sliding scale and periods when blood glucose is unstable and difficult to control.
> 13. Using alcohol to cleanse the skin before injection is not recommended for home care. If used, hold alcohol pad in place for a few seconds but do not massage.
> 14. Aspirating is not recommended for self-injection.
> 15. Check dose with another nurse before administering.

**Goal:** To return serum glucose to normal level.

A. Initially administer regular insulin on a proportional basis according to need (Box 15-2).
B. Administer rapid-acting insulin 15 minutes before and short-acting insulin 30 minutes before a meal or snack; do not administer insulin if there is no carbohydrate intake.
C. Maintain adequate fluid intake.
D. Evaluate serum electrolyte levels.
   1. Do not administer potassium unless client is voiding or if urine output begins to drop.
   2. Serum potassium levels will be misleading if the client is dehydrated or in a state of ketoacidosis.
E. Evaluate hydration status.
F. Evaluate for clinical manifestations of hypoglycemia and hyperglycemia.

> **TEST ALERT:** Monitor hydration status and electrolyte balance.

**Goal:** To plan and implement a teaching regimen.

A. Assess current level of knowledge regarding diabetes.
B. Evaluate cultural and socioeconomic parameters.
C. Evaluate client's support system (family, significant others).

**Box 15-3 DIABETIC "SICK DAY" GUIDELINES**

*If you do not feel well (are not eating regularly or have fever, lethargy, nausea, and vomiting, etc.):*

1. Check your blood glucose every 3 to 4 hours and urine ketones when voiding.
2. Increase your intake of fluids that are high in carbohydrates; every hour, drink fluids that replace electrolytes: fruit drinks, sports drinks, soups, regular soft drinks (not diet beverages).
3. If you cannot eat and you have replaced four to five meals with liquids, notify your health care provider.
4. Get plenty of rest; if possible, have someone stay with you.
5. Do not omit or skip your insulin injections or oral medications unless specifically directed to do so by your health care provider.
6. Follow your health care provider's instructions regarding blood glucose levels and insulin or oral hypoglycemic agents.
7. Stay warm, stay in bed, and do not overexert yourself.
8. Call your health care provider when:
    a. You have been ill for 1 to 2 days without getting any better.
    b. You have been vomiting or had diarrhea for more than 6 hours.
    c. Your urine self-testing shows moderate to large amounts of ketones.
    d. You are taking insulin and your blood glucose level continues to be greater than 240 mg/dL (13.32 mmol/L) after you have taken two to three supplemental doses of regular insulin (prearranged with your provider).
    e. You are taking insulin and your blood glucose level is less than 60 mg/dL (3.3 mmol/L).
    f. You have type 2 diabetes, you are taking oral diabetic medications, and your premeal blood glucose levels are 240 mg/dL (13.3 mmol/L) or greater for more than 24 hours.
    g. You have signs of severe hyperglycemia (very dry mouth or fruity odor to breath), dehydration, or confusion.
    h. You are sleepier or more tired than normal.
    i. You have stomach or chest pain or any difficulty breathing.
    j. You have any questions or concerns about what you need to do while ill.

D. Instruct regarding sick-day guidelines (Box 15-3).
E. Instruct to wear or carry medic alert information.

**TEST ALERT:** Determine ability of family/support systems to provide care for client. Identify client's and family's strengths.

F. Administration of insulin (see Box 15-2).
    1. Correct injection techniques.
    2. Rotate injection site within 1 inch from previous injection site (Figure 15-9).
    3. Check expiration date on the insulin.
    4. Duration and peak action of prescribed insulin.
    5. Allow for practice time and return demonstration.
    6. Administer at the same time each day.

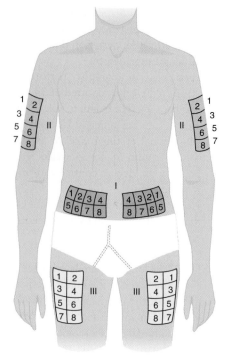

**FIGURE 15-9 Sites used for Insulin Injection.** The injection site can affect the onset, peak, and duration of action of the insulin. Insulin injected into the abdomen (area I) is absorbed fastest, followed by insulin injected into the arm (area II) and the leg (area III). (From Black, J. M., & Hawks, J. H. [2009]. *Medical-surgical nursing: Clinical management for positive outcomes* [8th ed.]. Philadelphia: Saunders.)

7. Clients following an intensive diabetes therapy program may choose to use an insulin pump or to monitor blood glucose levels at least four times a day and take injections at those times (Figure 15-10).
    a. The insulin pump is battery operated; insertion site is changed every 2 to 3 days; pump is refilled and reprogrammed when site is changed.
    b. Delivers continuous infusion of short-acting insulin over a 24-hour period, allowing for tight glucose control.
    c. Can deliver a bolus of insulin based on excessive carbohydrates ingested.
    d. Monitor the insertion site for redness and swelling.

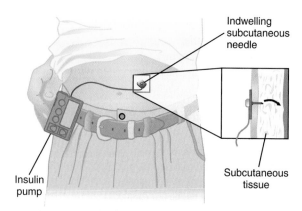

**FIGURE 15-10 Insulin Pump.** (From Black, J. M., & Hawks, J. H. [2009]. *Medical-surgical nursing: Clinical management for positive outcomes* [8th ed.]. Philadelphia: Saunders.)

8. Good handwashing is critical; destroy and dispose of single-use syringe safely.
9. Insulin pen is a compact portable device that is loaded with insulin and a good option for those who are visually impaired.
G. Oral hypoglycemic agents.
   1. Take medication as scheduled; do not skip or add doses.
   2. Signs and symptoms of hypoglycemia.
   3. Anticipate change in medication with pregnancy.
H. Monitoring blood glucose.
   1. Self-monitoring of blood glucose (SMBG)—use soap and water to cleanse site.
   2. Use side of finger pad rather than near the center. If alternative site is used (e.g., forearm), may require different equipment.
   3. Obtain blood drop needed for specific device.
I. Exercise.
   1. Establish an exercise program.
   2. Avoid sporadic exercise.
   3. Review instructions regarding adjustment of insulin and food intake to meet requirements of increased activity.
   4. Extremities involved in activity should not be used for insulin injection (e.g., arms when playing tennis).
J. Diet (Box 15-4).
   1. Regularly scheduled mealtimes.
   2. Understanding of food groups and balanced nutrition.
   3. Incorporate family tendencies and cultural patterns into prescribed dietary regimen.
   4. Provide client and family with written instructions regarding dietary needs.
K. Infection control.
   1. Report infections promptly.
   2. Insulin requirements may increase with severe infections.
   3. Increased problems with vaginitis, urinary tract infections, and skin irritation.
L. Avoid injury.
   1. Decreased healing capabilities, especially in lower extremities.

---

**Box 15-4  OLDER ADULT CARE FOCUS**

**Guidelines for Food Selection**
1. Avoid canned fruits that are in heavy syrup; select fruit packed in water.
2. Include fresh fruits and vegetables and whole-grain cereals and breads to provide adequate dietary fiber to prevent constipation.
3. Avoid casseroles, fried foods, sauces and gravies, and sweets.
4. Fats (oils, margarines) that are liquid at room temperature are better than those that are solid.
5. Read food labels; remember that the highest content ingredient is listed first.
6. Select foods in which the majority of calories do not come from a fat source.

2. Maintain adequate blood supply to extremities; avoid tight-fitting clothing around the legs.
3. Proper foot care (see Chapter 18).

**Goal:** To prepare the client with diabetes for surgery.

A. Obtain base serum laboratory values for postoperative comparison.
B. Surgery should be scheduled in early morning to decrease problems with diet and insulin replacement.
C. Oral hypoglycemic agents should not be given the morning of surgery.
D. For clients with NPO (nothing by mouth) status who require insulin, an IV of 5% dextrose in water ($D_5W$) is frequently started.
E. Obtain a blood glucose reading before sending the client to surgery to make sure he or she is not developing hypoglycemia.

> **NURSING PRIORITY:** Evaluate intake; do not give insulin to a client on NPO status unless an IV is in place.

**Goal:** To maintain control of diabetic condition in the client who has had surgery.

A. IV fluids and regular insulin until the client is able to take fluids orally.
B. Obtain blood glucose level four to six times a day to determine fluctuations.
C. After glucose levels stabilize, the client can usually resume taking his or her preoperative diabetic medication.
D. Observe for fluctuation of blood glucose immediately after surgery.
E. Avoid urinary bladder catheterization.
F. Evaluate peripheral circulation and prevent skin breakdown.
G. Assess for development of postoperative infections.

**Goal:** To identify diabetic ketoacidosis and help the client return to homeostasis.

A. Establish IV access.
B. Anticipate rapid infusion of normal saline solution or plasma expanders initially, then at a maintenance rate. Administer with caution to clients with cardiac conditions.
C. Administer insulin: use IV drip (regular insulin only) during the acute phase; then administer subcutaneously as blood glucose level begins to decrease.
D. Frequent monitoring of vital signs.
E. Frequent serum glucose checks.
F. Hourly urine measurements: do not administer potassium if urine output is low or dropping.
G. Monitor blood glucose levels frequently (normally every hour).
H. Cardiac monitor to determine presence of dysrhythmias secondary to potassium levels.
I. Monitor serum electrolyte levels, particularly potassium levels.
   1. Hyperkalemia may occur initially in response to the acidosis.

2. Hypokalemia occurs about 4 to 6 hours after treatment, as the acidosis is resolving.
J. Evaluate acid–base status.

**Goal:** To identify HHS and to help the client return to homeostasis.

A. Establish IV access.
B. IV infusion to rehydrate the client; normal saline solution is frequently used; closely monitor hydration status.
C. Low-dose insulin given intravenously at first to decrease blood glucose level slowly.
D. Evaluate urine output.
E. Monitor serum glucose level.
F. Evaluate acid–base status.
G. Assess the client for presence of other chronic health problems.

### Home Care

A. Maintain optimal weight.
B. Continue to receive long-term medical care (Box 15-5).
C. Notify all health care providers of diagnosis of diabetes; wear medical alert identification.
D. Recognize problems of the cardiovascular system.
   1. Peripheral vascular disease.
   2. Decreased healing.
   3. Increased risk for stroke.
   4. Increased risk for myocardial infarction.
   5. Presence of retinopathy.
   6. Increased risk for renal disease.
E. Recognize problems of peripheral neuropathy.
F. Help the client understand problems that diabetes imposes on pregnancy and the subsequent development of a high-risk pregnancy.
G. Help the client understand the problem of increased susceptibility to infections.

**Goal:** To help the client with diabetes maintain homeostasis throughout pregnancy.

A. Prevent infection.

---

**Box 15-5** "DO NOT" LIST FOR TEACHING CLIENTS WITH DIABETES MELLITUS

When teaching a client and family, the following should be included on the "do not" list.
**DO NOT:**
- Skip doses of insulin, especially when ill.
- Ignore symptoms of hypoglycemia or hyperglycemia—seek help.
- Forget that exercise will lower blood glucose levels.
- Drink excessive amounts of alcohol or drink lots of regular sodas or fruit juice.
- Smoke cigarettes or use nicotine products.
- Apply heat or cold directly to your feet.
- Go barefoot.
- Put oil or lotion between your toes.
- Forget to order your insulin, oral hypoglycemic medication, or glucose-monitoring supplies.

---

B. Frequent evaluation of glucose levels and monitoring of changes in insulin requirements.
C. Utilization of insulin rather than oral hypoglycemic agents for pregestational diabetic mother.
D. Maintain optimum level of weight gain; labor may be induced, or cesarean delivery may be required if complications are evident.

**NURSING PRIORITY:** Advise the client to stop exercising immediately if uterine contractions occur while exercising and to drink two to three glasses of water and lie down on her side for an hour. If contractions do not subside, have her contact her health care provider.

**Goal:** To help the client with diabetes maintain homeostasis throughout labor and delivery.

A. IV $D_{10}W$, Ringer's lactate, or $D_5$ Ringer's lactate to maintain homeostasis during labor along with continuous infusion of insulin.
B. Fetal monitoring to identify early stages of fetal distress.
C. X-ray pelvimetry to identify cephalopelvic disproportion.
D. Increased incidence of dystocia because of large infants.
E. Frequent evaluation of serum glucose levels (every 2–3 hours).

**Goal:** To help the client with diabetes return to homeostasis during the postpartum period.

A. Anticipate fluctuation in insulin requirements caused by:
   1. Loss of fetal insulin.
   2. Removal of placental influence on insulin.
   3. Changes in metabolic activity.
B. Observe and monitor for rapid fluctuations in serum glucose levels.
C. Prevent postpartum infection.

### Hypoglycemia (Insulin Reaction/Shock)

**Hypoglycemia is a condition characterized by a decreased serum glucose level, which results in decreased cerebral function.**

*Assessment*

A. Risk factors.
   1. Poorly controlled diabetes.
      a. Too little food.
      b. Increase in exercise without adequate food.
      c. Increase in insulin intake.
   2. Excessive alcohol intake with poor nutrition.
   3. Gastroenteritis or gastroparesis, which may impede absorption of food.
   4. Reflex action of insulin caused by increased carbohydrate intake (Somogyi effect).
B. Clinical manifestations.
   1. Lability of mood.
   2. Emotional changes, confusion.
   3. Headache, lightheadedness, seizures, coma.
   4. Impaired vision.
   5. Tachycardia, hypotension.
   6. Nervousness, tremors.
   7. Diaphoresis.

C. Diagnostics.
  1. Serum glucose below 70 mg/dL (3.89 mmol/L).

*Treatment*

A. Carbohydrates (15–20 g) by mouth if client is alert and can swallow.

  1. Milk preferred in children with a mild reaction; it provides immediate lactose, as well as protein and fat for prolonged action.
  2. Simple sugars for immediate response: orange juice, honey, candy, glucose tablets.
  3. If simple carbohydrates are taken to increase blood glucose, client should plan on eating protein or complex carbohydrates to prevent rebound hypoglycemia.
B. Glucagon can be given subcutaneously, intramuscularly, or intravenously if client is unconscious. In an acute care setting, hypoglycemia may be treated with 20 to 50 mL of 50% dextrose IV push.

*Nursing Interventions*

**Goal:** To increase serum glucose level.

A. Glucose/carbohydrate preparations as indicated.

---

**⚠ NURSING PRIORITY:** When in doubt of diagnosis of hypoglycemia versus hyperglycemia, administer carbohydrates; severe hypoglycemia can rapidly result in permanent brain damage, which is why hypoglycemia is considered an endocrine emergency.

---

B. Thorough assessment of the client with diabetes for the development of hypoglycemia.

**Goal:** To help the client identify precipitating causes and activities to prevent the development of hypoglycemia.

A. Instruct the client with diabetes to carry simple carbohydrates.
B. Administer between-meal snacks at the peak action of insulin.
C. Between-meal snacks should limit simple carbohydrates and increase complex carbohydrates and protein.
D. Evaluate the client's understanding of insulin and control of diabetes; reaffirm teaching as appropriate.

📋 **Metabolic Syndrome**

**Metabolic syndrome (syndrome X or insulin resistance syndrome) is a syndrome that increases a client's chance of developing cardiovascular disease and diabetes mellitus and is characterized by obesity, hypertension, abnormal lipid levels, and high blood glucose.**

*Assessment*

A. Risk factors.
  1. Insulin resistance related to excessive visceral fat.
  2. Obesity, inactivity.
B. Clinical manifestations (Figure 15-11).
C. Diagnostics.
  1. Elevated fasting blood glucose and triglycerides.
  2. Decreased high-density lipoprotein cholesterol.

# METABOLIC SYNDROME - SYNDROME X

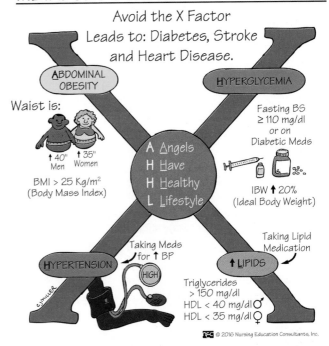

**FIGURE 15-11 Metabolic Syndrome.** (From Zerwekh, J., Garneau, A., & Miller, C. J. [2017]. *Digital collection of the memory notebooks of nursing* [4th ed.]. Chandler, AZ: Nursing Education Consultants, Inc.)

*Treatment*

A. Medications.
  1. Antihyperlipidemics.
  2. Antihypertensives.
  3. Metformin.

*Nursing Interventions*

A. To reduce risk factors—lifestyle modifications.
B. To promote healthy diet—low in saturated fats; promote weight loss.
C. To encourage regular physical activity.

📋 **Pancreatitis**

**Pancreatitis is an inflammatory condition of the pancreas (Figure 15-12).**

A. Acute: characterized by an acute inflammatory process; problems range from mild edema to severe hypotension and severe hemorrhagic necrosis.
B. Chronic: characterized by progressive destruction and fibrosis of the pancreas; condition may follow acute pancreatitis but may also occur alone.

*Assessment*

A. Risk factors/etiology.
  1. Biliary tract obstructive disease, causing reflux of bile secretions is most common cause.
  2. Smoking, hyperlipidemia.
  3. Alcohol intake precipitating an increase in the secretion of pancreatic enzymes.
B. Less common causes include trauma, viral infections, penetrating duodenal ulcer, cysts, abscesses, cystic fibrosis,

# PANCREATITIS
## (Inflammatory Condition of the Pancreas)

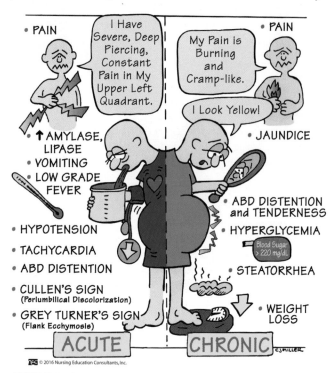

**FIGURE 15-12 Pancreatitis.** (From Zerwekh, J., Garneau, A., & Miller, C. J. [2017]. *Digital collection of the memory notebooks of nursing* [4th ed.]. Chandler, AZ: Nursing Education Consultants, Inc.)

Kaposi sarcoma, and certain drugs (corticosteroids, thiazide diuretics, oral contraceptives, sulfonamides, nonsteroidal antiinflammatories).

C. Clinical manifestations.
   1. Severe constant left upper quadrant or midepigastric pain.
      a. Radiates to the back or flank area.
      b. Exacerbated by eating.
   2. Acute.
      a. Persistent vomiting.
      b. Low-grade fever.
      c. Hypotension and tachycardia.
      d. Jaundice, if common bile duct is obstructed.
      e. Abdominal distention.
      f. Cullen sign: bluish periumbilical discoloration.
      g. Grey Turner sign: bluish flank discoloration.
      h. Hypoactive or absent bowel sounds.
   3. Chronic.
      a. Decrease in weight.
      b. Mild jaundice.
      c. Steatorrhea.
      d. Abdominal distention and tenderness.
      e. Hyperglycemia.
D. Diagnostics.
   1. Increase in serum amylase (hallmark) and lipase levels.
   2. Increase in urine amylase level.
   3. Hyperglycemia.
   4. Leukocytosis.
   5. Elevated C-reactive protein.
   6. Hypocalcemia.
   7. Ultrasonography.
   8. Computed tomography scan.

## Treatment

A. Medications.
   1. Analgesics, antispasmodics.
   2. Antibiotics, carbonic anhydrase inhibitors.
   3. Antacids, proton pump inhibitors.
   4. Chronic pancreatitis may include pancreatic enzyme products and insulin.
B. Decrease pancreatic stimulus.
   1. NPO status; IV fluids.
   2. Nasogastric suction.
   3. Bed rest.
   4. Diet: (if not NPO) low-fat, high-carbohydrate.
C. Surgical intervention to eliminate precipitating cause (biliary tract obstruction).

## Complications

A. Pseudocyst—cavity surrounding the pancreas filled with inflammatory exudate.
B. Abscess—large fluid cavity within the pancreas that results from extensive necrosis.

## Nursing Interventions

Nursing interventions are the same for the client with acute pancreatitis and for the client with chronic pancreatitis experiencing an acute episode.

**Goal:** To relieve pain.

A. Administer analgesics; pain control is essential (restlessness may cause pancreatic stimulation and further secretion of enzymes).
B. Place client in side-lying position with knees drawn up to chest or in semi-Fowler's position with knees flexed toward the chest.
C. Evaluate precipitating cause.

**Goal:** To decrease pancreatic stimulus.

A. Bed rest.
B. Maintain NPO status initially.
C. Maintain nasogastric suctioning.
D. Small frequent feedings when food is allowed.
E. Pain control.

**Goal:** To prevent complications.

A. Identify electrolyte imbalances, especially hypocalcemia.
B. Maintain adequate hydration.
C. Maintain respiratory status; problems occur because of pain and ascites.
D. Assess for hypoglycemia and development of diabetes.

## Home Care

A. Avoid all alcohol intake.
B. Know signs of hyperglycemia and development of diabetes; understand when to return for evaluation of blood glucose level.

C. Bland diet, low in fat, high in carbohydrates (protein recommendations vary).

D. Replacement of pancreatic enzymes.

## Cancer of the Pancreas

**The majority of pancreatic tumors occur in the head of the pancreas. As tumors grow, the bile ducts are obstructed, causing jaundice. Tumors in the body of the pancreas frequently do not cause symptoms until growth is advanced. Cancer of the pancreas has a poor prognosis.**

### Assessment

A. Risk factors/etiology.
  1. Peak incidence is between ages 65 and 80.
  2. History of chronic pancreatitis and diabetes mellitus is common.
  3. Cigarette smoke (2–3 times more common among smokers).
B. Clinical manifestations.
  1. Dull, aching abdominal pain.
  2. Nausea.
  3. Anorexia and progressive weight loss.
  4. Jaundice.
C. Diagnostics.
  1. Increased cancer-associated antigen 19-9 (CA 19-9) level.
  2. Abdominal or endoscopic ultrasonography.
  3. Spiral CT scan.
  4. Needle aspiration.
  5. Endoscopic retrograde cholangiopancreatography.
  6. MRI.

### Treatment

A. Surgery: Whipple's procedure (radical pancreatic duodenectomy).
B. Radiation therapy.
C. Chemotherapy.

### Nursing Interventions

**Goal:** To maintain homeostasis (see Nursing Interventions for pancreatitis).

**Goal:** To provide preoperative nursing measures if surgery is indicated.

A. Maintain nasogastric suctioning; assess for adequate hydration.
B. Control hyperglycemia.
C. Assess cardiac and respiratory stability.
D. Assess for development of thrombophlebitis.

**Goal:** To promote comfort, prevent complications, and maintain homeostasis in client who has undergone Whipple's procedure.

A. General postoperative care (see Chapter 3). Extensive surgical resection of the pancreas and surrounding tissue.
B. Evaluate for hypercoagulable state and bleeding tendencies.
C. Monitor for fluctuation in serum glucose levels.
D. Maintain NPO status and nasogastric suction until peristalsis returns.

E. Encourage adequate nutrition when appropriate.
  1. Decrease fats and increase carbohydrates.
  2. Small, frequent feedings.
F. Closely observe for development of problems from thromboemboli to coagulation problems; surgery and immobility.

### Home Care

A. Evaluate for bouts of anxiety and depression caused by severity of illness and prognosis (see Chapter 12).
B. Assist client in setting realistic goals.
C. Encourage venting of feelings.
D. Discuss methods for pain control.

## PHYSIOLOGY OF THE ADRENALS

The adrenal glands are located at the apex of each kidney.

A. Adrenal medulla: secretes catecholamines, epinephrine, and norepinephrine; under the influence of the sympathetic nervous system.
B. Adrenal cortex: main body of the adrenal gland; responsible for the secretion of glucocorticoids (cortisol, hydrocortisone), mineralocorticoids (aldosterone), and adrenal sex hormones (androgens and estrogen); adrenal cortical function is essential for life.
C. Function of the adrenal cortex is controlled by the negative feedback mechanisms regulating hormone release; pituitary gland secretes adrenocorticotropic hormone (ACTH), which in turn regulates hormone release of the adrenal cortex.

> **! NURSING PRIORITY:** Clients experiencing problems of the adrenal medulla have severe fluctuations in blood pressure related to the levels of catecholamines.

### System Assessment

A. Adrenal medulla.
  1. Evaluate changes in blood pressure.
  2. Assess for changes in metabolic rate.
B. Adrenal cortex.
  1. Evaluate changes in weight.
  2. Evaluate changes in skin color and texture and the presence and distribution of body hair.
  3. Assess cardiovascular system for instability, as evidenced by a labile blood pressure and cardiac output.
  4. Evaluate GI discomfort.
  5. Assess fluid and electrolyte changes from effects of mineralocorticoids and glucocorticoids.
  6. Assess for changes in glucose metabolism.
  7. Assess for changes in reproductive system and in sexual activity.
  8. Evaluate changes in muscle mass.

## DISORDERS OF THE ADRENALS

### Pheochromocytoma

Pheochromocytoma is a rare disorder of the adrenal medulla characterized by a tumor that secretes an excess of epinephrine and norepinephrine.

### Assessment

A. Clinical manifestations.
1. Persistent or paroxysmal hypertension.
2. Palpitations, tachycardia.
3. Hyperglycemia.
4. Diaphoresis.
5. Nervousness, apprehension.
6. Headache.
B. Diagnostics (see Appendix 15-1).
1. Increase in urinary excretion of total free catecholamine.
2. Increase in urinary excretion of vanillylmandelic acid and metanephrine.
3. Serum assay of catecholamine.
4. Magnetic resonance imaging, CT scan.
C. Treatment.
1. Medications.
a. Antihypertensive medications (alpha-adrenergic blockers to lower blood pressure quickly).
b. Antidysrhythmic medications.
c. Potassium replacement.
2. Surgery: removal of the tumor is the treatment of choice.

### Nursing Interventions

**Goal:** To decrease client's hypertension and provide preoperative nursing measures as appropriate (see Chapter 3).

A. Decrease intake of stimulants.
B. Sedate as indicated.
C. Maintain calm, quiet environment.
D. Assess vital signs frequently.

**Goal:** To help the client return to homeostasis after adrenalectomy.

A. Maintain normal blood pressure the first 24 to 48 hours after surgery; client is at increased risk for hemorrhage or severe hypotensive episode.
1. Assess for blood pressure changes caused by catecholamine imbalance (both hypertension and hypotension).
2. Administer analgesics judiciously.
3. Administer corticosteroids as indicated.
4. Maintain quiet, cool environment.
5. Maintain IV fluid administration.
B. Assess for hypoglycemia.
C. Tendency toward hemorrhagic problems.
D. Monitor renal perfusion and urinary output.
E. Assess for problems of adrenal insufficiency.

**Goal:** To maintain health after adrenalectomy.

A. Continued medical follow-up care.
B. If both adrenals are removed, the client will require lifelong replacement of adrenal hormones.

### Addison's Disease (Adrenocortical Insufficiency/Adrenal Hypofunction)

**Addison's disease is caused by a decrease in secretion of the adrenal cortex hormones.**

A. Decreased physiologic response to stress, vascular insufficiency, and hypoglycemia.

B. Decrease in aldosterone secretions (mineralocorticoids), which normally promote concentration of sodium and water and excretion of potassium.
C. May cause an alteration in adrenal androgen secretion necessary for secondary sex characteristics.

### Assessment

A. Risk factors/etiology.
1. An autoimmunity-induced problem.
2. Occurs after bilateral adrenalectomy.
3. Abrupt withdrawal from long-term corticosteroid therapy.
4. *Adrenal crisis* may be precipitated by stress, sudden withdrawal from corticosteroid therapy, adrenal surgery, or sudden pituitary gland destruction.
5. Tuberculosis, some fungal and viral infections.
6. Metastatic cancer.
B. Clinical manifestations (development of symptoms requires loss of 90% of both adrenal cortices) (Figure 15-13).
1. Onset is insidious; client may go for weeks to months before diagnosis is made.
2. Fatigue, weakness, weight loss.
3. GI disturbances, postural hypotension.
4. Bronze pigmentation of the skin.
5. Hyponatremia, hyperkalemia, hypoglycemia.
6. *Adrenal crisis* (Addisonian crisis).
a. Profound fatigue, dehydration.

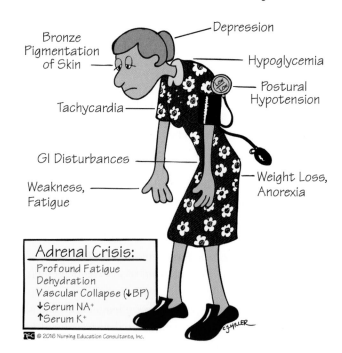

# ADDISON'S DISEASE
## Adrenocortical Insufficiency

**FIGURE 15-13 Addison's Disease.** (From Zerwekh, J., Garneau, A., & Miller, C. J. [2017]. *Digital collection of the memory notebooks of nursing* [4th ed.]. Chandler, AZ: Nursing Education Consultants, Inc.)

b. Vascular collapse (cyanosis and signs of shock: pallor, anxiety, weak/rapid pulse, tachypnea, and low blood pressure).

> **TEST ALERT:** Determine whether vital signs are abnormal (e.g., hypotension, hypertension); notify others of change in the client's condition.

C. Diagnostics (see Appendix 15-1).
   1. ACTH stimulation test, plasma ACTH level.
   2. Decreased serum sodium level and increased serum potassium and BUN levels.

### Treatment

Replace adrenal hormones.

### Nursing Interventions

**Goal:** To help the client return to homeostasis.

A. Initiate and maintain IV infusion of normal saline and dextrose solutions.
B. Administer large doses of corticosteroids through IV bolus initially, then titrate in a diluted solution.
C. Frequent evaluation of vital signs.
D. Assess sodium and water retention.
E. Evaluate serum potassium levels.
F. Protect client from noise, light, and temperature extremes.

> **⚠ NURSING PRIORITY:** If any client is experiencing difficulty with maintaining adequate blood pressure, do not move the client unless absolutely necessary. Avoid all unnecessary nursing procedures until the client's condition is stabilized.

**Goal:** To safely take steroid replacements (see Appendix 9-2).

A. Administer steroid preparations with food or an antacid.
B. Evaluate for edema and fluid retention.
C. Assess serum sodium and potassium levels.
D. Check daily weight.
E. Increase intake of protein and carbohydrates.
F. Evaluate for hypoglycemia.
G. Observe for cushingoid symptoms.

### 🔆 Home Care

A. Lifelong steroid therapy is necessary.
B. Dosage of steroids may need to be increased in times of additional stress.
C. Prevent infections and falls. Infection, diaphoresis, and injury will increase the need for steroids and may precipitate a crisis state.
D. Report gastric distress because it may be caused by steroids.
E. Carry a medical identification card.

### 📋 Cushing's Syndrome (Adrenal Cortex Hypersecretion/Hypercortisolism)

**Cushing's syndrome occurs as a result of excess levels of adrenal cortex hormones (primarily glucocorticoids) and, to a lesser extent, androgen and aldosterone.**

> **TEST ALERT:** Evaluate client's use of medications. Implement procedures to counteract adverse effects of medication. The most common cause of Cushing's syndrome is long-term steroid therapy for chronic conditions. Many chronic conditions necessitate the use of long-term steroid therapy.

### Assessment

A. Risk factors/etiology.
   1. More common in women.
   2. Pituitary hypersecretion.
   3. A benign pituitary tumor.
   4. Iatrogenic: most often a result of long-term steroid therapy.
B. Clinical manifestations (Figure 15-14).
   1. Marked change in personality (emotional lability), irritability.
   2. Changes in appearance.
      a. Moon face, deposit of fat on the back.
      b. Thin skin, purple striae.
      c. Truncal obesity with thin extremities.
      d. Bruises and petechiae.
   3. Persistent hyperglycemia, osteoporosis.
   4. GI distress from increased acid production.
   5. Increased susceptibility to infection.
   6. Sodium and fluid retention; potassium depletion.
   7. Hypertension.
   8. Changes in secondary sexual characteristics.
      a. Amenorrhea (females), hirsutism (females).
      b. Gynecomastia (males).
   9. Impotence or decreased libido.
C. Diagnostics (see Appendix 15-1).
   1. Increased serum sodium and decreased serum potassium levels.

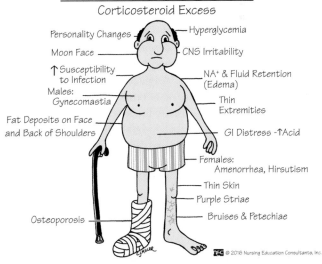

**FIGURE 15-14 Cushing's Syndrome.** *CNS,* Central nervous system; *GI,* gastrointestinal; *NA,* sodium. (From Zerwekh, J., Garneau, A., & Miller, C. J. [2017]. *Digital collection of the memory notebooks of nursing* [4th ed.]. Chandler, AZ: Nursing Education Consultants, Inc.)

2. Hyperglycemia.
3. Increased plasma cortisol levels.
4. Loss of diurnal variation in cortisone levels.
5. Low-dose and high-dose dexamethasone suppression test.
D. Complications.
  1. Heart failure, hypertension.
  2. Pathologic fractures, psychosis.

### Treatment

Treatment depends on the cause of the problem.

### Nursing Interventions

**Goal:** To assist the client to manage hormone imbalance.

A. Restrict sodium and water intake.
B. Monitor fluid and electrolyte levels.
C. Evaluate for hyperglycemia.
D. Assess for GI disturbances.
E. Prevent infection.

**Goal:** To prevent complications.

A. Excessive sodium and water retention: monitor for edema, hypertension, heart failure.
B. Potassium depletion: monitor for cardiac arrhythmias.
C. Evaluate the client's ability to cope with change in body image.
D. Evaluate for thromboembolic problems.
E. Predisposed to fractures; promote weight bearing; monitor for joint and bone pain; promote home safety.

### Home Care

A. Stress the need for continuous health care.
B. Encourage the continuation of activities.
C. Have the client demonstrate an understanding of the medication regimen.
D. Help the client identify methods of coping with problems of therapy.
E. Have the client demonstrate an understanding of specific problems for which he or she needs to notify the physician.

| Appendix 15-1 | ENDOCRINE DIAGNOSTICS | |
|---|---|---|

| Diagnostic Test | Normal | Clinical/Nursing Implications |
|---|---|---|
| **Thyroid** | | |
| Thyroxine ($T_4$) | 4.6–11 mcg/dL (59–142 nmol/L)<br>Increased in hyperthyroidism, decreased in hypothyroidism | 1. Stimulation of the thyroid gland by TSH will initiate the release of stored thyroid hormone. |
| Triiodothyronine ($T_3$) | 70–204 ng/dL (1.08–3.14 nmol/L)<br>Increased in hyperthyroidism, decreased in hypothyroidism | 1. When $T_3$ and $T_4$ are low, TSH secretion increases.<br>2. $T_3$ and $T_4$ are used to confirm abnormal TSH. |
| Thyroid-stimulating hormone (TSH) | 0.4–4.2 mU/L | 1. Most common test performed for clients with thyroid problems.<br>2. With hyperthyroidism the TSH is low, and with hypothyroidism the TSH is elevated. |
| Radioactive iodine uptake (RAIU) | 2–4 hr: 3%–19%<br>24 hr: 11%–30% | 1. PO dosing is not harmful.<br>2. No supplemental iodine for 5 weeks before test.<br>3. Thyroid medication can interfere with test results.<br>4. Instruct patient to increase fluid intake for 24–48 hours posttest. |
| Neonatal thyroxine ($T_4$) | Normal levels vary with age from 1 day to 120 days<br>1–3 days: 11–22 mcg/dL (188.03–376.07 nmol/L)<br>1–2 wk: 10–16 mcg/dL (170.94–273.50 nmol/L)<br>1–4 mo: 8–16 mcg/dL (136.75–273.50 nmol/L) | 1. Positive test result is associated with hypothyroidism.<br>2. Procedure is done by means of a heel puncture on infant.<br>3. Levels of neonatal $T_4$ are not interpreted in same terms as serum $T_4$ values; this is a completely different test. |
| **Pancreas** | | |
| Serum glucose<br>Oral glucose tolerance test | Maintains 70–100 mg/dL (3.9–5.6 mmol/L) (fasting)<br>1 hr: less than 200 mg/dL (11.1 mmol/L)<br>2 hr: less than 140 mg/dL (7.8 mmol/L) | 1. Test is timed to rule out diabetes by determining rate of glucose absorption from serum.<br>2. In healthy person, insulin response to large dose of glucose is immediate.<br>3. Insulin and oral hypoglycemic agents should not be administered before test. |

**Appendix 15-1    ENDOCRINE DIAGNOSTICS—cont'd**

| Diagnostic Test | Normal | Clinical/Nursing Implications |
|---|---|---|
| Glucose fasting blood sugar (FBS)<br>Also called fasting blood glucose (FBG) and fasting plasma glucose (FPG) | Same as serum glucose: 70–100 mg/dL (3.9–5.6 mmol/L)<br>—prediabetes: 101–125 mg/dL (5.6–6.9 mmol/L)<br>—>125 mg/dL (6.9 mmol/L) is diagnostic for diabetes | 1. Used as a screening test for problems of metabolism.<br>2. Maintain client in fasting state for 4–8 hours before blood draw.<br>3. If client is a known diabetic and experiences dizziness, weakness, or fainting, test glucose level.<br>4. If client is diabetic, withhold insulin or oral hypoglycemic agents until after blood is obtained. |
| Glycosylated hemoglobin (HbA$_{1c}$) | Nondiabetic range is usually 4%–6% (0.04–0.06); 2%–6.4% (0.02–0.06) considered good diabetic control (goal is 6.5% [0.07] or less); >7% (0.07) considered poor diabetic control | 1. More accurate test of diabetic control because it measures glucose attached to hemoglobin (indicates overall control for past 90–120 days, which is the life span of the RBC). |

**TEST ALERT:** Frequently, the level of the FBS is given in a question, and it is necessary to evaluate the level and determine the appropriate nursing intervention.

| Diagnostic Test | Normal | Clinical/Nursing Implications |
|---|---|---|
| Two-hour postprandial blood sugar | 65–139 mg/dL (3.6–7.7 mmol/L) | 1. Involves measuring the serum glucose 2 hours after a meal; results are significantly increased with diabetes. |
| Serum amylase | 30–122 U/L (0.53–2.04 ukat/L) | 1. Used to evaluate pancreatic cell damage.<br>2. Other intestinal conditions and inflammatory conditions cause increase. |
| Serum lipase | 31–186 U/L (0.52–3.11 ukat/L)<br>Normal values vary with method; elevated is abnormal | 1. Appears in serum after damage to pancreas. |
| Urine sugar | Negative for glucose | 1. Use fresh double-voided specimen.<br>2. A rough indicator of serum glucose levels.<br>3. Results may be altered by various medications. |
| Ketone bodies (acetone) | Negative | 1. Ketone bodies occur in the urine before there is significant increase in serum ketones.<br>2. Use freshly voided urine. |
| Urinary amylase | 2-hr specimen 2–34 U/hr<br>24-hr specimen 24–408 U/24 hr | 1. In pancreatic injury, more amylase enters blood and is excreted in urine.<br>2. May be done on a 2-hr or a 24-hr urine specimen. |
| **Pituitary**<br>Growth hormone (GH) | <4 ng/mL (ug/L) in men<br><18 ng/mL (ug/L) in women | 1. NPO after midnight.<br>2. Maintain bed rest until serum sample is drawn. |
| Osmolarity urine | 300–900 mOsm/kg (mmol/kg) of water | 1. Used in evaluating ADH. |
| Osmolarity serum | 285–295 mOsm/kg (mmol/kg) of water | 2. Do serum and urine tests at same time and compare results. |
| | | 3. Normally, urine osmolarity should be higher than serum. |
| **Adrenal Medulla**<br>Urinary vanillylmandelic acid (VMA) | <6.8 mg (34.31 μmol/day) in 24 hr<br>Increased with pheochromocytoma | 1. Client will need to be on VMA-restricted diet (no coffee, tea, chocolate, aspirin, vanilla, citrus fruits) 2–3 days before the test and during testing.<br>2. 24-hr urine collection. |
| **Urine Catecholamines**<br>Epinephrine, norepinephrine<br>Dopamine<br>Metanephrine<br>Normetanephrine<br>ACTH stimulation test | Increased in conditions that precipitate increase in catecholamine secretion<br>Increase in plasma cortisol levels by more than 7 mcg/dL (193.12 nmol/L) above baseline | 1. Same as for VMA.<br>2. ACTH is given as IM or IV bolus, and samples are drawn at 30 and 60 min to evaluate ability of adrenal glands to secrete steroids. |

*Continued*

## Appendix 15-1   ENDOCRINE DIAGNOSTICS—cont'd

| Diagnostic Test | Normal | Clinical/Nursing Implications |
|---|---|---|
| **Adrenal Cortex** | | |
| ACTH suppression (dexamethasone suppression test) | Normal suppression; 50% decrease in cortisone production (cortisol level <3 mcg/dL [82.76 nmol/L]) | 1. An overnight test: A small amount of dexamethasone is administered in the evening, and serum and urine are evaluated in the morning; extensive test may cover 6 days.<br>2. Cushing syndrome is ruled out if suppression is normal. |
| Plasma cortisol levels for diurnal variations | Secretion high in early morning, decreased in evening.<br>8:00 a.m.: 5–23 mcg/dL (137.94–634.52 nmo/L)<br>4:00 p.m.: 3–16 mcg/dL 83–441 nmol/L) | 1. Elevation in plasma cortisol levels occurs in the morning and significant decrease in evening and night—a diurnal variation. |
| 24-hour urine for 17-hydroxycorticosteroids and 17-ketosteroids | Male: 3–10 mg/24 hr (8.28–27.59 nmol/d)<br>Female: 2–8 mg/24 hr (5.51–22.07 nmol/d)<br>Child under 12 yr: <4.5 mg/24 hr (12.41 nmol/d) | 1. Increase in urine levels indicates hyperadrenal function. |

*ACTH,* Adrenocorticotropic hormone; *ADH,* antidiuretic hormone; *IM,* intramuscular; *IV,* intravenous; *NPO,* nothing by mouth; *PO,* by mouth; *RBC,* red blood cell.

## Appendix 15-2   MEDICATIONS USED IN ENDOCRINE DISORDERS

| Medications | Side Effects | Nursing Implications |
|---|---|---|
| **ADH Replacement** | | |
| Desmopressin: nasal spray, PO, IV, subQ | Excessive water retention, headache, nausea, flushing | 1. Monitor daily weight, intake and output, and urine specific gravity. |
| Vasopressin: IM, subQ | Vasoconstriction | 1. Vasopressin more likely to cause adverse cardiovascular and thromboembolic problems. |

**Antithyroid Agents:** Inhibit production of thyroid hormone; do not inactivate thyroid hormone in circulating blood. They are not reliable for long-term inhibition of thyroid hormone production.

| | | |
|---|---|---|
| Methimazole: PO<br>Propylthiouracil (PTU): PO | Agranulocytosis; abdominal discomfort; nausea, vomiting, diarrhea; crosses placenta<br>Same; crosses placenta more rapidly | 1. May increase anticoagulation effect of heparin and oral anticoagulants.<br>2. May be combined with iodine preparations.<br>3. Monitor CBC.<br>4. Store methimazole in light-sensitive container.<br>5. May be used before surgery or treatment with radioactive iodine. |
| Lugol's solution: PO | Inhibits synthesis and release of thyroid hormone | 1. Administer in fluid to decrease unpleasant taste.<br>2. May be used to decrease vascularity of thyroid gland before surgery. |

**Radioactive Iodine:** Accumulates in the thyroid gland; causes partial or total destruction of thyroid gland through radiation.

| | | |
|---|---|---|
| Radioactive iodine: PO | Discomfort in thyroid area; bone marrow depression<br>Desired effect: permanent hypothyroidism | 1. Increase fluids immediately after treatment because radioactive isotope is excreted in the urine.<br>2. Therapeutic dose of radioactive iodine is low; no radiation-safety precautions are required.<br>3. Contraindicated in pregnancy. |

**Thyroid Replacements:** Replace thyroid hormone.

| | | |
|---|---|---|
| Levothyroxine sodium: PO, IV<br>Liothyronine: PO, IV<br>Liotrix: PO<br>Thyroid: PO | Overdose may result in symptoms of hyperthyroidism: tachycardia, heat intolerance, nervousness | 1. Be careful in reading exact name on label of medications; micrograms and milligrams are used as units of measure.<br>2. Generally taken once a day on an empty stomach before breakfast.<br>3. Within 3–4 days, begin to see improvement; maximum effect in 4–6 weeks. |

| Appendix 15-2 MEDICATIONS USED IN ENDOCRINE DISORDERS—cont'd | | |

| Medications | Side Effects | Nursing Implications |
|---|---|---|
| **Pancreatic Enzymes:** Replacement enzymes to aid in digestion of starch, protein, and fat. | | |
| Pancrelipase: PO | GI upset and irritation of mucous membranes | 1. Client is usually on a high-protein, high-carbohydrate, low-fat diet.<br>2. Enteric-coated tablets should not be crushed or chewed.<br>3. Pancrelipase is given just before or with each meal or snack. |
| **Antihypoglycemic Agent:** Increases plasma glucose levels and relaxes smooth muscles. | | |
| Glucagon: IM, IV, subQ<br>Dextrose 50%: IV | None significant | 1. IV glucose is the preferred route.<br>2. Watch for symptoms of hypoglycemia and treat with food first, if conscious.<br>3. Client usually awakens 5–20 min after receiving glucagon. |
| **Oral Hypoglycemic Agents:** Stimulate beta cells to secrete more insulin; enhance body utilization of available insulin (see Table 15-1 for insulin). | | |

*General Nursing Implications*
- Dose should be decreased for older adults.
- Use with caution in clients with renal and hepatic impairment.
- All clients should be observed carefully for symptoms of hypoglycemia and hyperglycemia.
- Medications should be taken in the morning.
- Long-term therapy may result in decreased effectiveness.

| Medications | Side Effects | Nursing Implications |
|---|---|---|
| **Sulfonylureas:** Stimulate the pancreas to make more insulin. | | |
| Chlorpropamide: PO<br>Glipizide: PO<br>Glyburide: PO<br>Glimepiride: PO<br>Gliclazide: PO<br>Tolbutamide: PO<br>Tolazamide: PO | Hypoglycemia, jaundice, GI disturbance, skin reactions (fewer side effects with second-generation agents) | 1. Tolbutamide has shortest duration of action; requires multiple daily doses.<br>2. Glyburide has a long duration of action.<br>3. Interact with calcium channel blockers, oral contraceptives, glucocorticoids, phenothiazines, and thiazide diuretics.<br>4. Instruct client to avoid alcohol; disulfiram-like reaction may occur (nausea, vomiting, flushing). |
| **Biguanides:** Decrease sugar production in the liver and help the muscles use insulin to break down sugar. | | |
| Metformin: PO | Dizziness, nausea, back pain, possible metallic taste | 1. Administered with meals.<br>2. Has a beneficial effect on lowering lipids.<br>3. Weight gain may occur.<br>4. Do not use in clients with liver, kidney, or heart failure or clients who drink excessive amounts of alcohol. |
| **Alpha-Glucosidase Inhibitors:** Slow down body absorption of sugar after eating; also known as *starch blockers*. | | |
| Acarbose: PO<br>Miglitol: PO | Diarrhea, flatulence, abdominal pain | 1. Take at beginning of meals; not effective on an empty stomach.<br>2. Acarbose is contraindicated in clients with inflammatory bowel disease.<br>3. Frequently given with sulfonylureas to increase effectiveness of both medications. |
| **Thiazolidinediones (Glitazones):** Enhance insulin utilization at receptor sites (they do *not* increase insulin production); also referred to as *insulin sensitizers*. | | |
| Pioglitazone: PO | Weight gain, edema | 1. May affect liver function; monitor LFTs.<br>2. Postmenopausal women may resume ovulation; pregnancy may occur.<br>3. Increased risk of heart disease; should not be used in heart failure. |

*Continued*

**Appendix 15-2   MEDICATIONS USED IN ENDOCRINE DISORDERS—cont'd**

| Medications | Side Effects | Nursing Implications |
|---|---|---|
| **Meglitinides (Nonsulfonylurea Insulin Secretagogues) (Glinides):** Stimulate release of insulin from beta cells. | | |
| Nateglinide: PO<br>Repaglinide: PO | Weight gain, hypoglycemia | 1. Rapid onset and short duration.<br>2. Take 30 min before meals (or right at mealtime).<br>3. Do not take if meal is missed. |
| **Dipeptidyl Peptidase-4 (DDP-4) Inhibitors (Gliptins):** Enhance the incretin system, stimulate release of insulin for beta cells, and decrease hepatic glucose production. | | |
| Sitagliptin: PO<br>Linagliptin: PO<br>Saxagliptin: PO<br>Alogliptin: PO | Upper respiratory tract infection, sore throat, headache, diarrhea | 1. Should not be used in type 1 diabetes or for the treatment of diabetic ketoacidosis. |

### Injectable Drugs for Diabetes

| Medications | Side Effects | Nursing Implications |
|---|---|---|
| **Amylin Mimetics (Agonists):** Complement the effects of insulin by delaying gastric emptying and suppressing glucagon secretion. | | |
| Pramlintide: subQ | Hypoglycemia, nausea, injection site reactions | 1. Teach client to take other oral medications at least 1 hour before taking or 2 hours after because of delayed gastric emptying.<br>2. Injected into thigh or abdomen.<br>3. Cannot be mixed with insulin. |

> **⊞ NURSING PRIORITY:** Can cause severe hypoglycemia when used with insulin; usually occurs within 3 hours after injection.

| Medications | Side Effects | Nursing Implications |
|---|---|---|
| **Incretin Mimetics:** Stimulate release of insulin, decrease glucagon secretion, decrease gastric emptying, and suppress appetite. | | |
| Exenatide: subQ<br>Dulaglutide: subQ<br>Liraglutide: subQ<br>Albiglutide: subQ | Hypoglycemia, nausea, vomiting, diarrhea, headache, possible weight loss | 1. Used in conjunction with metformin.<br>2. Monitor weight.<br>3. Not indicated for use with insulin.<br>4. Monitor for pancreatitis and kidney problems. |
| **Sodium Glucose Cotransporter Inhibitors (Gliflozins):** Transport sodium and glucose into cells using sodium/potassium ATPase pumps. | | |
| Canagliflozin: PO<br>Dapagliflozin: PO<br>Empagliflozin: PO | Genital yeast infections, UTIs, polyuria.<br>Hypoglycemia when used with other antidiabetic drugs. | 1. Inhibit glucose reabsorption.<br>2. More currently under development.<br>3. Risk of ketoacidosis. |
| **Combination Therapy:** Two oral hypoglycemic medications are combined in one tablet. Most often the combination is metformin with a sulfonylurea. | | |
| Metformin/glyburide: PO<br>Metformin/repaglinide: PO<br>Pioglitazone/glimepiride: PO<br>Rosiglitazone/glimepiride: PO<br>Sitagliptin/simvastatin: PO | See individual drugs for side effects. | 1. Monitor for cardiac changes, congestive heart failure.<br>2. May cause GI disturbances. |

*CBC,* Complete blood count; *GI,* gastrointestinal; *IM,* intramuscularly; *IV,* intravenously; *LFTs,* liver function tests; *PO,* by mouth (orally); *subQ,* subcutaneously.

## Study Questions
## Endocrine: Care of Adult, Maternity, and Pediatric Clients

More questions on
evolve

1. A client is receiving NPH insulin 20 units subcutaneously at 0700 hours daily. At 3 pm, the nurse finds the client apparently asleep. What priority action should the nurse perform to assess for a hypoglycemic reaction?
   1. Feel the client and bed for dampness.
   2. Observe the client for Kussmaul respirations.
   3. Smell the client's breath for acetone odor.
   4. Note if the client is incontinent of urine.

2. The nurse is caring for a client postoperative thyroidectomy. What action should the nurse prioritize? **Select all that apply.**
   1. Have the client speak every 5 to 10 minutes if hoarseness is present.
   2. Support the head with pillows and avoid flexion of the neck.
   3. Check the breath sounds for stridor.
   4. Assess for tingling in the toes, fingers, and around the mouth or muscular twitching.
   5. Assess every 4 hours for the first 24 hours for signs of hemorrhage.
   6. Place with head of bed flat, in a side-lying position in case of vomiting.

3. The nurse is assigned to care for a newly admitted client with acute pancreatitis. Admitting assessment includes midepigastric pain of an 8 out of 10, low-grade fever, and elevated amylase and lipase levels with hypocalcemia and hyperglycemia. What should be the nurse's priority action?
   1. Deliver proton pump inhibitor.
   2. Place nasogastric (NG) tube.
   3. Administer IV calcium gluconate.
   4. Administer oral analgesic.

4. A client is found to be comatose with a blood glucose level of 50 mg/dL (2.8 mmol/L). What action should the nurse implement first?
   1. Infuse 1000 mL of D5W over a 12-hour period.
   2. Administer 50% glucose intravenously.
   3. Check the client's urine for the presence of sugar and acetone.
   4. Encourage the client to drink orange juice with added sugar.

5. A nurse is caring for a client with Addison's disease who has been in a car accident and presents to the emergency department with severe hypotension, fever, weakness, and confusion. Place the nurse's action in a priority order.
   1. Vital sign assessment.
   2. Delivery of 0.9% saline and 5% dextrose solution.
   3. Placement of an IV.
   4. Delivery of high-dose hydrocortisone replacement.
   5. Health history information.

6. A client is prescribed levothyroxine daily. What should the nurse include in the discharge teaching? **Select all that apply.**
   1. Taper the dose, never stop abruptly.
   2. Take it at bedtime to avoid the side effects.
   3. Call the health care provider if you experience palpitations or nervousness.
   4. Decrease the intake of juices and fruits with high potassium and calcium contents.
   5. Regular follow-up care will be required.

7. The nurse is creating a plan of care about exercise for a client newly diagnosed with diabetes. What should be included in the plan? **Select all that apply.**
   1. Exercise needs to be vigorous and daily.
   2. Properly fitting footwear is important.
   3. Exercise is best done after meals when glucose levels are rising.
   4. It is important to monitor glucose levels before, during, and after exercise.
   5. Exercise-induced hypoglycemia may occur several hours after exercise.

8. The nurse is caring for a client with thyroid disease who is experiencing a "racing heart," weight loss, exophthalmos, and heat intolerance. What additional actions should the nurse take? **Select all that apply.**
   1. Evaluate if the client is receiving a beta-blocker.
   2. Assess for hypotension.
   3. Request increased calories with three balanced meals a day.
   4. Apply lubricating eye drops throughout the day.
   5. Place a circulating fan in the room.

9. A nurse is urgently called to a homebound neighbor's house. The neighbor is found unconscious and has a history of insulin-dependent diabetes. After determining there is no functioning glucometer available, what should the nurse's next action be?
   1. Administer 10 units of regular insulin subcutaneously.
   2. Arouse the client to drink 4 to 6 ounces of orange juice.
   3. Administer glucagon 1 mg subcutaneously.
   4. Find a phone to call EMS.

10. A client is scheduled for a routine glycosylated hemoglobin A<sub></sub>$A_{1c}$. What needs to be included in the teaching about the test?
    1. Drink only water after midnight and come to the clinic early in the morning.
    2. Eat a normal breakfast and be at the clinic 2 hours later.
    3. Expect to be at the clinic for several hours because of the multiple blood draws.
    4. Come to the clinic at the earliest convenience to have blood drawn.

11. The nurse is caring for a client who began showing signs of diabetes insipidus 4 hours ago and was treated with IV fluids and one dose of nasal desmopressin (DDAVP). How will the nurse know the treatment is effective? **Select all that apply.**
    1. Urine output will decrease.
    2. Blood pressure will lower.
    3. Glucose level will normalize.
    4. Sodium level change from 128 mEq/L to 134 mEq/L.
    5. Urine specific gravity of 1.029.

12. A client with a diagnosis of type 2 diabetes has been prescribed a course of prednisone for severe arthritis pain. How should the nurse adjust the plan of care? **Select all that apply.**
    1. Monitor blood glucose levels more frequently.
    2. Monitor for signs of bleeding.
    3. Monitor urine output every 4 hours.
    4. Monitor for increased signs of infection.
    5. Monitor for increased confusion.

13. A client with Cushing's syndrome is admitted to the medical–surgical unit. During the admission assessment, the nurse notes that the client has a flat affect but is irritable when questioned, has a poor memory, reports a loss of appetite, wants to sleep all the time, and doesn't care if she gets well. What collaborative action should the nurse take in response to this information?
    1. Discuss with the health care provider a concern for depression.
    2. Request a neurology consult for a CT scan.
    3. Discuss with the dietitian a need for a nutritional consult.
    4. Request a social service consult for home evaluation.

14. A patient with a pituitary tumor is treated with a transsphenoidal hypophysectomy. What would be a priority postoperative action?
    1. Ensure that any clear nasal drainage is tested for glucose.
    2. Maintain the patient flat in bed to prevent cerebrospinal fluid (CSF) leak.
    3. Assist the patient with tooth brushing to keep the surgical area clean.
    4. Encourage deep breathing and coughing to prevent respiratory complications.

15. A nurse is planning care for a client with syndrome of inappropriate antidiuretic hormone (SIADH). What is a priority problem that the nurse should consider for the patient, based on an understanding of this condition?
    1. Disturbed sleep pattern related to nocturia.
    2. Risk for fall related to hypovolemia.
    3. Electrolyte imbalance related to metabolic acidosis.
    4. Risk for seizures related to hyponatremia.

16. When caring for a client with diabetes insipidus, which assessment changes require a priority action? **Select all that apply.**
    1. Urine output change from 270 mL/hr to 100 mL/hr.
    2. Finger stick glucose of 182 mg/dL.
    3. Weight decrease of 1 kg overnight.
    4. Urine becoming paler in color.
    5. Serum osmolality of 300 mOsm/kg

17. A client admitted with a pheochromocytoma returns from the operating room after adrenalectomy. Which assessment is most concerning?
    1. Glucose of 70 mg/dL.
    2. Potassium of 3.4 mEq/L.
    3. Blood pressure of 169/98 mm Hg.
    4. Sodium of 146 mEq/L.

18. The nurse receives the new orders below for a client admitted in thyroid crisis. Which order should the nurse question?

> Jane Johnson
> MR: 96837
> DOB: 6/5/1962
> Allergies: NKDA
>
> **Admission Orders – 5/20/19**
> 1. Admit to hospital for thyroid crisis
> 2. Cardiac monitor continuous
> 3. Hyperthermia blanket PRN
> 4. IV fluids 0.9% 50 mL/hr × 1 liter
> 5. Propranolol
> 6. Propylthiouracil
> 7. Stat $T_3$, $T_4$, and TSH serum level

1. IV fluids.
2. Serum blood tests.
3. Propylthiouracil.
4. A hyperthermia blanket.

19. The nurse is caring for a postoperative client who had a thyroidectomy. The client develops difficulty breathing from laryngospasms, muscular spasms, and twitching, Which medication should the nurse have available for emergency treatment in the client who has had a thyroidectomy?
    1. Calcium chloride.
    2. Potassium chloride.
    3. Magnesium sulfate.
    4. Propylthiouracil.

20. A client with diabetes receives a combination of regular and NPH insulin at 0700 hours. At what point in the day should the client be educated about peak incidence of hypoglycemia?
    1. 12 p.m. to 1 p.m. (1200–1300 hours).
    2. 9 a.m. and 5 p.m. (0900 and 1700 hours).
    3. 10 a.m. and 10 p.m. (1000 and 2200 hours).
    4. 8 a.m. and 11 a.m. (0800 and 1100 hours).

## Answers to Study Questions

1. *1*
When clients are sleeping, the only observable symptom of hypoglycemia is diaphoresis. Kussmaul breathing and acetone odor to breath are indicative of hyperglycemia. Incontinence is not associated with hypoglycemia, and polyuria may be associated with hyperglycemia. (Lewis et al., 10 ed., p. 1146)

2. *2,3,4*
It is anticipated that the client will be hoarse for 3 to 4 days after surgery. Increased hoarseness can be a sign of edema, but other signs of edema are more frequently seen, such as laryngeal stridor. Serum levels of calcium are important to monitor because of possible damage to the parathyroids during surgery and can be assessed by signs of tetany like tingling and twitching. Increased hoarseness can also be a sign of hypocalcemia, but assessment every 5 to 10 minutes is excessive. Hemorrhage after surgery is a great concern, and assessments should take place every 2 hours for the first 24 hours. Positioning should be semi-Fowler's, supporting the head with pillows to avoid flexion and tension on the suture lines. (Lewis et al., 10 ed., p. 1168)

3. *2*

With the management of acute pancreatitis, the pain is better controlled when the client is NPO and an NG tube with gastric suction is initiated. Pain medicine should be IV because patient is NPO. Although a PPT and IV calcium may be used, they are not the priority. (Lewis et al., 10 ed., p. 1001)

4. *2*

The unconscious, hypoglycemic client needs immediate treatment with 50% intravenous glucose (highly concentrated). Administering 1000 mL of D₅W over 12 hours does not provide enough glucose to treat the problem. Trying to give oral fluids to an unconscious client should never be done because it increases the risk for aspiration. Urine sugar does not need to be evaluated if the serum blood glucose is available. (Lewis et al., 10 ed., p. 1180)

5. *1, 3, 2, 4, 5* (listed in order of priority)

Addison's disease is due to a hypofunctioning of the adrenal cortex. This client is demonstrating signs of addisonian crisis. Since the client is known to have Addison's disease and is demonstrating signs of crisis, assessment of vital signs should be followed by the placement of an IV, IV fluids, and IV hydrocortisone to allow the body the hormone needed for the stress response. Circulatory collapse can occur in these clients, so there is urgency in the delivery of cortisol. They are often unresponsive to vasopressors and fluid replacement. (Lewis et al., 10 ed., p. 1178)

6. *3, 5*

Levothyroxine increases the metabolic rate of body tissues. Some serious side effects include cardiovascular collapse, dysrhythmias, and tachycardia. Because of these side effects, clients should be instructed not to take the medication if their pulse is greater than 100 beats/min and to notify their provider of headaches, nervousness, chest pain, palpitations, or any unusual symptoms. Therapy will be lifelong, and regular follow-up care is needed to monitor serum blood levels. The medication should be taken in the morning before food, and there are no dietary limitations. (Lewis et al., 10 ed., p. 1170)

7. *2,3,4,5*

Exercise for clients with diabetes mellitus should include regular and moderate activity with properly fitting footwear to prevent injury. Exercise sessions should include a warm-up and a cool-down period. The best time for exercise is after meals and should be individualized by the health care provider. Monitoring glucose is important before, during, and after exercise. The client needs to know that hypoglycemia can occur several hours after the exercise is completed. (Lewis et al., 10 ed., p. 1134)

8. *1,4,5*

Beta-blockers are used effectively for symptomatic relief of thyrotoxicosis. When the client feels palpitations or "heart racing," the nurse should evaluate for tachycardia and cardiac changes. The client with hyperthyroidism will experience hypertension, not hypotension. Because of the weight loss, a high-calorie diet of 4000 to 5000 cal/day is recommended with six full meals each day. Exophthalmos is the protrusion of the eyeballs from the orbits from fat deposits and fluid in the orbital tissues and ocular muscles from hyperthyroidism. When the eyelids do not close, corneal ulcers and loss of vision can occur. Eyedrops are helpful to prevent dryness. A fan in the client's room will provide comfort. (Lewis et al., 10 ed., pp. 1164–1166)

9. *3*

Hypoglycemia can be quickly reversed with effective treatment. Treatment should not be delayed, because permanent brain death can occur. If monitoring equipment is not available or the client has a history of fluctuating blood glucose levels, hypoglycemia should be assumed and treatment initiated. (Lewis et al., 10 ed., p. 1146)

10. *4*

Glucose attaches to the hemoglobin molecule of the red blood cell. A glycosylated hemoglobin test gives an average of blood glucose over the past 3 to 4 months, and a blood sample can be obtained at any time during the day. It is not used in the diagnosis of diabetes and does not need to be a fasting specimen. (Lewis et al., 10 ed., p. 1118)

11. *1,5*

Desmopressin (DDAVP) alleviates polyuria by acting as antidiuretic hormone (ADH). In the case of diabetes insipidus, urine output will decrease and urine specific gravity should return to a normal level of 1.010 to 1.030. The blood pressure should increase because more water is being retained in the bloodstream, which will lower sodium levels. Glucose is not affected by diabetes insipidus. (Lewis et al., 10 ed., p. 1161)

12. *1,4*

An adverse reaction to corticosteroids is hyperglycemia. A client with type 2 diabetes must monitor blood glucose levels closely while taking steroids. Clients taking corticosteroids are also at increased risk for infection due to suppressed immune response and not a decrease in white blood cells. Bleeding, confusion, and changes in urine output are not typical a concern. (Lehne, 8 ed., p. 874)

13. *1*

Cushing's syndrome develops because of an excess of cortisol, in this case from prolonged exogenous steroid administration. Depression and a marked change in personality are common. It is important that the client be taught how to deal with the emotional changes of the disease. (Lewis et al., 10 ed., 1174)

14. *1*

With a transsphenoidal hypophysectomy the pituitary gland is removed. CSF leaks and epistaxis are common postoperative complications, and it is important that any clear fluid draining from the nose is tested for glucose. Postoperative care includes elevating the head of the bed at all times to a 30-degree angle, and the client should avoid sneezing, coughing, and tooth brushing for at least 10 days to prevent a CSF leak. (Lewis et al., 10 ed., p. 1159)

15. *4*

SIADH occurs when excessive antidiuretic hormone (ADH) is released, even when the plasma (serum) osmolality is normal. The excess ADH increases the permeability of the renal tubules, causing reabsorption of water into the circulation. As a result of extracellular fluid expansion, serum osmolality decreases, and sodium levels decline (as a result of being diluted), leading to hyponatremia and a risk for seizures. (Lewis et al., 10 ed., p. 1106)

16. *4, 5*

Diabetes insipidus (DI) is associated with a decrease (or deficiency) in the secretion of antidiuretic hormone (ADH). Lack of ADH leads to increased urinary output (as much as 5–20 L/day). A concern would be demonstrated if the urine becomes more dilute, increases in quantity, blood pressure drops, or the blood becomes more viscous. (Lewis et al., 10 ed. p. 1160–1161)

17. *3*

Pheochromocytoma is a tumor in the adrenal medulla that produces excess catecholamines (epinephrine and norepinephrine). An excess of these catecholamines can cause severe hypertension. Surgery (adrenalectomy) alleviates the elevated blood pressure most of the time. In 10% to 30% of clients, hypertension remains and must be monitored and treated. Electrolyte imbalances and blood sugar are not typically affected. (Lewis et al., 10 ed., pp. 1107, 1181)

18. *4*

Fever (hyperthermia) is a symptom of thyroid storm. The correct treatment would be a hypothermia blanket to cool the client. All other choices (IV fluids, laboratory tests, and propylthiouracil) are appropriate prescriptions for this diagnosis. (Lewis et al., 10 ed., p. 1165)

19. *1*

Calcium chloride or calcium gluconate should be available to treat tetany caused by accidental removal of the parathyroid glands during surgery. The parathyroid glands regulate calcium metabolism. Potassium chloride replaces the electrolyte potassium. Magnesium sulfate is used in the treatment of preeclampsia (pregnancy-induced hypertension). Propylthiouracil is an antithyroid medication used to block production of thyroid hormone. (Lewis et al., 10 ed., p. 1173)

20. *2*

Regular insulin (a short-acting insulin) peaks in 2 to 3 hours, and NPH (an intermediate-acting insulin) peaks in 4 to 10 hours. Hypoglycemia would most likely occur between 9 a.m. and 5 p.m. (0900 and 1700 hours). (Lewis et al., 10 ed., p. 1126)

# CHAPTER SIXTEEN

# Hematology: Care of Adult and Pediatric Clients

# 16

## PHYSIOLOGY OF THE BLOOD

A. Components.
1. Plasma (does not contain cellular elements): clear, straw-colored liquid; accounts for about half of the total blood volume.
2. Formed elements (cells): account for about half of the volume.
   a. Erythrocytes (red blood cells [RBCs]).
   b. Leukocytes (white blood cells).
   c. Thrombocytes (platelets).
B. Characteristics of plasma (Figure 16-1).
1. Plasma is about 90% water.
2. Protein: 6% to 8% of the plasma.
   a. Albumin: most abundant protein; maintains colloid osmotic pressure of the plasma.
   b. Globulins.
      (1) Gamma globulins (immunoglobulins [Ig]) consist primarily of antibodies.
      (2) Alpha and beta globulins are essential factors in the clotting mechanism.
   c. Fibrinogen: inactive protein produced in the liver, activated to form fibrin; necessary for clot formation.
   d. Prothrombin: necessary element for coagulation produced in the liver; production is dependent on vitamin K.
   e. Normal body nutrients are carried by the plasma.
      (1) Carbohydrates in the form of glucose.
      (2) Proteins in the form of amino acids.
      (3) Fat in the form of lipids.
   f. Metabolic waste products are carried to organs of excretion by the plasma.
      (1) Urea, uric acid.
      (2) Lactic acid, creatinine.
C. Characteristics of erythrocytes (RBCs).
1. Formed in the red bone marrow; erythropoiesis is production of RBCs.
2. In early childhood, all bones contain red marrow; as child grows, red marrow is replaced with fatty, yellow marrow.
3. In the adult, only specific bones contain red marrow (flat and irregular bones such as pelvic bones, vertebrae, ribs, cranial bones, and scapula.)
4. Vitamin $B_{12}$ and folic acid are necessary for the production of erythrocytes.

5. Erythrocytes: primary function is transportation of oxygen and carbon dioxide.
   a. Hemoglobin is the primary component of the RBC.
      (1) Serves as a buffer in the acid–base balance.
      (2) Hemoglobin combines easily with oxygen to form oxyhemoglobin.
      (3) Iron is a major component of hemoglobin and is necessary for normal oxygen transport.
   b. Hematocrit is a percentage of the blood occupied by the erythrocytes.

> **NURSING PRIORITY:** As a general rule of thumb, the hematocrit is usually three times the hemoglobin value.

6. When RBCs are exposed to hypotonic solutions, water enters the cells, thus precipitating cellular wall rupture and destruction or hemolysis of the RBCs.
7. Hemolysis also occurs when cellular membranes are damaged, as in trauma and burns.
D. Characteristics of the leukocytes (white blood cells).
1. Function: primary work of the leukocytes is accomplished when the cells leave the circulating volume and enter the body tissue to remove pathogens.
2. Types of cells.
   a. Granulocytes (polymorphonuclear leukocytes) originate in the bone marrow.
      (1) Consist of neutrophils, eosinophils, and basophils.
      (2) Primary function is to destroy bacteria (phagocytosis).
   b. Agranular leukocytes (mononuclear) originate primarily in the lymphatic tissue.
      (1) Consist of lymphocytes and monocytes.
      (2) Assist in the removal of broken-down tissue cells.
      (3) Primarily involved in activating the immune response.
E. Characteristics of thrombocytes (platelets).
1. Function: primarily involved with hemostasis; when a vessel wall is damaged, platelets adhere to the area and eventually form a platelet plug to decrease bleeding.
F. Hemostasis.
1. Extrinsic mechanisms: clotting process initiated by tissue damage and blood loss.

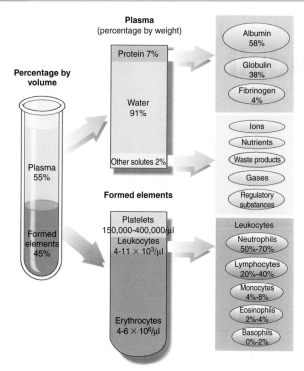

**FIGURE 16-1 Approximate Values for the Components of Blood in the Adult.** Normally, 45% of the blood is composed of blood cells, and 55% is composed of plasma. (From Patton, K. T., & Thibodeau, G. A. [2014]. *The human body in health and disease* [6th ed.]. St. Louis, MO: Mosby.)

2. Intrinsic mechanism: clotting mechanism within the vessel where blood loss and tissue trauma are not present.
3. Both mechanisms produce the same result: clot formation.
4. Three phases of hemostasis (coagulation).
   a. First phase: tissue injury precipitates release of platelet factor; in presence of calcium and accessory factors, thromboplastin is formed.
   b. Second phase: prothrombin is converted to thrombin; thromboplastin in phase 1 initiates the conversion of prothrombin.
   c. Third phase: thrombin converts soluble fibrinogen to insoluble fibrin (fibrin is an insoluble protein that looks like a fine network of thread like a mesh or a web).
5. Erythrocytes are not part of the actual coagulation process; RBCs are essentially trapped in the fibrin mesh and give the clot its characteristic color.
6. Fibrinolysis: process by which clots, formed in tissue and small vessels, are dissolved by fibrinolysin.
G. Blood classification.
   1. Major blood groups: A, B, AB, and O.
      a. Blood compatibility and systems of classification are based on the presence or absence of specific antigens present on RBCs, as well as specific antibodies in the plasma.
      b. RBC antigens are inherited and are cell surface proteins: A and B.
         (1) Neither A nor B antigens are present in type O blood (universal donor).
         (2) A antigen is present in type A blood.

(3) B antigen is present in type B blood.
(4) A and B antigens are both present in type AB blood (universal recipient).
   c. There are two antibodies present in the plasma: anti-A and anti-B.
      (1) Both plasma antibodies are present in type O blood.
      (2) Anti-B is present in type A blood.
      (3) Anti-A is present in type B blood.
      (4) Neither is present in type AB blood.
   d. If the antigen A on the RBCs of the donor comes in contact with the antibody A of the recipient and vice versa, agglutination and hemolysis will occur (e.g., type A blood transfused into type B recipient).
   e. Although "universal donor" and "universal recipient" types may be used to classify blood in an emergency, blood type tests are always done to prevent transfusion reactions.
      (1) O negative is called the *universal donor* because there are no antigens on the RBCs, and Rh (D) is not present.
      (2) AB positive is called the *universal recipient* because there are no antibodies in the serum, and Rh (D) is present.
2. Rh System.
   a. Rh system consists of a third antigen, D, which is present on the RBC.
   b. Rh-positive individuals have the D antigen present; this is represented with a (+) sign after the ABO group (e.g., A+).
   c. Rh-negative individuals do not have the D antigen present; this is represented with a (−) sign after the ABO group (e.g., B−).
   d. Normal plasma does not contain Rh antibodies (anti-D). Antibodies are formed in Rh-negative blood if transfused with Rh-positive blood; thus the recipient is sensitized to the Rh factor, and subsequent Rh-positive blood might result in a severe transfusion reaction.
   e. Problems of sensitization occur in the newborn when the mother is Rh negative and the infant is Rh positive (see Chapter 26).

## System Assessment

A. History.
   1. Disease of bone marrow and/or RBC-producing organs.
   2. Treatment that depressed bone marrow activity (especially chemotherapy or radiation therapy).
   3. Familial history and/or genetic predisposition of hematologic disorders (sickle cell anemia, hemophilia, thalassemia, and hemochromatosis).
   4. Prior blood transfusions and/or reactions.
B. Bleeding problems occurring during pregnancy, labor and delivery, or immediately after delivery in both mother and infant.
C. Presence of chronic disorders or disease processes (liver, kidney, or spleen disorders).
D. Effects of aging (Table 16-1).

**Table 16-1    AGE-RELATED ASSESSMENT FINDINGS FOR THE HEMATOLOGIC SYSTEM**

| Assessment Area | Hematologic System Findings | Older Adult Changes and Significance |
|---|---|---|
| Nail beds (assess capillary refill) | Pallor, cyanosis, and decreased capillary refill are often noted in hematologic disorders. | Nails are typically thickened and discolored. Use another body area such as the lips or mucous membrane to assess for pallor. |
| Hair distribution | Thin or absent hair on trunk and extremities may indicate poor oxygenation and blood supply to area. | Older adults are losing body hair but often in an even pattern distribution that has occurred slowly over time. Lack of hair only on lower legs and toes may indicate poor circulation. |
| Skin moisture and color | Skin dryness, pallor, flushing, and jaundice may occur with anemia, leukemia, rapid hemolysis, or liver disease. | Dry skin is a normal aspect of aging and thus becomes an unreliable indicator of skin moisture. Pigment loss and skin changes along with some yellowing occur with aging. |

E. Evaluate effect a hematologic disorder has on client's activities of daily living.
   1. How long has client experienced symptoms?
   2. What are the client's current activity levels and metabolic requirements?
   3. Presence or absence of bleeding episodes.
   4. Presence or absence of pain. If pain is present, how well is it controlled?
   5. Presence of appropriate coping/defense mechanisms.
F. Assess client's current nutritional status (especially iron, folic acid, and protein).
G. Evaluate current blood values—complete blood count (CBC).
H. Evaluate status of respiratory and cardiovascular systems in maintaining homeostasis.
I. Focused examination should include the liver, spleen, skin, and lymph nodes.
   1. Lymph nodes.
      a. Ordinarily, lymph nodes are not palpable in adults, but when a node is palpable, it should be small (0.5–1.0 cm).
      b. Abnormal findings include nodes that are tender, hard, fixed, or enlarged. Tender nodes are often a result of the inflammatory process, whereas hard or fixed nodes are associated with malignancy.
   2. Skin: abnormal findings include pallor, jaundice, purpura, petechiae, and ecchymosis.
   3. Liver and spleen: enlargement.

## Anemias

**Anemia is characterized by a low RBC count and decreased levels of hemoglobin and hematocrit.**

A. Origin (Figure 16-2).
   1. Defect in bone marrow production of RBCs.
   2. Loss of RBCs.
      a. Hemorrhage.
      b. Chronic bleeding.
      c. Hemolytic processes.
   3. Hereditary disorders of the RBCs.
   4. Inadequate nutritional intake of iron, folic acid.
B. The more rapidly an anemia occurs, the more severe the symptoms will be.

C. Healthy term infants have adequate iron storage for the first 5 to 6 months; premature infants may need iron supplementation at 2 to 3 months of age.
D. Common goal in treatment of all anemias is to identify the origin and correct the problem.

> **! NURSING PRIORITY:** Recognize signs of anemia in older adult clients: pallor, confusion, fatigue, peripheral edema, worsening heart failure (HF), and pulmonary congestion.

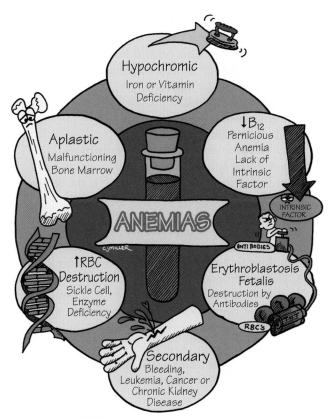

**FIGURE 16-2 Anemias.** (From Zerwekh, J., Garneau, A., & Miller, C. J. [2017]. *Digital collection of the memory notebooks of nursing* [4th ed.]. Chandler, AZ: Nursing Education Consultants, Inc.)

1. Assessment.
    a. Pale skin, delayed wound healing, brittle thinning hair, spoon-shaped fingernails, and generalized lymphadenopathy.
    b. Shortness of breath, dyspnea on exertion, tachypnea.
    c. Tachycardia, palpitations, postural hypotension: Cardiac complications can progress to cardiac decompensation.
    d. Chronic fatigue, weakness, and apathy.
    e. Anorexia, nausea, weight loss, constipation, and diarrhea.
    f. Beefy red tongue, stomatitis, hematemesis.
    g. Headache, dizziness, tingling in extremities.
    h. Chronic anemia may result in growth retardation in infants and children.

> **TEST ALERT:** Identify client's ability to maintain activities of daily living.

E. Iron deficiency anemia: characterized by inadequate intake of dietary iron or excessive loss of iron.
    1. Risk factors/etiology.
        a. Common in adolescents.
        b. Vegetarians and lacto–ovo vegetarians.
        c. Occurs in infants whose primary diet is milk.
        d. May occur in pregnancy.
        e. Heavy menstrual bleeding.
        f. Other blood loss states (e.g., peptic ulcer disease [PUD]).
    2. Older adults are more prone to iron deficiency anemia because of poor dietary iron intake and decreased absorption in the small intestine.
    3. Diagnostics: decreased iron, hemoglobin, and hematocrit values.
    4. Clinical manifestations.
        a. May be asymptomatic in the early stages.
        b. General symptoms of anemia.
        c. Pallor, glossitis, cheilitis (cracking at the corners of the mouth)—most common findings.
    5. Treatment: supplemental iron intake is necessary for several months to replenish body storage.
        a. Supplemental iron (see Appendix 16-2).
        b. Increased dietary iron intake (see Chapter 2).
        c. Supplemental folic acid (green leafy vegetables, fortified cereals, enriched rice and bread, liver, Great Northern beans, black-eyed and green peas, avocado, peas, tomatoes, oranges).

> **TEST ALERT:** Evaluate client's nutritional status; adapt a diet to meet special needs of the client; evaluate effect of nutritional status on condition.

F. Pernicious anemia: condition characterized by an inability to absorb vitamin $B_{12}$ (cobalamin). It may be associated with loss of intrinsic factor (e.g., gastrectomy, gastric bypass), or it may be an autoimmune problem.
    1. Risk factors/etiology.
        a. Generally not associated with inadequate dietary intake.
        b. More common in older adults; most common age at diagnosis is 60 years.
        c. Familial tendency.
        d. May be precipitated by gastrectomy, gastritis, Crohn disease, or chronic alcoholism.
        e. Long-term use of proton pump inhibitors and $H_2$-histamine receptor blockers prevent the release of the intrinsic factor.
        f. Gastric atrophy, especially in the older adult.
    2. Diagnostics (see Appendix 16-1).
        a. Homocysteine, cobalamin, and serum folate levels.
        b. Reduced number of RBCs and presence of abnormal RBCs.
        c. Gastric analysis for free hydrochloric acid.
    3. Clinical manifestations.
        a. General symptoms of anemia, confusion.
        b. Paresthesia in the extremities, weakness, reduced vibratory sense.
        c. Loss of sense of balance, ataxia.
        d. Smooth, beefy, red tongue (glossitis).
    4. Treatment.
        a. Injections of vitamin $B_{12}$ or intranasal cyanocobalamin may be required for life.
        b. Maintain good nutrition with adequate iron, vitamin C, and folic acid intake.
        c. Monitor for gastric cancer—there is increased potential with pernicious anemia.
G. Aplastic anemia: characterized by pancytopenia—depression of the bone marrow in production of all blood cell types: RBCs, WBCs, and platelets.
    1. Risk factors/etiology.
        a. Exposure to certain medications and chemicals can precipitate aplastic anemia.
            (1) Chemotherapeutic agents, radiation.
            (2) Sulfonamides, chloramphenicol, methotrexate.
            (3) Anticonvulsant medications (e.g., phenytoin).
            (4) Benzene, insecticides, arsenic.
        b. Radiation therapy.
        c. Up to 70% of cases are idiopathic in origin and are thought to have an autoimmune basis.
    2. Diagnostics: bone marrow biopsy reveals severe decrease in all marrow elements (pancytopenia; see Appendix 16-1).
    3. Clinical manifestations.
        a. General symptoms of anemia.
        b. Fever.
        c. Infections associated with neutropenia.
        d. Bleeding problems associated with thrombocytopenia.
    4. Treatment.
        a. Remove causative agent.
        b. Hematopoietic stem cell transplant (see Appendix 16-4).

c. Immunosuppressive therapy with antithymocytic globulin (ATG) and cyclosporine.

H. Folic acid deficiency anemia: associated with decreased dietary intake of folic acid.
1. Risk factors/etiology (origin very similar to that of vitamin $B_{12}$ deficiency).
    a. Poor nutrition due to decreased folic acid intake, alcoholism, anorexia.
    b. Malabsorption syndromes.
    c. Deficiency may occur with increased demands for folic acid: infancy, adolescence, and pregnancy.
    d. Drugs: anticonvulsants, methotrexate, and oral contraceptives.
    e. Hemodialysis.
2. Clinical manifestations.
    a. Slow, insidious onset.
    b. Weight loss, emaciated.
    c. May appear ill with malnourishment.
3. Diagnostics.
    a. Differentiate between folic acid deficiency and vitamin $B_{12}$ deficiency.
        (1) Both are dietary deficiencies.
        (2) Folic acid deficiency—malabsorption syndrome often caused by drugs (oral contraceptives, anticonvulsants, or methotrexate).
        (3) Vitamin $B_{12}$ deficiency—failure to absorb $B_{12}$ from gut as a result of partial gastrectomy, pernicious anemia, or malabsorption syndromes.
    b. Serum folate levels less than 3 ng/mL.
4. Treatment: oral replacement, 1 mg/day or 5 mg/day for malabsorption syndromes or chronic alcoholism; encourage increase dietary intake of folic acid (organ meats, green leafy vegetables, citrus fruits, whole grains, and beans).

### Nursing Interventions

For all clients with anemia.
**Goal:** To assist in establishing a diagnosis.

A. Complete nutritional evaluation.
B. Obtain history of possible causes.

**Goal:** To decrease body oxygen needs.

A. Assess client's tolerance to activity.
B. Provide diversional activities but also provide for adequate rest.
C. May need supplemental oxygen.
D. Monitor oxygenation with pulse oximetry.

**Goal:** To prevent infections.

A. Decrease exposure by frequent hand hygiene and limiting visitors.
B. Evaluate for temperature elevations frequently.
C. Observe for elevated WBC count.
D. Monitor absolute neutrophil count.
E. Maintain adequate hydration.

**Goal:** To assess for complications of chronic anemic state.

A. Evaluate ability of cardiovascular system to maintain adequate cardiac output.
B. Evaluate for symptoms of hypoxia (see Chapter 17).

**Goal:** To help client understand implications of disease and measures to maintain health.

A. Explain medical regimen.
B. Discuss importance of continuing medical follow-up.
C. Explain benefits and side effects of medications.
D. Identify foods high in vitamin $B_{12}$, iron, and folic acid (see Chapter 2).

## Sickle Cell Anemia

**Sickle cell anemia is a problem characterized by the sickling effect of the erythrocytes, an inherited autosomal recessive disorder.**

A. Basic defect of the erythrocyte is in the globulin portion of the hemoglobin.
B. Sickling problem is not apparent until around 6 months of age; the increased levels of fetal hemoglobin up to that age prevent serious sickling problems.
C. Predominantly a problem of children and adolescents. A child may be asymptomatic between crises. The problems from childhood may cause long-term complications as they become adults.
D. Pathologic changes of sickle cell (elongated, crescent shaped RBCs) disease result from:
1. Increased blood viscosity.
2. Increased RBC destruction.
3. Increased viscosity of the blood and sickling eventually precipitates ischemia and tissue necrosis caused by capillary stasis and thrombosis.
4. Cycle of occlusion, ischemia, and infarction to vascular organs, especially the spleen, liver, and kidneys.
E. Conditions precipitating sickling effect triggered by low oxygen tension in the blood.
1. Dehydration, acidosis, hypoxia.
2. Viral or bacterial infection (most common).
3. High altitude.
4. Emotional or physical stress or surgery.
F. Pathologic effects of sickle cell disease on pregnancy.
1. Mother.
    a. Increased anemia problems.
    b. Increase in thromboembolic problems.
    c. Increased risk for preeclampsia
2. Infant.
    a. Small for gestational age (SGA).
    b. Spontaneous abortion.
    c. Fetal distress caused by hypoxia.
G. Multiple body systems are involved.

> **⚠ NURSING PRIORITY:** Because pregnant women with sickle cell anemia are not iron deficient, they should avoid taking iron supplements, even those found in prenatal vitamins.

*Assessment*

A. Risk factors/etiology.
   1. Autosomal recessive disorder (see Chapter 26).
      a. Normal hemoglobin (HgbA) is replaced by abnormal sickle hemoglobin (HgbS).
      b. Presence of HgbS in 35% to 45% of hemoglobin indicates sickle cell trait.
   2. May occur in persons of African American, Mediterranean, Caribbean, Arabian, East Indian, and Hispanic descent.
B. Clinical manifestations: primarily the result of obstruction caused by sickled RBCs and by increased RBC destruction.
   1. Splenomegaly: caused by congestion and engorgement with sickled cells; decreases immune response.
   2. Liver failure, hepatomegaly, and necrosis from severe impairment of hepatic blood flow.
   3. Jaundice, pale mucous membranes, fatigue, fever, and intense pain.
   4. Kidney damage caused by the congestion of glomerular capillaries and tubular arterioles.
   5. Skeletal changes caused by hyperplasia and congestion of bone marrow.
C. Crisis: often precipitated by an infection or dehydration; can occur spontaneously (Figure 16-3).
   1. Vasoocclusive crisis: blood flow is impaired by sickled cells, causing ischemia and pain.
      a. Extremities: occlusions in the small distal vessels of the hands and the feet, characterized by pain, swelling, and decreased function (hand–foot syndrome).
      b. Abdomen: severe abdominal pain.
      c. Pulmonary: symptoms of pneumonia.
      d. Renal: hematuria.
      e. Central nervous system: visual problems.
   2. Sequestration crisis: pooling of the blood in the liver and spleen with decreased blood volume.

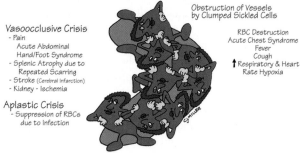

SICKLE CELL ANEMIA CRISIS
(Inherited Red Blood Cell Disorder)

**FIGURE 16-3 Sickle Cell Anemia Crisis.** (From Zerwekh, J., Garneau, A., & Miller, C. J. [2017]. *Digital collection of the memory notebooks of nursing* [4th ed.]. Chandler, AZ: Nursing Education Consultants, Inc.)

D. Diagnostics (see Appendix 16-1): early diagnosis, before 2 months of age, helps minimize complications.
   1. Hemoglobin electrophoresis indicates the presence and percentage of HgbS.
   2. Sickle turbidity tests (SICKLEDEX) used for screening.

*Treatment*

A. Prevention of the sickling problem.
   1. Adequate hydration.
   2. Prevent infections, especially respiratory tract infections; pneumococcal and influenza vaccines are recommended.
   3. Clients generally do not require iron because of increased resorption.
   4. Daily folic acid supplement.
   5. Hydroxyurea to increase the production of HgbF, thereby reducing hemolysis and the number of sickled cells.
   6. Oxygen: assists to prevent a crisis in clients with respiratory problems, but it does not reverse a sickling crisis or reduce pain; client should avoid high altitudes.
B. Treatment of crisis.
   1. Bed rest, deep vein thrombosis prophylaxis (using anticoagulants), hydration, antibiotics.
   2. Analgesics for pain; supplemental oxygen as needed.
   3. Blood transfusions and/or exchange transfusions (see Appendix 16-3).
C. Surgery: splenectomy for severe splenic sequestration.

*Complications*

A. With repeated sickling episodes, organs that have high need for oxygen are most affected.
B. Infection, especially pneumonia.

*Nursing Interventions*

**Goal:** To prevent sickle cell disease.

A. Participate in community screening programs and education for high-risk population.
B. Refer persons who are carriers (autosomal recessive trait) for genetic counseling (see Figure 26-1).

**Goal:** To prevent sickling crisis.

A. Maintain adequate hydration; intravenous (IV) fluids may be necessary.
B. Promote respiratory health and tissue oxygenation; avoiding crowds, inhaling irritants, and routine exercise.
C. Prevent infection; promote thorough hand hygiene.
D. Hydroxyurea: reduces sickling episodes; a long-term complication is leukemia.

**Goal:** To control pain.

A. Assessment of involved area (severity scale 1–10, location, quality).
B. Appropriate analgesics: meperidine is not recommended; morphine, hydromorphone, fentanyl, or methadone may be used; patient-controlled analgesia (PCA) devices are frequently used to control pain.
C. Nonsteroidal antiinflammatory agents and antiseizure medications may also be used for pain control.
D. Allow client to assume a position of comfort.
   1. Passive range of motion may be beneficial.
   2. No active or passive range of motion if patient is actively bleeding into joints.
E. Maintain rest if movement exacerbates pain.

> **TEST ALERT:** Determine effectiveness of pain control. Care of the child with sickle cell disease frequently centers around pain control (see Chapter 3).

**Goal:** To maintain adequate hydration and oxygenation.

A. Evaluate adequacy of hydration; assess skin turgor, monitor urine output, thirst mechanism.
B. Low urine specific gravity may not be indicative of fluid balance if there is renal involvement; monitor blood urea nitrogen (BUN), creatinine, and urine specific gravity.
C. Monitor IV fluid administration carefully; normal saline often given first in crises.
D. Maintain accurate intake and output records; assess daily weight, signs of fluid overload with replacement.
E. Evaluate electrolyte balance; monitor laboratory values, replace deficiencies.
F. Administer oxygen as indicated; monitor arterial blood gases (ABGs) and/or $O_2$ saturation.
G. Provide good pulmonary hygiene.
H. Assess for metabolic acidosis.

> **TEST ALERT:** Monitor hydration status; evaluate client's response to parenteral administration of fluids.

**Goal:** To identify complication of affected organs—systematic evaluation of client to identify problems discussed in section on clinical manifestations.

 **Home Care**

A. Increase fluids with physical activity and/or if living in excessively hot or cold climates.
B. Seek early intervention for symptoms of infection, especially respiratory tract infection; report temperature elevations, coughing, or pain.
C. Encourage normal growth and developmental activities as tolerated by the child.
D. Client with sickle cell disease should avoid situations that may precipitate hypoxia.
   1. Traveling to high-altitude areas.
   2. Flying in an unpressurized aircraft.
   3. Participating in overly strenuous exercise.

E. Inform all significant health care personnel that child should wear medical identification.

> **TEST ALERT:** Compare physical development of client with normal development. Chronically ill children frequently are slower in growth and development; care is provided for the developmental level, not the chronologic age.

 **Polycythemia Vera (Primary)**

**Polycythemia vera is a chronic disorder characterized by a proliferation of all red marrow cells due to a chromosomal mutation.**

*Assessment*

A. Risk factors: usually occurs during middle age; median age is 60 years and is more common in males.
B. Diagnostics.
   1. Complete blood count (CBC)—increased RBC, WBC, platelets, and hemoglobin (see Appendix 16-1).
   2. Erythropoietin level.
   3. Bone marrow biopsy demonstrates an increase in WBCs, RBCs, and platelets.
C. Clinical manifestations.
   1. Early: hypertension (that may lead to) headache, vertigo, tinnitus (especially fingers and toes), pruritus, and visual disturbances.
   2. Ruddy complexion (plethora).
   3. Hepatosplenomegaly; peptic ulcer, dyspepsia.
   4. Problems of decreased blood flow.
      a. Angina, hypoxia.
      b. Intermittent claudication (pain in muscles during activity, relieved with rest).
      c. Thrombophlebitis.
      d. Hypertension: increased blood viscosity or peripheral resistance.
   5. Complication: stroke secondary to thrombosis.

*Treatment*

A. Phlebotomy (2–3 times per week initially, then every 2–3 months).
B. Myelosuppressive agents (busulfan, hydroxycarbamide).
C. Symptom management: paroxetine for erythromelalgia (peripheral dilation of blood vessels), allopurinol for gout, interferon alpha for pruritus, and low-dose aspirin to decrease the risk of blood clots.

*Nursing Interventions*

**Goal:** To help client understand dietary implications to deal with inadequate food intake due to peptic ulcer pain, dyspepsia, and symptoms of hyperuricemia (gout).

A. Monitor intake and output; avoid fluid overload with rehydration.
B. Avoid foods high in purines—yeast, sweetbreads, some seafood, mutton, veal, liver, bacon, salmon, turkey, trout, and alcohol.

**Goal:** To help client understand implications of the disease and long-term health care needs (i.e., prevention of deep vein thrombosis [DVT] and stroke, monitoring for signs of leukemia and myelofibrosis as a result of long-term effects of chemotherapy drugs to treat disease).

## Leukemia

**Leukemia is an uncontrolled proliferation of abnormal white blood cells; eventual cellular destruction occurs as a result of the infiltration of the leukemic cells into the body tissue.**

A. Highly vascular organs of the reticuloendothelial system are primarily affected; spleen, liver, and lymph nodes show marked infiltration, enlargement, and eventually fibrosis.
B. Invasion of the bone marrow by the leukemic cells can precipitate pathologic fractures.
C. Three primary consequences of leukemia.
   1. Anemia from RBC destruction and bleeding.
   2. Infection associated with neutropenia.
   3. Bleeding tendencies caused by decreased platelets.
D. Types of leukemia.
   1. Acute lymphocytic leukemia (blast or stem cell) (ALL).
      a. Peak occurrences: around 4 years of age, then again around 65 years.
      b. Favorable prognosis with chemotherapy.
      c. Leukemic cells will infiltrate the meninges, precipitating increased intracranial pressure; leukemic meningitis.
   2. Acute myelogenous leukemia (AML).
      a. Most common in older adults.
      b. Peak incidence age 60 to 70 years.
   3. Chronic myelogenous leukemia (CML).
      a. Uncommon before the age of 20 years; peak incidence age 45 years.
      b. Onset is generally slow.
      c. Symptoms are less severe than those in acute stages of disease.
      d. Presence of Philadelphia chromosome in 90% of cases.
   4. Chronic lymphocytic leukemia (CLL).
      a. Common malignancy of older adults; rare before age 30, and more common in men.
      b. Frequently asymptomatic; often diagnosed in a chronic fatigue workup.

### Assessment

A. Clinical manifestations (Figure 16-4).
   1. Anemia, fever (infection), and bleeding tendencies occurring together.
   2. Anorexia, weight loss, cough.
   3. Central nervous system involvement: headache, confusion, increased irritability.
   4. Fatigue, lethargy.
   5. Petechiae, bruises easily, epistaxis.
   6. Complaints of bone and joint pain.
   7. Hepatomegaly and splenomegaly.

## SYMPTOMS OF LEUKEMIA

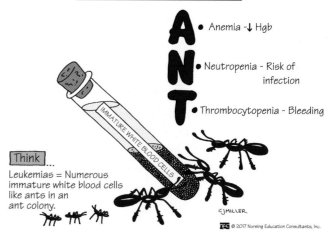

- Anemia -↓ Hgb
- Neutropenia - Risk of infection
- Thrombocytopenia - Bleeding

Think ...
Leukemias = Numerous immature white blood cells like ants in an ant colony.

**FIGURE 16-4 Symptoms of Leukemia.** (From Zerwekh, J., Garneau, A., & Miller, C. J. [2017]. *Digital collection of the memory notebooks of nursing* [4th ed.]. Chandler, AZ: Nursing Education Consultants, Inc.)

B. Diagnostics (see Appendix 16-1).
   1. Bone marrow aspiration: increased numbers of blast (immature) cells (see Appendix 16-1).
   2. Lumbar puncture to identify presence of leukemic cells in spinal fluid.
   3. Complete blood count.
   4. Studies to evaluate liver function (ALT, AST) and renal function studies (BUN, serum creatinine); most chemotherapy agents are detoxified in the liver and excreted by way of the renal system; these systems need to be evaluated before chemotherapy is initiated.

### Treatment

A. Medications.
   1. Corticosteroids.
   2. Antineoplastic agents (see Appendix 11-1).
   3. Xanthine–oxidase inhibitor: allopurinol decreases uric acid levels in clients receiving antineoplastic agents (see Appendix 25-2).
   4. Chemotherapy usually involves an induction phase, a consolidation phase, and a maintenance phase.
   5. A combination of chemotherapy agents is used initially to promote a remission.
   6. Majority of children with ALL will go into remission during the induction phase.
B. Hematopoietic stem cell transplantation [HSCT] (see Appendix 16-4).
C. Radiation therapy (see Chapter 11).
D. A remission is characterized by absence of leukemic cells and disappearance of all disease symptoms.

### Nursing Interventions

**Goal:** To prevent infection.

A. Systematically assess for evidence of infection: fever, inflammation, pain.
B. Monitor temperature elevation closely; notify health care provider of increase greater than 100.5°F (38°C).

C. Meticulous skin care, especially oral hygiene and around perianal area.

D. Neutropenic precautions—protect client from exposure to infection; degree of restriction depends on immunosuppression.

E. Initiate protective environment for HSCT clients.

F. Protect client from persons with communicable childhood diseases, especially those with chickenpox.

G. Polio (IPV), varicella, measles–mumps–rubella, and influenza immunizations are not recommended to be given to children or adults during immunosuppression.

H. Avoid urinary catheterization if possible.

I. Encourage adequate protein and calorie intake, low-bacteria diet (avoid unwashed fruit and vegetables).

J. Maintain adequate hydration.

> **⚠ NURSING PRIORITY:** Prevention and early treatment of common infections are a priority in the plan of care for this client.

**Goal:** To prevent or limit bleeding episodes (Box 16-1).

A. Use local measures to control bleeding (pressure to area; cold packs).

B. Restrict strenuous activity.

---

### Box 16-1 BLEEDING PRECAUTIONS

Indications: Clients diagnosed with leukemia, hemophilia, DIC, low platelets, or any condition that causes bleeding; clients receiving anticoagulants or thrombolytic medications.

- Limit number of venipunctures and intramuscular injections.
- Use smallest-size needle for all injections or IV infusions.
- Perform guaiac (occult blood) tests on stool as necessary.
- Oral hygiene:
  - Discourage flossing.
  - Use soft-bristle toothbrush; may need to use cotton-tipped swabs while gums are friable.
  - Avoid harsh mouthwashes with alcohol.
  - Rinse mouth frequently with mild nonalcoholic mouthwash.
- Use electric razor for shaving.
- Assess perianal area for fissures and bleeding daily.
- Discourage client from vigorous coughing or nose blowing.
- Prevent constipation.
- Avoid aspirin products; evaluate NSAIDs for bleeding properties.
- Avoid catheters (urinary and suctioning) when possible.
- Avoid enemas and suppositories when possible; use water-soluble lubricant if indicated.
- Avoid overinflation of blood pressure cuff or leaving cuff inflated for prolonged period of time.
- Provide safe environment and prevent injury according to age (padded side rails, soft toys, nonskid shoes, etc.).
- Monitor for bleeding episode: nosebleed, hematuria, increased bruising, and menstruation.

*DIC,* Disseminated intravascular coagulation; *NSAIDs,* nonsteroidal antiinflammatory drugs.

---

C. Involve client in evaluating level of activity; decrease activity when platelet counts are low and anemia is present.

**Goal:** To prevent renal complications associated with chemotherapy.

A. Maintain adequate hydration to flush chemicals from the kidneys.

B. Monitor levels of uricemia.

C. Monitor renal function before and during treatment.

**Goal:** To provide pain relief.

A. Use acetaminophen rather than aspirin or nonsteroidal antiinflammatory drugs (NSAIDs).

B. Maintain an environment conducive to rest.

C. Position carefully; may coordinate positioning with administration of analgesics.

D. Evaluate effectiveness of pain relief; administer analgesic before pain becomes severe.

E. Do not exercise affected joints.

**Goal:** To decrease adverse effects of chemotherapy (see Chapter 11).

**Goal:** To prevent and recognize complications of transfusions (see Appendix 16-3).

**Goal:** To demonstrate an understanding of the disease and its prognosis and to display an ability to cope with the diagnosis and its consequences (physical, psychological, social, and spiritual).

A. Assist client and family in maintaining realistic expectations.

B. Be honest in discussion of the outcome and possible side effects of anticipated therapy.

C. Provide emotional support and encourage venting of feelings.

> **TEST ALERT:** Care of client receiving chemotherapy, blood transfusions, client and family teaching, and pain relief are all components of the examination.

 **Home Care**

A. Do not take aspirin or medications that contain aspirin; caution in use of NSAIDS.

B. Monitor weight gain or loss.

C. Counseling to determine effect of client's or child's illness on family members.

D. Encourage family involvement in client's care.

E. Discourage pets (e.g., fish, birds, cats), fresh flowers, and houseplants because of the possibility of bacteria and virus transmission.

F. Teach family methods to stop bleeding.

G. Help parents prepare for their child's return to school.

H. Teach the importance of good handwashing and other infection prevention measures.

I. Teach family members to recognize the early signs of infection and importance of reporting these signs as soon as they are observed.

J. Provide information about community resources for the client and family (e.g., Leukemia & Lymphoma Society, American Cancer Society, Meals on Wheels).

> **TEST ALERT:** Help the family manage care of a client with long-term needs; determine the family's understanding of causes of illness; determine effectiveness of the client's support system.

## Lymphomas

**Lymphomas are characterized by malignant neoplasms originating in the bone marrow and lymphocytes.**

A. Hodgkin disease: characterized by painless enlargement of lymph nodes with progression to involve the liver and spleen. Common metastatic sites are the spleen, liver, bone marrow, and lungs. Disease is spread by extension along the lymphatic system. This is the most curable of the lymphomas.
  1. Assessment.
    a. Risk factors/etiology.
      (1) Familial tendency, more prevalent in men than in women.
      (2) May be caused by Epstein-Barr virus or exposure to occupational toxins.
      (3) Increased incidence in immunosuppressed clients (HIV infection).
    b. Clinical manifestations.
      (1) Initially, painless enlargement of cervical, axillary, inguinal, or mediastinal lymph nodes.
      (2) Symptoms result from pressure on adjacent organs.
      (3) Fever, malaise, night sweats.
      (4) Weight loss, fever, and night sweats are associated with a poor prognosis.
      (5) Ingestion of small amounts of alcohol cause pain at affected lymph node sites.
    c. Diagnostics: lymph node biopsy specimen showing presence of Reed-Sternberg cells (see Appendix 16-1).
  2. Treatment: chemotherapy and radiation.
B. Non-Hodgkin's disease (NHL): a neoplastic growth (derived from B and T cells) that originates in the lymphoid tissue. It spreads malignant cells unpredictably, infiltrating the lymphoid tissue.
  1. Assessment.
    a. Risk factors/etiology.
      (1) Increased incidence in clients with immunodeficiency or autoimmune conditions who have used immunosuppressant medications.
      (2) Associated with viral infections (Epstein-Barr, hepatitis B and C) and occupational exposure to carcinogens and chemicals (pesticides, herbicides, and solvents).
    b. Clinical manifestations.
      (1) Symptoms are highly variable, depending on where the disease has spread.
      (2) Lymphadenopathy that can wax and wane.

c. Diagnostics: based on classification system of the histopathology of malignant cells.
  (1) Magnetic resonance imaging (MRI), lymph node biopsy establishes the cell type and pattern.
  (2) Classification system—World Health Organization (WHO): NHL are categorized by the type of lymphocyte they originate in. The most common categories for classifying NHL are B-cell lymphomas and T-cell lymphomas.
  2. Treatment: chemotherapy and radiation.
    a. Treatment is directed by clinical behavior of NHL: low grade (indolent), intermediate or high grade (aggressive), and highly aggressive.
    b. The more aggressive forms respond better to chemotherapy than the low-grade forms of NHL.

### Nursing Interventions

**Goal:** To maintain physiologic equilibrium.

A. Maintain hydration and nutrition.
B. Maintain good pulmonary hygiene.
C. Evaluate for shortness of breath; maintain in semi-Fowler's position.
D. Decrease body needs for oxygen.
E. Assess ability of cardiovascular system to maintain cardiac output.
F. Manage pain and effects of therapy.

**Goal:** To prevent infection (see "Goal: To prevent infection" in previous Leukemia section).
**Goal:** To decrease adverse effects of chemotherapy and radiation therapy (see Chapter 11).
**Goal:** To help the client understand the implications of the disease and its prognosis; to have the client demonstrate the ability to cope with the diagnosis and its long-term implications (see Nursing Interventions in Chapter 11).

## Multiple Myeloma (Plasma Cell Myeloma)

**Multiple myeloma is a malignancy of plasma cells, specifically the B lymphocytes. Infiltration occurs in the bones and soft tissues.**

### Assessment

A. Clinical manifestations.
  1. Back pain, bone pain (pelvis, spine, and ribs most common).
  2. Pathologic fractures as a result of diffuse osteoporosis.
  3. Hypercalcemia, high serum protein levels.
  4. Renal failure.
B. Diagnostics.
  1. Serum and/or protein electrophoresis; increased Bence-Jones protein in urine.
  2. Bone marrow biopsy, showing increased numbers of plasma cells (see Appendix 16-1).
  3. Skeletal bone surveys, MRI, and/or positron emission tomography and computed tomography scans showing areas of bone erosions, thinning, and/or fractures caused by demineralization.
  4. Prognosis is based on beta$_2$-microglobulin and albumin levels.

### Treatment

A. Chemotherapy with corticosteroids (see Table 11-1) and immunomodulators (see Appendix 25-2).
B. Immunotherapy and targeted drug therapy.

### Nursing Interventions

**Goal:** To maintain physiologic equilibrium.

A. Careful ambulation to decrease hypercalcemia and improve pulmonary status.
B. Adequate hydration to prevent calcium from precipitating in the kidneys; careful monitoring of hydration status.
C. Comfort measures and analgesics for pain.
D. Safety measures to prevent pathologic fractures.
   1. Do not lift anything weighing more than 10 pounds.
   2. Use proper body mechanics.
E. Braces may be necessary to support the spine.
F. Prevention of infection.

**Goal:** To help the client understand implications of the disease and measures to maintain health.

## DISORDERS OF COAGULATION

### Hemophilia

**Hemophilia is a genetic disorder caused by a defect in the clotting mechanism. Classically, there are two types, distinguishable only by laboratory tests. Clinically, the two types are the same, but both may occur in varying degrees of severity. The disease is most often recognized during the toddler stage (Figure 16-5).**

A. Hemophilia A: factor VIII deficiency (classic hemophilia).
B. Hemophilia B: factor IX deficiency (Christmas disease).

### Assessment

A. Risk factors/etiology: both types of hemophilia are sex-linked recessive disorders.
   1. Family history of hemophilia.
   2. Primarily affects males; females are carriers.

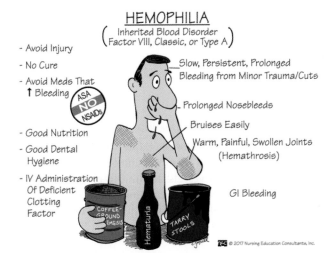

HEMOPHILIA
( Inherited Blood Disorder
Factor VIII, Classic, or Type A )

- Avoid Injury
- No Cure
- Avoid Meds That ↑ Bleeding 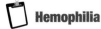 ASA NO NSAIDS
- Good Nutrition
- Good Dental Hygiene
- IV Administration Of Deficient Clotting Factor

Slow, Persistent, Prolonged Bleeding from Minor Trauma/Cuts
Prolonged Nosebleeds
Bruises Easily
Warm, Painful, Swollen Joints (Hemathrosis)
GI Bleeding
COFFEE-GROUND EMESIS
Hematuria
TARRY STOOLS
© 2017 Nursing Education Consultants, Inc.

**FIGURE 16-5 Hemophilia.** (From Zerwekh, J., Garneau, A., & Miller, C. J. [2017]. *Digital collection of the memory notebooks of nursing* [4th ed.]. Chandler, AZ: Nursing Education Consultants, Inc.)

B. Clinical manifestations.
   1. Persistent or prolonged bleeding that occurs from minor trauma/insults.
   2. Hemarthrosis: bleeding into joint cavities.
   3. Spontaneous hematuria.
   4. Hematoma.
   5. Intracranial hemorrhage may be fatal.
   6. Petechiae are uncommon, because platelet count is normal.
C. Diagnostics.
   1. History of bleeding episodes.
   2. Family inheritance pattern.
   3. Identification of deficient factor (factor assay).
   4. Partial thromboplastin time (PTT), bleeding time.

### Treatment

A. Intravenous administration of the specific coagulation factor the client is lacking. Monitor the client for signs and symptoms of possible mild or severe (anaphylactic) allergic reaction.
B. Desmopressin (DDAVP): synthetic vasopressin used to treat mild cases; given IV or intranasally.
C. Aminocaproic acid and tranexamic acid—antifibrinolytic agents used to prevent recurrent bleeds rather than treat acute, ongoing bleeds.
D. Treatment may be carried out at home.

### Nursing Interventions

**Goal:** To prevent spontaneous bleeding episodes (see Box 16-1).

A. Decrease risk for injury.
   1. Make environment as safe as possible without hampering motor development.
   2. Instruct client to avoid contact sports but encourage noncontact sports (e.g., swimming).
   3. Regular exercise and physical therapy to promote muscle strength around joints and decrease bleeding episodes.
B. Preventive dental care, and prevent oral infections.
C. Maintain normal weight; increased weight causes increased strain on the joints.
D. Avoid any aspirin compounds or NSAIDs.
E. Administer clotting factors before, during, and after invasive medical procedures.

**Goal:** To recognize and treat bleeding episodes.

A. Apply pressure to the area.
B. Immobilize and elevate the joints involved.
C. Do not perform passive range of motion on affected joints.
D. Apply cold pack to promote vasoconstriction.
E. Observe for signs of internal bleeding: tarry stools, slurred speech, headache.
F. Administer clotting factors in a timely manner.

**Goal:** To prepare client and family to administer clotting factors intravenously at home.

A. Correct technique for venipuncture.

B. Indications for use.

 C. Encourage child to learn self-administration, generally around age 9 to 12 years.

**Goal:** To prevent permanent joint degeneration.

A. Elevate joint and immobilize during acute bleeding episode.
B. Encourage active range of motion so child will limit movement based on pain tolerance.
C. Physical therapy after the acute phase, no weight bearing until swelling has resolved.
D. Maintain pain relief during physical therapy.

> ■ **NURSING PRIORITY:** Apply RICE to the affected joints: rest, ice, compression, elevation.

### Home Care

A. Have client and family demonstrate ability to perform IV initiation and administration.
B. Have client and family discuss situations that call for use of IV infusion of deficient factor: endoscopy, dental work, etc.
C. Discuss with family the importance of routine prophylactic dental checkups.
D. Encourage venting of feelings regarding diagnosis of the disease.
E. Encourage counseling for parents regarding concern and guilt over hereditary disorder.

> **TEST ALERT:** Modify approaches in care based on child's development; determine family's understanding of the causes and/or consequences of the client's illness and ability to provide care; assist family in crisis.

### Thrombocytopenia

**Thrombocytopenia refers to a reduction in platelet levels below 150,000/mL, leading to bleeding episodes that can occur after trauma or injury. Prolonged bleeding is the hallmark feature associated with thrombocytopenia. In some instances, spontaneous bleeding can occur without any precipitating cause or injury sustained to the client.**

A. Immune thrombocytopenic purpura (ITP)—most common; considered to be an autoimmune disorder caused by an infection, *H. pylori* or virus. Macrophages attack antibody-coated platelets, as these platelets are not recognized in the body; this leads to platelet destruction.
B. Thrombotic thrombocytopenic purpura (TTP)—closely linked with hemolytic–uremic syndrome; more common in females. May also be caused by certain drug therapies (chemotherapy, antiviral agents, oral contraceptives, platelet inhibitors), and is observed in pregnancy. Spontaneous bleeding and clotting occur concurrently. The reduction in platelets causes the prolonged bleeding, and circulating platelets in the bloodstream aggregate causing micro thrombi to travel to arterioles and capillaries.

C. Heparin-induced thrombocytopenia (HIT)—Complication associated with heparin therapy where thrombocytopenia develops 5 to 10 days after receiving heparin; venous and arterial thromboses are frequent complications associated with HIT.

### Assessment

A. Risk factors/etiology.
   1. Recent or excessive bleeding.
   2. Compromised immune function (HIV infection, cancer).
   3. Prior history of bleeding problems.
   4. Medications (loop diuretics, NSAIDs, aspirin and aspirin-containing products, antibiotics).
   5. Chemotherapy.
B. Clinical manifestations.
   1. Petechiae, ecchymosis on skin and mucous membranes.
   2. Epistaxis and gingival bleeding.
   3. Dizziness, hypotension, abdominal pain, tachycardia (internal bleeding).
   4. Internal or external hemorrhage.
C. Diagnostics (see Appendix 16-1).
   1. Low platelet levels.
   2. Specific blood studies to determine type of thrombocytopenia (ITP antigen-specific assay, PF4-heparin complex).
   3. Bone marrow biopsy.

### Treatment

A. Identify and treat the underlying problem.
B. Corticosteroids.
C. Immunosuppressant therapy.
D. Platelet transfusions and plasmapheresis, based on precipitating cause.
E. Splenectomy (ITP and TTP).
F. Warfarin and thrombolytic agents (HIT).

### Nursing Interventions

**Goal:** To identify the problem early and to decrease potential adverse effects.

A. Assess and monitor for bleeding.
B. Nursing measures to prevent bleeding episodes (see Box 16-1).
C. Assess and support all vital systems.
D. Monitor platelet count.

### Disseminated Intravascular Coagulation

**Disseminated intravascular coagulation (DIC) is a serious secondary coagulation disorder involving widespread clotting in the small vessels, leading to consumption of clotting factors, thereby precipitating a bleeding disorder. It is not a disease but a result of underlying conditions.**

### Assessment

A. Risk factors/etiology.
   1. Increase in release of coagulation factors into circulation: hemolytic processes, extensive tissue damage.

   2. Damage to the vascular endothelium (burns, transplant rejection).
   3. Shock, hemolytic processes (transfusion reactions).
   4. Infection: sepsis.
   5. Obstetric complications: hemorrhage.
   6. Malignancies: leukemia, lymphoma, tumor lysis syndrome.
B. Clinical manifestations.
   1. Thrombocytopenia: petechiae, ecchymosis on skin and mucous membranes.
   2. Prolonged bleeding from multiple body areas, such as venipuncture sites.
   3. Hypotension leading to shock.
   4. Multiple organ dysfunction syndrome.
C. Diagnostics (see Appendix 16-1).
   1. Low fibrin and platelet levels.
   2. Prolonged prothrombin time (PT), partial thromboplastin time (PTT), and activated partial thromboplastin time (aPTT).
   3. Elevated fibrin split products (FSPs) and D-dimer assay.

## Treatment

A. Correction of the underlying problem.
B. Platelets, fresh frozen plasma transfusions, cryoprecipitate based on precipitating cause.
C. Heparin or low-molecular-weight heparin (enoxaparin)—used only when the benefit of reduced clotting outweighs the risk of further bleeding.
D. Recombinant human activated protein C: drotrecogin alfa—anticoagulant and antiinflammatory effects.
E. Treatment of shock, as indicated.

## Nursing Interventions

**Goal:** To identify the problem early and to decrease potential adverse effects.

A. Thorough assessment of bleeding problems in clients severely compromised by other problems (shock and sepsis).
B. Nursing measures to prevent bleeding episodes (see Box 16-1).
C. Assess and support all vital systems.

**Goal:** To help the client's family understand the implications of the disease and demonstrate appropriate coping behaviors.

A. Provide emotional support and encourage visiting as intensive care policies and client's condition allow.
B. Encourage ventilation of feelings regarding critical illness of family member.
C. Be available to family members during visiting time.

## DISORDERS OF THE SPLEEN

The spleen is a part of the lymphatic system and can be affected by many disorders that result in splenomegaly (enlarged spleen). The spleen usually contains approximately 350 mL of blood and about one-third of the platelet volume.

## Assessment

A. Risk factors/etiology for splenomegaly.
   1. Chronic myelogenous leukemia.
   2. Heart failure.
   3. Systemic lupus erythematosus.
B. Clinical manifestations.
   1. Hypersplenism: splenomegaly with peripheral cytopenias (anemia, leukopenia, thrombocytopenia).
   2. Pain due to splenomegaly.
   3. Splenic rupture from trauma or inadvertent tearing during other surgical procedures.
C. Diagnostics (see Appendix 16-1).
   1. CBC, pitted or pocked RBCs or Howell-Jolly bodies.
   2. Abdominal ultrasound/CT.

## Treatment

A. Splenectomy.
B. Analgesics for pain.
C. Platelets, fresh frozen plasma transfusions.

## Nursing Interventions

**Goal:** To identify the problem early (splenomegaly, hypersplenism, or splenic rupture) and to decrease potential adverse effects.

A. Thorough assessment of spleen problem and management to address issues of splenomegaly (pain), hypersplenism, or splenic rupture (emergency surgery).
B. Nursing measures to prevent bleeding episodes in hypersplenism (see Box 16-1).
C. Assess and support all vital systems.
D. Monitor for complications after surgery—hemorrhage, shock, fever, abdominal distention, immunologic deficiencies (IgM), infection.

**Goal** To help the client's family understand the implications of the problem and demonstrate appropriate coping behavior.

A. Provide emotional support and encourage visiting as intensive care policies and client's condition allow.
B. Encourage venting of feelings regarding critical illness of family member.
C. Be available to family members during visiting time.
D. Teach about lifelong risk for infection after splenectomy; encourage vaccination for pneumococcus.

## Appendix 16-1   HEMATOLOGIC DIAGNOSTICS

| Test | Normal | Clinical and Nursing Implications |
|---|---|---|
| Bone marrow aspiration or biopsy | All formed cell elements within normal range<br>Erythrocytes: 4.5–6.0 $10^6$/mcL<br>Leukocytes: 4.0–11 $10^3$/mcL<br>Platelets: 150–400 × $10^3$ units/L | 1. Evaluates presence, absence, or ratio of cells characteristic of a suspected disease (e.g., hematopoiesis pathology, chromosomal abnormalities, staging cancers, anemias).<br>2. Used to diagnosis leukemia and myeloma.<br>3. Preferable site is posterior superior iliac spine of pelvis; and proximal tibia (in children).<br>4. Client preparation:<br>  • Position client prone or on the side.<br>  • Local anesthetic is used.<br>  • Feeling of pressure when bone marrow is entered; pain occurs as marrow is being withdrawn. |

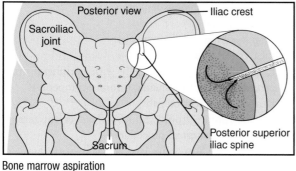

Bone marrow aspiration

| | | |
|---|---|---|
| | | After test:<br>1. Observe for bleeding at site.<br>2. Apply pressure to site 5–10 minutes or longer if client is thrombocytopenic.<br>3. Bed rest for approximately 30–60 min afterward.<br>4. Assess for signs of shock (tachycardia, hypotension).<br>5. Monitor for infection (redness and pain at puncture site). |
| Lymph node biopsy | No evidence of Reed-Sternberg cells | 1. Specimen showing presence of Reed-Sternberg cells indicates lymphoma. |
| Sickle cell test (SICKLEDEX) | No hemoglobin (Hgb) S present | 1. Routine screening test for sickle cell trait or disorder; does not distinguish between them.<br>2. False-negative result in infants aged less than 3 months.<br>3. False-positive result can occur for up to 3–4 months after a transfusion of RBCs that are positive for the trait. |
| Hemoglobin electrophoresis | Separates various hemoglobins and allows for identification of specific problem | 1. Differentiates between trait or disorder in sickle cell anemia.<br>2. Diagnosis of thalassemia and hemolytic anemia. |
| Partial thromboplastin time (PTT)<br>Activated partial thromboplastin time (aPTT) | Normal: 60–70 sec<br><br>Normal: 30–40 sec | 1. Sensitive in monitoring heparin; draw 30 minutes to 1 hour before next heparin dose.<br>2. May be used to detect circulating anticoagulants.<br>3. Prolonged in hemophilia because of deficiency of intrinsic clotting. |
| Prothrombin time (PT)<br>International normalized ratio (INR) | 11.0–12.5 sec or 85%–100% (each client will have a control value)<br>Normal INR: 0.8–1.0 | 1. Production of prothrombin depends on adequate intake and utilization of vitamin K.<br>2. Both tests may be used in management of warfarin therapy.<br>3. INR should be maintained at 2.0–3.0 for individuals with risk for clots (atrial fibrillation, history of recent DVT) and between 3.0 and 4.0 for individuals with mechanical heart valves or vascular stents.<br>4. Hemophilia does not alter PT because of no involvement of the extrinsic clotting system. |
| Homocysteine | Normal: 4–14 μmol/L | 1. An amino acid metabolized through pathways that require vitamin $B_{12}$.<br>2. Increased in $B_{12}$ and folic acid deficiency. |

## Appendix 16-1 HEMATOLOGIC DIAGNOSTICS—cont'd

| Test | Normal | Clinical and Nursing Implications |
|---|---|---|
| D-dimer | Normal: <0.4 mcg/mL | 1. Used to measure fibrin fragment created by fibrin degradation and clot lysis. 2. Used in management of low-molecular-weight heparin therapy, and for diagnosis of DIC and pulmonary embolism. 3. Client must be NPO for 10–12 hours before test, as meat contains increased levels of homocysteine. |
| Ferritin | Male: 12–300 ng/mL or 12–300 mcg/L (SI units) Female: 10–150 ng/mL or 10–150 mcg/L (SI units) Newborn: 25–200 ng/mL | 1. Major iron storage protein reflects iron storage. 2. Diagnoses iron deficiency anemia. |
| Bence-Jones protein | Negative | 1. Collection of a 24-hour urine specimen. 2. Presence of Bence-Jones protein is diagnostic for multiple myeloma. |
| Serum folate | 5–25 ng/mL or 11–57 mmol/L | 1. Needed for erythropoiesis. 2. Decreased in iron deficiency anemia, megaloblastic anemia. 3. Assesses nutritional status; decreased levels in clients with alcoholism. |
| Spleen scan | A method to evaluate splenic function | 1. Injection of a radioactive isotope to evaluate spleen. |
| Beta$_2$ microglobulin | Can be performed on blood, urine, or cerebrospinal fluid | 1. Generally, high beta$_2$ microglobulin and lower levels of albumin are associated with a poorer prognosis in malignancies (multiple myeloma, leukemia, or lymphoma). |
| Albumin | 3.5–5.0 g/dL (35–50 g/L) | 1. High albumin levels caused by the disease process in multiple myeloma can result in renal failure. |
| Serum and/or protein electrophoresis | Protein spike is abnormal | 1. Used to detect hyperglobulinemic states—multiple myeloma, lymphoma. |

DIC, Disseminated intravascular coagulation; DVT, deep vein thrombosis; INR, international normalized ratio; NPO, nothing by mouth, RBCs, red blood cells. Figure from Pagana, K., & Pagana, T. (2014). Mosby's manual of diagnostic and laboratory tests (5th ed.). St. Louis, MO: Mosby.

## Appendix 16-2 HEMATOLOGIC MEDICATIONS

| Medications | Side Effects | Nursing Implications |
|---|---|---|
| **Iron Preparations:** Replacement. | | |
| Ferrous fumarate: PO Ferrous gluconate: PO Ferrous sulfate: PO Iron dextran injection: IV, IM Epoetin alfa: IV, subQ | GI irritation Nausea Constipation Toxic reactions: Fever Urticaria | 1. Absorbed better on empty stomach; however, may give with meals if GI upset occurs. 2. Absorption increased if administered with vitamin C. 3. Liquid preparations should be diluted and given through a straw to prevent staining of the teeth. 4. Tell client stool may be black and iron may cause constipation. 5. Eggs, milk, cheese, and antacids inhibit oral iron absorption. 6. Iron preparations inhibit oral tetracycline absorption. IM/IV preparations may be used if on oral tetracycline. 7. Anaphylactic reaction can occur; test dose should be given. 8. IM should be avoided because of pain and tissue discoloration. 9. If given IM, use Z-track method to prevent tissue staining. 10. IV route recommended if oral route is not acceptable. |
| **Vitamin K:** Necessary for normal prothrombin activity. | | |
| Vitamin K: phytonadione: PO, subQ, IM, IV | GI upset, rash IV not recommended because of hypersensitivity reactions | 1. PO and subQ most common routes. 2. Antidote for warfarin. 3. Observe bleeding precautions. |

GI, Gastrointestinal; IM, intramuscularly; IV, intravenously; PO, by mouth (orally); SubQ, subcutaneously.

## Appendix 16-3 BLOOD TRANSFUSIONS

| Blood Component for Transfusion | Purpose of Administration | Nursing Implications |
| --- | --- | --- |
| Packed RBCs: 250–350 mL per unit. | To increase oxygen-carrying capacity<br>To decrease risk for incompatible antibodies from the plasma | 1. Chart:<br>• Type and amount of blood product infused.<br>• Time started and time completed.<br>• Blood unit identification number.<br>• Rate of infusion—slower rate in older adults.<br>2. Vital signs are taken immediately before transfusion, at 5 min and 15 min into transfusion, every hour during transfusion, and at completion of transfusion.<br>3. Closely observe older adult clients for indications of fluid overload. |
| Platelets: 30–60 mL per unit | To treat thrombocytopenia | 1. Chart amount and type of infusion.<br>2. Infuse rapidly—as fast as client tolerates. |
| Fresh frozen plasma: 250 mL per unit | Administered for clotting factors, proteins, fluid volume | 1. Chart amount and type infused.<br>2. Infuse immediately after thawing.<br>3. Infused for 30–60 minutes or as client tolerates. |
| Whole blood: 500 mL per unit | To provide volume replacement and increase oxygen-carrying capacity<br>Administered with greater than 25% blood loss | 1. Same as with packed RBCs.<br>2. Observations for fluid volume overload. |

**TEST ALERT:** Administer and discontinue blood and/or blood products; check blood products according to institution policies; evaluate appropriate IV access; evaluate client's response.

### Nursing Guidelines for Packed RBCS or Whole Blood Transfusions

1. Informed consent and alternatives should be explained to the client. Autologous (using client's own blood) and designated donor transfusions are options. If client is unable to give consent, consent should be obtained from family.
2. Obtain the type and cross-match records and the unit of blood to administer.
   Check:
   a. The ABO group on the unit against the cross-match records.
   b. The Rh type of the blood against the cross-match record.
   c. Have two licensed individuals, commonly two RNs, compare and match the patient identification with the labeled blood component and sign that they correspond.
   d. Check the client's name, date of birth, and hospital number on the unit of blood and on the cross-match records with another licensed nurse.
   e. If any of these do not match, DO NOT GIVE THE BLOOD.
   f. Check the expiration date on the unit of blood.
3. Administer the blood immediately after receiving it from the blood bank; blood should NEVER be stored in a unit refrigerator or allowed to sit out at room temperature. The maximum amount of time blood can be out of monitored storage is 30 min.
4. Do not add any medications to blood products.
5. Do not warm blood before transfusion unless there are several units to be infused rapidly and client is in danger of developing a hypothermic response. If blood must be warmed, use equipment that is specifically designed for this procedure.
6. Inspect the blood bag for leaks, abnormal color, excessive air, or bubbles.
7. The average rate of transfusion in an adult is 1 unit of blood over about 2 to 3 hours, depending on the condition of the client.
8. The blood administration set should be changed after 2 units have infused to decrease risk for bacterial contamination.
9. It is not recommended to use an infusion pump; the pump increases RBC hemolysis.
10. Multiple transfusions can result in hyperkalemia and hypocalcemia.
11. Administer blood through a Y-set with normal saline only, and a filter below the Y in the tubing.
12. Administer within 4 hours of starting the RBCs or whole blood transfusion.

### Nursing Guidelines for Platelets and Fresh Frozen Plasma

1. Obtain type and cross-match records; check client and unit identification in same way as for packed RBCs.
2. Unit should not contain any clumps or have unusual color.
3. Fresh frozen plasma must be administered immediately.
4. Infuse each unit normally over 15 to 30 minutes.

**! NURSING PRIORITY:** The majority of major adverse transfusion reactions are due to improper identification of the blood product and the recipient.

### ✓ KEY POINT: Guidelines for Performance Phase of Transfusion

• Check the prescriber's order; check the labels on the blood bag against the client identification at the bedside with another licensed nurse.
• Baseline vital signs must be obtained before hanging the blood; if the client has a temperature greater than 101°F (38.3°C), advise the health care provider before starting the transfusion.

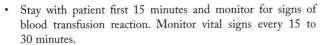

## Appendix 16-3  BLOOD TRANSFUSIONS—cont'd

- Stay with patient first 15 minutes and monitor for signs of blood transfusion reaction. Monitor vital signs every 15 to 30 minutes.
- Whole blood or RBCs should be administered with at least a 22-gauge cannula/needle. Slightly smaller needles can be used for platelets, albumin, and clotting factor replacement.
- Use only normal saline, NOT $D_5W$, to initiate the transfusion; it causes the blood to hemolyze and precipitate.
- Always use a standard blood administration set with a filter; DO NOT use straight IV tubing.

- Initiate infusion (rate of approximately 100–125 mL/hr, depending on client's condition) and remain with the client; the first 10 to 15 min is the most critical period; the majority of transfusion reactions occur during administration of the first 50 mL.
- During the transfusion, continue to monitor for circulatory overload or transfusion reaction.
- Blood deteriorates rapidly after about 2 hr or exposure to room temperature; a unit of blood should not hang longer than 4 hr.

| Transfusion Reactions | Nursing Management |
| --- | --- |

### Hemolytic Transfusion Reaction

1. Low back pain
2. Hypotension, tachycardia, tachypnea
3. Apprehension, sense of impending doom
4. Fever, chills, flushing
5. Chest pain
6. Dyspnea
7. Onset is rapid

1. Stop blood transfusion immediately and notify physician.
2. Change the IV tubing; do not allow blood in the tubing to infuse into the client; maintain IV access.
3. Obtain first-voided urine specimen to test for blood in the urine.
4. Anticipate blood samples to be drawn by the laboratory.
5. With suspected renal involvement, treatment with diuretics is initiated to promote diuresis.

### Allergic Reaction

1. Urticaria (hives)
2. Pruritus
3. Facial flushing
4. Severe shortness of breath, bronchospasm

1. If client has a history of allergic reactions, the antihistamine diphenhydramine may be given before starting the transfusion.
2. Stop transfusion until status of reaction can be determined; if symptoms are mild and transient, the transfusion may be resumed.
3. If anaphylactic/severe allergic reaction, initiate CPR if needed, have epinephrine ready for administration, and do not continue administration of transfusion.

### Febrile Reaction

1. Chills and fever
2. Headache, flushing
3. Muscle stiffness/pain
4. Increased anxiety

1. Keep client covered and warm during transfusion.
2. Give antipyretics as prescribed (acetaminophen). Avoid aspirin and NSAIDs in thrombocytopenic patients.
3. Stop the transfusion until status of reaction can be determined.
4. Transfusion with leukocyte-poor RBCs or frozen washed packed cells may prevent this reaction in clients susceptible to fever.
5. Most common reaction.

*CPR*, Cardiopulmonary resuscitation; *D₅W*, 5% dextrose in water; *IV*, intravenous; *NSAIDs*, nonsteroidal antiinflammatory drugs; *RBCs*, red blood cells; *RN*, registered nurse.

## Appendix 16-4  HEMATOPOIETIC STEM CELL TRANSPLANT[a]

**Goal:** To restore hematologic and immunologic function in clients with immunologic deficiencies, leukemia, congenital or acquired anemias.

### Procedure

In the adult client, approximately 400 to 800 mL of bone marrow or harvested stem cells are processed and transfused into the client. (See Appendix 16-1 for care of donor client for bone marrow aspiration.)

1. Typing:
   a. Allogenic: matching of a histocompatible donor, preferably a relative.
   b. Autologous: uses client's own bone marrow that has been collected from disease-free tissue and then frozen.
   c. Syngeneic: donor is an identical twin with perfect tissue match.

2. Immunoablative preparation pretransplant: chemotherapy and radiation to produce immunologically suppressed state before the hematopoietic transfusion; procedure takes 5 to 10 days.

### Complications

1. Bacterial, viral, or fungal infection from immunosuppressed state.
2. Severe thrombocytopenia resulting in bleeding problems.
3. Graft-versus-host disease (rejection).
   a. Acute rejection generally occurs in 7 to 30 days after transplantation; chronic rejection occurs in 100 days.
   b. Erythematous rash on the palms and feet, spreading to the trunk, may be an early symptom.
   c. Altered liver enzyme profiles with liver tenderness and jaundice.

*Continued*

d. Gastrointestinal disturbances: anorexia, nausea, vomiting, diarrhea.

## Nursing Implications

1. Preparation of the client for immunosuppression with chemotherapy and radiation therapy.

aIncludes bone marrow transplant and stem cell transplant.

2. Confirmation of rejection is by skin or oral mucosal biopsy.
3. Successful engraftment is indicated by formation of erythrocytes, leukocytes, and platelets, usually 2 to 5 weeks after transplantation.
4. Care of the immunosuppressed client (see Chapter 10).

# Study Questions
# Hematology: Care of Adult and Pediatric Clients

More questions on
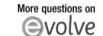

1. A client and her husband are positive for the sickle cell trait. The client asks the nurse about the chances of her children having sickle cell disease. The nurse understands that this genetic problem will reflect what pattern in the client's children?
   1. One of her children will have sickle cell disease.
   2. Only the male children will be affected.
   3. Each pregnancy carries a 25% chance of the child being affected.
   4. If she has four children, one of them will have the disease.

2. The nurse is preparing discharge teaching for a client with aplastic anemia. What will be important to include in the teaching plan? **Select all that apply.**
   1. Take your iron with meals every day and decrease the amount of green, leafy vegetables in your diet.
   2. Establish a balance between rest and activity; avoid excessive fatigue.
   3. Rest and supplemental oxygen may be required during periods of dyspnea.
   4. Drink a glass of wine in the evening to help increase your appetite.
   5. Notify your health care provider if you begin to experience frequent bruising.
   6. Increase your intake of dairy products (milk and cheese) and protein.

3. A client is experiencing a sickle cell crisis during labor and delivery. What is the best nursing action?
   1. Maintain IV fluid infusion and assess adequacy of hydration.
   2. Administer a high concentration of oxygen.
   3. Insert a Foley catheter and monitor hourly urine output.
   4. Provide continuous sedation for pain relief.

4. The nurse is preparing a teaching plan for a family with a child who has been diagnosed with sickle cell anemia and crisis. What will the nurse include in the teaching regarding the pathophysiology of sickle cell crisis?
   1. It results from altered metabolism and dehydration.
   2. Tissue hypoxia and vascular occlusion cause the primary problems.
   3. Increased bilirubin levels will cause hypertension.
   4. There are decreased clotting factors with an increase in white blood cells.

5. A young adult comes to the clinic complaining of dizziness, weakness, and palpitations. What will be important for the nurse to evaluate initially when obtaining the health history?
   1. Activity and exercise patterns
   2. Nutritional patterns
   3. Family health status
   4. Coping and stress tolerance

6. A child with leukemia is being discharged after beginning chemotherapy. What instructions will the nurse include in the teaching plan for the parents of this child?
   1. Provide a diet low in protein and high in carbohydrates.
   2. Avoid unwashed fruits and vegetables.
   3. Notify the doctor if the child's temperature exceeds 102°F (39°C).
   4. Increase the use of humidifiers throughout the house.

7. Which client is most likely to have iron deficiency anemia?
   1. A client with cancer receiving radiation therapy twice a week
   2. A toddler whose primary nutritional intake is milk
   3. A client with a peptic ulcer who had surgery 6 weeks ago
   4. A 15-year-old client in sickle cell crisis

8. A client with hemophilia comes to the emergency department after bumping his knee. The knee is rapidly swelling. What is the first nursing action?
   1. Initiate an IV site to begin administration of cryoprecipitate.
   2. Perform a type and cross-match for possible transfusion.
   3. Draw blood for determination of hemoglobin and hematocrit values.
   4. Apply an ice pack and compression dressings to the knee.

9. A client has an order for one unit of packed cells. What is a correct nursing action?
   1. Initiate the IV with 5% dextrose in water (D5W) to maintain a patent access site.
   2. Initiate the transfusion within 30 minutes of receiving the blood.
   3. Monitor the client's vital signs for the first 5 minutes.
   4. Monitor the client's vital signs every 2 hours during the transfusion.

10. A nurse is caring for a client who is receiving a blood transfusion. The transfusion was started 30 minutes ago at a rate of 100 mL/hr. The client begins to complain of low back pain and headache and is increasingly restless. What is the first nursing action?
    1. Slow the infusion and evaluate the vital signs and the client's history of transfusion reactions.
    2. Stop the transfusion, disconnect the blood tubing, and begin a primary infusion of normal saline solution.
    3. Stop the infusion of blood and begin infusion of normal saline solution from the Y connector.
    4. Recheck the unit of blood for correct identification numbers and cross-match information.

11. The nurse is caring for a client with leukemia who is experiencing bleeding into the knee joints. What is the best nursing care for this client regarding joint mobility and activity?
    1. Encourage short walks around the room every 2 hours.
    2. Keep the joint immobilized and maintain bed rest for the client.
    3. Gently put the legs through passive range of motion every 4 hours.
    4. Keep the legs wrapped with elastic bandages and immobilized in splints.

12. The nurse is providing discharge instructions to a client who has had a splenectomy. The teaching is based on the knowledge that splenectomy clients have:
    1. Decreased leukocytes
    2. Increased platelets
    3. Decreased hemoglobin
    4. Increased eosinophils

13. A client in sickle cell crisis is admitted to the emergency department. What are the priorities of care in order of importance?
    1. Nutrition, hydration, electrolyte balance
    2. Hydration, pain management, electrolyte balance
    3. Hydration, oxygenation, pain management
    4. Hydration, oxygenation, electrolyte balance

14. The nurse is providing teaching to a family whose child has been recently diagnosed with hemophilia. Which of the following would the nurse include in this discussion?
    1. Hemophilia is a genetic disease that is more common in females.
    2. Hemophilia is correctable through transfusions and bone marrow transplantation.
    3. Hemophilia is most often a sex-linked congenital disorder.
    4. Hemophilia is preventable through genetic counseling.

15. A client has been diagnosed with disseminated intravascular coagulopathy (DIC). The nurse will anticipate administering which of the following fluids?
    1. Packed red blood cells (PRBCs)
    2. Fresh frozen plasma (FFP)
    3. Volume expanders, such as D10W
    4. Whole blood

16. A client has been diagnosed with pernicious anemia. What will the nurse teach this client regarding the medication he will need to take after he goes home?
    1. Monthly vitamin B12 injections will be necessary.
    2. Daily ferrous sulfate (in oral form) will be prescribed.
    3. Coagulation studies are important to monitor the effect of medications.
    4. He should reduce his intake of leafy, green vegetables to decrease vitamin K.

17. The parents of a client with hemophilia are taking their child home. Which statement indicates a need for further education regarding hemophilia?
    1. "We should ensure that our child has regular dental appointments."
    2. "We need to wrap our child's limbs daily to prevent bleeding."
    3. "We should help our child select activities that minimize the risk of injury."
    4. "We should not give our child aspirin."

18. The nurse identifies which problems as risk factors for the development of a sickle cell crisis? **Select all that apply.**
    1. Recurrence of acute otitis media
    2. A fall with swelling at the kneecap and joint
    3. Fractured radius requiring internal fixation
    4. Recurrence of respiratory tract infection
    5. Traveling to a location of higher altitude
    6. Dehydration

19. The nurse is caring for a client who has hypersplenism. What laboratory test finding would indicate that the client has splenomegaly?
    1. Presence of Reed-Sternberg cells
    2. Elevated red blood cell count
    3. Increased Bence-Jones protein in urine
    4. Presence of Howell-Jolly bodies in a blood smear

20. Which of the following would be appropriate discharge instructions for the client that has just been diagnosed with polycythemia vera? **Select all that apply.**
    1. "You can expect to have repeated phlebotomies."
    2. "Take an iron supplement daily."
    3. "Low-dose aspirin may be prescribed by your health care provider."
    4. "A warm bath may be used to decrease generalized pruritus."
    5. "Avoid crowds due to increased risk of infection secondary to your low white blood cell (WBC) count."
    6. "Try to keep well hydrated by drinking at least 2 liters of fluid per day."

# Answers to Study Questions

**1.** *3*
In autosomal recessive traits, when both parents have the trait, there is a 25% chance with each pregnancy that the child will have the disease. When only males are affected, it is an X-linked recessive disease, such as hemophilia. Because there is a 1 in 4 chance of transmitting the trait, it is possible that none of the children would be affected. Frequently, there is a negative family history of the disease. (Lewis et al., 10 ed., p. 616)

**2.** *2, 3, 5*
Because clients who are anemic experience chronic fatigue, it is important to balance rest and activities to avoid problems with tachycardia and dyspnea. If a client has a problem with dyspnea during activities, supplemental oxygen may be necessary. The health care provider should be notified if bruising occurs, because this could indicate further problems in the hematologic system. Iron should be taken on an empty stomach, but if significant GI upset occurs, it can be taken with food. All alcoholic beverages should be avoided. There is no indication to increase the intake of dairy products and protein. A balanced diet should be followed. (Lewis et al., 10 ed., pp. 608)

**3.** *1*
Adequate hydration is critical during stress periods for the client with sickle cell disease, and this is particularly true of a client in labor. Oxygen may or may not be ordered in low concentrations. A urinary retention catheter is not necessary at this time and would be a potential cause of infection. Although pain relief is important for both the sickling issues and the labor pains, continuous sedation would not be indicated because this would be detrimental to the fetus. (Lewis, 10 ed., pp. 617–619; Lowdermilk et al., 10 ed., pp. 721–722)

**4.** *2*
When there is inadequate hydration, the sickled cells begin to clump together, which leads to vascular occlusion. Tissue hypoxia occurs as a result of the decreased oxygen-carrying capacity of the sickled red blood cells and from the vascular occlusion. Increased bilirubin from the hemolysis of the RBC does not cause hypertension, but jaundice and an increased incidence of cholelithiasis may occur. With sickle cell anemia, there is not a decrease in clotting factors. (Lewis et al., 10 ed., pp. 616–617)

**5.** *2*
Iron deficiency anemia is characterized by fatigue, dizziness, weakness, increased pulse, palpitations, and increased sensitivity to cold. The adult female often becomes anemic for a variety of reasons, such as poor nutrition and heavy menses. (Lewis et al., 10 ed., pp. 609–610)

**6.** *2*
Fresh fruits and vegetables harbor microorganisms, which can cause infections in the immunosuppressed client. Fruits and vegetables should either be peeled or cooked. The doctor should be notified of a temperature greater than 100°F because of immunosuppression. A diet low in protein is not indicated, and humidifiers may harbor fungi in the water containers. (Lewis et al., 10 ed., pp. 639–640)

**7.** *2*
The toddler will need to eat a balanced diet and may require an iron supplement. A diet based primarily on milk products will not cover the iron needs of a toddler. A client in sickle cell crisis may experience anemia, but it is due to the increased destruction of red blood cells, not poor iron intake. The client receiving radiation therapy may also develop anemia; however, it is not due to poor nutritional intake but to bone marrow suppression. The client who has had gastric surgery may develop anemia as a result of a lack of adequate utilization of vitamin $B_{12}$. (Lewis et al., 10 ed., p. 610)

**8.** *4*
Rest, ice, compression, and elevation (RICE) are the immediate treatments to reduce the swelling and bleeding into the joint. These are the priority actions for bleeding into the joint, regardless of the cause. The other options (administer cryoprecipitate, cross-match for blood, draw blood to check hemoglobin and hematocrit) may be done, but they are not the initial priority action. It will be important to rest the joint to prevent hemarthrosis. No weight bearing on joint until all swelling is resolved. (Lewis et al., 10 ed., p. 628)

**9.** *2*
The whole blood must be given within the first 30 minutes to prevent hemolysis and growth of bacteria in the blood. Vital signs are to be checked after administration of the first 50 mL and after the first 15 minutes. (Lewis et al., 10 ed., p. 649)

**10.** *2*
Stop the blood infusion and disconnect the line to decrease the further infusion of red blood cells. Begin administration of normal saline solution with new tubing. The remainder of the blood should be returned to the blood bank for evaluation regarding the reaction. (Lewis et al., 10 ed., pp. 650–652)

**11.** *2*
The knee joint should remain immobilized during the active bleeding phase; walking and passive range of motion may increase the bleeding. The legs are not wrapped, but compression dressings may be placed on the knee. (Lewis et al., 10 ed., p. 628)

**12.** *2*
Removing the spleen will lead to an increase in peripheral RBC, WBC, and platelet counts. In addition, after splenectomy, immunologic deficiencies may develop (IgM); however, IgG and IgA remain normal. There is always a lifelong risk for infection after a splenectomy. (Lewis et al., 10 ed., p. 647)

**13.** *3*
The priorities for care of a client in sickle cell crisis are focused on providing fluid, oxygen, and pain control during the crisis to reduce sickling and prevent complications. Electrolyte management is not a priority, nor is nutrition. (Lewis et al., 10 ed., pp. 617–619)

**14.** *3*
Hemophilia is a sex-linked genetic disorder carried by females but manifested in males. The female is a carrier and the male exhibits

the condition in a sex-linked disorder. Genetic counseling is important for a couple to identify the risks involved, but if a woman who is a carrier decides to have children, the risk of her children having the condition cannot be prevented. (Lewis et al., 10 ed., p. 626)

### 15. *2*

Fresh frozen plasma contains all coagulation factors including V and VIII. DIC results when the body can no longer create clotting factors; thus, fresh frozen plasma is the best answer. Packed red blood cells will be used to increase oxygenation, but this is second-line treatment in this situation. Whole blood is used less frequently, but it does not provide adequate clotting factors. Volume expanders will not help increase clotting factors. (Lewis et al., 10 ed., pp. 630–631)

### 16. *1*

Pernicious anemia is caused by lack of intrinsic factor to effectively utilize vitamin $B_{12}$ and is treated by monthly vitamin $B_{12}$ injections. Ferrous sulfate is given for iron deficiency anemia. Coagulation studies are not necessary because the client is not receiving anticoagulants. Decrease in vitamin K is not necessary because the client is not receiving warfarin. (Lewis et al., 10 ed., pp. 612)

### 17. *2*

Wrapping limbs does not prevent bleeding and does not stop bleeding during acute episodes. Regular dental appointments are necessary to prevent dental problems in a child with hemophilia. Children with hemophilia should be encouraged to participate in activities that are not contact sports and have minimal risk of injury. Aspirin, NSAIDs, and other blood thinners should be avoided. (Lewis et al., 10 ed., p. 628)

### 18. *4, 5, 6*

Recurrence of respiratory tract infections is associated with an increase in sickling crisis, not an acute case of otitis media. Respiratory infections generally involve fever, coughing, malaise, and anorexia. These factors contribute to dehydration. Dehydration may also precipitate an attack as the blood is thicker and more prone to clotting. Problems with oxygen saturation are also associated with sickling crisis, thus traveling to a higher altitude where there is less oxygen may precipitate a crisis. Injuries to joints or fractures needing surgical repair do not lead to a sickle cell crisis. (Lewis et al., 10 ed., p. 617)

### 19. *4*

The presence of pitted or packed RBCs or Howell-Jolly bodies in a peripheral blood smear is diagnostic of splenomegaly. The presence of Reed-Sternberg cells in a lymph node biopsy specimen is diagnostic for Hodgkin disease. Elevated Bence-Jones protein in the urine is found in multiple myeloma. With hypersplenism, you would find cytopenia characterized by anemia, leukopenia, and thrombocytopenia. An elevated RBC, WBC, or platelet count would occur after a splenectomy. (Lewis et al., 10 ed., p. 647)

### 20. *1, 3, 6*

Phlebotomy is the main method of treatment to reduce the hematocrit. Generally, the client will have 300 to 500 mL of blood removed each time, aimed at keeping the hematocrit level between 45% and 48%. Iron supplementation is to be avoided because it raises the hematocrit, and low-dose aspirin is often prescribed to help prevent clot formation. Warm baths may precipitate pruritus, not relieve it. Cool baths may be beneficial, and alpha-interferon is sometimes prescribed for severe itching. There is no risk of infection with crowds, as the WBC count is increased instead of decreased, and the client should maintain normal hydration, which helps decrease clot formation. (Lewis et al., 10 ed., p. 621)

# 17

# Respiratory: Care of Adult and Pediatric Clients

Gas Exchange, Perfusion

## PHYSIOLOGY OF THE RESPIRATORY SYSTEM

### Physiology of Respiration

Respiration is a process by which gas is exchanged between the circulating blood and the inhaled air.

A. Organs of the respiratory system. (Figure 17-1).
B. Gases flow from an area of high pressure to an area of low pressure; pressure below atmospheric pressure is designated as negative pressure.
C. Inspiration.
   1. Stimulus to the diaphragm and the intercostal muscles by way of the central nervous system.
   2. Diaphragm moves down, and intercostal muscles move outward, thereby increasing the capacity of the thoracic cavity and decreasing intrathoracic pressure to below atmospheric pressure.
   3. Through the airways, the lungs are open to atmospheric pressure; air will flow into the lungs to equalize intrathoracic pressure with atmospheric pressure.
D. Expiration.
   1. Diaphragm and intercostal muscles relax and return to a resting position; therefore lungs recoil, and capacity is decreased.
   2. Air will flow out until intrathoracic pressure is again equal to atmospheric pressure.
E. Negative pressure is greater during inspiration; therefore, air flows easily into the lungs.
F. Compliance describes how elastic the lungs are or how easily the lungs can be inflated; when compliance is decreased, the lungs are more difficult to inflate.
G. Control of respiration.
   1. Movement of the diaphragm and accessory muscles of respiration is controlled by the respiratory center located in the brainstem (medulla oblongata and pons).
      a. The respiratory center controls respirations by way of the spinal cord and phrenic nerve.
      b. Activity of the respiratory center is regulated by chemoreceptors. These receptors respond to changes in the chemical composition of the cerebrospinal fluid (CSF) and the blood (specifically the $Pao_2$, $Paco_2$, and pH).

2. The medulla contains the central chemoreceptors responsive to changes in $CO_2$ blood levels.

> **! NURSING PRIORITY:** The primary respiratory stimulus is $CO_2$; when the $Paco_2$ is increased, ventilation is initiated.

3. Carotid and aortic bodies contain the peripheral chemoreceptors for arterial $O_2$ levels.
   a. Primary function is to monitor arterial $O_2$ levels and stimulate the respiratory center when a decrease in $Pao_2$ occurs.
   b. When arterial $O_2$ decreases to less than 60 mmHg, stimulation to breathe is initiated by the chemoreceptors.
   c. In a person whose primary stimulus to breathe is hypoxia, this becomes the mechanism of ventilatory control (hypoxic drive).
H. The process of gas exchange.
   1. Ventilation: the process of moving air between the atmosphere and alveoli.
   2. Diffusion: the process of moving $O_2$ and $CO_2$ across the alveolar capillary membrane.
   3. Perfusion: the process of linking the venous blood flow to the alveoli.

### Oxygen and Carbon Dioxide Transport

A. Internal respiration is the exchange of gases between the blood and interstitial fluid. The gases are measured by an analysis of arterial blood (Table 17-1).
B. $O_2$ delivered to the tissue is dependent on cardiac output.
C. A decrease in the arterial $O_2$ tension ($PaO_2$) and a decrease in the saturation of the hemoglobin with oxygen ($SaO_2$) results in a state of hypoxemia.
D. At high levels (above 10,000 feet), there is reduced $O_2$ in the atmosphere, resulting in a lower inspired $O_2$ pressure and a lower $PaO_2$. Commercial planes are pressurized to an altitude of 8000 feet.

> **TEST ALERT:** Apply knowledge of pathophysiology to monitoring for complications; identify client status based on pathophysiology.

### System Assessment

A. History.
   1. Determine the frequency of upper respiratory problems and/or surgeries involving respiratory problems.

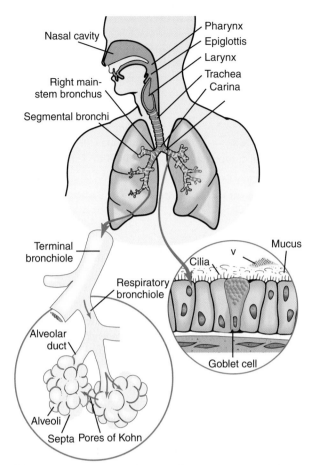

**FIGURE 17-1 Respiratory System.** (Redrawn from Price, S. A., & Wilson, L. M. (2003). *Pathophysiology: Clinical concepts of disease processes* [6th ed.]. St Louis, MO: Mosby.)

| Table 17-1 | NORMAL ARTERIAL BLOOD GAS VALUES | | |
|---|---|---|---|
| Acidity index | pH | 7.35–7.45 |
| Partial pressure of dissolved oxygen | $Pao_2$ | 80–100 mmHg |
| Percentage of hemoglobin saturated with oxygen | $Sao_2$ | 95% or greater |
| Partial pressure of dissolved carbon dioxide | $Paco_2$ | 35–45 mmHg |
| Bicarbonate | $HCO_3{}^2$ | 22–26 mEq/L (mmol/L) |

**NURSING PRIORITY:** An $Sao_2$ less than 95% indicates respiratory difficulty.

2. Status of immunizations.
   a. Tuberculin (TB) skin test (also known as PPD or Mantoux test).
   b. Pertussis, polio, pneumococcal pneumonia vaccine (Pneumovax).
   c. Influenza vaccination.

3. Medications (including over the counter, prescriptions, herbs, and vitamins).
4. Lifestyle and occupational environments.
5. Habits: smoking and alcohol intake.
6. Any change in activities of daily living and activity secondary to respiratory problems.
B. Physical assessment.

**TEST ALERT:** Monitor changes in the client's respiratory status. The primary indicators of respiratory disorders are sputum production, cough, dyspnea, hemoptysis, pleuritic chest pain, fatigue, change in voice, and wheezing.

1. Initially observe client's resting position.
   a. Appearance: comfortable or distressed?
   b. Assess client in the sitting position, if possible.
   c. Any dyspnea or respiratory discomfort?
2. Evaluate vital signs.
   a. Appropriate for age level?
   b. Establish database and compare with previous data.
   c. Assess client's pattern of vital signs; normal vital signs vary greatly from one individual to another (see Table 3-2).

**TEST ALERT:** Apply knowledge of client pathophysiology when measuring vital signs; intervene when vital signs are abnormal; interpret data that need to be reported immediately.

3. Assess upper airway passages and patency of the airway.
4. Inspect the neck for symmetry; check to see whether the trachea is in midline and observe for presence of jugular vein distention.
5. Assess the lungs.
   a. Visually evaluate the chest/thorax.
      (1) Do both sides move equally?
      (2) Observe characteristics of respirations and note whether retractions are present (Figure 17-2).
      (3) Note chest wall configuration (barrel chest, kyphosis, scoliosis).
   b. Palpate chest for tenderness, masses, and symmetry of motion.
   c. Auscultate breath sounds; begin at lung apices and end at the bases, comparing each area side to side. Breath sounds should be present and equal bilaterally.
   d. Determine presence of tactile fremitus: When client says "ninety-nine," there should be equal vibrations palpated bilaterally. Over areas of consolidation (pneumonia), there will be an increase in the vibrations.
   e. Determine presence of adventitious breath sounds (abnormal/extra breath sounds).
      (1) Crackles: usually heard during inspiration and do not clear with cough; occur when airway contains fluid (previously also known as *rales*); sounds are not continuous (early cardiac failure, pneumonia, and atelectasis).

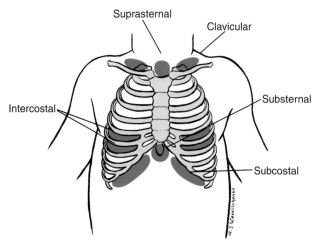

**FIGURE 17-2** **Location of Retractions.** (From Hockenberry, M. J., & Wilson, D. [2015]. *Wong's nursing care of infants and children* [10th ed.]. St. Louis, MO: Mosby.)

(2) Wheezes: may be heard during inspiration and/or expiration; are caused by air moving through narrowed passages; sound is music-like and continuous (asthma, bronchitis, chronic emphysema).

(3) Pleural friction rub: heard primarily on inspiration over an area of pleural inflammation; may be described as a grating sound (pleuritis accompanied by pain with breathing).

(4) Stridor: high-pitched, inspiratory, crowing sound (croup [laryngotracheobronchitis—LTB], acute epiglottitis).

6. Assess cough reflex and sputum production.
    a. Is cough associated with pain?
    b. What precipitates coughing episodes?
    c. Is cough productive or nonproductive?
    d. Characteristics of sputum.
        (1) Consistency, amount, presence of odor.
        (2) Color (should be clear or white); changes in color indicate infection.

> ⚠ **NURSING PRIORITY:** When mucus is retained and pools in the lungs, gas diffusion is decreased, providing a medium for bacteria growth.

    e. Presence of hemoptysis—duration and amount.
7. Assess for and evaluate dyspnea.
    a. Onset of dyspnea and precipitating causes.
    b. Presence of orthopnea.
    c. Presence of adventitious breath sounds.
    d. Noisy expiration.
    e. Level of tolerance of activity.
    f. Correlate vital signs with dyspnea.
    g. Cyanosis (a very late and unreliable sign of hypoxia).
        (1) For dark-skinned clients, assess less pigmented areas (oral cavity, nail beds, lips, palms).
        (2) Dark-skinned clients may exhibit cyanosis in the skin as a gray hue rather than blue.
        (3) Assess for prolonged capillary refill time, should be less than 3 seconds.

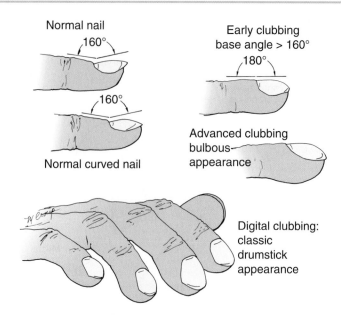

**FIGURE 17-3** **Digital Clubbing.** (Redrawn from Price, S. A., & Wilson, L. M. (2003). *Pathophysiology: Clinical concepts of disease processes* [6th ed.]. St. Louis, MO: Mosby.)

8. Assess for and evaluate chest pain.
    a. Location and character of pain.
    b. Pain associated with cough.
    c. Pain either increased or decreased with breathing.
9. Evaluate fingers for clubbing (characteristic in clients with chronic respiratory disorders) (Figure 17-3).
10. Evaluate pulmonary diagnostics (see Appendix 17-1).
    a. Hemoglobin and hematocrit (presence of polycythemia or anemia).
    b. Electrolyte imbalances.
    c. Arterial blood gases (ABGs).

## RESPIRATORY DISORDERS

### 📋 Hypoxia

Hypoxia is a condition characterized by an inadequate amount of $O_2$ available for cellular metabolism.

> **TEST ALERT:** Problems with respiratory status occur in all nursing disciplines. Questions may center around nursing priorities and nursing interventions in maintaining an airway and promoting ventilation in the client with respiratory difficulty. The questions may arise from any client situation (e.g., obstetrics, newborn, surgical, etc.).

A. Hypoxia occurs when signs and symptoms occur because of a decrease in $Pao_2$; hypoxemia occurs when the amount of $O_2$ in the arterial blood is less than normal.
    1. Decreased $O_2$ in inspired air.
    2. Disorders causing respiratory obstruction and alveolar hypoventilation.

B. Hypoxia may be caused by inadequate circulation.
1. Shock.
2. Cardiac failure.
C. Anemia precipitates hypoxia caused by a decrease in the $O_2$-carrying capacity of the blood.
1. Inadequate red blood cell production.
2. Deficient or abnormal hemoglobin.

### Assessment

A. Risk factors/etiology.
1. Chronic hypoxia.
a. Chronic obstructive pulmonary disease (COPD).
b. Cystic fibrosis, cancer of the respiratory tract.
c. Heart failure, chronic anemia.
2. Inflammatory problems affecting alveolar surface area and membrane integrity (e.g., pneumonia, bronchitis).
3. Acute hypoxia.
a. Acute respiratory failure, sudden airway obstruction.
b. Conditions affecting pulmonary expansion (e.g., respiratory paralysis).
c. Conditions causing decreased cardiac output (heart failure, shock, cardiac arrest, etc.).
d. Hypoventilation (brain attack or stroke, sedation, anesthesia, etc.).
B. Clinical manifestations: underlying respiratory problem, either chronic or acute (Table 17-2).
C. Diagnostics (see Appendix 17-1).
D. Compensatory mechanisms.
1. Increase in cardiac output (tachycardia).
2. Increase in extraction of $O_2$ from capillary blood.
3. Increase in level of hemoglobin.
E. Complications.
1. Acute.
a. Cardiac decompensation.
b. Progression to chronic hypoxia.

2. Chronic.
a. $CO_2$ narcosis (increase in $CO_2$ content of blood).
b. Cor pulmonale (right-sided heart failure due to respiratory NOT cardiac causes).
c. Cardiac failure.
3. Treatment: depends on underlying problem.

**NURSING PRIORITY:** In the client with chronic lung disease who is experiencing severe hypoxia, $O_2$ should never be withheld for fear of increasing the $Pao_2$ levels.

### Nursing Interventions

**Goal:** To maintain good pulmonary hygiene and prevent hypoxic episode.

A. Position client to maintain patent airway.
1. Unconscious client: position on side with the chin extended.
2. Conscious client: elevate the head of the bed and may position on side as well, or "tripod position" (leaning forward with mouth open).
B. Encourage coughing and deep breathing (Box 17-1).
C. Suction client as needed and as indicated by amount of sputum and ability to cough.
D. Maintain adequate fluid intake to keep secretions liquefied.
E. Encourage exercises and ambulation as indicated by condition.
F. Administer expectorants.
G. Administer $O_2$ if dyspnea is present (Appendix 17-7).

**NURSING PRIORITY:** Administer fluids very cautiously to a client who is having difficulty breathing. Begin with small sips of water to determine whether the client can swallow effectively—thickened liquids are easier to control. Do not begin with fluids that contain any fat (milk) or caloric value because of the increased risk for aspiration.

| Table 17-2 | SYMPTOMS OF RESPIRATORY DISTRESS AND HYPOXIA |
|---|---|
| **Early Symptoms** | **Late Symptoms** |
| Restlessness | Extreme restlessness to stupor |
| Tachycardia | Severe dyspnea |
| Tachypnea, exertional dyspnea | Slowing of respiratory rate |
| Orthopnea, tripod positioning | Bradycardia |
| Anxiety, difficulty speaking | Cyanosis (peripheral or central) |
| Poor judgment, confusion | |
| Disorientation | Intercostal retractions |
| **Pediatrics** | |
| Flaring nares (infants) | Mottling, pallor, and cyanosis |
| Substernal, suprasternal, supraclavicular and intercostal retractions (see Figure 17-2) | Sudden increase or sudden decrease in agitation |
| | Inaudible breath sounds |
| Stridor—expiratory and inspiratory | Altered level of consciousness |
| Increased agitation | Inability to cry or to speak |

### Box 17-1 EFFECTIVE COUGHING

- Increase activity before coughing: walking or turning from side to side.
- Place client in sitting position, preferably with feet on the floor.
- Client should turn his or her shoulders inward and bend head slightly forward.
- Take a gentle deep breath in through the nose and breathe out completely.
- Take two deep breaths through the nose and mouth and hold for 5 seconds.
- On the third deep breath, cough to clear secretions.
- Sips of warm liquids (coffee, tea, or water) may stimulate coughing.
- Demonstrate to client how to splint chest or incision during cough to decrease pain.
- Premedicate 30 to 60 minutes before activity/procedures if very painful (incisions, etc.).

**Respiratory Care Priorities**

- The older adult client may not present with respiratory symptoms but instead with restlessness, confusion, and disorientation.
- Age-related changes that may affect respiratory function include the following:
  - Decreased cough and laryngeal reflexes
  - Decreased mucociliary function
  - Decreased functioning alveoli
  - Decreased respiratory muscle strength
  - Increased anteroposterior diameter
  - Increased residual volume

**Respiratory Care Priorities for the Older Adult**

- Provide adequate rest periods between activities such as bathing, going for treatments, eating.
- Increase compliance with medications by scheduling medication administration with routine activities.
- Encourage annual flu vaccination.
- Evaluate client's response to changes in activity and therapy frequently.
- Position the client upright in a position of comfort to facilitate chest/lung expansion.
- Monitor response of oxygen therapy.
- Maintain adequate hydration but use caution with older adults because of increased tendency for fluid volume overload.

**Goal:** To implement nursing measures to decrease hypoxia (Box 17-2).

A. Assess patency of airway (first/highest priority).
1. Can client speak? If not, initiate emergency procedures (see Appendix 17-3).
2. If speaking is difficult because of level of hypoxia, place in semi-Fowler's position, begin oxygen, obtain assistance, and remain with client.
3. If client is coherent and able to speak in sentences, continue with assessment of the problem.
4. Evaluate amount of secretions and ability to cough; suction and administer $O_2$ as indicated.
B. Assess use of accessory muscles, presence of retractions.
C. Maintain calm approach, because increasing anxiety will potentiate hypoxia.

> **NURSING PRIORITY:** Increasing anxiety will accelerate dyspnea in a client who is experiencing severe difficulty breathing.

D. Place adult or older child in a semi-Fowler's position, if not contraindicated.
E. Place infant in an infant seat or elevate the mattress.

> **NURSING PRIORITY:** Position a client experiencing dyspnea with a pillow placed lengthwise behind the back and head. Do not flex the client's head forward or backward.

F. Assess color and presence of diaphoresis.
G. Evaluate vital signs: Are there significant changes from previous readings?

H. Evaluate for dysrhythmias.
1. If the client is on a cardiac monitor, check for presence of premature atrial or ventricular contractions.
2. Evaluate level of tachycardia.
I. Evaluate chest movements: Are they symmetric?
J. Evaluate anterior and posterior breath sounds.
K. Assess client for chest pain with dyspnea.
L. Notify physician of significant changes in respiratory function.
M. Remain with client experiencing acute dyspnea or hypoxic episodes.
N. Assess response to $O_2$ therapy.
O. Monitor ABGs and pulse oximetry.

## Sleep Apnea

**Sleep apnea is a disorder in which an individual frequently stops breathing during sleep (cessation of breathing for 10 seconds or longer occurring at least 5 times/hour). The individual may not be aware of snoring or apneic episodes. Apneic episodes cause recurrent arousals from sleep.**

### Types

- Obstructive sleep apnea results from an obstruction of the upper airway due to inadequate motor tone of the tongue.
- Central sleep apnea occurs when the brain does not send appropriate signals to the muscles that control breathing.

### Assessment

A. Cardinal symptoms (the 3 S's—snoring, sleepiness, and significant-other report of sleep apnea episodes).
B. Clinical manifestations.
1. Disruptive snoring, unrefreshing sleep.
2. Short-term memory loss, morning headaches.
3. Hypersomnia, witness apnea.
4. Gasping while sleeping, large neck, enlarged tonsils.
5. Nasal deformity/septal deviation.
6. Obesity, driving accidents (falling asleep).
7. Increasing irritability, personality changes, and depression.
C. Diagnostics: overnight polysomnography (PSG) to determine frequency and apneic events.
D. Comorbid conditions.
1. Resistant hypertension.
2. Recurrent atrial fibrillation, stroke.
3. Myocardial infarction, heart failure, coronary artery disease (CAD).

### Treatment

A. Lifestyle changes to include weight loss, smoking cessation, decreased consumption of alcohol, and avoidance of use of tranquilizers.
B. Oral appliances designed to keep the throat open during sleep.
C. Change in sleeping position.
D. Continuous positive airway pressure (CPAP) during sleep—pressure helps keep the upper airway open.
E. Uvulopalatopharyngoplasty to remove the tonsils and adenoids and resect the uvula, the posterior part of the soft palate, and any excessive pharyngeal tissue.

*Nursing Interventions*

**Goal:** To reinforce teaching about proper use of equipment.

A. Have client participate in the selection of mask and equipment.
   1. Teach client how to troubleshoot equipment.
   2. Include spouse or bed-partner in education.
B. If client is hospitalized, check hospital policy to see if client can use his or her own equipment.

## Pleural Effusion

**Pleural effusion is caused by a collection of fluid in the pleural space. It is generally associated with other disease processes.**

*Assessment*

A. Pathophysiology.
   1. Causes: heart failure, pneumonia, TB, malignancy, pulmonary embolism, acute pancreatitis, and connective tissue disease.
   2. If the pleural fluid becomes purulent, the condition is referred to as empyema.
B. Clinical manifestations.
   1. Symptoms of an underlying problem.
   2. Large quantities of fluid will cause shortness of breath and dyspnea.
   3. Decreased breath sounds.
   4. Pleuritic pain on inspiration.
   5. Asymmetric chest expansion.
C. Diagnostics (see Appendix 17-1).
   1. Malignancy may be determined by cytologic examination of the aspirated fluid.
   2. Culture and sensitivity on aspirated fluid.

*Treatment*

A. Thoracentesis (see Appendix 17-1) and pleurodesis (inflammation caused by instilling a sclerosing agent into the pleural cavity, which leads to pleura sticking to chest wall).
B. If empyema develops (purulent fluid in the pleural space), area may have to be opened and allowed to drain. Client will receive antibiotics.
C. Chest tube placement is necessary if fluid buildup is rapid, requiring removal to facilitate respirations.

*Nursing Interventions*

**Goal:** To recognize problems associated with chest tube placement and prevent an acute episode of hypoxia (see Hypoxia, Nursing Interventions).

## Home Care

A. Demonstrate to client and family the prescribed method of managing wound care.
B. Client is at increased risk for respiratory tract infections.
C. The purulent fluid is localized and will not be hazardous to other family members if the basic concepts of hand hygiene and sterile technique for dressing changes are used.

## Croup Syndromes

The term *croup* describes a group of conditions characterized by edema and inflammation of the upper respiratory tract.

A. Acute epiglottitis: a severe infection of the epiglottis characterized by rapid inflammation and edema of the area; generally occurs in children aged 2 to 7 years; may rapidly cause airway obstruction.
   1. Cause: most commonly *Haemophilus influenzae*.
   2. Clinical manifestations: hypoxia (see Table 17-2).
      a. Rapid, abrupt onset.
      b. Sore throat, difficulty swallowing.
      c. Inflamed epiglottis.
      d. Symptoms of increasing respiratory tract obstruction.
         (1) Characteristic position: sitting with the neck hyperextended (sniffing position) and mouth open (tripod position), drooling.
         (2) Inspiratory stridor (crowing).
         (3) Suprasternal and substernal retractions.
         (4) Increased restlessness and apprehension.
      e. High fever (greater than 102°F).

> **! NURSING PRIORITY:** The absence of spontaneous cough and the presence of drooling and agitation are cardinal signs distinctive of epiglottitis. Do not put tongue blade or culture swab into the mouth or throat; can cause airway obstruction.

   3. Treatment.
      a. Endotracheal intubation for obstruction (see Appendix 17-5).
      b. Humidified oxygen.
      c. Antibiotics: intravenous (IV) and then by mouth (PO).
B. Acute laryngotracheobronchitis (croup): inflammation of the larynx and trachea, most often in children under 5 years of age.
   1. Cause: viral agents (influenza and parainfluenza viruses, respiratory syncytial virus).
   2. Slow onset, frequently preceded by upper respiratory tract infection.
   3. Respiratory distress (see Table 17-2).
      a. Inspiratory stridor when disturbed, progressing to continuous stridor.
      b. Flaring of nares, use of accessory muscles of respiration.
      c. "Seal bark" cough is classic sign.
   4. Low-grade fever (usually less than 102°F [38.8°C]).
   5. Signs of impending obstruction.
      a. Retractions (intercostals, suprasternal, and substernal) at rest.
      b. Increased anxiety and restlessness.
      c. Tachypnea (rate may be greater than 60 breaths/min).
      d. Pallor and diaphoresis.
      e. Nasal flaring.

> **TEST ALERT:** Intervene when vital signs are abnormal; position client to prevent complications; interpret client data that need to be reported immediately.

6. Treatment.
    a. Maintain patent airway.
    b. Bronchodilators, racemic epinephrine (for moderate to severe croup) by inhalation.
    c. Cool mist humidification.
    d. No sedatives.
    e. Oxygen.
    f. Corticosteroids, administered intravenously, intramuscularly, or orally.
C. Acute spasmodic laryngitis: mildest form of croup; generally occurs in children 1 to 3 years old.
    1. Cause: viral with an allergy component.
    2. Clinical manifestations.
        a. Characterized by paroxysmal attacks.
        b. Characteristically occurs at night.
        c. Mild respiratory distress (see Table 17-2).
        d. No fever.
        e. After the attack, the child appears well.
    3. Treatment:
        a. Child is generally cared for at home.
        b. Usually self-limiting.
        c. Cool mist or humidity may decrease spasm.

### Nursing Interventions

**Goal:** To maintain patent airway in hospitalized child.

A. Tracheotomy set or endotracheal intubation equipment readily available.

> **⚠ NURSING PRIORITY:** For a child with suspected epiglottitis, do not examine the throat with a tongue depressor or take a throat culture; have child seen by primary care provider immediately. Resuscitation equipment and suction should be readily available.

B. Suction endotracheal tube or tracheotomy only as necessary.
C. Position for comfort; do not force child to lie down.
D. If child is intubated, do not leave unattended.
E. If obstruction is impending, maintain ventilation with a bag and valve mask resuscitator until child can be intubated.
F. If transport is required, allow the child to sit upright in parent's lap if possible.

**Goal:** To evaluate and maintain adequate ventilation.

A. Assess for increasing hypoxia.
B. Provide humidified $O_2$; closely evaluate, because cyanosis is a late sign of hypoxia.
C. Conserve energy; prevent crying.
D. Monitor pulse oximetry for adequate oxygenation.

**Goal:** To maintain hydration and nutrition.

A. Administer IV fluids.
B. Do not give oral fluids until danger of aspiration is past.

> **TEST ALERT:** Identify client potential for aspiration. In children with severe respiratory distress (rate greater than 60), do not give anything by mouth because of increased risk for aspiration.

C. Give IV fluids during acute episodes.
D. Provide high-calorie liquids when danger of aspiration is over.
E. Suction nares of infant before feeding.
F. Assess for adequate hydration.

### Home Care

A. Teach parents to recognize symptoms of increasing respiratory problems and when to notify physician.
B. Cool mist may assist to decrease edema and/or spasms of airway.
C. Maintain adequate fluid intake.
D. Immunization with *H. influenza* type B vaccine.

## Bronchiolitis (Respiratory Syncytial Virus)

Bronchiolitis is an inflammation of the bronchioles; alveoli are usually normal.

A. Respiratory syncytial virus (RSV) infection is most common in winter and spring (November to March); peaks in children 2 to 5 months old.
B. RSV is transmitted by direct contact with respiratory secretions.
C. RSV is considered the single most important respiratory pathogen of infancy and early childhood.

### Assessment

A. Cause: usually begins after an upper respiratory tract infection; incubation period of 5 to 8 days.
B. Reinfection is common; severity tends to decrease with age and repeated infections.
C. Clinical manifestations.
    1. Initial.
        a. Rhinorrhea and low-grade fever commonly occur first.
        b. Coughing, wheezing.
    2. Acute phase.
        a. Lethargic.
        b. Tachypnea, air hunger, retractions.
        c. Increased wheezing and coughing.
        d. Periods of apnea, poor air exchange.
D. Diagnostics: nasal secretions for RSV antigens.

### Treatment

A. Rest, fluids, and high-humidity environment.
B. $O_2$.
C. Prevention—medication: palivizumab.
D. Treatment—medication: ribavirin.

### Nursing Interventions

**Goal:** To promote effective breathing patterns.

A. Frequent assessment for development of hypoxia (see Table 17-2); close monitoring of $O_2$ saturation (oximetry) levels.
B. Increase in respiratory rate and audible crackles in the lungs are indications of cardiac failure and should be reported immediately.
C. Maintain airway via position and removal of secretions.

D. Maintain adequate hydration to facilitate removal of respiratory secretions.

E. Conserve energy; avoid unnecessary procedures but encourage parents to console and cuddle infant.

**Goal:** To prevent transmission of organisms.

A. If hospitalized, the child should be placed in a private room or a room with another RSV child, with contact precautions in place (see Appendix 9-3).

B. Decrease number of health care personnel in client's room.

C. Nurses assigned to care for these children should not be assigned the care of other children who are at high risk for respiratory tract infections.

D. Prophylaxis medication with palivizumab for high-risk infants.

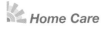 **Home Care**

A. Decreased energy level; will tire easily.

B. Small frequent feedings.

C. Teach parents how to assess for respiratory difficulty.

D. Teach parents care implications if child is receiving prophylactic medications (see Appendix 17-2).

## Tonsillitis

**Tonsillitis is an inflammation and infection of the palatine tonsils.**

### Assessment

A. Risk factors/etiology.
   1. More common in children.
   2. Increased severity in adults.

B. Clinical manifestations.
   1. Edematous, enlarged tonsils; exudate on tonsils.
   2. Difficulty swallowing and breathing.
   3. Frequently precipitates otitis media.
   4. Mouth breathing, persistent cough, fever.

C. Diagnostics: throat culture for group A beta-hemolytic streptococci.

### Treatment

A. Antibiotic for identified organism.

B. Surgery: tonsillectomy for severe repeated episodes of tonsillitis once acute infectious episode is resolved.

### Nursing Interventions

**Goal:** To promote comfort and healing in home environment (Figure 17-4).

A. Nonirritating soft or liquid diet.

B. Cool mist vaporizer to maintain moisture in mucous membranes.

C. Throat lozenges, warm gargles to soothe the throat.

D. Antibiotics: important to give child all of the medication prescribed to prevent reoccurrence.

E. Analgesics, antipyretic (acetaminophen).

**Goal:** To provide preoperative nursing measures if surgery is indicated (see Chapter 3).

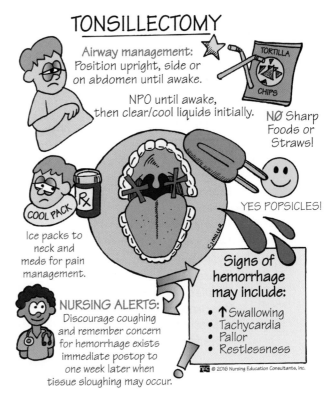

**FIGURE 17-4 Tonsillectomy.** (From Zerwekh, J., Garneau, A., & Miller, C. J. [2017]. *Digital collection of the memory notebooks of nursing* [4th ed.]. Chandler, AZ: Nursing Education Consultants, Inc.)

**Goal:** To maintain patent airway and evaluate for bleeding after tonsillectomy.

A. No fluids until child is fully awake; then cool, clear liquids initially. Avoid brown- or red-colored fluids and milk products.

B. Position child on side or abdomen to facilitate drainage until fully awake; when awake and alert, child may assume position of comfort but needs to remain in bed for the day.

C. Evaluate for frequent or continuous swallowing or clearing of throat caused by bleeding; check throat with flashlight for bleeding.

D. Have nasopharyngeal suction equipment available.

E. Monitor for tachycardia, pallor, and increasing restlessness.

F. Apply ice collar to decrease edema.

G. Give oral acetaminophen (with codeine or hydrocodone if needed) for pain; aspirin is contraindicated.

H. Discourage coughing.

I. Do not use straws for drinks.

> ⚠ **NURSING PRIORITY:** Before the child is fully awake, position him or her on side or abdomen to prevent aspiration from bloody drainage or vomitus. Always consider the client who has had a tonsillectomy to be nauseated as a result of swallowing blood.

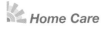 **Home Care**

A. Child will have sore throat for several days; discourage coughing and excessive activity.

# PNEUMONIA

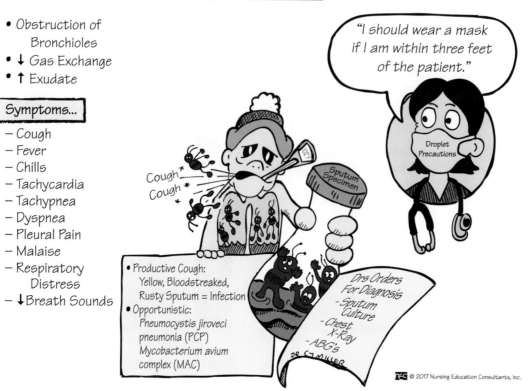

- Obstruction of Bronchioles
- ↓ Gas Exchange
- ↑ Exudate

Symptoms...

- Cough
- Fever
- Chills
- Tachycardia
- Tachypnea
- Dyspnea
- Pleural Pain
- Malaise
- Respiratory Distress
- ↓ Breath Sounds

Cough *
Cough *

• Productive Cough:
Yellow, Bloodstreaked,
Rusty Sputum = Infection
• Opportunistic:
Pneumocystis jiroveci
pneumonia (PCP)
Mycobacterium avium
complex (MAC)

Sputum Specimen

Drs Orders For Diagnosis
- Sputum Culture
- Chest X-Ray
- ABG's
DR CJ MILLER

"I should wear a mask if I am within three feet of the patient."

Droplet Precautions

© 2017 Nursing Education Consultants, Inc.

**FIGURE 17-5 Pneumonia.** (From Zerwekh, J., Garneau, A., & Miller, C. J. [2017]. *Digital collection of the memory notebooks of nursing* [4th ed.]. Chandler, AZ: Nursing Education Consultants, Inc.)

B. Symptoms of bleeding are especially significant on the fifth to tenth postoperative days, when tissue sloughing may occur as a result of healing and/or infection.

C. Maintain adequate hydration; encourage intake of soft foods and nonirritating fluids.

D. A gray membrane on the sides of the throat is normal and should disappear in 1 to 2 weeks.

## Pneumonia

**Pneumonia is an acute inflammatory process caused by a microbial agent; it involves the lung parenchyma, including the small airways and alveoli (Figure 17-5).**

### Assessment

A. Predisposing conditions.
  1. Chronic upper respiratory tract infection, prolonged immobility.
  2. Smoking, decreased immunity (disease and/or age).
  3. Aspiration of foreign material or gastric contents.
  4. Chronic health problems: cardiac, pulmonary, diabetes, cancer, stroke.
  5. Nosocomial pneumonia: caused by tracheal intubation, intestinal/gastric tube feedings, ventilator-associated pneumonia (VAP) (Box 17-3).

B. Etiology.
  1. Viral: influenza, parainfluenza, RSV (primarily infants and young children).
  2. Bacterial: *Streptococcus pneumoniae, Mycoplasma pneumoniae, Staphylococcus aureus.*
  3. Fungal (increased risk in immunocompromised clients).

C. Clinical manifestations.
  1. Fever, chills, tachycardia, tachypnea, dyspnea.
  2. Productive cough: thick, blood-streaked, yellow, purulent sputum.

---

**Box 17-3 STRATEGIES TO PREVENT VENTILATOR-ASSOCIATED PNEUMONIA**

Ventilator-associated pneumonia (VAP) is an airway infection that develops at least 48 hours after a patient is intubated.
- VAP is the leading cause of death related to hospital-acquired infections.
- VAP can develop as a result of aspiration of stomach contents or when bacterial colonies from the oral cavity, sinuses, and trachea develop on the endotracheal tube.

**Nursing Implications**
1. Handwashing.
2. Elevate head of bed between 30 to 45 degrees.
3. Provide oral care to prevent oral–tracheal contamination.
4. Use of continuous-suction endotracheal tube.
5. Daily assessment related to readiness to extubate.
6. Change ventilator circuit only if needed (no more often than every 48 hours).
7. Peptic ulcer disease (PUD) prophylaxis.
8. Deep venous thrombosis (DVT) prophylaxis, if appropriate.

Adapted from How-to Guide: Prevent Ventilator-Associated Pneumonia. Cambridge, MA: Institute for Healthcare Improvement; 2012. (Available at www.ihi.org).

3. Pleuritic chest pain, malaise, altered mental status.
4. Respiratory distress (hypoxia) (see Table 17-2).
5. Diminished breath sounds, wheezing, crackles, tactile fremitus, dullness to percussion.
6. Pediatrics.
   a. Feeding difficulty in infants.
   b. Cough nonproductive initially.
   c. Moderate to high fever.
   d. Adventitious breath sounds, tachypnea.
   e. Retractions, nasal flaring

D. Diagnostics (see Appendix 17-1).

> ◼ **OLDER ADULT PRIORITY:** An older adult client may initially present with mental confusion and volume depletion rather than respiratory symptoms and fever (see Box 17-2).

### Treatment

A. Antibiotic according to organism identified (see Appendix 9-2).

> **TEST ALERT:** Administration of medications: do not start antibiotics until a good sputum specimen (Appendix 17-9) has been collected. An accurate culture and sensitivity test cannot be done if client has already begun receiving antibiotics.

B. Respiratory precautions: transmitted via airborne droplets (see Appendix 9-3).
C. Inhalation therapy.
   1. Cool $O_2$ mist, incentive spirometer.
   2. Postural drainage, turn, cough, and deep breathe.
   3. Bronchodilators.
D. Chest physiotherapy (CPT)—suctioning, percussion, and postural drainage.

### Nursing Interventions

**Goal:** To prevent occurrence.

A. Encourage mobility and ambulation if possible.
B. Good respiratory hygiene; turn, cough, deep breathe, and incentive spirometry.
C. Identify high-risk clients.
D. Encourage pneumococcal vaccine for susceptible clients.

**Goal:** To decrease infection and remove secretions to facilitate $O_2$ and $CO_2$ exchange.

A. Antibiotics.
B. Have client turn, cough, and deep breathe.
C. Liquefy secretions.
   1. Adequate hydration (administer PO fluids cautiously to prevent aspiration).
   2. Cool mist inhalation.
D. Evaluate breath sounds and changes in sputum.
E. Position for comfort or place in semi-Fowler's position.
F. Nursing measures to prevent and evaluate levels of hypoxia (see Hypoxia, Nursing Interventions; also see Table 17-2).
G. Provide adequate pain control measures to facilitate coughing and deep breathing.

**Goal:** To teach client and family how to provide home care when appropriate.

A. Antibiotics.
B. Cool mist humidification.
C. Maintain high oral fluid intake.
D. Antipyretic: acetaminophen.
E. Frequent changes of position.
F. Understand symptoms of increasing respiratory problems and when to notify physician.

## 📋 Tuberculosis

**TB is a reportable communicable disease that is characterized by pulmonary manifestations.**

A. Characteristics.
   1. Organism is primarily transmitted through respiratory droplets; it is inhaled and implants on respiratory bronchioles or alveoli; predominately spread by repeated close contact.
   2. Latent TB infection (LTBI): a client in good health is frequently able to resist the primary infection and does not have active disease; these clients will continue to harbor the TB organism.
   3. The primary site or tubercle may undergo a process of degeneration or caseation; this area can erode into the bronchial tree, and TB organisms are active and present in the sputum, resulting in further spread of the disease.
   4. The area may never erode but may calcify and remain dormant after the primary infection. However, the tubercle may contain living organisms that can be reactivated several years later.
   5. The majority of people with a primary infection will harbor the TB bacilli in a tubercle in the lungs and will not exhibit any symptoms of an active infection.
   6. May occur as an opportunistic infection in clients who are immunocompromised.

### Assessment

A. Predisposing conditions.
   1. Frequent close or prolonged contact with infected individual.
   2. Debilitating conditions and diseases.
   3. Poor nutrition and crowded living conditions.
   4. Increasing age.
B. Cause: *Mycobacterium tuberculosis*, a gram-positive, acid-fast bacillus.
C. Clinical manifestations (up to 20% of clients may be asymptomatic).
   1. Fatigue, malaise, anorexia, weight loss.
   2. May have a chronic cough that progresses to more frequent and productive cough.
   3. Low-grade fever and night sweats.
   4. Hemoptysis is associated only with advanced condition.
   5. May present with acute symptoms.
   6. Clients with LTBI will have a positive skin test, but they are asymptomatic.
D. Diagnostics (see Appendix 17-1).

1. QuantiFERON-TB (QFT) rapid diagnostic: blood test to identify presence of antigens; does not take the place of sputum smears and cultures.
2. New rapid test: nucleic acid amplification test (NAAT); results in 2 hours.
3. Bacteriologic studies to identify acid-fast bacilli in the sputum (see Appendix 17-1).

E. Complications.
 1. Pleural effusion.
 2. Pneumonia.
 3. Other organ involvement.

## Treatment

A. Medication (see Appendix 17-2) (Figure 17-6).
 1. Medical regimen involves simultaneous administration of two or more medications; this increases the therapeutic effect of medication and decreases development of resistant bacteria.
 2. Sputum cultures are evaluated every 2 to 4 weeks initially; then monthly after sputum is negative. Sputum cultures should be negative within several weeks of beginning therapy; this depends on the medication regimen and the resistance of the bacteria.

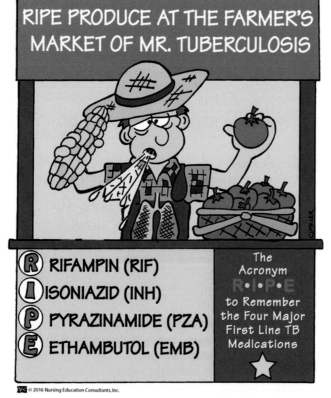

**FIGURE 17-6 Tuberculosis Medications: RIPE.** (From Zerwekh, J., Garneau, A., & Miller, C. J. [2017]. *Digital collection of the memory notebooks of nursing* [4th ed.]. Chandler, AZ: Nursing Education Consultants, Inc.)

3. Direct observed therapy (DOT): health care personnel provide the medications and observe that client swallows medication; preferred strategy for all clients.
4. Prophylaxis chemotherapy for LTBI.
 a. Close contact with a client with a new diagnosis of TB.
 b. Newly infected client with positive skin test reaction.
 c. Client with positive skin test reaction with conditions that decrease immune response (HIV infection, steroid therapy, chemotherapy).
 d. Isoniazid (INH) most often used for prophylaxis.

B. Most often treated on an outpatient basis.

## Nursing Interventions

**Goal:** To understand implications of the disease and measures to protect others and maintain own health.

A. Evaluate client's lifestyle and identify needs regarding compliance with treatment and long-term therapy.
B. Identify community resources available for client.

C. Understand medication schedule and importance of maintaining medication regimen.
 1. Nonadherence is a major contributor to the development of multidrug resistance and treatment failure.
 2. DOT recommended to guarantee adherence; may require client to come to public health clinic for nurse to administer medication.

D. Return for sputum checks every 2 to 4 weeks during therapy.
E. Balanced diet and good nutritional status.
F. Avoid alcohol and all medications that may damage the liver.
G. Avoid excessive fatigue; endurance will increase with treatment.
H. Identify family and close contacts who need to report to the public health department for TB screening.
I. Offer client HIV testing.

**Goal:** To prevent transmission of the disease.

A. When sputum is positive for the organism, implement airborne precautions for hospitalized client (see Appendix 9-3).
B. Wear an N95 or high-efficiency particulate air (HEPA) respirator when caring for the patient.
C. Home care: teach respiratory precautions.
 1. Cover mouth and nose when sneezing or coughing.
 2. Practice careful handwashing routine.
 3. Wear a surgical mask when in contact with other people.
 4. Discard all secretions (nose and mouth) in plastic ags.
 5. Reevaluate periodically for active disease or secondary infection.

## Chronic Obstructive Pulmonary Disease

**Chronic obstructive pulmonary disease (COPD) is a group of chronic respiratory disorders characterized by obstruction of airflow, primarily chronic bronchitis and emphysema.**

A. Although each of the disorders (chronic bronchitis, emphysema) may occur individually, it is more common for two or more problems to coexist and the symptoms to overlap (most commonly bronchitis and emphysema).

B. Clinical manifestations common to chronic airflow limitation (Figure 17-7).
   1. Distended neck veins, ankle edema.
   2. Orthopnea or tripod positioning, barrel chest (Figure 17-8).
   3. Prolonged expiratory time, pursed-lip breathing.
   4. Diminished breath sounds.
   5. Thorax is hyperresonant to percussion.
   6. Exertional dyspnea progressing to dyspnea at rest.
   7. Increased respiratory rate.

C. As a result of a prolonged increase in $Paco_2$ levels, the normal respiratory center in the medulla is affected; when this occurs, hypoxia will become the primary respiratory stimulus.

D. Emphysema: primarily a problem with the alveoli characterized by a loss of alveolar elasticity, overdistention, and destruction, with severe impairment of gas exchange across the alveolar membrane.
   1. Clinical manifestations of emphysema.
      a. Cough is not common; sensation of air hunger.
      b. Use of accessory muscles of respiration; expiratory wheezes.
      c. Anorexia with weight loss, thin in appearance; barrel chest.
      d. In general, no cardiac enlargement; cor pulmonale occurs late in disease; decreased $Pao_2$ with activity.

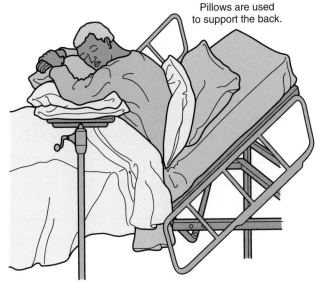

Pillows are used to support the back.

Other pillows are placed on an overbed table to support the weight of the arms, shoulders, and head.

**FIGURE 17-8 Orthopnea Position.** (From deWit, S., Stromberg, H., & Dallred, C. [2017]. *Medical-surgical nursing: Concepts and practice* [3rd ed.]. St. Louis, MO: Elsevier.)

   e. ABGs changes late in disease.
   f. Characteristic tripod position—leaning forward with arms braced on knees.

E. Chronic bronchitis: primarily a problem related irritation of airway characterized by excessive mucus production and impaired ciliary function, which decreases mucus clearance. Client may develop polycythemia as a result of the low $Pao_2$. History of productive cough lasting at least 3 months for 2 consecutive years.
   1. Clinical manifestations of chronic bronchitis.
      a. Excessive, chronic sputum production (generally not discolored unless infection is present).
      b. Impaired ventilation, resulting in decreased $Pao_2$ and symptoms of hypoxia; increased $Paco_2$ ($CO_2$ narcosis).
      c. Respiratory symptoms: productive cough, exercise intolerance, wheezing, and shortness of breath, progressing to cyanosis.
      d. Dependent edema.
      e. Generally normal weight or overweight.
      f. Cardiac enlargement with cor pulmonale.

### Assessment

A. Risk factors/etiology.
   1. Cigarette smoking (including passive smoking)—most common cause.
   2. Chronic infections.
   3. Inhaled irritants (from occupational exposure and air pollution).
   4. Alpha$_1$-antitrypsin deficiency: enzyme deficiency leading to decreased lung elasticity and COPD at an early age.
   5. Aging: changes in thoracic cage and respiratory muscles and loss of elastic recoil.

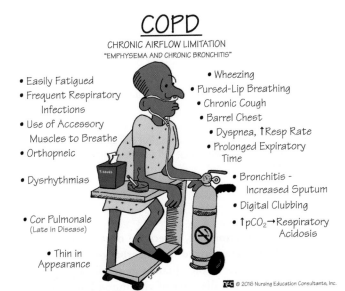

## COPD
### CHRONIC AIRFLOW LIMITATION
"EMPHYSEMA AND CHRONIC BRONCHITIS"

- Easily Fatigued
- Frequent Respiratory Infections
- Use of Accessory Muscles to Breathe
- Orthopneic
- Dysrhythmias
- Cor Pulmonale (Late in Disease)
- Thin in Appearance

- Wheezing
- Pursed-Lip Breathing
- Chronic Cough
- Barrel Chest
- Dyspnea, ↑Resp Rate
- Prolonged Expiratory Time
- Bronchitis - Increased Sputum
- Digital Clubbing
- ↑pCO$_2$→Respiratory Acidosis

© 2016 Nursing Education Consultants, Inc.

**FIGURE 17-7 Chronic Obstructive Pulmonary Disease.** (From Zerwekh, J., Garneau, A., & Miller, C. J. [2017]. *Digital collection of the memory notebooks of nursing* [4th ed.]. Chandler, AZ: Nursing Education Consultants, Inc.)

B. Diagnostics: see Appendix 17-1.
  1. Pulmonary function studies show increased residual volume (air trapping).
  2. ABGs (see Table 17-1).
     a. Changes in $Paco_2$: most often increased in bronchitis.
     b. Low $Pao_2$ more prominent in clients with bronchitis.
     c. Decompensated condition: decreased $Pao_2$, increased $Paco_2$, decreased pH—respiratory acidosis with hypoxia.
C. Complications.
  1. Cor pulmonale (right-side heart failure).
  2. Infections (pneumonia).
  3. Peptic ulcer and gastroesophageal reflux (GERD; see Chapter 20).
  4. Acute respiratory failure.

### Treatment

A. Prevention or treatment of respiratory tract infections.
B. Bronchodilators (see Appendix 17-2).
C. Mucolytics and expectorants (see Appendix 17-2).
D. Chest physiotherapy (suctioning, percussion, and postural drainage).
E. Breathing exercises, low-flow humidified $O_2$.
F. Exercise to maintain cardiovascular fitness; most common exercise is walking.
G. Corticosteroids (see Appendix 9-2).

> **NURSING PRIORITY:** Administer low-flow $O_2$ for clients with emphysema. High concentrations of $O_2$ would decrease the client's hypoxic drive and increase respiratory distress.

### Nursing Interventions

**Goal:** To improve ventilation.

A. Teach pursed-lip breathing: inhale through the nose and exhale against pursed lips.
B. Avoid activities increasing dyspnea.
C. Humidified $O_2$ (low flow via nasal cannula at a rate of 1–3 L/min) should be used when clients are experiencing exertional or resting hypoxemia.
  1. Monitor for hypercapnia, hypoxia, and acidosis.
  2. A significant increase in $Pao_2$ may decrease respiratory drive ($O_2$ toxicity).
  3. Administer $O_2$ via nasal cannula or Venturi mask (to deliver a more precise $Fio_2$).
  4. Assess for pressure ulcers on the nares with a nasal cannula and on the top of the client's ears where the elastic holds the mask.

> **NURSING PRIORITY:** Administer $O_2$ therapy and evaluate results; the risk for inducing hypoventilation should not prevent the administration of $O_2$ at low levels to the client with COPD who is experiencing respiratory distress.

D. Assess breath sounds before and after coughing.
E. Avoid cough suppressants.

F. Place client in high-Fowler's or sitting position.
G. Maintain adequate hydration to facilitate removal of secretions.

> **NURSING PRIORITY:** The optimal amount of $O_2$ is the concentration that reverses the hypoxemia without causing adverse effects.

**Goal:** To improve activity tolerance.

A. Balance activities and dyspnea: gradually increase activities; use portable $O_2$ tank when walking; avoid respiratory irritants.
B. Encourage pursed-lip and diaphragmatic breathing during exercise and as needed.
C. Schedule activities after respiratory therapy.
D. Assess for negative responses to activity.

**Goal:** To maintain adequate nutrition.

A. Soft, high-protein, high-calorie diet—especially for underweight clients with emphysema.
B. Postural drainage completed 30 minutes before meals or 3 hours after meals.
C. Good oral hygiene after postural drainage.
D. Small frequent meals; rest before and after meals.
E. Use a bronchodilator before meals.
F. Encourage at least 2000 to 3000 mL fluid daily unless contraindicated.

### Home Care

A. Encourage client and family to verbalize feelings about condition and lifelong restriction of activities.
B. Client teaching.
  1. Include client in active planning for home care.
  2. Instruct client regarding community resources.
  3. Instruct client regarding medication schedule and side effects of prescribed medications.
C. Recognize signs and symptoms of upper respiratory tract infection and know when to call physician.
D. Encourage activities such as walking—an increase in respiratory rate and shortness of breath will occur, but if respirations return to normal within 5 minutes of stopping activity, it is considered normal.

> **TEST ALERT:** Administer narcotics, tranquilizers, and sedatives with caution; instruct client about self-administration of prescribed medications.

### Asthma

**Asthma is an intermittent, reversible obstructive airway problem. It is characterized by exacerbations and remissions. Between attacks the client is generally asymptomatic. It is a common disorder of childhood but may also cause problems throughout adult life (Figure 17-9).**

A. A chronic inflammatory process producing bronchial wall edema and inflammation, increased mucus secretion, and smooth muscle contraction.

# ASTHMA
(Reactive Airway Disease)

**Triggers**
- Hypersensitivity
- URI
- Exercise
- Air Pollutants
- Respiratory Infections
- GERD

**Familial Tendency**

**Intermittent Reversible Airway Obstruction**

**Hypoxemia:**
Tachycardia
↑ Restlessness
Tachypnea

**Asthma Attack**
- Cough
- ↑ Mucus
- Shortness of Breath
- Chest Tightness
- Early - ↓Paco₂
- Late - ↑Paco₂
- Wheezing & Prolonged Expiration
- Retractions

**Emergency:**
If symptoms do not respond to usual treatment in 30 minutes, patient should seek medical attention.

**Status Asthmaticus**
Can be life threatening!

© 2016 Nursing Education Consultants, Inc.

**FIGURE 17-9 Asthma.** (From Zerwekh, J., Garneau, A., & Miller, C. J. [2017]. *Digital collection of the memory notebooks of nursing* [4th ed.]. Chandler, AZ: Nursing Education Consultants, Inc.)

B. Intermittent narrowing of the airway is caused by:
   1. Constriction of the smooth muscles of the bronchi and the bronchioles (bronchospasm).
   2. Excessive mucus production.
   3. Mucosal edema of the respiratory tract.
C. Constriction of the smooth muscle causes significant increase in airway resistance, thereby trapping air in the lungs.
D. Emotional factors are known to play an important role in precipitating childhood asthma attacks.
E. Exercise-induced asthma: initially after exercise there is an improvement in the respiratory status, followed by a significant decline; occurs in the majority of clients; may be worse in cold, dry air and better in warm, moist air.

## Assessment

A. Risk factors/etiology.
   1. Hypersensitivity (allergens) and airway inflammation.
   2. Exercise.
   3. Air pollutants and occupational factors.
   4. Pediatric implications.
      a. *Reactive airway disease* is the term used to describe asthma in children.
      b. General onset before age 3 years.
      c. Children are more likely to have airway obstruction.
B. Diagnostics (see Appendix 17-1).
   1. Pulmonary function studies/tests (PFTs).
   2. History of hypersensitivity reactions (history of eczema in children).
   3. Increased serum eosinophil count.
C. Clinical manifestations: *early-phase reactions* occur immediately and last about an hour; *late-phase reactions* do not begin until 4 to 8 hours after exposure and may last

for hours or as long as 2 days; attacks may begin gradually or abruptly.
   1. Episodic wheezing, chest tightness, shortness of breath, persistent cough.
   2. Use of accessory muscles in breathing, orthopnea.
   3. Symptoms of hypoxia (see Table 17-2); cyanosis occurs late.
   4. Increased anxiety, restlessness, diaphoresis.
   5. Difficulty speaking, thick tenacious sputum.

> **PEDIATRIC PRIORITY:** Children who are sweating profusely and refuse to lie down are more ill than children who lie quietly. Parents should seek immediate medical attention if a child does not respond to early treatment of an asthma attack.

D. Complications: status asthmaticus is severe asthma unresponsive to initial or conventional treatment.

## Treatment

A. Medications (see Appendix 17-2).
   1. Beta₂-adrenergic agonists (short-acting and long-acting) administered by nebulizer or metered-dose inhaler.
   2. Antibiotics, if infection is present.
   3. Bronchodilators, expectorants.
   4. Inhaled steroids and antiinflammatory drugs to prevent and/or decrease edema.
   5. Supplemental $O_2$ to maintain $Sao_2$ at 90%.
B. Status asthmaticus.
   1. Oxygen, IV fluids for hydration.
   2. May require intubation and mechanical ventilation (Appendix 17-8).
   3. IV bronchodilators and steroids.
C. Medications to avoid for the client with asthma.
   1. Beta-adrenergic blockers cause bronchoconstriction.
   2. Cough suppressants, antihistamines.

> **NURSING PRIORITY:** Using a spacer device allows more medication to reach its site of action in the lungs with less deposited in the mouth and throat.

## Nursing Interventions

See Hypoxia, Nursing Interventions.
**Goal:** To relieve asthma attacks.

A. Position for comfort: usually high-Fowler's position or tripod position.
B. Close monitoring of response to $O_2$ therapy: $Sao_2$ levels and changes in respiratory status.
C. Assess response to bronchodilators and aerosol therapy.
D. Carefully monitor ability to take PO fluids; risk for aspiration is increased.
E. Observe for sudden increase or decrease in restlessness; either may indicate an abrupt decrease in oxygenation.
F. Assess for side effects of medications, such as tremors and tachycardia.

> **NURSING PRIORITY:** Determine changes in a client's respiratory status: the *inability* to hear wheezing breath sounds in the client with asthma in acute respiratory distress may be an indication of impending respiratory obstruction.

### Home Care

A. Assess emotional factors precipitating asthma attacks.
B. Educate client and family regarding identifying and avoiding allergens.
C. Implement therapeutic measures before attack becomes severe.
D. Explain purposes of prescribed medications and how to use them correctly (see Appendix 17-2).
E. Administer bronchodilators before performing postural drainage.
F. Use bronchodilators and warm up before exercise to prevent exercise-induced asthma.
G. Encourage participation in "quiet" activities according to developmental level.

## Cystic Fibrosis

**Cystic fibrosis is a chromosomal abnormality characterized by a generalized dysfunction of the exocrine glands. The disease primarily affects the lungs, pancreas, and sweat glands.**

A. The factor responsible for the multiple clinical manifestations of the disease process is the mechanical obstruction caused by thick mucus secretions.
B. Effects of disease process.
   1. Pulmonary system: bronchial and bronchiolar obstruction by thick mucus, causing atelectasis and reduced area for gas exchange; the thick mucus provides an excellent medium for bacterial growth and secondary respiratory tract infections.
   2. Pancreas: decreased absorption of nutrients caused by the obstruction of pancreatic ducts and lack of adequate enzymes for digestion.
   3. Sweat glands: excretion of excess amounts of sodium and chloride.

### Assessment

A. Risk factors/etiology.
   1. Inherited as an autosomal recessive trait.
   2. Most common in Caucasians.
B. Clinical manifestations.
   1. Wide variation in severity and extent of manifestations, as well as period of onset.
   2. Gastrointestinal tract.
      a. May present with meconium ileus in the newborn.
      b. Increased bulk in feces from undigested foods.
      c. Increased fat in stools (steatorrhea); foul smelling.
      d. Decreased absorption of nutrients: weight loss or failure to thrive.
      e. Increased appetite caused by decreased absorption of nutrients.
      f. Abdominal distention.
      g. Rectal prolapse related to the large bulky stools and loss of supportive tissue around rectum.
      h. Vitamin A, D, E, and K deficiency.
   3. Genital tract.
      a. In females the increased viscosity of cervical mucus may lead to decreased fertility due to blockage of sperm.
      b. Males are generally sterile because of absence or obstruction of the vas deferens.
   4. Respiratory tract.
      a. Evidence of respiratory tract involvement generally occurs in early childhood.
      b. Increasing dyspnea, tachypnea.
      c. Paroxysmal, chronic productive cough.
      d. Pulmonary inflammation: chronic bronchiolitis and bronchitis.
      e. Symptoms of chronic hypoxia: clubbing, barrel chest.
      f. Mucus provides excellent medium for bacteria growth and chronic infections.
   5. Excessive salt on the skin: "salty taste when kissed."
C. Diagnostics (see Appendix 17-1).
   1. Sweat chloride test: normal chloride concentration range is less than 40 mEq/L (mmol/L), with a mean of 18 mEq/L (mmol/L); chloride concentration 40 to 60 mEq/L (mmol/L) is suggestive of a diagnosis of cystic fibrosis.
   2. Pancreatic enzymes: decrease or absence of trypsin and chymotrypsin.
   3. Fat absorption in intestines is impaired.
D. Complications.
   1. Frequent pulmonary infections, pneumothorax.
   2. Diabetes secondary to destruction of pancreatic tissue.
   3. Cor pulmonale and respiratory failure are late complications.
   4. Gastroesophageal reflux disease (GERD).

### Treatment

Child is usually cared for at home unless complications are present.

A. Diet: balanced, high-calorie, high-protein, fats as tolerated, increased salt intake.
B. Fat-soluble vitamins A, D, E, and K in water-soluble forms.
C. Pancreatic enzyme replacement with meals (see Appendix 15-2).
D. Antibiotics are given prophylactically and when there is evidence of infection; tobramycin.
E. Pulmonary therapy.
   1. Physical therapy: postural drainage, breathing exercises.
   2. Aerosol therapy and chest physiotherapy (CPT).
   3. Percussion and vibration.
   4. Expectorants (see Appendix 17-2).

### Nursing Interventions

**Goal:** To promote optimum home care for child (see Chapter 2 for care of chronically ill child).

A. Identify community resources for family.
B. Assist family to identify problems and solutions congruent with their lifestyle.
C. Encourage verbalization regarding effect of child's problem on the family and the family's ability to cope with the child at home.

D. When appropriate, teach child about disease and treatment and encourage active participation in planning of care.

E. Assist parents to identify activities to promote normal growth and development.

**Goal:** To maintain nutrition.

A. Minimum restriction of fats; need to increase intake of pancreatic enzyme with increased fat intake.

B. Pancreatic enzymes with meals and snacks.

C. Vitamins A, D, E, and K in water-soluble form.

D. Good oral hygiene after postural drainage.

E. Postural drainage 1 to 2 hours before meals or 3 hours after meals.

**Goal:** To prevent or minimize pulmonary complications.

A. Assist child to mobilize secretions.
   1. CPT: postural drainage, breathing exercises, nebulization treatments.
   2. Encourage active exercises appropriate to child's capacity and developmental level.

B. Prevent respiratory tract infections.

C. Prevent pneumothorax: no power lifting, intensive isometric exercises, scuba diving.

## Cancer of the Upper Airway

**Oral/pharyngeal cancer is uncontrollable growth of malignant cells invading and causing damage to areas around the mouth, including the lips, cheeks, gums, tongue, soft and hard palate, the floor of the mouth, tonsils, sinuses, and even the pharynx.**

Cancer of the larynx may involve the vocal cords or other areas of the larynx. The majority of lesions are squamous cell carcinomas and slow growing. If detected early, this type of cancer is curable by surgical resection of the lesion.

### Assessment

A. Risk factors/etiology.
   1. More common in older adult men.
   2. History of tobacco and alcohol use.

B. Clinical manifestations of oral cancer.
   1. Leukoplakia: whitish elevated patch on oral mucosa or tongue (premalignant lesion).
   2. Erythroplasia (erythroplakia): a red velvety patch on the mouth or tongue (premalignant lesion).
   3. A sore in the mouth that bleeds and does not heal.
   4. A lump or thickening in the cheek.
   5. Difficulty chewing or swallowing.

C. Clinical manifestations of laryngeal cancer (may be asymptomatic).
   1. Early changes.
      a. Voice changes, hoarseness, oral leukoplakia.
      b. Persistent unilateral sore throat, difficulty swallowing.
      c. Feeling of foreign body in throat.
   2. Late changes.
      a. Pain.
      b. Dysphagia and decreased tongue mobility.
      c. Airway compromise.

D. Diagnostics: direct laryngoscopic examination with biopsy.

### Treatment

Varies with the extent of the malignancy.

A. Radiation: brachytherapy—placing a radioactive source into or near the area of the tumor; may also be used with external radiation treatments (see Chapter 11).

B. Surgical intervention.
   1. Partial laryngectomy: preserves the normal airway and normal speech mechanism; if a tracheotomy is performed, it is removed after the risk for swelling and airway obstruction has subsided.
   2. Radical neck dissection or total laryngectomy, involves resection of the trachea, a permanent tracheotomy for breathing, and an alternative method of speaking (Figure 17-10).
   3. Depending on location of oral lesions, a glossectomy (removal of the tongue) and/or mandibulectomy (removal of mandible) may be performed; cancers of the oral cavity metastasize early to cervical lymph nodes.

### Complications

A. Airway obstruction.

B. Hemorrhage.

C. Fistula formation.

### Nursing Interventions

**Goal:** To prevent oral and laryngeal cancer.

A. Avoid chemical, physical, or thermal trauma to the mouth.

B. Maintain good oral hygiene: regular brushing and flossing.

C. Prevent constant irritation in the mouth; repair dentures or other dental problems.

D. See a doctor for any oral lesion that does not heal in 2 to 3 weeks.

**Goal:** To prepare client for surgery.

A. General preoperative preparation (see Chapter 3).

B. Consult with surgeon as to the anticipated extent of the surgery; determine how airway and nutritional needs will be addressed.

C. Discuss with client the possibility of a temporary tracheotomy or, if anticipated, a permanent tracheotomy.

D. Encourage venting of feelings regarding a temporary or permanent loss of voice after surgery and alteration in physical appearance.

E. If total laryngectomy is anticipated, schedule a visit from the speech pathologist or member of the laryngectomy club to reassure client of rehabilitation potential.

F. Establish a method of communication for immediate postoperative period.

G. Discuss nutritional considerations after surgery.

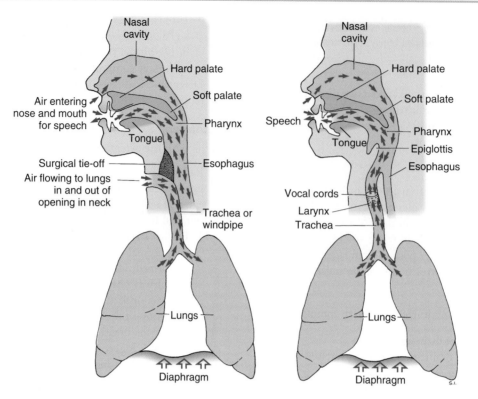

**FIGURE 17-10 Normal Airflow in and out of Lungs (Left) and Airflow in and out of the Lungs After Total Laryngectomy (Right).** Clients using esophageal speech trap air in the esophagus and release it to create sound. (From deWit, S., Stromberg, H., & Dallred, C. [2017]. *Medical-surgical nursing: Concepts and practice* [3rd ed.]. St. Louis, MO: Elsevier.)

**Goal:** To maintain patent airway after laryngectomy.

A. If tracheotomy is not performed, evaluate for hematoma and increasing edema of the incisional area precipitating respiratory distress.
B. Place in semi-Fowler's position.
C. Administer humidified $O_2$ therapy.
D. Closely monitor for respiratory compromise (hypoxia).
E. Monitor vital signs for hemorrhage.
F. Avoid analgesics that depress respiration.
G. Promote good pulmonary hygiene.
H. If tracheostomy is present, suction as indicated (see Appendix 17-6).

**Goal:** To maintain airway; to prevent complications after tracheotomy (see Appendix 17-5).
**Goal:** To promote nutrition postoperatively.

A. Method of nutritional intake depends on the extent of the surgical procedure (see Appendix 20-5 for tube feedings).
B. IV fluids for first 24 hours.
C. Gastrostomy, nasogastric, or nasointestinal tubes may be placed during surgery and used until edema has subsided.
D. Provide good oral hygiene; may need to suction oral cavity if client cannot swallow.
E. Evaluate tolerance of tube feedings; treat nausea quickly to prevent vomiting (see Appendix 20-5).

F. Closely observe for swallowing difficulty with initial oral feedings.
1. Bland, nonirritating foods.
2. Thicker foods allow more control over swallowing; thin, watery foods should be avoided.
G. For a partial laryngectomy, the possibility of aspiration is a primary concern during the first few days after surgery.

**TEST ALERT:** Identify clients at high risk for aspiration.

**Goal:** To promote wound healing.

A. Assess pressure dressings and presence of edema formation.
B. Monitor wound suction devices (Hemovac, Jackson-Pratt); drainage should be serosanguineous.
C. Monitor patency of drainage tubes every 3 to 4 hours; fluid should gradually decrease.
D. If skin flaps were used, the wound is often left uncovered for better visualization of flap and to prevent pressure on area.
E. When drainage tubes are removed, carefully observe area for increased swelling.
F. Type of oral hygiene is indicated by the extent of the procedure.
1. Mouth irrigations.
2. Soothing mouth rinses (cool normal saline or nonirritating antiseptic solutions).

3. If dentures are present, clean mouth well before replacing.
4. Oral hygiene before and after oral intake.
5. Avoid using stiff toothbrushes and metal-tipped suction catheters.

**Goal:** To identify resources for speech rehabilitation after laryngectomy.

A. If a partial laryngectomy was done, client should have gradual improvement in voice; client is generally allowed to begin whispering 2 to 3 days after surgery.
B. Follow-up visit from laryngectomy club member.
C. Arrange counseling with speech pathologist.
D. Identify different methods for speech management: esophageal speech, electric/artificial larynx, or tracheo-esophageal puncture (closest to normal speech).

### Home Care

A. Encourage client to begin own suctioning and caring for the tracheostomy before he or she leaves the hospital.
B. Assist the family in obtaining equipment for home use.
   1. System for humidification of air in home environment.
   2. Suction and equipment necessary for tracheostomy care.
C. Care of stoma.
   1. No swimming.
   2. Wear plastic collar over stoma while showering.
   3. Maintain high humidification at night to increase moisture in airway.
   4. Avoid use of aerosol sprays.
D. Nutritional considerations: client cannot smell; taste will also be affected.
E. Infection.
F. Increased secretions.
G. Client should carry appropriate medical identification.
H. Encourage client to put arm and shoulder on affected side through range-of-motion exercises to prevent functional disabilities of the shoulder and neck.

### Cancer of the Lung

**Cancer of the lung is a tumor arising from within the lung. It may represent the primary site or may be a metastatic site from a primary lesion elsewhere.**

#### Assessment

A. Risk factors.
   1. Smoking, including passive smoking.
   2. Occupational exposure to and/or inhalation of carcinogens.
B. Clinical manifestations: nonspecific; appear late in disease.
   1. Persistent chronic cough.
   2. Cough initially nonproductive; then may become productive of purulent and/or blood tinged.
   3. Dyspnea and wheezing with bronchial obstruction.
   4. Recurring fever.
   5. Common sites of metastasis.
      a. Liver, bones, brain, pancreas.
      b. Lymph nodes: mediastinum.
   6. Pain is a late manifestation.
   7. Paraneoplastic syndrome: hormone changes, skin changes, neuromuscular and vascular changes; symptoms are controlled with successful treatment of cancer.
C. Diagnostics: bronchoscopy with biopsy.

#### Treatment

Varies with the extent of the malignancy.
A. Radiation: may be used preoperatively to reduce tumor mass.
B. Surgery: treatment of choice early in condition.
   1. Lobectomy: removal of one lobe of the lung.
   2. Pneumonectomy: removal of the entire lung.
   3. Lung-conserving resection: removal of a small area (wedge) or a segment of the lung.
C. Chemotherapy (see Chapter 11).
D. Treatment may involve all three therapies.

#### Nursing Interventions

**Goal:** To prepare client for surgery.

A. General preoperative preparations (see Chapter 3).
B. Improve quality of ventilation before surgery.
   1. No smoking.
   2. Bronchodilators.
   3. Good pulmonary hygiene.
C. Discuss anticipated activities in the immediate postoperative period.
D. Encourage venting of feelings regarding diagnosis and impending surgery.
E. Establish baseline data for comparison after surgery.
F. Orient client to the intensive care unit, if indicated.

**Goal:** To maintain patent airway and promote ventilation after thoracotomy.

A. Removal of secretions from tracheobronchial tree, either by coughing or suctioning.
B. Have client cough frequently, deep breathe, and use incentive spirometer.
C. Assess vital signs; correlate with quality of respirations.
D. Provide supplemental $O_2$ as indicated.
E. Control pain so that client can take deep breaths and cough.
F. Do not position the client who has undergone a wedge resection or lobe resection on the affected side for extended periods of time; this will hinder the expansion of the lung remaining on that side. If client is in stable condition, place in semi-Fowler's position to promote optimal ventilation.

**NURSING PRIORITY:** Postoperative positioning of the client who has had thoracic surgery is important to remember, especially the client who has undergone pneumonectomy.

G. If the client who has undergone pneumonectomy experiences increased dyspnea, place him or her in semi-Fowler's position. If tolerated, positioning on the operative side is recommended to facilitate full expansion of lung on unaffected side.

H. Encourage ambulation as soon as possible.

I. Assess level of dyspnea at rest and with activity.

J. Maintain water-sealed drainage system (see Appendix 17-4). The client who has undergone pneumonectomy will not have chest tubes for lung reexpansion because there is no lung left in the pleural cavity, but chest tubes may be used for fluid drainage.

**Goal:** To assess and support cardiac function after thoracotomy.

A. Monitor for dysrhythmias; assess adequacy of cardiac output.

B. Evaluate urine output.

C. Administer fluids and transfusions with extreme caution; client's condition is very conducive to development of fluid overload.

D. Evaluate hydration and electrolyte status.

**Goal:** To maintain normal range of motion and function of the affected shoulder after thoracotomy.

A. Exercises to increase abduction and mobility of the shoulders.

B. Encourage progressive exercises.

**Goal:** To assist client to understand measures to promote health after thoracotomy.

A. No more smoking; avoid respiratory irritants.

B. Decreased strength is common.

C. Continue activities and exercises.

D. Stop any activity that causes shortness of breath, chest pain, or undue fatigue.

E. Avoid lifting heavy objects until complete healing has occurred.

F. Return for follow-up care as indicated.

## CRITICAL CARE

### PRIORITY CONCEPTS

Gas Exchange, Pain, Perfusion

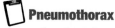 **Pneumothorax**

**Air in the pleural space results in the collapse or atelectasis of that portion of the lung. This condition is known as pneumothorax (Figure 17-11).**

A. Tension pneumothorax: the development of a pneumothorax that allows excessive buildup of pressure (due to air that cannot escape) in the pleural space, causing a shift in the mediastinum toward the unaffected side.

> **⚠ NURSING PRIORITY:** A tension pneumothorax can rapidly become an emergency situation. It is much easier to treat the client if the pneumothorax is identified *before* it begins to exert tension on the mediastinal area.

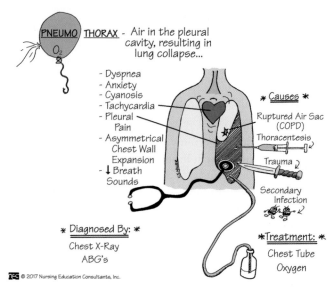

**FIGURE 17-11 Pneumothorax.** (From Zerwekh, J., Garneau, A., & Miller, C. J. [2017]. *Digital collection of the memory notebooks of nursing* [4th ed.]. Chandler, AZ: Nursing Education Consultants, Inc.)

### Assessment

A. Risk factors/etiology.
 1. Ruptured bleb (spontaneous).
 2. Thoracentesis.
 3. Infection.
 4. Trauma (penetrating or blunt chest injury).

B. Clinical manifestations.
 1. Diminished or absent breath sounds on the affected side.
 2. Dyspnea, hypoxia, tachycardia, tachypnea.
 3. Sudden onset of persistent chest pain, pain on affected side when breathing.
 4. Increasing anxiety.
 5. Asymmetric chest wall expansion.
 6. Hyperresonance on percussion of affected side.
 7. Possible development of a tension pneumothorax.
  a. Decreased cardiac filling, leading to decreased cardiac output.
  b. Tracheal shift from midline toward unaffected side.
  c. Increasing problems of hypoxia.

C. Diagnostics (see Appendix 17-1).

> **⚠ NURSING PRIORITY:** When atmospheric pressure is allowed to disrupt the negative pressure in the pleural space, it will cause the lung to collapse. This requires chest tube placement to reestablish negative pressure and reinflate the lung.

### Treatment

Placement of chest tubes connected to a water-sealed drainage system (see Appendix 17-4).

### Nursing Interventions

**Goal:** To recognize the problem and prevent a severe hypoxic episode (see Hypoxia, Nursing Interventions).

A. Begin $O_2$ therapy.

B. Place in semi-Fowler's position.
C. Notify physician and prepare client for insertion of chest tubes.

**Goal:** To reinflate lung without complications.

A. Have client cough and deep breathe every 2 hours.
B. Encourage exercise and ambulation.
C. Establish and maintain water-sealed chest drainage system (see Appendix 17-4).

## Open Chest Wound

**An open or "sucking" chest wound is frequently caused by a penetrating injury to the chest, such as a gunshot or knife wound. If a chest tube is inadvertently pulled out of the chest, a sucking chest wound may be created.**

### Assessment

A. Clinical manifestations.
1. Increase in dyspnea.
2. A chest wound with evidence of air moving in and out via the wound.

### Treatment

A. Have the client take a deep breath, hold it, and bear down against a closed glottis. Apply a light occlusive, vented dressing (taped/secured on three sides to allow air to escape) over the wound.

> **NURSING PRIORITY:** Immediately occlude the chest wound; do not leave the client to go find a dressing. If necessary, place a towel or whatever is at hand over the wound to stop the flow of air.

B. Prepare for insertion of chest tubes to water-sealed drainage system.
C. After covering the wound with a light occlusive dressing, carefully evaluate the client for development of a tension pneumothorax.

### Nursing Interventions

**Goal:** To prevent problems of hypoxia.
**Goal:** To assess for development of tension pneumothorax.

## Flail Chest

**Flail chest is the loss of stability of the chest wall with respiratory impairment as a result of multiple rib fractures (fractures at two or more points of the ribs involved).**

### Assessment

D. Clinical manifestations.
1. Paradoxical respirations: the movement of the fractured area (flailed segment) inward during inspiration and outward during expiration or opposite to the other areas of the chest wall.
2. Symptoms of hypoxia.
E. Diagnostics.
1. Chest x-ray film showing multiple rib fractures.
2. Crepitus over the ribs.

### Treatment

A. Maintain patent airway.
B. Adequate pain medication to enable client to breathe deeply.
C. $O_2$.
D. Endotracheal intubation with mechanical ventilation for severe respiratory distress (see Appendixes 17-5 and 17-8).
E. Chest tube placement if pneumothorax occurs as a result of puncture of the lung by the fractured rib.

> **TEST ALERT:** Determine changes in client's respiratory status.

### Nursing Interventions

**Goal:** To stabilize the chest wall and prevent complications.

A. Prepare client for endotracheal intubation and mechanical ventilation (see Appendixes 17-5 and 17-8).
B. Assess for symptoms of hypoxia.
C. Assess for symptoms of pneumothorax.

## Pulmonary Embolism

**A pulmonary embolism (PE) is an obstruction of a pulmonary artery, most often the result of an embolism caused by a blood clot (thrombus), air, fat, amniotic fluid, bone marrow, or sepsis. The severity of the problem depends on the size of the embolus.**

A. Of the clients that die of PE, the majority die because of failure to diagnose.
B. The majority of pulmonary emboli arise from thrombi in the deep veins of the legs.
C. A pulmonary embolism must originate from the venous circulation, or the right side of the heart.

### Assessment

A. Common risk factors/etiology.
1. Conditions or immobility predisposing to venous stasis and/or deep vein thrombosis: surgery within the past 3 months, stroke, spinal cord injury, and history of deep vein thrombosis (DVT), obesity, and advancing age.
2. Vascular injury: central venous catheters, thrombophlebitis, vascular disease, leg fractures.
3. DVT: the thrombus spontaneously dislodges secondary to jarring (turbulence) of the area—sudden standing, changes in rate of blood flow (Valsalva maneuver, increased blood pressure).
4. Hypercoagulability of blood.
B. Clinical manifestations.
1. Classic triad of symptoms: dyspnea, chest pain, and hemoptysis occur in only 20% of clients.
2. Other common symptoms.
a. Increased anxiety, cough.
b. Sudden, unexplained dyspnea, tachypnea.
c. Hypotension, tachycardia, syncope.
3. May result in sudden death if pulmonary embolism is large.

C. Diagnostics (see Appendix 17-1).
 1. Pulmonary angiography
 2. Enhanced spiral computed tomography (CT) scan (specific for PE).
 3. D-dimer test is elevated (greater than 250 mcg/L [1369 nmol/L]).
 4. Ventilation-perfusion scan (V/Q) is done for patients who cannot have contrast media.
 5. ABGs (establishes a baseline. Useful if client is high risk for PE).

## Treatment

A. Bed rest, high-Fowler's position if blood pressure permits.
B. Respiratory support: $O_2$, intubation if necessary, ventilator, etc.
C. Anticoagulants (heparin, low-molecular-weight heparin, or warfarin) to prevent further thrombus formation.
D. IV access for fluids and medications to maintain blood pressure.
E. Small doses of morphine sulfate may be used to decrease anxiety, alleviate chest pain, or improve tolerance to endotracheal tube.
F. Thrombolytics if unstable and PE confirmed.
G. Embolectomy or insertion of inferior vena cava filter.

**TEST ALERT:** Assess clients for complications caused by immobility. Immobilized clients have an increased risk for development of a pulmonary embolism. Questions require an understanding of principles for prevention of thrombophlebitis and subsequent embolism formation. It is far easier to prevent the problem than it is to treat the pulmonary embolism.

## Nursing Interventions

**Goal:** To identify clients at increased risk and prevent and/or decrease venous stasis (see Box 18-3).

**Goal:** To identify problem and implement nursing measures to alleviate hypoxia (see Hypoxia, Nursing Interventions).

**Goal:** To monitor client's respiratory function and response to treatment.

## Acute Respiratory Distress Syndrome (Adult Respiratory Distress Syndrome)

**Acute respiratory distress syndrome (ARDS) or noncardiogenic pulmonary edema, also referred to as shock lung and white lung, is a condition characterized by increased capillary permeability in the alveolar capillary membrane, resulting in fluid leaking into the interstitial spaces and the alveoli and a decrease in pulmonary compliance.**

## Assessment

A. Risk factors/etiology.
 1. Clients with multiple risk factors are more likely to develop ARDS.
 2. Risk factors.
  a. Direct lung injury: aspiration, pneumonia, chest trauma, embolism, inhalation injury.
  b. Indirect lung injury: sepsis (most common), severe massive trauma, acute pancreatitis, anaphylaxis, shock.
B. Clinical manifestations.
 1. Restlessness, confusion, tachypnea, and dyspnea.
 2. Refractory hypoxemia (increasing hypoxia not responding to increased levels of fraction of inspired $O_2$ [$Fio_2$]; see Table 17-2).
 3. Tachycardia, adventitious lung sounds, diaphoresis.
 4. Profound respiratory distress and use of accessory muscles.
 5. Cyanosis or mottling.
C. Diagnostics: chest x-ray, ABGs, and may include CT examination (see Appendix 17-1).

**❗ NURSING PRIORITY:** It is essential to closely monitor the ABGs in a client with ARDS. A decreasing $Pao_2$ and increasing difficulty breathing are indications that the client's condition is deteriorating.

## Treatment

Care is generally provided in an intensive care setting.

A. Maintain oxygenation.
 1. Endotracheal intubation and mechanical ventilation.
 2. Positive end-expiratory pressure (PEEP): used to decrease the effects of intrapulmonary shunting and to improve pulmonary compliance.
 3. Alternative ventilation strategies may include airway pressure-release ventilation (APRV) and high-frequency oscillatory (HFO) ventilation.
B. Hemodynamic pressure monitoring for evidence of cardiac failure (see Appendix 19-5).
C. Treatment of underlying condition.
D. Nutritional support: requires increased calories to meet metabolic demand.

**TEST ALERT:** Monitor client's gas exchange; increasing levels of $CO_2$ are generally not a problem with the client with ARDS; the problem exists with the diffusion of $O_2$ and the availability of the $O_2$ to the circulating hemoglobin.

## Nursing Interventions

**Goal:** To maintain airway patency and improve ventilation.

A. Frequent assessment for increasing respiratory difficulty; anticipate intubation or tracheotomy (see Appendix 17-5).
B. Endotracheal tube or tracheotomy suctioning.
C. Evaluate ABG reports, constant monitoring of $Sao_2$.
D. Sedation and paralytic agents are required for patients to tolerate alternative modes of ventilation (see Appendix 17-8).
E. Monitor hemoglobin levels and $Pao_2$ saturation levels.
F. Positioning (prone to assist with redistribution of blood flow to less damaged areas of the lungs).

**Goal:** To maintain fluid balance.

A. Fluid balance maintained with IV hydration; avoid fluid volume overload.
B. Evaluate serum electrolyte levels.
C. Strict intake and output, daily weights.

**Goal:** To assess and maintain cardiac output.

A. Assess for dysrhythmias, especially tachydysrhythmias.
B. Correlate vital signs with other assessment changes.
C. Evaluate cardiac output in relation to fluid intake.
D. Evaluate cardiac output when PEEP is initiated because it will compromise venous return (decreased preload).

**Goal:** To provide emotional support to client and family.

A. Careful repeated explanation of procedures to client and to family.
B. Calm, gentle approach to decrease anxiety.
C. Be available to family at visiting times to explain procedures and equipment.
D. If endotracheal tube or tracheotomy is in place, explain to family and client that speech is only temporarily interrupted.
E. Assist client to maintain communication.

## Pulmonary Edema

**Pulmonary edema or acute decompensated heart failure (ADHF) is caused by an abnormal accumulation of fluid in the lung in both the interstitial and alveolar spaces.**

A. Origin is most often cardiac: pulmonary congestion occurs when the pulmonary vascular bed receives more blood from the right side of the heart (venous return) than the left side of the heart (cardiac output) can accommodate.
B. Pulmonary edema results from severe impairment in the ability of the left side of the heart to maintain cardiac output, thereby causing an engorgement of the pulmonary vascular bed.

### Assessment

A. Risk factors/etiology.
  1. Alteration in capillary permeability (inhaled toxins, pneumonia, severe hypoxia).
  2. Cardiac myopathy, cardiac failure, overhydration.
B. Clinical manifestations: hypoxia (see Table 17-2).
  1. Decreasing $Pao_2$, dyspnea, tachypnea.
  2. Severe anxiety, restlessness, irritability, confusion.
  3. Cool, moist skin.
  4. Tachycardia, $S_3$, $S_4$ gallop, dependent edema.
  5. Severe coughing productive of frothy, blood-tinged sputum.
  6. Noisy, wet breath sounds that do not clear with coughing.

> **❗ OLDER ADULT PRIORITY:** Pulmonary edema can occur rapidly and become a medical emergency.

C. Diagnostics: B-type natriuretic peptide (BNP) levels measured to assess for heart failure (HF) (less than 100 pg/mL [ng/L] rules out HF).

### Treatment

Condition demands immediate attention; medications are administered intravenously.

A. $O_2$.
  1. $O_2$ in high concentration.
  2. Intubation and mechanical ventilation.
  3. Use of bilevel positive airway pressure (BiPAP).
B. Sedation (morphine) or muscle paralyzing agents to allow controlled ventilation: decreases preload/vasoconstriction, as well as decreasing anxiety and pain.
C. Diuretics to reduce the cardiac preload.
D. Dopamine/dobutamine to facilitate myocardial contractility.
E. Medications to increase cardiac contractility and cardiac output (see Appendix 17-2).
F. Vasodilators to decrease afterload.

### Nursing Interventions

**Goal:** To assess and decrease hypoxia (see Hypoxia, Nursing Interventions; also Table 17-2).

**Goal:** To improve ventilation.

A. Place in high-Fowler's position with legs dependent.
B. Administer high levels of $O_2$.
C. Evaluate level of hypoxia and dyspnea; may need endotracheal tube intubation and mechanical ventilation.
D. Problem may occur at night, especially in clients who are on bed rest.
E. IV sedatives/narcotics.
  1. To decrease anxiety and dyspnea and to decrease pressure in pulmonary capillary bed.
  2. Closely observe for respiratory depression.
  3. Administer a sedative to decrease anxiety if client has received a muscle-paralyzing agent.
  4. May be used to assist client to tolerate ventilator.

> **❗ NURSING PRIORITY:** Pulmonary edema is one of the few circumstances in which a client with respiratory distress may be given a narcotic. The fear of not being able to breathe is so strong that the client cannot cooperate. When a sedative/narcotic is administered, the nurse must be ready to support ventilation if respirations become severely depressed.

F. Administer bronchodilators and evaluate client's response and common side effects.
G. Closely monitor vital signs, pulse oximetry, hemodynamic changes, and cardiac dysrhythmias.

**Goal:** To reduce circulating volume (preload) and cardiac workload (afterload).

A. Diuretics (see Appendix 18-2).
B. Medications to decrease afterload and increase cardiac output (see Appendix 19-2).
C. Carefully monitor all IV fluids and evaluate tolerance of hydration status.
D. Maintain client in semi- to high-Fowler's position, but allow legs to remain dependent.

**Goal:** To provide psychological support and decrease anxiety.

A. Approach client in a calm manner.
B. Explain procedures.
C. Administer sedatives cautiously.
D. Remain with client in acute respiratory distress.

**Goal:** To prevent recurrence of problem.

A. Recognize early stages.
B. Maintain client in semi-Fowler's position.
C. Decrease levels of activity.
D. Use extreme caution in administration of fluids and transfusions.

---

### Appendix 17-1  PULMONARY DIAGNOSTICS

## X-Ray Studies

### Chest X-Ray Film

An x-ray film of the lungs and chest wall; no specific care is required before or after x-ray study.

### Bronchoscopy

Provides for direct visualization of larynx, trachea, and bronchi; client generally receives nothing by mouth (NPO status) for 6 hours before the examination; preoperative medication is given, and the client's upper airway is anesthetized topically.

#### Nursing Implications

1. After the examination, evaluate the client for return of gag reflex. Maintain client's NPO status until return of gag reflex.
2. Bronchial biopsy may be done to obtain cells for cytologic examination; observe client for development of pneumothorax or frank bleeding.

### Pulmonary Angiography

Contrast material (dye) is injected into the pulmonary arteries; the angiography permits visualization of the pulmonary vasculature; definitive diagnosis for pulmonary emboli.

#### Nursing Implications

1. Client should be well hydrated before procedure.
2. Increase fluid intake postprocedure to flush out the dye.
3. Check puncture site for bleeding, hematoma, or infection.

*Contraindications:* (1) dye or shellfish allergies, (2) unstable condition, (3) uncooperative client, (4) pregnancy, (5) bleeding disorders.

### Magnetic Resonance Imaging (MRI)

See Appendix 22-1.

### Computerized Tomography (CT Scan)

See Appendix 22-1.

## Pathology: Laboratory Studies

### Sputum Studies (see also Appendix 17-9)

Sputum specimen should come from deep in the lungs and not be contaminated with excessive amounts of saliva. It is best obtained in the morning upon arising; instruct client to rinse mouth out with water before collection to decrease contamination.

*Culture and Sensitivity Test:* Performed to determine presence of pathogenic bacteria and to determine which antibiotic the specific organism is sensitive to. Should be done before antimicrobial therapy is started.

*Acid-Fast Bacilli:* Sputum collection and analysis when tuberculosis (TB) is suspected; morning sputum may contain a higher concentration of organisms.

*Cytologic Examination:* Tumors in pulmonary system may slough cells into the sputum.

## Blood Work

*D-dimer:* Blood test to identify degradation of fibrin; degradation products not commonly found in healthy clients. Elevated in thromboembolism and in DIC. Normal is less than 0.4 mcg/mL.

## Pulmonary Function Studies

Studies may be done (1) to evaluate pulmonary function before surgery, (2) to evaluate response to bronchodilator therapy, (3) to differentiate diagnosis of pulmonary disease, and (4) to determine the cause of dyspnea.

Client must be alert and cooperative; client should not be sedated. Study is done in the pulmonary function laboratory; client directed to breathe into a cylinder from which a computer interprets and records data in specific values. Client should not smoke or use bronchodilating medications for 6 hours before the test.

## Pulse Oximetry

Measurement is made by placing a sensor on the finger or earlobe; a beam of light passes through the tissue and measures the amount of oxygen-saturated hemoglobin. If probe is placed on the finger, any nail polish should be removed. It provides a method for continuously evaluating the oxygen saturation levels ($SpO_2$). It is noninvasive, and there are no pre- or postoximetry preparations. Readings may be incorrect if severe vasoconstriction has occurred or if $PaO_2$ is less than 70%. Normal range is 95% or higher.

#### Nursing Implications

1. Pulse oximetry should be used:
   a. For the client who is on supplemental oxygen and is at increased risk for desaturation.
   b. For the chronically ill client who has a tracheotomy or is on mechanical ventilation for chronic respiratory problems.
   c. For the client who has a critical or unstable airway.
2. Pulse oximetry is not recommended to monitor oxygen saturation:
   a. For clients experiencing problems with hypovolemia or decreased blood flow to extremities.
   b. To evaluate respiratory status when ventilator changes are made.
   c. To monitor progress of client on high levels of oxygen.
   d. During cardiopulmonary resuscitation.

## Arterial Blood Gas Studies

ABGs are a measurement of the pH and partial pressures of dissolved gases (oxygen, carbon dioxide) of the arterial blood; it requires at least 0.6 mL of arterial blood obtained through an arterial puncture. If client's oxygen concentration or ventilatory settings have been changed or if a client has been suctioned, blood should not be drawn for at least 30 minutes (see Table 17-1). Perform Allen's test to assess collateral circulation before arterial puncture. Pressure should be maintained at the puncture site for a minimum

## Appendix 17-1 PULMONARY DIAGNOSTICS—cont'd

of 5 minutes. The arterial blood sample should be tightly sealed and placed on ice and taken to the laboratory immediately.

*Allen's Test:* Hold client's hand, palm up. While occluding both the radial and ulnar arteries, have the client clench and unclench his or her hand several times; the hand will become pale. While continuing to apply pressure to the radial artery, release pressure on ulnar artery. Brisk color return (5 to 7 seconds) to the hand should occur with the radial artery still occluded. If color does not return, then ulnar artery does not provide adequate blood flow, and cannulation or puncture of radial artery should not be done.

### Thoracentesis

Withdrawal of fluid from the pleural cavity/space; used for diagnostic and therapeutic purposes.

#### Nursing Implications

1. Explain procedure to client.
2. Position client.
   a. Preferably, client should sit upright on the side of the bed with the arms and head over the bedside table.
   b. If client is unable to assume sitting position, place on affected side with the head of the bed slightly elevated. Area containing fluid collection should be dependent.
   c. If client has a malignancy, cytotoxic drugs may be infused into the pleural space.
3. Support and reassure the client during the procedure.
4. After the procedure, position the client on his or her side with puncture side up (or in semi-Fowler's position). Monitor respiratory status and breath sounds for possible pneumothorax, and assess puncture site.

### Mantoux Skin Test (Tuberculin Test)

Mantoux test, or purified protein derivative (PPD) test, is a method of tuberculin skin testing. PPD is injected intradermally in the forearm. Results are read in 48 to 72 hours. A positive reaction means the individual has been exposed to *Mycobacterium tuberculosis* recently or in the past and has developed antibodies (sensitized). It does not differentiate between active or latent infection. It may take 2 to 12 weeks after exposure for sensitivity and a positive skin test reaction to develop.

#### Nursing Implications

1. Intradermal injection: A small (25-gauge) needle is used to inject 0.1 mL of PPD under the skin. The needle is inserted bevel up; a raised area or "wheal" (6 to 10 mm) will form under the skin. To avoid a false negative, a wheal needs to form.
2. The most common area for injection is the inside surface of the forearm.
3. Do not aspirate; do not massage area.
4. The client should be given specific directions to return, or plans should be made to read the test in 48 to 72 hours.
5. Interpretation: The area of induration (only the part of the reaction that can be felt; induration may not be visible) is measured, not the area of erythema or inflammation.
   a. An induration of 5 mm or more is a positive reaction in immunosuppressed clients who have been recently exposed to active TB.
   b. An induration of 10 mm is a positive reaction for all nonimmunocompromised persons.
   c. An induration of 15 mm is a positive reaction for individuals who are at low risk.

### Nuclear Medicine

*Lung Scan* (V/Q Scan): A procedure to determine defects in blood perfusion in the lung; particularly useful in the client believed to have a pulmonary embolus or a ventilation/perfusion problem. For the perfusion component, a radioactive dye is injected or is inhaled, and the specific uptake is recorded on x-ray film. For the ventilation component, the client breathes the tracer element through a face mask with a mouthpiece. The ventilation component requires the client's cooperation. Client is not sedated or on dietary restrictions for the examination.

> **TEST ALERT:** Monitor laboratory values and notify primary health care provider regarding results; recognize deviations from normal; use critical thinking when evaluating client's diagnostic values.

---

 ## Appendix 17-2 RESPIRATORY MEDICATIONS

**Bronchodilators:** Relax smooth muscle of the bronchi, promoting bronchodilation and reducing airway resistance; also inhibit the release of histamine.

### General Nursing Implications

- Metered-dose inhalers (MDIs): handheld pressurized devices that deliver a measured dose of drug with each "puff." When two puffs are needed, 1 minute should elapse between them. A spacer may be used to increase the delivery of the medication.
- Dry powder inhalers (DPIs) deliver more medication to lungs and do not require coordination as with an MDI; medication is delivered as a dry powder directly to the lungs; 1 minute should elapse between puffs.
- Bronchodilators: Beta$_2$ agonists and theophylline are given with caution to the client with cardiac disease because tachydysrhythmias and chest pain may occur.
- Aerosol delivery systems have fewer side effects and are more effective.

| Medications | Side Effects | Nursing Implications |
|---|---|---|
| **Beta$_1$ and Alpha Agonists** | | |
| ▲ Epinephrine: subQ, IV<br>Racemic (nebulized) epinephrine | Headache<br>Dizziness<br>Hypertension<br>Tremors<br>Dysrhythmias | 1. Do not administer to clients with hypertension or dysrhythmias.<br>2. Primarily used to treat acute asthma attacks and anaphylactic reactions.<br>3. With racemic epinephrine, results should be observed in less than 2 hours. |

*Continued*

**Appendix 17-2 RESPIRATORY MEDICATIONS—cont'd**

| Medications | Side Effects | Nursing Implications |
|---|---|---|
| Theophylline: PO, IV | Tachycardia<br>Hypotension<br>Nausea/vomiting<br>Seizures | 1. Theophylline blood levels should be determined for long-term use; therapeutic levels are between 10 and 20 mcg/mL (56–111 mmol/L); levels greater than 20 mcg/mL (111 mmol/L) are toxic.<br>2. IV administration may cause rapid changes in vital signs.<br>3. Considered to be a third-line drug for use with asthma.<br>4. Avoid caffeine.<br><br>**! NURSING PRIORITY:** Monitor blood levels of medications. |

**Rapid-Acting Control**

| ***Beta₂ Agonists*** | | |
|---|---|---|
| Albuterol: MDI, DPI, PO, aerosol<br>Terbutaline: aerosol, PO<br>Pirbuterol: MDI<br>Levalbuterol: nebulizer<br>Metaproterenol: nebulizer, MDI | Tachycardia, tremors, and angina can occur but are rare with inhaled preparations | 1. Used for short-term relief of acute reversible airway problems.<br>2. Not used on continuous basis in absence of symptoms.<br>3. Client teaching regarding proper use of MDI and/or DPI. |

| ***Anticholinergics*** | | |
|---|---|---|
| Ipratropium bromide: aerosol, MDI | Nasal drying and irritation<br>Minimal systemic effects | 1. Nasal spray may be used for clients with allergic rhinitis and asthma.<br>2. MDI used routinely, not with acute attacks to decrease bronchospasm associated with COPD.<br>3. Therapeutic effects begin within 30 seconds. |
| Tiotropium: inhalation | Dry mouth | 1. For long-term maintenance.<br>2. Takes effect in 20 minutes; lasts 24 hours.<br>3. Report immediately blurred vision, eye pain, halos. |

**Long-Acting Control**

| ***Beta₂ Agonists*** | | |
|---|---|---|
| Salmeterol: DPI | Headache, cough, tremors, dizziness | 1. Administered two times daily (every 12 hours).<br>2. *Not used for short-term relief:* effects begin slowly and last for up to 12 hours. |

| ***Corticosteroids*** | | |
|---|---|---|
| Beclomethasone: MDI<br>Triamcinolone acetonide: MDI<br>Fluticasone: MDI | Oropharyngeal candidiasis, hoarseness, throat irritation, bad taste, cough, minimal side effects<br>Can slow growth in children and adolescents<br>With prolonged use, can cause adrenal suppression and bone loss | 1. Works well with seasonal and exercise-induced asthma.<br>2. Prophylactic use decreases number and severity of attacks.<br>3. May be used with beta₂ agonist.<br>4. Gargle after each dose and use a spacer to decrease candidiasis.<br>5. Do NOT use with acute attacks.<br><br>**! NURSING PRIORITY:** Individuals on long-term corticosteroids need to be instructed on the importance of adequate calcium and vitamin D intake and weight-bearing exercise to minimize bone loss. |

| ***Mast Cell Stabilizers*** | | |
|---|---|---|
| Cromolyn sodium: MDI | Inhalation: cough, dry mouth, throat irritation, and bad taste | 1. Prophylactic use decreases number and severity of attacks.<br>2. Prevents bronchoconstriction before exposure to known precipitant (e.g., exercise).<br>3. Not used for an acute attack. |
| Nedocromil sodium: MDI | Unpleasant taste | 1. Given to children over 6 years old.<br>2. Maximal effects develop within 24 hours.<br>3. Does not treat an acute asthmatic attack. |

| **Leukotriene Modifiers** | | |
|---|---|---|
| Montelukast: PO<br>Zafirlukast: PO | Headache, GI disturbance | 1. Once daily dose in the evening.<br>2. Administer within 1 hour before or 2 hours after eating. |

**Appendix 17-2 RESPIRATORY MEDICATIONS—cont'd**

| Medications | Side Effects | Nursing Implications |
|---|---|---|

**Antitubercular:** Broad-spectrum antibiotic specific to TB bacilli.

**General Nursing Implications**
- Client is not contagious when sputum culture is negative for three consecutive cultures.
- Use airborne respiratory precautions when sputum is positive for bacilli.
- Treatment includes combination of medications for about 6 to 12 months.
- Monitor liver function studies for clients receiving combination therapy.
- After initial therapy, medications may be administered once daily or on a twice-weekly schedule.
- Teach clients they should not stop taking the medications when they begin to feel better.
- Advise clients to return to the doctor if they notice any yellowing of the skin or eyes or begin to experience pain or swelling in joints, especially the big toe.
- Medication regimens always contain at least two medications to which the infection is sensitive; inadequate treatment is primary cause of increased incidence.

| Medications | Side Effects | Nursing Implications |
|---|---|---|
| Isoniazid: PO, IM | Peripheral neuritis<br>Hypersensitivity<br>Hepatotoxicity<br>Gastric irritation<br>Weakness | 1. Administer with (pyridoxine) vitamin $B_6$ to prevent peripheral neuritis.<br>2. Primary medication used in prophylactic and active treatment of TB. |
| Rifampin: PO<br>Rifapentine: PO (a derivative of rifampin) | Hepatotoxicity—hepatitis<br>Hypersensitivity<br>Gastric upset | 1. May negate the effectiveness of birth control pills and warfarin.<br>2. May turn body secretions orange: urine, perspiration, tears—can stain soft contacts. |
| Rifabutin: PO | Rash, GI disturbances<br>Hepatotoxicity | 1. May turn body secretions orange: urine, perspiration, tears; can stain soft contacts.<br>2. Use with caution in pregnancy. |
| Ethambutol: PO | Optic neuritis<br>Allergic reactions—<br>  dermatitis, pruritus<br>Gastric upset<br>Hepatotoxicity<br>Elevated uric acid—acute gout | 1. Give with food if GI problems occur.<br>2. Observe for vision changes.<br>3. Do not use in children under age 7 years. |
| Pyrazinamide: PO | Hepatotoxicity<br>Increased uric acid levels | 1. May take with food to reduce GI upset. |

**Nasal Decongestants:** Produce decongestion by acting on sympathetic nerve endings to produce constriction of dilated arterioles.

| Medications | Side Effects | Nursing Implications |
|---|---|---|
| Phenylephrine hydrochloride:<br>  intranasal<br>Oxymetazoline: nasal spray<br>Pseudoephedrine: PO, nasal<br>  aerosol spray | Large dose will cause<br>  CNS stimulation,<br>  anxiety, insomnia,<br>  increased blood<br>  pressure, and<br>  tachycardia | 1. With long-term use of intranasal preparations, rebound congestion may occur.<br>2. Not recommended for children under 6 years old.<br>3. Medications are frequently found in OTC combination decongestants.<br>4. Caution clients with high blood pressure to check with their health care provider before using. |
| | | **TEST ALERT:** Evaluate client's use of home remedies and OTC medications. |

**Antihistamine:** Blocks histamine release at $H_1$ receptors (see Appendix 9-2).

**NURSING PRIORITY:** Monitor for safety concerns in the older adult related to dizziness and sedation.

**NURSING PRIORITY:** Antihistamines should be used with caution with clients with asthma because thickening of secretions could impair breathing.

*Continued*

## Appendix 17-2 RESPIRATORY MEDICATIONS—cont'd

| Medications | Side Effects | Nursing Implications |
|---|---|---|
| **Expectorant:** Stimulates removal of respiratory secretions; reduces viscosity of the mucus. | | |
| Guaifenesin: PO | Nausea<br>GI upset | 1. Increase fluid intake for effectiveness.<br>2. Expect increased cough. |
| **Mucolytic:** Breaks down and loosens excessive mucus from the airways. | | |
| Dornase Alfa: aerosol | Dyspnea<br>Chest pain<br>Fever<br>Voice alteration<br>Laryngitis<br>Nasal stuffiness or discharge | 1. Do not mix with any other drugs in the nebulizer.<br>2. Store in the refrigerator and protect from strong light. |
| **Antivirals:** Used for treatment of severe respiratory syncytial virus (RSV) in hospitalized children. | | |
| Ribavirin: aerosol | Anemia, increased respiratory problems | 1. Should not be used for infants receiving mechanical ventilation.<br>2. Carefully monitor respiratory status of infant.<br>3. Used on hospitalized infants.<br>4. Pregnant nurses should not have direct contact with medication (pregnancy category X). |
| **Prophylaxis:** RSV | | |
| Palivizumab: IM | Hypersensitivity | 1. IM injections required once a month (very expensive); pain and erythema at injection site.<br>2. Dosing for high-risk infants and children should begin in late fall (November) and continue through early spring (April). |

*CNS,* Central nervous system; *GI,* gastrointestinal; *IM,* intramuscularly; *IV,* intravenously; *OTC,* over the counter; *PO,* by mouth (orally); *subQ,* subcutaneously; *TB,* tuberculosis; *UTI,* urinary tract infection.

## Appendix 17-3 SUDDEN AIRWAY OBSTRUCTION

**❗ NURSING PRIORITY:** The procedure to remove airway obstruction is not effective in the child with epiglottitis or sudden airway obstruction caused by inflammation of the upper airways.

**Goal:** To identify foreign body airway obstruction.

**❗ NURSING PRIORITY:** If the individual is coughing forcefully, do not interfere with attempts to cough and expel the foreign body. Do not administer any forceful blows to the back.

1. If the victim can speak or cry, there is probably adequate air exchange.
2. If the victim cannot speak or cry but is conscious, proceed to implement abdominal thrusts to clear the obstructed airway.
3. If the victim is unconscious:
   a. Call for help: dial 911/announce code blue, etc.
   b. Place client supine.
   c. Open airway using head-tilt/chin-lift method.
   d. Observe for presence of foreign body; perform finger sweep to remove only if visible.
   e. Maintain open airway; if there is no evidence of breathing, deliver two effective breaths (breaths that cause visible chest rise) by mask or bag-valve mask (BVM).

   f. If effective breaths cannot be delivered, reposition head, reopen airway, and attempt to ventilate victim again.
   g. If still unable to ventilate, initiate procedure for relieving obstructed airway.

**TEST ALERT:** Identify and intervene in life-threatening situations; evaluate and document client's response to emergency procedures.

**Goal:** To clear obstructed airway—adult and child (conscious and unconscious).

1. Conscious: Perform Heimlich (abdominal thrusts) maneuver (chest thrusts if pregnant or obese) until obstruction is removed or client becomes unconscious.
   a. Stand behind client and wrap arms around waist.
   b. Make a fist and place thumb side against client's abdomen; place fist midline, just above the umbilicus and below the xiphoid.
   c. Place other hand over fist and press into client's abdomen using quick upward thrusts.
   d. Repeat upward thrusts until foreign body is dislodged or client becomes unconscious.
   e. When client becomes unconscious, evaluate for presence of foreign body in the airway, remove if identified, and attempt to ventilate.

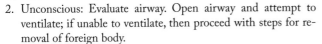

2. Unconscious: Evaluate airway. Open airway and attempt to ventilate; if unable to ventilate, then proceed with steps for removal of foreign body.
   a. Position client supine, kneel astride the client's thighs; with the heel of the hand, apply forceful upward thrust to the abdomen well below the xiphoid and above the umbilicus.
   b. Administer five abdominal thrusts, return to the client's head, open the airway, and assess for breathing; if absent, provide two effective breaths.

**Goal:** To clear obstructed airway—infant (conscious and unconscious).

1. Place the infant over the forearm with the head dependent.
2. Deliver up to five forceful back blows between the shoulder blades.

3. Supporting the head, turn the infant back over and administer up to five chest compressions (lower one-third of the sternum, approximately one finger breadth below the nipple line).
4. Attempt to remove foreign body only if it can be visualized.
5. If infant becomes unconscious, check the mouth before giving breaths to see if foreign body can be identified. Start CPR using CAB (compressions, airway, breathing).

> **! PEDIATRIC PRIORITY:** Do not do a blind sweep of the infant or child's mouth; the foreign body should be visualized before you attempt to sweep the mouth.

## Purposes

1. To remove air and/or fluid from the pleural cavity.
2. To restore negative pressure in the pleural cavity and promote reexpansion of the lung.

## Principle of Water-Sealed Chest Drainage

The water seal (or dry seal on some equipment) serves as a one-way valve; it prevents air, under atmospheric pressure, from reentering the pleural cavity. On inspiration, air and fluid leave the pleural cavity via the chest tube; the water or dry seal keeps the air and fluid from reentering (Figure 17-12).

> **! NURSING PRIORITY:** There must be a seal (either water or dry seal) between the client and the atmospheric pressure.

## Equipment

*Three-chamber disposable chest drainage system:* A molded plastic system that provides a collection chamber, a water-sealed chamber, and a suction-control chamber. When suction is applied, there should be a continuous, gentle bubbling in the water in the suction control chamber (Figure 17-13).

## Nursing Implications

### Assessment

1. Evaluate for hypoxia.
2. Evaluate character of respirations.
3. Assess for symmetric chest wall expansion.
4. Evaluate breath sounds bilaterally.
5. Palpate around insertion site for subcutaneous emphysema.

### Intervention

1. Perform range of motion of the affected arm and shoulder.
2. Encourage coughing and deep breathing every 2 hours.
3. Encourage ambulation if appropriate.
4. Administer pain medications as indicated.
5. Place in low Fowler's or semi-Fowler's position.

### Observe Drainage System for Proper Functioning

1. Water level in the water-seal chamber and in the tubing from the client should fluctuate (tidal): rise on inspiration and fall on

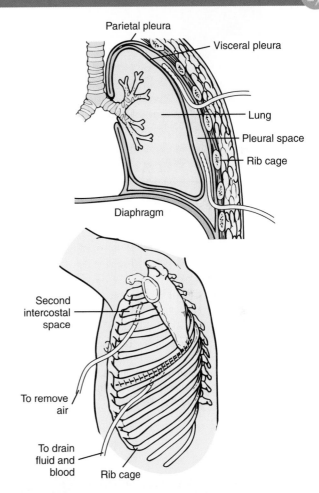

**FIGURE 17-12 Placement of Chest Tubes.** (From Lewis, S. L., et al. [2017]. *Medical-surgical nursing: Assessment and management of clinical problems* [10th ed.]. St. Louis, MO: Mosby.)

expiration. The opposite occurs with positive-pressure mechanical ventilation.

2. Continuous bubbling should not occur in the fluid where water seal is maintained; continuous bubbling indicates an air leak; continuous bubbling should occur only in the system that maintains a third chamber for suction control.

*Continued*

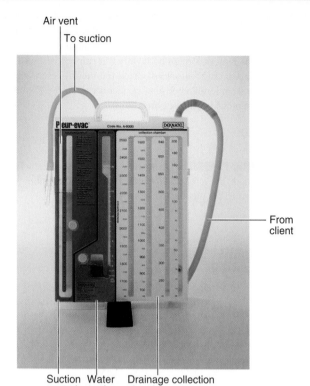

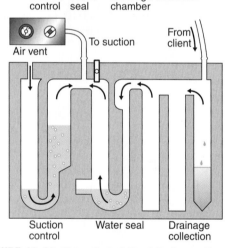

FIGURE 17-13 **Water-Sealed Chest Drainage.** (From Potter, P. A., & Perry, A. G. [2009]. *Fundamentals of nursing* [7th ed.]. St. Louis, MO: Mosby.) Recommend using Chest drainage unit.

3. Initial bubbling may occur in the water-sealed chamber with coughing or with deep respiration as air is moved out of the pleural cavity and intermittent bubbling with respirations until the lung is reexpanded.

Maintain Water-Sealed System

1. Keep all drainage equipment below the chest-tube insertion site.
2. Evaluate for dependent loops in the tubing; this increases resistance to drainage. All extra tubing should be coiled in the bed and flow in a straight line to the system.
3. Tape all connections.
4. Note characteristics and amount of drainage. Mark level on the collection chamber of the drainage system as needed and every 8 hours.
5. Vigorous "milking" or stripping of chest tubes should not be done routinely on clients because it increases pleural pressures.
6. Change the disposable chest drainage system when the collection chamber is approximately half full. The nurse can change the closed chest drainage system.
7. Do not clamp chest tubes during transport.

> **TEST ALERT:** Monitor effective functioning of therapeutic devices; determine whether chest drainage is functioning properly; adjust tubes to promote drainage; identify abnormal chest tube drainage; evaluate for achievement of goal of chest tubes; assess and intervene when unexpected responses to therapy occur.

## Chest Tube Removal

1. Criteria for removal of the tube:
   a. Less than 50 mL drainage per day.
   b. Fluctuations/tidaling/bubbling stop in the water-seal chamber.
   c. Chest x-ray film reveals expanded lung.
   d. Client has good breath sounds and is breathing comfortably.
2. Procedure.
   a. Provide appropriate analgesia about 30 minutes before procedure.
   b. Generally, the physician will want the client in a low Fowler's or semi-Fowler's position, unless contraindicated.
   c. The physician will ask the client to exhale and hold it or to exhale and bear down (a Valsalva maneuver). Either of these procedures will increase the intrathoracic pressure and prevent air from entering the pleural space.
   d. With the client holding his or her breath, the physician will quickly remove the tube and place an occlusive bandage over the area; the client can then breathe normally.
   e. Assess the client's tolerance of the procedure; check breath sounds, and a chest x-ray film may be obtained to determine that the lungs remain fully expanded.

## Endotracheal Intubation

Placement of an endotracheal (ET) tube through the mouth or nose into the trachea (Figure 17-14).

### Purpose

To provide an immediate airway; to maintain a patent airway; to facilitate removal of secretions and provide method for artificial ventilation.

### Nursing Interventions

1. Provide warm, humidified oxygen.
2. Establish method of communication because the client cannot speak; child is unable to cry.
3. Maintain safety measures.
   a. Prevent client from accidentally removing tube: soft hand/wrist restraints or mittens.

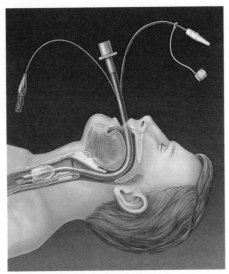

**FIGURE 17-14 Position of Endotracheal Tube.** (From Potter, P. A., & Perry, A. G. [2017]. *Fundamentals of nursing* [9th ed.]. St. Louis, MO: Mosby.)

b. Secure ET tube to the face.

c. Child with an ET tube requires constant attendance.

4. As soon as tube is inserted, assess symmetry of chest expansion and bilateral breath sounds. Assess for presence of bilateral breath sounds every 2 hours. If tube slips farther into the trachea, it may pass into the right mainstem bronchus, obliterating the left mainstem bronchus. Determine placement by checking breath sounds.

5. Cuff must remain inflated if client is on a volume ventilator. If the client has adequate spontaneous respiration and is not on a ventilator, the cuff may be left deflated.

6. Minimal occluding volume (MOV) should be used when inflating the cuff to prevent aspiration or to maintain mechanical ventilation. This is accomplished by placing a stethoscope over the trachea or by listening to the client's breath sounds to determine when air stops moving past the cuff. A safe pressure on the cuff is 20 to 25 mmHg.

7. Provide frequent oral hygiene; assess for pressure areas on the nose or the mouth.

8. Client's nothing-by-mouth (NPO) status is maintained as long as tube is in place.

9. Suction as indicated (see Appendix 17-6).

### Tracheostomy

A surgical opening in the trachea (Figure 17-15).

#### Purpose

To maintain airway over an extended period; to facilitate removal of secretions.

### Nursing Interventions

#### Initially After Tracheostomy

1. Provide warm, humidified oxygen.

2. Small amount of bleeding around the tube is expected.

3. Observe for pulsations of the tube; it may be resting on the innominate artery; notify physician of observation.

4. Maintain frequent contact and communication with client and provide reassurance.

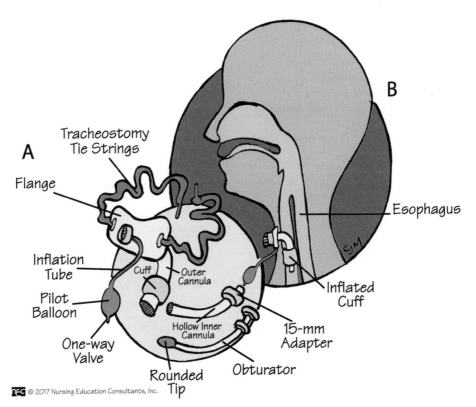

© 2017 Nursing Education Consultants, Inc.

**FIGURE 17-15 Tracheostomy Tube.** (From Zerwekh, J., Garneau, A., & Miller, C. J. [2017]. *Digital collection of the memory notebooks of nursing* [4th ed.]. Chandler, AZ: Nursing Education Consultants, Inc.)

*Continued*

**Appendix 17-5 ARTIFICIAL AIRWAYS—cont'd**

**Maintenance of Tracheostomy**

1. Provide warm, humidified oxygen.
2. Establish method of communication because client cannot speak; child is unable to cry.
3. Maintain safety measures.
   a. Secure tracheal tube to the client's neck.
   b. Use safety measures to prevent client from dislodging tube: soft restraints, tracheostomy ties.
   c. Prevent clothing or bed covers from occluding area of tracheal opening.
   d. Child with a tracheostomy requires continuous attendance.
4. Assess for symmetric expansion of chest wall and bilateral breath sounds.
5. Provide frequent oral hygiene; turn every 2 hours.
6. Inflate tracheostomy cuff during tube feedings or feedings by mouth (minimal occluding volume).
7. Cuff must remain inflated if client is on a ventilator. If the client has adequate spontaneous respiration, the cuff may be left deflated.
8. Suction as indicated (see Appendix 17-6).

> **TEST ALERT:** Provide tracheostomy care and suctioning as necessary/appropriate.

9. If tracheal tube has an obturator, it should be taped to the head of the bed. If the tracheostomy tube is accidentally removed, the obturator will be necessary for replacing the tube.
10. A fenestrated tracheostomy tube can be adapted so that air will flow throughout normal passages; frequently used when client is beginning to be weaned from the ventilator. If client has respiratory difficulty when the inner cannula is removed, immediately reinsert the cannula to provide a tracheal airway. The tube can also be plugged so that client can speak or cough through normal airway. Make sure the cuff is deflated before plugging the tracheostomy.
11. Establish means of communication; keep call light within easy reach of client.
12. If the client accidentally removes the tube, use the obturator to attempt to replace the tube in the tracheal opening. If unable to replace tracheotomy tube, hold the opening open with a hemostat until physician is available to replace the tube.

> **■ NURSING PRIORITY:** The purpose of the cuff on a tracheostomy tube or on an ET tube is to facilitate the delivery of air to the lungs, not to secure the tube position. Tracheostomy ties/straps secure the tube in position.

**Appendix 17-6 SUCTIONING THROUGH ARTIFICIAL AIRWAYS**

> **■ NURSING PRIORITY:** Suctioning the endotracheal tube or the tracheostomy is done to remove excess secretions and to maintain patent airway. Suctioning should always be done before a cuff is deflated.

1. Determine that the client needs to be suctioned.
   a. Auscultate lungs to detect presence of secretions.
   b. Observe to see whether client is experiencing immediate difficulty with removal of secretions.
   c. Monitor $O_2$ saturation (pulse oximetry) and arterial blood gases (ABGs).
   d. Monitor for increased anxiety and restlessness.
2. Explain procedure if client is not familiar with it, or simply indicate you are going to assist with the removal of the secretions.
3. All equipment introduced into the trachea or the endotracheal (ET) tube must be sterile.
4. Attach the suction catheter to the suction source while maintaining sterile technique.
5. If client is not in immediate danger of airway occlusion, hyperoxygenate with 100% $O_2$ for three to four hyperinflations.
6. Gently insert sterile catheter into the opening without applying suction. Insert catheter to the point of slight resistance, then pull catheter back 1 to 2 cm.
7. Apply suction as the catheter is withdrawn.
8. Each suctioning pass should not exceed 10 seconds in duration.
9. Reconnect client to oxygen source and evaluate whether one suctioning episode was sufficient to remove secretions.

10. Hyperoxygenate client for 1 to 5 minutes after suctioning; assess vital signs and $O_2$ saturation—values should return to normal or to the previous levels before suctioning.
11. Avoid suctioning client before drawing blood for determination of arterial blood gas values. Client should be allowed to stabilize for approximately 30 minutes before blood is drawn.
12. Monitor oximetry while suctioning; if oximetry does not come back to normal level immediately after suctioning, do not attempt to suction client again; replace oxygen and/or ventilatory connection and continue to monitor closely.

**Complications of Suctioning**

1. Hypoxia: If possible, preoxygenate with high percentage of $O_2$ before and after suctioning.
2. Dysrhythmias: Limit suctioning to 10 seconds; monitor rhythm during suctioning; if bradycardia or tachycardia develops, discontinue suctioning immediately.
3. Bronchospasm: Try to time the suctioning with client's own cycle; insert tube during inspiration.
4. Airway trauma: Maintain suction level below 120 mmHg. Never force the suction catheter.
5. Infection: Use sterile technique; assess the color and quantity of sputum suctioned.
6. Atelectasis: Use suction catheters that are approximately one-third or less of the diameter of tube.

> **TEST ALERT:** Intervene to improve respiratory status; suction client's respiratory tract (oral, nasal, tracheostomy, and ET tube).

# OXYGEN DELIVERY DEVICES

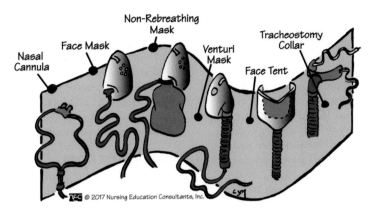

**FIGURE 17-16 Oxygen Delivery Devices.** (From Zerwekh, J., Garneau, A., & Miller, C. J. [2017]. *Digital collection of the memory notebooks of nursing* [4th ed.]. Chandler, AZ: Nursing Education Consultants, Inc.)

**Goal:** The goal of oxygen therapy is to maintain an optimum level of oxygenation at the lowest effective level of fraction of inspired oxygen ($FiO_2$) (Figure 17-16).

## Methods of Administration

Oxygen is measured in liters per minute (LPM) flow: a range of 2 to 8 LPM is the most common order.
1. *Low-flow systems:* nasal cannula, standard mask, nonrebreather mask.
2. *High-flow systems:* Venturi mask, nebulizer mask, and ventilators. Oxygen is measured as $FiO_2$ in concentrations from 24% to 100%: 10 LPM oxygen flow is required to obtain accurate percentage flow.

## Humidification

1. Adds water vapor to inspired gas.
2. Prevents drying and irritation of respiratory membranes.
3. Loosens thick secretions, allowing them to be more easily removed.

## Indications for Oxygen Administration

1. A decrease in oxygen in the arterial blood (hypoxemia).
2. An increase in the work of breathing.
3. To decrease the cardiac workload.

**TEST ALERT:** Monitor client receiving oxygen therapy. Evaluate response.

## Oxygen Safety in Administration

1. Properly ground all electrical equipment.
2. Do not permit any smoking by anyone in the area.
3. Use water-based, not oil-based, lubricants.
4. Use oxygen with caution in clients with chronic airway disease; most often administered via mask or nasal cannula at 2 to 4 LPM, unless client is in severe distress.
5. Oxygen supports combustion but is not explosive.

## Oxygen Toxicity

A medically induced condition produced by inhalation of high concentrations of oxygen over a prolonged period of time. Toxicity is directly related to concentration of oxygen, duration of therapy, and degree of lung disease present.
1. Tracheal irritation and cough.
2. Dyspnea and increasing cough.
3. Decrease in vital capacity.
4. The $PaO_2$ continues to decrease, even with an increasing $FiO_2$.
5. Atelectasis.

**TEST ALERT:** Monitor and maintain clients on a ventilator.

## Ventilators

Ventilators deliver air and/or oxygen at a predetermined tidal volume. The ventilator delivers the volume of air and/or oxygen within safe ranges of pressure. A pressure limit is set, and an alarm will sound if the tidal volume cannot be delivered within the set pressure limits. The intrathoracic pressure is increased with the ventilator; this decreases the venous blood return (preload) to the right side of the heart and subsequently decreases cardiac output.

### Patterns of Ventilation

1. **Control ventilation:** Delivers a predetermined rate and volume of gas (air/oxygen) independent of patient's effort. This mode of ventilation is rarely used.
2. **Assist-control ventilation (AC):** The client may initiate the cycle with inspiration. All initiated breaths are supported with the preset tidal volume or pressure.

*Continued*

3. **Synchronized intermittent mandatory ventilation (SIMV):** Delivers preset tidal volume or pressure and rate allowing for spontaneous breaths between; synchronizes with the patient's efforts. Used as a weaning mode.

4. **Positive end-expiratory pressure (PEEP):** Maintains positive pressure at alveolar level at end of expiration to facilitate the diffusion of oxygen. PEEP will increase the intrathoracic pressure, thus further decreasing the venous return and causing a decrease in preload.

5. **Indications for use:** Acute respiratory distress syndrome (ARDS); clients unable to maintain patent airway; neuromuscular diseases causing respiratory failure.

6. **Continuous positive airway pressure (CPAP):** Used to augment the functional residual capacity (FRC) during spontaneous breathing. Used to wean clients from ventilators and may be administered by face mask. Patients must have spontaneous respirations.

7. **High-frequency ventilation:** Small amounts of gas (air/oxygen) are delivered at a rapid rate. Requires sedation and pharmacologic paralysis.

> **TEST ALERT:** Identify changes in respiratory status and intervene to improve respiratory status; assess client for unexpected response to therapy.

### Nursing Implications

1. All alarms should be set and checked each shift, especially low pressure and low exhaled volume.
2. A bag and valve mask resuscitator is placed in the client's room in case of mechanical failure of equipment.
3. Central venous pressure (CVP) and pulmonary artery pressure readings will be affected by the ventilator; readings should be determined in a consistent manner.
4. Ventilator setting for fraction of inspired oxygen ($Fio_2$), tidal volume, respiratory rate, pattern of control (AC/SIMV, etc.), and PEEP should be checked and charted in the nurses' notes.
5. Assess client's tolerance of the ventilator; intravenous medications such as propofol, a short-acting hypnotic that produces amnesia, or fentanyl, a central nervous system depressant, may be used. If weaning or removal of the ventilator is anticipated, do not medicate the client.
6. The client frequently experiences a high level of anxiety and fear. Explain equipment and alarms to the client and to the family. Maintain a calm, reassuring approach to the client.

7. When ventilator changes are made, carefully assess the client's response (pulse oximetry, arterial blood gas [ABGs], and vital signs).
8. Never allow the condensation in the tubing to flow back into fluid reservoir.
9. Adequate nutrition is mandatory and will facilitate weaning. The gastrointestinal (GI) tract is preferred if functioning.
   a. Nutritional support provided via the GI tract preserves mucosal integrity, improves intestinal blood, and decreases the incidences of sepsis.
   b. The use of a small-bore transpyloric tube emptying in the duodenum is the recommended route to administer either bolus or continuous feedings. (Elevate the head of the bed 30 degrees during feeding.)

### Common Ventilator Alarms

1. High pressure alarm: Sounds when tidal volume cannot be delivered at set pressure limit.
   **Nursing Care:** Increased secretions—suction; client biting tube—place oral airway; coughing and increased anxiety—administer sedative.
2. Low pressure alarm: Sounds when the machine cannot deliver the tidal volume because of a leak or break in the system.
   **Nursing Care:** Disconnection—check all connections for break in system; client stops breathing on the SIMV mode—evaluate client's tolerance; tracheostomy or endotracheal (ET) tube cuff is leaking—check for air escaping around cuff, may need to replace tracheostomy tube if cuff is ruptured.

### Weaning From Ventilators

Weaning may be done via a spontaneous breathing trial using a T-piece with heated mist and oxygen, or by SIMV mode on the ventilator or using continuous positive airway pressure (CPAP) via the ventilator. During weaning, it is imperative for the nurse to maintain close observation for increasing fatigue, dyspnea, and hypoxia. If client experiences dyspnea, he or she should be returned to the ventilator at whatever parameters were being used, and the doctor should be notified; anticipate drawing blood for determination of ABG values.

> **⚠ NURSING PRIORITY:** Focus on the client, not on the ventilator. In case of problems with the ventilator, assess the client; if adequate ventilation is not being achieved, take client off the ventilator, maintain respirations via a bag and valve mask resuscitator, and call for assistance.

---

**Appendix 17-9** **NURSING PROCEDURE: SPUTUM SPECIMEN COLLECTION**

## Sputum Specimen Collection

This test analyzes sputum samples (material expectorated from client's lungs and bronchi during deep coughing) to diagnose respiratory disease, identify the cause of pulmonary infections, identify abnormal lung cells, and assist in managing pulmonary disease.

### Nursing Implications

1. Sputum for culture and sensitivity should be collected as soon as possible (before administration of antibiotics if possible) to facilitate identification of bacteria and treatment.

2. Specimens for cytology and for acid-fast bacilli for TB diagnostics should be collected in the morning when bacteria and cells are most concentrated.
3. No mouthwash should be used before collection of specimen; have client rinse his mouth with water or brush his teeth with water, but do not use toothpaste.
4. Aerosol mist will assist in decreasing thickness of sputum and increasing effectiveness of coughing.
5. Maintain strict asepsis and standard precautions in collecting and transporting specimen; use sterile specimen collection container.

**Appendix 17-9 NURSING PROCEDURE: SPUTUM SPECIMEN COLLECTION—cont'd**

6. Acid-fast bacillus: Sputum collection should be done on 3 consecutive days.
7. Culture and sensitivity: Initial specimen should be obtained before antibiotics are administered.

### Clinical Tips for Problem Solving

If client experiences pain while coughing:
• Support painful area with roll pillows to minimize pain and discomfort.

• Encourage client to take several deep breaths before beginning. This assists in triggering the cough reflex and aerates the lungs (see Box 17-1).
• If client is unable to produce sputum specimen:
    • Attempt procedure early in the morning, when mucus production is greatest.
    • Notify physician to obtain orders for a bronchodilator or nebulization therapy.

# Study Questions
# Respiratory: Care of Adult and Pediatric Clients

More questions on
evolve

1. On the first postoperative day after a right lower lobe (RLL) lobectomy, the client deep breathes and coughs but has difficulty raising mucus. What nursing observation would indicate the client is not adequately clearing secretions?
    1. Chest x-ray film showing right-sided pleural fluid
    2. A few scattered crackles on RLL on auscultation
    3. Increase in $Paco_2$ from 35 to 45 mmHg
    4. Decrease in forced vital capacity

2. What nursing observation indicates that an unplanned extubation of an endotracheal tube has occurred?
    1. The high-pressure ventilator alarm activates
    2. Client is able to speak
    3. Increased swallowing efforts by client
    4. Increased crackles (rales) over left lung field

3. The client with COPD is to be discharged home while receiving continuous oxygen at a rate of 2 L/min via cannula. What information does the nurse provide to the client and his wife regarding the use of oxygen at home?
    1. Because of his need for oxygen, the client will have to limit activity at home.
    2. The use of oxygen will eliminate the client's shortness of breath.
    3. Precautions are necessary because oxygen can spontaneously ignite and explode.
    4. Use oxygen during activity to relieve the strain on the client's heart.

4. The nurse is caring for a client who is experiencing an acute asthma attack. He is dyspneic and experiencing orthopnea; his pulse rate is 120 beats/min. In what order will the nurse provide care to this client? Number the following options in the order in which they will be performed, with 1 being the first action and 4 being the last action.
    1. _____ Administer humidified oxygen.
    2. _____ Place in semi-Fowler's position.
    3. _____ Provide nebulizer treatment with bronchodilator.
    4. _____ Discuss factors that precipitate attack.

5. The wife of a client with COPD is worried about caring for her husband at home. Which statement by the nurse provides the most valid information?
    1. "You should avoid emotional situations that increase his shortness of breath."
    2. "Help your husband arrange activities so that he does as little walking as possible."
    3. "Arrange a schedule so your husband does all necessary activities before noon; then he can rest during the afternoon and evening."
    4. "Your husband will be more short of breath when he walks, but that will not hurt him."

6. Which statement correctly describes suctioning through an endotracheal tube?
    1. The catheter is inserted into the endotracheal tube; intermittent suction is applied until no further secretions are retrieved; the catheter is then withdrawn.
    2. The catheter is inserted through the nose, and the upper airway is suctioned; the catheter is then removed from the upper airway and inserted into the endotracheal tube to suction the lower airway.
    3. With suction applied, the catheter is inserted into the endotracheal tube; when resistance is met, the catheter is slowly withdrawn.
    4. The catheter is inserted into the endotracheal tube to a point of resistance, and intermittent suction is applied during withdrawal.

7. While a client's wife is visiting, she observes the client's chest drainage system and begins to nervously question the nurse regarding the amount of bloody drainage in the system. What is the best response from the nurse?
    1. "Your husband has been really sick; this must be a very difficult time. Let's sit down and talk about it."
    2. "I have checked all of the equipment, and it is working fine; you do not need to worry about it."
    3. "The system is draining collected fluid from around the lungs. The drainage is expected and does not mean that he is bleeding."
    4. "The chest tube is draining the secretions from his chest; it is important for him to deep breathe frequently."

8. The nurse is caring for an infant who is experiencing respiratory distress and being treated with continuous positive airway pressure (CPAP). The nurse knows that for this treatment to be most effective, the infant must be:
   1. Intubated with respiration maintained by controlled ventilation
   2. Able to breathe spontaneously
   3. Frequently stimulated to maintain respiratory rate
   4. Suctioned frequently to maintain alveolar ventilation

9. The nurse is assessing a client who is on a ventilator and has an endotracheal tube in place. What information confirms that the tube has migrated too far into the trachea?
   1. Decreased breath sounds are heard over the left side of the chest.
   2. Increased rhonchi are present at the lung bases bilaterally.
   3. Client is able to speak and coughs excessively.
   4. Ventilator pressure alarm continues to sound.

10. A 6-year-old client is admitted to the postoperative recovery area after a tonsillectomy. In what position will the nurse place the client?
    1. Semi-Fowler's position, with the head turned to the side
    2. Prone position, with the head of the bed slightly elevated
    3. On the back, with the head turned to the right side
    4. On the abdomen, with the head turned to the side

11. The nurse understands clamping a chest tube may cause what problem?
    1. Atelectasis
    2. Tension pneumothorax
    3. Bacterial infections in the pleural cavity
    4. Decrease in the rate and depth of respirations

12. On auscultation, the nurse hears wheezing in a client with asthma. Considering the pathophysiology of asthma, what would the nurse identify as the primary cause of this type of lung sound?
    1. Increased inspiratory pressure in the upper airways
    2. Dilation of the respiratory bronchioles and increased mucus
    3. Movement of air through narrowed airways
    4. Increased pulmonary compliance

13. What finding on the nursing assessment would be associated with a diagnosis of pneumonia in the older adult?
    1. Acute confusion
    2. Hypertension
    3. Hematemesis in the morning
    4. Dry hacking cough at night

14. The nurse is monitoring a client who is experiencing an acute asthma attack. What observations would indicate an improvement in the client's condition?
    1. Respiratory rate of 18 breaths/min
    2. Pulse oximetry of 88%
    3. Pulse rate of 110 beats/min
    4. Productive cough with rapid breathing

15. Clients with COPD usually receive low-dose oxygen via nasal cannula. The nurse understands that which problem may occur if the client receives too much oxygen?
    1. Hyperventilation
    2. Tachypnea
    3. Hypoventilation or apnea
    4. Increased snoring

16. A client has a diagnosis of right-sided empyema. Thoracentesis is to be performed in the client's room. The nurse will place the client in what position for this procedure?
    1. Prone position with feet elevated
    2. Sitting with upper torso over bedside table
    3. Lying on left side with right knee bent
    4. Semi-Fowler's position with lower torso flat

17. For a client with COPD, what is the main risk factor for pulmonary infection?
    1. Fluid imbalance with pitting edema
    2. Pooling of respiratory secretions
    3. Decreased fluid intake and loss of body weight
    4. Decreased anterior–posterior diameter of the chest

18. A client has a history of atherosclerotic heart disease with a sustained increase in his blood pressure. What is important to discuss with this client before he uses an over-the-counter decongestant?
    1. Urinary frequency and diuresis
    2. Bradycardia and diarrhea
    3. Vasoconstriction and increased arterial pressure
    4. Headache and dysrhythmias

19. What symptoms would the nurse expect to observe in a 19-month-old client with a diagnosis of laryngotracheobronchitis (LTB)?
    1. Stridor on inspiration
    2. Expiratory wheezing
    3. Paroxysmal coughing
    4. Hemoptysis

# Answers to Study Questions

1. *3*

Retained secretions may cause hypoventilation; this results in an increase in the Paco₂. The other options do not as effectively reflect a problem with clearing mucus. Pleural fluid is not removed via coughing; the fluid is in the pleural space, not in the lung. Although the Paco₂ is within the normal limits, there is still an increase noted, which is due to the hypoventilation. The nurse cannot easily measure the forced vital capacity at the bedside. (Ignatavicius & Workman, 8 ed., pp. 579, 581)

2. *2*

An unplanned extubation, which would be accidental removal of the endotracheal tube from the trachea, would allow air to pass through the trachea and vocal cords, allowing the client to make a noise—or to speak. Activation of the low-pressure alarm on the ventilator will be noted, along with diminished or absent breath sounds, signs of significant respiratory distress, and gastric distention. Increased swallowing is indicative of irritation in the throat or bleeding. Increase in adventitious sounds indicates excessive mucus in the lungs. (Lewis et al., 10 ed., p. 1573)

**3.** *4*
The primary purpose of oxygen therapy is to decrease the workload of the heart in clients with chronic pulmonary diseases and to assist in preventing right-sided heart failure. Use of oxygen may help relieve shortness of breath but will not eliminate it. Oxygen supports combustion but is not explosive; supplemental oxygen will allow more activity for the client, not less. (Ignatavicius & Workman, 8 ed., pp. 515)

**4.** *2, 1, 3, 4*
1___2___ Because oxygen is a priority, begin administration of oxygen.
2___1___ The first action is to place the client in semi-Fowler's position. Oxygen or inhalation therapy cannot be effective with severe orthopnea if the client is not in a sitting or upright position.
3___3___ Then administer the nebulizer treatment, which would include bronchodilators.
4___4___ Physiologic needs must be addressed before teaching or psychosocial needs are considered. (Ignatavicius & Workman, 8 ed., pp. 548–557)

**5.** *4*
Physical conditioning is important for clients with COPD. Activity needs to be paced so that undue fatigue does not occur. Some increase in shortness of breath with exercise is to be expected but will not damage the lungs. If the client stops exercising before an increase in shortness of breath, he will not experience a training effect. (Ignatavicius & Workman, 8 ed., p. 565)

**6.** *4*
The catheter must be advanced to an adequate depth (to prevent secretion buildup at the end of the tube and to clear the airway as much as possible). To minimize trauma, suction is applied only during catheter withdrawal. If the upper airway is suctioned, another sterile catheter must be obtained to suction the endotracheal tube. (Ignatavicius & Workman, 8 ed., pp. 525–526)

**7.** *3*
This is important information to explain to the client's wife regarding the bloody drainage in the chest tube collection system. After the nurse has explained the reason for the drainage, it would then be appropriate to sit down and talk with the wife. Checking the equipment may be appropriate, but telling the wife not to worry is a communication block (false reassurance). Having the client breathe deeply does not answer the question or address the wife's concern. (Ignatavicius & Workman, 8 ed., pp. 578–579)

**8.** *2*
CPAP only works when the infant is breathing on his own. When the airway is opened for a breath, the CPAP increases the pressure in the airway, which increases airflow to the lungs and oxygenation. CPAP is not used when a child requires controlled ventilation. Stimulating the infant may be appropriate, but the child must be able to breathe spontaneously for this to be effective. The child is not suctioned unless an excessive amount of mucus must be removed. (Hockenberry & Wilson, 10 ed., pp. 373–374)

**9.** *1*
An endotracheal tube that is inserted too far—beyond the carina—is most likely to enter the right main stem bronchus. The volume of air from the ventilator is only delivered to the right lung; breath sounds are decreased or absent over the left lung. The pressure alarm indicates that the current pressure is not adequate to deliver the tidal volume prescribed. This may occur but does not confirm the migration of the tube. (Ignatavicius & Workman, 8 ed., p. 615)

**10.** *4*
Before the child is fully awake, he or she should be placed on the abdomen with the head turned to one side to facilitate the drainage of secretions and to prevent aspiration. When alert, the child may sit up or assume a position of comfort. The other options are not appropriate because they do not allow for drainage of secretions from the mouth and throat after a tonsillectomy while the child is in early recovery. (Hockenberry & Wilson, 10 ed., p. 1174)

**11.** *2*
Tension pneumothorax occurs when air enters the pleural space with each inspiration, becomes trapped there, and is not expelled during expiration (i.e., one-way valve effect). Pressure builds in the chest as the accumulation of air in the pleural space increases. This can lead to a mediastinal shift. Atelectasis occurs when the atmospheric pressure enters the pleural cavity. This procedure has nothing to do with an infection or pulmonary consolidation. (Ignatavicius & Workman, 8 ed., pp. 623–624)

**12.** *3*
The wheezing is due to narrowing of the airway caused by bronchospasm. Increased mucus production hinders the airway as well; this also results in trapping of air in the alveoli. Increased pulmonary compliance indicates the lungs have good recoil and expansion. (Ignatavicius & Workman, 8 ed., pp. 550–551)

**13.** *1*
Confusion in the older adult is related to hypoxemia, which occurs with pneumonia. Vasodilation and dehydration cause hypotension and orthostatic changes. Crackles are typically heard when fluid is in the alveolar area. The cough is generally productive. The breathing is rapid and shallow without the use of accessory muscles. Hemoptysis may occur but not hematemesis (blood from the gastrointestinal tract). (Ignatavicius & Workman, 8 ed., pp. 591–592)

**14.** *1*
The respiratory rate is within normal limits at 18 breaths per minute. The option for the pulse oximetry is too low. The pulse rate is too high to indicate improvement, and the productive cough with rapid breathing is not as significant as the decrease in respiratory rate. (Ignatavicius & Workman, 8 ed., pp. 550–556)

**15.** *3*
In clients with chronic high $Pco_2$ levels (COPD), the administration of oxygen at a flow rate that increases the $Pao_2$ may cause apnea and require the use of a bag valve mask resuscitator to ventilate the client. When the $Pao_2$ increases significantly, it can decrease the client's stimulus to breathe and may cause carbon dioxide narcosis. (Ignatavicius & Workman, 8 ed., pp. 515, 563)

16. *2*

Positioning over the bedside table allows the ribs to separate, which assists the physician in positioning the needle into the pleural cavity. If the client is unable to assume a sitting position, he or she is placed on the affected side with head of bed slightly elevated. The area containing the fluid should be dependent. (Ignatavicius & Workman, 8 ed., p. 511 )

17. *2*

The ineffective clearing of secretions with resultant pooling can lead to an increased risk for infection. The client's appetite is usually decreased. The client has an increased anteroposterior diameter of the chest. (Ignatavicius & Workman, 8 ed., p. 566 )

18. *3*

Decongestants should be avoided by clients with hypertension because these medications often contain pseudoephedrine and phenylephrine, which cause central nervous system stimulation with vasoconstriction and increased blood pressure. They also precipitate anxiety and insomnia. Decongestants do not cause urinary frequency, diuresis, or dysrhythmias. (Lehne, 8 ed., p. 981)

19. *1*

Because croup causes upper airway obstruction, inspiratory stridor is a predominant symptom. Expiratory wheezing is heard in the asthmatic client. Paroxysmal coughing occurs more with spasmodic laryngitis. Hemoptysis is not common with croup syndromes. (Hockenberry & Wilson, 10 ed., p. 1186)

# CHAPTER EIGHTEEN

# Vascular: Care of Adult Clients 18

## PRIORITY CONCEPTS

Clotting, Health Promotion, Perfusion

## PHYSIOLOGY OF THE VASCULAR SYSTEM

### Vessels

A. Arteries: primary function is to transport nutrients and oxygen to the cellular level.
B. Capillaries: allow the exchange of fluid and nutrient between the blood and the interstitial fluid.
C. Veins: primary function is to return blood to the heart.
D. Lymphatic system: primary function is to return fluid and protein to the blood from the interstitial fluid.

### Blood Pressure (BP)

A. Baroreceptors are located in aortic arch and in carotid sinuses (carotid bodies) and are very sensitive to changes in pressure within vessel walls. An increase in pressure causes stimulation of the vagus nerve, which in turn decreases the heart rate.
B. Peripheral resistance is resistance of arterioles to flow of blood.
   1. Dilation decreases peripheral resistance, thereby decreasing BP.
   2. Vasoconstriction increases peripheral resistance, thereby increasing BP.
C. Systolic pressure represents the ejection of blood from the heart.
D. Diastolic pressure represents the pressure remaining in the arteries at the end of systole.
E. Pulse pressure is the difference between the systolic and diastolic pressures.
F. Mean arterial pressure (MAP) is the average pressure within the arterial system.
G. Autonomic nervous system influence on BP.
   1. Parasympathetic system: stimulates the vagus nerve.
   2. Sympathetic nervous system controls BP by:
      a. Maintaining peripheral resistance through constriction and dilation of the vessels.
      b. Increasing heart rate and force of contraction.
      c. Causing constriction of the large veins, which promotes an increase in venous return to the heart, thereby increasing cardiac output.
H. Renal influence on BP.
   1. Renin is an enzyme released by the kidneys when there is a decrease in renal blood flow.

2. Renin, a strong vasoconstrictor, increases BP.
3. Activation of the renin–angiotensin system increases secretion of aldosterone, thus precipitating sodium and water retention and increasing vascular volume.
I. Vasopressin (antidiuretic hormone) is released when BP falls below normal; this increases the blood volume, which increases BP.

### System Assessment

A. Health history.
   1. Identify risk factors for peripheral vascular disease and shock.
   2. Determine coping strategies.
B. Physical assessment.
   1. Inspection.
      a. Inspect extremities for edema, color changes, varicosities, ulcers, hair distribution.
      b. Monitor for jugular venous distention (JVD).
   2. Palpation.
      a. Monitor temperature, moisture, pulses, and edema in extremities.
      b. Neurovascular assessment (Figure 18-1).
   3. Auscultation.
      a. Evaluate BP (Box 18-1).
      b. Monitor for bruit (buzzing or humming heard over blood vessel).

---

**TEST ALERT:** Perform focused assessment or reassessment. Respond to changes in client vital signs.

---

## DISORDERS OF THE VASCULAR SYSTEM

### Atherosclerosis

**A gradual thickening and narrowing of the arterial lumen; sometimes referred to as "hardening of the arteries"** (Figure 18-2).

A. Process is slow and can gradually lead to a significant decrease in blood supply to tissue.
B. Arteries commonly affected by atherosclerosis and the ensuing problems:
   1. Coronary arteries: myocardial infarction.
   2. Cerebrovascular arteries: stroke, brain attack.
   3. Aorta: aortic aneurysm, peripheral vascular disease.
   4. Renal arteries: hypertension, renal failure.
   5. Peripheral arteries: peripheral vascular disease.

# NEUROVASCULAR ASSESSMENT

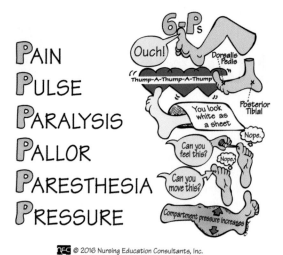

**FIGURE 18-1 Neurovascular Assessment.** (From Zerwekh, J., Garneau, A., & Miller, C. J. [2017]. *Digital collection of the memory notebooks of nursing* [4th ed.]. Chandler, AZ: Nursing Education Consultants, Inc.)

---

**Box 18-1   OLDER ADULT CARE FOCUS**

**Evaluation of Blood Pressure**

- If a client has had hypertension for a long time, the client's "normal" BP may need to be higher to maintain adequate blood flow and allow client to perform ADLs.
- Teach client how to avoid problems with orthostatic hypotension.
- Obtain BP while client is standing, lying, and sitting. Make sure client has not had any nicotine or caffeine for about 1 hour before BP is measured.
- Palpate for disappearance of the brachial or radial pulse when assessing BP to avoid the auscultatory gap.
- Compliance problems occur when client must take several medications for BP and cope with other chronic health problems.

*ADLs,* Activities of daily living; *BP,* blood pressure.

---

## Assessment

A. Modifiable risk factors.
  1. Elevated serum cholesterol (low-density lipoprotein [LDL] greater than 100 mg/dL, low high-density lipoprotein cholesterol [HDL-C] ("good" cholesterol) levels females greater than 55 mg/dL and males greater than 45 mg/dL with older adults' ranges increasing with age) and triglyceride (females 35–135 mg/dL and males 40–160 mg/dL) levels.
  2. Sedentary lifestyle, obesity.
  3. Stress, smoking.
B. Nonmodifiable risk factors.
  1. Familial tendencies, age.
  2. Race, gender (men at greater risk than women until age 60).
C. Conditions accelerating atherosclerotic development.
  1. Diabetes mellitus (DM).

# PROGRESSION OF ATHEROSCLEROSIS

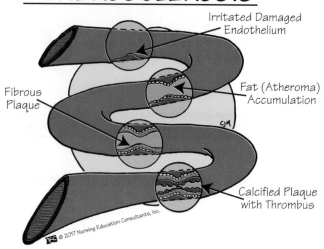

**FIGURE 18-2 Progression of Atherosclerosis.** (From Zerwekh, J., Garneau, A., & Miller, C. J. [2017]. *Digital collection of the memory notebooks of nursing* [4th ed.]. Chandler, AZ: Nursing Education Consultants, Inc.)

  2. Hypertension (HTN).
  3. High cholesterol/triglyceride levels.
D. Clinical manifestations: depends on artery involved.
E. Diagnostics (see Appendix 18-1).

---

**TEST ALERT:** Conduct cholesterol screening sessions and adapt a diet to meet the special needs of a client.

---

## Treatment

A. Decrease risk factors (exercise, stop smoking, decrease weight, decrease stress, decrease fat in diet).
B. Antihyperlipidemic and peripheral vasodilating medications (see Appendix 18-2).
C. Vascular surgery.

**Goal:** To identify individuals at high risk.

A. Screen for and recognize modifiable and nonmodifiable risk factors.
B. Recognize significant deviations of laboratory values (Table 18-1).
C. Identify and control conditions that accelerate atherosclerotic development.
D. Recognize common signs and symptoms of atherosclerosis.

## Hypertension (HTN)

**Hypertension or high blood pressure is an elevation above the normal limit.**

A. Definitions.
  1. Prehypertenstion is a systolic BP of 120 to 139 mmHg or diastolic BP of 80 to 89 mmHg.
  2. Hypertension is the persistent systolic BP of 140 mmHg or more, a diastolic BP of 90 mmHg or more, or current use of antihypertensive medications.

## Table 18-1 CHOLESTEROL AND LIPOPROTEIN LEVELS

| | |
|---|---|
| Cholesterol (total) | Less than 200 mg/dL (5.18 mmol/L) |
| Low-density lipoprotein (LDL) | Less than 130 mg/dL (3.37 mmol/L) |
| High-density lipoprotein (HDL) | Greater than 40 mg/dL (1.04 mmol/L) in males; greater than 50 mg/dL (1.30 mmol/L) in females |
| Triglycerides | Less than 150 mg/dL (1.69 mmol/L) |

3. The goal BP for patients 18 to 59 years without major comorbidities is less than 140/90.
4. The general population aged 60 years and older a desired blood pressure should be below 150/90. If this group has diabetes, chronic kidney disease, or both, the new goal is less than 140/90.

B. Classification (Figure 18-3).
1. Primary hypertension (essential or idiopathic): accounts for approximately 90% to 95% of cases of hypertension; exact cause unknown.

# HYPERTENSION

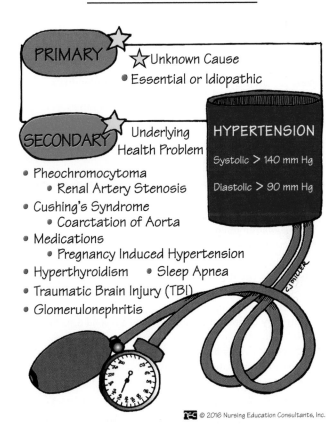

**FIGURE 18-3 Hypertension.** (From Zerwekh, J., Garneau, A., & Miller, C. J. [2017]. *Digital collection of the memory notebooks of nursing* [4th ed.]. Chandler, AZ: Nursing Education Consultants, Inc.)

2. Secondary hypertension: elevated BP with a specific cause that can be identified and corrected; accounts for 5% to 10% of cases of hypertension.
3. Hypertensive crisis or emergency: a sudden and severely elevated BP (often above 180/110 mmHg) with clinical evidence of target organ disease, which may be life threatening (addressed under Critical Care section of this chapter).

## Assessment

A. Risk factors (Table 18-2).
B. Clinical manifestations of primary hypertension.

> ❗ **NURSING PRIORITY:** BP should be evaluated with the client lying, sitting, and standing; readings should be obtained from both arms. Legs should not be crossed.

1. Most often asymptomatic (called "the silent killer").
2. Increase in blood pressure.

## Table 18-2 RISK FACTORS IN ESSENTIAL HYPERTENSION

**Nonmodifiable Factors**

| | |
|---|---|
| Age | Develops between 30 and 50 years of age. Poorer prognosis when developed at younger age. |
| Gender | More prevalent in men under 55 years; after age 55, it is more prevalent in women. |
| Ethnic group | The incidence of hypertension is twice as high among African Americans as among whites. |
| Family history | Clients with parents or siblings who have hypertension are at greater risk for high BP at a younger age. |

**Modifiable Factors**

| | |
|---|---|
| Obesity | Weight gain is associated with increased frequency of hypertension. Central abdominal obesity poses greatest risk. |
| Stress | Sustained or repeated stressors. |
| Substance abuse | Drug abuse, drinking more than 1 oz (30 mL) of alcohol per day, use of tobacco products. |
| Excess sodium intake | Can cause water retention and hypertension, especially in those who are already overweight. |
| Elevated serum lipids | Elevated levels of cholesterol and triglycerides are primary risk factors in atherosclerosis, which is a contributing factor to hypertension. |
| Sedentary lifestyle | Regular physical activity helps decrease risk. |
| Diabetes mellitus | Blood vessel disease associated with diabetes mellitus leads to high risk for hypertension. |
| Diet | Diet high in saturated fats and salt leads to atherosclerotic plaque buildup. |

*BP,* Blood pressure.
Modified from Joint National Committee: *The Eighth Report of the Joint National Committee on Prevention, Detection, Evaluation and Treatment of High Blood Pressure.* Retrieved from http://www.nmhs.net/documents/27JNC8HTNGuidelinesBookBooklet.pdf

**Table 18-3   COMPARISON OF ARTERIAL AND VENOUS PERIPHERAL DISEASE**

| Characteristic | Arterial | Venous |
|---|---|---|
| Peripheral pulses | Decreased or absent | Present; may be difficult to palpate with edema |
| Capillary refill | Greater than 3 sec | Less than 3 sec |
| Ankle-brachial index | Less than/equal to 0.90 | Greater than 0.90 |
| Edema | Absent unless leg constantly in dependent position | Lower leg edema |
| Hair growth | Loss of hair on legs, feet, toes | Hair may be present or absent |
| Ulcer location | Tips of toes, foot or lateral malleolus | Near medial malleolus |
| Ulcer margin | Rounded, smooth, looks "punched out" | Irregularly shaped |
| Ulcer drainage | Minimal | Moderate to large amount |
| Ulcer tissue | Black eschar or pale pink granulation | Yellow slough or dark red, "ruddy" granulation |
| Pain | Intermittent claudication or rest pain in foot; ulcer may or may not be painful | Dull ache or heaviness in calf or thigh; ulcer often painful |
| Nails | Thickened; brittle | Normal or thickened |
| Skin color | Dependent rubor; elevation pallor | Bronze-brown pigmentation; varicose veins may be visible |
| Skin texture | Thin, shiny, taut | Skin thick, hardened, and indurated |
| Skin temperature | Cool, temperature gradient down the leg | Warm, no temperature gradient |
| Dermatitis | Rarely occurs | Frequently occurs |
| Pruritus | Rarely occurs | Frequently occurs |

Adapted from Lewis, S. L., et al. (2017). *Medical-surgical nursing: Assessment and management of clinical problems* (10th ed.). St. Louis, MO: Elsevier/Mosby.

3. Cardiac effects.
   a. Angina, fatigue, activity intolerance
   b. Acute coronary syndrome (ACS)/coronary artery disease (CAD), heart failure.
   c. Left ventricular hypertrophy, palpitations.
4. Cerebrovascular effects.
   a. Transient ischemic attack.
   b. Stroke (cerebrovascular accident (CVA), brain attack).
   c. Dizziness, visual disturbances.
5. Peripheral vascular effects.
   a. Dizziness, visual disturbances.
   b. Atherosclerosis, intermittent claudication.
   c. Arterial insufficiency, venous stasis.
C. Diagnostics.
   1. Increase in blood pressure (utilizing correct blood pressure cuff size) on two separate occasions, even repeated readings at the same visit (Table 18-3).
   2. Diagnostic tests to rule out problem of secondary hypertension.

*Treatment*

A. Dietary management.
   1. Decrease sodium (no more than 2400 mg per day), cholesterol, and saturated fats.
   2. Reduce calories and sweets, use low-fat dairy products.
   3. Limit alcohol and caffeine consumption along with sugar-sweetened beverages.
   4. Consume vegetables, fruits, and whole grains.
B. Regular exercise (walking, jogging, or swimming): 30 to 45 minutes per day, 3 to 5 times a week.

C. Stress management.
D. Avoid all forms of tobacco products.
E. Antihypertensive and diuretic medications (Box 18-2; Appendix 18-2).
F. Control diabetes.

*Nursing Interventions*

**Goal:** To identify and educate high-risk individuals.

A. Conduct community BP screening programs.

**Box 18-2   BLOOD PRESSURE MEDICATION MANAGEMENT**

**Initial Drugs of Choice for Hypertension**
- ACE inhibitor (ACEI)
- Angiotensin receptor blocker (ARB)
- Thiazide diuretic
- Calcium channel blocker (CCB)

**Strategies for Administration**
- Strategy A: Start one drug, titrate to maximum dose, and then add a second drug.
- Strategy B: Start one drug, then add a second drug before achieving max dose of first.
- Strategy C: Begin two drugs at same time, as separate pills or combination pill. Initial combination therapy is recommended if BP is greater than 20/10 mmHg above goal.

*(Note: A strategy is selected based on client's clinical problems and comorbidities.)*
Modified from Joint National Committee: *The Eighth Report of the Joint National Committee on Prevention, Detection, Evaluation and Treatment of High Blood Pressure.* Retrieved from http://www.nmhs.net/documents/27JNC8HTNGuidelinesBookBooklet.pdf

B. Educate the public regarding risk factors (see Table 18-2).
C. Identify health-promoting behavior for high-risk individuals.
  1. Decrease weight; regular BP checkups.
  2. Avoid all tobacco products; limit alcohol and caffeine intake.
  3. Control diabetes; engage in regular exercise.
  4. Teach to take and record BP daily including any symptoms.
  5. Take medications as prescribed especially if BP is within normal limits.

**Goal:** To reduce BP and assist client to maintain control.

A. Assess response to medication regimen.
  1. Educate client and family members on how to take BP.
    a. Client should be seated with arm at heart level.
    b. No tobacco products or caffeine 30 minutes before measurement of BP.
    c. Use appropriate cuff size.
    d. Can use either upper arm or forearm for accurate readings.
    e. Do not cross legs.
  2. BP should be monitored frequently during initial medication dosage adjustments and at least twice a week thereafter, if not daily.
  3. Instruct client regarding possible side effects (Figure 18-4).
    a. Do not suddenly stop taking medications; report side effects to health care provider.
    b. Assure client that side effects are often temporary.
    c. Sexual problems, impotence should be reported.
  4. When BP is initially decreased, evaluate client for:
    a. Postural (orthostatic) hypotension.
    b. Decreased urinary output.
    c. Decrease in energy level and mental alertness.
  5. Assess factors contributing to noncompliance with medications.
    a. Cost of the medication.
    b. Failure to remember or to understand medication schedule or regimen.

### Home Care

A. DASH (**D**ietary **A**pproaches to **S**top **H**ypertension) diet; low-sodium/low-cholesterol diet.
B. Maintain optimum weight.

## ANTIHYPERTENSIVES

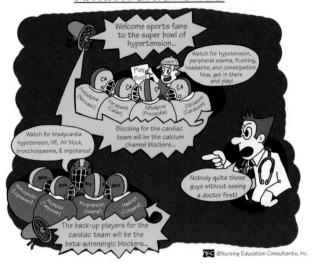

**FIGURE 18-4 Antihypertensives.** (From Zerwekh, J., Garneau, A., & Miller, C. J. [2017]. *Digital collection of the memory notebooks of nursing* [4th ed.]. Chandler, AZ: Nursing Education Consultants, Inc.)

C. Assist to identify an appropriate, consistent, regular exercise program.
  1. A gradually increasing exercise program.
  2. Episodic strenuous activity should be avoided.
  3. Walking, swimming, slow jogging.
  4. Avoid weight lifting and heavy isometric exercises.
D. Limit alcohol intake: 1 drink a day for women and 2 drinks a day for men (1 drink = 12 oz. [360 mL] beer, 5 oz. [150 mL] wine, or 1.5 oz. [45 mL] liquor such as vodka or gin).
E. Stop smoking.
F. Adhere to medication regimen.
  1. Take medication at regular times.
  2. Do not suddenly stop taking medications; call health care provider if experiencing problems with medication regimen; continue taking despite BP within normal ranges and check with physician for further recommendations.
  3. Plan with client a method to keep track of medications (e.g., using daily pill box or marking on calendar).
  4. Notify health care provider if unable to afford medications.
  5. Learn to recognize and report the most common side effects of medications.

G. Avoid hot baths, steam rooms, and spas (increases vasodilation).
H. Decrease and or prevent problems of orthostatic hypotension.
  1. Get up slowly, sit at the bedside to regain equilibrium, and then stand slowly.

2. Wear elastic support hose.
3. Lie or sit down when dizziness occurs.
4. Do not stand or sit for prolonged periods of time.
I. Monitor and record BP regularly; take records to physician visits.

## Aneurysm

**An aneurysm is a dilation or sac formed within the wall of an arterial vessel. The aneurysm may involve only one layer or all layers of the arterial wall.**

A. Types of aneurysms.
  1. Abdominal aortic aneurysm (AAA): occurs primarily in the abdominal aorta below the renal arteries.
  2. Thoracic aortic aneurysm: located in the thoracic area.
  3. Dissecting aneurysm: bleeding between the layers of the vessel wall.

*Assessment*

A. Risk factors.
  1. Atherosclerosis, nicotine use.
  2. Acute coronary syndrome (ACS), coronary artery disease (CAD), peripheral arterial disease (PAD), hypertension (HTN).
  3. Genetic predisposition; male gender.
  4. Obesity.
B. Clinical manifestations.
  1. Abdominal aortic aneurysm (AAA).
    a. May be asymptomatic.
    b. Epigastric, back, flank, or abdominal pain.
    c. Pulsating abdominal mass may be palpable.
    d. Signs of rupture or dissection.
      (1) Severe back pain.
      (2) Rapid hypotension and shock.
      (3) Abdominal distention and tenderness.
      (4) Hematoma formation in the flank region.
  2. Thoracic aortic aneurysm.
    a. Frequently asymptomatic.
    b. Compression of structures in the adjacent area.
    c. Dysphagia due to pressure on the esophagus.
    d. Hoarseness due to pressure on the laryngeal nerve.
    e. Pressure on the vena cava may cause edema of head and arms.
    f. Signs of rupture or dissection.
      (1) Sudden, constant, and excruciating back and chest pain.
      (2) Rapid hypotension, progressing to shock.
D. Diagnostics (see Appendix 18-1).

*Treatment*

A. Medical: risk factor modification.
B. Close monitoring of the aneurysm.

C. Surgical repair of aneurysm as soon as possible.
  1. Endovascular stent graft.
  2. Surgical resection and graft.

*Nursing Interventions*

**Goal:** To prepare client and family for surgery.

A. Provide perioperative care (see Chapter 3).
B. Identify other chronic health problems that will have implications postoperatively (hypertension, diabetes, peripheral vascular disease).
C. Evaluate characteristics of pulses in the lower extremities and mark for evaluation and comparison after surgery (see Figure 18-1 and Table 18-3).
D. Do not vigorously palpate the abdomen.
E. Monitor for indications of dissection or rupture.
F. Maintain BP at level low enough to decrease risk for rupture yet high enough to maintain perfusion.

**Goal:** To promote graft patency and circulation postoperatively.

A. General perioperative care (see Chapter 3).
B. Maintain adequate BP to facilitate tissue perfusion and filling of the graft.
C. Monitor for hemorrhage.
  1. Increasing abdominal girth, back pain.
  2. Symptoms of hypovolemia or shock.
D. Check peripheral circulation, sensation, and movement hourly for first 24 hours.
E. Symptoms of graft occlusion include:
  1. Changes or decrease in quality of pulse.
  2. Extremity cool below level of graft.
  3. Change in color of extremity.
  4. Increase in abdominal distention and increased severity of pain in extremities.
E. If chest tubes are present, monitor function and drainage (see Appendix 17-4).
F. Hourly urine output; hemodynamic monitoring.
G. Evaluate blood urea nitrogen and serum creatinine levels to assess renal function.

 *Home Care*

A. Activity restrictions.
  1. No heavy lifting for 6 to 12 weeks.
  2. Avoid activities that involve pushing, pulling, or straining.
B. Report any signs of infection, redness, swelling, drainage, or fever.

 **Peripheral Artery Disease**

**Also known as peripheral vascular disease (PVD), this disorder involves narrowing and obstruction of the**

arteries, especially the lower extremities. The chronic arterial obstruction progressively leads to decreased oxygen delivery to the tissues.

A. Lesions are predominantly found in the lower aorta below the renal arteries and extend through the popliteal area. Bifurcations at the renal, femoral, popliteal, and aortic iliac arteries are the most commonly affected.
B. By the time symptoms occur, the artery is approximately 85% to 95% occluded.
C. Leads to an increased risk for angina, myocardial infarction, and stroke.

### Assessment

A. Risk factors: see Atherosclerosis.
B. Clinical manifestations (Figure 18-5; and see Table 18-3).
   1. Intermittent claudication.
      a. Muscle pain and cramping with exercise; relieved with rest.
      b. Pain that occurs while resting or at night is indication of advanced stages.
   2. Paresthesia of the feet/lower extremities.
C. Diagnostics (see Appendix 18-1).
D. Complications.
   1. Delayed healing, infection.
   2. Necrosis, ulcerations.
   3. Gangrene/amputation.

## PERIPHERAL VASCULAR DISEASE (PVD)
### ARTERIAL vs VENOUS ULCERS

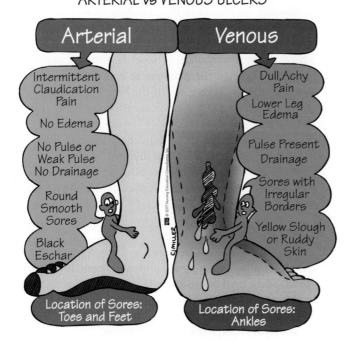

**Arterial**
- Intermittent Claudication Pain
- No Edema
- No Pulse or Weak Pulse No Drainage
- Round Smooth Sores
- Black Eschar
- Location of Sores: Toes and Feet

**Venous**
- Dull, Achy Pain
- Lower Leg Edema
- Pulse Present Drainage
- Sores with Irregular Borders
- Yellow Slough or Ruddy Skin
- Location of Sores: Ankles

**FIGURE 18-5 Peripheral Vascular Disease (PVD).** (From Zerwekh, J., Garneau, A., & Miller, C. J. [2017]. *Digital collection of the memory notebooks of nursing* [4th ed.]. Chandler, AZ: Nursing Education Consultants, Inc.)

### Treatment

A. Medical.
   1. Medication therapy—antihyperlipidemic, anticoagulant, antiplatelet, antihypertensive.
   2. Decrease progression of atherosclerosis.
      a. Stop all tobacco products.
      b. Decrease cholesterol and triglyceride intake.
      c. Reduce weight if needed.
      d. Control sodium intake.
      e. Exercise program as tolerated (especially walking).
      f. Control diabetes and hypertension.
   3. Prevent and control infection.
   4. Proper foot care.
B. Surgical: Procedures are performed when intermittent claudication interferes with the client's activities of daily living or when the circulation must be restored to salvage the limb.
   1. Peripheral atherectomy: removal of plaque within the artery.
   2. Bypass graft: bypass of an obstruction by suturing a graft proximally and distally to the obstruction.
   3. Patch graft angioplasty: artery is opened, plaque is removed, and a patch is sutured in the opening to widen the lumen.
   4. Amputation: used as a last resort when other therapies have failed and gangrene or infection is extensive.
C. Nonsurgical.
   1. Percutaneous transluminal balloon angioplasty (PTCA): use of a balloon catheter to compress the plaque against the arterial wall.
   2. Laser-assisted angioplasty: a probe is advanced through a cannula to the area of occlusion; a laser is used to vaporize the atherosclerotic plaque.
   3. Intravascular stent: placement of a stent within a narrowed vessel to maintain patency.

### Nursing Interventions

**TEST ALERT:** Identify client with a condition that increases the risk for insufficient vascular perfusion; assess client for abnormal peripheral pulses.

**Goal:** To assess for characteristics of arterial versus venous disease (see Table 18-3).

A. Assess and compare quality of peripheral pulses (see Figure 18-1, Figure 18-6).
B. Evaluate skin of the affected extremity.
   1. Color, warmth, capillary refill.
   2. Condition of the skin and nail beds.
   3. Presence of ulcers or lesions, and stages of healing.
C. Assess tolerance to activity; determine at what point claudication occurs and whether pain at rest is present.

**TEST ALERT:** Interpret client data that need to be reported immediately.

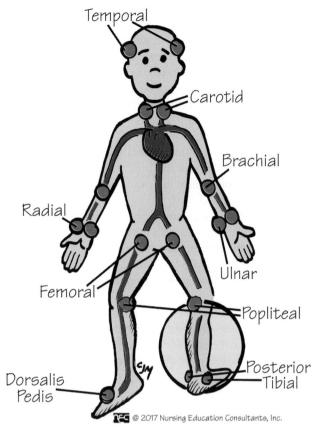

Temporal
Carotid
Brachial
Radial
Ulnar
Femoral
Popliteal
Dorsalis Pedis
Posterior Tibial

© 2017 Nursing Education Consultants, Inc.

**FIGURE 18-6** Common Sites for Palpating Arteries. (From Zerwekh, J., Garneau, A., & Miller, C. J. [2017]. *Digital collection of the memory notebooks of nursing* [4th ed.]. Chandler, AZ: Nursing Education Consultants, Inc.)

**Goal:** To prevent injury and infection.

A. Avoid vigorous rubbing of the extremity.
B. Prevent skin breakdown at pressure sites. Use heel covers and bed cradle to prevent pressure on the toes and heels.
C. Visually inspect extremities for discolored areas, breaks in skin, and signs of infection.
D. Maintain good skin hygiene and proper care of toenails.
   1. Encourage patients to see a podiatrist to trim toenails rather than doing this themselves.
   2. Do not trim calluses or corns.
   3. Seek treatment immediately for ingrown toenail or ulceration formation.
   4. Keep feet clean and dry, do not soak feet, use lubricating lotion to prevent skin cracks.
   5. Teach client to always wear well-fitting shoes; wear cotton socks, avoid shoes or socks that are too tight.

**Goal:** To increase arterial blood supply.

A. Encourage moderate exercise (e.g., walking).
   1. Level of pain should be a guide to exercise; activity should be stopped when pain occurs.
   2. Goal is 30 to 60 minutes per day, 3 to 5 days a week.
B. Promote blood flow to legs.
   1. Avoid standing in one position for prolonged periods.
   2. Avoid crossing legs at the knees or ankles while in bed. Do not raise knee gatch of the bed without

raising the foot of the bed to eliminate pressure behind the knee.
   3. Swelling may develop. Teach to avoid raising legs above the heart level as it decreases arterial blood flow to the feet. Hanging affected leg from the bed or sitting in an upright chair may decrease discomfort.
   4. Provide warmth (room temperature, extra clothing, blankets). Never apply external heat or cold to the extremities.
   5. Avoid pressure in the posterior popliteal area; avoid positions, clothing, or bandages that restrict circulation to the lower extremities (hose, girdles, elastic bandages, etc.).
   6. When client is sitting in a chair, make sure the feet are flat on the floor to decrease pressure from the edge of the chair behind the knee.
   7. Inspect feet daily for color changes or development of skin irritation/sores.
C. Prevent vasoconstriction.
   1. Decrease caffeine intake.
   2. Stop all tobacco use.
   3. Avoid becoming chilled, keep lower extremities warm.

**Goal:** To evaluate and promote circulation in affected extremity after vascular surgery.

A. Frequent assessment to determine adequacy of circulation and patency of graft.
   1. Circulation checks distal to the graft every 15 minutes × 4, then hourly × 24 hour; notify health care provider immediately of any changes in neurocirculatory status of extremities.
   2. Monitor ankle-brachial index (ABI) measurements.
   3. Assess for compartmental syndrome (see Chapter 23) and graft thrombosis.
B. Encourage movement of the extremity as soon as client is awake; avoid flexion in the area of the graft (femoral or popliteal area).
C. Assist client to ambulate as soon as possible; perform pulse checks when client returns to bed.
D. Do not raise the knee gatch of the bed.
E. Monitor anticoagulation medications; maintain bleeding precautions.
F. Assess for development of dependent edema; may require compression dressings or diuretic.
G. Notify surgeon or health care provider immediately of any symptoms suggestive of a further decrease in circulation or occlusion of graft.

## Home Care

A. Decrease weight if appropriate.
B. Avoid standing or sitting for prolonged periods of time.
C. Teach client methods to increase circulation during normal workday (do not cross legs; use a good chair; get up and walk every hour if working at a desk).
D. Avoid tight socks, stockings, or clothing.
E. Avoid trauma to the extremities—always wear shoes.
F. Avoid tobacco products and caffeine.
G. Wash and visually inspect feet daily; dry well between toes. Use a mirror to observe bottoms of feet.

H. Do not apply any type of direct heat or cold to the legs.

I. Lubricate dry skin; do not use lotions on open lesions or between the toes.

J. Seek professional care for calluses, corns, blisters, ulcers, etc.

K. File toenails straight across or see podiatrist for nail care and feet assessment.

L. Wear cotton socks and shoes that fit well; avoid shoes/nylon socks that cause feet to perspire.

M. Notify health care provider of:
1. Presence of lesions or blisters that do not heal, or infections on an extremity.
2. Increase in pain or decrease in exercise tolerance.

N. Instruct client and family on use of prescribed medications and common side effects.

## Raynaud's Phenomenon

**Raynaud's phenomenon consists of intermittent episodic spasms of the arterioles, most frequently in the fingers, toes, ears, and tip of the nose. Spasms are not necessarily correlated with other peripheral vascular problems.**

### *Assessment*

A. Risk factors/etiology.
1. Women 20 to 40 years of age.
2. Occupation related.
3. Tobacco use.
4. Associated with connective tissue diseases such as systemic lupus erythematosus and rheumatoid arthritis.

B. Clinical manifestations (Figure 18-7).
1. Symptoms are precipitated by:
   a. Exposure to cold.
   b. Emotional upset.
   c. Nicotine and caffeine intake.
2. Decreased perfusion leads to:
   a. Pallor and waxy appearance of tissue in the vasoconstrictive phase.
   b. Numbness and tingling.
   c. Throbbing, aching, tingling, and burning in the hyperemic phase.

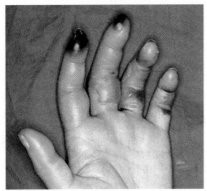

**FIGURE 18-7 Raynaud's Disease.** (From Kamal, A., & Brockelhurst, J. C. [1991]. *Color atlas of geriatric medicine* [2nd ed.]. St. Louis, MO: Mosby.)

3. Pulses usually unaffected.
4. Involvement bilateral.
5. Attacks are intermittent and last only a few minutes.

C. Diagnostics.
1. Based on history.
2. Presence of clinical manifestations.

D. Complications: may progress to ulceration/gangrene in severe cases.

### *Treatment*

A. Medical.
1. No cure; treatment is based on symptoms.
2. Medications: vasodilators, calcium channel blockers.

B. Surgical: sympathectomy.

### *Nursing Interventions*

**Goal:** To assist client in understanding disease implications and measures to decrease episodic attacks.

A. Prevent vasospasms.
1. Wear gloves when handling cold objects (items from the refrigerator or freezer).
2. Protect feet, hands, nose, and ears when exposed to cold weather.
3. Maintain warm environment.
4. Avoid caffeine and tobacco products.
5. Stress management.
6. Avoid vasoconstrictive drugs.

## Thromboangiitis Obliterans (Buerger's Disease)

**Thromboangiitis obliterans is a condition that causes vasculitis of the small and medium-size arteries and veins of the extremities.**

### *Assessment*

A. Risk factors.
1. Very strong relationship with tobacco use.
2. A type of arteritis that damages arterial walls.

B. Clinical manifestations.
1. Intermittent claudication; pain at rest in advanced stages; pain is the predominant symptom.
2. Ischemic ulcerations and gangrene may develop in fingers, toes, and then progress upward.
3. Temperature changes in affected limb.
4. Increased sensitivity to cold in the extremity.
5. Peripheral pulses may be diminished or absent.
6. Cyanosis and redness of the extremity.

C. Diagnostics.
1. Based on clinical manifestations.
2. Sometimes difficult to distinguish from PAD.

D. Complications: ulcerations and gangrene.

### *Treatment*

A. No cure; treatment is based on symptoms. Cessation of all tobacco use early in the disease can stop symptoms and progression of the disease. Exercise is also recommended to promote circulation in the lower extremities.

B. Medications: vasodilators, antiplatelets, calcium channel blockers.

C. Surgical therapy.
   1. Sympathectomy, revascularization.
   2. Amputation in extreme cases.

### Nursing Interventions

**Goal:** To evaluate level of involvement and increase circulation to the extremity.

A. Decrease or stop all tobacco use (also exposure to secondhand smoke).

B. Evaluate tolerance to activity.

C. Inspect feet for vascular changes.

D. Avoid extreme cold.

E. Perform circulatory checks of the affected extremity.

> **!** **NURSING PRIORITY:** The vascular problem has a direct relationship to cigarette smoking. For the condition to be controlled, the client must quit smoking.

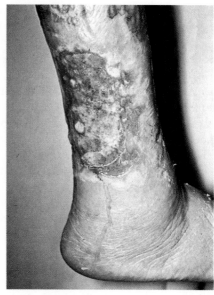

**FIGURE 18-8  Venous Leg Ulcer.** (From Kamal, A., & Brockelhurst, J. C. [1991]. *Color atlas of geriatric medicine* [2nd ed.]. St. Louis: Mosby.)

### Peripheral Venous Disease/(PVD) (Chronic Venous Insufficiency (CVI)/Venous Stasis Ulcers)

**Peripheral venous disease (PVD)/chronic venous insufficiency (CVI) is an alteration of the natural flow of blood through the veins of the peripheral circulation. Caused by thrombus formation and/or defective valves, this leads to regurgitation of blood, venous pooling, and edema in the lower extremities, eventually resulting in development of venous leg ulcers.**

### Assessment

A. Risk factors.
   1. Advancing age, increased venous pressure.
   2. Diabetes, obesity.
   3. Varicosities, prolonged immobility.
   4. Virchow triad (Box 18-3).
   5. Previous episode of DVT.
   6. Incompetence of the valves in the lower extremities.

B. Clinical manifestations (see Table 18-3; Figure 18-8).
   1. Stasis eczema leading to chronic itching. Trauma to the skin from scratching leads to breakdown and ulceration.
   2. "Brawny," leathery appearance to skin of lower leg.
   3. Sclerosis occurs as a result of long-standing edema; leg becomes larger at the calf.

   4. Ulcerations more commonly near the outer ankle.
   5. Ulcer appearance: irregular margins, copious exudate.
   6. Very painful.

C. Diagnostics: history and clinical manifestations.

> **!** **NURSING PRIORITY:** It is essential to distinguish between arterial and venous ulcers, as treatment methods are different.

D. Complications.
   1. Infection, cellulitis.
   2. Delayed or poor healing due to stasis of blood in the lower extremities.

### Treatment

A. Medical therapy.
   1. Compression therapy.
      a. Elastic compression stockings.
      b. Sequential compression devices.
      c. Unna boot (a paste bandage).
   2. Moist dressings.
   3. Good nutritional status.
   4. Treatment of varicose veins.
   5. Use of a wound vacuum in difficult cases.

B. Surgical therapy: excision of ulcer with skin grafting.

### Nursing Interventions

**Goal:** To prevent and treat venous stasis (Box 18-4).

A. Compression devices: prevention of venous stasis is the key to healing.
   1. Compression boots/stockings: extremity may be covered with continuous compression bandage, boot, or stocking.

---

**Box 18-3  VIRCHOW TRIAD**

**Three factors contributing to venous thrombosis.**
- Venous stasis
- Damage of endothelium of vein
- Hypercoagulability of the blood

- Encourage mobility; even standing at the bedside promotes venous tone.
- Elastic support stockings:
  - Hospitalized clients should wear them all the time.
  - Home clients generally wear them during the day. They should be put on before getting out of bed and removed when going to bed.
  - Toe hole should be under the toes and heel patch over the heel.
  - Make sure stockings are not causing increased pressure behind the knee, and do not allow stocking to bunch up and cause constriction behind the knee.
  - Do not hang feet dependently when putting stockings on; elevate the legs or put them parallel on the bed.
  - Make sure that stockings are the correct fit by measuring the legs and ordering the appropriate size and length.
- Teach client to elevate legs for about 20 minutes every 4 or 5 hours.
- Avoid prolonged sitting; walk around every 1 to 2 hours.
- Do not cross legs when sitting or lying in bed.
- Do not wear restrictive clothing.
- Maintain adequate fluid intake; avoid dehydration.
- Pneumatic sequential compression devices (SCDs) may be used in the hospital on clients at increased risk for complications secondary to venous stasis.
  - Remove every 8 hours to inspect skin.
  - If client is at high risk for development of thrombophlebitis, measure area to determine whether there is an increase in size of calf or thigh.
  - Assess legs for areas of warmth, tenderness, or inflammation.

2. Intermittent or sequential pneumatic compression devices: always check arterial circulation with any type of compression device.
3. Always assess adequacy of arterial circulation before compression therapy.

**TEST ALERT:** Implement measures to promote venous return, to manage potential circulatory complications, and to monitor wounds for signs and symptoms of infection.

**Goal:** To prevent infection and promote healing.

A. Keep feet clean and dry; assess for development of venous ulcers.
B. Apply moist oxygen-permeable dressings (e.g., hydrocolloids, foams).
C. Change dressings as necessary due to excessive wound drainage.
D. Prevent itching and breaks in skin from scratching.

E. Encourage increase in protein and vitamins to promote healing.
F. Maintain adequate blood perfusion and oxygen levels to tissue.

**TEST ALERT:** Perform or assist with dressing changes; provide wound care (e.g., central line dressing or wound dressings).

## Venous Thromboembolism/(VTE) (Thrombophlebitis)

**Venous thromboembolism (VTE) is the presence of a clot in a vein; it may be a superficial (SVT) or a deep vein thrombosis (DVT). Phlebitis is inflammation of a superficial vein without the presence of a clot (thrombus).**

*Assessment*

A. Risk factors (Virchow triad—see Box 18-3).
  1. Venous stasis.
    a. Surgery (especially hip, pelvic, and orthopedic surgery).
    b. Pregnancy, obesity, prolonged immobility.
    c. Heart disease (atrial fibrillation, heart failure).
  2. Hypercoagulability.
    a. Malignancies, dehydration.
    b. Blood dyscrasias.
    c. Oral contraceptives, hormone replacement therapy.
    d. Pregnancy and postpartum.
  3. Endothelial damage.
    a. IV fluids and drugs (IV catheterization, drug abuse, caustic solutions, or drugs).
    b. Fractures and dislocations (especially of the pelvis, hip, or leg).
    c. History of VTE/diabetes.

**TEST ALERT:** Provide measures to prevent complications of immobility.

B. Clinical manifestations.
  1. Firm, palpable, cordlike vein.
  2. Area around vein is tender to touch, reddened, and warm.
  3. Temperature elevation (greater than 100.4°F [38.0°C]).
  4. Extremity pain and edema.
  5. Elevated white blood cell count and positive blood culture.
C. Diagnostics (see Appendix 18-1).
D. Complications.
  1. Pulmonary emboli.
  2. Chronic venous insufficiency, venous stasis ulcers.

*Treatment*

A. Medical.
  1. Bed rest with elevation of the affected extremity.
  2. Anticoagulant, antiinflammatory, and fibrinolytic medications.

3. Warm moist packs.
4. Elastic support stockings only on unaffected leg during period of bed rest.
5. Prevent complications of immobility.

B. Surgical (done to prevent formation of pulmonary emboli).
   1. Venous thrombectomy.
   2. Vena cava interruption device.

*Nursing Interventions*

**Goal:** To prevent VTE.

> ⚠ **NURSING PRIORITY:** The most effective way to prevent the development of a pulmonary embolus is to prevent the development of VTE.

A. Nursing measures to decrease venous stasis (see Box 18-4).
B. Prevent complications of immobilization (see Chapter 3).
C. Prophylactic anticoagulation for the high-risk client.
D. Intermittent compression devices for high-risk clients.

> **TEST ALERT:** Identify client with condition that increases risk for insufficient vascular perfusion; intervene to promote venous return.

### 🗲 Home Care

A. Avoid oral contraceptives or oral hormone replacement therapy (HRT).
B. Avoid all nicotine products.
C. Use methods to decrease venous stasis (see Box 18-4).
D. Exercise regularly (especially walking).
E. Decrease weight, if appropriate.
F. Decrease sodium in diet if edema is present.
G. Follow instructions regarding anticoagulation therapy at home.
H. Recognize and respond to signs and symptoms of pulmonary emboli.

###  Varicose Veins

**Varicose veins occur when veins in the lower trunk and extremities become congested and dilated as a result of incompetent valves in the vessels and loss of elasticity of the vessel walls.**

*Assessment*

A. Risk factors/etiology.
   1. Congenital weakness of the vein wall.
   2. Obesity, pregnancy.
   3. Increasing age.
   4. Work settings requiring prolonged sitting or standing.
B. Clinical manifestations.
   1. Dilated, tortuous subcutaneous veins.

2. Objectionable cosmetic appearance of the vein.
3. Aching leg pain after prolonged standing.
4. Pain is generally relieved by elevating the extremity.
5. Nocturnal leg cramps.

C. Diagnostics:
   1. Positive Trendelenburg test.
   2. Physical appearance, duplex ultrasound

## TREATMENT

A. Medical: prevent venous stasis (see Box 18-4).
B. Surgical.
   1. Noninvasive laser therapy or high-intensity pulsed-light therapy.
   2. Sclerotherapy: injection of sclerosing agent into the affected vein.
   3. Surgical ligation of the veins; may be combined with vein stripping as well.
   4. Endovenous ablation—collapse and sclerosis of vein.

*Nursing Interventions*

**Goal:** To improve circulation and prevent complications.

A. Decrease venous stasis.
B. Facilitate venous return.
   1. Elastic stockings or compression wraps.
   2. Sequential compression devices.
   3. Frequent contraction of calf muscles.
C. Avoid constrictive clothing.
D. Avoid prolonged standing or sitting.

## CRITICAL CARE

### PRIORITY CONCEPTS

Gas Exchange, Perfusion

### 🗒 Hypertensive Crisis

**Hypertensive crisis is a term used to indicate either a hypertensive urgency (develops over days to weeks; no target organ damage) or a hypertensive emergency (develops over hours to days). BP is severely elevated over 180/110 (often greater than 220/140 mmHg) (Figure 18-9).**

*Assessment*

A. Risk factors/etiology.
   1. History of hypertension and noncompliance with or nonappropriate medication therapy.
   2. Cocaine or crack use; amphetamines; phencyclidine (PCP), lysergic acid diethylamide (LSD).
   3. Pheochromocytoma.
   4. Head injury, acute aortic dissection.
B. Clinical manifestations.
   1. Hypertensive emergency—sudden rise in BP with severe headache, nausea, vomiting, seizures, confusion, coma.
   2. Renal insufficiency to renal failure.

# HYPERTENSIVE CRISIS

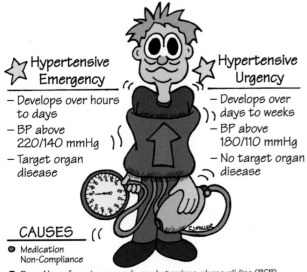

**Hypertensive Emergency**
- Develops over hours to days
- BP above 220/140 mmHg
- Target organ disease

**Hypertensive Urgency**
- Develops over days to weeks
- BP above 180/110 mmHg
- No target organ disease

## CAUSES
- Medication Non-Compliance
- Drug Abuse [cocaine or crack, amphetamines, phencyclidine (PCP), lysergic acid diethylamide (LSD)]
- Head Injury
- Preeclampsia/Eclampsia
- Pheochromocytoma
- MAOI Meds with Tyramine-Containing Foods
- Acute Aortic Dissection

© 2016 Nursing Education Consultants, Inc.

**FIGURE 18-9 Hypertensive Crisis.** (From Zerwekh, J., Garneau, A., & Miller, C. J. [2017]. *Digital collection of the memory notebooks of nursing* [4th ed.]. Chandler, AZ: Nursing Education Consultants, Inc.)

3. Rapid cardiac decompensation—unstable angina, myocardial infarction, pulmonary edema possible.
4. Neurologic symptoms similar to a stroke (typical no focal or lateralizing signs).

## Treatment
A. Medical: IV antihypertensive medications (vasodilators, nitroglycerin).

## Nursing Interventions
**Goal:** To reduce BP in hypertensive crisis.

A. Administer oxygen.
B. Administer antihypertensive drugs via intravenous (IV) drip.
   1. Monitor BP every 5 to 15 minutes until diastolic is below 90.
   2. Monitor BP closely to ensure that BP is not lowered too quickly. Lowering BP too rapidly may compromise cerebral, renal, or coronary circulation.
C. BP should be monitored via an intraarterial line; titrate medication accordingly.
D. Hourly urine output to monitor renal perfusion.
E. Frequent neurologic checks.
F. Maintain client on bed rest while receiving IV antihypertensive medications.

## Shock

**Shock is a failure of the circulatory system to maintain adequate perfusion of vital organs.**

### Assessment

Signs and symptoms of shock are essentially the same, regardless of the precipitating cause.

A. Risk factors.
   1. Increased incidence in the very young and very old.
   2. Increased incidence in clients with chronic progressive disease states.
   3. Trauma, hemorrhage.
B. Classifications of shock (Table 18-4).
C. Clinical manifestations.
   1. Compensatory stage (early). The body is able to compensate by vasoconstriction or shunting of blood. BP is low but sufficient to perfuse vital organs.
      a. Client is oriented but may be restless or apprehensive with increased anxiety.
      b. BP—low normal; pulse—increased or normal; respirations—increased; temperature—normal or subnormal.

| Table 18-4 | CLASSIFICATION OF SHOCK | | |
|---|---|---|---|
| **Classification** | **Pathophysiology** | **Conditions** | **Treatment and Clinical Implications** |
| Hypovolemic | Reduced venous return due to reduced blood volume; 15%–25% reduction in volume. | Hemorrhage, burns, severe fluid loss, severe dehydration, ascites | 1. Administer volume replacement: blood transfusion and volume expanders. 2. Administer oxygen. 3. Will have decreased CVP/BP. |
| Cardiogenic | Heart unable to effectively circulate volume needed to meet tissue demands. | Dysrhythmias, MI, HF cardiomyopathy | 1. Administer oxygen 2. Monitor ECG/BP continuously. 3. Medications to increase cardiac output. 4. Evaluate hemodynamic parameters (see Appendix 19-5). 5. Treat dysrhythmias. |

*Continued*

**Table 18-4    CLASSIFICATION OF SHOCK—cont'd**

| Classification | Pathophysiology | Conditions | Treatment and Clinical Implications |
|---|---|---|---|
| Obstructive | Physical impediment to the flow of blood. | Pericardial tamponade, pulmonary embolism, vena cava compression, tension pneumothorax | 1. Will have increased CVP.<br>2. Treatment directed toward release of obstruction. |
| **Distributive (Three Types):** | | | |
| Neurogenic | Caused by widespread vasodilation.<br>Cardiac function and blood volume may be normal. | Spinal cord injury (T5 or higher), drug overdose, hypoglycemia, spinal anesthesia | 1. Administer vasoconstrictor medications.<br>2. Evaluate closely for fluid overload.<br>3. Bradycardia may require treatment (atropine). |
| Septic | Dilation of blood vessels by humoral or vasoactive substances. | Overwhelming infection; generally gram-negative organism | 1. Evaluate for origin of infection.<br>2. IV fluids, volume expanders.<br>3. Cardiotonics.<br>4. Administer oxygen. |
| Anaphylactic | Antigen–antibody reaction with release of histamine, causing vasodilation and relative hypovolemia. | Transfusion reactions, insect bites, side effect of medications, dye/food allergies | 1. Maintain airway: problem with laryngeal edema.<br>2. Oxygen as indicated.<br>3. Epinephrine and diphenhydramine, IV. |

> ⏹ **NURSING PRIORITY:** Shock is a dynamic condition. The client's status is constantly changing, either improving or deteriorating.

*CVP,* Central venous pressure; *ECG,* electrocardiogram; *HF,* heart failure; *IV,* intravenous; *MI,* myocardial infarction.

c. Urine output may be slightly decreased but within normal range.

d. Mean arterial pressure (MAP) may decrease 10 to 15 mmHg from baseline; poor perfusion of extremities with decreasing pulse pressure; vital organs are perfused.

e. Complaints of thirst and feeling cool; skin pale and cool.

f. Nausea/vomiting common as BP decreases.

2. Progressive stage (intermediate). The body can no longer maintain an adequate supply of oxygenated blood to the tissues and vital organs. Worsening of symptoms associated with decreased tissue perfusion.

a. Decreasing sensory perception; decreased responsiveness to stimuli.

b. Vital signs.

(1) Decrease in MAP of 20 mmHg or more.

(2) Pulse rate increased with weak or thready, peripheral pulses.

(3) Respirations—rate is increased with dyspnea.

c. Cold, moist skin; pallor.

d. Decrease in urine to oliguric levels.

3. Refractory (irreversible, late). Cellular ischemia and necrosis lead to organ failure and death.

a. Progressively decreasing level of consciousness to unresponsiveness, then death.

b. BP—not measurable (unable to perfuse vital organs); pulse—slow and irregular; respirations—irregular, labored.

c. Anuria.

d. Hypoxia, develops metabolic acidosis; unlikely to recover.

D. Diagnostics: based on the clinical manifestations and history of underlying problems.

### Treatment

Depends on the underlying problem and promptness of intervention.

A. Treat underlying cause.

B. IV access and fluid resuscitation to restore intravascular volume.

C. Position supine to increase venous return but not compromise pulmonary status.

D. Medication therapy to restore vasomotor tone and cardiac function (see Appendix 18-2).

E. Supplemental oxygen therapy and mechanical ventilation.

F. Hemodynamic monitoring (see Appendix 19-5).

### Nursing Interventions

**Goal:** To identify and correct cause of shock.

A. Rapid response to developing signs or symptoms.

1. Maintain bed rest.

2. Position supine; may elevate legs.

3. Maintain airway; provide supplemental oxygen.

4. Keep warm; no chilling.

5. Protect from falls and injury.

B. Evaluate for progression of shock—compensating to noncompensating.

**Goal:** To maintain adequate respiratory function.

A. Administer high-flow oxygen (100%).
  1. Nonrebreather mask, bag and valve mask.
  2. Mechanical ventilation as indicated.
B. Monitor oxygenation.
  1. Pulse oximetry, ABGs.
  2. Breath sounds.
  3. Orientation level, presence of confusion.

**Goal:** To maintain adequate circulation and/or tissue perfusion.

A. Control bleeding.
B. Maintain fluid volume.
  1. Blood and/or blood products.
  2. IV fluids, volume expanders (colloid solutions).
  3. Monitor intake and output.
C. Ensure venous access.
  1. Two large-bore (14- to 16-gauge) peripheral lines or central line for IV medications and fluid resuscitation.
  2. Intramuscular (IM), subcutaneous, and oral medications generally not given because of inadequate and/or unpredictable absorption.
D. Cardiogenic shock and neurogenic shock do not involve decreased circulating blood volume; monitor closely for fluid overload.

**Goal:** To maintain cardiac output and vascular tone.

A. Monitor hemodynamic changes.
  1. Monitor central venous pressure (CVP), MAP, pulmonary artery wedge pressure (PAWP); integrate data with assessment data and infusion of vasopressor drugs (see Appendix 19-5).
  2. Administer fluids to increase circulating volume.
  3. Assess adequacy of end organ perfusion (urine output, orientation, peripheral pulses).
B. Medication therapy (see Appendix 18-2).

**TEST ALERT:** Adjust/titrate dosage of medications based on assessment of physiologic parameters (e.g., titrating medication to maintain a specific BP). Assess client for continued decreased cardiac output; interpret data that need to be reported immediately.

C. Monitor renal response and urinary output.
  1. Urinary catheter, hourly output measurements.
  2. Maintain output greater than 30 mL/hr.
  3. Monitor blood urea nitrogen and creatinine.

**Goal:** To maintain homeostasis.

A. Ongoing neurologic evaluation.
  1. Check orientation status and loss of consciousness frequently. Reorient as needed.
  2. Minimize sensory overload caused by hospital environment.
B. Evaluate gastrointestinal (GI) status.
  1. Maintain nothing by mouth (NPO) status and provide frequent oral hygiene.
  2. Monitor bowel sounds and distention.
  3. Possible nasogastric tube in presence of paralytic ileus and/or visceral ischemia.
C. Provide emotional support.
  1. Keep client informed of procedures and tests.
  2. Solicit support for family members (i.e., social worker, clergy, etc.).
  3. Keep family members informed of client's condition.

| Appendix 18-1 | VASCULAR DIAGNOSTICS | | |
|---|---|---|---|
| Test | Normal Value | Therapeutic Value | Nursing Implications |
| **Serum Studies** | | | |
| Fragment D-dimer (D-dimer test) | <250 ng/mL | <250 ng/mL | 1. Produced by the action of plasma on fibrin, verifies fibrinolysis has occurred. 2. Used in diagnosis of DIC and to screen for venous thromboembolism, acute MI, and PE. |
| PT (prothrombin time) | 10–13 sec range | 1.5–2.5 times normal | 1. Sensitive to alterations in vitamin K. 2. Limit intake of foods with vitamin K. 3. Used to evaluate liver function and response to warfarin medications. 4. Watch for blood dyscrasias. |
| aPTT (activated partial thromboplastin time) | Activated: 24–36 sec | 1.5–2.5 times normal | 1. Indicator of adequacy of anticoagulation with heparin. 2. Do not draw sample from extremity with a heparin lock or infusion. 3. Watch for blood dyscrasias. |
| INR (international normalized ratio) | | 2–3 (anticoagulation) | 1. Calculated level based on PT; method of standardizing values. 2. Used to evaluate warfarin. |
| ACT (activated coagulation time) | 80–135 sec | 180–240 sec or 2 times normal | 1. Used to evaluate anticoagulation with heparin. |

## Appendix 18-1 VASCULAR DIAGNOSTICS—cont'd

### Invasive Studies

**Magnetic Resonance Angiography (MRA):** Involves contrast medium injected to help visualize blood flow through peripheral arteries. Most common test used.

See Appendix 19-1 for nursing care.

**Venography (Phlebography):** Involves injection of a radiopaque dye into either the artery or the vein; x-ray films are obtained to identify atherosclerotic plaque, occlusion, injury, or presence of an aneurysm.

Nursing care should include:
1. Explain procedure to client. Mild sedative may be indicated.
2. Requires an informed consent to be signed.
3. Postprocedure:
   a. Frequent circulatory checks distal to the puncture site.
   b. Monitor for allergic reactions to the dye.
   c. Apply pressure dressing to arterial puncture site and monitor for bleeding.

### Noninvasive Studies

**Doppler Ultrasonography:** Handheld Doppler device used to detect flow of blood in peripheral arterial disease; is not sensitive to early disease changes.

**Ankle-Brachial Index (ABI):** Calculated index using a handheld Doppler; divide the ankle SBP by the highest brachial SBP; normal = 1.00 to 1.30; moderate PAD = 0.41 to 0.70.

**Venous/Arterial Duplex Scan:** Uses a color Doppler to trace blood flow through an artery or vein. Has become the primary diagnostic tool for VTE because it allows for visualization of the vein.

**Computed Tomography (CT):** Allows for visualization of the arterial wall and adjacent structures; used for diagnosis of abdominal aortic aneurysm, graft occlusions.

**Trendelenburg Test:** To test for venous incompetence. Client lies supine with leg elevated to promote venous drainage; a tourniquet is applied at midthigh, and client is asked to stand. Veins normally fill from below or distally; a varicose vein will fill from above or proximally because of the incompetent valves. Do not leave tourniquet in place longer than 1 minute.

*DIC,* Diffuse intravascular coagulation; *MI,* myocardial infarction; *PAD,* peripheral artery disease; *PE,* pulmonary embolism; *SBP,* systolic blood pressure; *VTE,* venous thromboembolism.

## Appendix 18-2 MEDICATIONS

**Antihyperlipidemic Medications:** Decrease LDL cholesterol but preferably not the HDL cholesterol. Used in combination with dietary restrictions, exercise, and smoking cessation to reduce blood lipid levels.

### General Nursing Implications
- Serum liver enzymes should be monitored throughout therapy.
- Medications should be taken before evening meal or at bedtime.
- Medications should be used in conjunction with other lipid-lowering therapies (exercise, low-cholesterol diet, smoking cessation).
- Serum cholesterol and triglyceride levels should be monitored before and periodically throughout therapy.
- When taking statins, avoid grapefruit and grapefruit juice in the diet.

**Primary Prevention Guidelines**
- LDL-C levels equal to or greater than 190 mg/dL should be evaluated for secondary causes.
- Diabetics age 40 to 75 should be treated with high-intensity statin therapy.
- Adults 40 to 75 with LDL-C of 70 to 189 mg/dL without clinical signs of ASCVD or DM should be treated with moderate- to high-intensity statins.

| Appendix 18-2 | MEDICATIONS—cont'd | |
|---|---|---|

| Medications | Side Effects | Nursing Implications |
|---|---|---|
| Colesevelam: PO<br>Colestipol: PO<br>Cholestyramine: PO | Constipation<br>Bloating<br>Indigestion | 1. Increase fiber and fluid intake to prevent constipation.<br>2. Administer other medications 1 hour before or 6 hours after these meds. |
| Nicotinic acid: PO | Flushing<br>GI disturbances<br>Hyperglycemia<br>Gouty arthritis | 1. Immediately report signs of hepatotoxicity (darkening of urine, light-colored stools, anorexia).<br>2. Flushing can be decreased by premedicating with a NSAID 30 min before administration. |
| Gemfibrozil: PO<br>Fenofibrate: PO | Diarrhea<br>GI disturbances<br>Hematuria<br>Gallstones | 1. Assess for increase in muscle pain.<br>2. Will potentiate warfarin-derivative anticoagulants. |
| Lovastatin: PO<br>Simvastatin: PO<br>Fluvastatin: PO<br>Atorvastatin: PO<br>Pravastatin: PO<br>Rosuvastatin: PO<br>Pitavastatin: PO | Rhabdomyolysis<br>Elevated liver enzymes<br>GI disturbances | 1. Give with evening meal.<br>2. Should not be given to clients with preexisting liver disease.<br>3. Assess for increase in muscle pain.<br>4. Monitor liver enzymes closely.<br>5. Do not confuse pravastatin with lansoprazole.<br>6. Simvastatin has multiple drug interactions. |
| Ezetimibe: PO | Hepatotoxic<br>Cholecystitis | 1. Assess for increase in muscle pain.<br>2. Monitor liver enzymes closely. |
| Combination drugs-<br>Ezetimibe and simvastatin: PO<br>Amlodipine and atorvastatin: PO<br>Niacin and lovastatin: PO | Hepatotoxic<br>May interact with other drugs such as warfarin, cyclosporine, and some antibiotics<br>Watch for drug combinations and potential effects not related to lipids (for example BP) | 1. Combination drugs may assist with compliance to drug regime.<br>2. Monitor liver enzymes, BP, and muscle discomfort depending on drug combination. |
| Icosapent ethyl: PO | Arthralgias | 1. Used for patients with hypertriglyceridemia levels greater than 500 |
| Evolocumab: SQ<br>Alirocumab: SQ<br>Taken every 2-4 weeks | Injection site discomfort, muscle/limb pain, Icosapent ethyl fatigue | 1. Used with familial hypercholesterolemia to lower LDL in patients who cannot take statins |

▲ **Anticoagulants:** Prolong coagulation by inactivation of clotting factors (heparin) and by decreasing synthesis of clotting factors (warfarin).

### General Nursing Implications

- Increased risk for bleeding when used concurrently with other drugs, herbal remedies, or foods affecting coagulation.
- Maintain bleeding precautions.
- Review laboratory results – CBC with attention to Hb & Hct and platelets.
- Second health care provider should always check order, calculation of dosage, and/or infusion pump settings when being administered intravenously.
- Do not automatically discontinue according to automatic stop policies (procedures, surgery) without verifying the order; reevaluate all clients whose anticoagulants are being held for procedures and assess the need to reorder the anticoagulant therapy.
- Patient should wear a medical alert bracelet.

**NURSING PRIORITY:** Clarify all anticoagulant dosing for clients. Caution to be taken with reading labels for heparin concentrations especially for IV bolus doses.

*Continued*

**Appendix 18-2   MEDICATIONS—cont'd**

R x

| Medications | Side Effects | Nursing Implications |
|---|---|---|
| Heparin: IV, subQ<br>May not be given PO<br>Short-term anticoagulation | Visible or occult blood in emesis, urine, stool, or sputum<br>Bleeding from trauma site, surgical site, or intracranially<br>Heparin-induced thrombocytopenia: associated with increase in thrombosis | 1. Check the APTT for normal levels versus therapeutic levels.<br>2. Protamine sulfate is the antidote.<br>3. IV administration should be administered via infusion pump to ensure accurate dosage.<br>4. Will not dissolve established clots.<br>5. Evaluate client for decreased platelets.<br>6. Effective immediately after administration; anticoagulation effect has short half-life.<br>7. Before starting infusion, and with each change of the container or rate of infusion, have second practitioner check drug, dosage, route, and rate.<br>8. Do not store in same area as insulin; both are given by units. |
| **Low-Molecular-Weight Heparin (LMWH)** | | |
| Enoxaparin: subQ<br>Dalteparin: subQ<br>Tinzaparin: subQ | Similar to those with heparin | 1. Use: prophylaxis for thromboembolic problems in high-risk clients (immobility, hip or knee replacement).<br>2. Dosage *is not* interchangeable with heparin.<br>3. Leave the air lock in the prefilled syringe to prevent leakage.<br>4. Should be injected into the "love handles" of the abdomen. |
| Warfarin sodium: PO<br>Long-term anticoagulation | Bleeding ranging from bruising to major hemorrhage | 1. Check the PT and INR to evaluate level of anticoagulation; INR greater than 3 may indicate adverse drug reaction.<br>2. Vitamin K is the antidote.<br>3. Client teaching:<br>  a. Bleeding precautions (see Box 16-1).<br>  b. Advise all health care providers of medication.<br>  c. Not recommended if pregnant or lactating.<br>  d. Maintain routine checks on coagulation studies.<br>  e. Do not stop taking medication unless told to do so by health care provider.<br>4. Check drug literature when administering with other medications; drug interactions are common.<br>5. Oral contraceptives may decrease effectiveness.<br>6. Half-life is 3–5 days; discontinue 3 days before an invasive procedure. |
| Dabigatran: PO<br>Apixaban: PO<br>Argatroban: IV<br>Direct thrombin inhibitor<br>Rivaroxaban: PO | Has same potential for bleeding, as with warfarin<br>Does not have the dietary and drug interactions that warfarin has | 1. Due to potential breakdown and loss of potency from moisture, should not be stored in pillboxes or organizers.<br>2. Inform health care provider if having surgery or dental surgery.<br>3. Does not require INR/PT monitoring.<br>4. High risk for stroke if abrupt discontinuation |

**TEST ALERT:** Questions about anticoagulant medications are consistently found on the examination.

| Appendix 18-2 | MEDICATIONS—cont'd |
|---|---|

| Medications | Side Effects | Nursing Implications |
|---|---|---|

### Antiplatelet Medications: Inhibit platelet aggregation and prolong bleeding time. Used to prevent and treat thromboembolism events such as stroke, MI, and peripheral artery disease.

#### General Nursing Implications

- Use with caution in patients at risk for bleeding.
- Concurrent use with NSAIDs, heparin, thrombolytics, or warfarin may increase risk of bleeding.
- Teach bleeding precautions to client and family.
- Monitor bleeding times throughout therapy.

| Medications | Side Effects | Nursing Implications |
|---|---|---|
| Aspirin: PO | GI bleeding, hemorrhagic stroke, ecchymosis<br>Tinnitus | 1. Given in small doses (e.g., 81 mg daily).<br>2. Prophylactic therapy for prevention of MI and thrombotic stroke in clients with TIAs.<br>3. Take with food. |
| Clopidogrel: PO<br>Prasugrel: PO<br>Ticagrelor: PO<br>Vorapaxar: PO | Abdominal pain, dyspepsia, diarrhea<br>Blood dyscrasias | 1. Prophylactic treatment for prevention of MI, strokes in clients with established peripheral artery disease, or after stent placement.<br>2. Effect is decreased significantly when combined with omeprazole.<br>3. Take with food. |
| Cilostazol: PO | Headache, dizziness, GI bleeding, flatus, diarrhea | 1. Monitor for relief of intermittent claudication.<br>2. Grapefruit juice inhibits metabolism.<br>3. Administer on an empty stomach. |
| Ticlopidine: PO | Diarrhea, bleeding, aplastic anemia | 1. Monitor coagulation studies throughout therapy.<br>2. Monitor cholesterol/triglyceride levels.<br>3. Older adult clients may have increased sensitivity. |

#### Blood Viscosity Reducing Agent

| Medications | Side Effects | Nursing Implications |
|---|---|---|
| Pentoxifylline: PO | GI disturbances, dizziness | 1. Monitor for relief of intermittent claudication in lower extremities.<br>2. Therapeutic effect may not be noted for 2–4 weeks.<br>3. Do not chew, crush, or break tablets. |

### Antihypertensive Medications

#### General Nursing Implications

- Advise client that postural hypotension may occur and explain how to decrease effects.
  - Sit on side of bed before standing.
  - Do not stand for prolonged periods of time.
  - Older clients are at increased risk.
  - Symptoms may occur with first dose or subsequent doses.
  - Problem is most often temporary.
- Hypotension may be increased by hot weather, hot showers, hot tubs, and alcohol ingestion.
- Client should not abruptly discontinue medication or change dosage without consulting health care provider. Abrupt withdrawal can cause rebound hypertension.
- Encourage a low-sodium diet, weight maintenance or reduction, and limitations of caffeine.
- Discourage use of all tobacco products.
- Have client report unpleasant side effects related to sexual dysfunction.
- Advise client not to take over-the-counter cough medications or decongestants that contain pseudoephedrine; these medications cause an increase in BP.
- Administer with meals to enhance absorption.
- Monitor BP and pulse frequently during initial dosage adjustments and daily/weekly during therapy, record results, and take when visiting health care provider.

*Continued*

## Appendix 18-2   MEDICATIONS—cont'd

| Medications | Side Effects | Nursing Implications |
|---|---|---|
| **Vasodilators:** Act directly on vascular smooth muscle to produce vasodilation. | | |
| Hydralazine HCl: PO, IM, IV | Tachycardia, headache, sodium retention, drug-induced lupus syndrome | 1. Advise client that postural hypotension may occur.<br>2. Vitamin $B_6$ may be used to prevent peripheral neuritis with long-term therapy.<br>3. May be used in combination with other antihypertensive medications. |
| Nitroprusside: IV | Nausea/vomiting, headache, abdominal pain, dizziness, excessive hypotension | 1. Used to treat hypertensive crisis; very rapid response.<br>2. Solution must be prepared immediately before use and protected from light during administration; use within 24 hours.<br>3. Administer via infusion pump to ensure accurate flow rate.<br>4. Maintain continuous ECG and BP monitoring, preferably in a critical care setting. |
| Minoxidil: PO | Tachycardia, fluid retention, nausea, headache, fatigue | 1. Used to treat severe hypertension, unresponsive to other antihypertensives. |
| Nitroglycerin: PO, SL, topical, IV, spray | Hypotension, headache, flushing, skin irritation | (see Box 19-2)<br>1. Evaluate BP prior to administration.<br>2. If given IV, use an infusion pump and dosage to titrate for BP or chest pain per health care provider's guidelines.<br>3. SL/spray given for episodes of angina. Administer one dose every 5 minutes for a total of three doses. If no relief, transport to health care facility for further treatment and evaluation. |
| **Centrally Acting Inhibitors (Antiadrenergics):** Decrease sympathetic effect (norepinephrine), resulting in decreased BP and peripheral resistance, decrease in heart rate, and no change in cardiac output. | | |
| Methyldopa: PO<br>Methyldopate: IV<br>Clonidine: PO or topical<br>Guanabenz: PO<br>Guanfacine: PO | Hepatotoxicity, hemolytic anemia sexual dysfunction, orthostatic hypotension, dry mouth, sedation | 1. If withdrawn abruptly, may precipitate a hypertensive crisis.<br>2. Do not confuse methyldopa with levodopa or L-dopa.<br>3. Appears on Beers list*: Older adult clients may have increased sensitivity to methyldopa. Monitor for depression or altered mental status. |
| **ACE Inhibitors:** Reduce peripheral resistance without increasing cardiac output, rate, or contractility; angiotensin antagonists. | | |
| Captopril: PO<br>Enalapril: PO, IV<br>Lisinopril: PO<br>Ramipril: PO<br>Moexipril: PO<br>Trandolapril: PO | Postural hypotension, hyperkalemia, insomnia, nonproductive cough, loss of taste | 1. Monitor closely on first dose; hypotension and first-dose syncope may occur.<br>2. Can cause hyperkalemia; *may not need* a potassium supplement when given with a diuretic.<br>3. Skipping doses or stopping drug may result in rebound hypertension.<br>4. Aspirin and NSAIDs may reduce effectiveness.<br>5. Not to be used with potassium-sparing diuretics. |

| *Medications* | *Side Effects* | *Nursing Implications* |
|---|---|---|

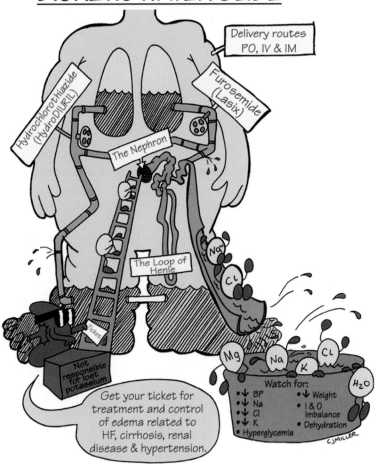

**FIGURE 18-10 Diuretic Water Slide.** *HF,* Heart failure; *PO,* by mouth; *IM,* intramuscular *IV,* intravenous. (From Zerwekh, J., Garneau, A., & Miller, C. J. [2017]. *Digital collection of the memory notebooks of nursing* [4th ed.]. Chandler, AZ: Nursing Education Consultants, Inc.)

**Beta-Adrenergic Blockers:** See Appendix 19-2.

**Calcium Channel Blockers:** See Appendix 19-2.

### Diuretics (Figure 18-10)

*General Nursing Implications*

- In hospitalized clients, evaluate daily weights for fluid loss or gain.
- Maintain intake and output ratios.
- Monitor for hypokalemia, anorexia, muscle weakness, numbness, tingling, paresthesia, confusion, and excessive thirst.
- Advise client of foods that are rich in potassium.
- Administer medications in the morning to allow diuresis to occur during the day.
- Teach client how to decrease effects of postural hypotension.
- Monitor BP response to medication.
- Interactions:
  - Digitalis action is increased in presence of hypokalemia.
  - Lithium levels may be increased in presence of hyponatremia.

*Continued*

**Appendix 18-2** MEDICATIONS—cont'd

| Medications | Side Effects | Nursing Implications |
|---|---|---|

**Loop Diuretics:** Block sodium and chloride reabsorption, which causes water and solutes to be retained in the nephrons. Prevention of reabsorption of water back into the circulation causes an increase in excretion of the water and, thus, diuresis.

| Medications | Side Effects | Nursing Implications |
|---|---|---|
| Furosemide: PO, IM, IV<br>Bumetanide: PO, IM, IV<br>Torsemide: PO, IV | Dehydration, hypotension; excessive loss of potassium, sodium, chloride; hyperglycemia, hyperuricemia; muscle weakness | 1. Furosemide is a strong diuretic that provides rapid diuresis.<br>2. Use with caution in older adults; CNS problems of confusion, headache.<br>3. Monitor closely for tinnitus/hearing loss.<br>4. Do not confuse Bumex (trade name for bumetanide) with buprenorphine (Buprenex).<br>5. Do not confuse furosemide with torsemide.<br>6. IV push should be over 1–2 minutes. |

**Thiazide Diuretics:** Increase renal excretion of NaCl, K, and water. Require adequate urine output to be effective.

| Medications | Side Effects | Nursing Implications |
|---|---|---|
| Chlorothiazide: IV, PO<br>Chlorthalidone: PO<br>Hydrochlorothiazide: PO<br>Metolazone: PO (a thiazide-like diuretic; may give 2–4 times per week depending on patient need and tolerance) | Dehydration, hypotension; excessive loss of potassium, hyperglycemia, hyperuricemia; muscle weakness, dry mouth, lethargy | 1. Frequently used as first-line drug to control essential hypertension.<br>2. Increased risk for digitalis toxicity if taking digoxin products.<br>3. If allergic to thiazides or sulfonamides, metolazone may be contraindicated.<br>4. May need potassium supplements. |

**Aldosterone Antagonist (Potassium-Sparing Diuretics):** Blocks the effect of aldosterone; inhibits the renal–angiotensin–aldosterone system (RAAS); blocks receptors in the renal tubules, heart, and blood vessels. Used in treatment of heart failure and hypertension.

| Medications | Side Effects | Nursing Implications |
|---|---|---|
| Spironolactone: PO<br>Triamterene: PO | Hyperkalemia, hyponatremia, impotence, hypotension | 1. May be used in combination with other diuretics to reduce potassium loss.<br>2. Potassium-sparing effects may result in hyperkalemia.<br>3. Not used for clients experiencing renal failure.<br>4. Avoid salt substitutes and foods containing large amounts of sodium or potassium. |

**Osmotic Diuretic:** Increases osmotic pressure of the fluid in the renal tubules, preventing reabsorption of sodium and water.

| Medications | Side Effects | Nursing Implications |
|---|---|---|
| Mannitol: IV | Pulmonary edema, HF, tissue dehydration, nausea, vomiting | 1. Stop infusion if client begins to show symptoms of CHF or pulmonary edema.<br>2. Use an IV filter to prevent infusion of crystals; warm vial and shake vigorously to dissolve crystals.<br>3. Monitor infusion site closely for infiltration and/or extravasation. |

## Medications Used for Treatment of Shock

### General Nursing Implications

- Most often limited to critical care settings; constant monitoring is required.
- Administered IV in diluted solution by infusion pump.
- Monitor IV infusion site closely; leakage into tissue may cause tissue sloughing.
- Administer via central line if possible.
- Continuous ECG/BP monitoring; observe client closely for cardiac dysrhythmias.
- Monitor urinary output every hour.
- Medications should not be administered to clients receiving MAOIs or tricyclic antidepressants.

## Appendix 18-2   MEDICATIONS—cont'd

| Medications | Side Effects | Nursing Implications |
|---|---|---|
| **Adrenergics:** Increases myocardial contractility, thereby improving cardiac output, BP, and urine output. | | |
| ▲ Dopamine: IV[a] | Dysrhythmias (tachycardia), angina, hypertension, headaches | 1. Should not be given to clients with tachydys-rhythmias or ventricular fibrillation. <br> 2. Have second practitioner check drug, dosage, route, etc. <br> 3. If extravasation occurs, stop infusion immediately |
| Dobutamine: IV[a] | Tachycardia, dysrhythmias, hypertension | 1. If extravasation occurs, stop infusion; area may be infused with phentolamine mesylate. |
| Epinephrine hydrochloride: IV[a] | Nervousness, restlessness, tremors, angina, dysrhythmias, tachycardia, hypertension. | 1. Be sure to read label correctly and use correct strength/concentration. <br> 2. Use in treatment of anaphylactic shock and cardiac arrest. |

[a]Infusion pumps MUST be utilized to infuse these medications.
▲ High-alert medications;
*ACE,* Angiotensin-converting enzyme; *APTT,* activated prothrombin time; *BP,* blood pressure; *ECG,* electrocardiogram; *CNS,* central nervous system; *GI,* gastrointestinal; *HDL,* high-density lipoprotein; *HF,* heart failure; *IM,* intramuscularly; *IV,* intravenously; *LDL,* low-density lipoprotein; *INR,* international normalized ratio; *MAOI,* monoamine oxidase inhibitor; *MI,* myocardial infarction; *NSAID,* nonsteroidal antiinflammatory drug; *PO,* by mouth (orally); *PT,* prothrombin time; *subQ,* subcutaneously. *TIA,* transient ischemic attack; VS, vital signs.
*Beers List: A list of potentially inappropriate medications for the older adult. (See https://www.americangeriatrics.org/files/documents/beers/PrintableBeersPocketCard.pdf for a listing.)

## Study Questions
## Vascular: Care of Adult Clients

More questions on
evolve

1. What is an important nursing action in the safe administration of heparin?
   1. Check the prothrombin time (PT) and administer the medication if it is less than 20 seconds.
   2. Use a 20-gauge, 1-inch (2.5 cm) needle and inject into the deltoid muscle and gently massage the area.
   3. Dilute in 50 mL 5% dextrose in water ($D_5W$) and infuse by intravenous piggyback (IVPB) over 15 minutes.
   4. Use a 25-gauge, ½-inch (1.25 cm) needle and inject the medication into the subcutaneous tissue of the abdomen.

2. While discussing her diagnosis of hypertension, a client asks the nurse how long she is going to have to take all of the medications that have been prescribed. On what principle is the nurse's response based?
   1. The client will be scheduled for an appointment in 2 months; the doctor will decrease her medications at that time.
   2. As soon as her blood pressure (BP) returns to normal levels, the client will be able to stop taking her medications.
   3. To maintain stable control of her BP, the client will have to take the medications indefinitely.
   4. The nurse cannot discuss the medications with the client; the client will need to talk with the doctor.

3. The nurse is teaching a client about home care and treatment of venous stasis ulcers on his leg. What should be included in the nurse's instructions? Select all that apply:
   1. Dressings do not need to be changed frequently because there is minimal drainage.
   2. Healing will be facilitated by wearing leg compression devices.
   3. When the client is in the sitting position, he should keep his legs elevated.
   4. Avoid standing for prolonged periods of time.
   5. Cool packs can be applied to the ulcers to decrease inflammation.
   6. Soak the affected extremity in warm water every evening.

4. The nurse is caring for a client who is 6 hours postpartum. What nursing actions are directed toward the prevention of postpartum thrombophlebitis?
   1. Encourage early ambulation and increased fluid intake.
   2. Allow bathroom privileges only and elevate the lower extremities.
   3. Administer anticoagulants and evaluate the clotting factors.
   4. Encourage the client to breastfeed the infant as soon as possible.

5. The nurse is preparing to administer spironolactone to a client. After assessing the client, what data indicate the need to withhold the medication?
   1. Potassium level of 5.8 mEq/L (mmol/L)
   2. Apical pulse rate of 58 beats/min
   3. BP of 130/90 mmHg
   4. Urine output of 30 mL/hr

6. Which nursing action would be most effective in preventing venous stasis in the postoperative surgical client?
   1. Raise the foot of the bed for 1 hour, then lower it to stimulate blood flow.
   2. Massage the lower extremities every 6 hours.
   3. Facilitate active range of motion of the upper body to stimulate cardiac output.
   4. Help the client walk as soon as permitted and as often as possible.

7. A client has had her blood pressure evaluated weekly for month. At the end of the month, the nurse averages out the weekly blood pressures at 150/96 mmHg. The client is 20 pounds (9.1 kg) overweight, and her cholesterol is 240 mg/dL (6.22 mmol/L). What is important information for the nurse to include in the teaching plan for this client?
   1. Refer her to the doctor for further follow-up and medications.
   2. Increase the fiber in her diet and begin a daily 30-minute workout.
   3. Reduce her sodium intake and decrease the dietary calories that come from fat.
   4. Reduce her cholesterol intake for 1 month and check her BP 3 times a week.

8. Four hours after aortic–femoral bypass graft surgery, the nurse assesses the client and is unable to palpate pulses in the operative leg. The client complains of pain in the leg. What is the first nursing action?
   1. Massage the leg and apply warm towels.
   2. Elevate the leg and recheck the pulse.
   3. Call the physician immediately.
   4. Help the client ambulate.

9. What is the desired action of dopamine when administered in the treatment of shock?
   1. It increases myocardial contractility.
   2. It is associated with fewer severe allergic reactions.
   3. It causes rapid vasodilation of the vascular bed.
   4. It supports renal perfusion by dilation of the renal arteries.

10. The client returns to his room after a thoracotomy. What will the nursing assessment reveal if hypovolemia from excessive blood loss is present?
    1. CVP of 3 cm $H_2O$ and urine output of 20 mL/hr
    2. Jugular vein distention with the head elevated 45 degrees
    3. Chest tube drainage of 50 mL/hr in the first 2 hours
    4. Increased BP and increased pulse pressure

11. A client with hypertension asks the nurse what type of exercise she should do each day. What is the nurse's best response?
    1. "Exercise for an hour, but only three times a week."
    2. "Walk on the treadmill for 45 minutes every morning."
    3. "Begin walking and increase your distance as you can tolerate it."
    4. "Exercise only in the morning and stop when you get tired."

12. The nurse is preparing discharge teaching for a client with hypertension who is being treated with furosemide and clonidine. The nurse would caution the client about which over-the-counter medications?
    1. Antihistamines
    2. Acetaminophen
    3. Topical corticosteroid cream
    4. Decongestant cough preparations

13. The nurse is monitoring an IV infusion of sodium nitroprusside. Fifteen minutes after the infusion is started, the client's blood pressure goes from 190/120 mmHg to 120/90 mmHg. What is a priority nursing action?
    1. Recheck the BP and call the doctor.
    2. Decrease the infusion rate and recheck the blood pressure in 5 minutes.
    3. Stop the medication and keep the IV open with $D_5W$.
    4. Assess the client's tolerance of the current level of BP.

14. The nurse is teaching a client with hypertension about his antihypertensive medications, hydrochlorothiazide (HCTZ) and enalapril. What is important to include in this teaching?
    1. "Stand up slowly to decrease problem with dizziness."
    2. "Increase fluid intake because of increased loss of body fluids."
    3. "When you begin to feel better, the doctor will decrease your medications."
    4. "Stay out of the sunshine, and make sure you have adequate sodium intake."

15. The nurse is administering propranolol to a client who is being treated for hypertension. What is the desired response to this medication?
    1. Vasodilation occurs, resulting in a decrease in the cardiac afterload.
    2. The cardiac rate is decreased, with a resulting decrease in the cardiac output.
    3. Cardiac output is decreased, and the arterial BP rises.
    4. Pericardial fluid is decreased, thus decreasing the cardiac workload.

16. Which instruction should be included in discharge teaching for the client with a new prescription for simvastatin?
    1. Flushing occurs in almost all individuals.
    2. Sedation is common but will decrease with time.
    3. Liver enzyme levels should be monitored every few months.
    4. Watch closely for occurrence of postural hypotension.

17. The nurse is caring for a client with venous blood pooling in the lower extremities caused by chronic venous insufficiency. The nurse would identify what assessment data that would correlate with this diagnosis? Select all that apply.
    1. Stasis dermatitis
    2. Diminished peripheral pulses
    3. Peripheral edema
    4. Gangrenous wounds
    5. Venous stasis ulcers
    6. Skin hyperpigmentation

# Answers to Study Questions

**1. 4**

Medication should be administered with a small-gauge (25 gauge) needle into the subcutaneous tissue without aspirating or massaging the area. Partial thromboplastin time (PTT) is used to monitor the effects of heparin. Although heparin may be administered IV, it must be diluted in more than 50 mL $D_5W$ and would be administered over a longer period of time than 15 minutes. (Lewis et al., 10th ed., p. 820)

**2. 3**

Noncompliance with blood pressure medications is a common problem in the treatment of hypertension. The client must understand that the only way to keep her blood pressure under control is to continue to take her medications, potentially for the rest of her life. She will not be able to discontinue the medications unless there is a significant change in her condition as a result of weight loss, an exercise program, and/or decreased stress. Patients usually require follow-up and adjustments at monthly intervals until the goal BP is reached. Antihypertensives control BP but do not cure hypertension, therefore the medication cannot be stopped once the target reading is reached. (Ignatavicius & Workman, 8th ed., pp. 712–713, 717–718)

**3. 2, 3, 4**

Healing of venous stasis ulcers is dependent on relieving the venous congestion in the extremity. Compression devices and elevation of the extremity are the most effective methods. The client should avoid standing for long periods because this increases venous stasis. Moist cool and/or warm packs are not used, but moist environment dressings are utilized. Dressings need to be changed as frequently as necessary because there may be excessive drainage. (Ignatavicius & Workman, 8th ed., pp. 734–735)

**4. 1**

Early ambulation is the most effective and safe way to prevent thrombophlebitis with any type of client. This promotes venous return and prevents venous stasis. Anticoagulants (heparin and warfarin) are administered as ordered postpartum with a diagnosis of thrombophlebitis; they are not used for prevention. The legs should be elevated when the client is in a sitting position. There is no evidence that breastfeeding affects blood coagulation in any way. (Ignatavicius & Workman, 8th ed., pp. 730–731)

**5. 1**

Aldactone is a potassium-sparing diuretic. The client's potassium level is high; therefore the medication should be held and the doctor should be notified. Urine output of 30 mL/hr is normal output. The BP is elevated, which is the reason the client is receiving the medication. The pulse rate is not affected by this medication. (Igntavicius & Workman, 8th ed., pp. 262, 712, 714)

**6. 4**

The postoperative client has decreased mobility, which may create an environment in which clotting can be caused by venous stasis. Active exercise, such as having the client ambulate as soon as possible, will stimulate circulation and venous return. This reduces the possibility of clot formation. The lower extremities should not be massaged because this may disrupt a clot and cause a pulmonary embolism. (Ignatavicius & Workman, 8th ed., pp. 730–731)

**7. 1**

The client should be referred for further evaluation of blood pressure. The blood pressure is definitely elevated, the client is overweight, and she has an increased level of cholesterol. A multifocal approach is necessary to control the blood pressure. Because of the multiple risk factors, increasing fiber in the diet and exercise would not likely be sufficient to reduce the hypertension. Neither would dietary changes. This patient needs a multifocal approach. (Ignatavicius & Workman, 8th ed., pp. 710–712)

**8. 3**

Occlusion to the aortic/femoral bypass graft is considered a medical emergency, and physician notification is imperative. No other nursing options would alleviate the problem. Massaging the leg and having the client ambulate would be contraindicated. If the pulses cannot be palpated and the client is experiencing pain, the nurse should not wait to call the physician. (Ignatavicius & Workman, 8th ed., pp. 723–724)

**9. 4**

Dopamine will support renal perfusion when administered in low doses in the initial stages of shock. At higher doses and as the client becomes more decompensated, the effect of the dopamine on the renal perfusion decreases. Vasodilation would further complicate the shock situation, and allergies are not a common problem. Vasoconstriction is not a primary property of dopamine in low doses. Dopamine increases cardiac rate, but that is not the desired therapeutic action for a client in shock. (Ignatavicius & Workman, 8th ed., pp. 748; Lewis et al., 10th ed., p. 1599)

**10. 1**

A low-range CVP reading and the decrease in urine output would be associated with hypovolemia caused by hemorrhage. Normal CVP is 2 to 6 cm $H_2O$. The decrease in urine output is reflective of poor renal perfusion. Jugular vein distention is indicative of increased CVP, which does not occur with hypovolemia. Chest tube drainage is within the normal expectations. The blood pressure decreases with hemorrhage. (Lewis et al., 10th ed., p. 1564)

**11. 3**

When any client begins exercising, it should be gradually, with increasing activity as the client tolerates it. A complication of hypertension is heart failure, which may first be seen as dyspnea on exertion. The client should exercise as tolerated and stop when she gets tired or begins to have shortness of breath, regardless of the amount of time she has already exercised. (Lewis et al., 10th ed., p. 689).

**12. 4**

Decongestants and over-the-counter cough medicines frequently contain pseudoephedrine. These medications will cause an increase in blood pressure and interfere with the effectiveness of the antihypertensive medications. (Lewis et al., 10th ed., p. 697)

**13. 2**

Nipride is a powerful, rapid vasodilator. The nurse should decrease the infusion first before the pressure drops further, then assess the client's response to the decreased rate. If the client's urinary output remains adequate and there is no dizziness or neurologic change, then the client is probably tolerating the blood pressure level. (Lewis et al., 10th ed., p. 692).

**14.** *1*
A common side effect of a combination of antihypertensive and diuretic medications is postural hypotension. It is important to teach the client how to deal with it. The client should not increase intake of fluids, because the diuretics are being given to decrease excess fluid. The client should decrease his intake of sodium. When the client is feeling better, the medication is working and will probably not be decreased. (Lewis et al., 10th ed., p. 697)

**15.** *2*
The primary action of the beta-blocker, propranolol, is to slow the cardiac rate. The medication is effective in the treatment of hypertension or dysrhythmias that result in tachycardia. With a decrease in cardiac rate, there is also a decrease in cardiac output. The beta-blockers do not cause vasodilation. A decrease in cardiac output

would cause a decrease in arterial BP, not an increase. Beta-blockers do not have an effect on pericardial fluid. (Lewis et al., 10th ed., pp. 691–692)

**16.** *3*
Most of the "statin" drugs used for hyperlipidemia are hepatotoxic. Liver enzyme levels should be determined as a baseline before administration of the drug is started and then checked periodically throughout therapy. (Lewis et al., 10th ed., pp. 709–711)

**17.** *1, 3, 5, 6*
Long-term impairment of venous return leads to chronic venous insufficiency that is characterized by leathery, brawny appearance from erythrocyte extravasation to the extremity, persistent edema, stasis dermatitis, and pruritus. Venous leg (stasis) ulcers characteristically form near the ankle on the medial aspect, with wound margins that are irregularly shaped with tissue that is a ruddy color. Gangrenous wounds and diminished peripheral pulses are associated with arterial occlusive disease. (Lewis et al., 10th ed., pp. 826–828)

# CHAPTER NINETEEN

# Cardiac: Care of Adult, Maternity, and Pediatric Clients

# 19

## PRIORITY CONCEPTS

Health Promotion, Pain, Perfusion

## PHYSIOLOGY OF THE CARDIAC SYSTEM

### Structure of the Heart

A. The heart is located on the left side of the mediastinum.
B. The apex of the heart points downward and to the left at about the fifth to sixth intercostal space, midclavicular line. In a healthy individual, the point of maximum impulse (PMI) may be palpated here; this is also the area to auscultate when evaluating the apical heart rate.
C. The heart is contained in a loose sac called the pericardium.
   1. There is a space between the visceral and parietal layers of the pericardium.
   2. The pericardial space contains about 5 to 20 mL of pericardial fluid to lubricate the sac and cushions the heart.
D. Myocardial wall.
   1. Epicardium: the outer surface.
   2. Myocardium: the middle layer of cardiac muscle.
   3. Endocardium: the lining of the inner surface of the cardiac chambers.
E. Cardiac chambers – four of them (Figure 19-1).
   1. The right side of the heart has a thinner myocardium than the left side and is a low-pressure system.
   2. The left ventricle is composed of a thicker muscle, is a high-pressure system, and is capable of generating enough force to eject blood through the aortic valve and through the systemic circulation.
F. Cardiac valves: maintain the directional flow of blood.
   1. Atrioventricular valves are controlled and supported by papillary muscle and chordae tendineae.
      a. The tricuspid valve lies between the right atrium (RA) and the right ventricle (RV).
      b. The mitral valve lies between the left atrium (LA) and the left ventricle (LV).
      c. Both valves prevent backflow of blood from the ventricles into the atria during systole.
   2. Semilunar valves (cusp valves) are controlled by the backward pressure of blood flow at the end of systole.
      a. Pulmonic valve: the outflow valve of the RV into the pulmonary circulation.
      b. Aortic valve: the outflow valve of the LV into the aorta.
      c. Both valves prevent the backflow of blood from the pulmonary artery and the aortic arch into the ventricle during diastole.
G. Direction of blood flow through the heart structure (see Figure 19-1).

### Cardiac Function

A. One complete cardiac cycle consists of contraction of the myocardium (systole) and subsequent relaxation of the myocardium (diastole).
B. The amount of blood ejected with ventricular contraction is the stroke volume.
C. Starling's law of the heart: the greater the cardiac muscles are stretched, the more forceful the contraction. If an increased amount of blood flows into the heart, the heart will increase the force of contraction and eject a larger amount of blood.
D. Cardiac output ($CO = SV \times HR$).
   1. The cardiac output (CO) can be determined by multiplying the stroke volume (SV) by the heart rate (HR) in beats per minute ($CO = SV \times HR$).
   2. The heart pumps approximately 4 to 8 L of blood every minute in a healthy individual.
   3. Factors regulating stroke volume.
      a. Degree of stretch of the cardiac muscle before contraction (Starling's law).
      b. Contractility: ability of the myocardium to contract.
      c. Preload.
      d. Afterload. (Figure 19-2).
E. Autonomic nervous system.
   1. Parasympathetic (vagus nerve) stimulation.
      a. Slows the heart rate by decreasing impulses at the sinoatrial (SA) node.
      b. Slows transmission of the impulse through the atrioventricular (AV) node.
   2. Sympathetic stimulation.
      a. Increases heart rate.
      b. Increases force of contraction.
F. Factors that increase myocardial oxygen demands.
   1. Increased heart rate.
   2. Increased force of contractions.
   3. Increased afterload.

### Myocardial Blood Supply

A. Coronary arteries.
   1. Left coronary artery divides into the left anterior descending (LAD) and left circumflex artery and

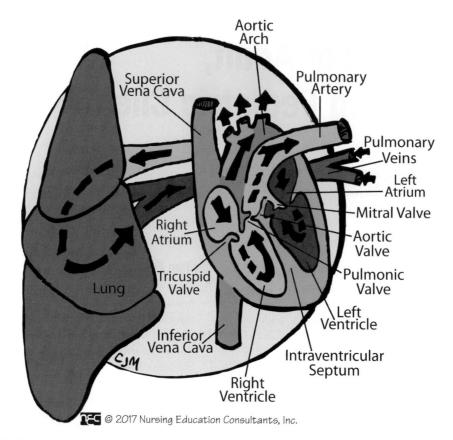

**FIGURE 19-1 Blood Flow Through the Heart.** (From Zerwekh, J., Garneau, A., & Miller, C. J. [2017]. *Digital collection of the memory notebooks of nursing* [4th ed.]. Chandler, AZ: Nursing Education Consultants, Inc.)

## PRELOAD AND AFTERLOAD

**Preload:**

Pressure from volume of blood in ventricles at end of diastole (end diastolic pressure)

Increased in:
  Hypervolemia
  Regurgitation of cardiac valves
  Heart Failure

**Afterload:**

Resistance left ventricle must overcome to circulate blood

Increased in:
Hypertension
Vasoconstriction

↑Afterload =
↑Cardiac workload

© 2016 Nursing Education Consultants, Inc.

**FIGURE 19-2 Preload and Afterload.** (From Zerwekh, J., Garneau, A., & Miller, C. J. [2017]. *Digital collection of the memory notebooks of nursing* [4th ed.]. Chandler, AZ: Nursing Education Consultants, Inc.)

supplies the LA, LV, interventricular septum, and a portion of the RV.

2. Right coronary artery branches supply the RA, RV, and portion of posterior wall of the LV.

3. Require a diastolic pressure of 60 mmHg to adequately perfuse the heart, kidneys, and brain.

B. Collateral circulation.

1. When gradual occlusion of large coronary vessels occurs as a result of arteriosclerotic heart disease (ASHD), the smaller vessels increase in size to provide perfusion by an alternative blood flow.

2. Because of the development of collateral circulation, coronary artery disease may be well advanced before the client experiences symptoms.

## Conduction System

A. Controls the rate and rhythm of the heart by creating and transporting electrical impulses.

B. Electrical impulses initiate depolarization of the myocardium, which triggers a cardiac contraction.

1. Electrical impulse starts at the SA node (located in the right atrium), travels to the AV node (located at the atrioventricular junction), through the bundle of His, down the right and left bundle branches (located in the ventricular septum), and ends in the Purkinje fibers.

2. Electrical activity of the heart is recorded on an electrocardiogram (ECG).

E. Relationship of conducting pathways to the electrocardiogram (ECG) (Figure 19-3).

1. P wave: indicative of the impulse generated from the sinoatrial node (SA node); initiates atrial depolarization.

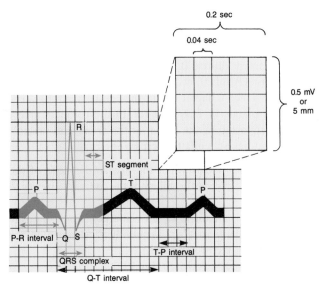

**FIGURE 19-3  Normal Electrocardiogram (ECG).** (From Hockenberry, M. J., & Wilson, D. [2015]. *Wong's nursing care of infants and children* [10th ed.]. St. Louis, MO: Mosby.)

2. PR interval: delay of the impulse at the atrioventricular node (AV node) and bundle of His to promote ventricular filling.
3. QRS complex: passage of the impulse through the bundle of His, down the bundle branches, through the Purkinje fibers; depolarization of the ventricle occurs.
4. T wave: ventricular repolarization and return to the resting state.
5. ST segment: above the baseline in cardiac injury (ST elevation) and below the baseline with ischemia (ST depression).

### System Assessment

A. Health history.
   1. Identify presence of risk factors for the development of arteriosclerotic disease.
   2. Coping strategies.

3. Respiratory.
   a. History of difficulty breathing.
   b. Medications taken for respiratory problems.
   c. Determine normal activity level.
4. Circulation.
   a. History of chest discomfort (Table 19-1).
   b. History of edema, weight gain, syncope.
   c. Skin temperature and pulses.
5. Medications taken for the heart or for high blood pressure.

B. Physical assessment.
   1. What is the general appearance of the client: Is there any evidence of distress? What is the client's level of orientation and ability to think clearly?
   2. Evaluate blood pressure.
      a. Pulse pressure: the difference between systolic and diastolic pressure.
      b. Assess for postural (orthostatic) hypotension (decrease in blood pressure when client stands).
      c. Take blood pressure sitting, standing, and lying if client is having problems with pressure changes (see Chapter 3 for accurate blood pressure measurement).
      d. Paradoxical blood pressure (paradoxical pulse): a decrease in systolic blood pressure of at least 10 mmHg that occurs during inspiration.
   3. Evaluate quality and rate of pulse; assess for dysrhythmias (see Appendix 19-3 for determining dysrhythmias).
      a. Pulse deficit: the radial pulse rate is less than the apical pulse rate; occurs in atrial fibrillation and atrial flutter.
      b. Pulsus alternans: regular rhythm but quality of pulse alternates with strong beats and weak beats.
      c. Thready pulse: weak and rapid; difficult to count.
   4. Assess quality and pattern of respirations and evidence of respiratory difficulty.
   5. Auscultation of the heart (Figure 19-4).
      a. Heart sounds heard during the cardiac cycle.
         (1) $S_1$: closure of the atrioventricular (AV) valves—mitral and tricuspid.

| Table 19-1 | ASSESSING CHEST PAIN (PQRST) | | | |
|---|---|---|---|---|
| **P—Precipitating Factors** | **Q—Quality of Pain** | **R—Region and Radiation of Pain** | **S—Severity Symptoms/Signs (associated with chest pain)** | **T—Timing and Response to Treatment** |
| May occur without precipitators | Pressure | Substernal or retrosternal | Severity—scale from 1–10 | Sudden onset |
| Physical exertion | Squeezing | Spreads across the chest | Diaphoresis, cold clammy skin | Constant |
| Emotional stress | Heaviness | Radiates to the inside of either or both arms, the neck, jaw, back, upper abdomen | Nausea, vomiting | Duration more than 30 min |
| Eating a large meal | Smothering | | Dyspnea | Not relieved with nitrates or rest |
| | Burning | | Orthopnea | Relief with narcotics |
| | Severe pain | | Syncope | |
| | Increases with movement | | Apprehension | |
| | | | Dysrhythmias | |
| | | | Palpitations | |
| | | | Auscultation of extra heart sounds | |
| | | | Auscultation of crackles | |
| | | | Weakness | |

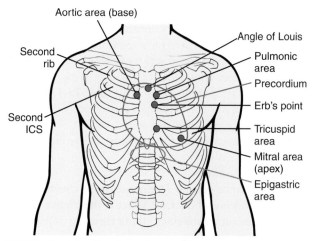

**FIGURE 19-4 Cardiac Auscultatory Sites.** (From McCance, K., & Huether, S. [2014] *Pathophysiology: The biologic basis for disease in adults and children* [7th ed.]. St. Louis, MO: Elsevier.)

(2) $S_2$: closure of the semilunar valves—aortic and pulmonic.

(3) $S_3$: represents rapid ventricular filling; normal in children and young adults; in adults older than 30 years, it may be an indication of volume overload, ventricular dysfunction secondary to hypertension.

(4) $S_4$: caused by the atria contracting forcefully in an effort to overcome an abnormally stiff or hypertrophic ventricle.

b. Presence of murmurs created by turbulent blood flow: graded on a scale of loudness from 1 to 6.

   (1) Abnormal flow through diseased valves: stenosis and insufficiency.

   (2) Abnormal flow of blood between cardiac chambers (congenital heart disease).

c. Presence of a pericardial friction rub: a scratchy, high-pitched sound usually heard over the left lower sternal border during $S_1$ and $S_2$; can be heard best with client sitting and leaning forward.

> **TEST ALERT:** Identify common abnormal heart sounds (e.g., $S_3$, $S_4$).

6. Evaluate adequacy of peripheral vascular circulation and check for presence of peripheral edema.
7. Evaluate for presence of chest pain or discomfort (see Table 19-1).
   a. Location.
   b. Intensity of pain.
   c. Precipitating causes.

> **TEST ALERT:** Perform focused assessment or reassessment; interpret data that need to be reported immediately (Box 19-1).

# DISORDERS OF THE CARDIAC SYSTEM

## Coronary Artery Disease (CAD)

Coronary artery disease (CAD), also called arteriosclerotic heart disease (ASHD), occurs as a result of the atherosclerotic process (see Chapter 18) in the coronary arteries. The buildup of plaque or fatty material in the coronary artery causes a narrowing of the lumen of the artery and precipitates myocardial ischemia that causes chest pain.

A. Pain (angina) occurs when the oxygen demands of the heart muscle exceed the ability of the coronary arteries to deliver it.
B. Temporary ischemia does not cause permanent damage to the myocardium. Pain frequently subsides when the precipitating factor is removed.
C. Risk factors for CAD (see Box 19-1).
D. CAD treatment: health promotion, physical activity, nutritional therapy, lipid-lowering drug therapy, antiplatelet therapy.

## 📋 Chronic Stable Angina

**Chest pain that occurs intermittently over a long period with a similar pattern of onset, duration, and intensity of symptoms.**

---

### Box 19-1   RISK FACTORS FOR CORONARY ARTERY DISEASE (CAD)

**Major Modifiable Risk Factors**
Elevated lipids
- Total cholesterol greater than 200 mg/dL (5.18 mmol/L)
- Triglycerides greater than or equal to 150 mg/dL (1.7 mmol/L)
- LDL greater than 160 mg/dL (4.14 mmol/L)
- HDL less than 40 mg/dL (1.0 mmol/L) in men or 50 mg/dL (1.3 mmol/L) in women

Blood pressure greater than or equal to 140/90 mmHg
Tobacco use
Physical inactivity
Obesity: waist circumference greater than or equal to 102 cm (40 inches) in men and 88 cm (35 inches) in women
**Contributing Modifiable Risk Factors:** diabetes mellitus, metabolic syndrome, psychosocial (stress, anger, hostility, depression), fasting blood glucose greater than or equal to 100 mg/dL (5.5 mmol/L), elevated homocysteine levels

**Nonmodifiable Risk Factors**
Genetic predisposition
Positive family history of heart disease
Increasing age
Gender: more common in men than women until age 75
Ethnicity: more common in white men than in African Americans

> **TEST ALERT:** Teach health promotion information. Know the CAD risk factors and be able to teach the client how to effectively reduce his or her risk factors.

## Types

A. Prinzmetal angina–variant angina is pain that tends to be cyclic caused by coronary spasms and occurs at rest.
B. Microvascular angina—ischemia secondary to microvascular disease affecting the small distal branches of the coronary arteries, referred to as Syndrome X.

## Assessment

A. Episodic pain lasting a few minutes relieved by rest or nitroglycerin.
B. Provoked by a stressor.
   1. Physical exertion, temperature extremes.
   2. Strong emotions, consumption of heavy meal.
   3. Tobacco use, sexual activity.
   4. Stimulants (cocaine, amphetamines).
   5. Circadian rhythm patterns.

## Treatment – Chronic Stable Angina

A. Short- and long-acting nitrates.
B. Angiotensin-converting enzyme (ACE) inhibitors and angiotensin receptor blockers (ARB).
C. Beta adrenergic blockers, calcium channel blockers.
D. Lipid-lowering drugs.
E. Sodium current inhibitor.
F. Cardiac catheterization.

## Acute Coronary Syndrome (ACS)

**Prolonged ischemia that is not immediately reversible. ACS includes unstable angina, non–ST-segment-elevation myocardial infarction (NSTEMI), and ST-segment-elevation myocar-dial infarction (STEMI) (Figure 19-5).**

A. Unstable angina is chest pain that is new in onset, occurs at rest, or occurs with increasing frequency, duration, or with less effort then chronic stable angina.
B. Myocardial infarction (MI): NSTEMI: nonocclusive thrombus without ST segment elevation on the 12-lead ECG. Interventional procedures usually occur within 12 to 72 hours if there are no contraindications. Thrombolytic therapy is not indicated.
C. Myocardial infarction: STEMI: occurs from an abrupt stoppage of blood flow through a coronary artery from a thrombus caused by platelet aggregation. There will be ST-segment elevation in the ECG leading to areas of infarction. STEMIs are emergent and must be opened within 90 minutes of presentation.
D. MI is a dynamic process occurring over several hours and most often occurs in the area of the left ventricle.
E. The severity of the situation depends on the area of the heart involved and the size of the infarction.

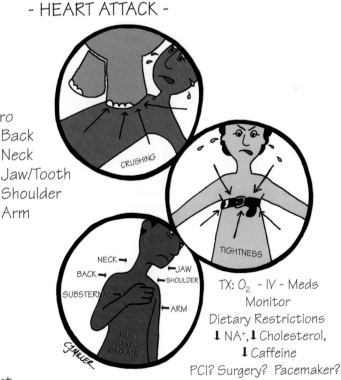

# - MYOCARDIAL INFARCTION (MI) -
## - CORONARY OCCLUSION -
### - HEART ATTACK -

- Pain:
   Sudden Onset
   Substernal
   Crushing
   Tightness
   Severe
   Unrelieved by Nitro
   May Radiate To: Back
                    Neck
                    Jaw/Tooth
                    Shoulder
                    Arm
- Dyspnea
- Syncope (↓ BP)
- Nausea
- Vomiting
- Extreme Weakness
- Diaphoresis
- Denial is
   Common
- ↑ Pulse
- Changes in ST Segment

TX: O$_2$ - IV - Meds
Monitor
Dietary Restrictions
↓ NA⁺, ↓ Cholesterol,
↓ Caffeine
PCI? Surgery? Pacemaker?

© 2016 Nursing Education Consultants, Inc.

**FIGURE 19-5 Myocardial Infarction.** (From Zerwekh, J., Garneau, A., & Miller, C. J. [2017]. *Digital collection of the memory notebooks of nursing* [4th ed.]. Chandler, AZ: Nursing Education Consultants, Inc.)

F. Clients with occlusion of the left anterior descending (LAD) artery (anterior or septal MI) have the highest mortality rate because of development of LVF and dysrhythmias.

G. Healing process.
   1. In the first 24 hours, the inflammatory process is well established; leukocytes invade the area, and cardiac enzymes are released from the damaged cells.
   2. In 4 to 10 days: necrotic zone is well defined.
   3. In 10 to 14 days: the formation of scar tissue foundation begins.
   4. The presence of preestablished collateral circulation will assist in decreasing the size of the necrotic area.

> **! NURSING PRIORITY:** Clients with diabetes who have CAD may not experience chest pain because of diabetic neuropathy. New-onset atrial fibrillation should be explored as a sign of an MI.

### Assessment

A. Risk factors/etiology: coronary artery disease
B. Clinical manifestations of MI.
   1. Pain in varying levels of severity (PQRST) (see Table 19-1).
   2. Pain not relieved by rest, position changes, or nitrate administration.
   3. Pain most often located behind or just to the left of the sternum or epigastric area.
   4. Pain may radiate to neck, jaw, and shoulders.
   5. Client may describe pain as squeezing, choking, or constricting or as a vague feeling of pressure and indigestion.
   6. Client will frequently deny seriousness of the pain.
   7. Accompanying symptoms may include diaphoresis, weakness, dyspnea, pallor, anxiety, nausea, and/or vomiting.
   8. Women's typical clinical manifestations.
      a. Indigestion, interscapular pain, aching jaw, choking sensation with exertion.
      b. Fatigue, sleep disturbance, and dyspnea.

> **! OLDER ADULT PRIORITY:** The only symptom of an MI in older adults may be shortness of breath or indigestion. Those older than 80 years of age may present with acute confusion or disorientation, which can indicate inadequate cardiac output and tissue perfusion.

C. Diagnostics—see Appendix 19-1.
   1. 12-lead ECG.
      a. ST-segment elevation MI (STEMI), traditional.
      b. Non–ST elevation MI (NSTEMI), common in women.
   2. Elevated cardiac troponin I.
   3. Elevated creatinine kinase isoenzyme MB (CK-MB).

### Treatment—Acute Coronary Syndrome

A. Immediate treatment of an MI (Figure 19-6).
B. Restricted activity, supplemental oxygen.

## IMMEDIATE TREATMENT OF AN M.I.

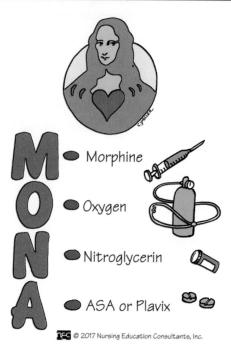

**FIGURE 19-6  MONA: Immediate Treatment of an MI.** (From Zerwekh, J., Garneau, A., & Miller, C. J. [2017]. *Digital collection of the memory notebooks of nursing* [4th ed.]. Chandler, AZ: Nursing Education Consultants, Inc.)

C. Fibrinolytic (reperfusion) therapy (Appendix 19-2).
D. Procedures/surgical interventions.
   1. Percutaneous coronary intervention (PCI).
      a. Balloon angioplasty: a balloon-tipped catheter is inserted into an artery in the groin to the affected coronary artery. The balloon is then inflated in an effort to compress the plaque and dilate the narrowed artery, reestablishing blood flow to the myocardium.
      b. Stent: expandable wire mesh that can be inserted during a PCI. A stent serves as a scaffold to maintain patency of the coronary artery. Stents may be bare metal or drug-clotting types and will require extended treatment with aspirin and clopidogrel after they are placed.
   2. Cardiac revascularization: coronary artery bypass graft (CABG) surgery, open heart surgery.
      a. Transmyocardial laser revascularization (TMR): laser probe is inserted into the wall of the left ventricle; channels are created to promote the development of revascularization. Used for patients with advanced CAD who are not candidates for CABG surgery.

> **! NURSING PRIORITY:** Immediate reperfusion with an invasive intervention (stent or CABG) is used to save the life of the client in cardiogenic shock.

E. Control of the modifiable risk factors (see Box 19-1).

## Complications of MI

A. Dysrhythmias (see Appendix 19-3).

> **! NURSING PRIORITY:** Dysrhythmia, especially ventricular fibrillation, is the most frequent cause of death in the client with an MI. The greatest risk for death from an MI is during the first 2 hours.

B. Heart failure, cardiogenic shock.

> **! NURSING PRIORITY:** Occurring with necrosis of more than 40% of the ventricle, cardiogenic shock has a high mortality rate, making early detection essential. Most clients have a "stop-and-start" pattern of chest pain, resulting in piecemeal extension of damage. Monitor for and report immediately: restlessness or confusion; tachycardia; continued chest discomfort; tachypnea, hypotension; systolic blood pressure less than 90 mmHg or 30 mmHg less than baseline, low urine output; weak pulses; and cold, clammy skin.

C. Papillary muscle dysfunction or rupture.
D. Left ventricular aneurysm, ventricular septal wall rupture.
E. Dressler syndrome.

## Nursing Interventions for Angina and Acute Coronary Syndrome

> **TEST ALERT:** Intervene to improve client's cardiovascular status; assess client for decreased cardiac output; meet client's pain management needs; use critical thinking when addressing pain management.

**Goal:** To decrease pain and increase perfusion and myocardial oxygenation.

A. Begin supplemental oxygen.
B. Position client in reclining position with head elevated.
C. Assess characteristics of pain: administer morphine for pain control.
D. Administer medications.
   1. Administer nitroglycerin (sublingually, IV, or spray; see Appendix 19-2): evaluate client's response; pain from chronic angina is usually relieved; pain from acute angina may not be relieved.
   2. Narcotic analgesics (IV morphine in small increments until pain subsides).
   3. Antiplatelet agent (see Appendix 18-2).
E. Maintain calm, reassuring atmosphere.
F. Establish venous access for fluids and IV medications.
G. Notify physician if pain does not respond to medication or if vital signs deteriorate.

> **! NURSING PRIORITY:** To relieve chest pain and to decrease cardiac damage resulting from an inadequate blood and oxygen supply to the myocardium, there must be an immediate reduction in the workload of the heart that results in a decrease in oxygen consumption: rest, nitroglycerin, oxygen therapy.

**Goal:** To evaluate characteristics of anginal pain and client's overall response.

A. Does pain increase with breathing? (Anginal pain is generally not affected by breathing or changes of position.)
B. Assess activity tolerance or precipitating factor.
C. Assess changes in characteristics of pain (see Table 19-1).
D. Evaluate response of pain to treatment or progression to more severe level.
E. Obtain a 12-lead ECG within 10 minutes of onset of client presentation with chest discomfort.
F. Evaluate vital signs.
   1. Presence of $S_3$ gallop, a ventricular gallop rhythm, which may indicate heart failure in clients over 30 years old.
   2. Presence of jugular vein distention; peripheral edema (right heart failure—RHF).
   3. Presence of frothy sputum or wet breath sounds (left heart failure—LHF).
   4. Adequacy of cardiac output: peripheral pulses, urinary output, level of consciousness.
G. Continuous ECG monitoring: assess for presence of dysrhythmia and effect on cardiac output.
H. Monitor troponin levels (see Appendix 19-1).
I. Assess client's psychosocial response: denial is common; anger, fear, and depression occur in both client and family.

> **TEST ALERT:** Intervene to improve client's cardiovascular status; provide client with strategies to manage decreased cardiac output.

**Goal:** To provide care after percutaneous coronary intervention (with or without stent).

A. Monitor for chest pain and hypotension; reocclusion is a primary complication.
B. Assess for bleeding or hematoma formation.
C. Frequently assess status of circulation distal to area of cannulation.
D. A sheath may be left in place; monitor area for bleeding; if bleeding occurs, put manual pressure on the area and notify the physician.
E. Prevent flexion of affected extremity and maintain bed rest for 6 to 8 hours.
F. Client is to avoid heavy lifting; may return to work in 1 to 2 weeks.
G. Notify the doctor of any chest pain, syncope, or bleeding at the site.
H. Assess ECG for evidence of ST-segment changes.

**! NURSING PRIORITY:** As long as chest pain persists, cardiac ischemia continues. If client experiences tachycardia, decrease activity whether client has chest pain or not.

**Goal:** To evaluate characteristics of cardiac pain and client's overall response.

A. Continuous cardiac monitoring to identify and treat dysrhythmias affecting cardiac output.
B. Frequent assessment for dysrhythmias, murmurs, and presence of $S_3$, $S_4$.
C. Maintain IV access.
D. Maintain bed rest for the first 24 hours.

**TEST ALERT:** Meet client's pain management needs; provide medication for pain relief; use clinical decision making when administering medications; monitor for effects of pain medication.

E. Frequent assessment of chest pain.
F. Evaluate urinary output and renal response.
G. Assess respiratory system for pulmonary congestion.
H. Evaluate peripheral circulation; assess for dependent edema.
I. Maintain NPO (nothing by mouth) status initially; then allow clear liquids; progress to light meals that are low in sodium and cholesterol.
J. Promote normal bowel pattern.
   1. Stool softeners, bedside commode.
   2. Caution against stimulation of the vagus nerve (Valsalva maneuver).
   3. Increase fiber in diet.

**TEST ALERT:** Identify potential/actual stressors for the client; implement measures to reduce environmental stress; promote methods to reduce stress.

K. Decrease anxiety.
   1. Keep client informed regarding progress and immediate plan of care.
   2. Decrease sensory overload.
   3. Encourage verbalization of concerns and fears.
L. Monitor for changes in neurologic status: confusion, disorientation, etc.
M. Monitor progressive activity.
   1. Encourage progressive activity: walking in hallway three to four times a day with gradual increasing increments.
   2. Decrease of 20 mmHg in systolic BP, changes in heart rate greater than 20 beats per minute, shortness of breath, nausea, and/or chest pain indicate poor tolerance to activity.
   3. Assess heart rhythm, fatigue, and blood pressure after each activity.
   4. Resting tachycardia is a contraindication to activity.

**TEST ALERT:** Determine changes in client's cardiovascular system. Monitor progress of client with cardiac disease and evaluate tolerance to changes in activity.

### Home Care

A. Participate in organized cardiac rehabilitation program.
   1. Progressive monitored exercise.
   2. Dietary modifications.
   3. Stress management.
   4. Continued education regarding ACS and decreasing personal risk factors.
B. Understand medication regimen.
C. Teach client how to take his or her pulse and check for rate and regularity.
D. Teach client how to evaluate response to exercise (dyspnea, tachycardia, chest pain, etc.).
   1. Remain close to home to begin walking program.
   2. Client should always carry nitroglycerin when walking or exercising.
   3. Client should check pulse rate before, halfway through, and at the end of activity.
   4. Stop activity for pulse increase of more than 20 beats per minute, shortness of breath, chest pain, nausea, or dizziness.
E. Call the doctor for pain not controlled by nitroglycerin, significant changes in pulse rate, decreased tolerance to activity, syncope, or an increase in dyspnea.
F. Sexual intercourse can generally be resumed in 4 to 6 weeks after MI or when the client can walk one block or climb two flights of stairs without difficulty.
   1. Do not drink any alcohol before sexual activity.
   2. Take nitroglycerin before sexual activity.
   3. Do not have sex after a heavy meal.
   4. Position for intercourse does not influence cardiac workload but considered for client comfort.
   5. Do not take erectile dysfunction medications (see Appendix 24-2) if taking nitrates.

**TEST ALERT:** Assess client's ability to perform self-care. Determine whether the client with cardiac disease understands the illness and whether he or she can demonstrate knowledge of care.

### Heart Failure (HF)

**Heart failure includes cardiac decompensation, cardiac insufficiency, ventricular failure, and ultimately results in the inability of the heart to pump adequate amounts of blood into the systemic circulation resulting in impaired tissue perfusion.**

#### Physiology of Ventricular Failure

A. Systolic (left-sided) failure.
   1. Left ventricle (LV) unable to maintain adequate CO and generate needed pressure to eject blood through the aorta effectively.
   2. Left ventricular hypertrophy (LVH) develops; increasing pressure in pulmonary capillary bed causes

lungs to become congested, resulting in impaired gas exchange.

3. Hallmark is decrease in LV ejection fraction (EF).
4. Precipitating factors.
   a. MI (left ventricular infarct)—contractile dysfunction.
   b. Hypertension—increased afterload.
   c. Mechanical abnormalities—aortic and mitral valve disease.
   d. Cardiomyopathy.

B. Diastolic failure.
   1. Ventricles unable to relax during diastole (filling).
   2. Stroke volume and cardiac output is decreased.
   3. Venous engorgement in both systemic and pulmonary systems.
   4. Precipitating factors.
      a. LVH secondary to chronic hypertension most common.
      b. Aortic stenosis or hypertrophic cardiomyopathy.
      c. More common in older adults, women, and those who are obese.

C. Mixed systolic and diastolic failure.
   1. Poor systolic function compromised with dilated LV walls.
   2. Low ejection fractions (less than 35%), high pulmonary artery pressures, and failure of both sides of the heart.
   3. Seen in dilated cardiomyopathy.

D. Cardiac compensatory mechanisms will attempt to maintain the body requirements for cardiac output; when these mechanisms become ineffective, cardiac decompensation or failure will occur.

E. Edema development in heart failure.
   1. Decreased cardiac output leads to decrease in renal perfusion, the kidneys respond by stimulating the adrenal cortex to increase the secretion of aldosterone, thus increasing the retention of sodium and water.
   2. With an increase in the venous pressure from the increased circulating volume, there is an increase in the capillary pressure, and dependent, pitting edema occurs.

F. In children, HF occurs most often as the result of a structural problem of the heart. Ventricular function may not be impaired, but symptoms occur because of increased pulmonary artery pressure and pulmonary venous congestion.

G. Particularly in older adults, decreased poor cardiac output and reduction in cerebral perfusion can cause confusion, memory loss, and slow verbal responses.

**Assessment**

A. Risk factors/etiology.
   1. MI, CAD, valvular disease.
   2. Hypertension, congenital heart disease.
B. Clinical manifestations.
   1. Types of HF (Figure 19-7 , Figure 19-8).
      a. Left sided failure—pulmonary symptoms.
      b. Right sided failure—systemic symptoms.

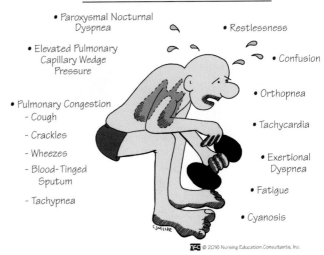

FIGURE 19-7 **Left Sided Heart Failure.** (From Zerwekh, J., & Garneau, A., J., Miller, C. J. [2017]. *Digital collection of the memory notebooks of nursing* [4th ed.]. Chandler, AZ: Nursing Education Consultants, Inc.)

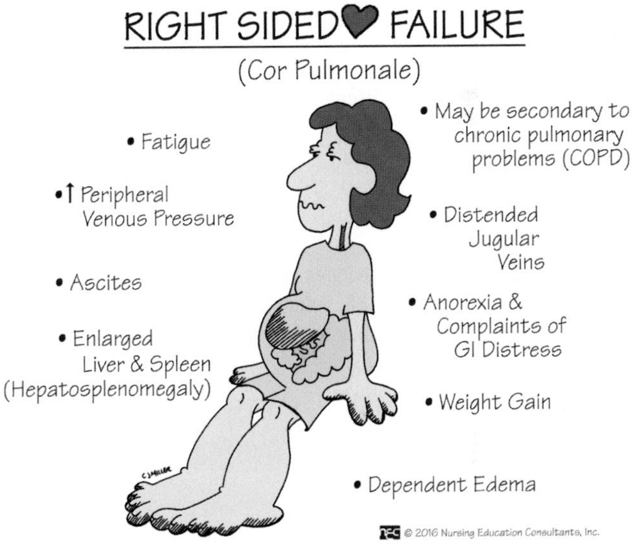

FIGURE 19-8 **Right Sided Heart Failure.** (From Zerwekh, J., Garneau, A., & Miller, C. J. [2017]. *Digital collection of the memory notebooks of nursing* [4th ed.]. Chandler, AZ: Nursing Education Consultants, Inc.)

2. Acute decompensated heart failure (ADHF)—pulmonary edema due to left ventricular failure secondary to CAD.
3. Chronic heart failure.
   a. FACES acronym (Figure 19-9).
   b. Tachycardia, nocturia, chest pain, weight changes.
   c. Skin changes: cool, damp, diaphoretic, absent hair growth and a brown or brawny skin discoloration on lower extremities.
   d. In infants, difficulty with feeding causes failure to thrive and failure to gain adequate weight.

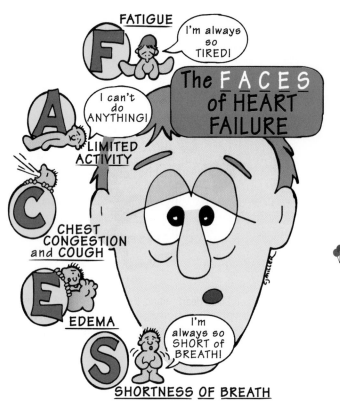

**FIGURE 19-9 FACES of Chronic Heart Failure.** (From Zerwekh, J., Garneau, A., & Miller, C. J. [2017]. *Digital collection of the memory notebooks of nursing* [4th ed.]. Chandler, AZ: Nursing Education Consultants, Inc.)

**TEST ALERT:** Determine changes in client's cardiovascular status as related to the client's HF; interpret which data need to be reported immediately; reevaluate the client with abnormal heart sounds.

C. Diagnostics (see Appendix 19-1).

### Treatment

A. Treatment of the underlying problem.
B. Prevention.
  1. Administration of prophylactic antibiotics to clients with rheumatic heart disease before medical procedures to prevent mitral valve damage.
  2. Effective early treatment of hypertension.
  3. Early treatment of dysrhythmia.
C. Position client in high Fowler's with feet horizontal in bed or dangling at beside.
D. Oxygen.
E. Activity limitations.
F. Medications: treatment for HF includes reduction of the preload and afterload and improvement of the contractility of the myocardium.
  1. Positive inotropic agents: cardiac glycosides; beta-adrenergic agonists (see Appendix 19-2).
  2. Diuretics (see Appendix 18-2).
  3. Aldosterone antagonists (see Appendix 18-2).

4. Vasodilators (see Appendix 18-2).
5. Morphine.
6. Angiotensin-converting enzyme (ACE) inhibitors (see Appendix 18-2).
7. Classified as high-alert drugs, beta-blockers are contraindicated in acute heart failure, and when used for chronic HF are started slowly at a very slow dose. Carvedilol, metoprolol, and bisoprolol are approved for treatment of chronic HF. Do not give with bradycardia (HR less than 60) or hypotension (SBP less than 100 mmHg) (see Appendix 19-2).
8. Electrolyte replacement; carefully monitor serum potassium levels.
9. Antidysrhythmic drugs (see Appendix 19-2).
10. Anticoagulants (see Appendix 18-2).
G. Dietary restriction of sodium; fluid restriction for moderate to severe HF and renal insufficiency. Sodium and fluids may not be restricted for infants and children; infants seldom need fluid restriction because of difficulty feeding.

### Complications

A. Pleural effusion, cardiogenic shock, renal failure.
B. Left ventricular thrombus, hepatomegaly.

**! NURSING PRIORITY:** The goals for therapeutic intervention in clients with HF are to:
• Decrease symptoms—dyspnea and fatigue.
• Improve cardiac output: digitalis and oxygen.
• Decrease cardiac afterload: decrease activity, administer vasodilator.
• Decrease cardiac preload: diuretics, decrease sodium, and fluid intake.

### Nursing Interventions

**Goal:** To decrease cardiac demands and improve cardiac output.

A. Assess vital signs and compare with other physical assessment data.
B. Conserve energy.
  1. Encourage rest alternated with activity.
  2. Monitor pulse, respiratory rate, and dysrhythmias during periods of activity.
C. Avoid chilling; it increases oxygen consumption, especially in infants.
D. Supplemental oxygen, especially when needed with increased activity.
E. Provide uninterrupted sleep, when possible.
F. Minimize crying in children and infants.
G. Decrease stress and anxiety; encourage parents to remain with child.

**TEST ALERT:** Check for interactions among client's drugs, foods, and fluids. For clients receiving digitalis and diuretics, it is very important to monitor the serum potassium level. A significant decrease in the serum potassium level may affect cardiac rhythm and can precipitate digitalis toxicity.

**Goal:** To decrease circulating volume.

A. Assess breath sounds; check for distended neck veins and peripheral edema.

B. Low-sodium diet and fluid restriction in adults and older children.

C. Evaluate fluid retention by determining accurate daily weight (1-kg or 2.2-lb weight gain = 1 L of fluid loss or retention).

D. Accurate intake and output; monitor electrolyte balance and therapeutic effect of fluid loss.

**Goal:** To reduce respiratory distress.

A. Position.
  1. An adult may be placed in Fowler or semi-Fowler position or may sit in an armchair.
  2. When in semi-Fowler position, do not elevate client's legs; doing so increases venous return (preload).
  3. An infant or small child may breathe better in a side-lying position with the knees drawn up to the chest.
  4. An infant may be placed in an infant seat, especially after feeding.
  5. Make sure diapers are loosely pinned and safety re-straints do not hinder maximum expansion of the chest.
  6. Hold infant upright over the shoulder with knees flexed (knee-chest position).

B. Administer oxygen: use oxygen hood for infants and nasal cannula for adults and older children; supplemental oxygen to keep saturation levels at or greater than 90%.

C. Evaluate breath sounds, evaluate adventitious breath sounds and presence of congestion.

D. Do not allow infants to cry for extend periods.

E. For clients who smoke, encourage them to stop and/or provide smoking cessation advice.

> **⊞ PEDIATRIC NURSING PRIORITY:** Infants: if cyanosis decreases with crying, the problem is usually pulmonary; if cyanosis increases with crying, the problem is usually cardiac.

**Goal:** To monitor for development of hypoxia (see Chapter 17).

**Goal:** To maintain nutrition.

A. Provide small, frequent meals of easily digestible foods; allow client adequate time to eat.

B. Assist client with cultural implications in dietary management.

C. An infant will require increased calories because of increased metabolic rate.
  1. May require tube feedings.
  2. An infant does not generally require fluid restriction because of decreased fluid intake secondary to the dyspnea.
  3. Do not prop the bottle; burp the infant frequently.
  4. Decreased calorie intake will result in decreased strength, decreased weight gain, and failure to meet developmental motor skills.

### Home Care

A. Client should begin walking short distances, 250 to 300 feet (72–91 meters), at least 3 to 4 times per week; distance can be increased as tolerated (no shortness of breath, dizziness, chest pain, or tachycardia).

B. Teach client how to count his or her pulse.

C. Teach client to do daily weigh-ins every morning, before breakfast and with similar clothes on (nightgown, pajamas, etc.).

D. Discuss use of and safety factors for home oxygen.

E. Contact health care provider for:
  1. Weight gain of 3 to 5 pounds (1.4–2.3 kg) over a week or 1 to 2 pounds overnight (0.5–0.9 kg).
  2. Increase in dyspnea or angina, especially with decreased activity or at rest.
  3. Waking up breathless at night.
  4. Nausea with abdominal swelling, pain, and tenderness.
  5. Increased urination at night; presence of or increase in peripheral edema.
  6. Cough (especially when lying down) or respiratory congestion.
  7. Fatigue or weakness.

F. Provide written instructions for medications, especially if they are on digitalis.

G. Assess client's home situation and ability of caregivers.

### ⊞ Rheumatic Fever and Heart Disease

**Rheumatic fever is an inflammatory disease that is usually self-limiting. Rheumatic heart disease is the term used to describe the cardiac value damage that occurs as a complication from rheumatic fever.**

A. Usually preceded by a group A beta-hemolytic streptococcal (GABHS) infection.

> **⊞ NURSING PRIORITY:** Prevention and adequate treatment of streptococcal (GABHS) infections prevent the development of rheumatic heart disease.

B. Inflammatory hemorrhagic lesions called *Aschoff bodies* form, causing swelling, fragmentation, and alterations of connective tissue in the heart, joints, skin, and the central nervous system (CNS).

C. Myocardial involvement is characterized by the development of valvulitis, pericarditis, and myocarditis.
  1. Valvulitis produces scarring of the cardiac valves.
  2. Rheumatic carditis is the only symptom that produces permanent damage; most often involves damage to the endocardium and primarily to the mitral valve.
  3. Rheumatic fever usually occurs during childhood, but manifestations of cardiac damage may not be evident for years.

### Assessment

A. Risk factors/etiology: previous infection by GABHS.

B. Clinical manifestations: symptoms vary; no specific symptom or laboratory test is diagnostic of rheumatic fever. Criteria for the diagnosis require a combination of symptoms to be present.

1. Carditis.
   a. Tachycardia out of proportion to fever.
   b. Long, high-pitched apical systolic murmur beginning with $S_1$ and continuing throughout cycle.
   c. Pericarditis, pericardial friction rub, and complaints of chest pain.
2. Migratory polyarthritis.
3. Chorea—of gradual onset, a sudden aimless, irregular movement of the extremities, involuntary facial grimacing, speech disturbance, weakness.
4. Erythema marginatum—nonpruritic macule found on trunk and proximal portion of extremities.
5. Subcutaneous nodules over bony prominences.
6. History of a recent streptococcal infection.

### Treatment

A. Adequate antibiotic treatment of initial streptococcal infection.
B. Rest and decreased activity until tachycardia subsides.
C. Salicylates to reduce fever and discomfort and control the inflammatory process, especially in the joints.
D. Prophylactic treatment: client is susceptible to reoccurrence of rheumatic fever.
   1. Begin after immediate therapy is complete.
   2. Monthly administration of penicillin over extended period, depending on extent of cardiac involvement.
   3. Additional prophylactic antibiotics are given when invasive procedures are necessary (genitourinary procedures, dental work, etc.).

### Complications

A. Severe valvular damage precipitates the development of HF and may require open heart surgery for replacement of diseased valve.
B. Heart failure.

### Nursing Interventions

*Child is generally cared for in the home environment.*

**Goal:** To assist parents and family to provide home environment conducive to healing and recovery.

A. Decrease activity if pulse rate is increased or if child is febrile.
B. Friends may visit for short periods; child is not contagious.
C. Maintain adequate nutrition.
   1. May be anorexic during the febrile phase.
   2. Provide soft or liquid foods as tolerated.
   3. Assist child with feeding if choreiform movements are severe.
   4. Maintain adequate hydration.
D. Salicylates to control inflammatory process and as analgesics for arthralgia.
E. Reassure child that chorea and joint involvement are only temporary and there will be no residual damage.
F. Teach signs of heart failure and when to seek medical attention.

**Goal:** To help parents understand need for long-term prophylactic antibiotic therapy.

A. Importance of preventing recurring infections.
B. Include child in planning, especially when numerous injections are involved.
C. Importance of prophylactic therapy before invasive procedures.
D. Continued medical follow-up for the development of valvular problems as child grows.
E. Follow-up required with females; cardiac problems may not be manifested until woman is pregnant.

## Infective Endocarditis

**Infective endocarditis (IE) is an infection of the valves and inner lining or endocardium of the heart.**

A. Organisms tend to grow on the endocardium in an area of increased turbulence of blood flow or in areas of previous cardiac damage (rheumatic heart disease, congenital malformations).
B. Bacteria may enter from any site of localized infection; most common are *Staphylococcus aureus* and *Streptococcus viridans*.
C. Organisms grow on the endocardium and produce characteristic vegetation consisting of fibrin deposits, leukocytes, and microbes; vegetation may then invade adjacent valves.
D. Vegetation is fragile and may break off, resulting in emboli.

### Assessment

A. Risk factors/etiology.
   1. Most often bacterial but may be fungal or viral.
   2. History of endocarditis, prosthetic valves, or acquired valvular disease.
   3. Aging, renal dialysis, IV drug abuse.
   4. History of recent invasive procedures.
   5. Hospital-acquired bacteremia.
B. Clinical manifestations.
   1. Symptoms of systemic infection: low-grade, intermittent fever; chills; weakness; malaise.
   2. Murmur develops, or changes in previous murmurs occur.
   3. Symptoms associated with heart failure.
   4. Vascular symptoms.
      a. Splinter hemorrhages causing black longitudinal streaks in the nailbeds.
      b. Petechiae in conjunctiva, lips, buccal mucosa, on the ankle, and in the antecubital and popliteal areas.
      c. Red and painful Osler's nodes on fingertips.
      d. Janeway lesions: small, flat, painless red spots on the palm and soles.
      e. Infants may have feeding difficulties, respiratory distress, tachypnea, tachycardia, HF, or septicemia.
   5. Symptoms associated with emboli.
      a. Spleen: splenomegaly, upper left quadrant pain.
      b. Kidney: flank pain, hematuria.
      c. Brain: hemiplegia, decreased level of consciousness, visual changes.

C. Diagnostics.
  1. Echocardiography, ECG.
  2. Blood cultures, drawn 30 minutes apart from two sites.

*Treatment*

A. IV antibiotic therapy for 4 to 6 weeks (see Appendix 9-2).
B. Bed rest if high fever or evidence of HF is present.
C. IV antibiotic therapy for 2 to 8 weeks and only prophylactic antibiotics for high-risk children having congenital heart disease, prosthetic heart valve, cardiac transplant, or previous IE infection.
D. Surgical intervention for severe valvular damage.

*Complications*

A. HF secondary to valve damage.
B. General systemic emboli.

*Nursing Interventions*

**Goal:** To help parents understand the need for long-term prophylactic therapy (see Nursing Interventions under Rheumatic Heart Disease).
**Goal:** To maintain homeostasis and prevent complications.

A. IV antibiotic medications.
B. Assess activity tolerance; activities may be restricted until:
  1. Temperature is normal.
  2. Resting pulse is less than 100 beats/min.
  3. ECG is stable.
C. Evaluate for occurrence of emboli and heart failure.

**Home Care**

A. Good oral hygiene: daily care and regular dental visits.
B. Avoid excessive fatigue; plan rest periods and activity.
C. Client and family must understand the need for continued antibiotics.
D. Report temperature elevations, fever, chills, anorexia, weight loss, and increased fatigue.
E. Advise all health care providers of history of endocarditis.
F. Teach parents of high-risk children to receive prophylactic antibiotic treatment 1 hour before dental procedures, invasive procedures, or when there is an infection of the skin.

**Pericarditis**

**Pericarditis is an inflammation of the pericardium. The pericardial space is a cavity between the inner and the outer layer of the pericardium.**

A. Acute pericarditis: may be dry or may cause excessive fluid accumulation in the pericardial space.
B. Chronic constrictive pericarditis: results from scarring and causes a loss of elasticity; the scarring and thickening of the pericardium prevent adequate cardiac filling during diastole.

*Assessment*

A. Risk factors/etiology.
  1. Acute pericarditis.
    a. Infection.

  b. Myocardial infarction.
    (1) Acute pericarditis may occur within 48 to 72 hours after an MI.
    (2) Dressler syndrome occurs about 4 to 6 weeks after an MI.
  2. Chronic constrictive pericarditis: usually begins with acute episode; fluid is gradually absorbed with scarring and thickening.
B. Clinical manifestations.
  1. Acute.
    a. Pericardial friction rub caused by myocardium rubbing against inflamed pericardium.
    b. Pain increases with deep inspiration and lying supine; sitting may relieve pain; pain may radiate, making it difficult to differentiate from angina.
  2. Chronic: symptoms are characteristic of gradually occurring HF and decreased cardiac output; chest pain is not a prominent symptom.

**NURSING PRIORITY:** Have the client lean forward and hold his or her breath momentarily while assessing heart sounds. If a pericardial friction rub is present, the scratchy, leathery sound auscultated continues with no air exchange and can be determined to be cardiac rather than pleural in origin.

C. Diagnostics: acute and chronic (see Appendix 19-1).
  1. Increased leukocytes.
  2. Inflammation: increased C-reactive protein (CRP), increased erythrocyte sedimentation rate (ESR).

*Complications*

Pericardial effusion (fluid in pericardial space) can result in cardiac tamponade.

*Treatment*

A. Acute episode.
  1. Treat underlying problem.
  2. Bed rest.
  3. Antiinflammatory medications (NSAIDs and corticosteroids).
  4. If pleural effusion and tamponade occur, pericardiocentesis (aspiration of fluid from the pericardial sac) is performed.

*Nursing Interventions*

**Goal:** To maintain homeostasis and promote comfort.

A. Assess characteristics of pain; administer appropriate analgesics.
B. Upright position, with client leaning forward, may relieve the pain.
C. Decrease anxiety, because client often associates problem with an MI; help client distinguish the difference.
D. Observe for symptoms of cardiac tamponade.
  1. Paradoxical blood pressure: precipitous decrease in systolic blood pressure on inspiration.

2. CVP increased; presence of jugular venous distention.
3. Muffled or distant heart sounds.
4. Narrowing pulse pressure.
5. Tachypnea, tachycardia, decrease in cardiac output.
E. In a client with chronic pericarditis, evaluate for symptoms of HF and initiate appropriate nursing interventions.

## Kawasaki Disease

**Kawasaki disease (mucocutaneous lymph node syndrome) is an acute systemic vasculitis of unknown cause that is self-limiting but can lead to a complication of coronary artery aneurysm** (Figure 19-10).

### Assessment

A. Clinical manifestations.
1. High fever unresponsive to antipyretics and antibiotics.
2. Conjunctiva of eye reddened.
3. Inflammation of pharynx.
4. Red cracked lips, "strawberry tongue"—sloughing of outer coating of tongue, leaving large papillae exposed.
5. Rash, cervical lymphadenopathy.
6. Erythema of palms and soles; edema of hands and feet.
7. Myocarditis, tachycardia, gallop rhythm.
B. Diagnostics.
1. Anemia, leukocytosis (shift to the left).
2. Elevated sedimentation rate, CRP.
3. Echocardiogram to monitor cardiac function.

### Treatment

A. High-dose IV immunoglobulin G (IVIG) for 7 to 10 days.
B. Salicylate therapy initially at higher dosages followed by low-dose therapy.
C. Anticoagulant therapy for heart enlargement or with coronary aneurysms.

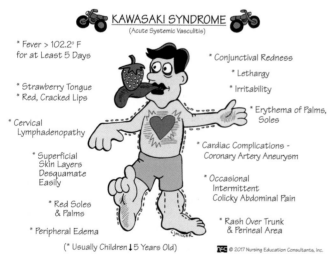

**KAWASAKI SYNDROME**
(Acute Systemic Vasculitis)

* Fever > 102.2° F for at Least 5 Days
* Strawberry Tongue
* Red, Cracked Lips
* Cervical Lymphadenopathy
* Superficial Skin Layers Desquamate Easily
* Red Soles & Palms
* Peripheral Edema
* Conjunctival Redness
* Lethargy
* Irritability
* Erythema of Palms, Soles
* Cardiac Complications - Coronary Artery Aneurysm
* Occasional Intermittent Colicky Abdominal Pain
* Rash Over Trunk & Perineal Area

(* Usually Children ↓5 Years Old)

© 2017 Nursing Education Consultants, Inc.

**FIGURE 19-10 Kawasaki Syndrome.** (From Zerwekh, J., Garneau, A., & Miller, C. J. [2017]. *Digital collection of the memory notebooks of nursing* [4th ed.]. Chandler, AZ: Nursing Education Consultants, Inc.)

### Complications

A. Coronary artery aneurysm.
B. Myocardial infarction.

### Nursing Interventions

**Goal:** To ensure early diagnosis and treatment.
**Goal:** To prevent cardiovascular complications.
**Goal:** To provide discharge teaching regarding medications, potential complication of MI and signs of cardiac ischemia, delay of measles–mumps–rubella (MMR) and varicella vaccine for 11 months after IVIG administration.

## Cardiac Valve Disorders

A. Causes of valve disease.
1. Congenital heart disease.
2. Rheumatic heart disease.
3. Infective endocarditis.
4. Ischemia caused by ACS.
B. Mitral valve is the most common area of involvement because of high pressures in left side of heart, followed by the aortic valve.
C. Valvular stenosis: a narrowing of the valve opening and progressive obstruction to blood flow; increase in workload of the cardiac chamber pumping through the stenosed valve.
D. Valvular insufficiency (incompetency, regurgitation): impaired closure of the valve allows blood to flow back into the cardiac chamber, thereby increasing the workload of the heart.
E. Mitral valve.
1. Stenosis: mitral valve thickens and calcifies, which increases workload on the left atrium as it attempts to force blood through the narrowed valve. Rheumatic fever progressing to rheumatic carditis is most common cause.
2. Mitral insufficiency (regurgitation): with each cardiac contraction, the left ventricle forces blood back into the left atrium.
3. With both conditions, the left atrium dilates and hypertrophies because of an increase in workload. This causes an increase in pulmonary pressure and right ventricular hypertrophy with the subsequent development of HF.
F. Aortic valve.
1. Aortic stenosis: increased (afterload) work of the left ventricle as it attempts to propel blood through the narrowed valve. Considered a disease of "wear and tear" with aging.
2. Aortic insufficiency: increased (afterload) work of the left ventricle as blood leaks back into the left ventricle after contraction.
3. With both conditions, the left ventricle dilates and hypertrophies as a result of increased pressure; this precipitates left ventricular failure.

### Assessment

A. Risk factors: associated with history of rheumatic fever, endocarditis, cardiovascular disease.

B. Clinical manifestations—mitral valve disorders.
1. Exertional dyspnea progressing to orthopnea.
2. Progressive fatigue caused by decrease in cardiac output.
3. Cardiac murmur (diastolic), palpitations.
4. Systemic embolization.
5. Atrial fibrillation (concern is maintaining cardiac output).
C. Clinical manifestations—aortic valve disorders.
1. Syncope and vertigo.
2. Nocturnal angina with diaphoresis (condition interferes with coronary artery filling).
3. Dysrhythmia, systolic murmur in stenosis.
4. Dyspnea and increasing fatigue, heart failure (exertional dyspnea, orthopnea, and paroxysmal nocturnal dyspnea).
5. With severe disease, the nurse notes a "bounding" arterial pulse and widened pulse pressure; client feels palpitations and may have nocturnal angina with diaphoresis.
6. Upon auscultation, a high-pitched, blowing, decrescendo diastolic murmur with aortic regurgitation can be noted.
D. Diagnostics (see Appendix 19-1).

*Treatment*

A. Prevention of HF, pulmonary edema, thromboembolism, and endocarditis.
1. Oxygen as needed to maintain $O_2$ saturation at 95%.
2. Digitalis (see Appendix 19-2).
3. Diuretics.
4. Beta-blockers to decrease cardiac rate.
B. Prophylactic anticoagulation to prevent thrombus formation.
C. Prophylactic antibiotics before invasive procedures.
D. Open heart surgery for valve replacement when there is evidence of progressive cardiac failure. Two types: mechanical or biologic (tissue).
E. Percutaneous transluminal balloon valvuloplasty (PTBV): performed in cardiac catheterization laboratory; balloon is threaded through the affected valve in an attempt to separate the valve leaflets

> **■ NURSING PRIORITY:** Monitor respiratory status closely with clients with mitral stenosis who often have pulmonary hypertension and stiff lungs. Postop clients with aortic valve replacements are at high risk for hemorrhage. Carefully monitor heart rate and blood pressure.

*Nursing Interventions*

**Goal:** To prevent development of rheumatic heart disease and provide prophylactic treatment to individuals with history of rheumatic heart disease.

**Goal:** To teach importance of recommended long-term anticoagulant therapy for clients with mechanical valve replacement or clients with biologic valve replacement who have atrial fibrillation.

**Goal:** To prevent and/or to identify early development of HF (see Heart Failure, Nursing Interventions).

> **■ NURSING PRIORITY:** Primary care for the client with cardiac valve disease consists of maintaining homeostasis and preventing the development of HF. The client should be advised to avoid excessive fatigue and should be assessed according to the level of activity tolerance.

> **TEST ALERT:** Client education for valvular disease includes the importance of taking prophylactic antibiotic therapy before invasive dental or respiratory procedures but is *not* recommended before gastrointestinal procedures.

## 📋 Cardiovascular Disease in Pregnancy

**Rheumatic heart disease (mitral valve problems) and congenital heart defects account for the greatest incidence of cardiac disease in pregnancy.**

A. Normal physiologic alterations of pregnancy that increase cardiovascular stress.
1. Increase in oxygen requirements.
2. Thirty percent to 50% increase in cardiac output; peaks at 20 to 26 weeks' gestation.
3. Increase in plasma volume.
4. Weight gain.
5. Hemodynamic changes during delivery.
B. As normal pregnancy advances, the cardiovascular system is unable to maintain adequate output to meet increasing demands. Classification of the severity of cardiac disease in pregnancy (including relation to prescription of physical activity) is presented in Table 19-2.

> **■ NURSING PRIORITY:** Be familiar with policy and procedures and emergency management of the pregnant client who develops cardiac decompensation or arrest. Document carefully what nursing actions were taken in an emergency situation.

### Table 19-2 CLASSIFICATION OF HEART FAILURE

| Class | Description |
|---|---|
| I | Clients with no limitations on activities; they suffer no symptoms from ordinary activities |
| II | Clients with slight, mild limitation of activity; they are comfortable at rest or with mild exertion |
| III | Clients with marked limitation of activity; they are comfortable only at rest |
| IV | Clients who should be at complete rest, confined to a bed or chair; any physical activity brings on discomfort, and symptoms occur even at rest |

> **■ NURSING PRIORITY:** The functional classification of the disease is determined at 3 months' gestation and again at 7 to 8 months' gestation. Pregnant women may progress from class I or II to III or IV during pregnancy. Women with cyanotic congenital heart disease do not fit into the New York Heart Association (NYHA) classifications because the causes of their exercise-induced symptoms are not related to heart failure.

Adapted from the Criteria Committee, New York Heart Association (NYHA), Boston, 2017.

## Assessment

Clinical manifestations indicative of cardiac decompensation are those of impending HF.

A. Frequent cough, progressive dyspnea with usual activities; orthopnea.
B. Progressive general edema, jugular venous distension (JVD).
C. Palpitations.
D. Excessive fatigue for level of activity.
E. Dysrhythmia, atrial fibrillation, and tachycardia.
F. Congested breath sounds, cyanosis, tachypnea.
G. Cardiac decompensation increases with length of gestation; *highest incidence* of HF is observed at 28 to 32 weeks' gestation.

## Treatment

A. Management of the pregnant client.
1. Balanced nutritional intake; iron and folic acid supplements.
2. Limited physical activity; stop any activity that increases shortness of breath.
3. Diuretics, digitalis, anticoagulants, and antidysrhythmics may be given.
4. May be hospitalized at 28 to 32 weeks' gestation because of impending HF.
5. If coagulation problems occur, heparin is usually used because it does not cross the placenta.
B. Management of the client during labor and delivery.
1. Supplemental oxygen.
2. Epidural regional anesthesia is generally used for delivery.
C. Management of the client during the postpartum period: treated symptomatically according to status of cardiovascular system; the first 24 to 48 hours postpartum is period of *highest risk* for HF in the mother.

## Nursing Interventions

**Goal:** To assist client to maintain homeostasis during pregnancy.

A. Written information regarding nutritional needs.
B. Nursing assessment and client education regarding early symptoms of HF.
C. Frequent rest periods; activity may be severely restricted during the last trimester.

> ❗ **NURSING PRIORITY:** One of the most effective means of decreasing the cardiac workload is to decrease activity; therefore the pregnant client needs to avoid excessive fatigue to prevent or decrease cardiac decompensation.

D. Decrease stress by keeping client informed of progress.

**Goal:** To help client maintain homeostasis during labor and delivery.

A. Position client on side with head and shoulders elevated.
B. Observe for increasing dyspnea, cough, or adventitious breath sounds during labor.
C. Evaluate information from continuous fetal and maternal monitoring.
D. Encourage open glottis pushing during labor; prevent Valsalva maneuver.
E. Prepare for vaginal delivery.
F. Provide pain relief as indicated.
1. Pain increases cardiac work.
2. Evaluate effects of analgesia on fetus.

> **TEST ALERT:** Interpret what data from a client need to be reported immediately.

**Goal:** To maintain homeostasis in the postpartum period.

A. Assessment of cardiac adaptation to changes in hemodynamics.
1. Increased blood flow due to decreased abdominal pressure may precipitate reflux bradycardia.
2. Assess for chest pain and adequacy of cardiac output.
B. Maintain semi-Fowler's position or side-lying position with the head elevated.
C. Gradual progression of activities (depending on cardiac status) as indicated by:
1. Pulse rate.
2. Respiratory status.
3. Activity tolerance.
D. Progressive ambulation as soon as tolerated to prevent venous thrombosis.
E. Assist mother and family to prepare for discharge.

> **TEST ALERT:** Immediately after birth, the woman with cardiac dysfunction is at risk for HF, as blood volume increases significantly when extravascular fluid moves into the vascular compartment and creates a significant increase in the workload of the heart.

## Congenital Heart Disease

A. Clinical manifestations depend on the severity of the defect and the adequacy of pulmonary blood flow.
B. Normal pressure in the right side of the heart is significantly lower than pressure in the left side; there is an increased blood flow from an area of high pressure to an area of low pressure.
1. When there is an opening between the right and left sides of the heart, oxygenated blood will shunt from the left side of the heart to the right side (right-to-left shunt).
2. When the pressures on the right side of the heart exceed the pressure on the left side of the heart, unoxygenated blood from the right side will flow into the left side and unoxygenated blood will flow into the systemic circulation (left-to-right shunt).
C. Physical consequences of congenital heart defects.
1. Delayed physical development.
a. Failure to gain weight, caused by anorexia and/or inability to maintain adequate caloric intake to meet increased metabolic demands.

b. Tachycardia and tachypnea precipitate increase in caloric requirements.

2. Excessive fatigue, especially during feedings.
3. Frequent upper respiratory tract infections.
4. Dyspnea, tachycardia, tachypnea.
5. Hypercyanotic spells (called "blue" spells or "tet" spells): infant suddenly becomes acutely cyanotic and hyperpneic; occur most often in children 2 months to 1 year of age.

D. Diagnostics (see Appendix 19-1).

> **⚠ NURSING PRIORITY:** Infants and children less than 2 years with congenital heart disease should receive a monthly respiratory syncytial virus (RSV) vaccination during RSV season.

## Defects With Increased Pulmonary Artery Blood Flow

Increased blood volume on the right side of the heart increases the flow of blood through the pulmonary artery. This may decrease the systemic blood flow.

A. Atrial septal defect (ASD): opening in the septum between the atrium; blood shunts from left to right; often caused by failure of foramen ovale to close (Figure 19-11).
B. Ventricular septal defect (VSD): opening in the septum between the ventricles; blood shunts from left side to right side, allowing oxygenated blood to mix with unoxygenated blood (Figure 19-12).
C. Patent ductus arteriosus (PDA): failure of the fetal ductus arteriosus to close after birth; blood is shunted from the left side to the right side; may be treated with indomethacin (prostag-landin inhibitor) or ibuprofen, NSAIDs that change the oxygen concentration of the tissue and en-hance tissue changes that close the defect (Figure 19-13).

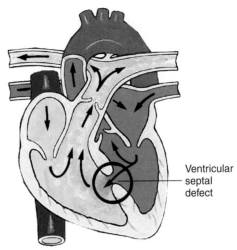

**FIGURE 19-12  Ventricular Septal Defect.** (From Hockenberry, M. J., & Wilson, D. [2015]. *Wong's nursing care of infants and children* [10th ed.]. St. Louis, MO: Mosby.)

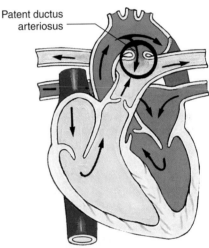

**FIGURE 19-13  Patent Ductus Arteriosus.** (From Hockenberry, M. J., & Wilson, D. [2015]. *Wong's nursing care of infants and children* [10th ed.]. St. Louis, MO: Mosby.)

D. Clinical manifestations.
   1. May be asymptomatic.
   2. Signs of HF are common.
   3. Characteristics "machinery type" murmurs.

## 🌸 Obstructive Defects With Decreased Pulmonary Artery Blood Flow

Problems occur when the normal blood flow through the heart meets an obstruction. The pressure in the ventricle and in the artery before the obstruction is increased; pressure beyond the obstruction is decreased.

A. Coarctation of the aorta (narrowing of the aortic arch); specific symptoms depend on the location of the coarctation in relation to arteries coming off the aortic arch (Figure 19-14).
   1. Clinical manifestations.
      a. Marked differences in blood pressure in the upper and lower extremities; area proximal to the defect

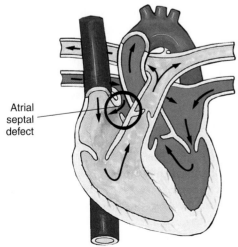

**FIGURE 19-11  Atrial Septal Defect.** (From Hockenberry, M. J., & Wilson, D. [2015]. *Wong's nursing care of infants and children* [10th ed.]. St. Louis, MO: Mosby.)

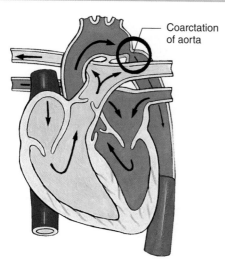

**FIGURE 19-14 Coarctation of the Aorta.** (From Hockenberry, M. J., & Wilson, D. [2015]. *Wong's nursing care of infants and children* [10th ed.]. St. Louis, MO: Mosby.)

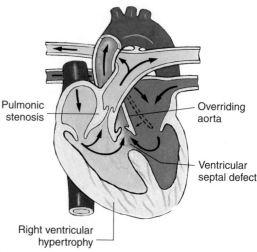

**FIGURE 19-15 Tetralogy of Fallot.** (From Hockenberry, M. J., & Wilson, D. [2015]. *Wong's nursing care of infants and children* [10th ed.]. St. Louis, MO: Mosby.)

(upper extremities) has high pressure and a bounding pulse.
  (1) Epistaxis.
  (2) Headaches.
  (3) Bounding radial and temporal pulses.
  (4) Dizziness and fainting.
  b. Area distal to defect has decreased blood pressure and weaker pulse.
    (1) Lower extremities are cooler; mottling is present.
    (2) Weak peripheral and femoral pulses.
  c. May develop HF especially in infants.
 2. Increased risk for hypertension, ruptured aorta, aortic aneurysm, and stroke.
B. Aortic stenosis: a narrowing or constriction of the aortic valve that increases resistance to ejection of blood from the left ventricle into systemic circulation; increases pulmonary vascular congestion.
 1. Clinical manifestations.
  a. Decreased cardiac output, faint pulses, hypotension, tachycardia.
  b. Children have exercise intolerance and may have chest pain.
  c. Characteristic murmur.
 2. At risk for infective endocarditis, coronary insufficiency, ventricular dysfunction.

### Defects With Decreased Pulmonary Blood Flow

An anatomic defect is present between the right and left sides of the heart (ASD or VSD). There is increased pulmonary artery resistance to blood flow, therefore pressure increases in the right side of the heart. As the resistance in the pulmonary circulation increases, pressure in the right ventricle increases. This pressure increases until it is greater than pressure on the left side of the heart and unoxygenated (unsaturated)

blood moves into the left side of the heart (right-to-left shunt).
A. Tetralogy of Fallot: consists of four defects—VSD, pulmonic stenosis, overriding aorta, and right ventricular hypertrophy (Figure 19-15).
 1. Clinical manifestations depend on the size of the VSD and the pressures in the heart.
  a. May be acutely cyanotic at birth or may have minimal cyanosis due to patent ductus arteriosus.
  b. Child may have mild cyanosis that progresses.
  c. Infant may experience acute episodes of hypoxia (blue spells, tet spells); may occur during agitation or crying.
  d. Posturing or squatting in the older child.
  e. HF does not usually develop because overload of right ventricle flows into the aorta and the left ventricle; therefore pulmonary congestion does not occur. HR may occur postoperatively.
 2. At risk for emboli, seizures, changes in level of consciousness, or sudden death from anoxia.
B. Tricuspid atresia: tricuspid valve does not develop, and there is no opening from the right atrium to the right ventricle; an ASD, or patent foramen ovale, is present and provides mixing of oxygenated and unoxygenated blood; results in decreased pulmonary blood flow.
 1. Clinical manifestations.
  a. Cyanosis usually occurs during newborn period.
  b. Tachycardia, dyspnea.
  c. Older children have chronic hypoxemia and clubbing.
 2. Continuous infusion of prostaglandin E₁ may be used to maintain a patent ductus arteriosus until surgery can be performed.

### Mixed Defects

Mixed defects are present when the survival of the infant depends on the mixing of oxygenated and unoxygenated

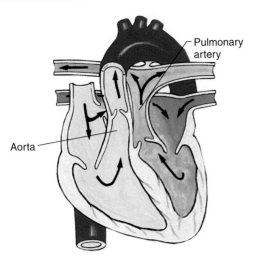

**FIGURE 19-16 Transposition of the Great Vessels.** (From Hockenberry, M. J., & Wilson, D. [2015]. *Wong's nursing care of infants and children* [10th ed.]. St. Louis, MO: Mosby.)

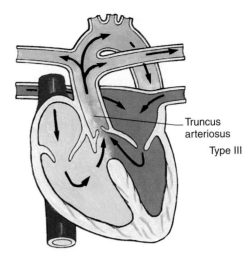

**FIGURE 19-17 Truncus Arteriosus.** (From Hockenberry, M. J., & Wilson, D. [2015]. *Wong's nursing care of infants and children* [10th ed.]. St. Louis, MO: Mosby.)

blood for survival. Pulmonary congestion occurs as a result of the increased flow of blood into pulmonary vasculature.

A. Transposition of great vessels: the pulmonary artery receives blood from the left ventricle, and the aorta receives blood from the right ventricle. A communicated defect—ASD, VSD, or patent ductus arteriosus—must be present to provide for mixing of oxygenated and un-oxygenated blood (Figure 19-16).
   1. Clinical manifestations depend on size of associated defects and mixing of blood.
      a. Newborns with minimal communication defects are cyanotic at birth.
      b. Symptoms of HF.
      c. Cardiomegaly develops shortly after birth.
   2. Prostaglandins may be given to maintain patency of ductus arteriosus to promote mixing of blood.
B. Truncus arteriosus: the pulmonary artery and aorta fail to separate; results in a single vessel that receives blood from both ventricles (Figure 19-17).
   1. Clinical manifestations.
      a. Cyanosis and HF develop in infancy.
      b. Characteristic murmur.
   2. Multiple surgical repairs are necessary to replace conduits as child grows.

### Nursing Interventions

**Goal:** To evaluate infant's response to cardiac defect.

A. Evaluate infant's Apgar scores at birth.
B. Evaluate adequacy of weight gain in first few months.
C. Assess feeding problems.
   1. Poor sucking reflex.
   2. Poor coordination of sucking, swallowing, and breathing.
   3. Fatigues easily during feeding.
D. Frequency of upper respiratory tract infections.
E. Determine whether cyanosis occurs at rest or is precipitated by activity.

F. Presence and quality of pulses in extremities.
G. Bacterial endocarditis is a primary concern before and after correction of a congenital defect; all fevers should be reported.

**Goal:** To promote oxygenation.

A. Effectively cope with hypercyanotic spells (blue spells, tet spells).
   1. Occurs suddenly, often when the infant is agitated.
   2. Hold the infant upright in a knee-chest position; this reduces the venous return and increases systemic vascular resistance, which increases pressure on the right side of the heart and diverts more blood flow through the pulmonary artery.
   3. Administer 100% O₂ via a face mask until respirations are improved.
   4. Maintain good hydration and carefully monitor hemoglobin levels.
   5. Older child may assume squatting position to increase peripheral resistance and decrease right-to-left shunting.
B. Supplemental oxygen, good pulmonary hygiene, and chest physiotherapy to maintain oxygen saturation levels.
C. Prevent overexertion, decrease excessive crying, and promote rest to conserve energy and caloric expenditure.
D. Maintain hydration for pulmonary hygiene and to prevent embolic problems and stroke.
E. Infants may require gavage feeding if respiratory distress limits oral feeding.

**Goal:** To assist parents in adjusting to diagnosis.

A. Allow family to grieve over loss of perfect infant.
B. Evaluate parents' level of understanding of the child's problem.
C. Foster early parent–infant attachment; encourage touching, holding, feeding, and general physical contact.
D. Help the family develop a relationship that fosters optimum growth and development of all family members.

(See Chapter 2 for psychosocial aspects of caring for chronically ill children.)

E. Discharge teaching subjects should include: medication administration (digoxin), activity level, diet, wound care, prophylaxis for infective endocarditis, follow-up appointments, and instructions when to contact health care provider.

---

**TEST ALERT:** Provide emotional support to family; assist family members in managing care of a child with a chronic illness.

---

**Goal:** To detect, prevent, and treat HF.

**Goal:** To provide appropriate nursing interventions for the client undergoing open heart surgery for repair of a defect.

## CRITICAL CARE

### PRIORITY CONCEPTS

Infection, Pain, Perfusion

### Cardiac Surgery

A. CABG, aortic and mitral valve replacements: open heart surgery is performed with the use of the cardiopulmonary bypass machine; this machine allows for full visualization of the heart while maintaining perfusion and oxygenation.

B. Closed heart surgery is performed without the use of the bypass machine.
   1. Minimally invasive direct coronary artery bypass grafts (MIDCABG): one of the most common procedures; these are grafts to the left anterior descending artery.
   2. Aortic and mitral balloon valvuloplasty.

C. Intensive care unit for 24 to 36 hours after surgery for intensive monitoring of client's hemodynamic status.

### Nursing Interventions

For preoperative and postoperative care, see Chapter 3.

**Goal:** To prepare the client psychologically and physiologically for surgery.

A. Evaluate client's history for other chronic health problems.

B. Establish baseline data for postoperative comparison.

C. Provide appropriate preoperative teaching according to age level; frequently includes a visit to the intensive care unit (parents should accompany the child on the visit).

D. Discuss immediate postoperative nursing care and anticipated nursing procedures.

E. Correct metabolic and electrolyte imbalances.

F. Establish and maintain adequate hydration.

G. Anticipate adjustments in medication schedule before surgery.
   1. Digitalis dosage is usually decreased.

   2. Diuretics may be discontinued 48 hours before surgery.
   3. Long-acting insulin will be changed to regular insulin.
   4. Antihypertensive medication dosage may be modified.

H. Eliminate possible sources of infection.

**Goal:** To evaluate and promote cardiovascular function after surgery.

A. Maintain adequate blood pressure.

B. Evaluate for dysrhythmia; document and treat accordingly (see Appendix 19-3).

C. Maintain client in semi-Fowler's position.

D. Evaluate fluid and electrolyte balances.
   1. Record daily weight and compare with previous weight.
   2. Evaluate electrolyte balance, especially potassium levels.
   3. Assess for adequate hemoglobin, hematocrit, and prothrombin time (PTT) values.
   4. Evaluate hemodynamic levels for adequate volume (see Appendix 19-5).
   5. Measure urine output hourly to evaluate adequacy of renal perfusion.
   6. Administer IV fluids, as indicated.

E. Observe for hemorrhage: most often identified by an increase in mediastinal chest tube drainage.

F. Evaluate adequacy of peripheral circulation.
   1. Mark location of pedal pulses preoperatively, assess postoperatively.
   2. If saphenous vein is harvested, monitor incision for wound edge approximation, drainage, and signs of infection. Keep incision clean; apply antibacterial ointment to site.

G. Mediastinal chest tubes are frequently placed in the pericardial sac to prevent tamponade.

H. Bedside hemodynamic monitoring as indicated (see Appendix 19-5).

**Goal:** To evaluate and promote respiratory function.

A. Mechanical ventilation via an endotracheal tube may be used for approximately 12 to 24 hours after surgery. Generally, children are extubated sooner than adults.

B. Maintain water-sealed drainage for mediastinal/chest tubes (see Appendix 17-4).

C. Pulmonary hygiene via endotracheal tube; carefully assess pulse oximetry during suctioning.

D. Promote good respiratory hygiene after extubation (fluids, incentive spirometry, activity).

E. Evaluate arterial blood gases for adequate oxygenation, as well as acid–base balance.

F. Encourage activity as soon as possible; client should be out of bed on the first postoperative day.

G. Monitor pulse oximetry levels.

**Goal:** To evaluate neurologic status for complications after surgery.

A. Recovery from anesthesia within appropriate time frame.

B. Able to move all extremities equally.

C. Appropriate response to verbal command.

D. Assess for changes in neurologic status.

**Goal:** To prevent complications of immobility (see Chapter 3) after surgery.

**Goal:** To decrease anxiety and promote comfort after surgery.

A. Frequent orientation to surroundings.

B. Careful explanation of all procedures.

C. Prevent sensory overload.

D. Promote uninterrupted sleep.

E. Administer pain medications as appropriate.

## Common Complications After Cardiac Surgery

A. Dysrhythmia (see Appendix 19-5).
  1. Premature ventricular contractions.
  2. Ventricular tachycardia.
  3. Atrial dysrhythmias are most common the first 3 days after surgery.
  4. Conduction blocks.

B. Hypovolemia.
  1. Low cardiac output may be due to hypovolemia.
  2. Frequently, vasoconstriction is present immediately after surgery. Vasodilation occurs as client's body temperature increases and precipitates hypovolemia.
  3. Evaluate hemodynamic parameters for adequacy of cardiac output.
  4. Observe client closely for response to fluid replacement, because fluid overload occurs very rapidly, especially in children and older adults.

C. Emboli.
  1. Pulmonary emboli.
  2. Arterial emboli.
    a. Occur most frequently after valvular surgery.
    b. Client may be receiving prophylactic anticoagulants.
    c. Evaluate neurologic system for evidence of cerebral emboli.

D. Cardiac tamponade.
  1. Pressure on the heart caused by a collection of fluid in pericardial sac.

  2. May be caused by fluid collecting postoperatively or from pericarditis; be sure pericardial chest drainage system is functioning. Report output that is greater than 150 mL/hr.
  3. Pressure prevents adequate filling of ventricles, thereby decreasing cardiac output.
  4. Pulsus paradoxus: precipitous decrease in systolic blood pressure on inspiration; diagnostic for tamponade.
  5. Client may become confused and restless and have new-onset chest pain; JVD and CVP are frequently increased; blood pressure is decreased.
  6. Heart sounds are described as muffled or distant.
  7. A decrease in drainage may occur in the mediastinal tubes.
  8. Treatment involves reestablishing patency of mediastinal tube, surgical exploration of bleeding areas, or pericardiocentesis with pericarditis.

E. Intensive care unit (ICU) delirium (most common in adults); incorrectly called ICU psychosis, because client is *not* psychotic.
  1. Characteristics.
    a. Alterations in mentation (delusions, short attention span, loss of memory).
    b. Psychomotor behavior (restlessness, lethargy).
    c. Sleep–wake cycle (daytime sleepiness, nighttime agitation).
  2. Prevention of ICU delirium.
    a. Ensure adequate oxygenation.
    b. Maintain orientation to time and place.
    c. Reduce sensory overload—limit noise on alarms, overhead paging, conversations at bedside about the client but without their participation.
    d. Get client out of bed as soon as possible; position client to look out window if available.
    e. Maintain continuity in nursing staff.
    f. Carefully explain all procedures.
    g. Encourage expression of feelings.

---

## Appendix 19-1  CARDIAC DIAGNOSTICS

### Serum Laboratory Studies

#### Cardiac Markers

The contents of the injured cells are released into the bloodstream.

**Creatinine Kinase Isoenzyme MB (CK-MB):**
CK-MB is specific to heart muscle. Increases greater than 5% of total CK are highly indicative of MI. Increases occur within 4 to 6 hours after an MI, peak in 12 to 24 hours, and return to normal in 24 to 36 hours.

**Cardiac Troponin T and Cardiac Troponin I:**
A myocardial muscle protein released into the bloodstream with myocardial muscle damage; normal level is less than 0.2 ng/mL (mg/L) for T and less than 0.03 ng/dL (mg/L) for I. Levels are elevated early—within 4 to 6 hours after an MI—and peak within 10 to 24 hours. Any rise in values indicates cardiac necrosis or acute MI.

**Myoglobin:**
A low-molecular-weight heme protein found in cardiac and skeletal muscles; *myoglobin* is the earliest cardiac marker detected, within 2 hours after an MI, rapidly declining after 7 hours. Because it is nonspecific for cardiac muscle, it has limited clinical usefulness.

#### Nursing Implications

1. Enzymes must be drawn on admission and obtained in a serial manner thereafter. There is a characteristic pattern to the increases and decreases of enzyme levels in a client with an MI.
2. The larger the infarction, the larger the enzyme response.
3. Evaluate serial levels of the enzymes; increased levels of troponin are the most significant and diagnostic of myocardial damage.
4. Cardiac-specific troponin helps discriminate from other tissue injury.

*Continued*

> **! NURSING PRIORITY:** For a client with an increase in CK-MB (CK$_2$) and an increase in cardiac troponin levels, it is important to monitor closely for symptoms of acute coronary syndrome (ACS). In a client with ACS, serum levels may be checked every 6 to 8 hours during the acute phase.

### C-Reactive Protein (CRP), Highly Sensitive C-Reactive Protein (hs-CRP)

Identification of the protein that is synthesized by the liver and not normally present in the blood except when there is inflammation from tissue trauma. The response to the test assists in evaluating the severity and course of inflammatory conditions. Highly sensitive CRP (hs-CRP) is an independent risk factor for the development of CAD and ACS.

Normal: Less than 1 mg/L (9.52 nmol/L); a level greater than 3 mg/L (28.57 nmol/L) is significant and may indicate some degree of inflammatory response caused by plaque formation. It is used to determine treatment options for those at risk for CAD and to manage statin therapy after an acute MI.

### Serum Electrolytes

ECG changes with potassium levels.

### Hyperkalemia

1. Tall, peaked T wave, widening of the QRS.
2. Cardiac arrest.

### Hypokalemia

1. U wave that occurs after the T wave.
2. Premature ventricular contractions (PVCs).
3. Ventricular tachycardia, ventricular fibrillation.

### Erythrocyte Sedimentation Rate

Used as a gauge for evaluating progression of inflammatory conditions; inflammatory process precipitates a rapid settling of the red blood cells.

Normal values vary greatly, depending on the laboratory method used.

### B-Type Natriuretic Peptide (BNP)

Natriuretic peptides promote vasodilation and diuresis through sodium loss. Fluid overload caused by heart failure stretches the ventricles leading to a release of the B-type natriuretic peptide (BNP). Serial BNP values may be determined to evaluate left ventricular function; assists to identify heart failure versus respiratory failure as cause of dyspnea. Normal is less than 100 pg/mL (ng/L). Values increase with age and in women and are lower in people who are obese.

## Noninvasive Diagnostics

### Electrocardiogram (ECG)

A graphic representation of the electrical activity of the heart, generally conducted by using a 12-lead format. Test to identify conduction in rhythm disorders and the occurrence of ischemia, injury, or death of myocardial tissue.

### Holter Monitor

Client is connected to a small portable ECG unit with recorder that records the client's heart activity for approximately 24 to 48 hours. The client keeps a log of activity, pain, and palpitations. Client should not remove leads but is encouraged to maintain normal activity; client should not shower or bathe while the monitor is in place. The recording is analyzed and compared with the client's activity log.

### Event Monitor (Transtelephonic Event Recorder)

Client is connected to portable ECG unit with a recorder. The client can activate the recorder whenever he or she feels any type of dizziness or palpitations. Monitor may be worn for extended periods. Monitor leads and battery are removed for showering but should be reconnected immediately. Recordings are transmitted over the phone.

### Exercise Stress Test

This test involves the client exercising, usually on a treadmill that increases speed and incline to increase the heart rate. ECG leads are attached to the client, and the response of the heart to exercise is evaluated. If the client is unable to walk on the treadmill, medications may be administered to simulate the exercise.

#### Nursing Implications

1. Provide appropriate pretest preparation; establish baseline vital signs and cardiac rhythm.
2. Client should:
   a. Avoid smoking, eating, or drinking any caffeine beverages for 3 hours before the test.
   b. Avoid stimulants, eating, and extreme temperature changes immediately after the test.
3. Cardiac monitoring is done constantly during test.
4. Reasons for terminating an exercise stress test: chest pain, significant increase or decrease in blood pressure, or significant ECG changes.
5. If any of these changes occur, the test is terminated and the stress test result is said to be positive.

### Echocardiogram

An ultrasound procedure to evaluate valvular function, cardiac chamber size, ventricular muscle, and septal motion. The ultrasound waves are displayed on a graph and interpreted.

### Transesophageal Echocardiography

Provides a higher-quality picture than regular echocardiogram. The throat is anesthetized, and a flexible endoscope is passed into the esophagus to the level of the heart. Sedation is used during the procedure.

#### Nursing Implications

1. Maintain NPO for 4 to 8 hours before test.
2. Check for gag and swallow reflex before client resumes oral intake of fluids.

## Invasive Diagnostics

### Cardiac Catheterization

An invasive procedure in which a catheter is passed through the brachial or femoral artery for left-side cardiac catheterization; the

## Appendix 19-1 CARDIAC DIAGNOSTICS—cont'd

brachial or femoral vein for right-side cardiac catheterization. Cardiac catheterization will provide data regarding status of the coronary arteries, as well as cardiac muscle function, valvular functions, and left ventricular function (ejection fraction).

### Nursing Implications

1. Pretest preparation.
   a. Maintain NPO status for 6 hours before test.
   b. Check for dye allergy, especially allergy to iodine and contrast media.
   c. Record quality of distal pulses for comparison after test.
   d. Determine whether any medications need to be withheld.
   e. Appropriate client education (feeling of warmth when dye is injected; will be awake during procedure; report any chest pain; need to lie still).
2. After the test.
   a. Evaluate catheterization entry site (most often femoral) for hematoma formation. Notify physician immediately for

excessive bleeding at the site, dramatic changes in blood pressure.
   b. Evaluate neurovascular status (pulses distal to catheterization site, color, sensation of the extremity). Notify physician immediately for a decrease in peripheral circulation or neurovascular changes in affected extremity.
   c. Assess for dysrhythmias.
   d. Maintain bed rest; avoid flexion; keep extremity straight for 3 to 6 hours.
   e. Keep head of bed elevated at 30 degrees or less.
   f. Encourage oral intake of fluids; IV access may be maintained.

### Positron Emission Tomography (PET)

Very sensitive in identifying viable and nonviable cardiac tissue. The procedure takes about 2 to 3 hours, and a radioactive dye is injected intravenously, followed by glucose. A client's glucose must be between 60 and 140 mg/dL (3.3–7.8 mmol/L) before the test.

*NPO,* Nothing by mouth; *IV,* intravenously.

## Appendix 19-2 CARDIAC MEDICATIONS

**Nitrates:** Increase blood supply to the heart by dilating the large coronary arteries; cardiac workload is reduced due to decrease in venous return because of peripheral vasodilation (decreases preload).

| Medications | Side Effects | Nursing Implications |
|---|---|---|
| Nitroglycerin: sublingual<br>Nitroglycerin extended release: buccal tablets<br>Nitroglycerin: topical (patch)<br>Nitroglycerin IV<br>Nitroglycerin ointment: topical, by the inch<br>Nitroglycerin translingual spray<br>Isosorbide dinitrate: PO, extended release | Headaches (will diminish with therapy), postural hypotension, syncope, blurred vision, dry mouth, reflex tachycardia | 1. Advise client that alcohol will potentiate postural hypotension.<br>2. Educate client regarding self-medication (Box 19-2).<br>3. Do not take with erectile dysfunction drugs.<br>4. Topical or transdermal application is used for sustained protection against anginal attacks.<br>5. Avoid skin contact with topical form; remove all previous applications when applying topical form.<br>6. Sublingual tablets and translingual spray given for an immediate response. |

*IV,* Intravenously; *PO,* by mouth (orally).

## Box 19-2 CLIENT EDUCATION FOR NITROGLYCERIN ADMINISTRATION

1. Keep in a tightly closed, dark glass container.
2. Carry supply at all times—either sublingual (SL) tablets or translingual spray; do not swallow sublingual tablets or inhale the translingual spray.
3. Fresh tablets should cause a slight tingling under the tongue.
4. Date all opened containers and discard all medication that is 6 months old.
5. Take nitroglycerin prophylactically to avoid pain—before sexual intercourse, exercise, walking, etc.
6. Take nitroglycerin when pain begins; stop all activity.
7. If pain is not relieved in 5 minutes, call 911 and activate EMS.
8. While waiting for EMS response, if chest pain remains unrelieved, take another SL pill and then a third 5 minutes later.
9. Remain lying down; orthostatic hypotension can be a problem.
10. Long-acting preparations should not be abruptly discontinued; this may precipitate vasospasm.
11. To decrease development of tolerance in long-acting preparations, schedule an 8-hour nitro-free period each day, preferably at night.
12. Do not take erectile dysfunction drugs with nitroglycerin.

**TEST ALERT:** Instruct clients about self-administration of medications.

*Continued*

**Appendix 19-2 CARDIAC MEDICATIONS—cont'd**

| Medications | Side Effects | Nursing Implications |
|---|---|---|

**Calcium Channel Blockers:** Blockade of calcium channel receptors in the heart causes decreased cardiac contractility and a decreased rate of sinus and AV node conduction. Used to treat chronic stable angina, hypertension, Prinzmetal angina, and supraventricular dysrhythmias (paroxysmal supraventricular tachycardia [PSVT], atrial fibrillation, and atrial flutter).

| Medications | Side Effects | Nursing Implications |
|---|---|---|
| Diltiazem: PO, IV<br>Nifedipine: PO<br>Clevidipine: IV for severe hypertension<br>Verapamil: IV, PO | Constipation (Verapamil—especially in older adults), exacerbation of HF, hypotension, bradycardia, peripheral dilation and edema, and headaches. | 1. Monitor heart rate and blood pressure.<br>2. Nifedipine is less likely to exacerbate preexisting cardiac conditions; is not effective in treating dysrhythmias.<br>3. Intensifies cardio-suppressant effects of beta-blocker medications.<br>4. Client education includes reporting dyspnea, orthopnea, JVD, or swelling of the legs; changing positions slowly. |

**Beta-Adrenergic Blocking Agents (Adrenergic Antagonists):** Blockade of beta₁ receptors in the heart causes decreased heart rate and decreased rate of AV conduction. Used to treat hypertension and angina. Beta-blockers should be administered to all clients experiencing unstable angina or having an MI, unless contraindicated. Consider using a cardioselective beta-blocker for clients with a history of bronchospasm.

| Medications | Side Effects | Nursing Implications |
|---|---|---|
| ▲ Labetalol: PO, IV<br>Metoprolol: PO, IV<br>Propranolol: PO, IV<br>Atenolol: PO, IV<br>▲ High-Alert Medications: all IV preparations.<br>Carvedilol: PO<br>*Note: Carvedilol, bisoprolol, and metoprolol sustained release are used to treat HF.*<br>Cardioselective—atenolol, carteolol, metoprolol, betaxolol, bisoprolol, nebivolol at low dose | Bradycardia, hypotension, depression, lethargy, and fatigue | 1. High-alert medications.<br>2. Closely monitor cardiac client—may precipitate heart failure but is also used to treat heart failure.<br>3. Teach client how to decrease effects of postural hypotension.<br>4. Teach client not to stop taking medication when he or she feels better.<br>5. Bradycardia is common adverse effect.<br>6. If client has diabetes, blood glucose control may be impaired.<br>7. No longer considered first-line therapy for essential HTN (diuretics, ACE inhibitors, ARBs, and CCBs perform more effectively). |

▲ High-alert medications; *ACE,* angiotensin-converting enzyme; *ARBs,* angiotensin receptor blockers; *AV,* atrioventricular; *CCBs,* calcium channel blockers; *HF,* heart failure; *HTN,* hypertension; *IM,* intramuscularly; *IV,* intravenously; *MI,* myocardial infarction; *PO,* by mouth (orally).

**Antidysrhythmics:** Decrease cardiac excitability; delay cardiac conduction in either the atrium or ventricle. Atropine is cardiac stimulant for bradycardia.

**General Nursing Implications**
- Assess client for changes in cardiac rhythm and affect cardiac output.
- Evaluate effect of medication on dysrhythmia and resulting effects on cardiac output.
- Client should be on bed rest and have a cardiac monitor attached during IV administration.
- Have atropine available for cardiac depression resulting in symptomatic bradycardia.
- All cardiac depressant medications are contraindicated in clients with sinus node or AV node blocks.
- Digitalis will enhance cardiac depressant effects.
- Closely monitor for dysrhythmias that are precipitated by the treatment.
- See Appendix 19-3: Cardiac Dysrhythmias.

| Medications | Side Effects | Nursing Implications |
|---|---|---|
| Quinidine sulfate: PO | Hypotension<br>Diarrhea, nausea, vomiting | 1. Administer with food.<br>2. Monitor for ECG changes for toxicity—widened QRS and prolonged QT.<br>3. *Use:* supraventricular tachycardia and ventricular dysrhythmias. |
| Atropine: subQ, IV | Tachycardia<br>Dry mouth, blurred vision, dilated pupils, urinary retention | 1. *Use:* symptomatic bradycardia<br>2. Monitor heart rate and rhythm after administration.<br>3. Can cause chest pain in clients with ischemic CAD.<br>4. Contraindicated in clients with acute angle-closure glaucoma. |

**Appendix 19-2   CARDIAC MEDICATIONS—cont'd**

| Medications | Side Effects | Nursing Implications |
|---|---|---|
| Adenosine: IV | Common—facial flushing, shortness of breath, dyspnea, and chest pain<br>Significant hypotension<br>AV heart block | 1. *Use:* first drug for PSVT, WPW.<br>2. **Not** used for irregular wide complex tachycardias because it can degenerate to VF and has a rapid half-life, therefore must be given rapidly undiluted over 1–3 sec followed by bolus of 20 mL of normal saline.<br>3. Causes a brief period of asystole after administration; monitor for bradycardia and hypotension.<br>4. Monitor heart rate and rhythm closely after administration.<br>5. PVCs and recurrence of PSVT may occur. |
| Amiodarone hydrochloride: PO, IV<br>▲ High-Alert Medication: IV route | Bradycardia, AV heart block, hypotension, worsening dysrhythmias<br>Toxicity—lung, visual, liver, and thyroid<br>Muscle-related side effects usually develop early in treatment. | 1. *Use:* life-threatening ventricular arrhythmias (pulseless VT/Vfib), atrial fibrillation, PAF, PSVT.<br>2. Do not administer with other drugs that prolong the QT interval.<br>3. Continually monitor ECG during IV infusion.<br>4. Slow infusion rate if bradycardia and AV block occur; pacemaker therapy, if necessary.<br>5. Can cause cardiac and respiratory arrest. |
| Lidocaine hydrochloride: IV<br>▲ High-Alert Medication: IV route | Drowsiness, confusion, paresthesias, slurred speech, seizures, severe depression of cardiac conduction | 1. *Use:* ventricular dysrhythmias (PVCs, VT, VF).<br>2. Must use IV preparation for IV infusion.<br>3. Given as a bolus loading dose then continual-drip 1–4 mg/min drip. |
| Mexiletine hydrochloride: PO | Hypotension and bradycardia<br>CNS (common): blurred vision, dizziness, ataxia, confusion.<br>GI disturbances—nausea/vomiting, diarrhea; CNS disturbances—tremor, dizziness | 1. *Use:* prevent/control ventricular dysrhythmias (PVCs, VT, VF).<br>2. Monitor blood pressure and heart rate. |
| Procainamide: PO, IV | Abdominal pain, cramping, hypotension, prolonged QT interval<br>Long-term use: systemic lupus erythematosus–like syndrome (pain and inflammation of joints)<br>Blood dyscrasias | 1. *Use:* short- and long-term control of ventricular and supraventricular dysrhythmias.<br>2. Client should report any joint pain and inflammation.<br>3. Closely monitor for bradycardia and hypotension.<br>4. Do not take OTC cold preparations. |
| Propranolol hydrochloride: PO, IV<br>▲ High-Alert Medication: IV route | See previous discussion of beta-adrenergic blockers | 1. *Use:* long- and short-term treatment and prevention of tachycardia (AF, atrial flutter, PSVT, PVCs). |

▲ High-alert medications; *AF,* atrial fibrillation; *AV,* atrioventricular; *CNS,* central nervous system; *ECG,* electrocardiogram; *GI,* gastrointestinal; *IV,* intravenously; *OTC,* over-the-counter; *PAF,* paroxysmal atrial tachycardia; *PSVT,* paroxysmal supraventricular tachycardia; *PEA,* pulseless electrical activity; *PO,* by mouth (orally); *PVC,* premature ventricular complex; *subQ,* subcutaneously; *VF,* ventricular fibrillation; *VT,* ventricular tachycardia.

▲ **Fibrinolytics:** Work by different actions to initiate fibrinolysis of a clot. Medications are not clot specific; they will break up a clot on a surgical incision and a clot from an MI.

*General Nursing Implications*
- Therapy should begin as soon as the MI is diagnosed or when there is a history of prolonged angina. For best results, from admission in the ED until medication is administered is 30 min (door-to-needle) or within 60 min of onset of symptoms.
- Fibrinolytics can be given within 6 hr from onset of symptoms for client with an MI and a 3-hr time frame for clients with a nonhemorrhagic CVA.
- "Door-to-needle goal" of 30 min for most optimum results.
- If a client has any of the following, fibrinolytic therapy may be contraindicated:
  - Systolic BP greater than 180 mmHg or diastolic BP greater than 110 mmHg.
  - Significant closed head or facial trauma within the past 3 months.
  - History of intracranial hemorrhage, currently on anticoagulants, CPR longer than 10 min.
  - Pregnancy, serious systemic disease (liver, kidney).
- Bleeding precautions (see Box 16-1).

*Continued*

| Appendix 19-2 | CARDIAC MEDICATIONS—cont'd | |
| --- | --- | --- |
| ▲ **Medications** | **Side Effects** | **Nursing Implications** |
| Alteplase: IV<br>Reteplase: IV<br>Tenecteplase (TNKase): IV | Bleeding and hypotension | 1. First-line therapy for clots caused by an MI, limited arterial thrombosis, and thrombotic strokes.<br>2. Given within the first 2–4 hours after the onset of an MI and within 3 hours following a stroke.<br>3. Obtain base vital signs and coagulation studies.<br>4. Avoid venipunctures during and after infusion.<br>*Use:* MI, PE, DVT; contraindicated in clients with active bleeding. |

▲ High-alert medications; *DVT,* deep vein thrombosis; *IV,* intravenously; *MI,* myocardial infarction; *PE,* pulmonary embolism.

## ▲ Cardiac Glycosides: Increase myocardial contractility, thereby increasing cardiac output. Decrease heart rate by slowing conduction of impulses through the AV node. Enhance diuresis by increasing renal perfusion.

### General Nursing Implications

- Take the apical pulse for a full minute; if the rate is less than 60 beats/min in an adult, less than 90 to 110 beats/min in infants and young children, or less than 70 beats/min in a child, hold the medication and notify the physician.
- Evaluate for tachycardia, bradycardia, and irregular pulse. If there is significant change in rate and rhythm, hold the medication and notify the physician.
- Evaluate serum potassium levels and response to diuretics; hypokalemia potentiates action of digitalis.
- Gastrointestinal symptoms are frequently the first indication of digitalis toxicity.
- Teach client not to increase or double a dose in the case of a missed dose; if client vomits, do not give an additional dose.
- Quinidine, verapamil, and ACE inhibitors increase plasma levels of digitalis.
- To achieve maximum results rapidly, an initial loading dose is administered; then dose is reduced to a maintenance dose.
- Digibind is a digitalis antagonist and may be used for digitalis toxicity; watch for decreased potassium levels and client's response to decreased digitalis levels.

| **Medication** | **Side Effects** | **Nursing Implications** |
| --- | --- | --- |
| ▲ Digoxin: PO, IV | Most common: anorexia, nausea, vomiting<br>Most serious: drug-induced dysrhythmias<br>Visual disturbances, fatigue<br>Children/infants: frequent vomiting, poor feeding, or slow heart rate may indicate toxicity | 1. Therapeutic plasma levels of digoxin are 0.5–2.0 ng/mL (0.64–2.56 nmol/L).<br>2. First sign of toxicity is usually GI symptoms.<br>3. Slowed heart rate or rhythm changes may indicate toxicity.<br>4. Withhold digoxin for up to 48 hours before elective cardioversion, as it increases the risk for VF.<br>5. Increased risk of digitalis toxicity when client has hypokalemia.<br>6. *Use:* supraventricular tachycardia, HF. |

▲ High-alert medications; *HF,* Heart failure; *IV,* intravenously; *PO,* by mouth (orally).

| Appendix 19-3 | CARDIAC DYSRHYTHMIAS |
| --- | --- |

A dysrhythmia is defined as an interruption in the normal conduction of the heart, either in the rate or the rhythm.

> **TEST ALERT:** Initiate, maintain, and/or evaluate telemetry monitoring; identify abnormal cardiac rhythms; and initiate protocols to manage cardiac arrhythmias.

### Characteristics of Normal Sinus Rhythm

Rate: 60 to 100 beats/min
Rhythm: regular
P waves: present, precede each QRS complex
P-R interval: 0.12 to 0.20 sec
QRS complex: present and under 0.10 sec

Dysrhythmias may be classified according to rate—either bradycardia or tachycardia. They are also classified according to their origin—atrial or ventricular. Ventricular dysrhythmias are more life threatening than atrial dysrhythmias are. (See Common Dysrhythmias later.)

### Nursing Implications

1. Identify dysrhythmia and evaluate client's tolerance.
2. Monitor adequacy of cardiac output, keep on bed rest and oxygen.
3. Convert abnormal rhythm to normal sinus rhythm—medications or cardioversion.
4. Prevent complications.

### Interpretation of Electrocardiogram

1. Determine heart rate. Count the P waves in a 6-sec strip to determine the atrial rate and count the R or Q waves to determine the ventricular rate.

2. Are the QRS complexes occurring at regular intervals?
3. Are P waves present for each QRS complex?
4. Measure the P-R interval.
5. Measure the QRS interval.
6. Identify the T wave and ST segment.
7. Analyze any abnormalities.
8. Correlate findings with characteristics of normal sinus rhythm.

> **TEST ALERT:** Identify cardiac rhythm strip abnormalities (sinus tachycardia, premature ventricular contractions, V-tach, atrial fibrillation, and ventricular fibrillation); initiate, maintain, and/or evaluate telemetry monitoring; intervene to improve client cardiovascular status; initiate protocol to manage cardiac dysrhythmias.

**Common Dysrhythmias**

| Rhythm | Characteristics | Interventions/Implications |
|---|---|---|
| Sinus bradycardia | Sinus rhythm less than a rate of 60 beats/min | Assess client for tolerance of the rate. If hypotension or decreasing LOC occurs, the rhythm is treated. *Treatment:* atropine (can be given via endotracheal tube). If atropine is effective, chronotropic drug infusions are recommended as alternative to external transcutaneous pacing. |
| Sinus tachycardia | Regular rhythm; P waves present. Rate: 100–150 beats/min | Assess client for tolerance of the rate. Most often caused by caffeine, alcohol, or physiologic response to stimuli. Treatment based on underlying cause. *Treatment:* vagal maneuvers, adenosine, beta-blockers, calcium channel blockers, synchronized cardioversion. |
| Paroxysmal supraventricular tachycardia (PSVT) | Rhythm is intermittent and is initiated suddenly; terminates suddenly with or without treatment. Monitor for sustained rapid ventricular response: palpitations, chest pain, weakness, fatigue, dyspnea, anxiety, hypotension, and syncope. Signs of heart failure: angina, heart failure, cardiogenic shock. Nonsustained ventricular response: asymptomatic, occasional palpitations | *Treatment:* vagal stimulation, adenosine, beta-blockers, calcium channel blockers, synchronized cardioversion. |

*Continued*

| Rhythm | Characteristics | Interventions/Implications |
|---|---|---|
| Atrial fibrillation (AF) 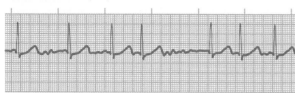 | Grossly irregular rate; cannot identify P waves or P-R interval on ECG<br><br>Controlled rate: 60–100 beats/min<br><br>Uncontrolled rate: greater than 100 beats/min | Assess client for tolerance to rapid cardiac rate.<br><br>Most common dysrhythmia. Evaluate client for systemic emboli (pulmonary emboli or an embolic stroke) from clots that tend to form in fibrillating atrium; a decrease in cardiac output will occur with tachycardia; maintain bed rest until rate is controlled. Pulse deficit will occur with rapid rate. Anticoagulation before cardioversion if client is in AF for longer than 48 hours.<br><br>*Treatment:* digitalis, calcium channel blockers, beta-blockers, cardioversion, or dronedarone.<br><br>Anticoagulants such as warfarin, dabigatran, rivaroxaban, or apixaban. |

**AV Block**

| Rhythm | Characteristics | Interventions/Implications |
|---|---|---|
| First-degree block 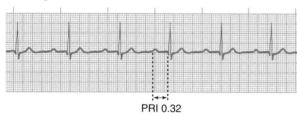<br>PRI 0.32 | Prolonged P-R interval; all P waves are followed by a QRS complex<br><br>May result from digitalis toxicity, electrolyte imbalance, or myocardial ischemia | Identify and treat the underlying cause.<br><br>Must have an ECG tracing to identify.<br><br>*Treatment:* no treatment, usually asymptomatic |
| Third-degree or complete block 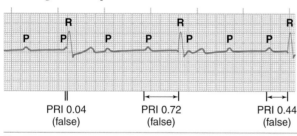<br>PRI 0.04 (false)   PRI 0.72 (false)   PRI 0.44 (false) | No correlation between atrial impulses and ventricular response<br><br>Rate: atrial rate 80–90 beats/min, with ventricular rate around 30 beats/min | May occur after an MI; symptoms depend on client's tolerance to rhythm; very unstable and may lead to asystole.<br><br>*Treatment:* dopamine and epinephrine until pacing can be established with a pacemaker. |
| Premature ventricular contractions or beats (PVCs, PVBs) 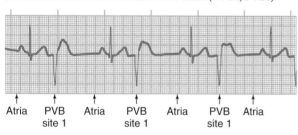<br>Atria   PVB site 1   Atria   PVB site 1   Atria   PVB site 1   Atria | Premature ectopic beats; occur within a basic rhythm; are of ventricular origin; no P waves; wide, bizarre QRS complex | Indicative of ventricular irritability; considered to be significant and should be treated if they:<br>1. Occur in excess of 6 beats/min.<br>2. Occur in a consecutive manner or in pairs.<br>3. Occur on a T wave of a preceding complex ("R" on "T" phenomenon).<br>*Treatment:* oxygen, electrolyte replacement, amiodarone, and/or procainamide; PVCs frequently precede ventricular tachycardia. |

## Appendix 19-3   CARDIAC DYSRHYTHMIAS—cont'd

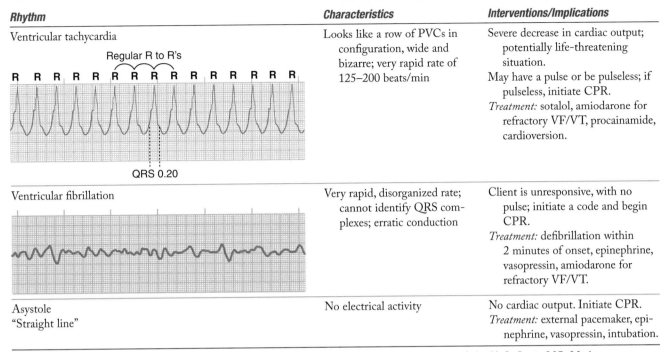

| Rhythm | Characteristics | Interventions/Implications |
|---|---|---|
| Ventricular tachycardia | Looks like a row of PVCs in configuration, wide and bizarre; very rapid rate of 125–200 beats/min | Severe decrease in cardiac output; potentially life-threatening situation. May have a pulse or be pulseless; if pulseless, initiate CPR. *Treatment:* sotalol, amiodarone for refractory VF/VT, procainamide, cardioversion. |
| Ventricular fibrillation | Very rapid, disorganized rate; cannot identify QRS complexes; erratic conduction | Client is unresponsive, with no pulse; initiate a code and begin CPR. *Treatment:* defibrillation within 2 minutes of onset, epinephrine, vasopressin, amiodarone for refractory VF/VT. |
| Asystole "Straight line" | No electrical activity | No cardiac output. Initiate CPR. *Treatment:* external pacemaker, epinephrine, vasopressin, intubation. |

Illustrations from Monahan, F. D., et al. (2007). *Phipps' medical-surgical nursing: Health and illness perspectives* (8th ed.). St. Louis, MO: Mosby.
*AF,* Atrial fibrillation; *AV,* atrioventricular; *CPR,* cardiopulmonary resuscitation; *ECG,* electrocardiogram; *LOC,* level of consciousness; *MI,* myocardial infarction; *PVCs,* premature ventricular contractions; *VF,* ventricular fibrillation, *VT,* ventricular tachycardia.

## Appendix 19-4   PACEMAKERS

### Temporary Pacing

*Noninvasive:* Application of two large external electrodes attached to an external pulse generator.

*Invasive:* Wire electrodes are in contact with the heart and are attached to a battery-operated pulse generator. Wires may be placed on the epicardium during heart surgery; leads are passed through the chest wall. Wires may also be placed via a catheter inserted in the antecubital vein and lodged in the right atrium and/or ventricle. Used in emergency situations and in severe cases of bradycardia. Anticipate placement of permanent pacemaker (PM).

*Permanent:* An internal generator is inserted into soft tissue of upper chest or abdomen, and electrodes are positioned in the atrium and ventricles. PM may synchronize pacing between atrium and ventricle (Figure 19-18). Procedure is planned and conducted under optimal conditions; used in persistent chronic heart block, dysrhythmias, and/or severe bradycardia.

### Pacing Modes

*Synchronous demand:* The heart is stimulated to beat when the client's pulse rate falls below a set value or rate (majority of pacemakers have a set rate between 60 and 72 beats/min; if client's pulse rate falls below the set value, the pacemaker initiates a heartbeat). The pacemaker "senses" the normal heartbeat and the following conduction. If a normal cardiac beat is initiated and conducted, the pacemaker does not initiate an impulse.

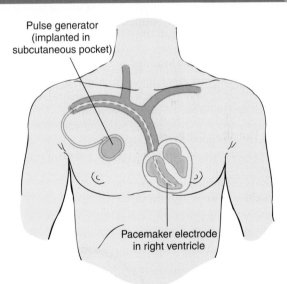

**FIGURE 19-18  Permanent Pacemaker Placement.** (From Monahan, F. D., et al. [2007]. *Phipps' medical-surgical nursing: Health and illness perspectives* [8th ed.]. St. Louis, MO: Mosby.)

*Atrioventricular:* The ventricle is sensed, and the atrium is paced. If the ventricle does not depolarize, then it is also paced.

*Universal atrioventricular:* Both the atrial and ventricular circuits sense and pace in the respective chambers. This most closely resembles the normal conduction system.

*Continued*

**Appendix 19-4 PACEMAKERS—cont'd**

## Pacemaker Failure

A cardiac monitor or an electrocardiogram (ECG) must be available to verify pacemaker failure.

*Failure to sense:* The pacemaker fails to recognize spontaneous heartbeats and will fire inappropriately. This is dangerous because the pacer impulse may be discharged during a critical time in the cardiac cycle and cause a lethal arrhythmia.

*Failure to pace:* A malfunction in the pacemaker generator; it may also be due to dislodgment of the leads.

*Failure to capture:* May occur with a low battery or poor connection. The pacemaker is discharging the impulse, but there is no responding cardiac contraction.

### Nursing Implications

1. Assess for dysrhythmias; rate should not fall below preset level.
2. Maintain bed rest if pulse rate drops below preset level.
3. Hypotension, syncope, and bradycardia should not occur.

### Client Education

1. Notify all health care providers of pacemaker placement and parameters; wear a medical alert identification.

2. Avoid constrictive clothing that puts pressure on or irritates the site; report any signs of infection.
3. Safe environment: Avoid areas of high voltage, magnetic force fields (MRIs), or arc welding equipment.
4. Avoid activity that requires vigorous movement of arms and shoulders or any direct blows to PM site.
5. Teach client to check his pulse and report if pulse rate is less than 60 and client is experiencing symptoms; if this occurs, the pacemaker is not functioning properly, and this needs to be reported immediately.
6. Advise client to report immediately episodes of dizziness or syncope, difficulty breathing, chest pain, weight gain, and prolonged hiccupping.
7. Follow-up care and monitoring of pacemaker are important.
8. Client may travel without restrictions.

> **TEST ALERT:** Connect and maintain pacing devices; monitor pacemaker and implantable cardioverter defibrillator functions.

---

**Appendix 19-5 BEDSIDE HEMODYNAMIC MONITORING**

## Central Venous Pressure Monitoring

Central venous pressure (CVP) is an indication of the pressure within the right atrium or within the large veins in the thoracic cavity. An intravenous (IV) catheter is placed in the superior vena cava or in the right atrium via the subclavian vein or jugular vein. A CVP reading may also be obtained from the proximal lumen of the pulmonary artery catheter (Figure 19-19).

### Interpretation of Pressure Readings

Normal response may range from 2 to 6 mm of $H_2O$ pressure. CVP is a dynamic measurement; it must be correlated with client's overall clinical status for correct interpretation.

### Factors That Affect CVP Reading

1. Venous return to the heart (venous tone and vascular volume).
2. Intrathoracic pressure.
3. Function of the left side of the heart.
4. Coughing or straining (increase CVP).

> **NURSING PRIORITY:** The CVP is an index of the ability of the right side of the heart to handle venous return. Rising CVP may indicate hypervolemia or poor cardiac contractility. Decreasing CVP may indicate a state of hypovolemia or vasodilation.

### Nursing Implications

1. Each CVP reading should be measured from the same zero level point (level of the right atrium or the phlebostatic axis). The zero level on the manometer or the transducer should be placed at this level to obtain the reading. Client should be supine when the measurements are obtained; head may be slightly elevated, but the position should be consistent for all measurements.
2. If the CVP catheter is patent within the thoracic cavity, the fluid in the manometer or the digital readout will fluctuate with respirations or changes in thoracic pressure when the reading is obtained.

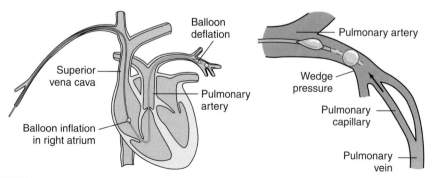

**FIGURE 19-19 Pulmonary Artery Catheter.** (Redrawn from Daily, E. K., & Schroeder, J. S. [1994]. *Techniques in bedside hemodynamic monitoring* [5th ed.]. St. Louis, MO: Mosby. In Monahan, F. D., et al. [2007]. *Phipps' medical-surgical nursing: Health and illness perspectives* [8th ed.]. St. Louis, MO: Mosby.)

3. Patency of the CVP line is maintained via IV infusion drip.
4. Catheter should be stabilized on the skin at the insertion site, and an occlusive sterile dressing should be applied.

## Complications

Air emboli and infections

> **⚠ NURSING PRIORITY:** To obtain hemodynamic measurements, the zero point of the transducer must be at the level of the right atrium, which is the midaxillary line at the fourth or fifth intercostal space.

## Critical Care

### Pulmonary Artery Pressure Monitoring (Swan-Ganz Catheter)

A multilumen catheter (Figure 19-20) is inserted and advanced through the right atrium and right ventricle into the pulmonary artery. The flow of blood carries the catheter into the pulmonary artery. Heparinized saline solution is infused under pressure to maintain the patency of the line.

### Interpretation of Pressure Readings

Pressure, flow, and oxygenation readings are obtained via a transducer; for readings to be accurate, the zero level of the transducer must be at the level of the right atrium or the phlebostatic axis (see CVP).

*Right atrial (RA) pressure:* Normal is 2 to 6 mmHg; a direct measurement of the pressure in the right atrium.

*Pulmonary artery pressure (PAP):* Normal is 15 to 25 mmHg systolic and 5 to 15 mmHg diastolic, with a mean pressure around 12 to 15 mmHg. Mean PAP is increased in clients with chronic pulmonary diseases and those with HF.

*Pulmonary capillary wedge pressure (PAWP or PCWP):* Normal is 4 to 12 mmHg. It is determined as a mean pressure and is obtained by inflating or wedging a small balloon on the catheter tip in a distal branch of the pulmonary artery. The wedge pressure is a direct reflection of pressure in the left cardiac chambers and reflects left ventricular end diastolic pressure (LVED). An upward trend is indicative of increases in pressures and/or fluid, whereas a downward trend indicates fluid, dehydration, or severe vasodilation.

*Cardiac output (CO):* amount of blood pumped in 1 minute. Normal range: 4 to 8 L/min

*Cardiac index (CI):* measurement of CO that includes BSA—a more precise measurement of CO.

*Systemic vascular resistance index (SVR):* the resistance the LV must eject against.

$Sao_2$: saturation of hemoglobin in arterial blood

$SvO_2$: mixed venous oxygen saturation

### Nursing Implications

1. Maintain patency of line via a heparinized flush solution administered under pressure.
2. The transducer should be at the level of the right atrium to ensure accurate measurements. Catheter should be secured to the skin and covered with an occlusive dressing. Each time the PCWP is evaluated, it is imperative that the balloon or the wedge be deflated to prevent pulmonary infarction, which is validated on the pressure monitor.

> **TEST ALERT:** Evaluate invasive monitoring data obtained with a pulmonary artery pressure.

## Complications

Infections, sepsis, ventricular dysrhythmias particularly during insertion, pulmonary infarction, air emboli.

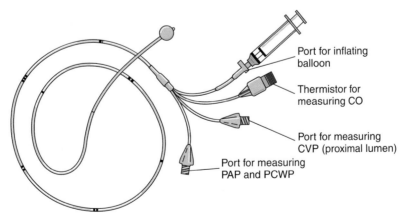

**FIGURE 19-20 Four-Lumen Thermodilution Pulmonary Artery Catheter.** (From Monahan F. D., et al. [2007]. *Phipps' medical-surgical nursing: Health and illness perspectives* [8th ed.]. St. Louis, MO: Mosby.)

Port for inflating balloon

Thermistor for measuring CO

Port for measuring CVP (proximal lumen)

Port for measuring PAP and PCWP

## Appendix 19-6 CARDIOPULMONARY RESUSCITATION (CPR) FOR HEALTH CARE PROVIDERS

The American Heart Association (AHA) has established standards for cardiopulmonary resuscitation for the health care provider. For further delineation of the procedure, consult the AHA Cardiopulmonary Resuscitation Guidelines. For health care providers, the AHA uses the term *infant* to refer to individuals between birth and 1 year of age; *child* is used to refer to those who are between 1 year of age and the onset of puberty.

1. Recognition.
   - Identify that the victim is unconscious.
   - Check the person for no breathing, abnormal breathing (adult), or only gasping.
   - Check the pulse for no more than 10 seconds.
   - Adult and child: check the carotid pulse.
   - Infant: check the brachial or femoral pulse.
   - Place victim in position to begin CPR.
   - Shout for help and activate the emergency medical services (EMS) system.
   - Attach monitor.
2. "C" External cardiac compressions.
   - Place the victim on a firm surface. If the client is in a bed, put a cardiac board behind him or her. DO NOT attempt to remove the victim from the bed.
   - Locate the lower half of the sternum in the adult. For the adult, place one hand over the lower sternum; place the other hand on top of the previous hand. For a child (age 1 year to puberty), use the heel of one hand, or two hands based on the size of the child, and press on the center of the chest at the nipple line. For an infant, locate the nipple line; the area for compression is one finger's width below the line.
   - Depress the sternum at least 2 inches (5 cm) in the adult; in children, at least ½ anterior-posterior (AP) diameter, about 2 inches (5 cm); in infants, at least ¼ diameter, about ½ inches (1.3 cm).
   - Push hard and fast—allow complete chest recoil.
   - If the pulse is absent, begin chest compressions—cycles of 30 compressions and 2 breaths.
   - If the pulse is present, continue rescue breathing, and recheck pulse every 2 min. If, despite adequate ventilation, the heart rate of an infant or child remains under 60 beats per min, chest compressions should be started.
   - Minimize interruptions to less than 10 seconds.
   - Rotate health care provider compressors every 2 minutes.
   *Adult and child:* One rescuer and two rescuers: 30 compressions (rate of 100 per min) to 2 ventilations.
   *Infant:* One rescuer: 30 compressions (rate of 100 per min) to 2 ventilations.
   *Two rescuers:* 15 compressions to 2 ventilations.
3. "A" Airway.
   - Open the airway: head-tilt/chin-lift maneuver. Use jaw thrust if trauma is suspected.
   - If victim is not breathing, give 2 rescue breaths using mouth-to-mouth or a pocket mask or bag mask.
   - Adult: 1 breath every 5 to 6 secs, 10 to 12 breaths per min.
   - Child and infant: 1 breath every 3 to 5 secs, 12 to 20 breaths per min.
   - Advanced airway present (laryngeal mask airway, endotracheal tube): 1 breath every 6 to 8 secs without trying to synchronize breaths with compressions, 8 to 10 breaths per min.
4. "B" Breathing.
   - Maintain the open airway.
   - Pinch nostrils closed.
   - Do not give "extra" breaths; do not give large, forceful breaths.
   - When an advanced airway is present, ventilate at the rate of 8 to 10 per min; do not pause for compressions.

> **!** PEDIATRIC NURSING PRIORITY: Be careful not to hyperextend the infant's head; this may block the airway. Don't pinch the infant's nose shut; cover the nose with your mouth instead. Breathe slowly, just enough to make the chest rise.

*Defibrillation:* Obtain automated external defibrillator (AED). Use AED as soon as available for sudden collapse (VF/pulseless VT).
   - Emphasis has been placed on delivery of high-quality CPR "push fast and hard" at a rate of 100 compressions per minute and early defibrillation for lethal dysrhythmias
   Steps for using an automated external defibrillator (AED):
1. Provide CPR until the AED arrives.
2. On arrival, open the case and turn the power on.
3. Select the correct pads for the size and age of the victim (only use the child pads/system for children less than 8 years old).
4. Attach the adhesive electrodes—one on the upper right side of the chest directly below the clavicle, the other below the left nipple below the left armpit.
5. Attach the connecting cable to the AED.
6. Compressions will need to be discontinued while the rhythm is analyzed.
7. If shock is indicated, loudly state "Clear!" and visually check to ensure that no one is touching the client.
8. Press the SHOCK button.
9. Resume CPR immediately with cycles of 30 compressions to 2 breaths.
10. Termination of CPR. A rescuer who is not a physician should continue resuscitation efforts until one of the following occurs:
    - Spontaneous circulation and ventilation have been restored.
    - Resuscitation efforts are transferred to another equally responsible person who continues the resuscitation procedure.
    - A physician, or physician-directed person, assumes responsibility for resuscitation procedure.
    - The victim is transferred to an emergency medical service (e.g., paramedics and ambulance).
    - The rescuer is exhausted and unable to continue resuscitation.

> **TEST ALERT:** Identify and intervene in life-threatening client situations. Notify primary health care provider about unexpected response/emergency situation of client.

**Appendix 19-7 NONDRUG TREATMENT OF DYSRHYTHMIAS**

Defibrillation is depolarization of the electrical impulses in the heart to allow the heart's own intrinsic pacemaker to regain control of cardiac rhythm.

## Defibrillation (Unsynchronized)

Depolarization of cardiac cells in an emergency situation with a life-threatening dysrhythmia:

1. Always begin cardiopulmonary resuscitation (CPR) if client has no pulse and is unconscious; do not wait for a defibrillator.
2. Make sure everyone is clear of the bed and the client is not lying in fluids.
3. Make sure everyone is clear from touching the bed or client.
4. Synchronization is turned off.
5. Shock energy—Biphasic: recommended by manufacturer (120–200 J); if unknown, use highest available. Second and third shocks should be at least initial shock, higher doses may be considered. Evidence shows single stacked shocks provide better outcomes than stack shocks because of less interruption with chest compressions.
6. Monophasic: 360 J.
7. If necessary, resume chest compressions immediately after the shock.
8. Minimize interruptions in chest compressions.
9. Document rhythm after defibrillation.
10. Remain with client and closely assess for adequacy and stability of cardiac output and cardiac rhythm.

## Synchronized Cardioversion

Depolarization of cardiac cells to allow the sinus node to regain control of cardiac rhythm:

1. An elective, planned procedure or used when client has a tachycardic rhythm with a pulse rate greater than 150 (unstable ventricular, supraventricular tachydysrhythmias, or stable tachydysrhythmias resistant to medical intervention).
2. Requires client teaching and informed consent when it is an elective procedure.
3. Document rhythm before synchronized cardioversion and immediately afterward.
4. The defibrillator is set (synchronized) to deliver a countershock during the QRS complex; this prevents the discharge from occurring on the T wave. Look for the sync markers on the R wave. Turn off and remove the oxygen from the client to prevent a fire.
5. Charge the defibrillator.
6. Shout "Clear!" and validate that no one is touching the client or bed before administering the shock for electrical safety.
7. Cardioversion is started at 50 J to 100 J, depending on the client's weight.
8. Remain with client and closely assess for adequacy and stability of cardiac output and cardiac rhythm.
9. If cardioversion is unsuccessful and the client's condition worsens into VF, ensure the synchronizer is turned off for immediate defibrillation.

## Implantable Cardioverter Defibrillators (ICD)

- Used in clients who have survived one or more episodes of sudden death from ventricular dysrhythmias or from refractory ventricular dysrhythmias not associated with a myocardial infarction.
- Implantable device can also be used as a pacemaker.
- Inserted in a subcutaneous pocket in the subclavicular or abdominal area.
- Client should avoid contact sports, increase activity gradually, and carry ICD identification information.
- Client should avoid working over large motors and should move away from devices if dizziness occurs; client should avoid magnets directly over area of ICD.
- Common response to device is anxiety and fear.
- Assess for fluid hazards; intravenous fluids and urine may conduct voltage.
- Clients should sit or lie down if they become dizzy or if they feel the ICD discharge.

## Radiofrequency Catheter Ablation

1. Used in clients who experience atrial tachycardia or AV nodal reentrant tachycardia. Electrophysiologic testing identifies the small region of the myocardium generating the dysrhythmia. A radiofrequency catheter is placed at the site, and the catheter is activated to generate RF energy. This energy destroys the tissue eliminating the dysrhythmia.
2. Complications are minimal but can include AV blocks and myocardial perforation.

# Study Questions
# Cardiac: Care of Adult, Maternity, and Pediatric Clients

More questions on

1. A client with chest pain is on a cardiac monitor. The monitor is showing ventricular tachycardia at a rate of 150 beats/min with multiple PVCs. The client is awake and coherent, and oxygen is being administered at a rate of 6 L/min via a nasal cannula. What is the nurse's next action?
   1. Immediately defibrillate.
   2. Administer adenosine IV push.
   3. Assess the blood pressure.
   4. Auscultation lung sounds.

2. The nurse is caring for a client with a history of heart failure. Which statements by the client require additional inquiry? **Select all that apply.**
   1. "I've noticed that I've gained 3 lbs. This week."
   2. "I sleep best in my recliner chair."
   3. "I've noticed that the swelling in my feet seems less."
   4. "I cannot make it through the grocery store without resting."
   5. "I often have to use the restroom at night."

3. The nurse is administering nitroglycerin intravenously to a client experiencing chest pain of an 8 on a 1 to 10 scale. What assessment changes would cause the nurse to decrease the infusion rate?
   1. Pain drops from an 8 to a 4.
   2. Heart rate increases from 110 to 115 beats per minute.
   3. Blood pressure drops from 110/65 (80) to 89/44 (59) mmHg.
   4. Client verbalizes his head is pounding.

4. In discharge planning for the client with heart failure, the nurse discusses the importance of adequate rest. What information is most important?
   1. A warm, quiet room is necessary.
   2. Bed rest promotes venous return.
   3. A hospital bed is necessary.
   4. Adequate rest decreases cardiac workload.

5. The nurse is assessing a client whose condition is being stabilized after experiencing a ST-segment-elevation myocardial infarction. Which assessment is most indicative of inadequate renal perfusion?
   1. Increasing serum blood urea nitrogen (BUN) level
   2. Urine specific gravity of less than 1.010
   3. Urine output of less than 30 mL/hr
   4. Low urine creatinine clearance

6. The nurse applies a nitroglycerin patch on a client who has undergone cardiac surgery. What nursing observation indicates that a nitroglycerin patch is achieving the desired effect?
   1. Chest pain is completely relieved.
   2. Client performs activities of daily living without chest pain.
   3. Pain is controlled with frequent changes of patch.
   4. Client tolerates increased activity without pain.

7. The nurse has been assigned a group of cardiac clients. What would be the most important information for the nurse to assess during the initial visit? **Select all that apply.**
   1. Presence of cardiac discomfort
   2. Medications taken before hospitalization
   3. Presence of jugular vein distention
   4. Heart sounds and apical rate
   5. Presence of diaphoresis
   6. History of difficulty breathing

8. During the night, a client with a diagnosis of acute coronary syndrome is found to be restless and diaphoretic. What is the best nursing action?
   1. Check his temperature and determine his serum blood glucose level.
   2. Turn the alarms low and promote sleep by decreasing the number of interruptions.
   3. Check the monitor to determine his cardiac rhythm and evaluate vital signs.
   4. Call the physician to obtain an order for sedation.

9. The nurse is providing preoperative care for client who is scheduled for cardiac surgery. During the preoperative preparation, what is an important nursing action?
   1. Perform a thorough nursing assessment to provide an accurate baseline for evaluation after surgery.
   2. Discuss with the client the steps of myocardial cellular metabolism and the anticipated surgical response.
   3. Provide preoperative education regarding the mechanics of the cardiopulmonary bypass machine.
   4. Discuss with the client and family the anticipated amount of postoperative chest tube drainage.

10. An older adult client is taking digoxin 0.25 mg once a day and furosemide 40 mg daily. She states having increasing lethargy and nausea over the past 2 days, but she is still able to take her medication. Her blood pressure is 150/98 mmHg; pulse is 110 beats/min and irregular; respiratory rate is 18 breaths/min. What laboratory information is most important for the nurse to evaluate?
    1. Hemoglobin, hematocrit, and white blood cell count
    2. Arterial blood gases and acid–base balance
    3. Blood urea nitrogen (BUN) and serum creatinine levels
    4. Serum electrolyte level.

11. During the shift handoff report, the nurse learns that one of the assigned clients is in first-degree heart block. What action should the nurse take?
    1. Count the radial pulse for 1 full minute.
    2. Determine the cardiac rate at the point of maximum impulse.
    3. Evaluate an ECG or monitor strip.
    4. Take hourly pulse checks and correlate with blood pressure.

12. The nurse is preparing a client for a cardiac catheterization. Which nursing interventions are necessary in preparing the client for this procedure? **Select all that apply.**
    1. Verify consent form has been signed.
    2. Explain procedure to client.
    3. Provide clear liquid, no caffeine diet.
    4. Evaluate peripheral pulses.
    5. Obtain a 12-lead ECG.
    6. Obtain history for shellfish allergy.

13. A client is admitted for evaluation of his permanent pacemaker. Which assessment is most concerning?
    1. Pulse rate of 96 beats/min with regular rate and rhythm
    2. Irregular pulse rate with premature ventricular beats
    3. Atrial premature beats shown on the monitor
    4. Pulse rate of 48 beats/min with premature ventricular beats

14. The nurse is assessing the pulse of a client in atrial fibrillation. Based on the graphic below, where should the stethoscope be placed to correctly auscultate this client's pulse?

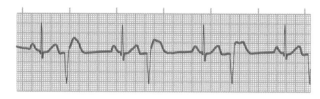

15. The vital signs of a client with cardiac disease are as follows: blood pressure of 102/76 mmHg, pulse of 52 beats/min, and respiratory rate of 16 breaths/min. Atropine sulfate is administered IV push. What nursing assessment indicates a therapeutic response to the medication?
    1. Pulse rate has increased to 70 beats/min.
    2. Systolic blood pressure has increased by 20 mmHg.
    3. Pupils are dilated.
    4. Oral secretions have decreased.

16. The nurse is taking the history of a client with heart failure caused by chronic hypertension. Which statement by the client is most concerning?
    1. "I get short of breath after walking about half a block."
    2. "My weight has dropped 15 pounds over the past 3 months."
    3. "My legs get swollen in the evenings."
    4. "Sometimes I get dizziness when I get up too quickly."

17. The nurse received handoff for a client returning from a cardiac angiogram and begins the initial assessment. The right femoral groin dressing has a dime-sized area of blood. What additional actions should the nurse perform? **Select all that apply.**
    1. Assess peripheral pulses in both legs and feet.
    2. Mark the dressing with a pen, circling the bloody drainage.
    3. Hold pressure on the dressing site for 20 minutes.
    4. Assess blood pressure.
    5. Place the client in a high-Fowler position.

18. The nurse is caring for a client being discharged after experiencing infective endocarditis. What is most important to include with the discharge teaching?
    1. Begin an exercise regimen as soon as possible, progressively increasing intensity each day.
    2. Monitor urinary output daily and report a change in color or quantity.
    3. Continue antibiotic therapy until the prescription is completed.
    4. Track and monitor heart rate and blood pressure daily upon arising.

19. The nurse is monitoring a client after thrombolytic therapy has been initiated. Shortly after the infusion is started, the client becomes confused, disoriented, cool, and clammy. The heart rate progressively increases to 120 and blood pressure drops to 60/40. What actions should the nurse take? **Select all that apply.**
    1. Stop the thrombolytic
    2. Apply oxygen
    3. Raise the head of the bed
    4. Call for assistance
    5. Reorient the client

20. The nurse is caring for a client who begins to exhibit the cardiac rhythm shown in the illustration below. As the nurse observes, the rhythm remains the same. What is the best nursing actions? **Select all that apply.**

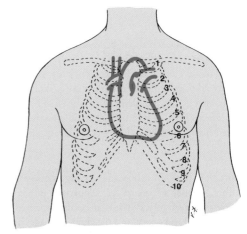

1. Call an emergency code and begin resuscitation.
2. Assess apical pulse, comparing to distal pulse.
3. Apply oxygen.
4. Assess for chest pain or shortness of breath.
5. Have the client cough.
6. Assess the blood pressure.

## Answers to Study Questions

**1.** *3*
The client is having chest pain; it is a priority to evaluate their blood pressure to determine whether they are tolerating the rhythm. Adenosine is given for supraventricular tachycardia. Defibrillation will be necessary if the client loses consciousness. Lung sounds are not a priority at this time. (Lewis et al., 10 ed., p. 769)

**2.** *1, 2, 4, 5*
Symptoms of heart failure include weight gain, orthopnea, fatigue, edema, and nocturia. Additionally the client can experience tachycardia, skin changes, behavioral changes, and chest pain. (Lewis et al., 10 ed., pp. 742–743)

**3.** *3*
Nitroglycerin is a vasodilator. It dilates the coronary arteries, thereby increasing myocardial blood supply; vasodilation of the peripheral circulation decreases the pressure against which the heart must pump (decreases afterload) and, by dilating the venous system, allows blood to pool in the venous system (decreases preload). It is important to continue the delivery of nitroglycerin until the client is pain free, since pain means coronary ischemia in the cardiac client. A headache is anticipated, as is tachycardia. Hypotension is expected with a vasodilator, but a drop this significant since the mean arterial pressure is below 60 mmHg. (Lehene, 9 ed., p. 593)

**4.** *4*
To help decrease pulmonary congestion and dyspnea, the nurse should encourage adequate rest to decrease cardiac workload; the client should not exert himself to the point of fatigue. Bed rest does promote venous return, but that is not the purpose of bed rest in the client with heart failure. A hospital bed is not necessary, and a quiet room is important if that is what promotes rest for the client. (Lewis et al., 10 ed., p. 752)

**5.** *3*
A sustained low cardiac output decreases renal perfusion and results in oliguria and impaired renal function. Oliguria is marked by output of less than 30 mL/hr. Increased BUN, changes in specific gravity (osmolarity), and creatinine clearance will be affected if the client develops renal failure. (Lewis et al., 10 ed., p. 1070)

**6.** *2*
Nitroglycerin is used to prevent angina so that the client can perform the normal activities of daily living without chest pain. Sublingual nitroglycerin or translingual spray is used to treat immediate-onset chest pain. (Lehne, 9 ed., p. 591)

**7.** *1, 3, 4, 5*
A focused cardiac assessment is directed toward assessing physiologic symptoms (cardiac pain, JVD distention, heart sounds and rate, presence of diaphoresis) that provide immediate information

regarding the client's condition, which is appropriate for the nurse to do at the beginning of each shift. After the physiologic parameters have been evaluated, the nurse can determine any history of difficulty breathing and a list of medications the client was taking before admission. (Lewis et al., 10 ed., p. 663)

8. *3*

Restlessness and diaphoresis may be indicative of decreased cardiac output, frequently originating from a dysrhythmia. Checking temperature and blood glucose levels is not a priority. Turning the alarm sound to low and reducing interruptions to facilitate sleep will be done when all physical problems are resolved. Physiologic needs must be addressed first. It is important to obtain critical assessment data before calling the doctor. (Lewis et al., 10 ed., pp. 742)

9. *1*

It is important to perform a thorough nursing assessment before the surgery. This provides a baseline for comparison of physiologic assessment data after surgery. Physiologic needs come first. The client and family do need to know about the chest drainage; however, this is client education. Providing a discussion about cellular metabolism and the mechanics of the cardiopulmonary bypass machine are not part of preoperative preparation. (Lewis et al., 10 ed., p. 739)

10. *4*

A low potassium level can precipitate digitalis toxicity. The client has been taking her medications and not eating regularly. She also has an irregular heartbeat and increased lethargy along with nausea, all of which can be signs of digitalis toxicity. She is taking a diuretic, which increases the excretion of potassium, and a low potassium level can cause digitalis toxicity. (Lehne, 9 ed., p. 524)

11. *3*

First-degree heart block can only be evaluated with an ECG or monitor tracing because the distinguishing factor is a prolonged P-R interval; all beats are being conducted. Other options are appropriate (determine cardiac rate, counting radial pulse for a full minute, and hourly pulse checks with blood pressure assessment) for this client; however, they do not assess first-degree block. (Lewis et al., 10 ed., p. 767)

12. *1, 4, 6*

In cardiac catheterization with angiography, contrast dye is injected into the coronary arteries, which allows visualization of the coronary arteries and provides information on patency. Informed consent is required before any invasive procedure. The physician is responsible for explaining the procedure to the client, and the nurse can reinforce the information. The client should be NPO for 6 to 18 hours before the procedure. A 12-lead ECG would be done, but this procedure is reflective of the conduction system, instead of the perfusion of the coronary arteries. Evaluating peripheral pulses is a nursing measure after the cardiac catheterization. It is important to check for iodine sensitivity or shellfish allergy because the procedure involves injecting contrast medium. (Lewis et al., 10 ed., pp. 677–678)

13. *4*

Most demand pacemakers are set somewhere between 60 and 72. A pulse rate of 48 is too slow for a properly functioning pacemaker. If the client's pulse rate falls below the preset pacemaker rate, the pacemaker should take over the pacing. With bradycardia, ventricular escape beats occur. A pulse rate of 96 beats/min is within normal limits. An irregular pulse rate with PVCs or atrial contractions are related to irritable foci in the heart and not indicative of pacemaker problems. (Lewis et al., 10 ed., p.775)

14. *4*

The nurse needs to auscultate the apical pulse when a client is in atrial fibrillation. The point of maximal impulse is the correct location for auscultation of the apical pulse. It is located at the fifth intercostal space, at the midclavicular line. This is the apex of the heart. It is noted with a black dot on the correct area in the illustration. (Lewis et al., 10 ed., p. 667)

15. *1*

Atropine is administered for symptomatic bradycardia. An increase in pulse rate is the therapeutic response for this client. All other options (increase in BP, dilated pupils, and dry mouth) are characteristic of atropine but are not desired actions for this client. (Lewis et al., 10 ed., p. 763)

16. *1*

Dyspnea on exertion is a classic sign of left ventricular problems, regardless of the precipitating cause. Lower extremity edema is also characteristic, but it is not as significant as dyspnea on exertion. Dizziness and fainting on standing are indicative of postural (orthostatic) hypotension. (Lewis et al., 10 ed., p. 664)

17. *1, 2, 4*

A cardiac catheterization includes the insertion of a large sheath into the femoral artery. There is a risk of hemorrhage after the procedure along with a loss of circulation distal to the insertion site. Priority care includes frequent assessment of circulation to the extremity. Peripheral pulses, color, and sensation should be evaluated in both feet as a comparison. Observation of the insertion site for hematoma and bleeding is also important. The nurse should mark the site, and if it enlarges, pressure should be applied. Monitor of the ECG and vital signs in important for evaluation of instability. The head of bed should remain flat until the groin site has developed hemostasis. (Lewis et al., 10 ed., pp. 677, 729)

18. *3*

Antibiotics (usually administered by IV piggyback [IVPB]) are indicated for infective endocarditis. This may continue at home with the assistance of a home care nurse to administer the IVPBs, or the client may be changed to oral antibiotics. The continued antibiotic is critical to the prevention of vegetation growth on the valves. The other options are not specific for managing a client with infective endocarditis. (Lewis et al., 10 ed., p. 780)

19. *1, 2, 4*

The symptoms the client is demonstrating support that he/she is hemorrhaging, the most common complication of thrombolytic therapy. The nurse needs to support oxygenation and perfusion by applying oxygen, lowering the head of the bed, and increasing fluids. The thrombolytics should be stopped and additional help given if needed since the client is very unstable. (Lewis et al., 10 ed., p. 724)

20. *2, 3, 4, 6*

The rhythm is premature ventricular beats or contractions (PVCs). Treatment is related to the cause, which may be hypoxia or from electrolyte replacement. Assessment of the client's hemodynamic status is important to determine whether treatment with drug therapy is needed. Drug therapy includes beta-blockers, procainamide, or amiodarone. (Lewis et al., 10 ed., p. 769)

# CHAPTER TWENTY

# Gastrointestinal: Care of Adult and Pediatric Clients

# 20

## PRIORITY CONCEPTS

Elimination, Inflammation, Nutrition

## PHYSIOLOGY OF THE GASTROINTESTINAL SYSTEM

### Digestion, Absorption, and Elimination Process

A. Digestion: physical and chemical breakdown of food.
  1. Length of time food remains in stomach depends on type of food, gastric motility, and psychological factors; average time is 3 to 4 hours.
  2. The pH of the stomach is acidic, which promotes production of pepsin to begin the initial breakdown of proteins.
  3. Chyme (food mixed with gastric secretions) moves through the pylorus into the small intestine.
  4. Intestinal digestive enzymes are released from the villi in the small intestine.
B. Absorption: transfer of food products into circulation.
  1. Occurs primarily in small intestine, where villi provide absorptive surface area; minimal amount of nutrients are absorbed in the stomach.
  2. Carbohydrates are broken down into monosaccharides, fats to glycerol and fatty acids, and proteins to amino acids; all are absorbed through the villi of the small intestine.
  3. Intrinsic factor is secreted in the stomach and promotes absorption of vitamin $B_{12}$ (cobalamin) in the small intestine.
  4. Presence of chyme in small intestine stimulates contraction of the gallbladder and relaxation of the sphincter of Oddi; this process releases bile for digestion of fats.
C. Elimination: excretion of waste products.
  1. Large intestine absorbs water and electrolytes and forms feces.
  2. Serves as a reservoir for fecal mass until defecation occurs.

### System Assessment

A. Evaluate client's history.
  1. Dietary and bowel habits.
  2. Nausea, vomiting, diarrhea, indigestion, constipation, flatulence: precipitating and alleviating factors. Does eating make it better or worse?
  3. Pain related to gastrointestinal (GI) tract.

  4. Previous problems associated with GI tract, including gastritis, hepatitis, colitis, gallbladder disease, peptic or duodenal ulcer, hernia, and hemorrhoids.
  5. Unexplained or unplanned weight gain or loss.
  6. Medication history, including over-the-counter (OTC) and prescription drugs.
  7. Previous surgeries related to GI system.
B. Assess vital signs for client's overall status.
C. Assess for presence and characteristics of abdominal pain.
D. Assess client's mouth.
  1. Presence of adequate saliva, condition of teeth and tongue.
  2. Presence of the gag reflex.
  3. Presence of oral lesions.
E. Evaluate the abdomen (client should be lying flat).
  1. Inspect: divide the abdomen into four quadrants and perform visual inspection for contour, scars, masses, and movement (aortic pulsation may be visible). Figure 20-1 shows anatomic divisions of the abdomen.
  2. Auscultate: each quadrant should be auscultated for bowel sounds before palpation.
    a. Bowel sounds are considered absent if no sound is heard for 5 minutes in any one quadrant.
    b. Normally, soft gurgles should be heard every 5 to 20 seconds.
    c. Borborygmi: loud, gurgling bowel sounds; may precede diarrhea.

**TEST ALERT:** To determine characteristics of bowel sounds, note presence in each quadrant, as well as frequency and pitch.

  3. Percussion: purpose is to determine presence of fluid, distention, and/or masses.
    a. Tympany is a high-pitched hollow sound commonly heard over areas distended with air.
    b. Dullness is a short high-pitched sound with little resonance; heard over fluid or solid masses.
  4. Palpation: purpose is to determine areas of tenderness, resistance, and swelling; deep palpation is used to identify organs and possible masses.
    a. Begin with light palpation of each quadrant; observe facial expression for any area of discomfort and/or guarding.
    b. Begin in area of least discomfort; if there is a problem area, palpate it last.

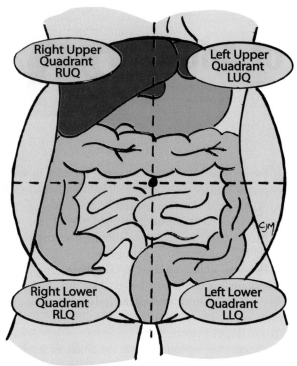

© 2017 Nursing Education Consultants, Inc.

**FIGURE 20-1 Abdominal Quadrants.** (From Zerwekh, J., & Miller, C. J. [2017]. *NCLEX review course.* Chandler, AZ: Nursing Education Consultants, Inc.)

---

### Box 20-1   OLDER ADULT CARE FOCUS

**Changes in Gastrointestinal System Related to Aging**
- Decreased hydrochloric acid and decreased absorption of vitamins; encourage frequent small feedings that are high in vitamins.
- Decreased peristalsis and decreased sensation to defecate; encourage diet high in fiber and minimum of 2000 mL of fluid daily; encourage physical activity.
- Decreased lipase from pancreas to aid in fat digestion; encourage smaller meals because diarrhea may be caused by increased fat intake.
- Decreased liver activity with decreased production of enzymes for drug metabolism, tendency toward accumulation of medications; instruct clients not to double up on their medications, especially cardiac medications.
- Increased disorders causing acute and/or chronic pain such as osteoarthritis may lead to increased use of aspirin, NSAIDs, and/or opioid medications as analgesics; monitor for side effects such as GI bleeding or constipation/fecal impaction.

---

    c. Check for rebound tenderness by pressing two fingers firmly over painful site and withdraw them rapidly; pain occurs on release of pressure.
F. Assess rectal area for lesions, hemorrhoids, or ulcerations.
G. Assess stool specimen.
    1. Color, consistency, odor.
    2. Presence of blood or mucus.
H. Evaluate elimination patterns and effects of aging on GI tract (Box 20-1).

# DISORDERS OF THE GASTROINTESTINAL SYSTEM

## Nausea and Vomiting

**Nausea is an unpleasant feeling that vomiting is imminent. Vomiting is an involuntary act in which the stomach contracts and forcefully expels gastric contents.**

A. Loss of fluid and electrolytes is the primary consequence of repeated vomiting; the very young and the older adult are more susceptible to complications of fluid imbalances.
B. Prolonged vomiting will precipitate a metabolic problem.
    1. Metabolic alkalosis is associated with prolonged vomiting and loss of hydrochloric acid.
    2. Metabolic acidosis occurs with *severe* prolonged vomiting of contents of the small intestine, resulting in loss of bicarbonate.

### Assessment

A. Precipitating causes.
    1. Pathogenic: related to a disease process (GI obstruction, toxic substances, etc.).
    2. Iatrogenic: resulting from a disease treatment.
        a. Chemotherapy/radiation.
        b. Medications.
        c. Surgery (postoperative complication).
    3. Pregnancy: vomiting most often occurs in the morning.

**TEST ALERT:** Monitor client's hydration status; modify client's care based on results of diagnostic tests.

B. Assessment.
    1. Identify precipitating cause.
    2. Assess frequency of vomiting, amount of vomiting, and contents of vomitus.
    3. Vomiting in children is common.
    4. Further investigation and intervention are needed for progressively severe vomiting, persistent vomiting over 24 hours, and/or symptoms of dehydration.
    5. Hematemesis: presence of blood in vomitus.
        a. Bright red blood is indicative of active bleeding.
        b. Coffee-ground material is indicative of blood retained in the stomach; the digestive process has broken down the hemoglobin.
    6. Projectile vomiting: vomiting not preceded by nausea in which vomitus is expelled with excessive force; often seen with increased intracranial pressure.
    7. Presence of fecal odor and bile in vomitus indicates a backflow of intestinal contents into stomach.
    8. Vomiting in children is usually self-limiting; assess for fever, diarrhea, and abdominal pain accompanying nausea and vomiting.
C. Diagnostics: clinical manifestations.

### Treatment

A. Eliminate the precipitating cause.
B. Antiemetics (see Appendix 20-2).
C. Parenteral replacement of fluid if loss is excessive (see Chapter 9).

*Nursing Interventions*

**Goal:** To prevent recurrence of nausea and vomiting and ensuing complications.

A. Prophylactic antiemetics for the client with a tendency to vomit.
B. Prompt removal of unpleasant odors, used emesis container, and soiled linens.
C. Good oral hygiene.
D. Place conscious client on side or in semi-Fowler's position; place unconscious client on side with head of bed slightly elevated to promote drainage of oral cavity.
E. Withhold food and beverages initially after client vomits; begin oral intake slowly; for adults, begin with tea, water, or oral rehydrating solutions at room temperature; for infants and children, begin with oral rehydrating solutions.
F. Assess surgical client for presence of bowel sounds and distention; do not begin oral administration of fluids if abdomen is tender or distended or no bowel sounds are present.
G. Support abdominal and thoracic incisions during vomiting.

> **TEST ALERT:** Identify client potential for aspiration; intervene to prevent aspiration.

**Goal:** To relieve nausea and vomiting.

A. Administer antiemetics.
B. Evaluate precipitating causes; relieve if possible.
C. Gastric decompression with a nasogastric (NG) tube may be used for prolonged vomiting.

**Goal:** To assess client's response to prolonged vomiting.

A. Monitor fluid and electrolyte status (see Chapter 9).
B. Assess for continued presence of gastric distention.
C. Assess for adequate hydration.

## Constipation

**Constipation exists when there is a decrease in frequency of bowel movements; stool is hard and difficult to pass, and there is less than one bowel movement every 3 days.**

*Assessment*

A. Precipitating causes.
   1. Decreased fiber and fluid intake.
   2. Immobility, inadequate exercise.
   3. Medications: opioids, antidepressants, iron supplements, anticonvulsants.
   4. Older adult client.
   5. Overuse of laxatives or enemas.
   6. Ignoring the urge to defecate.
   7. Diverticulosis, tumors, intestinal obstructions, irritable bowel syndrome.

> **TEST ALERT:** Evaluate client's use of home remedies and OTC drugs. Assess what the client is using to treat constipation; frequently, the older adult client is using harsh laxatives.

B. Clinical manifestations.
   1. Abdominal distention.
   2. Decreased amount and/or frequency of stool.
   3. Dry, hard stool; straining to pass stool.
   4. Impaction.
      a. Constipation, rectal discomfort.
      b. Anorexia, nausea, vomiting.
      c. Diarrhea around impacted stool.
C. Diagnostics: clinical manifestations, colonoscopy.

*Treatment*

A. Change dietary intake: increase intake of high-fiber foods and fluids.
B. Bulk laxatives, stool softeners, or enemas for occasional constipation problem (see Appendix 20-2).
C. Instruct client to maintain normal bowel schedule and not to ignore urge to defecate.
D. Discourage overuse or misuse of laxatives and enemas.
E. Encourage regular exercise.

*Nursing Interventions*

> **TEST ALERT:** Assess and intervene when client has a problem with elimination.

**Goal:** To identify client at risk for developing constipation and institute preventive measures (Box 20-2).
**Goal:** To implement treatment measures for fecal impaction removal.

A. An impaction may be present if client has had no bowel movement for 3 days or has passed only small amounts of semisoft or liquid stool.
B. Steps in removing impaction:
   1. Follow facility policy and procedure.

---

**Box 20-2  OLDER ADULT CARE FOCUS**

**Preventing Fecal Impaction**
- Increase intake of high-fiber foods: raw vegetables, whole-grain breads and cereals, fresh fruits.
- Increase fluid intake.
- Maintain regular activity: daily walking, swimming, or biking. If confined to wheelchair, change position frequently, perform leg raises and abdominal muscle contractions.
- Avoid overuse and misuse of laxatives and enemas.
- Encourage use of bulk-forming products to provide increased fiber (methylcellulose, psyllium).
- Encourage bowel movement at same time each day.
- Try to position client on bedside commode rather than on a bedpan to facilitate defecation.
- If client is experiencing diarrhea, check to see if stool is oozing around an impaction.

2. Manually check for presence of impaction with non-sterile, lubricated gloved finger.
3. Gently attempt to break up impaction using a scissor motion with the fingers.
4. Emphasis is on *prevention* of impaction (see Box 20-2).
5. Suppositories inserted into rectum may be given between attempts to clear the stool.

> ⚠ **NURSING PRIORITY:** Monitor client's heart rate during and after digital removal of feces; vagal stimulation can precipitate bradycardia.

## Diarrhea

**Diarrhea is the rapid movement of intestinal contents through the small bowel.**

A. Significant increase in number of stools, along with an increase in looseness of stool.
B. Infants and older adults are most susceptible to complications of dehydration and hypovolemia.
C. Acute diarrhea is most often caused by an infection and is self-limiting when all causative agents or irritants have been evacuated.
D. Rotavirus is the most common pathogen in young children hospitalized for treatment of diarrhea.
   1. Affects all age groups and is most common in cool weather.
   2. Incubation period is 48 hours.
   3. Important source of nosocomial infections in hospital.
   4. Children 6 to 24 months old are at increased risk for complications.

### Assessment

A. Precipitating causes.
   1. Bacteria (*Escherichia coli, Salmonella, Clostridium difficile,* Vancomycin-resistant enterococcus), viruses (rotavirus), and parasites *(Giardia lamblia).*
   2. Food poisoning (frequently, infection by bacteria).
   3. Medications (antibiotics and antacids).
   4. Food intolerance (lactose intolerance) or allergies to certain foods.
   5. Malabsorption problems: celiac disease and cystic fibrosis.
B. Clinical manifestations.
   1. Frequent, loose, watery bowel movements; sense of urgency.
   2. Stools may contain undigested food, mucus, pus, or blood; frequently are foul smelling.
   3. May experience abdominal bloating, cramping, distention, and vomiting with diarrhea, fatigue, weight loss.
   4. Hyperactive bowel sounds.
   5. May precipitate dehydration, hypokalemia, and hypovolemia, progressing to shock.
C. Diagnostics: stool examination; enzyme immunoassay (EIA) for rotavirus.

### Treatment

A. Identify and treat the underlying problem.
B. Decrease activity and irritation of the GI tract by decreasing intake.
C. Parenteral replacement of fluids and electrolytes if diarrhea is severe.
D. Do not administer antidiarrheal medications if causative agent is bacterial or parasitic. Antidiarrheals prevent client from purging the bacteria or parasite and traps the causative organism(s) in the intestines and prolongs the problem (see Appendix 20-2).
E. Viral infections are either treated with medication or left to run their course, depending on the severity and type of virus.
F. Probiotics, especially *Saccharomyces boulardii* and *Lactobacillus,* may be helpful in preventing antibiotic-induced diarrhea in clients receiving broad-spectrum antibiotics.
G. Rotavirus vaccine should not be given to severely immunocompromised infants.

### Nursing Interventions

**Goal:** To decrease diarrhea and prevent complications.

A. Identify precipitating causes and eliminate, if possible.
B. Offer soft, easily digestible food; does not have to be clear liquids.
C. Fluid and electrolyte replacement.
   1. Administer oral rehydrating solutions (ORSs); progress fluids and diet as tolerated.
   2. Frequently offer ORSs in small amounts at room temperature; do not offer high-carbohydrate fluids (juices), carbonated fluids, broth, or sports drinks.
   3. Nausea and vomiting are not contraindications to offering ORSs.
D. Keep rectal area clean and use barrier creams to protect skin.

**Goal:** To evaluate client's response to diarrhea.

A. Evaluate changes in vital signs correlating with fluid loss and hydration status (see Chapter 9).
B. Evaluate electrolyte changes and urine specific gravity.
C. Record intake and output and daily weight if diarrhea is progressive.
D. Inspect abdomen for distention, auscultate for bowel sounds, and palpate for areas of tenderness.

**Goal:** To prevent spread of diarrhea.

A. Good hand hygiene.
B. Initiate contact precautions (see Appendix 9-3).
   1. Proper disposal of diapers and soiled linens close to bedside.
   2. Instruct family regarding hand hygiene techniques.
   3. Maintain separate clean and dirty areas in the room; keep bedpans, soiled linens, and soiled diapers away from clean areas.
C. Instruct parents regarding importance of hand hygiene and how to care for infant or child at home.

⚠ **NURSING PRIORITY:** Consider acute-onset diarrhea as infectious until the cause is determined.

## 📋 Abdominal Pain

Abdominal pain may be acute or chronic. Acute pain may indicate a life-threatening problem within the abdomen that requires immediate attention.

A. The term *acute abdomen* is sometimes used to denote a broad spectrum of urgent pathologies.
B. Chronic abdominal pain is of long-term duration and may be referred from another area with similar nerve supply.

### Assessment

A. Precipitating causes for acute abdominal pain.
  1. Inflammation—gastroenteritis, appendicitis, pancreatitis, diverticulitis, cholecystitis.
  2. Peritonitis—perforated peptic ulcers, ruptured diverticula and appendix, intestinal perforation.
  3. Obstruction—bowel, biliary, and mesenteric occlusion.
  4. Internal bleeding—trauma, ruptured abdominal aortic aneurysm, GI bleeding, ruptured ectopic pregnancy.
B. Chronic abdominal pain.
  1. Irritable bowel syndrome (IBS).
  2. Peptic ulcer disease.
  3. Chronic pancreatitis and hepatitis.
  4. Pelvic inflammatory disease.
  5. Vascular insufficiency.
C. Clinical manifestations.
  1. Acute abdominal pain.
    a. Sudden, severe abdominal pain that is usually less than 24 hours in duration.
    b. Abdominal tenderness and distention.
    c. Elevated temperature.
    d. Nausea, vomiting, diarrhea.
  2. Chronic abdominal pain.
    a. Dull, aching, or diffuse pain across the abdomen.

### Nursing Interventions

**Goal:** To relieve abdominal pain.

A. Provide pain medication.
B. Nasogastric tube for abdominal decompression to relieve distention.
C. Preoperative preparation for client to go to surgery, if indicated.

**Goal:** To resolve inflammation.

A. Administration of antibiotics to alleviate infection.
B. Monitor complete blood count (CBC), electrolytes.

**Goal:** To monitor for complications (especially hypovolemic shock).

A. Monitor vital signs, level of consciousness, input and output, and $O_2$ saturation for indications of hypovolemic shock.

## 📋 Gastroesophageal Reflux Disease

Gastroesophageal reflux disease (GERD) is caused by the backward flow or reflux of gastric contents into the esophagus (esophageal reflux). Amount of damage depends on the amount and composition of gastric contents and the ability of the esophagus to remove the acidic fluids.

A. Gastric contents are able to move from area of increased pressure (stomach) to area of lower pressure (esophagus) through the malfunctioning lower esophageal sphincter (LES), reflux occurs, and the esophagus is exposed to acid (Figure 20-2).
B. The acid breaks down the esophageal mucosa, and an inflammatory response is initiated.
C. Hiatal hernia: a herniation of a portion of the stomach into the esophagus; frequently presents with same symptoms as GERD; clinical course and management are the same.

### Assessment

A. Risk factors (Figure 20-3).
  1. Lifestyle factors: obesity, smoking, excessive alcohol intake, consumption of high-fat or acidic foods, eating large meals, consumption of caffeine and carbonated beverages, stress.
  2. Pathologic predisposing factors: peptic ulcer disease (PUD), asthma, obstructive sleep apnea, cystic fibrosis, cancer.
  3. Medications decreasing LES pressure: calcium channel blockers, nitrates, anticholinergics.
  4. Other factors: scoliosis, poor esophageal sphincter tone (exacerbated by eating excessive amounts of food, lying down after a heavy meal, or strenuous exercise after eating).
  5. Clients with prolonged chronic GERD are at increased risk for cancer.

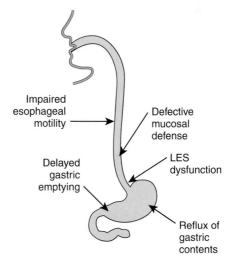

**FIGURE 20-2 Factors Involved in the Pathogenesis of Gastroesophageal Reflux Disease (GERD).** (From Lewis, S. L. et al. [2017]. *Medical-surgical nursing: Assessment and management of clinical problems* [10th ed.]. St. Louis, MO: Mosby.)

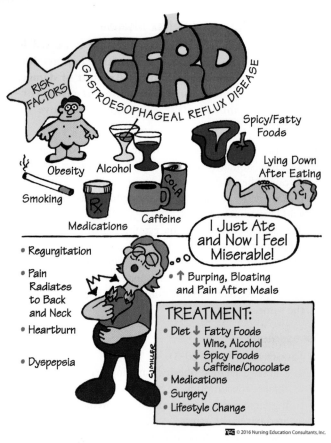

**FIGURE 20-3 Gastroesophageal Reflux Disease (GERD).** (From Zerwekh, J., Garneau, A., & Miller, C. J. [2017]. *Digital collection of the memory notebooks of nursing* [4th ed.]. Chandler, AZ: Nursing Education Consultants, Inc.)

B. Clinical manifestations.
  1. Reflux esophagitis (heartburn, dyspepsia).
  2. Increased pain after meals; may be relieved by antacids.
  3. Activities that increase intraabdominal pressure increase esophageal discomfort.
  4. Pain may radiate to back and neck.
  5. Regurgitation not associated with belching or nausea.
C. Complications.
  1. Aspiration of gastric contents: pneumonia, chronic bronchitis, esophageal strictures, Barrett's esophagus, a precancerous lesion that may predispose the client to develop esophageal adenocarcinoma.
  2. Dental erosion.
D. Diagnostics: 24-hour pH monitoring, esophageal manometry, esophagoscopy (see Appendix 20-1).

*Treatment*

A. Medical.
  1. Diet therapy: avoid intake of fatty foods; eat small, frequent meals; try chewing gum after and between meals.
  2. Avoid wine and other alcoholic beverages, caffeinated drinks, chocolate.
  3. Medications: histamine₂-receptor antagonists (H₂R blockers), proton pump inhibitors (PPIs) (see

Appendix 20-2), and GI stimulants or promotility drugs (see Appendix 20-2).
B. Surgical: fundoplication or antireflux surgery.
C. Endoscopic intervention at lower esophagus and gastroesophageal sphincter (fundoplication, radiofrequency, sclerosing agents).

*Nursing Interventions*

**Goal:** To decrease esophageal reflux.

A. Dietary
  1. Avoid drinking beverages during meals, including alcohol and carbonated drinks.
  2. Avoid drinking fluids 3 hours before bedtime.
  3. Eat 4 to 6 small meals per day (at 3-hour intervals) and avoid foods that precipitate discomfort (fats, caffeine, chocolate, spicy food, tomato products).
  4. Consume a high-protein, low-fat diet and avoid temperature extremes in foods.
B. Lifestyle
  1. If overweight, lose weight to decrease abdominal pressure gradient.
  2. Do not lie down for 2 to 3 hours after eating.
  3. Elevate the head of the bed on 4- to 6-inch (10–15 cm) blocks.
  4. Avoid tobacco, nonsteroidal antiinflammatory drugs (NSAIDs), and salicylates.

📋 **Gastritis**

**Gastritis is an inflammation and breakdown of the normal gastric mucosa barrier.**

A. Acute gastritis is generally self-limiting with no residual damage.
B. May be chronic or acute, diffuse or localized.

*Assessment*

A. Risk factors/etiology.
  1. Often caused by dietary indiscretion (gastric irritants: coffee, aspirin, alcohol).
  2. Smoking or exposure to radiation, psychological stress.
  3. Microorganisms: *Helicobacter pylori*, contaminated foods (*Staphylococcus* or *Salmonella* organisms).
  4. Medications causing gastric irritation (aspirin, corticosteroids, chemotherapy, NSAIDs).
  5. Prolonged alcohol abuse, binge drinking.
  6. Acute gastritis is a common problem in intensive care units because of stress. Clients with burns, uremia, sepsis, shock, mechanical ventilation, or multiorgan dysfunction who are not receiving enteral feeding are at significantly increased risk.

❗ **NURSING PRIORITY:** Best practice for the prevention of gastritis in clients who are ventilator dependent is the routine administration of antiulcerative medication (see Appendix 20-2).

B. Clinical manifestations (may be asymptomatic).
  1. Epigastric tenderness.

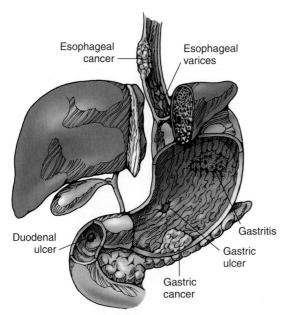

Esophageal cancer — Esophageal varices

Duodenal ulcer —

— Gastritis

— Gastric ulcer

Gastric cancer

**FIGURE 20-4 Common Causes of Gastrointestinal Bleeding.** (From Ignatavicius, D. D., & Workman, M. L. [2016]. *Medical-surgical nursing: Patient-centered collaborative care* [9th ed.]. Philadelphia: Saunders.)

2. Anorexia, nausea, vomiting, bloating, dyspepsia.
3. Chronic gastritis: frequently caused by the *H. pylori*.
   a. May precipitate pernicious anemia.
   b. Associated with peptic ulcer disease.
C. Diagnostics (see Appendix 20-1).
   1. Endoscopy with biopsy to rule out gastric carcinoma.
   2. Stool examination for occult blood.
   3. Gastric analysis for decreased acid production (achlorhydria).
   4. Serum, stool, and gastric biopsy for *H. pylori*.
D. Complications.
   1. Ulceration and hemorrhaging (Figure 20-4).
   2. Cancer of the stomach.

### Treatment

A. Eliminate cause.
B. Medical management.
   1. Antiemetics, antacids, PPIs, and $H_2R$ blockers (see Appendix 20-2).
   2. Treatment for *H. pylori* with antibiotics and PPIs.
C. Surgical intervention if medical treatment fails or hemorrhage occurs.

### Nursing Interventions

**Goal:** To decrease gastric irritation.

A. Nothing by mouth (NPO status) initially, with intravenous (IV) fluid and electrolyte replacement.
B. Plan of care for nausea and vomiting.
C. Begin ORSs as client tolerates them.

**Goal:** To monitor fluid status and prevent dehydration (see Chapter 7).
**Goal:** To assist client to identify and avoid precipitating causes.

## Gastroenteritis

**Gastroenteritis is the irritation and inflammation of the mucosa of the stomach and small bowel.**

### Assessment

A. Risk factors/etiology.
   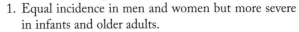
   1. Equal incidence in men and women but more severe in infants and older adults.
   2. Salmonella: fecal–oral transmission by direct contact or via contaminated food.
   3. Staphylococcal: transmission via foods that were handled by contaminated carrier.
   4. Dysentery: *E. coli* and *Shigella*.
B. Clinical manifestations.
   1. Abdominal cramping, distention, and pain.
   2. Nausea, vomiting, and diarrhea.
   3. Anorexia, fever, and chills.
C. Diagnostics: stool culture.

### Treatment

A. Nothing by mouth until nausea subsides.
B. Rehydrate with water and ORSs.
C. Client resumes eating with bland, easily digestible foods.
D. Appropriate medication for causative agents.

### Nursing Interventions

See Nursing Interventions section under Nausea and Vomiting.

##  Obesity

**Obesity is an imbalance between energy expenditure and caloric intake that results in an abnormal increase in fat cells.**

A. According to the Centers for Disease Control and Prevention, approximately 39% of people in the United States over age 20 are obese.
B. Children are considered overweight if their weight is in the 95th percentile or higher for their age, gender, and height on the growth chart.
C. Classified according to the body mass index (BMI).

### Assessment

A. Risk factors.
   1. Genetic predisposition.
   2. Sedentary lifestyle: energy intake (food) exceeds energy expenditure.
   3. Sociocultural: environment conducive to excessive caloric intake.
   4. Obesity puts client at increased risk for cardiovascular, respiratory, and musculoskeletal problems and increased risk for development of diabetes.
B. Clinical manifestations.
   1. A BMI of 25 to 29.9 $kg/m^2$ is considered overweight, a BMI of more than 30 $kg/m^2$ is considered obese, and a BMI greater than 40 $kg/m^2$ is considered severe/morbid obesity.
   2. Android obesity: fat is distributed over the abdomen and upper body (apple-shaped).

3. Gynecoid obesity: fat is distributed over the upper legs and hips (pear-shaped).
4. Android obesity is considered to be a higher risk for obesity-related problems, especially elevated triglycerides, hypertension, and type 2 diabetes.

### Treatment

A. Lifestyle changes and modification of dietary intake.
B. Bariatric surgery.
   1. Restrictive surgery.
      a. Vertical banded gastroplasty (VBG): adjustable gastric banding (AGB) involves placing a band around the fundus of the stomach; band may or may not be inflatable.
      b. Vertical sleeve gastrectomy (VSG): removes up to 85% of the stomach.
   2. Malabsorptive: biliopancreatic diversion (BPD) 70% of stomach removed; stomach and small intestine connected.
   3. Combination of restrictive and malabsorptive surgery: Roux-en-Y gastric bypass (RYGB) connects a small stomach pouch with the jejunum; first part of small intestine is bypassed.

### Nursing Interventions

**Goal:** To prepare client for surgery (see Chapter 3).

A. Discuss the importance of early ambulation to reduce complications.
B. Length of time in hospital depends on procedure.
C. Dietary changes.

**Goal:** To maintain homeostasis postoperatively (see Chapter 3).

A. Immediately postoperative airway may be a problem; maintain good pulmonary hygiene; ventilator support may be necessary.
   1. If continuous positive airway pressure (CPAP) was used at home, client will need it in hospital.
   2. Elevate the client's upper body at a 35- to 45-degree angle to reduce abdominal pressure and increase lung expansion.
B. Increased risks for thromboembolic problems: sequential compression stockings; encourage early ambulation and administer thromboprophylaxis with low-molecular-weight heparin.
C. Do not adjust an NG tube, and do not insert NG tube even if there is protocol to do so for nausea and vomiting; notify surgeon.
D. Observe client for development of anastomotic leaks: increasing back, shoulder, and/or abdominal pain; unexplained tachycardia or decrease urine output. Notify surgeon of these findings.
E. Extra attention is needed for skin care because of large folds of skin and extra weight.
F. In client with diabetes, assess for fluctuations in serum blood glucose; may require less hypoglycemics.
G. Client with malabsorption surgery may experience dumping syndrome (Box 20-3).

---

### Box 20-3 DUMPING SYNDROME

Condition occurs when a large bolus of gastric chyme and hypertonic fluid enter the intestine in an abnormally fast manner. Common after gastric or esophageal surgery.

**Goal:**
To assess for symptoms of condition.
- Weakness, dizziness, tachycardia.
- Epigastric fullness, abdominal cramping, hyperactive bowel sounds.
- Diaphoresis, cold, clammy skin.
- Generally occurs within 15–30 minutes after eating.
- Usually self-limiting and resolves in about 6–12 months but may become a chronic disorder.

**Goal:**
To prevent dumping syndrome.
- Decrease amount of food eaten at one meal; eat small meals at 3-hour intervals.
- Decrease simple carbohydrates; increase proteins and high-fiber foods as tolerated.
- No added fluid with meal; fluids can be taken 30–35 minutes before meals or 1 hour after meals.
- Decrease concentrated sweets; add fruits high in pectin to diet (peaches, plums, apples) to slow carbohydrate absorption in small intestine.
- Position client in semirecumbent position during meals; client may lie down on the left side for 20–30 minutes after meals to delay stomach emptying.
- Hypoglycemia may occur 2–3 hours after eating, caused by rapid entry of carbohydrates into jejunum.

**TEST ALERT:** Implement measures to improve client's nutritional intake. Prevent dumping syndrome and/or care for client experiencing dumping syndrome.

---

 **Home Care**

A. Diet.
   1. Eat at least four to six small meals a day; chew food completely.
   2. Drink fluids throughout the day, but do not drink fluids with meals.
   3. Avoid high-calorie, high-sugar, high-carbohydrate, and high-fat foods.
   4. Stop eating when you feel full.
   5. Try to get 50 to 60 g of protein daily; may need to take a protein supplement.
   6. Learn how to avoid dumping syndrome (see Box 20-3).
B. Take a chewable or liquid multivitamin with iron.
C. For women, do not try to get pregnant for about 18 months after surgery.
D. Join a support group for long-term psychosocial implications.
E. Develop a daily routine for exercise.

 **Peptic Ulcer Disease**

**Peptic ulcer disease (PUD) is an erosion of the GI mucosa by hydrochloric acid and pepsin. Any location in the GI**

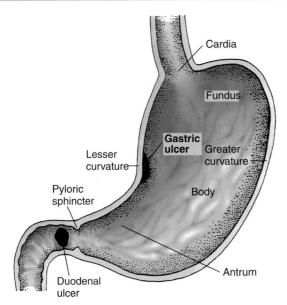

**FIGURE 20-5 The Most Common Sites for Peptic Ulcers.** (From Ignatavicius, D. D., & Workman, M. L. [2016]. *Medical-surgical nursing: Patient-centered collaborative care* [9th ed.]. Philadelphia: Saunders.)

tract that comes in contact with gastric secretions is susceptible to ulcer development.

A. Types of peptic ulcers (Figure 20-5).
  1. Duodenal (most common).
  2. Gastric.
  3. Physiologic stress ulcers.
B. Histamine release occurs with the erosion of the gastric mucosa in both duodenal and gastric ulcers. This results in vasodilation and increased capillary permeability, which further stimulates the secretion of gastric acid and pepsin. The continued erosion will eventually damage the blood vessels, leading to hemorrhage or erosion through gastric mucosa.
C. Characteristics.
  1. Risk factors.
    a. *H. pylori:* most common factor in both types of ulcers.
    b. Medications: aspirin, NSAIDs, corticosteroids, bisphosphonates.
    c. Alcohol abuse, smoking.
    d. Chronic gastritis.
    e. Hot, rough, or spicy foods are not a factor.
    f. Duodenal ulcers are associated with high secretion of HCl acid.
    g. Physiologic stress ulcers are associated with physical stress: burns, sepsis, and trauma.
  2. Clinical manifestations.
    a. Burning pain lasting minutes to hours; the pain associated with ulcers may be confusing, and symptoms may overlap from one type of ulcer to another.
      (1) Gastric ulcers: pain is high in epigastric area; occurs 1 to 2 hours after eating.
      (2) Duodenal ulcers: pain is in midepigastric area, just below the xiphoid process or in the back; occurs 2 to 4 hours after eating and is relieved by antacids or eating.

> **! NURSING PRIORITY:** Be careful to avoid confusing ulcer pain and indigestion with angina; do not administer antacids to cardiac clients complaining of midepigastric distress or "heartburn."

### Diagnostics

A. *H. pylori:* breath test; serum and stool analysis; differentiation is made between colonization and infection.
B. Gastric analysis (esophagogastroduodenoscopy [EGD]) with possible biopsy.

### Treatment

A. Medications (see Appendix 20-2).
  1. Medications to eliminate *H. pylori* bacteria.
    a. Metronidazole.
    b. Omeprazole.
    c. Clarithromycin, amoxicillin, tetracycline.
  2. Antacids.
  3. Histamine$_2$-receptor (H$_2$R) antagonists.
  4. Prostaglandin analogs and proton pump inhibitors (PPIs).
B. Lifestyle modifications.
  1. Eat a nonirritating or bland diet. Although hot, rough, or spicy foods do not cause PUD, avoid them if they cause discomfort.
  2. Minimize use of NSAIDs and antiinflammatory medications.
  3. Decrease or eliminate alcohol consumption and smoking.

### Complications

A. Frequently result in an emergency situation; initially treated conservatively, but surgery may be necessary.
B. Hemorrhage: bleeding when ulcer erodes through a vessel (see Figure 20-4).
  1. Clinical manifestations.
    a. Pain, nausea, vomiting.
    b. Hematemesis, melena, or both.
    c. More common in duodenal ulcers.
    d. Vital signs may reveal symptoms of shock (see Chapter 18).
  2. Treatment.
    a. Fluid volume replacement: blood, normal saline, Ringer's lactate.
    b. Medications to decrease acid production (see Appendix 20-2).
    c. NPO, NG tube; saline lavage may be done.
    d. Surgery if unresponsive to conservative therapy.

> **! NURSING PRIORITY:** Recognize and implement measures to manage potential circulatory complications (e.g., occurrence of a hemorrhage); carefully evaluate the client's blood pressure. Orthostatic hypotension (a blood pressure decrease of 20 mmHg or more in systolic blood pressure, a decrease of 10 mmHg or more in diastolic blood pressure, and/or an increase in the heart rate of 20 beats/min. from supine to standing) may be indicative of hypovolemia.

C. Perforation.
  1. Clinical manifestations.
    a. Sudden, severe, unrelenting abdominal pain.
    b. Rigid, "boardlike" abdomen.
    c. Hyperactive to absent bowel sounds.
    d. Severity of peritonitis is proportional to size of perforation and amount of gastric spillage.
  2. Treatment.
    a. Antibiotics.
    b. Perforation may seal; if not, laparoscopic or surgical closure.
    c. Fluid volume replacement.
D. Gastric outlet obstruction: more common in duodenal ulcers in the area of the pyloric valve.
  1. Clinical manifestations.
    a. Gradual onset of symptoms.
    b. History of PUD.
    c. Swelling, dilation of stomach.
    d. Vomiting: foul smelling and frequently projectile.
    e. Relief may be obtained by vomiting.
  2. Treatment.
    a. Decompress the stomach with NG suctioning; maintain continuous decompression to allow for healing.
    b. Fluid volume replacement.
    c. Antiulcer medications.
    d. Pyloroplasty to enlarge opening of pyloric valve.
E. Surgical interventions for intractable ulcers and/or complications.
  1. Partial gastrectomy: removal of majority of stomach (antrum and pylorus) with anastomosis to either the duodenum or the jejunum.
  2. Vagotomy: severing of the vagus nerve to decrease acid-secreting stimulus to gastric cells.
  3. Pyloroplasty (pyloric stenosis repair): enlargement of pyloric valve to facilitate passage of gastric contents into the small intestine; may be done in combination with vagotomy.
F. Postoperative complications.
  1. Dumping syndrome: affects up to half of clients who have undergone gastrectomy (see Box 20-3).
  2. Postprandial hypoglycemia: results from dumping syndrome; concentrated carbohydrates cause hyperglycemia, and excessive insulin is released, causing hypoglycemia about 2 hours after meals.

**TEST ALERT:** Teach client methods to prevent and/or manage complications associated with diagnosis.

### Nursing Interventions
**Goal:** To promote health and prevent reoccurrence of PUD.

A. Identify factors in lifestyle contributing to development of ulcer.
B. Identify factors that precipitate pain and discomfort.
C. Avoid aspirin compounds and NSAIDs.

D. Identify presence of *H. pylori* and follow therapy; ulcers tend to reoccur, so discontinuation or interruption of therapy can be detrimental.
E. Client should not take any other medications or OTC drugs that are not prescribed.

**TEST ALERT:** Evaluate use of home remedies and OTC drugs. The client with PUD may have been using antacids for a prolonged time.

**Goal:** To relieve acute pain and promote healing.

A. Dietary modifications.
  1. May be NPO with NG suctioning (decompression) for acute episode of gastric pain with nausea and vomiting (see Appendix 20-4).
  2. Nonirritating, bland foods are generally tolerated better during healing of acute episodes.
  3. Encourage small, frequent meals.
  4. Help client identify specific dietary habits that exacerbate or precipitate pain.
B. Identify characteristics of pain and activities that increase or decrease pain.

**Goal:** To promote homeostasis for client with gastric obstruction.

A. Nasogastric suctioning and careful assessment of hydration status; IV fluid replacement.
B. Reposition client from side to side to maintain effective gastric suctioning.
C. After several days of decompression, NG tube may be clamped for short periods and gastric residual measured; less than 200 mL residual is within normal range.
D. When gastric residual is within normal amount, oral feedings may begin at 30 mL per hour and be gradually increased; closely monitor for signs of obstruction.

**Goal:** To promote homeostasis when client is hemorrhaging.

A. Assess client response to hemorrhage.
  1. Evaluate hemoglobin and hematocrit levels.
  2. Assess for distention, increase in pain, and tenderness.
  3. Correlate vital signs with changes in client's overall condition.
  4. Assess stools and nasogastric drainage for presence of blood.
B. Maintain nasogastric decompression and suctioning (see Appendix 20-4).
  1. Insert NG tube for removal of gastric contents and maintain gastric suction.
  2. May implement saline solution lavage.
C. Monitor for hypovolemia and maintain hydration status (see Chapter 9).
  1. Establish peripheral infusion line, preferably with large-gauge needle for blood infusion.
  2. Insert indwelling urinary catheter, if indicated, to monitor urinary output; evaluate urine specific gravity.
  3. Prepare to administer whole blood transfusion (see Appendix 16-3) and IV fluids.

D. Hemodynamic monitoring (see Appendix 19-5).
E. Maintain NPO status, begin oxygen administration, maintain bed rest, and position client supine with legs slightly elevated.

**Goal:** To assess for complications of perforation and peritonitis (see Abdominal Pain section).
**Goal:** To assist client to return to homeostasis after gastric resection.

A. Provide general postoperative care as indicated (see Chapter 3).
B. Maintain nasogastric suction until peristalsis returns (see Appendix 20-4).

**TEST ALERT:** Monitor and maintain GI drainage. Distention and obstruction of the NG tube is a common problem for this client.

C. Assess continuously for:
   1. Increasing abdominal distention.
   2. Nausea, vomiting.
   3. Changes in bowel sounds.
D. No oral fluids until client tolerates clamping and/or removal of NG tube.
E. Begin oral fluids slowly: clear liquids first; then progress to bland, soft diet.
F. Based on client's condition, total parenteral nutrition may be necessary to maintain adequate nutrition (see Appendix 20-3).
G. Encourage ambulation to promote peristalsis.

**Goal:** To identify dumping syndrome (see Box 20-3).
**Goal:** To prevent the development of pernicious anemia after total gastric resection (see discussion of vitamin $B_{12}$ deficiency, Chapter 16).

### Appendicitis

**Appendicitis is the inflammation and obstruction of the appendix, leading to bacterial infection. If appendicitis is not treated, the appendix can become gangrenous and burst, causing peritonitis and septicemia, which could progress to death. It is the most common cause of acute abdominal pain.**

#### Assessment
A. Risk factors/etiology.
   1. Age: peak at 10 to 12 years of age; uncommon in children younger than 2 years.
   2. Diet: risk associated with a diet low in fiber and high in refined sugars and carbohydrates.
   3. Obstruction to opening of appendix: hardened fecal matter, foreign bodies, or microorganisms.
B. Clinical manifestations (Figure 20-6).
   1. Abdominal cramping and pain, beginning near the navel and then migrating toward McBurney's point (right lower quadrant); pain worsens with time.
   2. Rovsing's sign: pain in right lower quadrant when palpating or percussing other quadrants.

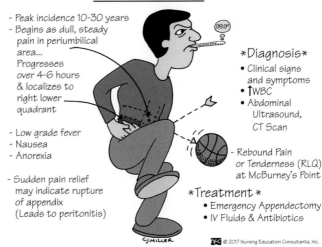

FIGURE 20-6 Appendicitis. (From Zerwekh, J., Garneau, A., & Miller, C. J. [2017]. *Digital collection of the memory notebooks of nursing* [4th ed.]. Chandler, AZ: Nursing Education Consultants, Inc.)

   3. Anorexia, nausea, vomiting, diarrhea.
   4. Low-grade fever.
   5. Side-lying position with knees flexed.
   6. Client complains of pain when asked to cough; asking client to cough is a better assessment method than palpating for rebound tenderness.
   7. Sudden, temporary relief from pain may indicate rupture of appendix.
C. Diagnostics: no specific diagnostic tool; diagnosis made from compilation of findings.
   1. Clinical manifestations.
   2. Urinalysis to rule out urinary tract infection.
   3. Abdominal ultrasonography and computed tomography (CT) to differentiate from other abdominal problems.
   4. CBC with differential reveals elevated white blood cell (WBC) count.
   5. Pregnancy test for adolescent females to rule out ectopic pregnancy.
D. Complications: rupture and peritonitis.

#### Treatment
A. Presurgery: NPO, fluid resuscitation, prophylactic antibiotic therapy; after diagnosis of appendicitis has been established, pain management with analgesics.
B. Open appendectomy or laparoscopic appendectomy.
C. Abdominal laparotomy and peritoneal lavage if appendix has ruptured.

#### Nursing Interventions
**Goal:** To assess clinical manifestations and to prepare for surgery.

A. Careful nursing assessment for clinical manifestations (Box 20-4).
B. Maintain NPO status until otherwise indicated.
C. Maintain bed rest in position of comfort.

**Box 20-4 UNDIAGNOSED ABDOMINAL PAIN**

**DO NOT**
- Give anything by mouth.
- Put any heat on the abdomen.
- Give an enema.
- Give strong narcotics.
- Give a laxative.

**DO**
- Maintain bed rest.
- Place in a position of comfort.
- Assess hydration.
- Assess abdominal status: distention, bowel sounds, passage of stool or flatus, generalized or local pain.

**Keep client NPO until notified otherwise.**

---

**TEST ALERT:** Determine need for administration of pain medications. Do not give opioids for pain control before a diagnosis of appendicitis is confirmed because this could mask symptoms.

---

D. Do not apply heat to the abdomen; cold applications may provide some relief or comfort.
E. Do not administer enemas.
F. Avoid unnecessary palpation of abdomen.

---

**⚠ PEDIATRIC NURSING PRIORITY:** Because children associate the stethoscope with listening, use the bell piece for initial palpation of the abdomen for tenderness. Children tolerate this type of pressure rather than palpation and probing with the fingers. Follow this initial approach, with manual palpation while carefully watching child's face for signs of discomfort.

---

**TEST ALERT:** Determine whether client is prepared for surgery or procedures. Appendicitis is a common problem; know how to care for client during diagnostic phase.

---

**Goal:** To maintain homeostasis and healing after appendectomy (see Chapter 3).

**Goal:** To prevent abdominal distention and to assess bowel function after abdominal laparotomy.

A. Maintain NPO status; then begin clear liquid diet, progressing to soft diet as tolerated.
B. Gastric decompression by NG tube; maintain patency and suction (see Appendix 20-4).
C. Monitor abdomen for distention and increased pain.
D. Assess peristaltic activity.
E. Evaluate and record character of bowel movements.

**Goal:** To decrease infection and promote healing after abdominal laparotomy.

A. Place client in semi-Fowler's position to localize and prevent spread of infection and reduce abdominal tension.

B. Antibiotics are usually administered via IV infusion; monitor response to antibiotics and status of IV infusion site.
C. Monitor vital signs frequently (every 2–4 hours) and evaluate for escalation of infectious process.
D. Provide appropriate wound care; evaluate drainage from abdominal Penrose drains and incisional area.

**Goal:** To maintain adequate hydration and nutrition and to promote comfort after abdominal laparotomy.

A. Maintain adequate hydration via IV infusion.
B. Evaluate tolerance of oral liquids when NG tube is removed.
C. Begin oral administration of clear liquids when peristalsis returns.
D. Progress diet as tolerated.
E. Administer analgesics as indicated.

---

**TEST ALERT:** Identify infection; peritonitis is common after surgery for a ruptured appendix.

---

 **Peritonitis**

**Peritonitis results from a localized or generalized inflammatory process of the peritoneum. It may occur when abdominal organs perforate or rupture and release their contents (bile, enzymes, hydrochloric acid, and bacteria) into the normal sterile peritoneal cavity.**

*Assessment*

A. Risk factors/etiology.
   1. Chemical peritonitis may result from an infection, the perforation of peptic ulcer, or a ruptured ectopic pregnancy.
   2. Bacterial peritonitis results from traumatic injury (abdominal trauma, ruptured appendix).
   3. Chemical peritonitis is rapidly followed by bacterial peritonitis.
   4. Pancreatic necrosis, pyelonephritis, ectopic pregnancy, malignancy, bile duct obstruction, and duodenal ulcer may cause peritonitis.

---

**TEST ALERT:** Monitor status of client who has undergone surgery; identify infection. Peritonitis is a potential complication any time the abdomen is entered either through trauma or for surgery.

---

B. Clinical manifestations (Figure 20-7).
   1. Presence of precipitating cause.
   2. Sharp or knifelike pain and/or dull and deep-seated pain over involved area; rebound tenderness; pain may radiate to back, shoulder, or scapula.
   3. Sudden, excruciating pain suggests the possibility of rupture.
   4. Abdominal mass or distention: note color and contour of abdomen.
   5. Abdominal muscle rigidity ("board-like" abdomen), guarding.
   6. Unexplained persistent or labile fever.

# PERITONITIS

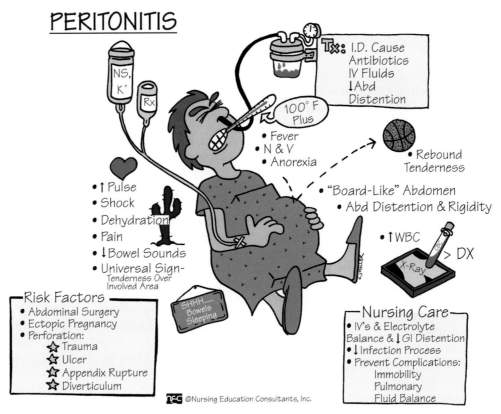

**FIGURE 20-7** Peritonitis. (From Zerwekh, J., Garneau, A., & Miller, C. J. [2017]. *Digital collection of the memory notebooks of nursing* [4th ed.]. Chandler, AZ: Nursing Education Consultants, Inc.)

7. Anorexia, nausea, vomiting.
8. Tachycardia, hypotension, shallow respirations: signs of impending or actual shock.
9. Decreased or absent bowel sounds.
10. Hypovolemia, dehydration.
11. Shallow respirations in attempt to avoid pain.
C. Diagnostics.
1. CBC for elevated WBC count and hemoconcentration of fluid shifts (see Chapter 9).
2. Abdominal x-ray, CT, and ultrasonography to evaluate for free air or fluid in the peritoneal cavity
3. Peritoneal lavage (aspiration) to evaluate abdominal fluid.

## Treatment

A. Identify and treat precipitating cause; frequently requires surgical intervention.
B. Opioid analgesic may be administered during diagnostic phase to ensure client cooperation.
C. Antibiotics.
D. IV fluids and electrolyte replacement.
E. Decrease abdominal distention: NPO, NG tube.

## Nursing Interventions

**Goal:** To provide pain control, wound care, prevent complications of immobility, and monitor postoperative progress (see Chapter 3).

**Goal:** To maintain fluid and electrolyte balances and reduce gastric distention.

A. Maintain nasogastric suction (see Appendix 20-4).
B. Maintain IV fluid replacement: normal saline or lactated Ringer's solution to maintain hydration and urine output of 30 mL/hr; assess urine specific gravity.
C. Administer potassium supplements with caution because of possible renal complications.
D. Assess level of distention and return of peristalsis and bowel function.
E. Maintain intake and output records.
F. Assess for problems of dehydration and hypovolemia (see Chapter 9).
G. Encourage activities to facilitate return of bowel function.
1. Encourage ambulation.
2. Attempt to decrease analgesics and maintain adequate pain control.
3. Maintain adequate hydration.

**Goal:** To reduce infectious process.

A. Administer antibiotics via IV infusion; assess client's tolerance of antibiotics and status of infusion site.
B. Evaluate vital signs and correlate with progress of infectious process.
C. Assess wound for signs of infection, purulent/foul-smelling drainage.

D. Maintain in semi-Fowler's position to enhance respirations and to localize drainage and prevent formation of subdiaphragmatic abscess.

## Diverticular Disease

**When a diverticulum (a pouch-like herniation of superficial layers of the colon through weakened muscle of the bowel wall) becomes inflamed, it is known as diverticulitis. Multiple diverticula are known as diverticulosis.**

**Meckel's diverticulum is a congenital diverticulum present in about 2% of the population, usually presenting with symptoms before age 2 years.**

### Assessment

A. Risk factors/etiology.
  1. Diet.
     a. Low-fiber, high refined-carbohydrate diet.
     b. Constipation.
     c. Indigestible fibers (corn, seeds, etc.) may precipitate diverticulitis, but they do not contribute to the development of diverticula.
  2. Age: 50% of adults are affected by age 80 years.
  3. As diverticula form, the colon wall becomes thickened; diverticulitis results from retention of stool and bacteria in the diverticulum.
  4. Inactivity and constipation.
B. Clinical manifestations.
  1. Diverticular disease is frequently asymptomatic; symptoms vary with degree of inflammation.
  2. Diverticulitis occurs when undigested food and bacteria are trapped in the diverticula.
     a. Symptoms of infection (fever, leukocytosis, and increased C-reactive protein).
     b. Acute left lower quadrant pain; may be accompanied by nausea and vomiting.
     c. Abdominal distention and increased pain on palpation.
     d. May progress to abscess, intestinal obstruction, and/or perforation.
C. Diagnostics (see Appendix 20-1).
  1. Computed tomography and/or ultrasound.
  2. Barium enema or colonoscopy is contraindicated in acute diverticulitis.

### Treatment

A. Management of uncomplicated diverticulum.
  1. High-fiber diet, mainly fruits and vegetables.
  2. Decreased intake of fat and red meat.
  3. Stool softeners, bulk laxatives.
  4. Increased activity: walking, exercise.
B. Diverticulitis.
  1. Oral antibiotics when symptoms are mild.
  2. Antispasmodic medications.
  3. Liquid diet and progress to semisolids as the diverticulitis resolves.
C. Severe diverticulitis.
  1. Broad-spectrum antibiotics.
  2. Bowel rest: NPO; may have an NG tube; hydration with IV fluids.

  3. Pain management with opioids; avoid morphine (decreases peristalsis).
  4. Assess for signs of bleeding and peritonitis.
  5. Surgery for obstruction, abscess, hemorrhage, or perforation.

**Goal:** To help client understand dietary implications and maintain prescribed therapy to prevent exacerbations.

A. Teach client to gradually reintroduce fiber after an acute episode of diverticulitis; aim for 25 g of fiber per day for women and 38 g for men.
B. Maintain high fluid intake.

**TEST ALERT:** Adapt the diet to the special needs of the client; determine client's ability to perform self-care.

C. Weight reduction if overweight or obese.
D. During acute diverticulitis, avoid activities that increase intraabdominal pressure (e.g., straining at stool, bending, lifting); avoid wearing tight restrictive clothing.
E. Use bulk laxatives to prevent acute episodes of diverticulitis but not during an episode; avoid enemas and harsh laxatives.

**Goal:** To decrease colon activity in client with diverticulitis.

A. Maintain clear liquids or NPO status.
B. Bed rest.
C. Adequate hydration via parenteral fluids.
D. As attack subsides, gradually introduce food and fluids.

### Home Care

A. High-fiber diet to prevent diverticulitis.
B. If client has any abdominal distress, all fiber should be avoided until tenderness resolves.
C. Report fevers, constant abdominal pain, and dark, tarry stools.

## Inflammatory Bowel Disease (IBD)

**IBD is an autoimmune disease characterized by chronic inflammation of the GI tract with periods of remission and exacerbation. It is considered an autoimmune disease; tissue damage is due to overactive sustained inflammatory response.**

A. *Crohn's disease* (ileitis or enteritis) is inflammation occurring anywhere along the GI tract, from the mouth to the anus; patches of inflammation occur next to healthy bowel tissue; most frequently affecting the terminal ileum and colon.
B. *Ulcerative colitis* is an inflammation and ulceration that most commonly occurs in the sigmoid colon and rectum; inflammation frequently begins in the rectum and spreads in a continuous manner up the colon; seldom is the small intestine involved.
C. Clients frequently experience periods of complete remission that alternate with exacerbations.
D. Even though the two conditions have different criteria for diagnosis, a clear differentiation cannot be made between them in about one-third of the cases.

## Assessment

A. Risk factors/etiology.
1. Familial tendency.
2. Commonly occur in the teenage years, with a second peak in occurrence in clients 60 years old and older.
3. Altered inflammatory response.
B. Clinical manifestations—Crohn's disease.
1. Diarrhea, bloody stools.
2. Weight loss; nutritional deficiencies; impaired absorption of vitamin $B_{12}$ (cobalamin).
3. Intermittent fever.
4. Entire thickness of bowel wall is involved; fistulas are not uncommon.
5. Nausea, abdominal pain, flatulence.
C. Clinical manifestations—ulcerative colitis.
1. Abdominal pain.
2. Bloody diarrhea.
3. Number of stools increases with exacerbation of condition; 10 to 20 stools per day in acute exacerbation.
4. Increased in systemic symptoms (fever, malaise, anorexia) with exacerbation.
5. Anemia.
6. Minimal small bowel involvement.
D. Diagnostics (see Appendix 20-1).

## Complications

A. Crohn's disease.
1. Perirectal and intraabdominal fistulas; fissures and rectal abscesses.
2. Perforation and peritonitis.
3. Nutritional deficiencies, especially of fat-soluble vitamins.
B. Ulcerative colitis.
1. Perforation and peritonitis with toxic megacolon.
2. Increased risk for cancer after 10 years.

## Treatment

A. Dietary modifications: increased calories, protein, and fluids. Encourage client to eat small servings several times a day.
B. Medications for Crohn's disease.
1. Antiinflammatory: aminosalicylates (sulfasalazine; see Appendix 9-2) and corticosteroids (see Appendix 9-2).
2. Antimicrobials: prevent or treat infection.
3. Immunosuppressants to decrease or suppress the immune response (see Appendix 23-2).
4. Biologic and targeted medications: infliximab, adalimumab, and certolizumab pegol (see Appendix 20-2).
5. Antidiarrheals.
C. Medications for ulcerative colitis: aminosalicylates and corticosteroids to decrease inflammation.
D. Surgical intervention may be necessary if client fails to respond to medical management and if fistulas, perforation, bleeding, or intestinal obstruction occur.
1. Total removal of colon, rectum, and anus with formation of permanent ileostomy (see Appendix 20-8).
2. Total removal of colon, rectum, and anus with formation of continent ileostomy (Kock's pouch).
3. Total removal of colon with formation of an ileoanal reservoir (J pouch).
4. Minimally invasive surgery (MIS) involves a laparoscopy to remove small areas of diseased tissue in the ileum and ileocecal areas.

## Nursing Interventions

**Goal:** To promote hemodynamic stability and hydration.

A. Evaluate and maintain adequate hydration status; monitor weight.
B. Encourage fluid intake of 2500 to 3000 mL/day.
C. Evaluate electrolyte status; monitor potassium level if on corticosteroids.
D. Assess characteristics and number of stools.

**Goal:** To promote nutrition.

A. Balanced diet with increased protein and calories.
B. Assess for iron deficiency anemia due to blood loss and reduced intake of iron.
C. Assess for anemia due to lack of absorption of vitamin $B_{12}$ (cobalamin); monthly injections or daily oral or nasal spray may be necessary.
D. Help client identify and avoid foods that precipitate diarrhea.
E. Parenteral nutrition or enteral feeding may be necessary because of malabsorption (see Appendixes 20-3 and 20-5).
F. Supplemental folic acid for clients on long-term sulfasalazine treatment.
G. Supplemental liquid nutrition.

**Goal:** To promote emotional and psychosocial stability.

A. Frequent bowel movements, rectal discomfort, and uncontrollable disease result in anxiety, frustration, and depression; promote comfort by keeping anal area clean and keeping room clear of offensive odors.
B. Establish trust, encourage self-care strategies, and refer to support groups.
C. Encourage rest to prevent fatigue.
D. Symptoms of reoccurrence of the problem—call the physician if these occur:
1. Continued diarrhea and weight loss.
2. Chills, fever, malaise.

## Home Care

A. Dietary modifications, avoidance of foods that cause diarrhea.
B. Medication regimen: precautions regarding steroids or immunosuppressive medications.
C. Dressings and wound care if fistula is present.
D. Identify appropriate measures to decrease stress in lifestyle.
E. Acute symptoms may be exacerbated or, as disease progresses, become chronic.

## Intestinal Obstruction

**Interference with normal peristalsis and impairment to forward flow of intestinal contents is known as intestinal obstruction.**

A. Types of obstruction (Figure 20-8).
   1. Mechanical obstruction.
      a. Strangulated hernia.
      b. Intussusception: the telescoping of one portion of the intestine into another (occurs most often in infants and small children).
      c. Volvulus: twisting of the bowel.
      d. Tumors: cancer (most frequent cause of obstruction in older adults).
      e. Adhesions (fibrous bands between tissues and organs after surgery).
   2. Neurogenic: interference with nerve supply in the intestine.
      a. Paralytic ileus or adynamic ileus occurring as a result of abdominal surgery or inflammatory process.
      b. Potential sequelae from spinal cord injury.
   3. Vascular obstruction: interference with the blood supply to the bowel.
      a. Infarction of superior mesenteric artery.
      b. Bowel obstructions related to intestinal ischemia may occur rapidly and may be life threatening.
B. Regardless of the precipitating cause, the ensuing problems are a result of the obstructive process.
C. The higher the obstruction in the intestine, the more rapidly symptoms will occur.
D. Fluid, gas, and intestinal contents accumulate proximal to the obstruction. This causes distention proximal to the obstruction and bowel collapse distal to the obstruction.
E. As fluid accumulation increases, so does pressure against the bowel. This precipitates extravasation of fluids and electrolytes into the peritoneal cavity. Increased pressure may cause the bowel to rupture.
F. Increased pressure causes an increase in capillary permeability and leakage of fluids and electrolytes into peritoneal fluid; this leads to a severe reduction in circulating volume.
G. Intussusception is the most common cause of intestinal obstruction in children from ages 3 months to 6 years.
H. The location of the obstruction determines the extent of fluid and electrolyte imbalance and acid–base imbalance.
   1. Dehydration and electrolyte imbalance do not occur rapidly if obstruction is in the large intestine.
   2. If the obstruction is located high in the intestine, dehydration occurs rapidly because of the inability of the intestine to reabsorb fluids; metabolic alkalosis develops from loss of gastric acid due to vomiting or NG suctioning.

### Assessment

A. Risk factors/etiology: identify type of obstruction and precipitating cause.
B. Clinical manifestations.
   1. Vomiting.
      a. Occurs early and is more severe if the obstruction is high.
      b. Higher obstruction may contain bile, and vomiting may be projectile.
      c. Vomiting caused by lower obstructions occurs more slowly and may be foul smelling due to the presence of bacteria and fecal material.
   2. Abdominal distention.
   3. Bowel sounds initially may be hyperactive proximal to the obstruction and decreased or absent distal to the obstruction; eventually, all bowel sounds will be absent.
   4. Colicky-type abdominal pain.
   5. Fluid and electrolyte imbalances, dehydration.
   6. Intussusception.
      a. Child is healthy with sudden occurrence of acute abdominal pain, vomiting, and fever.
      b. Child may pass one normal stool; then as condition deteriorates, the child may pass a stool described as "currant jelly" (a mixture of blood and mucus).
      c. A "sausage-shaped" mass may be palpated in the abdomen.

**TEST ALERT:** Determine characteristics of bowel sounds. This is particularly important for the client with intestinal problems.

C. Diagnostics (see Appendix 20-1).
   1. Abdominal x-ray or CT scan to differentiate obstruction from perforation.
   2. Barium enema to identify area of obstruction; only done after a bowel perforation has been ruled out.

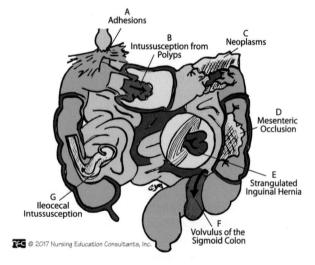

## TYPES OF BOWEL OBSTRUCTIONS

A
Adhesions

B
Intussusception from Polyps

C
Neoplasms

D
Mesenteric Occlusion

E
Strangulated Inguinal Hernia

G
Ileocecal Intussusception

F
Volvulus of the Sigmoid Colon

© 2017 Nursing Education Consultants, Inc.

**FIGURE 20-8  Bowel Obstructions.** (From Zerwekh, J., Garneau, A., & Miller, C. J. [2017]. *Digital collection of the memory notebooks of nursing* [4th ed.]. Chandler, AZ: Nursing Education Consultants, Inc.)

## Complications

A. Infection/septicemia.
B. Gangrene of the bowel.
C. Perforation of the bowel.
D. Severe dehydration and electrolyte imbalances.

## Treatment

A. Mechanical and vascular intestinal obstructions are generally treated surgically; ileostomy or colostomy may be necessary.
B. Conservative treatment includes nasogastric suctioning and decompression (see Appendix 20-4).
C. Fluid and electrolyte replacement; antibiotic therapy.
D. Intussusception: pneumoenema (air enema) with or without water-soluble contrast or ultrasound-guided hydrostatic (saline) reduction.
   1. Risk of intestinal perforation exists with hydrostatic reduction.
   2. Emergency surgical repair if hydrostatic reduction is not successful.

## Nursing Interventions

**Goal:** To prepare client for diagnostic evaluation and to maintain ongoing nursing assessment for pertinent data (see Appendix 20-1).

A. Monitor all stools; passage of normal stool may indicate reduction of the obstruction, especially an intussusception.
B. Classic signs and symptoms of intussusception may not be present; observe child for diarrhea, anorexia, vomiting, and episodic abdominal pain.

**Goal:** To decrease gastric distention and to maintain hydration and electrolyte balance.

A. Maintain NPO status.
B. Maintain nasogastric suction (see Appendix 20-4).
C. Monitor IV fluid replacement: most often normal saline or lactated Ringer's solution.
D. Administer potassium supplements with caution because of complications of decreased renal function.
E. Evaluate peristalsis, presence of any bowel function.
F. Maintain accurate intake and output records.
G. Assess for dehydration, hypovolemia, and electrolyte imbalance (see Chapter 9).
H. Measure abdominal girth to determine whether distention is increasing.
I. Encourage activities to facilitate return of bowel function.
   1. Encourage physical activity as tolerated.
   2. Attempt to decrease amount of medication (especially opioids) required for effective pain control.
   3. Maintain hydration.
J. Frequently, the position of comfort is side-lying with knees flexed.

**Goal:** To provide appropriate preoperative preparation when surgery is indicated (see Chapter 3).
**Goal:** To maintain homeostasis and promote healing after abdominal laparotomy (see Chapter 3).

**Goal:** To decrease infection and promote healing after surgery.

A. Monitor client's response to antibiotics.
B. Monitor vital signs frequently and evaluate for presence or escalation of infectious process.
C. Provide wound care. Evaluate drainage and healing from abdominal drains and from abdominal incisional area.

**TEST ALERT:** Empty and reestablish negative pressure of portable wound suction devices (Hemovac and Jackson-Pratt drains).

**Goal:** To reestablish normal nutrition and promote comfort after abdominal laparotomy.

A. Evaluate tolerance of liquids when NG tube is removed.
B. Begin administration of clear liquids initially and continue to evaluate for peristalsis and/or distention, nausea, and vomiting.
C. Progress diet as tolerated.
D. Administer analgesics as needed.
E. Promote psychological comfort.
   1. Respond promptly to requests.
   2. Carefully explain procedures.
   3. Encourage questions and ventilation of feelings regarding status of illness.
   4. Encourage parents to ask questions and to room-in with infant or child; rapidity of the onset of child's condition challenges parents' ability to cope.

## Hernia

**A hernia is a protrusion of the intestine through an abnormal opening or weakened area of the abdominal wall.**

A. Types.
   1. Inguinal: a weakness in which the spermatic cord in men and the round ligament in women passes through the abdominal wall in the groin area; more common in men; most common type of hernia in children.
   2. Femoral: protrusion of the intestine through the femoral ring; more common in women.
   3. Incisional or ventral: weakness in the abdominal wall caused by a previous incision.
   4. Umbilical: occurs most often in children when the umbilical opening fails to close adequately; most common hernia in infants; may occur in adults when the rectus muscle is weak from surgical incision.
   5. Classification. (Figure 20-9)
      a. Reducible: hernia may be replaced into the abdominal cavity by manual manipulation.
      b. Incarcerated or irreducible: hernia cannot be pushed back into place.
      c. Strangulated: blood supply and intestinal flow in the herniated area are obstructed; strangulated hernia leads to intestinal obstruction and possible perforation or necrosis.
B. Risk factors.
   1. Chronic cough, such as smoker's cough or cough associated with cystic fibrosis.

# "SIR" HERNIA

**S**trangulated...
  Blood supply is cut off, emergency surgery situation.

**I**ncarcerated...
  Hernia is trapped outside peritoneal cavity.

**R**educible...
  Hernia moves back into peritoneal cavity.

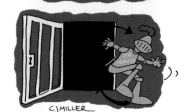

CJMILLER

© 2017 Nursing Education Consultants, Inc.

**FIGURE 20-9 Hernia.** (From Zerwekh, J., Garneau, A., & Miller, C. J. [2017]. *Digital collection of the memory notebooks of nursing* [4th ed.]. Chandler, AZ: Nursing Education Consultants, Inc.)

2. Obesity or weakened abdominal musculature.
3. Straining during bowel movement or lifting heavy objects.
4. Pregnancy.

## Assessment

A. Clinical manifestations.
  1. Hernia protrudes over the involved area when the client stands or strains, or when the infant cries.
  2. Severe pain occurs if hernia becomes strangulated.
  3. Strangulated hernia produces symptoms of intestinal obstruction.
B. Diagnostics (see Appendix 20-1).

## Treatment

A. Preferably elective surgery through abdominal incision.
B. Laparoscopic hernia repair.
C. Emergency surgery for strangulated hernias producing intestinal obstruction.

## Nursing Interventions

**Goal:** To prepare client for surgery, if indicated (see Chapter 3).
**Goal:** To maintain homeostasis and promote healing after herniorrhaphy.

A. General postoperative nursing care (see Chapter 3).
B. Repair of an indirect inguinal hernia: assess male clients for development of scrotal edema; may require the use of a scrotal support with application of an ice bag.
C. Encourage deep breathing and activity.
D. If coughing occurs, teach client how to splint the incision.

E. Refrain from heavy lifting for approximately 6 to 8 weeks after surgery.
F. Wound care.
  1. Keep wound clean and dry: use occlusive dressing or leave open to air.
  2. Change diapers frequently and/or prevent irritation and contamination in incisional area.

## Hypertrophic Pyloric Stenosis

**Hypertrophic pyloric stenosis (HPS) is the obstruction of the pyloric sphincter by hypertrophy and hyperplasia of the circular muscle of the pylorus. Symptoms usually present in the first few weeks of life.**

### Assessment

A. Risk factors/etiology.
  1. Occurs most often in firstborn, full-term male infants (infantile hypertrophic pyloric stenosis).
  2. Seen more frequently in Caucasian infants.
B. Clinical manifestations.
  1. Onset of vomiting may be gradual, usually occurs at 3 weeks or as late as 5 months; is progressive and may be projectile.
  2. Emesis is not bile stained but may be curdled or bloody.
  3. Vomiting occurs shortly after feeding.
  4. Infant is hungry and irritable; wants to eat after vomiting.
  5. Infant does not appear to be in pain or acute distress.
  6. Weight loss occurs, if untreated.
  7. Stools decrease in number and in size.
  8. Dehydration occurs as condition progresses; hypochloremia and hypokalemia occur as vomiting continues.
  9. Upper abdomen is distended, and an "olive-shaped" mass may be palpated in the right epigastric area.
C. Diagnostics (see Appendix 20-1).
D. Treatment: surgical release of the pyloric muscle (pyloromyotomy).

### Nursing Interventions

**Goal:** To maintain hydration and gastric decompression; to initiate appropriate preoperative nursing activities (see Appendix 20-4).

A. Maintain nasogastric decompression if NG tube is in place and record type and amount of drainage.
B. Assess hydration status and electrolyte balance, especially serum calcium, sodium, and potassium levels.
C. NPO status with continuous IV infusion (most often saline solutions) may be required.
D. Accurate intake and output records: complete description of all vomitus and stools.
E. Monitor vital signs and check for signs of peritonitis.
F. Preoperative teaching for parents.

**Goal:** To maintain adequate hydration and promote healing after pyloromyotomy.

A. Postoperative vomiting in the first 24 to 48 hours is not uncommon; maintain IV fluids until infant tolerates adequate oral intake.

B. Continue to monitor infant in the same manner as in the preoperative period.

C. Feedings are initiated early; bottle-fed infant may begin with clear liquids containing glucose and electrolytes, small amounts offered frequently.

D. Breastfed infants: mother can express breast milk and offer small amounts in a bottle or initially limit nursing time.

**Goal:** To help parents provide appropriate home care after pyloromyotomy.

A. No residual problems are anticipated after surgery.

B. Instruct parents regarding care of the incisional area.

## Cancer of the Stomach

**Stomach or gastric cancer is an adenocarcinoma of the stomach wall.**

A. Tumors in the cardia and fundus of the stomach are associated with a poor prognosis.

B. Metastasis generally occurs by direct extension of the malignant growth into adjacent organs and structures (esophagus, spleen, pancreas, etc.).

C. Because of the ability of the stomach to accommodate the growing tumor, symptoms may not be evident until metastasis has occurred.

### Assessment

A. Risk factors/etiology.
 1. Increased incidence in men.
 2. Peak incidence in seventh decade.
 3. Presence of *H. pylori* is considered an increased risk factor.
 4. Increased incidence in presence of other chronic gastric problems.
 5. Diet including smoked foods, salted fish and meat, and pickled vegetables.

B. Clinical manifestations.
 1. Early symptoms.
  a. Loss of appetite, persistent indigestion.
  b. Early satiety, dyspepsia.
  c. Nausea, vomiting, fatigue, and weakness.
  d. Blood in stool.
 2. Later symptoms.
  a. Pain often exacerbated by eating.
  b. Weight loss, anemia.
  c. Nausea and vomiting due to impending GI obstruction.
  d. Presence of a palpable mass in the stomach; ascites from involvement of peritoneal cavity.

C. Diagnostics (see Appendix 20-1).
 1. Gastroscopy and biopsy.
 2. CT and full-body imaging for metastasis.

### Treatment

Partial or complete gastrectomy is the preferred method of treatment. Chemotherapy and radiation usually follow surgery.

### Nursing Interventions

See Nursing Interventions for gastric resection under Peptic Ulcer Disease.

## Cancer of the Colon and Rectum (Colorectal Cancer)

**Colorectal cancer (cancer of the colon and/or the rectum) is the third most common cancer in the United States and the second leading cause of cancer-related deaths.**

A. Eighty-five percent of colorectal cancers arise from adenomatous polyps that can be detected and removed by sigmoidoscopy or colonoscopy.

B. Symptoms frequently do not appear until condition is advanced with metastatic sites.

C. Most common areas of metastasis include regional lymph nodes, liver, lungs, and peritoneum.

### Assessment

A. Risk factors/etiology.
 1. Family history (first-degree relative) of colorectal cancer.
 2. Incidence increases significantly after age 50.
 3. History of inflammatory bowel disease.
 4. High-fat, high-calorie, low-residue diet with high intake of red meat increases anaerobic bacteria in bowel, which convert bile acids into carcinogens.
 5. Alcohol, tobacco use, and obesity are also associated with increased risk.

B. Clinical manifestations.
 1. Symptoms are vague early in disease state and may take years to present.
 2. Bloody stools, melena (dark tarry) stools.
 3. Change in bowel habits: constipation and diarrhea.
 4. Change in shape of stool (pencil- or ribbon-shaped in sigmoid or rectal cancer).
 5. Weakness and fatigue from iron deficiency anemia and chronic blood loss.
 6. Pain, anorexia, and unexpected weight loss are late symptoms.
 7. Bowel obstruction may lead to perforation and peritonitis.

C. Diagnostics (see Appendix 20-1).
 1. Sigmoidoscopy and colonoscopy with biopsies.
 2. Carcinoembryonic antigen (CEA) tumor marker detected in blood.

### Treatment

A. Colon resection: may have resection with or without a colostomy or may have an abdominal-perineal resection that includes resection of the sigmoid colon, rectum, and anus.

B. Laser photocoagulation: destroys small tumors and palliative for large tumors obstructing bowel.

C. Endoscopic excision or electrocoagulation for small, localized tumors or for clients who are poor surgical candidates.

D. Radiation therapy: external, intracavity, or implanted; may be used preoperatively to shrink tumor size.

E. Chemotherapy: reduces recurrence and prolongs survival in stage II and III rectal tumors.

### Nursing Interventions

**Goal:** To provide information to high-risk clients.

A. Diet: high-fiber, low-fat diet with a decreased intake of red meat.

B. Digital rectal examinations yearly after age 40.

C. Annual fecal occult blood testing after age 50.

D. Colonoscopy every 3 or 5 years after age 40 for high risk; otherwise every 10 years for average risk.

**Goal:** To provide preoperative care.

A. Determine extent of surgery anticipated; colostomy is not always done.

B. Bowel preparation: low-residue diet, cathartics 24 hours before surgery.

C. Oral neomycin to decrease bacteria in the bowel.

D. If colostomy is to be done, discuss implications and identify appropriate area for stoma on abdomen (see Appendix 20-8).

E. Prepare client for change in body image if colostomy is indicated.

**Goal:** To provide appropriate wound care after abdominal–perineal resection.

A. Client will have three incisional areas:
   1. Abdominal incision.
   2. Incisional area for colostomy.
   3. Perineal incision.

> **TEST ALERT:** Identify factors interfering with wound healing and/or symptoms of infection.

B. Perineal wound.
   1. Wound may be left open to heal by secondary intention: provide warm sitz baths (100.4°–100.6°F [38.0–38.1°C]) for 10 to 20 minutes to promote debridement, increase circulation to the area, and promote comfort.
   2. Wound may be partially closed with drains (Jackson-Pratt and/or Hemovac) in place: assess the wound for integrity of suture line and presence of infection; drainage should be serosanguineous; drains remain in place until drainage is less than 50 mL/24 hour (see Chapter 3).
   3. Wound may be open and packed: drainage is profuse first several hours after surgery; may require frequent reinforcement and dressing change; drainage is serosanguineous.

C. Position client with a perineal wound on his or her side; do not allow client to sit for prolonged period until wound is healed.

D. Assess status of stoma and healing of abdominal incision (see Appendix 20-8).

**Goal:** To maintain homeostasis and promote healing after abdominal–perineal resection or colon resection (see Chapter 3).

A. Infections, hemorrhage, wound disruption, thrombophlebitis, and stoma problems are the most common complications.

B. Help client begin to become independent with colostomy care early in recovery period (see Appendix 20-8).

**Goal:** To provide psychosocial support.

A. Emotional support is essential with cancer diagnosis; recovery is long and frequently painful.

B. Sexual dysfunction may occur; determine from physician if nerve paths for erection and ejaculation were in area of resection; provide opportunity for questions.

C. Keep room clean and free of offensive smells; client may be self-conscious regarding open wound and/or stoma; provide opportunity for questions and discussion.

### Home Care

A. Recovery period is long; help client and family identify community resources.

B. Help client and family identify resources and obtain equipment for colostomy care (see Appendix 20-8).

C. Instruct client in care of perineal wound if it is not healed.
   1. Sitz baths: always check temperature of water; wound tissue can be easily damaged.
   2. Presence of continuous drainage may indicate a fistula.

D. Identify community resources for client: home health visits, social services, etc.

E. Assess client's ability to care for stoma; help client begin self-care before discharge (see Appendix 20-8). Refer to wound ostomy continence nurse if indicated.

### Celiac Disease

**Celiac disease is a type of malabsorption syndrome also known as sprue or gluten-sensitive enteropathy. This disease is an immune reaction to rye, wheat, barley, and oat grains that leads to an inflammatory response, causing damage to the villi of the small intestines and resulting in the inability to absorb nutrients (malabsorption).**

A. Previously considered a disease of childhood, with symptoms beginning between the ages of 1 year and 5 years; celiac disease is now commonly seen at all ages, with mean age of diagnosis being 40 years.

B. Symptoms frequently begin in early childhood but condition may not be diagnosed until client is an adult.

C. Development of celiac disease is dependent on genetic predisposition, ingestion of gluten, and immune-mediated response.

### Assessment

A. Cause: congenital defect or an autoimmune response in gluten metabolism.

B. Clinical manifestations.
  1. Symptoms may begin when child has increased intake of foods containing gluten: cereals, crackers, breads, cookies, pastas, etc.
  2. Foul-smelling diarrhea with abdominal distention and anorexia in infants and toddlers.
  3. Poor weight gain in children, failure to thrive.
  4. Constipation, vomiting, and abdominal pain may be the initial presenting symptoms in adults.
  5. Vitamin deficiency leads to central nervous system impairment and bone malformation or decreased bone density and osteoporosis.
  6. May be associated with other autoimmune conditions (rheumatoid arthritis, type 1 diabetes, thyroid disease).
C. Diagnostics: biopsy of duodenum and small intestine.

*Treatment*

Primarily dietary management: gluten-free diet.

*Nursing Interventions*

**Goal:** To help client and family understand diet therapy and promote optimal nutrition intake.

A. Written information regarding a gluten-free diet; corn, rice, potato, flax, and soy products may be substituted for wheat in diet.
B. Diet should be well balanced and high in protein.
C. Teach client and/or family how to read food and medication labels for gluten content; thickenings, soups, instant foods, and some medications may contain hidden sources of gluten.
D. Important to discuss the necessity of maintaining a lifelong gluten-restricted diet; problems may occur in clients who relax their diet and experience an exacerbation of the disease state.
E. Lack of adherence to dietary restrictions may precipitate growth retardation, anemia, bone deformities, and lymphomas.

**TEST ALERT:** Adapt the diet to meet client's specific needs.

## Hirschsprung's Disease

**Hirschsprung's disease (congenital aganglionic megacolon) is characterized by a congenital absence of ganglionic cells that innervate a segment of the colon wall.**

A. Clinical symptoms vary depending on the age when symptoms are recognized, the length of the affected bowel, and presence of inflammation.
B. Most common site is the rectosigmoid colon; colon proximal to the area dilates (i.e., megacolon).

*Assessment*

A. Risk factors/etiology: congenital anomaly.
B. Clinical manifestations.
  1. May be acute and life threatening or may be a chronic presentation.

2. Internal sphincter loses ability to relax for defecation.
3. Newborn.
  a. Failure to pass meconium within 48 hours after birth.
  b. Vomiting, abdominal distention.
  c. Reluctance to take fluids.
4. Older infant and child.
  a. Chronic constipation, impactions.
  b. Passage of ribbon-like, foul-smelling stools and diarrhea.
  c. Failure to thrive.
  d. Lack of appetite.
C. Diagnostics: rectal biopsy to confirm.

*Treatment*

A. Surgical correction usually involves resection of aganglionic bowel with creation of a temporary colostomy to relieve the obstruction.
B. The final repair closes the colostomy, and the bowel is reanastomosed.

*Nursing Interventions*

**Goal:** To promote normal attachment and prepare infant and parents for surgery.

A. Allow parents to vent feelings regarding congenital defect of infant.
B. Foster infant–parent attachment.
C. General preoperative preparation of the infant; neonate does not require any bowel preparation.
D. Careful explanation of colostomy to parents.

**Goal:** See Nursing Interventions for client who has undergone abdominal surgery in the Intestinal Obstruction section of this chapter.
**Goal:** To help parents understand and provide appropriate home care for their infant/child after colostomy (see Appendix 20-8).

A. Colostomy is most often temporary.
B. Parents should be actively involved in colostomy care before discharge.

## Hemorrhoids

**Dilated hemorrhoidal veins of the anus and rectum; may be internal (above the internal sphincter) or external (outside of the external sphincter).**

*Assessment*

A. Risk factors/etiology: conditions that increase anorectal pressure.
  1. Pregnancy, obesity, prolonged constipation.
  2. Prolonged standing or sitting.
  3. Portal hypertension.
  4. Straining at bowel movement.
B. Clinical manifestations.
  1. External hemorrhoids appear as protrusions at the anus.
  2. Prolapsed hemorrhoids may bleed or become thrombosed.

3. Thrombosed hemorrhoid: a blood clot in a hemorrhoid that causes inflammation and pain.
4. Rectal bleeding during defecation.
C. Diagnostics: rectal examination.

### Treatment

A. Conservative treatment.
1. Sitz baths, stool softeners, ointments, topical anesthetics.
2. Prevent constipation: diet high in fiber (bran) and roughage with increased water intake.
3. Avoid straining with bowel movement; keep anal area clean.
B. Aggressive treatment.
1. Ligation of prolapsed, thrombosed hemorrhoids with small rubber band.
2. Infrared coagulation for bleeding hemorrhoids.
3. Surgery for painful, large, bleeding hemorrhoids.

### Nursing Interventions

**Goal:** To provide appropriate information to help client manage problem at home.

A. Avoid prolonged standing or sitting.
B. Take sitz baths to decrease discomfort.
C. Use OTC ointments to decrease discomfort.
D. Apply ice pack, followed by a warm sitz bath, if severe discomfort occurs.
E. Avoid constipation and straining at stool.

### Home Care

A. Encourage bulk laxatives and increased fluid intake to promote soft stool for first bowel movement.
B. Rectal pain may be severe; analgesics and local application of moist heat may be used.
C. Review preventive techniques; weight loss and avoidance of constipation.

---

## Appendix 20-1   GASTROINTESTINAL SYSTEM DIAGNOSTICS

### X-Ray

#### Upper Gastrointestinal Series or Barium Swallow

X-ray examination in which barium or Gastrografin is used as a contrast material; used to diagnose structural abnormalities and problems of the esophagus, stomach, and small intestine. As the client swallows the barium, x-ray films are obtained to show the structures, function, position, and abnormalities of organs from mouth through jejunum.

#### Nursing Implications

1. Explain procedure to client (usually not done on client with acute abdomen until possibility of perforation has been ruled out).
2. Maintain client's nothing by mouth (NPO) status 8 hours before procedure.
3. Client will swallow barium to coat the GI tract for visualization of various landmarks and structures and assume various positions on the x-ray table.
4. After examination, promote normal excretion of barium to prevent impaction. Barium can cause constipation, so encourage extra fluid. It may be necessary to use a stool softener or laxative to promote evacuation of barium.
5. Stool should return to normal color within 72 hours.

#### Lower Gastrointestinal Series or Barium Enema

X-ray examination of the colon in which barium is used as a contrast medium; barium is administered rectally.

#### Nursing Implications

1. Maintain client's NPO status for 8 hours before test. Client may have clear liquids the evening before the test.
2. Colon must be free of stool; laxatives and enemas are administered the evening before the test.
3. Explain to client that he or she may experience cramping and the urge to defecate during the procedure.
4. After the procedure, increase fluids and administer a laxative to assist in expelling the barium.

### Endoscopy

#### Gastroscopy, Esophagogastroduodenoscopy (EGD), Colonoscopy, Sigmoidoscopy, Capsule Endoscopy

*Endoscopy* is the direct visualization of the gastrointestinal tract (GI) via a flexible, fiber optic, lighted scope.

*Upper GI:* inflammation, ulcerations, tumors; evaluation and treatment of esophageal varices.
*Lower GI:* evaluation of diverticular disease or irritable bowel syndrome; treatment of active bleeding or ulceration; identification of polyps, tumors, inflammation, fissures, or hemorrhoids.
The endoscope is capable of obtaining biopsy specimens and clipping benign polyps.

#### Nursing Implications Before Procedure

1. Upper GI: NPO for up to 12 hours before procedure.
2. Lower GI: bowel prep—cathartics and/or enemas, clear liquid diet for 24 hours before test.
3. Client should avoid aspirin, NSAIDs, iron supplements, and gelatin containing red coloring for a week before procedure.
4. May give preoperative medication for relaxation and to decrease secretions.
5. For upper GI studies, a topical anesthesia will be used to anesthetize the throat before insertion of the scope.
6. Upper GI studies: assess client's mouth for dentures and removable bridges.
7. Lower GI studies: help client into the left side-lying, knee-chest position; explain the need to take a deep breath during the insertion of the scope; client may feel urge to defecate as scope is passed.
8. Conscious sedation frequently used for upper and lower GI studies or colonoscopy.

#### Nursing Implications During Procedure

1. Verify informed consent and client identification.
2. For upper GI studies, confirm NPO status for past 8 hours; for lower GI studies, confirm bowel preparation.
3. Assess for presence of GI bleeding; notify physician if any bleeding is present.
4. Maintain safety: airway precautions during sedation; positioning, monitor level of sedation (see Chapter 3).

#### Nursing Implications After Procedure

1. Upper GI: *maintain client's NPO status until the gag reflex returns;* position client on his or her side to prevent aspiration until gag or cough reflex returns; use throat lozenges or warm saline solution gargles for relief of sore throat.
2. Monitor vital signs and $O_2$ saturation during recovery.

3. Observe for signs of perforation: upper GI bleeding—dysphagia, substernal or epigastric pain; lower GI bleeding—rectal bleeding, increasing abdominal distention.
4. Assist client to upright position: observe for orthostatic hypotension.
5. Warm sitz bath for any anal discomfort.

### Analysis of Specimens

Capsule endoscopy requires client to swallow a capsule with a camera that transmits photos of the GI tract.

#### Nursing Implications Before Procedure
1. Bowel prep according to physician.
2. Explain client will swallow capsule and wear an external monitor to capture pictures.

#### Nursing Implications During Procedure
1. Keep client NPO for 4 to 6 hours.
2. Remove monitoring device after 8 hours.

### Paracentesis; Diagnostic Peritoneal Lavage

*Procedure:* A catheter is inserted into the peritoneal cavity, most often just below the umbilicus.

**Purposes**
1. To determine effect of blunt abdominal trauma.
2. To assess for presence of ascites.
3. To identify cause of acute abdominal problems (e.g., perforation, hemorrhage).
   - To assess for intraabdominal bleeding after a blunt trauma to the abdomen. If no blood is aspirated, normal saline is infused into the peritoneal cavity. The fluid is aspirated or allowed to drain by gravity. Fluid should return clear with a slight yellow cast if there is no injury. Bloody fluids, presence of bacterial or fecal material, high white or red blood cell count occur with a positive test result; immediate surgery may be required.
   - If client has abdominal fluid from ascites or other abdominal pathologic conditions, a specimen of the fluid is obtained without instilling fluid.

### Nursing Implications
1. An NG tube may be used to maintain gastric decompression during procedure.
2. Have the client void before the procedure; if client has a full bladder at the time of insertion of the catheter, risk for bladder perforation and peritonitis is increased.
3. In clients with chronic liver problems, assess coagulation laboratory values before procedure.
4. Place client in semi-Fowler's position.
5. Maintain sterile field for puncture.
6. Weigh the client before and after the paracentesis and document the weights.
7. Measure the drainage and record accurately.

**Complications**
1. Perforation of bowel: peritonitis.
2. Introduction of air into abdominal cavity; client may complain of right referred shoulder pain (caused by air under the diaphragm).
3. Contraindicated in pregnancy and in clients with coagulation defects or possible bowel obstruction.
4. Hypotension/hypovolemia if too much fluid is removed.

### Stool Examination

Stool is examined for form and consistency and to determine whether it contains mucus, blood, pus, parasites, or fat. Stool will be examined for presence of occult blood.

#### Nursing Implications
1. Collect stool in sterile container if examining for pathologic organisms.
2. A fresh, warm stool is required for evaluation of parasites or pathogenic organisms.
3. Collect the sample from various areas of the stool.
4. The result of the guaiac test for occult blood is positive when the paper turns blue.
5. Document medications and over-the-counter drugs client is taking when sample is obtained.
6. Sample should be approximately the size of a walnut or 30 mL, if soft.

## Antiemetics

| Medications | Side Effects | Nursing Implications |
|---|---|---|
| **Dopamine Antagonists:** Depress or block dopamine receptors chemoreceptor trigger zone of the brain | | |
| *Phenothiazines*—suppress emesis<br>Chlorpromazine hydrochloride: PO, suppository, IM<br>Promethazine: PO, IM, suppository<br>▲ High-Alert Medication for IV route<br>Prochlorperazine: PO, suppository, IM<br>Thiethylperazine maleate: PO, suppository, IM | Central nervous system depression, drowsiness, dizziness, blurred vision, hypotension, photosensitivity | 1. Subcutaneous injection or intravenous administration may cause tissue irritation and necrosis.<br>2. Use with caution in children; do not administer chlorpromazine to infants less than 6 months old, prochlorperazine to children weighing less than 20 lb (9 kg) or less than 2 years old, or thiethylperazine to children less than 12 years old.<br>3. Thorazine should be used only in situations of severe nausea or vomiting. Can also be used for intractable hiccups.<br>4. Thiethylperazine: cautious use in clients with liver and kidney diseases.<br>5. Promethazine can cause fatal respiratory depression, especially in the young. Do not give promethazine to children under 2 years of age, and use it with caution in children older than 2 years. |

*Continued*

| Medications | Side Effects | Nursing Implications |
|---|---|---|
| ***Prokinetics***—stimulate motility<br>Metoclopramide: PO, IM, IV | Restlessness, drowsiness, fatigue, anxiety, headache | 1. Used to decrease problems with esophageal reflux, gastroparesis, and nausea and vomiting associated with chemotherapy.<br>2. Contraindicated in GI obstruction, perforation, or hemorrhage. |

**Antihistamines:** Depress the chemoreceptor trigger zone, block histamine receptors.

| | | |
|---|---|---|
| Hydroxyzine: PO, IM<br>Dimenhydrinate: PO, suppository, IM | Sedation; anticholinergic effects—blurred vision, dry mouth, difficulty in urination, and constipation; paradoxical excitation may occur in children | 1. Caution client regarding sedation: should avoid activities that require mental alertness.<br>2. Administer early to prevent vomiting.<br>3. Use with caution in clients with glaucoma and asthma.<br>4. Subcutaneous injection may cause tissue irritation and necrosis; use Z-track injection technique. |

**Serotonin Receptor Antagonists:** Act on specific serotonin (5-HT) receptors to decrease nausea and vomiting.

| | | |
|---|---|---|
| Ondansetron: IV, PO<br>Granisetron: IV<br>Dolasetron: PO | Headache, diarrhea, rash, bronchospasm | 1. Assess baseline vitals.<br>2. Use caution in clients with liver dysfunction.<br>3. Ondansetron prolongs the QT interval and poses a risk of torsades de pointes, a potentially life-threatening dysrhythmia.<br>4. Use cautiously in clients with electrolyte abnormalities, heart failure, or bradydysrhythmias. |

## Laxatives

### General Nursing Implications

- Laxatives should be avoided in clients who have nausea, vomiting, undiagnosed abdominal pain and cramping, and/or any indications of appendicitis or peritonitis.
- Dietary fiber should be taken for prevention of, and as first-line treatment for, constipation.
- Daily intake of fluids should be increased.
- Constipation is determined by stool firmness and frequency.
- Increasing activity will increase peristalsis and decrease constipation.
- Opioid analgesics and anticholinergics will cause constipation.
- A laxative should be used only briefly and in the smallest amount necessary.
- Use laxatives with caution during pregnancy.

| Medications | Side Effects | Nursing Implications |
|---|---|---|
| ***Bulk-forming***—stimulate peristalsis and passage of soft stool<br>Methylcellulose<br>Psyllium<br>Fibercon<br>Bran | Esophageal irritation, impaction, abdominal fullness, flatulence | 1. Not immediately effective; 12–24 hours before effects are apparent.<br>2. Use with caution in clients with difficulty swallowing.<br>3. Administer with full glass of fluid to prevent problems with irritation and impaction. |
| ***Surfactants***—decrease surface tension, allowing water to penetrate feces<br>Docusate sodium | Occasional mild abdominal cramping | 1. Do not use concurrently with mineral oil.<br>2. Not recommended for children less than 6 years old. |
| ***Stimulants***—stimulate and irritate the large intestine to promote peristalsis and defecation<br>Bisacodyl: PO, suppository,<br>Senna concentrate: PO, suppository | Diarrhea, abdominal cramping | 1. Use for short period of time.<br>2. Do not use in presence of undiagnosed abdominal pain or GI bleeding. |
| ***Osmotics***—osmotic agents that pull fluid into the bowel<br>Polyethylene glycol: PO, NG<br>Magnesium hydroxide: PO | Nausea, bloating, abdominal fullness | 1. Primary use is in preparing the bowel for examination.<br>2. Clear liquids only (no gelatin with red coloring) after administration.<br>3. Polyethylene glycol requires the client to drink a large amount of fluid (4 L); provide 8–10 oz (240–300 mL) chilled at a time to increase client consumption and enhance taste.<br>4. Best if consumed over 3–4 hours.<br>5. Hyperosmotics and saline cause frequent bowel movements; advise client to plan accordingly.<br>6. Most osmotic laxatives cause problems with loss of water, whereas sodium phosphate can lead to fluid retention. |

## Appendix 20-2 MEDICATIONS—cont'd

### Antidiarrheal Agents

| Medications | Side Effects | Nursing Implications |
|---|---|---|
| Anhydrous morphine: PO | Lightheadedness, dizziness, sedation, nausea, vomiting, paralytic ileus, abdominal cramping | 1. Opioid derivatives, suppress peristalsis.<br>2. Not recommended during pregnancy or breastfeeding.<br>3. Can produce drug dependence and mild withdrawal symptoms.<br>4. Encourage increased fluids.<br>5. Avoid activities that require mental alertness. |
| Diphenoxylate/Atropine: PO<br>Loperamide HCl: PO<br>Bismuth subsalicylate: PO | May precipitate constipation and an impaction | 1. Absorbent, has soothing effect, and absorbs toxic substances.<br>2. May interfere with absorption of oral medications.<br>3. Should not be given to clients with fever >101°F (38.3°C).<br>4. Do not give in presence of bloody diarrhea. |

### Antiulcer Agents

**Antacid:** An alkaline substance that will neutralize gastric acid secretions; nonsystemic. Some combination antacids also relieve gas, and some work as laxatives. Several antacids form a protective coating on the stomach and upper GI tract.

| | | |
|---|---|---|
| Aluminum hydroxide: PO<br>Aluminum hydroxide and magnesium salt combinations: PO | Constipation, phosphorus depletion with long-term use<br>Constipation or diarrhea, hypercalcemia, renal calculi | 1. Avoid administration within 1–2 hours of other oral medications; should be taken frequently—before and after meals and at bedtime.<br>2. Instruct clients to take medication even if they do not experience discomfort.<br>3. Clients on low-sodium diets should evaluate sodium content of various antacids.<br>4. Administer with caution to the client with cardiac disease because GI symptoms may be indicative of cardiac problems. |
| Sodium preparations<br>Sodium bicarbonate: PO | Rebound acid production, alkalosis | 1. Discourage use of sodium bicarbonate because of occurrence of metabolic alkalosis and rebound acid production. |

### Histamine H₂ Receptor Antagonists: Reduce volume and concentration of gastric acid secretion.

| | | |
|---|---|---|
| Cimetidine: PO, IV, IM | Rash, confusion, lethargy, diarrhea, dysrhythmias, gynecomastia, reduced libido and impotence (binds to androgen receptors), and pneumonia (decreased gastric pH leads to bacterial colonization of respiratory tract). | 1. Take 30 minutes before or after meals.<br>2. May be used prophylactically or for treatment of PUD.<br>3. Do not take with oral antacids. |
| Ranitidine: PO, IM, IV | Headache, GI discomfort, jaundice, hepatitis | 1. Use with caution in clients with liver and renal disorders.<br>2. Do not take with aspirin products.<br>3. Wait 1 hour after administration of antacids. |
| Nizatidine: PO<br>Famotidine: PO, IV | Anemia, dizziness<br>Headache, dizziness, constipation, diarrhea | 1. Use with caution in clients with renal or hepatic problems.<br>2. Dosing may be done without regard to food or to meal time.<br>3. Caution clients to avoid aspirin and other NSAIDs. |

*Continued*

| Appendix 20-2 | MEDICATIONS—cont'd |
| --- | --- |

| Medications | Side Effects | Nursing Implications |
| --- | --- | --- |
| **Proton Pump Inhibitors:** Inhibit the enzyme that produces gastric acid. | | |
| Omeprazole: PO<br>Lansoprazole: PO<br>Pantoprazole: PO, IV<br>Esomeprazole: PO | Headache, diarrhea, dizziness | 1. Administer before meals.<br>2. Do not crush or chew; do not open capsules.<br>3. Sprinkle granules of lansoprazole over food; do not chew granules.<br>4. The combination of omeprazole with clarithromycin effectively treats clients with *Helicobacter pylori* infection in duodenal ulcer. |
| **Cytoprotective Agents:** Bind to diseased tissue to provide a protective barrier to acid. | | |
| Sucralfate: PO | Constipation, GI discomfort | 1. Avoid antacids.<br>2. Used for prevention and treatment of stress ulcers, gastric ulceration, and PUD.<br>3. May impede the absorption of medications that require an acid medium (phenytoin, digoxin, warfarin, and fluoroquinolone antibiotics). |
| **Prostaglandin Analogs:** Suppress gastric acid secretion; increase protective mucus and mucosal blood flow. | | |
| Misoprostol | GI problems, headache | 1. Contraindicated in pregnancy.<br>2. Indicated for prevention of NSAID-induced ulcers. |
| **Intestinal Medications** | | |
| **Intestinal Antibiotics:** Decrease bacteria in the GI tract; used to sterilize bowel before surgery. | | |
| Kanamycin sulfate: PO<br>Neomycin sulfate: PO | Nephrotoxicity, neurotoxicity and ototoxicity | 1. Monitor kidney function.<br>2. If on warfarin monitor clotting times. |
| Paromomycin: PO | Vomiting and diarrhea | 1. Administer with meals.<br>2. Administer with caution in clients with ulcerative bowel disease. |
| **5 Aminosalicylates (5 ASA):** Antiinflammatory effect in small bowel and colon; used to treat ulcerative colitis and Crohn's disease. | | |
| Sulfasalazine: PO | Nausea, fever rash, arthralgia, agranulo-cytosis, and hemolytic anemia | 1. Assess client for allergy to sulfur.<br>2. Should not be used with thiazide diuretics.<br>3. Monitor CBC; maintain adequate hydration.<br>4. May continue on medication to maintain remission. |
| Mesalamine: PO, PO enteric coated tablet, suppository or enema | GI symptoms, headache | 1. Suppository or enema has minimal systemic effects.<br>2. Rectal administration is usually at night. |
| Balsalazide: PO | Abdominal pain, headache, nausea and diarrhea. | 1. Monitor for renal and hepatic function. |
| **Immunomodulators (monoclonal antibodies):** Synthesized from recombinant DNA technology, used to target specific cell receptors; mainly used in cancer treatment but now being used to treat Crohn's disease. | | |
| Infliximab: IV<br>Adalimumab: IV | Fever, chills, rash, headache, joint pain, GI symptoms, infections, infusion reactions, lymphoma | 1. Control allergic and flulike symptoms with antihistamines and acetaminophen. |

*CBC,* Complete blood count; *GI,* gastrointestinal; *IM,* intramuscular; *IV,* intravenous; *PO,* by mouth (orally); *NSAID,* nonsteroidal antiinflammatory drug; *PUD,* peptic ulcer disease.

## Parenteral Nutrition (PN)

PN is an intravenous (IV) delivery of highly concentrated nutrients and vitamins; it is used when the process of nutrition—ingestion, digestion, and absorption— is impaired. Parenteral nutrition is also referred to as total parenteral nutrition (TPN) or hyperalimentation and can be administered through either a peripheral vein or central vein. It provides complete nutritional support.

**Goal:** To provide adequate nutrition and to facilitate healing and growth of new body tissue.

**Goal:** To maintain client in positive nitrogen balance and promote healing.

### Routes of Administration

1. *Peripheral:* Peripheral total parenteral nutrition (PPN) is administered via a large peripheral vein or peripherally inserted midline catheter when nutritional support is needed for a short period (less than 14 days). Solution is less concentrated than total parenteral nutrition (TPN) and may include IV lipid emulsions.
2. *Central:* Central total parenteral nutrition (TPN) is administered via a central venous catheter (CVC) line inserted into the jugular or subclavian vein or via a peripherally inserted central catheter (PICC) placed into the basilic or cephalic vein and advanced to the distal end of the superior vena cava where nutrients are directly delivered into the client's circulation. It is used in clients who need long-term nutritional support or when a client has high protein and caloric requirements. Solutions used are hypertonic with high glucose content and require rapid dilution via a central venous line or a PICC.

### Nursing Implications

1. PN may be commercially prepared and then customized in the hospital pharmacy specifically for the client's most recent blood analysis findings; *nothing should be added to solution after it has been prepared in the pharmacy.*
2. Orders are written daily, based on the current electrolyte and protein status; always check the doctor's order for correct fluid for the day.
3. Solution may be refrigerated for up to 24 hours, but solution should be taken out of refrigeration 30 minutes before infusion. If solution has been hanging for 24 hours, it should be discarded and a new bag of solution hung. Tubing changes need to occur every time a new bag is added to the infusion and daily with each new infusion.
4. Begin PN at a slow rate (40–60 mL per hour) and then gradually increase to prescribed infusion rate. Maintain constant flow rate; if infusion of solution is behind, determine how much, divide that amount over about 24 hours, and gradually increase rate to level of previous infusion order. Do not randomly accelerate the infusion to "catch up" over an hour; *PN must be administered via an infusion pump.*
5. Monitor serum blood glucose levels on a regular basis; some institutions require glucose testing every 4 to 6 hours. May be less frequent after first week of administration.

6. Infusion is initiated and discontinued on a gradual basis to allow the pancreas to compensate for increased glucose intake. If PN is temporarily unavailable, give $D_{10}W$ or $D_{20}W$ until PN solution is available.
7. Monitor intake and output and compare daily trends. Body weight is an indication of the adequacy of hydration. Tissue healing is an indication of adequacy of protein and positive nitrogen balance.
8. Check label on bag of solution against orders; check solution for leaks, clarity, or color changes.

### Maintenance

1. A sterile occlusive dressing should be used at the catheter site; change site dressing every 48 to 72 hours or per facility protocol.
2. Change filter and IV tubing every 24 hours for PN containing lipids and every 72 hours for PN containing amino acids or dextrose or per facility protocol.
3. Do not draw blood or measure central venous pressure (CVP) from the PN line.
4. Maintain record of daily weight; desired weight gain is approximately 2 pounds (1 kg) per week.

**TEST ALERT:** Evaluate client's nutritional status: monitor client's response to PN.

### Complications

1. Hyperglycemia may be caused by too rapid infusion of solution or by solutions containing dextrose. Blood glucose is monitored every 4 to 6 hours during initial infusion or per facility protocol, and insulin replacement may be ordered.
2. Fat emulsion syndrome may occur in clients receiving IV fat (lipid) emulsion. Monitor for fever, increased triglycerides, and clotting problems.
3. Refeeding syndrome is characterized by fluid retention, electrolyte imbalances (hypophosphatemia, hypokalemia, hypomagnesemia), and hyperglycemia; occurs in clients with chronic malnutrition states that are started on aggressive nutritional support. Observe closely for cardiac dysrhythmias, respiratory arrest, and neurologic disturbances such as paresthesias.
4. Catheter-related infection: Monitor site and change dressing according to policy; clients may be immunosuppressed and signs of infection may be masked. If infection is suspected (erythema, tenderness, exudates), a culture should be done and health care provider notified immediately.

   Septicemia: Strong glucose solutions provide good media for bacteria; observe strict aseptic techniques in dressing changes. The client may exhibit signs of a systemic infection (fever, nausea, vomiting, lethargy, elevated WBC count).
5. Air embolus or risk for pneumothorax (central line): Increased tendency to occur during insertion of central catheter line and during dressing changes for central line care). If air embolism is suspected, administer oxygen, clamp tubing, and place client in left lateral Trendelenburg position.

**Appendix 20-4   NURSING PROCEDURE: NASOGASTRIC AND NASOINTESTINAL TUBES**

1. *Nasogastric (Levin) or NG tube:* Single lumen.
   A. Used for gastric decompression; may connect to intermittent suction.
   B. Administer tube feedings.
2. *Nasointestinal tubes.*
   A. Inserted the same as NG tube but reaches the small intestine.
   B. After initial insertion, if possible, have client lie on right side until proper placement is confirmed.
   C. Requires x-ray confirmation of placement before use. Leave guide wire in place until placement is confirmed.

> **⚠ NURSING PRIORITY:** Never attempt to reinsert the stylet (partially or completely) once it is removed.

   D. More comfortable for client but easier to clog with meds or kink with movement.
   E. Not attached to suction.

## ✓ KEY POINTS

- Before insertion, position the client in high-Fowler's position, if possible. (If client cannot tolerate high-Fowler's, place in left lateral position.)
- Use a water-soluble lubricant to facilitate insertion.
- Measure the tube from the tip of the client's nose to the earlobe and from the nose to the xiphoid process to determine the approximate amount of tube to insert to reach the stomach.
- Insert the tube through the nose into the nasopharyngeal area; flex the client's head slightly forward.
- Secure the tube to the nose; do not allow the tube to exert pressure on the upper inner portion of the nares.
- Validating placement of tube:
   A. Always validate correct placement upon initial insertion with a chest x-ray.

   B. After initial insertion and chest x-ray, may validate by aspiration of gastric contents. Measure pH of aspirated fluid (pH of gastric secretions is usually less than 4). Note that this method may not be accurate if the client is on medications that alter the pH of gastric secretions.
   C. It is *no longer recommended to* determine placement by injecting air and listening with a stethoscope for sound of air in the stomach.
   D. Always validate placement of an NG tube before instilling anything into tube.
- Once tube placement is validated, mark the tube to indicate where the tube exits the nose.
- Label the tube for use only for enteral feedings and/or oral medication administration.

### Clinical Tips for Problem Solving

- *Abdominal distention:* Check for patency and adequacy of drainage, determine position of tube, assess presence of bowel sounds, and assess for respiratory compromise from distention.
- *Nausea and vomiting around tube:* Place client in semi-Fowler's position or turn to side to prevent aspiration; suction oral pharyngeal area. Attempt to aspirate gastric contents and validate placement of tube. Tube may not be far enough into stomach for adequate decompression and suction; try repositioning. If tube patency cannot be established, tube may need to be replaced.
- *Inadequate or minimal drainage:* Validate placement and patency; tube may be in too far and be past pyloric valve or not in far enough and in the upper portion of the stomach. Reassess length of tube insertion and characteristics of drainage; request x-ray for validation.

> **TEST ALERT:** ALWAYS check the placement of an NG tube before injecting or irrigating it; placement should be checked each shift; do not adjust or irrigate the NG tube on a client after a gastric resection because of the risk of disruption of the anastomosis or staple line.

**Appendix 20-5 NURSING PROCEDURE: ENTERAL FEEDING**

### Short-Term

1. *Nasogastric:* Provides alternative means of ingesting nutrients for clients.
2. *Nasointestinal:* A weighted tube of soft material is placed in the small intestine to decrease chance of regurgitation. A stylet or guide wire is used to progress the tube into the intestine. Do not remove stylet until tube placement has been verified via x-ray. Do not attempt to reinsert stylet while tube is in place; this could result in perforation of the tube.

### Long-Term

1. *Percutaneous endoscopic gastrostomy (PEG):* A tube is inserted percutaneously into the stomach; local anesthesia and sedation are used for tube placement.

2. *Percutaneous endoscopic jejunostomy (PEJ):* A tube is inserted percutaneously into the jejunum.
3. *Gastrostomy:* A surgical opening is made into the stomach, and a gastrostomy tube is positioned with sutures.

### Methods of Administering Enteral Feedings

- Continuous: controlled with a feeding pump. Decreases nausea and diarrhea and deceases the risk of aspiration.
- Intermittent/bolus: prescribed amount of fluid infuses via a gravity drip or feeding pump over specific time. For example, 350 mL is given over 30 minutes.
- Cyclic: involves feeding solution infused via a pump for a part of a day, usually 12 to 16 hours. This method may be used for weaning from feedings.

## Appendix 20-5 NURSING PROCEDURE: ENTERAL FEEDING—cont'd

### *Nursing Implications*

- The client should be sitting or lying with the head elevated 30 to 45 degrees. Head of bed should remain elevated for 30 to 60 minutes after feeding if intermittent or cyclic feeding is used; for continuous feeding maintain semi-Fowler's position at all times.
- If feedings are intermittent, tube should be irrigated with water before and after feedings.
- Aspirate gastric contents to determine residual. If residual is more than 200 mL and there are signs of intolerance (nausea, vomiting, distention), hold next feeding for 1 hour and recheck residual; or if residual is greater than half of last feeding, delay next feeding for 1 to 2 hours and recheck the residual volume. If gastric residual volume remains high after the second residual check, consider a promotility agent.
- Return aspirated contents to stomach to prevent electrolyte imbalance.
- Flush the tube with 30 to 50 mL of water:
  A. After each intermittent feeding.
  B. Every 4 to 6 hours for continuous feeding.
  C. Before and after each medication administration.
- When a PEG or PEJ tube is placed, immediately after insertion, measure the length of the tube from the insertion site to the distal end and mark the tube at the skin insertion site. This tube should be routinely checked to determine whether the tube is migrating from the original insertion point.
- For continuous or cyclic feeding, add only 4 hours of product to the bag at a time to prevent bacterial growth. A closed system is preferred, with each set being used no longer than 24 hours.
- Prevent diarrhea:
  A. Slow, constant rate of infusion.
  B. Keep equipment clean to prevent bacterial contamination.
  C. Check for fecal impaction; diarrhea may be flowing around impaction.
  D. Identify medical conditions that would precipitate diarrhea.
- For continuous feeding, change feeding reservoir every 24 hours.

> **⚠ NURSING PRIORITY:** If in doubt of a tube's placement or position, stop or hold the feeding and obtain x-ray confirmation of location.

> **TEST ALERT:** Change rate and amount of tube feeding based on client's response.

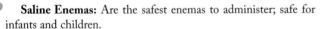

## Appendix 20-6 NURSING PROCEDURE: ENEMAS

### Types of Enemas

**Soap Suds Enema:** Castile soap is added to tap water or normal saline. Dilute 5 mL of Castile soap in 1 L of water.

**Tap Water Enema:** Request order for specific quantity when administered to infants or children; should not be repeated because of risk for water toxicity. Use caution when administering to adults with altered cardiac and renal reserve.

**Saline Enemas:** Are the safest enemas to administer; safe for infants and children.

**Retention Enema:** An oil-based solution that will soften the stool. Should be retained by client for 30 to 60 minutes. Typically 150 to 200 mL. May be mineral oil or similar oil or may include antibiotics or nutritive solution.

**Hypertonic Enema:** Used when only a small amount of fluid is tolerated (120–180 mL). Commercially prepared Fleet enema.

**Carminative Enema:** An agent used to expel gas from the GI tract. Example is magnesium sulfate/glycerin/water (MGW).

### ✓ KEY POINTS: Administering an Enema

- Fill enema container with warmed solution.
- Allow solution to run through the tubing before inserting into rectum so that air is removed.
- Place client in the left lateral Sims' position.
- Generously lubricate the tip of the tubing with water-soluble lubricant.
- Gently insert tubing into client's rectum (3–4 inches (8–10 cm) for adults, 1 inch (2.5 cm) for infants, 2 to 3 inches (5–8 cm) for children), past the external and internal sphincters.
- Raise the solution container no more than 12 to 18 inches (30–46 cm) above the client.
- Allow solution to flow slowly. If the flow is slow, the client will experience fewer cramps. The client will also be able to tolerate and retain a greater volume of solution.

### Clinical Tips for Problem Solving

If client expels solution prematurely:

- Place client in supine position with knees flexed.
- Slow the water flow and continue with the enema.
- If the enema returns contain fecal material before surgery or diagnostic testing, repeat enema. If, after three enemas, returns still contain fecal material, notify physician.
- If client complains of abdominal cramping during instillation of fluid, slow the infusion rate by lowering the fluid bag.

> **TEST ALERT:** Assist and intervene with client who has an alteration in elimination.

**Appendix 20-7 NURSING PROCEDURE: STOOL SPECIMEN**

## Types of Stool

- Normal: semisoft to semisolid, brown color
- Narrow, ribbon-like stool: spastic or irritable bowel, or obstruction
- Diarrhea: spastic bowel, viral infection
- Blood and mucus, soft stool: bacterial infection
- Mixed blood or pus: colitis
- Yellow or green stool: severe, prolonged diarrhea; rapid transit through bowel
- Black stool: gastrointestinal bleeding or intake of iron supplements
- Tan, clay-colored, or white stool: liver or gallbladder problems
- Red stool: colon or rectal bleeding; some medications and foods may also cause a red coloration
- Fatty stool, pasty or greasy: intestinal malabsorption, pancreatic disease

## ✓ KEY POINTS: Collecting the Specimen

- Always wear gloves during procedure.
- Use clean bedpan or bedside commode to collect stool; do not use stool that has been in contact with toilet bowl water or urine.
- Collect stool specimen in a clean, dry container. If stool is to be evaluated for organisms, use a sterile container. Use a tongue blade to obtain specimens from several areas of the stool and place in the stool collection container.
- The client collecting a stool specimen for an occult blood test needs to follow directions regarding diet restrictions (no red meat, beets, or foods that may cause the stool to turn red or lead to a false-positive result).
- Stool specimen should be approximately size of a walnut. If stool is liquid, approximately 30 mL is needed.
- Take the specimen immediately to the laboratory. Do not allow it to remain on the unit.

**TEST ALERT:** Obtain specimens for laboratory tests.

---

**Appendix 20-8 NURSING PROCEDURE: CARE OF THE CLIENT WITH AN OSTOMY**

## Types of Ostomies (Figure 20-10)

**Colostomy:** Opening of the colon through the abdominal wall; stool is generally semisoft, and bowel control may be achieved.
**Ileostomy:** Opening of the ileum through the abdominal wall; stool drainage is liquid and excoriating; drainage is frequently continuous; it is therefore difficult to establish bowel control. Fluid and electrolyte imbalances are common complications.
**Kock's Ileostomy:** May be referred to as a "continent" ileostomy; an internal reservoir for stool is surgically formed. Decreases problem of skin care caused by frequent irritation of stoma by drainage. Primary complications are leakage at the stoma site and peritonitis; rarely used today.

**Goals:**
1. Maintain physiologic and psychological equilibrium.
2. Assist client to maintain total care of colostomy or ileostomy before discharge.

### Preoperative Care

1. Preoperative education: Actively involve family and client; encourage questions concerning the procedure.
2. Placement of stoma is evaluated, and site is selected with client standing. Select a site that is easily seen and accessible to client; select a flat area of the abdomen, avoiding skin creases and folds; select site that does not interfere with clothing, such as the waist area.

## ✓ KEY POINTS: Postoperative Nursing Implications—Initial Care

- Evaluate stoma every 8 hours after surgery. It should remain pink and moist; dark blue stoma indicates ischemia.
- Measure the stoma and select an appropriately sized appliance. Mild to moderate swelling is common for the first 2 to 3 weeks after surgery, which necessitates changes in size of the appliance.
- Appliance should fit easily around the stoma and cover all healthy, abdominal skin.

- Keep the skin around the stoma clean, dry, and free of stool and intestinal secretions. Prevent contamination of the abdominal incision.
- Ostomy bags should be changed when about one-third full to avoid weight of bag dislodging skin barrier.

## ✓ KEY POINTS: Pouching an Ostomy

- A pouching system consists of a pouch and skin barrier.
  - Pouches come in one- and two-piece systems and are flat or convex.
  - Pouches may have the opening precut by the manufacturer; others require the stoma opening to be cut by the nurse or client to fit stoma.
  - Pouch may have an integrated closure or may need a clip (older types).
- Change the pouching system approximately every 3 to 7 days.
- Carefully remove used pouch and skin barrier gently by pushing skin away from barrier; may need to use an adhesive remover to facilitate removal of skin barrier.
- Measure stoma by using measurement tool provided with pouch.

**⚠ Nursing Priority:** Stoma measurement may change, especially 2 to 4 weeks after surgery, so remeasurement will be required.

- Trace measured stoma pattern from tool onto pouch/skin barrier and cut the opening.
- Remove protective backing and apply pouch over stoma.

## ✓ KEY POINTS: Irrigation

- Do not irrigate an ileostomy or maintain regular irrigations in child with colostomy.
- Irrigate colostomy at same time each day to assist in establishing a normal pattern of elimination.
- Involve client in care as early as possible.
- In adults, irrigate with 500 to 1000 mL of warm tap water.

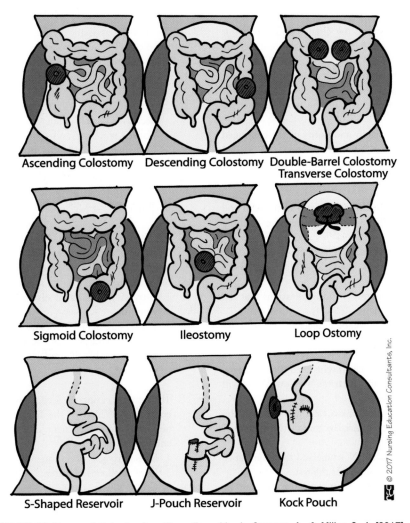

**FIGURE 20-10  Types of Colostomies.** (From Zerwekh, J., Garneau, A., & Miller, C. J. [2017]. *Digital collection of the memory notebooks of nursing* [4th ed.]. Chandler, AZ: Nursing Education Consultants, Inc.)

**! NURSING PRIORITY:** Use a cone-tipped ostomy irrigator; do not use an enema tube/catheter.

- Do not irrigate more than once a day.
- Do not irrigate in the presence of diarrhea or severe abdominal pain.
- Place the client in a sitting position for irrigation, preferably in the bathroom with the irrigation sleeve in the toilet.
- Elevate the solution container approximately 12 to 20 inches (30–51 cm) and allow solution to flow in gently. If cramping occurs, lower fluid or clamp the tubing.
- Allow 25 to 45 minutes for return flow. Client may want to walk around before the return starts.
- Encourage client to participate in care of his or her own colostomy. Have client perform return demonstration of colostomy irrigation before leaving the hospital.
- Assist the client to control odors: diet and odor control tablets.
- Kock's ileostomy is drained when client experiences fullness. A nipple valve is created in surgery and drained by insertion of a catheter.

**Clinical Tips for Problem Solving**

If water does not flow easily into colostomy stoma:
- Check for kinks in tubing from container.
- Check height of irrigating container.
- Encourage client to change positions, relax, and take a few deep breaths.

If client experiences cramping, nausea, or dizziness during irrigation:
- Stop flow of water, leaving irrigation cone in place.
- Do not resume until cramping has passed.
- Check water temperature and height of water bag; if water is too hot or flows too rapidly, it can cause dizziness.

If client has no return of stool or water from irrigation:
- Be sure to apply drainable pouch; solution may drain as client moves around.
- Have client increase fluid intake; he or she may be dehydrated.
- Repeat irrigation next day.

If diarrhea occurs:
- Do not irrigate colostomy.
- Check client's medications; sometimes they may cause diarrhea.
- If diarrhea is excessive and/or prolonged, notify physician.

**TEST ALERT:** Provide ostomy care.

## Study Questions
## Gastrointestinal: Care of Adult and Pediatric Clients

More questions on
evolve

1. Six hours after gastric resection, the client's NG aspirate is continuing to drain bright red fluid. What is the best nursing action?
   1. Continue to monitor the amount of drainage and correlate it with any change in vital signs.
   2. Reposition the NG tube and irrigate the tube with normal saline solution.
   3. Call the physician immediately and notify of the continued bright red aspirate.
   4. Irrigate the NG tube with iced saline solution and attach the tube to gravity drainage.

2. The nurse is providing preoperative care for a client who will have a gastric resection. What will the preoperative teaching include?
   1. An NG tube will be in place several days after surgery.
   2. The client will be started on a low-residue, bland diet about 2 days after the surgery.
   3. Explain the anticipated prognosis and implications that the client may have a malignancy.
   4. A urinary retention catheter will be in place for 1 week after surgery.

3. The nurse is planning care for a client scheduled for esophago-gastroduodenoscopy (EGD) and a barium swallow. What will the nursing care plan include?
   1. Anticipating the client will receive a clear liquid diet in the evening and then receive nothing by mouth (NPO status) 8 hours before the test.
   2. Discussing with the client the NG tube and the importance of gastric drainage for 24 hours after the test.
   3. Explaining to the client that he will receive nothing by mouth (NPO status) for 24 hours after the test to make sure his stomach can tolerate food.
   4. Discussing the general anesthesia and explaining to the client that he will wake up in the recovery room.

4. In preparing a pediatric client for an appendectomy, the nurse would question which doctor's orders?
   1. Penicillin 600,000 units IV piggyback, now.
   2. Obtain signed consent form from parents.
   3. Administer enemas until clear.
   4. 500 mL Ringer's lactate solution at 50 mL/hr.

5. In planning discharge teaching for the client who has undergone a gastrectomy, the nurse includes what information regarding dumping syndrome? Select all that apply.
   1. Symptoms may include nausea, vomiting, weakness, and abdominal cramping.
   2. The client should eat three to four small meals per day.
   3. Consumption of fluids should be very limited with the meal.
   4. The client should increase the amount of complex carbohydrates and fiber in the diet.
   5. Activity will decrease the problem; it should be scheduled about 1 hour after meals.
   6. You may need to take a multivitamin with calcium and iron supplements.

6. The nurse is assessing a child with a tentative diagnosis of appendicitis. The nursing assessment is most likely to reveal what characteristics concerning the pain? Select all that apply.
   1. Colicky, cramping abdominal pain located around the umbilicus
   2. Tenderness in the left lower quadrant, associated with decreased bowel sounds
   3. Nausea, vomiting, and anorexia after onset of pain
   4. Gnawing pain radiating through to the lower back, with severe abdominal distention
   5. Sharp pain with severe gastric distention, frequently associated with hemoptysis
   6. Tenderness at McBurney's point

7. The nurse is caring for a client who has been diagnosed with a bleeding duodenal ulcer. Which data identified on a nursing assessment would indicate a possible intestinal perforation and require immediate nursing action?
   1. Increasing abdominal distention, with increased pain and vomiting
   2. Decreasing hemoglobin and hematocrit with bloody stools
   3. Diarrhea with increased bowel sounds and hypovolemia
   4. Decreasing blood pressure with tachycardia and disorientation

8. The nurse is caring for a client who is scheduled for a gastric endoscopy. Which of the following actions must the nurse perform before the client is able to eat or drink after the endoscopy?
   1. Check oxygen saturation.
   2. Give small sips of water.
   3. Check all vital signs.
   4. Assess the client's gag reflex.

9. A client is admitted with duodenal ulcers. What will the nurse anticipate the client's history to include?
   1. Recent weight loss
   2. Frequent acetaminophen use
   3. Burning pain 2 to 5 hours after a meal
   4. Episodes of vomiting

10. The nurse is preparing discharge teaching for a client with a diagnosis of gastroesophageal reflux disease (GERD). What would be important for the nurse to include in this teaching plan? Select all that apply.
    1. Elevate the head of the bed.
    2. Decrease intake of caffeine products.
    3. Discuss strategies for weight loss if overweight.
    4. Increase fluid intake with meals.
    5. Take omeprazole at bedtime.
    6. Eat a bedtime snack of milk and protein.

11. The nurse is conducting discharge dietary teaching for a client with diverticulosis who is recovering from an acute episode of diverticulitis. Which statement by the client would indicate to the nurse that the client understood his dietary teaching?
    1. "I will need to increase my intake of protein and complex carbohydrates to increase healing."
    2. "I need to progress my diet from liquids to soft, low-fiber foods until the diverticulitis is completely resolved."
    3. "I will not put any added salt on my food, and I will decrease intake of foods that are high in saturated fat."
    4. "Milk and milk products can cause a lactose intolerance. If this occurs, I need to decrease my intake of these products."

12. What is the priority nursing action for the client who is complaining of nausea in the recovery room after gastric resection?
    1. Evaluate the NG tube for patency.
    2. Call the physician for an antiemetic order.
    3. Place client in semi-Fowler's position so that he will not aspirate.
    4. Medicate the client with a narcotic analgesic.

13. The nurse is assisting a client immediately before a colonoscopy. The nurse will direct the client and help him move into what position?
    1. Prone
    2. Sims' lateral
    3. Slight Trendelenburg
    4. Flat with lithotomy stirrups

14. What will be important for the nurse to do when collecting a stool specimen for an occult blood (Hemoccult) test?
    1. Samples should be taken from two areas of the stool.
    2. Three separate stool samples will be required for accuracy of test.
    3. The nurse should collect about 20 mL of stool sample.
    4. Any red color on or near the specimen is considered positive.

15. A school-age child with a diagnosis of celiac disease asks the nurse, "Which foods will make me sick?" Which food items would the nurse teach the child to avoid?
    1. Rice cereals, milk, and tapioca
    2. Corn cereals, milk, and fruit
    3. Corn or potato bread and peanut butter
    4. Malted milk, white bread, and spaghetti

16. The nurse practitioner orders an enteral formula at a rate of 50 mL/hr. A can holds 250 mL. How many cans would the nurse need for the next 24 hours?
    Answer: _____ cans

17. What are the best nursing actions in caring for a young client with appendicitis before surgery? Select all that apply:
    1. Maintain bed rest.
    2. Offer full liquids to maintain hydration.
    3. Keep patient still and position with right leg flexed
    4. Position on left side, apply a warm K-Pad to the abdomen.
    5. Administer morphine intravenously to relieve pain.
    6. Keep the client NPO and maintain a peripheral IV for fluid replacement.

18. The nurse would identify which of the following clients to be at an increased risk for the development of a fecal impaction? Select all that apply:
    1. Post barium enema
    2. Obese client in traction
    3. Poorly hydrated older adult
    4. Client receiving opioid medications
    5. Three days after colostomy
    6. Acute appendicitis

## Answers to Study Questions

**1.** *1*
After gastric surgery, the aspirate is usually bright red at first, gradually darkening within the first 24 hours after surgery. Normally the color changes to yellow-green within 36 to 48 hours. This is a normal occurrence on the first postoperative day and should be correlated with the vital signs. The tube is in the correct position because it is draining gastric secretions. There is no indication to notify anyone or to irrigate the NG tube. (Lewis et al., 10 ed., p. 918)

**2.** *1*
NG tubes are left in place for several days after gastric resection. It is important to prevent the stomach from becoming distended and putting pressure on the suture line. A diet will be started after there is evidence of good bowel function. Diet will be clear liquids until client tolerance is determined. It is not a nursing responsibility to advise the client regarding prognosis and status of malignancy. A urinary retention catheter may or may not be in place; preferably, the client will be voiding. (Lewis et al., 10 ed., p. 918)

**3.** *1*
NPO status before a barium swallow and an esophagogastroduodenoscopy (EGD) and a clear liquid diet the evening before the procedures are routine orders for these tests. There is no general anesthesia. The client can eat or drink as tolerated after procedure once the gag reflex returns, and there is no routine placement of NG tubes. (Lewis et al., 10 ed., p. 845)

**4.** *3*
Enemas or laxatives are not administered before surgery in clients with an acute abdomen. If gastric motility is stimulated, there is an increased danger of appendiceal rupture. All other orders are appropriate before an appendectomy. (Lewis et al., 10 ed., pp. 942–943)

**5.** *1, 3, 6*
Dumping syndrome is not uncommon after a combination bariatric surgery. Common symptoms include nausea, vomiting, abdominal cramping, weakness, palpitations, diaphoresis, and dizziness. Precautions such as limiting the amount of fluids taken with a meal should be implemented. The intake of foods high in iron,

calcium, and $B_{12}$ may not prevent the vitamin or mineral deficiencies, because the problem is with the absorption of these elements; supplements may be necessary. The client should plan to eat six small meals a day to decrease distention of the remaining stomach and limit the ingestion of carbohydrates, which may cause hyperglycemia. Rest after a meal, rather than activity, is helpful because it may prevent gastric contents from emptying too rapidly into the small intestine, thus generating the symptoms. (Lewis et al., 10 ed., pp. 917–918)

6. *1, 3, 6*
Colicky, cramping abdominal pain located around the umbilicus often noted as "referred pain" for its vague periumbilical localization is characteristic of appendicitis. The most common point of tenderness is over the area known as McBurney's point. Typically, nausea, vomiting, and anorexia follow onset of pain. Diarrhea, poor feeding, lethargy, and irritability may accompany peritonitis. Tenderness in the right lower quadrant (not the left) that occurs during palpation or percussion is called Rovsing's sign. Gastric distention and gnawing radiating pain are not common signs of appendicitis; gnawing pain is more characteristic of ulcers. Hemoptysis is not seen in appendicitis but in pulmonary edema. Remember, all the items in an option have to be correct if it is the correct answer. (Hockenberry & Wilson, 10 ed., p. 1079)

7. *1*
Perforation is characterized by increasing distention and board-like abdomen. There is frequently increasing pain with fever and guarding of the abdomen. Peritonitis occurs rapidly. The nurse should maintain the client NPO, keep the client on bed rest, and immediately notify the physician. Decreasing hemoglobin and hematocrit and decreasing blood pressure are associated with hemorrhage rather than perforation. Remember to select an answer that reflects what the question is specifically asking. (Lewis et al., 10 ed., p. 912)

8. *4*
Topical sedation during endoscopy helps block the gag reflex and numbs the esophagus, eliminating the discomfort of the tube. The nurse would know the dangers of allowing the client to eat or drink before the sedation has lost its effect. The nurse will test for the return of the client's gag reflex before allowing sips of water to be taken, to avoid aspiration. (Lewis et al., 10 ed., p. 849)

9. *3*
Duodenal ulcers are characterized by high gastric acid secretion and rapid gastric emptying. Food buffers the effect of the acid; consequently, pain increases when the stomach is empty. Pain does not characteristically occur immediately after eating but 2 to 5 hours after a meal because the presence of food helps buffer the acid. The client does not usually have bouts of nausea unless bleeding or obstruction is a problem. Duodenal ulcers are associated with aspirin and NSAID use but not acetaminophen. (Lewis et al., 10 ed., p. 911)

10. *1, 2, 3, 5*
Each of these actions will help either neutralize the acid in the stomach or decrease the physiologic reflux. Proton pump inhibitors will decrease the amount of acid produced in the stomach. Increased fluids with meals will exacerbate the problem, as will eating before going to bed. (Lewis et al., 10 ed., pp. 901–902)

11. *2*
Constipation increases problems with diverticula. Upon discharge, the client should continue fluids, progressing to soft foods that are low in fiber. A diet high in fiber is recommended once the acute diverticulitis is resolved completely. The other options do not have any specific relevance to diverticula disease. (Lewis et al., 10 ed., p. 964)

12. *1*
Evaluate the NG tube patency; it is important to prevent the nausea and vomiting. The next action would be to put the client in semi-Fowler's position. It is important to assess the client and take nursing measures to determine the source of the nausea and to decrease the nausea before calling the doctor. (Lewis et al., 10 ed., p. 918)

13. *2*
Sims' lateral position is most commonly used for best access and visualization during the procedure and for the client's comfort. Lithotomy position with stirrups is used for gynecologic examinations and prostate surgery. (Ignatavicius & Workman, 8 ed., p. 1095)

14. *1*
Stool samples should be taken from different areas of the stool to more accurately reflect the presence of occult blood. The nurse only needs to collect a small sample of stool for the test. The test is done on the nursing unit and is not sent to the laboratory for further evaluation. Three separate samples will more accurately validate the presence of blood, but it is not required. Diets rich in red meat may cause a false-positive result. (Potter & Perry, 9 ed., p. 1156)

15. *4*
The child with celiac disease will need a gluten-free diet, eliminating foods such as pastas and breads that are made from wheat or dessert foods made from malt whey. Remember BROW—barley, rye, oats, and wheat. Foods that would be appropriate include rice and corn cereals, milk, corn and potato breads, tapioca, peanut butter, and honey. (Lewis et al., 10 ed., p. 967)

16. *5 cans*
50 × mL/hr × 24 hours/day = 1200 total mL for 24 hours
1200 mL/24 hr ÷ 250 mL/can = 4.8 cans or 5 cans. (Potter & Perry, 9 ed., p. 617)

17. *1, 3, 6*
Before surgery, keep the patient still, minimize movement, and offer to flex the right leg, which may increase comfort. Keep the client NPO because of the impending surgery; initiate IV fluid replacement. Maintain the client on bed rest; do not apply any type of heat to the abdomen. Narcotics are given cautiously if at all because the analgesic may mask the symptoms of rupture. (Lewis et al., 10 ed., p. 942)

18. *1, 2, 3, 4*
A barium enema procedure can lead to fecal impaction caused by barium left in the colon. An obese client in traction who is immobile and a poorly hydrated older adult (decreased motility and fluid intake) may also experience fecal impaction. These three conditions can contribute to the development of an impaction that may require manual removal. Opioid medications are central nervous system depressants, thus slowing peristalsis and contributing to constipation and fecal impaction. Acute appendicitis would be a condition in which no rectal enemas or manipulation would be indicated. (Lewis et al., 10 ed., pp. 934–935)

# CHAPTER TWENTY-ONE

# Hepatic and Biliary: Care of Adult and Pediatric Clients

## 21

Infection, Inflammation, Pain

## PHYSIOLOGY OF THE HEPATIC AND BILIARY SYSTEM

### Organs of the Hepatic and Biliary System

A. Liver.
  1. The liver produces approximately 600 to 1200 mL of bile daily.
    a. Bile drains from the liver via the common bile duct.
    b. The common bile duct enters the duodenum, either close to or in conjunction with the pancreatic duct.
  2. It can sustain 90% damage with loss of tissue and still remain functional.
B. Gallbladder.
  1. The gallbladder is capable of storing 20 to 50 mL of bile. When food enters the duodenum, the gallbladder contracts; the sphincter of Oddi, which controls the release of bile, relaxes, and bile enters the intestine via the common duct.
  2. When the sphincter of Oddi closes, bile flows back into the gallbladder for storage.
  3. The primary function of the gallbladder is concentration and storage of bile.

### Functions of the Liver

A. Synthesis of absorbed nutrients.
  1. Serum glucose regulation.
  2. Lipid (fat) metabolism.
  3. Protein metabolism.
B. Synthesis of prothrombin for normal clotting mechanisms. Vitamin K is necessary for adequate prothrombin production.
C. Vitamin and mineral storage.
  1. Produces and stores vitamins A and D.
  2. Vitamin $B_{12}$ and iron are stored in the liver.
D. Drug metabolism: barbiturates, amphetamines, and alcohol are metabolized by the liver.
E. Production of bile and bile salts.
  1. Bile is continuously formed in the liver.
  2. Bilirubin, a bile pigment, is excreted by the liver.
    a. The spleen removes and breaks down the hemoglobin in worn-out red blood cells. This results in the production of bilirubin.
    b. Bilirubin is carried from the spleen to the liver for excretion.
    c. Bilirubin is conjugated in the liver (made water soluble) and secreted into the bile.

### System Assessment (Box 21-1)

A. History.
  1. History of liver, gallbladder, or jaundice problems.
  2. History of bleeding problems.
  3. History of reproductive problems.
  4. Medication intake, alcohol consumption.
  5. Recent association with anyone with jaundice.
B. Physical assessment.
  1. Inspection.
    a. Skin.
      (1) Presence of vascular angiomas, skin lesions, or petechiae.
      (2) Hydration status.
      (3) Color of the skin (jaundiced).
      (4) Presence of peripheral edema.
    b. Abdomen.
      (1) Evidence of jaundice.
      (2) Contour of the abdomen.
      (3) Presence of visible abdominal wall veins.
  2. Palpation of the abdomen.
    a. Pain, tenderness, presence of distention.
    b. Hepatomegaly, splenomegaly.
C. Nutritional assessment.
  1. Weight gain or loss; dietary intake.
  2. Problems of anorexia, nausea, and vomiting.

### Pathophysiology of Jaundice

A. Jaundice may begin so gradually that it is not noticed immediately.
B. Increased levels of bilirubin cause a yellowish discoloration of the skin. It may be first observed as a yellow color in the sclera of the eyes. Serum bilirubin levels must be three times normal level (2–3 mg/dL [34-51 mmol/L]) for jaundice to occur. The yellow discoloration is due to deposits of bilirubin in the skin and body tissue.
C. Types of jaundice.
  1. Hemolytic jaundice.
    a. Occurs with an increase in the breakdown of red blood cells, which causes an increase in the amount of unconjugated bilirubin in the blood.
    b. Causes of hemolytic jaundice.
      (1) Blood transfusion reactions.

**Box 21-1 FOCUSED ASSESSMENT: LIVER AND BILIARY**

- Skin color: jaundice
- Changes in abdominal girth
- Changes in stool: pale, frothy, fatty
- History of contact with infectious individuals
- Issues with indigestion and food intolerance
- Type of pain
- Psychosocial problems associated with alcohol use

(2) Sickle cell crisis, hemolytic anemias.
(3) Hemolytic disease of the newborn.
2. Hepatocellular jaundice.
   a. Results from the inability of the liver to clear normal amounts of bilirubin from the blood.
   b. Causes of hepatocellular jaundice.
      (1) Hepatitis, cirrhosis.
      (2) Hepatocellular cancer.
3. Obstructive jaundice.
   a. Results from an impediment to bile flow through the liver and the biliary system.
   b. Obstruction may be within the liver or it may be outside the liver.
   c. Causes of obstructive jaundice.
      (1) Hepatitis, cirrhosis.
      (2) Liver or pancreatic cancer.
      (3) Obstruction of the common bile duct by a stone.

## DISORDERS OF THE HEPATIC SYSTEM

 **Hepatitis**

**Widespread inflammation of the liver tissue is called hepatitis.**

A. Types of hepatitis. (Table 21-1; Figure 21-1)
   1. Toxic and drug-induced hepatitis.
      a. Toxic: systemic poisons: carbon tetrachloride, gold compounds.
      b. Drug-induced: isoniazid (INH), chlorothiazide, methotrexate, methyldopa, acetaminophen.
   2. Autoimmune hepatitis.
      a. Cause is unknown; associated with other autoimmune diseases.
      b. Requires different treatment from viral hepatitis; treated with corticosteroids and immunosuppressants.
B. The inflammatory process causes hepatic cell degeneration and necrosis.

**TEST ALERT:** Teach health promotion information; follow infection control guidelines/protocols. Prevent transmission in the hospital in addition to teaching the importance of personal hygiene.

**Assessment**

Regardless of the type of hepatitis, the clinical picture is similar.

A. Risk factors/etiology and sources/spread of disease (see Table 21-1).
B. Clinical manifestations: all clients experience inflammation of the liver tissue and exhibit similar symptoms.
   1. Anicteric phase.
      a. Anorexia, nausea, malaise, headache.
      b. Upper right quadrant discomfort.
      c. Low-grade fever, hepatomegaly.
   2. Icteric phase (jaundiced).
      a. Dark urine caused by increased excretion of bilirubin.
      b. Pruritus due to accumulation of bile salts beneath the skin.
      c. Stools light and clay colored.
      d. Liver remains enlarged and tender.
   3. Posticteric phase (after jaundice).
      a. Malaise, easily fatigued.
      b. Hepatomegaly remains for several weeks.
   4. Anicteric hepatitis (absence of jaundice).
      a. Frequently occurs in children.
      b. Many clients with hepatitis A and hepatitis C (non-A, non-B) may not show clinical jaundice.
      c. Unexplained fever, general GI disturbances.
      d. Anorexia and malaise.

 **PEDIATRIC PRIORITY:** Typical symptoms noted along with arthralgia and skin rashes with hepatitis B rather than hepatitis A. Jaundice is seldom noted.

   5. Onset of hepatitis A (HAV) is more acute; symptoms are generally less severe.
   6. Onset of hepatitis B (HBV) is more insidious; symptoms are more severe.
   7. Most cases of hepatitis C are asymptomatic or mild, but they tend to be persistent and lead to chronic liver disease.
C. Diagnostics (see Appendix 21-1).
   1. Antigen and antibody markers (see Table 21-1).
   2. Increased alanine aminotransferase (ALT), aspartate aminotransferase (AST), and serum bilirubin levels.

**Treatment**

 A. Prevention—routine immunizations for HAV and HBV for children.
B. Medications (see Table 21-1; Appendix 21-2).
C. HBV prevention—administer hepatitis B immune globulin (HBIG) for one-time or acute exposure.
D. Encourage good nutrition; no specific dietary modifications; clients will probably not tolerate a high-fat diet.
E. Decreased activity; promote rest.

**Complications**

A. Chronic, active hepatitis.
B. Fulminant hepatitis: severe, acute case of hepatitis.

**Table 21-1  TYPES OF HEPATITIS**

| Characteristics | Sources of Infection | Spread of Infection | Diagnostic Tests and Drug Therapy |
|---|---|---|---|
| **Hepatitis A Virus (HAV)**<br>*Incubation:* 15–50 days (peak incidence 25–30)<br>• Fecal–oral (primarily fecal contamination and oral ingestion) | • Crowded conditions (e.g., daycare, nursing home)<br>• Poor personal hygiene<br>• Poor sanitation<br>• Contaminated food, milk, water, shellfish<br>• Clients with subclinical infections, infected food handlers, sexual contact, IV drug users | • Most infectious during 2 wk before onset of symptoms<br>• Infectious until 1–2 wk after the start of symptoms<br>• Disease and recovery uneventful<br>• Vaccination available | • Anti-HAV immunoglobulin M (IgM)—indicates acute infection<br>• Anti-HAV immunoglobulin G (IgG)—not routinely done<br>• No drug therapy available |
| **Hepatitis B Virus (HBV)**<br>*Incubation:* 60–150 days (average 90 days)<br>• Percutaneous (parenteral) or permucosal exposure to blood or blood products<br>• Sexual contact<br>• Perinatal transmission | • Unprotected sexual intercourse with an infected partner<br>• Contaminated needles, syringes, and blood products<br>• Asymptomatic carriers<br>• Tattoos or body piercing with contaminated needles<br>• HBV-infected mother (perinatal transmission)<br>• Contact with blood or open sores of an infected person | • Before and after symptoms appear<br>• Infectious for 4–6 mo<br>• Carriers continue to be infectious for life<br>• Vaccination available | • HBsAg (hepatitis B surface antigen)—marker of infectivity; positive in chronic carriers<br>• Anti-HBs (hepatitis B surface antibody)—previous infection or immunization<br>• HBeAg (hepatitis B e antigen)—marker of high infectivity<br>• Anti-HBe (hepatitis B e antibody)—indicates previous infection<br>• Drug therapy—nucleoside and nucleotide analogs; interferon. |
| **Hepatitis C Virus (HCV)**<br>*Incubation:* 14–180 days (average 56)<br>• Percutaneous (parenteral) or mucosal exposure to blood or blood products<br>• High-risk sexual contact<br>• Perinatal contact | • Needles and syringes<br>• Blood and blood products<br>• Sexual activity with infected partners<br>• Birth to an HCV-infected mother | • Begins 1–2 wk before symptoms appear<br>• Continues during clinical course and throughout life for chronic carriers<br>• Majority go on to develop chronic hepatitis C and remain infectious<br>• No vaccination available | • Anti-HCV (antibody to HCV)—acute or chronic infection marker<br>• Drug therapy—direct-acting antivirals (DAAs) |
| **Hepatitis D Virus (HDV)**<br>*Incubation:* same as HBV<br>• HBV must precede HDV<br>• Chronic carriers of HBV always at risk<br>• Uncommon in the US | • Same as HBV<br>• Coinfection only with HBV<br>• Routes of transmission same as for HBV | • Blood infectious at all stages of HDV infection<br>• No vaccination available | • Anti-HDV—indicates past or current infection<br>• HDV Ag (hepatitis D antigen)—marker present with a few days of infection<br>• No drug therapy available |
| **Hepatitis E Virus (HEV)**<br>*Incubation:* 14–60 days (average 40 days)<br>• Fecal–oral route<br>• Outbreaks associated with contaminated water supply in developing countries<br>• Uncommon in US | • Contaminated water, poor sanitation<br>• Found in Asia, Africa, and Mexico | • May be similar to HAV<br>• Self-limited, acute illness<br>• No vaccination available | • Not known<br>• Anti-HEV IgM and IgG—present 1 wk–2 mo after onset of illness<br>• No drug therapy available |

**TEST ALERT:** Follow infection control guidelines; standard precautions include blood and body fluids.

# HEPATITIS A & E

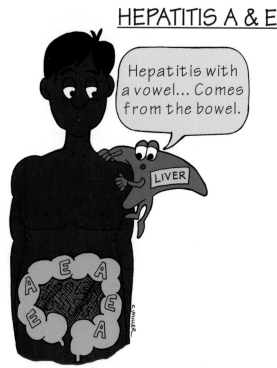

*Hepatitis with a vowel... Comes from the bowel.*

LIVER

© 2016 Nursing Education Consultants, Inc.

**FIGURE 21-1 Hepatitis with a Vowel Mnemonic.** (From Zerwekh, J., Garneau, A., & Miller, C. J. [2017]. *Digital collection of the memory notebooks of nursing* [4th ed.]. Chandler, AZ: Nursing Education Consultants, Inc.)

C. Permanent destruction of liver cells, leading to cirrhosis.
D. Hepatocellular carcinoma.

## Nursing Interventions

**Goal:** To control and prevent hepatitis.

A. Understand characteristics of transmission and preventive measures for hepatitis A.
  1. Good personal hygiene, especially handwashing.
  2. Participate in community activities for health education (e.g., environmental sanitation, food preparation, etc.).
  3. Identify individuals at increased risk for exposure: those with household contact, intimate sexual contact, daycare centers, schools, travel to areas with increased rates of hepatitis A, and/or institutional contact with those with active disease.
  4. Administer immune serum globulin (immunoglobulin G) within 2 weeks of exposure, if they do not have presence of anti-HAV antibodies (antibody to HAV).
  5. Preexposure prophylaxis: hepatitis A vaccine (single dose).
  6. Implement standard precautions.
  7. Clients should abstain from sexual activity during periods of communicability.

**OLDER ADULT PRIORITY:** Older adult clients are at higher risk for liver damage and complications of hepatitis.

B. Understand characteristics of transmission and preventive measures for hepatitis B.
  1. Identify individuals at increased risk for exposure: those with oral or percutaneous contact with HBsAg-positive fluid and those who have had sexual contact with carriers within 4 weeks of the appearance of jaundice.
  2. Administration of HBV vaccine.
  3. Postexposure prophylaxis: HBV vaccine series started and hepatitis B immune globulin (HBIG) given within 24 hours of exposure.
C. Understand characteristics of transmission and preventive measures for hepatitis C.
  1. No vaccine for HCV.
  2. Long-acting interferon is administered (pegylated interferon), along with antivirals (ribavirin).
D. Maintain strict contact-based standard precautions for hospitalized client with questionable diagnosis of hepatitis (see Appendix 9-3).

**Goal:** To promote healing and regeneration of liver tissue.

A. Bed rest with bathroom privileges initially; progressive activity according to liver function test results.
B. Promote psychological and emotional rest.
  1. Strict bed rest may increase anxiety.
  2. Frequently, young adults are concerned about body image; encourage verbalization and emphasize temporary nature of symptoms.
  3. Maintain communication and frequent contact.
C. Promote nutritional intake.
  1. Anorexia and decreased taste for food potentiate nutritional deficits.
  2. Small frequent feedings of favorite foods, good oral hygiene, and food served in a pleasant atmosphere.
D. Encourage increased fluid intake.

### Home Care

A. Continued need for adequate rest and nutrition until liver function test results are normal.
B. Avoid alcohol and over-the-counter medications, especially those containing acetaminophen and phenothiazine.

**TEST ALERT:** Evaluate client's use of over-the-counter medications for potential interactions that may affect therapeutic treatment.

C. Clients with HBV should avoid intimate and sexual contact until antibodies to the HBsAg are present and the client is no longer contagious.
D. If possible, client should have his or her own bathroom.
E. Client and family must understand importance of personal hygiene and good handwashing.
F. Client should not donate blood.

### Hepatic Cirrhosis

**Hepatic cirrhosis is a chronic, progressive disease of the liver characterized by degeneration and destruction of liver cells.**

A. Liver regeneration is disorganized and results in the formation of scar tissue, which in time will exceed the amount of normal liver tissue.

B. Types of cirrhosis.
  1. Alcoholic (previously called Laennec's): also called portal or nutritional cirrhosis; associated with alcohol abuse; accumulation of fat in liver cells leading to widespread inflammation and destruction of liver cells, which results in widespread scar formation.
  2. Postnecrotic: can follow hepatitis or exposure to hepatotoxin.
  3. Biliary: diffuse fibrosis and scarring caused by chronic biliary obstruction and infection.
  4. Cardiac: increase in venous pressure associated with long-term right-sided heart failure.
C. Complications of cirrhosis.
  1. Portal hypertension.
    a. Structural changes in the liver result in obstruction of normal hepatic blood flow, which causes increased pressure in the portal circulation.
    b. Collateral circulation develops as the body attempts to reduce the increased portal pressure. Common areas for collateral channels are:
      (1) Lower esophagus at the area of the gastric vein.
      (2) Anterior abdominal wall.
      (3) Parietal peritoneum.
      (4) Rectum.
    c. Esophageal varices form from collateral vessels in the lower esophagus.
    d. Gastric varices from collateral vessels in upper portion of stomach.
    e. Splenomegaly occurs from the increase of congestion in the splenic bed; may lead to leukopenia and splenomegaly.
    f. Caput medusae: dilated veins around the umbilical area.
  2. Peripheral edema and ascites.
    a. Edema results from:
      (1) Impaired liver synthesis of protein, resulting in decreased colloid osmotic pressure (hypoalbuminemia).
      (2) Portal hypertension, malnutrition.
    b. Ascites: accumulation of serous fluid in the peritoneal cavity.
      (1) With increased pressure in the liver, excessive protein and water leak out of the liver into the abdomen.
      (2) The presence of hypoalbuminemia results in decreased colloid osmotic pressure, which facilitates movement of fluid and protein into the abdominal cavity.
      (3) Hyperaldosteronism causes increased amounts of sodium and water to be retained.
  3. Hepatic encephalopathy (coma) results from the inability of the liver to detoxify ammonia.
    a. Ammonia is a by-product of protein metabolism.
    b. Large quantities of ammonia remain in the systemic circulation and cross the blood–brain barrier, producing toxic neurologic effects.

  4. Hepatorenal syndrome: characterized by functional renal failure with advancing azotemia, oliguria, and intractable ascites.

**TEST ALERT:** Identify changes in mental status.

*Assessment*
A. Risk factors/etiology.
  1. Excessive, prolonged alcohol consumption.
  2. Nutritional deficiencies.
  3. Typically these occur in combination of alcoholism and nutritional deficiency leading to a poorer prognosis.
  4. Predisposing chronic hepatic and biliary infections.
B. Clinical manifestations.
  1. GI disturbances: anorexia, indigestion, change in bowel habits, weight loss.
  2. Changes in the skin.
    a. Jaundice (hepatocellular and biliary), pruritus.
    b. Spider angiomas on the face, neck, and shoulders.
    c. Palmar erythema: reddened areas on the palms that blanch with pressure.
  3. Blood disorders: anemia.
  4. Coagulation disorders: spontaneous bruising from thrombocytopenia.
  5. Changes in sexual characteristics: gynecomastia, impotence in males; amenorrhea, vaginal bleeding in females.
  6. Peripheral neuropathy: probably caused by inadequate intake of vitamin B complex.
  7. Hepatomegaly, splenomegaly.
  8. Portal hypertension.
    a. Esophageal varices that bleed easily.
    b. Hemorrhoids.
    c. Collateral veins visible on abdominal wall.
    d. Development of edema and ascites.
    e. Edema generally located in feet, ankles, and presacral area.
    f. Severe abdominal distention and weight gain with ascites.
    g. Presence of fluid waves in the abdomen.
  9. Portal-systemic encephalopathy (Figure 21-2).
    a. Changes in mental responsiveness.
    b. Level of concentration: ask client to repeat a series of numbers; if client has encephalopathy, he or she will be unable to repeat a four- to six-digit sequence.
    c. Memory: determine client's ability to recall recent events (yesterday or past week) and remote events (last year).
    d. Apraxia: deterioration in writing and drawing; inability to construct or draw a figure.
    e. Asterixis (flapping tremors): clients with asterixis are unable to hold their hands out in front of them when asked; a flapping of the hands will occur.
    f. Fetor hepaticus: musty, sweet odor to breath due to inability of liver to degrade digestive products.
C. Diagnostics (see Appendix 21-1).

# HEPATIC ENCEPHALOPATHY
## HEPATIC COMA

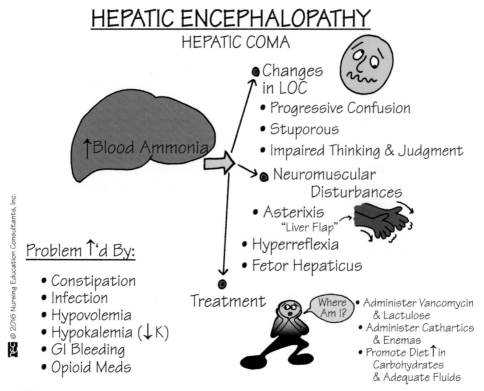

**FIGURE 21-2 Hepatic Encephalopathy.** (From Zerwekh, J., Garneau, A., & Miller, C. J. [2017]. *Digital collection of the memory notebooks of nursing* [4th ed.]. Chandler, AZ: Nursing Education Consultants, Inc.)

## Treatment

A. Cirrhosis.
  1. Rest.
  2. Dietary modification: increase calories and carbohydrates; protein and fat may be consumed as tolerated.
  3. Vitamin supplement, especially vitamin B complex.
  4. Abstinence from alcohol.
B. Ascites.
  1. IV albumin or other volume replacement after a high-volume paracentesis.
  2. Sodium restriction in diet.
  3. Fluid restriction for cases of severe ascites.
  4. Diuretics. Usually a combination of a K+ sparing and a loop diuretic.
  5. Paracentesis for temporary relief.
  6. Nonsurgical procedures to decrease portal hypertension by shunting portal blood flow: transjugular intrahepatic portosystemic shunt (TIPS).
  7. Peritoneovenous shunt (LeVeen shunt): a surgical procedure for reinfusion of ascitic fluid into venous system; rarely used due to high rate of complications.
C. Esophageal varices.
  1. Blood transfusions to restore volume from bleeding varices; vitamin K to correct coagulation abnormalities; proton pump inhibitors to decrease gastric acidity.
  2. Administration of IV vasopressin produces vasoconstriction of the splanchnic arterial bed, decreases portal

blood flow, and portal hypertension; somatostatin analog therapy may also be administered.
  3. Endoscopic sclerotherapy: injection of a sclerosing agent directly into esophageal varices; bleeding may recur because there has been no reduction in portal hypertension.
  4. Endoscopic variceal ligation (EVL) or banding of the varices: often used in combination with sclerotherapy.
  5. Balloon tamponade: mechanical compression of bleeding varices via esophageal gastric balloon tamponade (Minnesota tube; Linton-Nachlas tube; Sengstaken-Blakemore tube).
  6. Shunting surgical procedures: decrease portal hypertension by shunting portal blood flow; usually performed after second major bleeding episode.
  7. Management to prevent bleeding: beta-adrenergic blockers (propranolol), repeated sclerotherapy, endoscopic ligation, and portosystemic shunts.
D. Decrease portal systemic encephalopathy.
  1. Restriction of dietary protein intake.
  2. Neomycin: decreases the normal flora in the intestines to reduce bacterial activity on protein.
  3. Lactulose: used to reduce the amount of ammonia in the blood of clients with liver disease by drawing ammonia from the blood into the colon where it is removed from the body. May also be used to treat constipation because it pulls water into the colon to facilitate movement of waste through the GI system.
  4. Control of GI hemorrhage to decrease protein available in the intestine.

*Nursing Interventions*

**Goal:** To promote health in the client with cirrhosis.

A. Proper diet: increased protein as tolerated, adequate carbohydrates, vitamin supplements.
B. Adequate rest.

> **TEST ALERT:** Monitor client's hydration and nutritional status.

C. Avoid potential hepatotoxic over-the-counter drugs (aspirin and acetaminophen).
D. Check all body secretions for frank or occult blood.
E. Abstinence from alcohol.
F. Attention and care should be given the alcoholic client without being judgmental or moralizing.
G. Client should understand symptoms indicative of complications and when to seek medical advice.
H. Regular medical checkups.

**Goal:** To maintain homeostasis and promote liver function.

A. Rest and activity schedule based on clinical manifestations and laboratory data.
B. Measures to prevent complications of immobility (see Chapter 3).
C. Assist client to maintain self-esteem.
   1. Maintain positive, accepting atmosphere in the delivery of care.
   2. Encourage venting of feelings regarding disease.
D. Assist in activities of daily living, as necessary, to prevent undue fatigue.
E. Promote nutritional intake.
   1. Good oral hygiene; between-meal nourishment.
   2. Provide food preferences when possible.
   3. Administer antiemetic before meals, if necessary.
   4. Iron and vitamin supplements, especially vitamin B complex.
   5. Nasogastric or parenteral feeding if client is unable to maintain adequate intake.
F. Decrease discomfort of pruritus caused by jaundice: cool rather than warm baths, avoid excessive soap.
G. Maintain proper skin care to prevent breakdown.
H. Evaluate serum electrolyte levels, especially potassium and sodium levels, because of the use of diuretics to decrease ascites and edema.
I. Monitor temperature closely because of increased susceptibility to infection.
J. Assess for bleeding tendencies and prevent trauma to the mucous membranes.
K. Measure abdominal girth to determine whether it is increasing from ascitic fluid (Figure 21-3).

**Goal:** If esophageal varices are present, decrease risk for active bleeding by implementing the following measures.

A. Soft, nonirritating foods.
B. Discourage straining at stool.
C. Decrease esophageal reflux.
D. No salicylate compounds (aspirin).

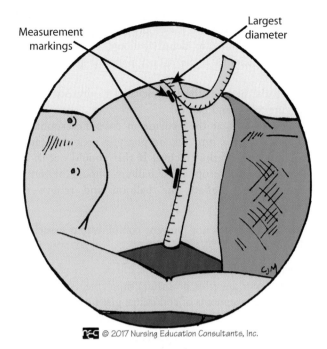

**FIGURE 21-3 Measuring Abdominal Girth.** (From Zerwekh, J., Garneau, A., & Miller, C. J. [2017]. *Digital collection of the memory notebooks of nursing* [4th ed.]. Chandler, AZ: Nursing Education Consultants, Inc.)

E. Evaluate sources of active bleeding.
   1. Monitor vital signs.
   2. Assess for melena and hematemesis.

**Goal:** To decrease bleeding from esophageal and gastric varices.

A. Gastric lavage with iced saline solution.
B. Assess and prevent complications associated with sclerotherapy.
   1. Client is sedated and the throat is anesthetized before the procedure.
   2. By means of endoscopy, the physician injects the sclerosing agent into the varices.
   3. Bleeding from the varices should stop within minutes.
   4. Client may experience chest discomfort for 2 to 3 days; administer an analgesic.
   5. Esophageal perforation and ulceration are complications associated with treatment; observe client for development of severe chest pain.
   6. Observe for return of active bleeding.

**Goal:** To decrease esophageal bleeding by using an esophageal tamponade balloon.

A. Constant observation is required while the balloon is inflated.
B. The client is to receive *absolutely* nothing by mouth; unable to swallow saliva; provide frequent oral and nasal hygiene.
C. Constant tension/traction is applied to maintain the pressure against the esophageal sphincter by the gastric

balloon. The gastric balloon is *not* to be deflated while tension is present and the esophageal balloon is inflated. Label each lumen to identify balloon.
D. Deflate balloons as per agency policy to prevent tissue necrosis.
E. Keep the head of the bed elevated to decrease gastric regurgitation and nausea.
F. Keep scissors at the bedside in case the esophageal balloon moves into the oropharynx area and causes obstruction of the trachea. If this should occur, the lumen to the esophageal balloon should be cut to immediately deflate the balloon and relieve the obstruction.

**Goal:** To assess for and prevent complications associated with ascites.

A. Decrease sodium intake.
B. Administer diuretics, potassium supplements.
C. Daily measurements of abdominal girth.
D. Maintain semi-Fowler's position to decrease pressure on the diaphragm.
E. Assess weight daily.
F. Monitor pulse oximetry for indications of respiratory distress.

**Goal:** To assess for and prevent complications of hepatic encephalopathy.

A. Frequent assessment of responsiveness.
B. Assess for changes in level of orientation and motor abnormalities (asterixis).
C. Provide and maintain a safe environment
D. Decrease production of ammonia.
 1. Increase carbohydrates and fluids.
 2. Decrease activity because ammonia is a by-product of metabolism.
 3. GI bleeding will increase ammonia levels as a result of the breakdown of red blood cells.
 4. Lactulose is used to promote excretion of ammonia in the stool; therapy must be titrated, as diarrhea may occur.
 5. Nonabsorbable intestinal antibiotics (see Appendix 9-2) will decrease protein breakdown.
E. Prompt treatment of hypokalemia.

**Goal:** To provide appropriate preoperative and postoperative care if surgical procedure is indicated (see Chapter 3).

A. Anastomosis of the high-pressure portal system to the low-pressure systemic venous system to create a shunt to decrease portal hypertension (portosystemic shunt), thereby decreasing problems with esophageal varices and ascites.
B. Client is at increased risk for postoperative complications.
 1. Hemorrhage, electrolyte imbalance.
 2. Seizures, delirium.
C. Surgical procedures do not alter course of progressive hepatic disease.

# Cancer of the Liver
**Metastatic cancer of the liver is more common than primary cancer of the liver.**

A. Liver is a common site for metastases because of increased rate of blood flow and capillary network.
B. Metastases are found in the liver in approximately one-half of all clients with late-stage cancer.
C. Prognosis is poor.

*Assessment*
A. Risk factors/etiology: malignancy elsewhere in the body.
B. Clinical manifestations.
 1. Anorexia, weight loss, fatigue, anemia, peripheral edema, nausea, vomiting.
 2. Right upper quadrant pain, ascites, jaundice.
C. Diagnostics (see Appendix 21-1).

*Treatment*
Treatment is primarily palliative.

A. Surgical excision of tumor if it is localized.
B. Chemotherapy: poor response.
C. Radiofrequency ablation (RFA) uses electrical energy to create heat to burn tumor (percutaneous approach).
D. Cryosurgery (cryoablation) uses liquid nitrogen to freeze liver tissue; not used for metastatic disease.
E. Percutaneous ethanol injection (PEI) or percutaneous acetic acid injection (PAI) is used to treat unresectable liver cancer.
F. Chemoembolization, sometimes called transarterial chemoembolization (TACE), uses an embolic agent mixed with other medications to reduce the blood supply to the tumor.
G. Systemic chemotherapy is not used, but sorafenib (Nexavar) is used to treat metastatic liver cancer because it inhibits new blood vessel growth in tumors.

*Nursing Interventions*
Focused on maintaining comfort; nursing care is the same as that for the client with advanced cirrhosis.

## DISORDERS OF THE BILIARY TRACT
# Cholelithiasis and Cholecystitis
**Cholelithiasis is the presence of stones in the gallbladder; this is the most common form of biliary disease. Cholecystitis is an inflammation of the gallbladder, which is frequently associated with stones; this condition may be acute or chronic.**

*Assessment*
A. Risk factors/etiology.
 1. Cholelithiasis. (Figure 21-4)
  a. Supersaturation of bile with cholesterol causes precipitate to occur.
  b. Conditions upsetting cholesterol and bile balance include infection and disturbances of cholesterol metabolism.

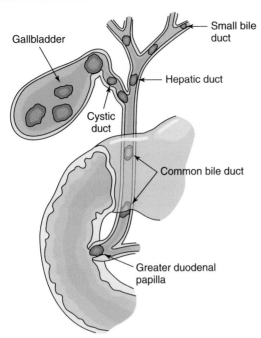

**FIGURE 21-4 Common Sites of Gallstones.** (From Monahan, F. D., et al. [2007]. *Medical-surgical nursing: Health and illness perspectives* [8th ed.]. St. Louis, MO: Mosby.)

c. Increased incidence in females, especially during pregnancy.
d. Increased incidence after age 40; obesity.
2. Cholecystitis. (Figure 21-5)
  a. Associated with stone formation.
  b. *Escherichia coli* is common bacteria involved.
  c. May also be associated with neoplasms, anesthesia, or adhesions.

## CHOLECYSTITIS

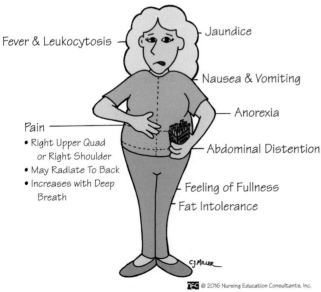

Fever & Leukocytosis

Jaundice

Nausea & Vomiting

Anorexia

Pain
• Right Upper Quad or Right Shoulder
• May Radiate To Back
• Increases with Deep Breath

Abdominal Distention

Feeling of Fullness

Fat Intolerance

© 2016 Nursing Education Consultants, Inc.

**FIGURE 21-5 Cholecystitis.** (From Zerwekh, J., Garneau, A., & Miller, C. J. [2017]. *Digital collection of the memory notebooks of nursing* [4th ed.]. Chandler, AZ: Nursing Education Consultants, Inc.)

**⚠ OLDER ADULT PRIORITY:** Incidence of gallstone increases with age. Older adults are more likely to go from asymptomatic gallstones to serious complications of gallstones without biliary colic.

B. Clinical manifestations.
  1. Cholelithiasis: severity of symptoms depends on the mobility of the stone and whether obstruction occurs.
    a. Epigastric distress, feeling of fullness.
    b. Abdominal distention.
    c. Vague pain in the right upper quadrant after consumption of meals high in fat.
  2. Obstruction of cystic ducts by stones, precipitating biliary colic.
    a. Severe abdominal pain radiating to the back and shoulder.
    b. Nausea, vomiting, tachycardia, diaphoresis.
    c. Pain occurs 3 to 6 hours after consumption of a heavy meal, especially if high in fat.
    d. Jaundice may occur with obstruction of bile flow.
    e. Urine may become very dark, and stools may be clay colored.
  3. Cholecystitis.
    a. Abdominal guarding, rigidity, rebound tenderness.
    b. Fever.
    c. Pain exacerbated by deep breathing.
    d. Onset may be sudden with severe pain.
C. Diagnostics (see Appendix 21-1).

### Treatment

A. Cholecystectomy for cholelithiasis: surgical removal of the stones.
B. Cholecystitis.
  1. Anticholinergics to decrease secretions and promote relaxation of the gallbladder.
  2. Analgesics: hydromorphone or morphine.
  3. Antibiotics for potential infection, if indicated.
  4. Atropine and dicyclomine will relieve spasms and decrease pain.
  5. Ketorolac may be used to decrease spasms and pain in older adults.
C. Laparoscopic cholecystectomy.
  1. One to four small incisions are made.
  2. Decreased surgical risk to client, as minimal incisions are used.
  3. Day surgery or overnight stay.
  4. Early ambulation and decreased pain.

**⚠ NURSING PRIORITY:** Common post-op problem of referred pain to the shoulder due to $CO_2$ that was not released or absorbed by body, which can irritate the phrenic nerve and diaphragm causing difficulty breathing.

D. Decrease dietary fat intake.

### Nursing Interventions

**Goal:** To decrease pain and inflammatory response.

A. Low-fat liquid diet during an acute attack.
B. Low-fat solids added as tolerated.

C. IV fluids and gastric decompression if nausea and vomiting are severe.

D. Antibiotics and analgesics.

E. Assess for indications of infection.

**Goal:** To provide appropriate preoperative nursing care if surgery is indicated (see Chapter 3).

**Goal:** To maintain homeostasis and prevent complications after cholecystectomy.

A. General postoperative care for clients having abdominal surgery (see Chapter 3).

B. Evaluate tolerance to diet and progress diet gradually to low-fat solids.

C. Penrose drain may be in place; client will frequently have large amounts of serosanguineous drainage; change dressing as indicated.

D. Sims' position to facilitate the movement of $CO_2$ gas pocket away from the diaphragm.

E. T-tube may be used to maintain patency of bile duct and to facilitate bile drainage until edema subsides (Figure 21-6).
1. Maintain tube to gravity drainage.
2. Observe amount and color of bile drainage.
3. Do not irrigate or clamp tube; do not raise tube above the level of the gallbladder.
4. Observe for bile drainage around the tube.
5. Observe and record drainage (bloody initially, then greenish brown).
6. Drainage is usually around 500 mL per day for several days after surgery; drainage will gradually decrease, and the doctor will remove the tube.
7. Drains and/or tubes are typically not placed or used after a laparoscopic cholecystectomy.

F. Monitor urine and stool for changes in color.

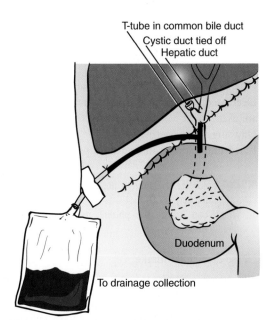

T-tube in common bile duct
Cystic duct tied off
Hepatic duct
Duodenum
To drainage collection

**FIGURE 21-6  Placement of a T-Tube.** (From Black, J. M., & Hawks, J. H. [2009]. *Medical-surgical nursing: Clinical management for positive outcomes* [8th ed.]. St. Louis, MO: Mosby.)

**Goal:** To assist client to understand implications of disease process and measures to maintain health after cholecystectomy.

A. Dietary teaching regarding low-fat diet.

B. Weight reduction, if appropriate.

C. Avoid heavy lifting for 4 to 6 weeks.

D. Understand symptoms indicating bile obstruction (i.e., stool and urine changes) and advise physician accordingly.

# CRITICAL CARE

## PRIORITY CONCEPTS

Immunity, Inflammation, Pain

### Acute Liver Failure

*A rapid onset of severe liver dysfunction in clients without a previous history of liver disease.*

#### Assessment

A. Risk factors/etiology.
1. Use of acetaminophen with excess alcohol consumption.
2. Drugs that have a toxic effect on the liver (isoniazid, sulfa-containing drugs, and NSAIDs).
3. Viral hepatitis (HBV); less commonly with hepatitis A (HAV).

B. Clinical manifestations.
1. Changes in mentation—often first sign.
2. Jaundice.
3. Coagulation abnormalities.
4. Encephalopathy.

C. Diagnostics (elevated bilirubin, liver enzymes; see Appendix 21-1).

D. Complications.
1. Renal failure.
2. Cerebral edema.

#### Treatment

A. Liver transplant, especially with clients who have severe encephalopathy.

#### Nursing Interventions

**Goal:** To monitor for worsening of symptoms and complications.

A. Early transfer to intensive care unit.

B. Maintain adequate fluid balance to protect renal function.

C. Monitor for cerebral edema; frequent neurologic checks.

D. Position head of bed elevated 30 degrees.

E. Avoid stimulating client and any straining or Valsalva maneuvers that may increase intracranial pressure.

**Goal:** To prepare client for liver transplant.

### Liver Transplantation

**Therapeutic option for clients with end-stage liver disease; not recommended for widespread malignant disease.**

#### Assessment

A. Rigorous prescreening process.

B. Rejection less common than with kidney transplants.

## Treatment

A. Live liver transplant: portion of liver is donated.
B. Split liver transplant: donor liver is divided and given to two recipients.

## Nursing Interventions

**Goal:** To monitor for postoperative complications.

A. Assess neurologic status, monitor for hemorrhage and common respiratory problems of pneumonia, atelectasis, and pleural effusion.

B. Monitor IV fluids, nasogastric tube drainage, Jackson-Pratt drain, and T-tube drainage.
C. Administer antibiotics and analgesics.
D. Critical to monitor for infection the first 2 months after surgery; fever may be the only sign.

**Goal:** To provide nursing care of the immunocompromised client (see Chapter 10).

---

### Appendix 21-1 DIAGNOSTICS OF THE HEPATIC AND BILIARY SYSTEM

| Laboratory Tests | Normal | Nursing Implications |
|---|---|---|
| **Serum Laboratory Tests** | | |
| **Bilirubin** | | |
| Direct | 0.1–0.3 mg/dL (1.7–5.1 umol/L) | 1. A rise in the serum level of bilirubin will occur if there is excessive destruction of red blood cells or if the liver is unable to excrete normal amounts of bilirubin. |
| Indirect | 0.1–1.0 mg/dL 1.7–17.1 umol/L) | |
| Total | 0.2–1.3 mg/dL (5–21 umol/L) | |
| **Protein Studies** | | |
| Total serum protein | 6.0–8.0 g/dL (60–80 g/L) | 1. Proteins are responsible for maintaining the colloid oncotic pressure in the serum. |
| Serum albumin | 3.5–5.0 g/dL (35–50 g/L) | 2. Synthesis of protein and normal serum protein levels are affected by various liver impairments. |
| Serum globulin | 2.0–3.5 g/dL (20–35 g/L) | |
| **Serum Enzymes** | | |
| Lactic dehydrogenase (LDH) | 140–280 units/L (0.83–2.5 μkat/L) | 1. Elevated in heart failure, hemolytic disorders, hepatitis, liver damage. |
| LDH$_5$ | 10–26 units (0.10–0.26 μkat/L)— | 1. LDH$_5$ isoenzyme elevated in hepatitis. |
| Aspartate aminotransferase (AST) | | 2. Elevated in liver disease, acute hepatitis, myocardial infarction, pulmonary infarction. |
| Alanine aminotransferase (ALT) | 10–40 unit/L (0.17–0.68 μkat/L) | 1. Elevated in liver disease, shock. |
| Alkaline phosphatase (ALP) | 38–126 units/L (0.65–2.14 μkat/L) | 1. Primary sources of ALP in body are bone and liver. Abnormally high readings may be associated with either liver or bone disease and must be correlated with presenting clinical symptoms. |
| Serum blood ammonia | 30–70 mcg/dL (21.42–50 μmol/L) | 1. Increasing blood ammonia is indicative of the inability of the liver to convert ammonia to urea. |
| Hepatitis antigens and antibodies | Negative for antigens | 1. Antigens indicate hepatitis (hepatitis B surface antigen [HBsAg] elevated in hepatitis B). Antibodies indicate exposure, current disease, or hepatitis B immunization. |
| **Biopsy** | | |
| **Liver Biopsy** | | |
| Percutaneous needle aspiration of liver tissue | | 1. Informed consent procedure. |
| | | 2. Client's status is NPO for 6 hours before procedure. |
| | | 3. Blood coagulation study results should be available on the chart before biopsy procedure. |
| | | 4. Immediately before needle insertion, have client take a deep breath, exhale completely, and hold breath. This immobilizes the chest wall and decreases the risk for penetration of the diaphragm with the needle. |
| | | 5. Keep client on bed rest for 12–14 hours. Client should be positioned on the right side for 2 hours postprocedure to apply pressure and decrease risk for hemorrhage. |
| | | 6. Assess for complications of pneumothorax and hemorrhage immediately after biopsy; assess for right upper abdominal pain or referred shoulder pain; observe for development of bile peritonitis. |

**TEST ALERT:** Monitor status of client after a procedure: Position the client on right side with a pillow under the costal margin to facilitate compression of the liver.

*Continued*

**Appendix 21-1    DIAGNOSTICS OF THE HEPATIC AND BILIARY SYSTEM—cont'd**

| Laboratory Tests | Normal | Nursing Implications |
|---|---|---|
| **Cholangiography** | | |
| ***Percutaneous Transhepatic Cholangiography (PTC)*** | | |
| IV injection of radiopaque dye to visualize the biliary duct system | | 1. Client's status is NPO for 8 hours before the test.<br>2. Assess for sensitivity to iodine.<br>3. Administer prophylactic IV antibiotic 1 hr before surgery.<br>4. Evaluate for iodine reaction after the test.<br>5. Client should drink large amounts of fluid after test to increase excretion of dye. |
| **Nuclear Imaging Scans (Scintigraphy)** | | |
| ***Hepatobiliary Scintigraphy (HIDA)*** | | |
| Shows size, shape, and position of biliary system. Radionuclide (Tc-99m) injected IV; client positioned under a camera or counter to record distribution of tracer | | 1. Explain to client that traces of radionuclide pose minimal danger.<br>2. Needs to lie flat during scanning procedure. |
| **Ultrasound** | | |
| ***Gallbladder Ultrasound*** | | |
| Uses high-frequency sound waves to examine the gallbladder; provides information about presence of tumors and patency of vessels and detects gallstones<br>Hepatobiliary ultrasound<br>Detects abscesses, cysts, tumors, and cirrhosis | | 1. Client is NPO for 8–12 hours because gas can reduce quality of images and food can cause gallbladder contraction.<br>2. Explain to client that a conductive gel (lubricant) will be applied to the skin and a transducer placed on the area. |
| **Endoscopy** | | |
| ***Endoscopic Retrograde Cholangiopancreatography (ERCP)*** | | |
| Fiber-optic endoscope and fluoroscopy inserted orally, descended into duodenum, then into common bile duct and pancreatic ducts, where contrast medium is injected for visualization of the structures. | | 1. Client is NPO for 8 hours before procedure.<br>2. Explain that sedative will be given before and during procedure.<br>3. Check for allergy to contrast medium.<br>4. Informed consent must be signed.<br>5. Check vital signs—monitor for perforation or infection; pancreatitis is most common complication.<br>6. Check for return of gag reflex before giving fluids. |

*ALP,* Alkaline phosphatase; *ALT,* alanine aminotransferase; *AST,* aspartate aminotransferase; *INR,* international normalized ratio; *IV,* intravenous; *NPO,* nothing by mouth.

| Appendix 21-2 | HEPATITIS DRUG THERAPIES |
|---|---|

**Acute Viral Hepatitis:** No specific drug therapy, only supportive therapy with antiemetics but not phenothiazines. Preventive immunizations (see Figures 2-1, 2-2).

| *Medication* | *Side Effects* | *Nursing Implications* |
|---|---|---|
| **Chronic Hepatitis B Therapies:** Do not eradicate the virus; produce a decrease in viral load, liver enzymes, and rates of disease progression drug resistance. | | |
| *First-Line Therapies:*<br>Pegylated interferon: subQ 3 ×<br>    per week<br>α-interferon: subQ once per week<br>*Nucleoside and Nucleotide Analogs:*<br>Entecavir: PO<br>Tenofovir: PO | Flulike symptoms: aches, fatigue, headache, nausea, anorexia, fever; insomnia, hair thinning, diarrhea, weight loss<br>Possible nephrotoxicity | 1. Monitor and teach to anticipate flulike symptoms.<br>2. Rest, drink fluids; eat small, frequent, light meals.<br>3. Administer in p.m. to reduce discomfort and sleep through side effects.<br>4. Use two forms of contraception.<br>5. Teach that entecavir is not to be used with pregnancy.<br>6. Monitor laboratory work for potential nephrotoxicity and lactic acidosis.<br>7. Monitor closely for acute exacerbation if drugs are discontinued. |
| **Chronic Hepatitis C Therapies:** First-line therapies used: pegylated interferon; α-interferon along with ribavirin. | | |
| Ribavirin: PO twice daily | Hemolytic anemia, anorexia, cough, dyspnea, insomnia, pruritus, rash, teratogenicity, conjunctivitis | 1. Frequent rest periods.<br>2. Small, frequent, light meals. |

*PO,* By mouth; *subQ,* subcutaneous.

# Study Questions
# Hepatic and Biliary: Care of Adult and Pediatric Clients

More questions on

1. After administering diuretics to a client with ascites, which of the following nursing actions most ensures safe care?
   1. Monitoring serum potassium for hyperkalemia
   2. Assessing the client for hypervolemia
   3. Weighing client weekly
   4. Documenting accurate intake and output

2. An obese 44-year-old woman with a history of chronic cholecystitis is to receive vitamin K before surgery. What is the purpose of this medication?
   1. To increase the digestion and utilization of fats
   2. To support the immune system and promote healing
   3. To aid in the emptying of bile from the gallbladder
   4. To facilitate coagulation activities of the blood

3. A client with cirrhosis is receiving neomycin sulfate. The nurse understands that the purpose of this medication is to:
   1. Decrease gastric acidity.
   2. Acidify feces and trap ammonia in the bowel.
   3. Decrease bacterial flora.
   4. Reduce portal hypertension.

4. What statement would indicate to the nurse that the client understands the discharge teaching regarding his cirrhosis?
   1. "I will decrease vitamin B intake."
   2. "I need to continue Tylenol daily."
   3. "I will weigh myself every day in the morning."
   4. "I can eat my regular diet."

5. The nurse is caring for a client with chronic hepatitis B virus (HBV). What will the teaching plan for this client include?
   1. Use a condom for sexual intercourse.
   2. Report any clay-colored stools.
   3. Eat a high-protein diet.
   4. Perform daily urine bilirubin checks.

6. The client returns to his room after liver biopsy. The nurse positions the client on his right side and assesses for bleeding. What is a priority nursing assessment?
   1. Assess the vital signs.
   2. Observe for frank bleeding.
   3. Check pretest prothrombin time and partial thromboplastin time values.
   4. Determine adequacy of urinary output.

7. A client with portal hypertension and ascites has had a paracentesis to relieve respiratory compromise. What medication will the nurse anticipate the client will receive?
   1. D10W
   2. Morphine
   3. IV salt-poor albumin
   4. Furosemide

8. The nurse is making a home visit to a client with hepatitis A virus (HAV). Before assessing the client, the nurse will gather the equipment and perform what action next?
   1. Wipe the bedside table with alcohol preps.
   2. Place the supplies on a clean, convenient work area.
   3. Maintain standard precautions before and after client contact.
   4. Put on a gown, mask, and gloves.

9. While talking with a client with a diagnosis of end-stage liver disease, the nurse notices the client is unable to stay awake and seems to fall asleep in the middle of a sentence. The nurse recognizes these symptoms to be indicative of what condition?
   1. Hyperglycemia
   2. Increased bile production
   3. Increased blood ammonia levels
   4. Hypocalcemia

10. What is the primary purpose of giving lactulose to a client with advanced liver disease?
    1. To ensure regular bowel movements
    2. To prevent bowel obstruction
    3. To decrease ammonia levels in the blood
    4. To promote clotting

11. Which position is best for the client who has undergone a traditional abdominal cholecystectomy?
    1. Side-lying position, to prevent aspiration
    2. Semi-Fowler's position, to facilitate breathing
    3. Supine, to decrease strain on the incision line
    4. Prone, to reduce nausea

12. A client who underwent cholecystectomy 3 days ago has a T-tube that has stopped draining. What is the best nursing action?
    1. Flush the tube with 5 mL of normal saline solution.
    2. Reposition the client.
    3. Continue to monitor.
    4. Assess for tube placement.

13. The nurse is caring for a client with hepatitis A. Which type of infection precaution is appropriate for this client?
    1. Standard precautions
    2. Droplet precautions
    3. Contact precautions
    4. Bloodborne precautions

14. A new employee at a facility needs to receive the hepatitis vaccine. Which statement reflects accurate understanding of the immunization?
    1. "I need to receive six shots—once a month until I show positive antibodies to hepatitis."
    2. "Once I receive the hepatitis vaccine, I will be immune to all types of hepatitis."
    3. "I will receive three injections over a period of months, which should protect me from hepatitis B."
    4. "The hepatitis vaccine is an oral vaccine with live attenuated virus."

15. What important teaching instructions should the nurse relay to the client before discharge following a laparoscopic cholecystectomy?
    1. Avoid dietary fat for at least 1 year.
    2. Avoid heavy lifting for at least 2 weeks.
    3. Expect bile-colored drainage from the incision.
    4. Resume all activities gradually.

16. Clients with liver disease frequently develop a problem with jaundice. What would the nurse identify as the physiologic cause of jaundice?
    1. Increased levels of ammonia
    2. Increased alanine aminotransferase (ALT) level
    3. Bilirubin levels above 4 mg/dL (68.4 umol/L)
    4. Increased red blood cell production

17. The client who has undergone a traditional cholecystectomy has a T-tube in place after surgery. What is the purpose of the T-tube in the care of this client?
    1. To remove bile leaking from the incision
    2. To provide a means of wound irrigation
    3. To drain bile from the common bile duct
    4. To prevent rupture of the inflamed gallbladder

18. What is the most important nursing intervention for the safety of a client with altered clotting mechanisms caused by hepatic cirrhosis?
    1. Promote independence in the client's activities of daily living.
    2. Administer antibiotics to decrease ammonia.
    3. Implement bleeding precautions.
    4. Increase vitamin supplements and nutritional intake.

19. A client has been diagnosed with cholecystitis. What menu selection would be appropriate for this client?
    1. Eggs, bacon, whole grain toast, and decaffeinated tea
    2. Fresh fruit, oatmeal, and decaffeinated coffee
    3. Roast beef sandwich with Swiss cheese and cranberry juice
    4. Cottage cheese, avocado, bagel, and tea

## Answers to Study Questions

1. *4*
Accurate intake and output measurements are essential for clients receiving diuretics. Hypokalemia, not hyperkalemia, is a frequent occurrence with diuretic therapy. Hypovolemia is a greater risk with an increased urine output. Clients should be weighed daily. (Lewis et al., 10 ed., p. 994)

2. *4*
Vitamin K is necessary for normal clotting. Cholecystitis can decrease the absorption of fat-soluble vitamins (A, D, E, and K) by interfering with fat metabolism, which can lead to potential difficulties with clotting. (Lewis et al., 10 ed., pp. 992, 1008)

3. *3*
Neomycin sulfate decreases bacterial flora in the bowel, thus decreasing ammonia. Proton pump inhibitors and H$_2$ blockers decrease gastric acidity in the treatment of cirrhosis. Lactulose acidifies feces in the bowel and traps ammonia, causing its elimination in the feces. Propranolol reduces portal venous pressure. (Lewis et al., 10 ed., p. 992)

**4.** *3*

Daily weight measurement is essential to monitor for volume overload. Clients with cirrhosis need increased vitamin B, especially B$_6$ (pyridoxine). Acetaminophen is hepatotoxic. The diet should be high in carbohydrates, include adequate amounts of protein to build tissue, and be moderate to low in fat intake. (Lewis et al., 10 ed., p. 994)

**5.** *1*

HBV is spread by sexual contact, so it is important to teach patients to use a condom for sexual intercourse, and the partner should be vaccinated. There will be no bilirubin in the urine or stools; clay-colored stools are expected, so they would not be reported. Client would not be told specifically to eat a high-protein diet. (Lewis et al., 10 ed., p. 982)

**6.** *1*

Vital signs must be assessed first if the nurse is monitoring the client for bleeding or shock. The nurse would do all of the assessments with vital signs as the priority. (Lewis et al., 10 ed., p. 845)

**7.** *3*

IV salt-poor albumin is given to replace protein lost in the ascites fluid and to restore oncotic pressure in the vascular bed. D$_{10}$W is an IV fluid, not a medication. Furosemide will diminish the ascitic fluid. The client has respiratory compromise and would not be given a narcotic pain medication (morphine). (Lewis et al., 10 ed., p. 991)

**8.** *3*

Hepatitis A is transmitted via fecal contamination and oral ingestion. It is important to maintain standard precautions before and after client contact. The use of standard precautions should prevent transmission of HAV to the health care worker. Paper towels are used to create a clean area surface. Alcohol preps are not effective. The mask is not appropriate because hepatitis is not spread by respiratory secretions. (Lewis et al., 10 ed., p. 982)

**9.** *3*

In end-stage liver disease, the liver cannot break down ammonia byproducts of protein metabolism. The increased ammonia levels in the serum cross the blood–brain barrier, causing uncontrolled drowsiness and confusion. Hyperglycemia is characterized by polyphagia, polydipsia, and polyuria, along with fatigue, weight loss, excessive thirst, and abdominal pain. Hypocalcemia is characterized by tetany symptoms. Increased bile production does not cause neurologic symptoms; it is related more to digestion. (Lewis et al., 10 ed., p. 990)

**10.** *3*

In a client with end-stage liver disease, lactulose is used to decrease ammonia levels in the blood, thus improving cognition and alertness. The ammonia is eliminated through the regular bowel movements that the medication promotes, preventing obstructions. Lactulose is not involved in blood clotting. (Lewis et al., 10 ed., p. 992)

**11.** *2*

A semi-Fowler's position improves lung expansion. The incision for a cholecystectomy is high and may interfere with respiratory exchange. The other positions would probably interfere with respirations. (Lewis et al., 10 ed., p. 1011)

**12.** *3*

Continue monitoring, as T-tube drainage decreases after day 2 and may stop between days 3 and 5. T-tubes are not irrigated. Placement is not checked. Repositioning will not change the drainage. (Lewis et al., 10 ed., p. 1009)

**13.** *1*

Standard precautions are the appropriate type of infection precautions for all clients with hepatitis. Droplet precautions are not necessary for clients with hepatitis. Because hepatitis A is transmitted through the oral–fecal route, contact precautions are not necessary, except for the methods provided by standard precautions. Bloodborne precautions (part of standard precautions) are necessary for clients with hepatitis B and C (which are bloodborne), as well as for clients with hepatitis D and G. (Lewis et al., 10 ed., p. 982)

**14.** *3*

The hepatitis vaccine is used to protect health care workers and other individuals from hepatitis B. The series consists of three intramuscular injections, the first two given at least 1 month apart and the third given 4 to 6 months later to provide long-lasting protection from hepatitis B only. (Lewis et al., 10 ed., p. 982)

**15.** *4*

Resuming all activities gradually is correct. A diet low in fat is usually ordered, and the client needs to avoid heavy lifting for 4 to 6 weeks. Bile-colored drainage is not to be expected postoperatively. (Lewis et al., 10 ed., p. 1009)

**16.** *3*

Increased levels of bilirubin (greater than 2.0 mg/dL [34 umol/L]) cause a discoloration of the skin called jaundice. The bilirubin value needs to be two to three times the normal level for jaundice to be manifested. Normal value of total bilirubin is 0.2 to 1.3 mg/dL (5–21 umol/L). Jaundice occurs because of an alteration in normal bilirubin metabolism or flow of bile into the hepatic or biliary system. Increased ammonia and ALT levels do not cause jaundice; they are problems associated with the malfunctioning liver. Hemolytic jaundice is due to an increased RBC production. (Lewis et al., 10 ed., pp. 977, 986)

**17.** *3*

A T-tube is used after a common bile duct exploration to drain bile and maintain patency of the duct until healing can occur. A T-tube should never be irrigated by the nurse. (Lewis et al., 10 ed., p. 1007)

**18.** *3*

The altered clotting mechanisms in a client with hepatic cirrhosis mean that the client has fewer clotting factors available to assist in the clotting process. Bleeding precautions should be in place. Although the client may be able to be independent in ADLs, for reasons of safety, supervision should be provided. Antibiotics and increased nutritional intake will not speed clotting times. (Lewis et al., 10 ed., pp. 994, 1008)

**19.** *2*

A low-fat diet is appropriate for the client with cholecystitis. Eggs, bacon, cheese, and avocados are high in fat and should be avoided. Other foods to avoid include whole milk, cream, butter, ice cream, fried foods, rich pastries, gravies, and nuts. (Lewis et al., 10 ed., p. 1008)

# 22 Neurology: Care of Adult and Pediatric Clients

## PRIORITY CONCEPTS

Functional Ability, Infection, Intracranial Regulation, Safety

## PHYSIOLOGY OF THE NERVOUS SYSTEM

A. Central nervous system (CNS): consists of brain and spinal cord.

B. Peripheral nervous system; consists of the 12 cranial and 31 spinal nerves and the autonomic nervous system (ANS). (Figure 22-1; Table 22-1)
   1. Autonomic nervous system (ANS). (Figure 22-2; Table 22-2)

C. Neuron: the functional cell of the nervous system.

D. Supporting cells (neuroglia cells) provide support, nourishment, and protection to the neuron.

E. Myelin sheath – dense membrane or insulator around the axon.

F. Nerve regeneration: entire neuron is unable to undergo complete regeneration.

G. Chemical neurotransmitters (neuromediators) facilitate the transmission of an impulse across the synapse to the next neuron.
   1. Acetylcholine.
   2. Norepinephrine.
   3. Dopamine.
   4. Serotonin.

H. Meninges: protective membranes that cover the brain and spinal cord.
   1. Pia mater: a delicate vascular connective tissue.
   2. Arachnoid: a delicate nonvascular, waterproof membrane that contains the cerebrospinal fluid.
   3. Dura mater: a tough white fibrous outer layer of protection.

I. Cerebrospinal fluid (CSF).
   1. Serves to cushion and protect the brain and spinal cord; brain literally floats in CSF.
   2. CSF is clear, colorless, watery fluid, approximately 100 to 200 mL in total volume, with a normal fluid pressure of 60 to 100 mmH$_2$O.

J. Cerebrum: the largest portion of the brain; separated into hemispheres; the cerebral cortex is the surface layer of each hemisphere.
   1. Frontal – controls higher cognitive function, memory retention, voluntary eye movements, voluntary motor movement, and expressive speech (Broca's area).
   2. Parietal – controls and interprets spatial information.
   3. Temporal – contains Wernicke's area, which is responsible for receptive speech and for integration of somatic, visual, and auditory data.
   4. Occipital: interprets vision.

K. Cerebellum: works with cerebrum to coordinate muscle movement and maintain balance.

L. Brainstem: consists of the midbrain, pons, and the medulla.
   1. Midbrain: responsible for motor coordination and visual and auditory relay centers.
   2. Pons: helps regulate respiration.
   3. Medulla: Has vital centers concerned with respiratory, vasomotor, and cardiac functions.

M. Diencephalon: part of the brain located between the cerebrum and midbrain.
   1. Thalamus: relays sensory messages; pain gateway.
   2. Hypothalamus.
      a. Regulation of visceral activities, including body temperature, fluid and electrolyte regulation, motility and secretions of the gastrointestinal tract, and arterial blood pressure.
      b. Regulation of endocrine glands via influence on the pituitary gland.
      c. Neurosecretion of antidiuretic hormone, which is stored in the pituitary gland.

N. Spinal cord.
   1. Ascending (afferent) tracts: sensory pathways.
   2. Descending (efferent) tracts: motor pathways.
   3. Intervertebral disks lie between the vertebrae to provide flexibility to the spinal column.
   4. Nucleus pulposus is the fibrocartilaginous portion of the intravertebral disk; acts as shock absorber for the spinal cord.
   5. Upper motor neurons: originate in the brain; transmit impulses from the brain to the lower motor neurons.
   6. Lower motor neurons: originate in the spinal cord; transmit impulses to the muscles and organs. These neurons form the reflex arc.

**TEST ALERT:** Identify pathophysiology related to an acute or chronic condition (e.g., signs and symptoms).

## System Assessment

A. History.
   1. Neurologic history.
      a. Avoid suggesting symptoms to the client.
      b. How the problems first presented and the overall course of the illness are important.

## LEVELS OF SPINAL NERVES

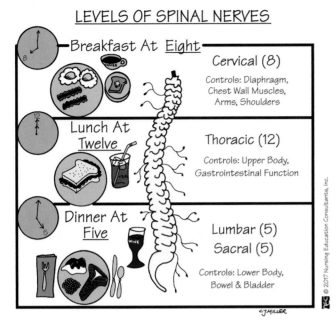

**FIGURE 22-1 Levels of Spinal Nerves.** (From Zerwekh, J., Garneau, A., & Miller, C. J. [2017]. *Digital collection of the memory notebooks of nursing* [4th ed.]. Chandler, AZ: Nursing Education Consultants, Inc.)

   c. Mental status must be assessed before the history data from the client can be assumed to be accurate.

> **⚠ NURSING PRIORITY:** In the older adult client, assess orientation and mental status before continuing assessment of neurologic function (Box 22-1).

   2. Medical history.
      a. Assess comorbidities (Box 22-2).
      b. Complete medication profile including complementary medications.
      c. Birth (or delivery) history: was client a difficult delivery?
      d. Sequence of growth and development.
   3. Family history: presence of hereditary or congenital problems.
   4. Personal history: activities of daily living (ADLs), any change in routine.
   5. History and symptoms of current problem.
      a. Paralysis or paresthesia, syncope.
      b. Headache, dizziness, speech problems.
      c. Visual problems, changes in personality.
      d. Memory loss, nausea, vomiting.
   B. Physical assessment.
      1. General observation of client.
         a. Posture, gait, coordination; perform Romberg test (have client stand with feet together, arms at sides; stand next to client to prevent falls; ask client to close eyes and continue to stand still). Positive if client loses balance and starts to fall.
         b. Position of rest for the infant or young child.
         c. Personal hygiene, grooming.

**Table 22-1   CRANIAL NERVES**

| No. | Name | Function |
|---|---|---|
| I | Olfactory | Sense of smell |
| II | Optic | Vision: conducts information from the retina |
| III | Oculomotor | Eye movement: up, down, and in (medial) Pupillary constriction and accommodation Muscle of the upper eyelid (ability to keep the eye open) |
| IV | Trochlear | Eye movement: downward and medial (cross eyes and look at nose) |
| V | Trigeminal: Ophthalmic Maxillary Mandibular | Corneal reflex Sensory fibers of the face Motor nerves for chewing and swallowing |
| VI | Abducens | Eye movement: lateral |
| VII | Facial | Facial expression Sense of taste on anterior tongue Muscle of the eyelid (ability to close the eye) |
| VIII | Acoustic (vestibulo-cochlear) | Reception of hearing and maintenance of equilibrium |
| IX | Glossopha-ryngeal | Sense of taste on posterior tongue Salivation Swallowing or gag reflex |
| X | Vagus nerve | Assists in swallowing action Motor fibers to larynx for speech Innervation of organs in thorax and abdomen Important in respiratory, cardiac, and circulatory reflexes |
| XI | Accessory (spinal) | Ability to rotate the head and raise the shoulder |
| XII | Hypoglossal | Muscles of the tongue |

## "AUTONOMIC NERVOUS SYSTEM RESPONSE"

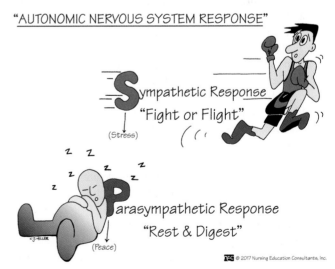

**FIGURE 22-2 Autonomic Nervous System Response.** (From Zerwekh, J., Garneau, A., & Miller, C. J. [2017]. *Digital collection of the memory notebooks of nursing* [4th ed.]. Chandler, AZ: Nursing Education Consultants, Inc.)

## Table 22-2 AUTONOMIC NERVOUS SYSTEM

| Area Affected | Sympathetic | Parasympathetic |
|---|---|---|
| Pupil | Dilates | Constricts |
| Bronchi | Dilates | Constricts |
| Heart | Increases rate and contractility | Decreases rate and contractility |
| Gastrointestinal | Inhibits peristalsis Stimulates sphincter | Stimulates peristalsis Inhibits sphincters |
| Bladder | Relaxes bladder muscle Constricts sphincter | Contracts bladder muscle Relaxes sphincter |
| Adrenal glands | Increases secretion of epinephrine and norepinephrine | |

## Box 22-1 OLDER ADULT CARE FOCUS

**Assessing Neurologic Function in Older Adults**
*Signs of Cognitive Impairment*
- Significant memory loss (person, place, time, and situation).
- Person: Does client know who he or she is, and can client give you his or her full name?
- Place: Can client identify his or her home address and where he or she is now?
- Time: What was the most recent holiday; what month, time of day, day of the week is it now?
- Situation: Can the client explain why he or she is in the health care facility?
- Does client show a lack of judgment?
- Is client agitated and/or suspicious?
- As determined from client's appearance and family's response, does client have problems with activities of daily living (ADLs)?
- Short-term memory: Can the client recall your name, name of the current president, or name of his or her doctor?
- Short-term recall: Ask the client to name three or four common objects; then ask client to recall them within the next 5 minutes.
- Does the client have sensory deficits (hearing and vision) of which he or she is not aware?

    d. Evaluate speech and ability to communicate.
      (1) Pace of speech: rapid, slow, halting.
      (2) Clarity: slurred or distinct.
      (3) Tone: high-pitched, rough.
      (4) Vocabulary: appropriate choice of words.
 2. Mental status (must take into consideration the client's culture and educational background).

!**NURSING PRIORITY:** Level of consciousness and mental status are critical assessment data for the client with neurologic deficits.

    a. Level of consciousness.
      (1) Oriented to person, place, time, and situation (in order of importance).

## Box 22-2 OLDER ADULT CARE FOCUS

**Causes of Confusion in the Older Adult Client**
*Decreased Cardiac Output*
- Myocardial infarction
- Dysrhythmias
- Heart failure

*Hypoxia/Respiratory Acidosis*
- Pneumonia
- Infection
- Hypoventilation

*Neurologic*
- Vascular insufficiency
- Infections
- Cerebral edema

*Metabolic—Altered Homeostasis*
- Electrolyte imbalance
- Hypoglycemia/hyperglycemia
- Dehydration
- Urinary tract infections

*Environmental*
- Strange surroundings
- Hypothermia/hyperthermia

      (2) Appropriate response to verbal and tactile stimuli.
      (3) Memory, problem-solving abilities.
    b. Mood.
    c. Thought content and intellectual capacity.
    d. General appearance and behavior.
 3. Assess pupillary status and eye movements (Figure 22-3).
    a. Size of pupils should be equal.
    b. Reaction of pupils.
      (1) Accommodation: pupillary constriction to accommodate near vision.
      (2) Direct light reflex: constriction of pupil when light is shone directly into eye.
      (3) Consensual reflex: constriction of the pupil in the opposite eye when the direct light reflex is tested.
    c. Evaluate ability to move eye.
      (1) Note nystagmus: fine, jerking eye movement.
      (2) Ability of eyes to move together.
      (3) Resting position of the iris should be at mid-position of the eye socket.
      (4) Assess for lid droop (ptosis).
    d. PERRLA: indicates that **P**upils are **E**qual, **R**ound, and **R**eactive to **L**ight and that **A**ccommodation is present.

!**NURSING PRIORITY:** When assessing a client's neurologic status, always evaluate symmetry. If asymmetric findings are detected, refine examination to determine CNS versus peripheral nervous system as origin of asymmetry.

## ASSESSMENT OF THE NEUROLOGIC SYSTEM—PUPILLARY CHECK

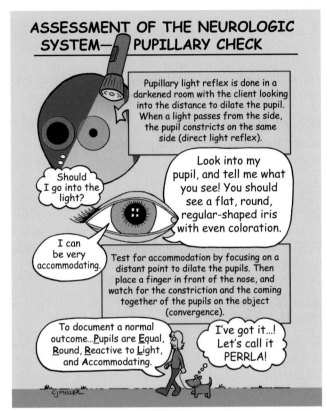

**FIGURE 22-3 Assessment of the Neurologic System: Pupillary Check.** (From Zerwekh, J., & Gaglione, T. [2011]. *Mosby's assessment memory notecards: Visual, mnemonic, and memory aids for nurses* [2nd ed.]. St. Louis, MO: Mosby.)

## ABNORMAL POSTURING

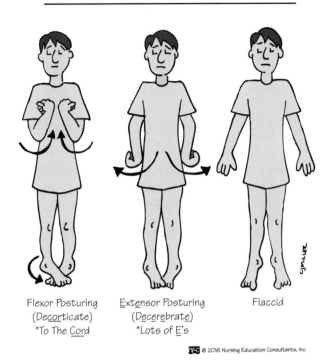

Flexor Posturing (Decorticate) *To The Cord    Extensor Posturing (Decerebrate) *Lots of E's    Flaccid

© 2016 Nursing Education Consultants, Inc.

**FIGURE 22-4 Abnormal Posturing.** (From Zerwekh, J., Garneau, A., & Miller, C. J. [2017]. *Digital collection of the memory notebooks of nursing* [4th ed.]. Chandler, AZ: Nursing Education Consultants, Inc.)

4. Evaluate motor function.
   a. Assess face and upper extremities for equality of movement and sensation.
   b. Evaluate appropriateness of motor movement—spontaneous and on command.
   c. Movement of extremities should always be evaluated bilaterally; tone, strength, and muscle movement of each side should be compared (e.g., bilateral hand grips of equal strength).
   d. Presence of inappropriate, nonpurposeful movement (e.g., posturing) (Figure 22-4).
      (1) Presence of nonpurposeful involuntary movements such as tremors, jerking, twitching, tics, or muscle fasciculation.
      (2) Decorticate: flexion, internal rotation of the arms, extension of the legs.
      (3) Decerebrate: extension and adduction of the arms, hyperextension of the legs.
      (4) Opisthotonos: extreme hyperextension of the head and dorsal arching.
      (5) Flaccid: limp, no movement
   e. Ability of an infant to suck and to swallow.
   f. Asymmetric contraction of facial muscles.
5. Evaluate reflexes.
   a. Gag or cough reflex.
   b. Swallow reflex.
   c. Corneal reflex.

   d. Babinski reflex: normal is negative in adults and children older than 2 years; positive sign is dorsiflexion of the foot and large toe with fanning of the other toes.
   e. Deep tendon reflexes (simple stretch reflex).
6. Assess vital signs and correlate with other data; changes often occur slowly, and the overall trend needs to be evaluated.
   a. Blood pressure and pulse: intracranial problems precipitate changes; systolic blood pressure may increase, and pulse rate may decrease.
   b. Respirations: rate, depth, and rhythm are sensitive indicators of intracranial problems.
      (1) Cheyne-Stokes respiration: periodic breathing in which hyperpnea alternates with apnea.
      (2) Neurogenic hyperventilation: regular, rapid, deep breathing.
      (3) Ataxic: completely irregular pattern with random deep and shallow respirations.
   c. Temperature: evaluate changes in temperature as related to neurologic control versus infection.

## DISORDERS OF THE NEUROLOGIC SYSTEM

### Brain Tumors

A. Brain tumors may be primary (originate from tissue within the brain) or secondary (metastasized from other areas of the body).

B. Supratentorial: tumors occurring above the tentorium, primarily the cerebrum.

C. Infratentorial: tumors occurring below the tentorium, primarily in the cerebellum or the brainstem.

D. Regardless of the origin, site, or presence of malignancy, problems of increased intracranial pressure (ICP) occur because of the limited area in the brain to accommodate an increase in the intracranial contents.

## Assessment

A. Risk factors/etiology.
   1. Age: highest incidence in people older than 70 years; common in children younger than 8 years.
   2. Presence of metastatic cancer of the lung or breast.
   3. Family history: gliomas tend to occur in other family members.
   4. Occupation: people who work with high levels of radiation, formaldehyde (pathologists), vinyl chloride (plastics manufacturers), and other chemicals are at increased risk for brain tumors.

B. Clinical manifestations: symptoms correlate with the location and growth rate of the tumor.
   1. Headache.
      a. Recurrent. May vomit on arising and then feel better.
      b. More severe in the morning, affected by position.
      c. Headache in infant may be identified by persistent, irritated crying and head rolling.
   2. Vomiting: with or without nausea; can be projectile.
   3. Papilledema (edema of the optic disc).
   4. Seizures (focal or generalized).
   5. Dizziness and vertigo.
   6. Mental status changes: lethargy and drowsiness, confusion, disorientation, and personality changes.
   7. Localized manifestations.
      a. Focal weakness: hemiparesis.
   8. Sensory disturbances: language, coordination, visual.
   9. Head tilt: child may tilt the head because of damage to extraocular muscles; may be first indication of a decrease in visual acuity.
   10. Changes in vital signs indicative of increasing ICP (Cushing's triad—severe systolic hypertension with widening pulse pressure and bradycardia).
   11. Cranial enlargement in the infant younger than 18 months.

C. Diagnostics (see Appendix 22-1).

## Treatment

A. Medical.
   1. Corticosteroids (see Appendix 9-2).
   2. Antiemetics (Appendix 20-2).
   3. Anticonvulsants (see Appendix 22-2).
   4. Complementary and alternative medicine.

B. Chemotherapy: oral, intravenous (IV), intrathecal, implanted.

C. Radiation: x-rays, gamma knife, stereotactic radiosurgery, brachytherapy.

D. Surgical intervention: craniotomy/craniectomy, biopsy, shunt placement, reservoir placement, laser removal.

## Complications

A. Meningitis, brainstem herniation, diabetes insipidus, and syndrome of inappropriate antidiuretic hormone secretion (SIADH, see Chapter 15).

B. Residual effects may include: seizures, dysarthria, dysphasia, disequilibrium, and permanent brain damage.

## Nursing Interventions

**Goal:** To provide appropriate preoperative nursing interventions.

A. General preoperative care with exceptions, as noted (see Chapter 3).

B. Prepare client and family for appearance of the client after surgery, location of waiting room, contact information.

C. Encourage verbalization regarding concerns about surgery.

D. Skin preparation is usually done in the operating room.

**Goal:** To monitor changes in ICP after craniotomy (Box 22-3).

A. Obtain frequent vital signs, neurologic checks, and cranial nerve assessments.

B. Carefully evaluate level of consciousness; increasing lethargy or irritability may be indicative of increasing ICP.

C. Discourage coughing (elevates intracranial pressure)

**Goal:** To prevent postop complications.

A. Monitor respiratory status.
   1. Monitor breath sounds, respiratory pattern, $O_2$ saturation, arterial blood gases (ABGs) as ordered.
   2. Head of bed (HOB) elevation (unless contraindicated) and turn every 2 hours, have client deep breathe.
   3. Suction as necessary. Suction increases ICP; hyperoxygenate and limit suction to less than 10 seconds.

B. Evaluate dressing.
   1. Location and amount of drainage.
   2. Clarify with surgeon whether the nurse or the surgeon will change dressing.
   3. Evaluate for CSF leak through the incision.

---

### Box 22-3 INCREASING INTRACRANIAL PRESSURE

**Adult**
Early: Restless, irritable, lethargic
Intermediate: unequal pupil response, projectile vomiting, vital signs changes
Late: decreased level of consciousness, decreased reflexes, hypoventilation, dilated pupils, posturing

**Infant/Child**
Early: Poor feeding, tense fontanel, headache, nausea and vomiting, increased pitch of cry, unsteady gait
Intermediate (younger than 18 months): Increased head circumference, altered consciousness, bulging fontanel; shrill cry, severe headache, blurred vision, stiff neck
Late: Same as adult

C. Maintain semi-Fowler's position and monitor for signs and symptoms of meningitis if there is a CSF leak from ears or nose.

D. Postoperative positioning for client who has had infratentorial surgery is as follows:
 1. Bed generally kept flat with gradual HOB elevation (as prescribed).
 2. Position client on either side; avoid supine position.
 3. Maintain head and neck in midline.

E. Keep nothing by mouth (NPO) for 24 hours.

F. Postoperative position for client who has had supratentorial surgery: semi- to low-Fowler's position.

G. Trendelenburg position is contraindicated for clients who have had either infratentorial or supratentorial surgery.

H. Do not position craniectomy patient on the operative side.

I. Maintain fluid and electrolyte balance.
 1. After client is awake and the swallow and gag reflexes have returned, begin offering clear liquids by mouth.
 2. Closely monitor intake and output, electrolytes, and osmolarity levels.

J. Evaluate changes in temperature: may be due to respiratory complications (infection) or to alteration in the function of the hypothalamus.

K. Provide appropriate postoperative pain relief.
 1. Administer short-acting opioids, acetaminophen.
 2. Maintain quiet, dim atmosphere.
 3. Avoid sudden movements.

L. Prevent complications of immobility (see Chapter 3).

M. Maintain seizure precautions (see Appendix 22-3).

### Home Care

See home care for clients with increasing ICP.

## Hydrocephalus

**Hydrocephalus is a condition caused by an imbalance in the production and absorption of CSF in the ventricles of the brain.**

### Classification: Primary

A. Noncommunicating (obstructive): circulation of CSF is blocked within the ventricular system of the brain.

B. Communicating: CSF flows freely within the ventricular system but is not adequately absorbed by arachnoid villi.

### Classification: Secondary

A. Congenital.

B. Acquired—possibly from trauma, infection, or tumor.

### Assessment

A. Risk factors/etiology.
 1. Neonate: usually the result of a congenital malformation.
 2. Older child, adult.
  a. Space-occupying lesion.
  b. Preexisting developmental defects.

B. Clinical manifestations: infant.
 1. Head enlargement: increasing circumference in excess of normal 2 cm per month for first 3 months.
 2. Separation of cranial suture lines.
 3. Fontanel becomes tense and bulging.
 4. Dilated scalp veins.
 5. Frontal enlargement, bulging "sunset eyes."
 6. Symptoms of increasing ICP.

C. Clinical manifestations: older child, adult.
 1. Symptoms of increasing ICP.
 2. Specific manifestations related to site of the lesion.

D. Diagnostics (see Appendix 22-1).
 1. Increasing head circumference is diagnostic in infants.

### Treatment

A. Noncommunicating and communicating: ventriculo-peritoneal shunt; CSF is shunted into the peritoneum.

B. Obstructive: removal of the obstruction (cyst, hematoma, tumor).

### Nursing Interventions

**Goal:** To monitor for the development of increasing ICP.

A. Daily measurement of the frontal–occipital circumference of the head in infants.

B. Assess for symptoms of increasing ICP (see Box 22-3).

C. Infant is often difficult to feed; administer small feedings at frequent intervals because vomiting may be a problem.

**Goal:** To maintain patency of the shunt and monitor ICP after shunt procedure.

A. Position supine, with head turned opposite side up to prevent pressure on the shunt valve and to prevent too-rapid depletion of CSF.

B. Position is not a problem with children who are having a shunt revision; they have not had an increase in ventricular pressure.

C. Monitor for increasing ICP and compare with previous data.

D. Monitor for infection, especially meningitis or encephalitis.

### Home Care

A. Teach parents symptoms of increasing ICP.

B. Have parents participate in care of the shunt before client's discharge.

C. Encourage parents and family to express feelings regarding client's condition.

D. Refer client to appropriate community agencies.

## Reye's Syndrome

**Reye's syndrome is a rare acute illness occurring after a viral illness (frequently after aspirin has been consumed) and results in fatty infiltration of the liver and subsequent liver degeneration and increased ICP.**

A. Damaged liver cells no longer adequately convert ammonia to urea for excretion from the body.

B. Circulating ammonia crosses the blood–brain barrier to produce acute neurologic effects.

*Assessment*

A. Risk factors/etiology.
   1. Most often preceded by an acute viral infection.
   2. Primarily affects children from the age of 6 months to adolescence.
   3. Frequently, the affected child has received salicylate (aspirin) for control of fever during the preceding viral infection.
   4. With warning labels now on aspirin, problem has significantly decreased.
B. Clinical manifestations.
   1. Stage 1.
      a. Initial symptom may be severe persistent vomiting.
      b. Lethargy, listlessness.
   2. Stage 2.
      a. Irritability, disorientation.
      b. Progresses to state of increased ICP with deepening coma and posturing.
C. Diagnostics (see Appendix 22-1).
   1. Definitive diagnosis is a liver biopsy.
   2. Prolonged prothrombin time.
   3. Elevated blood ammonia levels.
   4. Elevated serum aspartate aminotransferase (AST) and alanine aminotransferase (ALT) levels.

*Treatment*

A. Primarily supportive, based on stage of the disease; mechanical ventilation, fluid, and electrolyte balance.
B. Measures to decrease ICP.
C. Early intervention critical to successful treatment.

*Nursing Interventions*

**Goal:** To monitor progress of disease state and maintain homeostasis.

A. IV fluids.
B. Monitor serum electrolytes and liver function studies.
C. Maintain respiratory status; prevent hypoxia.
D. Assess for problems of impaired coagulation.
E. Decrease stress, anxiety: child may not remember events before the critical phase.

**Goal:** To monitor for and implement nursing actions appropriate for increasing ICP.

## Stroke (Brain Attack)

**Stroke, or brain attack, is the disruption of the blood supply to an area of the brain, resulting in tissue necrosis and sudden loss of brain function. Strokes are the leading cause of adult disability in the United States.**

A. Risk factors/etiology (Box 22-4).
B. Transient ischemic attack (TIA).
   1. Brief episode of neurologic dysfunction; usually resolves within 60 minutes.
   2. Considered a warning sign of an impending stroke.
   3. Teach client to seek immediate treatment for any stroke symptoms. Impossible to predict whether symptoms are TIA or stroke. Time is crucial!

---

**Box 22-4 RISK FACTORS ASSOCIATED WITH STROKE**

**Modifiable**
- Smoking
- Obesity
- Increased salt intake
- Sedentary lifestyle
- Increased stress
- Oral contraceptives

**Partially Modifiable**
- Hypertension
- Cardiac valve disease
- Dysrhythmias
- Diabetes mellitus
- Hypercholesterolemia

**Nonmodifiable**
- Gender: increased incidence in men
- Age
- Race: Increased incidence in the African American population
- Hereditary predisposition

---

C. Types of stroke.
   1. Ischemic stroke.
      a. Thrombotic stroke: formation of a clot that results in the narrowing of a vessel lumen and eventual occlusion.
         (1) Associated with hypertension and diabetes (i.e., conditions that accelerate the atherosclerotic process).
         (2) Produces ischemia of the cerebral tissue distal to occlusion and edema to the surrounding areas.
      b. Embolic stroke: occlusion of a cerebral artery by an embolus.
         (1) Common site of origin is the endocardium.
         (2) May affect any age group; associated with atrial fibrillation, endocarditis, and prosthetic cardiac valves.
   2. Hemorrhagic stroke.
      a. Bleeding into brain tissue, subarachnoid space, or ventricles.
      b. Resultant clot compresses brain tissue.
      c. The area of edema resulting from tissue damage may precipitate more damage than the vascular damage itself.
D. Neuromuscular deficits.
   1. Damage to the left side of the brain will result in paralysis of the right side of the body (Figures 22-5 and 22-6).
   2. Both upper and lower extremities of the involved side are weakened or paralyzed.
   3. With a stroke, the client has neurologic deficits related to mobility, sensation, and cognition.

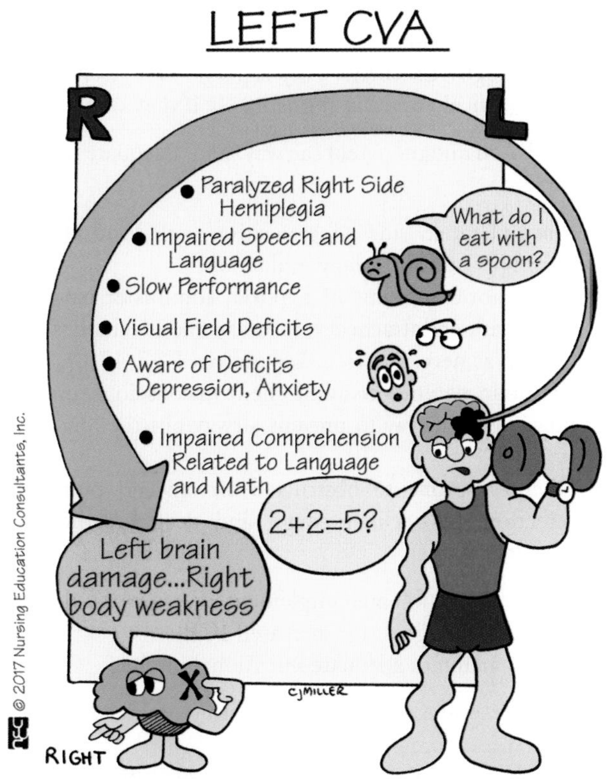

## LEFT CVA

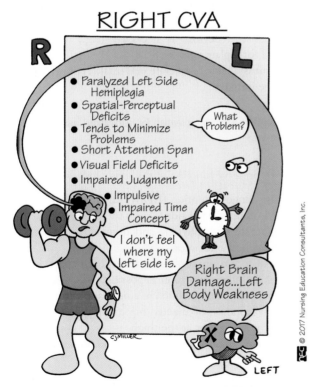

**FIGURE 22-5 Left CVA.** (From Zerwekh, J., Garneau, A., & Miller, C. J. [2017]. *Digital collection of the memory notebooks of nursing* [4th ed.]. Chandler, AZ: Nursing Education Consultants, Inc.)

## RIGHT CVA

**FIGURE 22-6 Right CVA.** (From Zerwekh, J., Garneau, A., & Miller, C. J. [2017]. *Digital collection of the memory notebooks of nursing* [4th ed.]. Chandler, AZ: Nursing Education Consultants, Inc.)

*Assessment*

A. Risk factors/etiology (Box 22-4).

B. Rapid assessment and diagnosis of stroke is critical—time is brain! (Figure 22-7).

   1. Evaluate airway, breathing, circulation (ABCs), neuro assessment, time of symptom onset within 10 minutes on arrival to emergency department.

   2. Noncontrast computed tomography (CT) scan within 25 minutes of arrival (rule out hemorrhagic stroke).

C. Clinical manifestations.

   1. TIA.

      a. Visual defects: blurred vision, diplopia, blindness of one eye, tunnel vision.

      b. Transient hemiparesis, gait problems, ataxia.

      c. Slurred speech, confusion.

      d. Transient numbness of an extremity.

   2. Stroke symptoms may occur suddenly with an embolism, more gradually with hemorrhage or thrombosis; manifestations vary according to which cerebral vessels are involved.

      a. Hemiplegia: loss of voluntary movement; damage to the right side of the brain will result in left-sided weakness and paralysis.

      b. Aphasia: defect in using and interpreting the symbols of language; may include written, printed, or spoken words; most common with left-brain damage.

      c. May be unaware of the affected side; neglect syndrome ensues.

      d. Cranial nerve impairment: chewing, gag reflex, dysphagia, impaired tongue movement, facial droop, ptosis, pupillary changes, abnormal eye movements.

      e. May be incontinent initially.

## FAST RECOGNITION OF A STROKE

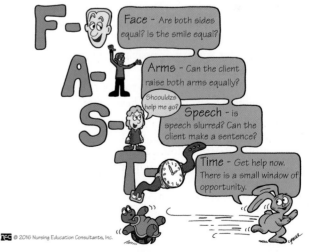

**FIGURE 22-7 FAST Recognition of Stroke.** (From Zerwekh, J., Garneau, A., & Miller, C. J. [2017]. *Digital collection of the memory notebooks of nursing* [4th ed.]. Chandler, AZ: Nursing Education Consultants, Inc.)

f. Agnosia: a perceptual defect that causes a disturbance in interpreting sensory information; client may not be able to recognize previously familiar objects.

g. Cognitive impairment of memory, judgment, proprioception (awareness of one's body position).

h. Hypotonia (flaccidity) for days to weeks, followed by hypertonia (spasticity).

i. Visual defects.
   (1) Homonymous hemianopia: loss of same half of visual field in each eye; client has only half of normal vision.
   (2) Horner's syndrome: ptosis of the upper eyelid, constriction of the pupil, and lack of tearing in the eye.

j. Apraxia: can move the affected limb but is unable to carry out learned movements.

k. Increased ICP, drowsiness to coma.

l. Gait disturbances.

D. Diagnostics (see Appendix 22-1). Client with signs and symptoms suggestive of stroke should have noncontrast CT to rule out hemorrhagic stroke.

### Treatment

Immediate treatment (differs depending on whether thrombotic or hemorrhagic stroke).

A. Prevent stroke.
   1. Aspirin, platelet inhibitors.
   2. Antihypertensives, anticoagulants if appropriate.

B. Ischemic stroke.
   1. IV recombinant tissue activator (tPA) to fibrinolyse clot and reestablish blood flow.
   2. Blood pressure maintained less than 185/110; informed consent.
   3. Monitor neuro status, monitor for bleeding or other complications.
   4. No antiplatelet therapy for 24 to 48 hours following tPA infusion.

C. Hemorrhagic stroke.
   1. Manage blood pressure (if elevated, increased risk of rebleed; if hypotensive decreased cerebral perfusion).
   2. Prepare for surgery—possible craniotomy for aneurysm repair.
   3. Administer nimodipine to reduce risk of vasospasm. Monitor blood pressure, heart rate, and level of consciousness (LOC).

D. Surgical interventions.
   1. Carotid endarterectomy.
   2. Craniotomy for evacuation of hematoma, aneurysm clipping.

E. Specific therapies to resolve physical, speech, or occupational complications, including use of assistive devices.

### Nursing Interventions

**Goal:** To prevent stroke through client education (see Box 22-4).

A. Identification of individuals with reversible risk factors and measures to reduce them.

B. Appropriate medical attention for control of chronic conditions conducive to the development of stroke.

C. Teach high-risk clients early signs of TIA/stroke and to seek medical attention immediately if they occur.

**Goal:** To maintain patent airway and adequate cerebral oxygenation.

A. Place client in side-lying position with head elevated; keep NPO until swallow evaluation.

B. Assess for symptoms of hypoxia; administer oxygen or assist with endotracheal intubation and mechanical ventilation as necessary (see Appendices 17-7, 17-8).

C. Maintain patent airway; if client unconscious, use oropharyngeal airway to prevent airway obstruction by the tongue.

D. Client is prone to obstructed airway and pulmonary infection; have client cough and deep breathe every 2 hours.

**Goal:** To assess for and implement measures to decrease ICP (see nursing goals for increased ICP).

**Goal:** To maintain adequate nutritional intake.

A. Swallow evaluation prior to initiating oral feedings; dysphagia is common after stroke.

B. Administer oral feedings with caution; check for presence of gag and swallowing reflexes before feeding.

C. Place food on the unaffected side of the mouth.

D. Select foods that are easy to control in the mouth (thick liquids) and easy to swallow; thin liquids often promote coughing because client is unable to control them.

E. Maintain high-Fowler's position for feeding.

F. Maintain privacy and unrushed atmosphere.

G. Use assistive devices as necessary (e.g., rocker knife, curved fork, plate guards).

H. If client is unable to tolerate oral intake, enteral feedings may be initiated.

> **TEST ALERT:** Identify potential for aspiration; assess client's ability to eat.

**Goal:** To preserve function of the musculoskeletal system.

A. Passive range of motion (ROM) on affected side; active ROM on unaffected side.

B. Collaborate with physical and occupational therapy to promote best outcomes.

C. Prevent foot drop: passive exercises; high-topped tennis shoes; ambulation as soon as possible.

D. Legs should be maintained in a neutral position; prevent external rotation of affected hip by placing a trochanter roll or rolled pillow at the thigh.

E. Reposition every 2 hours but limit the time spent on the affected side.

> **NURSING PRIORITY:** Protect the client's affected side: do not give injections on that side, watch for pressure areas when positioning, have client spend less time on affected side than in other positions.

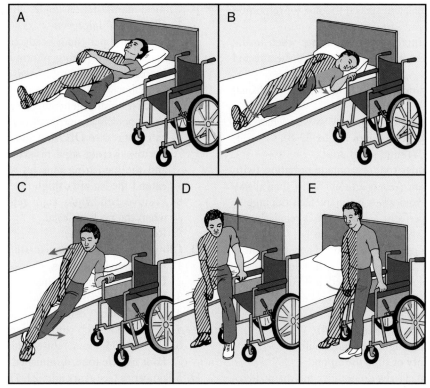

**FIGURE 22-8** **Transfer from Bed to Wheelchair by Client with Hemiplegia.** (From Black, J. M., & Hawks, J. H. [2005]. *Medical-surgical nursing: Clinical management for positive outcomes* [7th ed.]. Philadelphia: Saunders.)

F. Assess for adduction and internal rotation of the affected arm; maintain arm in a neutral (slightly flexed) position with each joint slightly higher than the preceding one.

G. Restraints should be avoided because they often increase agitation.

H. Maintain joints in position of normal function to prevent flexion contractures.

I. Assist client out of bed on the unaffected side; this allows client to provide some stabilization and balance with the good side (Figure 22-8).

> **TEST ALERT:** Mobility: assist client to ambulate, perform active and passive ROM exercises, assess for complications of immobility, prevent deep vein thrombosis (DVT), prevent skin breakdown, and encourage independence.

**Goal:** To maintain homeostasis.

A. Monitor vital signs, cardiac rhythms, heart and lung sounds.

B. Monitor hydration status.
1. Maintain euvolemia; assess skin turgor.
2. Monitor I & O and daily weight.
3. Assess for the development of peripheral edema.

C. Determine previous bowel patterns and promote normal elimination.
1. Avoid use of urinary catheter, if possible; if catheter is necessary, remove as soon as possible.
2. Offer bedpan or urinal every 2 hours; help establish a schedule.

3. Allow client to sit upright (bedside commode or toilet) to facilitate passage of stool.
4. Prevent constipation: provide increased bulk in diet, stool softeners, etc.
5. Provide privacy and decrease emotional trauma related to incontinence.

> **TEST ALERT:** Assess and manage a client with an alteration in elimination. Establish a toileting schedule; the client who has had a stroke will need assistance in reestablishing a normal bowel and bladder routine.

D. Prevent problems of skin breakdown through proper positioning, good skin hygiene, and adequate nutrition.

E. Assist client to identify problems of vision.

F. Maintain psychological homeostasis.
1. Client may be very anxious because of a lack of understanding of what has happened and his or her inability to communicate.
2. Speak slowly and clearly and explain what has happened.
3. Assess client's communication abilities and identify methods to promote communication.

### Home Care

A. Encourage independence in ADLs.

B. Identify clothing that is easy to get in and out of.

C. Active participation in ROM; have client do his or her own ROM on affected side.

D. Physical, occupational, and speech therapy for retraining of lost function.

E. Assist client to maintain sense of balance when in the sitting position; client will frequently fall to the affected side.

F. Encourage participation in carrying out daily personal hygiene.

G. Teach client safe transfer from bed to wheelchair and provide assistance as needed (see Figure 22-8).

H. Bowel and bladder training program.
1. To promote bladder tone, encourage urination (with or without assistance) every 2 hours rather than allowing the client to void when he or she feels the urge.
2. Teach client to perform Kegel exercises regularly.
3. Advise client to avoid caffeine intake.
4. Increased bulk in diet will help avoid constipation.
5. Increase fluids to 2000 mL per day as tolerated.
6. Administer stool softeners as needed (PRN).
7. Establish regular daily time for bowel movements.

I. Encourage social interaction.
1. Speech therapy (see Appendix 22-4).
2. Frequent and meaningful verbal stimuli.
3. Allow client plenty of time to respond.
4. Speak slowly and clearly; do not give too many directions at one time. Use short sentences.
5. Do not "talk down to" client or treat client as a child (elder speak).
6. Client's mental status may be normal; do not assume it is impaired.
7. Nonverbal clients do not lose their hearing ability.

J. Evaluate family support and the need for home health services.

> **TEST ALERT:** Assist family to manage care of a client with long-term care needs; determine needs of family regarding ability to provide home care after discharge.

## Meningitis

**Meningitis is an acute viral or bacterial infection causing inflammation of the meningeal tissue covering the brain and spinal cord.**

A. Bacterial meningitis increases permeability of protective membrane and results in an increased protein concentration in the CSF.

B. Inflammatory process results in the development of cerebral edema.

C. Bacterial meningitis is less common but more severe than viral meningitis.

### Assessment

A. Risk factors/etiology.
1. Pathogenic organism most often gains entry from an infection elsewhere in the body (bacterial, viral, fungal).
2. Meningococcal meningitis is the only form readily contagious; transmitted by direct contact with droplets from the airway of an infected person.

3. Increased mortality rate among infants.

B. Clinical manifestations: older child and adult.
1. Chills and high fever.
2. Severe and persistent headache.
3. Nausea and vomiting, photophobia.
4. Increasing irritability, malaise, changes in level of consciousness, listlessness.
5. Nuchal rigidity, generalized seizures.
6. Rash, petechiae, purpura (meningococcus infection—can progress to DIC and shock.
7. Positive Kernig sign: resistance or pain at the knee and the hamstring muscles when client attempts to extend the leg after thigh flexion.
8. Positive Brudzinski sign: reflex flexion of the hips when the neck is flexed.
9. Respiratory distress.

C. Clinical manifestations: neonate and infant.
1. Fever, apneic episodes.
2. Bulging fontanel, seizures.
3. Crying with position change, irritability.
4. Opisthotonos positioning: a dorsal arched position.
5. Changes in sleep pattern, increasing irritability.
6. Poor sucking; may refuse feedings.
7. Poor muscle tone, diminished movement.

D. Diagnostics (see Appendix 22-1).
1. Lumbar puncture with CSF analysis. If ICP is suspected, a CT scan is done before lumbar puncture to rule out obstructed arachnoid villi causing hydrocephalus; could result in herniation.
2. Elevated white blood cell (WBC) count.
3. CSF and blood cultures positive for bacterial meningitis.

### Treatment

A. Respiratory isolation (droplet precautions) until positive organism is identified.

B. IV antibiotics, possible steroids (see Appendix 9-2).

C. Optimum hydration.

D. Anticonvulsant medications (see Appendix 22-2).

E. Antivirals (see Appendix 10-1).

F. Maintain ventilation.

### Complications

A. Increasing ICP resulting in permanent brain damage.

B. Visual and hearing deficits, paralysis.

### Nursing Interventions

**Goal:** To identify the causative organism, control spread, and initiate therapy.

A. Maintain respiratory droplet precautions until organism is identified; place client in a private room (see Appendix 9-3).

B. Begin administration of IV antibiotics after lumbar puncture and CSF sampling.

C. Identify family members and close contacts who may require prophylactic treatment.

**Goal:** To monitor course of infection and prevent complications.

A. Frequent vital signs, neuro checks, monitor for increased ICP (see Box 22-3).

B. Maintain adequate hydration; monitor I & O, electrolytes.

C. Decrease stimuli in environment: dim lights, quiet environment, no loud noises.

D. Manage pain; analgesia, position of comfort generally side-lying with slight HOB elevation.

E. Seizure precautions. Treat fever; increased fever increases risk of seizure.

F. Monitor vascular status, septic emboli may block circulation in distal extremities.

G. Prevent complications of immobility.

H. Good respiratory hygiene.

## Encephalitis

**Encephalitis is an inflammatory process of the CNS, or "inflammation of the brain."**

### Assessment

A. Risk factors/etiology.
1. Most commonly occurs as a complication after a viral infection (measles, chickenpox, mumps).
2. May be herpes simplex virus in middle-aged adults.
3. May be transmitted by a vector such as a mosquito or tick.

B. Clinical manifestations.
1. Severe headache, nuchal rigidity.
2. Sudden fever, nausea/vomiting.
3. Seizures, irritability.
4. Decreased level of consciousness.
5. Motor involvement: ataxia, dysphasia, tremor, seizures.
6. Drowsiness, confusion, disorientation.
7. Bulging fontanels in infants.

C. Diagnostics.
1. Lumbar puncture and CSF analysis.
2. Viral studies to isolate the virus.
3. Electroencephalogram (EEG) for seizure activity.
4. Blood test for West Nile virus.

### Treatment

A. Anticonvulsants; antivirals
B. Treatment to decrease ICP.
C. Hydration, bed rest, proper nutrition.

### Nursing Interventions

Nursing interventions for encephalitis are the same as those for meningitis, with the exception of antibiotic therapy. Encephalitis is usually caused by a viral agent and is not responsive to antibiotic therapy; antibiotic therapy may be ordered to prevent bacterial infection.

**TEST ALERT:** Identify changes in client's mental status; treat client with seizures.

## Myasthenia Gravis

**Myasthenia gravis (MG) is a sporadic, neuromuscular disease characterized by fatigue and fluctuating muscle weakness. It is most often caused by an autoimmune attack on acetylcholine receptors at the neuromuscular junction. Nerve impulses are not transmitted and muscles do not contract.**

### Assessment

A. Risk factors/etiology.
1. Autoimmune disease; antiacetylcholine antibodies detected in serum of most clients with MG.
2. More common in women than men.
3. Tends to affect women at a younger age than men.

B. Clinical manifestations.
1. Primary problem is fluctuating skeletal muscle weakness and fatigue. Muscular fatigue increases with activity; worse at the end of the day.
   a. Ptosis (drooping of the eyelids) and diplopia (double vision) are frequently the first symptoms. (Ophthalmologist may be first contact regarding dysfunction.)
   b. Impairment of facial mobility and expression.
   c. Impairment of chewing and swallowing.
   d. Speech impairment; voice weakens after long conversations.
   e. No sensory deficit, loss of reflexes, or muscular atrophy.
   f. Poor bowel and bladder control.
2. Course is variable.
   a. May stabilize, short-term remission or severe progression.
   b. Exacerbations may occur; precipitated by stress (physical or emotional).
4. Myasthenic crisis: an acute exacerbation of muscle weakness that may require intubation and mechanical ventilation to support respiratory effort.
   a. Severe respiratory distress and hypoxia.
   b. Increased pulse and blood pressure.
   c. Decreased or absent cough or swallow reflex.
5. Cholinergic crisis: a toxic response to the anticholinesterase medications; anticholinesterase medications must be withheld—this response is rare with proper dosing of pyridostigmine.
   a. Nausea, vomiting, and diarrhea.
   b. Weakness with difficulty in swallowing, chewing, and speaking.
   c. Increased secretions and saliva.
   d. Muscle fasciculation, constricted pupils.

C. Diagnostics (see Appendix 22-1).
1. Electromyography: shows a decreasing response of muscles to stimuli.
2. Tensilon test.
   a. Used for diagnosing MG.
   b. Used to differentiate cholinergic crisis from myasthenic crisis.
   c. IV injection of edrophonium causes immediate, although short-lived, relief of muscle weakness.

### Treatment

A. Anticholinesterase (cholinergic) medications (see Appendix 22-2).
1. Neostigmine.
2. Pyridostigmine.
B. Corticosteroids (see Appendix 9-2).
C. Plasma electrophoresis (plasmapheresis): separation of plasma to remove autoantibodies from the bloodstream.

D. Immunosuppressive therapy.
E. Surgical removal of the thymus (thymectomy).

*Nursing Interventions*

Client may be hospitalized for acute myasthenic crisis, cholinergic crisis, or respiratory tract infection.
**Goal:** To maintain respiratory function.

A. Assess for increasing problems of difficulty breathing. Measure forced vital capacity frequently to assess respiratory status.
B. Determine client's medication schedule.
C. Assess ability to swallow; prevent problems of aspiration.

**TEST ALERT:** Identify clients at high risk for aspiration; do not give the client experiencing a myasthenic crisis anything to eat or drink.

D. Evaluate effectiveness of cough reflex.
E. Be prepared to intubate or provide ventilatory assistance.

**Goal:** To distinguish between a myasthenic crisis and a cholinergic crisis.

A. Maintain adequate ventilatory support during crisis.
B. Assist in administration of Tensilon test to differentiate crisis.
  1. Myasthenic crisis: client's condition will improve.
  2. Cholinergic crisis: client's condition will temporarily worsen.
C. If myasthenic crisis occurs, neostigmine may be administered.
D. If cholinergic crisis occurs, atropine may be administered and cholinergic medications may be reevaluated.
E. Avoid use of sedatives and tranquilizers, can cause respiratory depression.
F. Provide psychological support during crisis.

**Home Care**

A. Teach client importance of taking medication on a regular basis; peak effect of the medication should coincide with mealtimes.
B. If ptosis becomes severe, client may need to wear an eye patch to protect cornea (alternate eye patches if problem is bilateral).
C. Emotional upset, severe fatigue, infections, and exposure to extreme temperatures may precipitate a myasthenic crisis.

**Multiple Sclerosis**

**Multiple sclerosis (MS) is characterized by multiple areas of demyelination from inflammatory scarring of the myelin sheath surrounding neurons in the brain and spinal cord (CNS).**

A. The progression of the disease results in total destruction of the myelin, and the nerve fibers become involved.
  1. Loss of myelin sheath causes decreased impulse conduction, destruction of the nerve axon, and disruption of the impulse conduction.

  2. The demyelination occurs in irregular scattered patches throughout the CNS.
  3. Theories as to cause include autoimmunity and exposure to viruses.
B. Clinical course.
  1. Relapsing-remitting MS: most common initial course, causing sporadic attacks with exacerbations and remissions (partial or complete recovery) lasting days to months.
  2. Primary-progressive MS: client experiences a slow, steady worsening of symptoms without remission. Plateaus of severity may occur, but baseline function progressively worsens.
  3. Secondary-progressive MS: starts with relapsing-remitting course that later becomes steadily progressive.
  4. Progressive-relapsing MS: progressive from the start with relapse (worsening neurologic functioning).

*Assessment*

A. Risk factors/etiology: cause is unknown.
  1. More common in women; onset usually 20 to 50 years of age.
  2. More common in cooler climates.
B. Clinical manifestations (Figure 22-9).
  1. Signs and symptoms vary from person to person, as well as within the same individual, depending on the area of involvement.
  2. Cerebellar dysfunction: tremors, inability to direct movement, clumsy, loss of balance, ataxia, dysarthria (slurred speech), dysphagia (difficulty swallowing).
  3. Motor dysfunction: weakness of eye muscles, nystagmus, weakness or spasticity of muscles in extremities.
  4. Sensory: vertigo, blurred vision, diplopia (double vision), decreased hearing, tinnitus, paresthesias, numbness, tingling.
  5. Bowel and bladder dysfunction.
  6. Sexual dysfunction, impotence.
  7. Psychosocial.
    a. Intellectual functioning remains intact, but short-term memory, attention, information processing may become difficult.
    b. Emotional lability: increased excitability and inappropriate euphoria.
    c. Emotional effects of the chronic illness and changes in body image.
C. Diagnostics: no definitive diagnostic test. MRI may show plaques.

*Treatment*

A. No cure; medical treatment is directed toward slowing of the disease process and relief of symptoms.
B. Medications to decrease edema and inflammation of the nerve sites.
  1. Antiinflammatory agents.
  2. Immunomodulator agents: interferons.
  3. Adrenocorticotropic hormone for acute exacerbations.

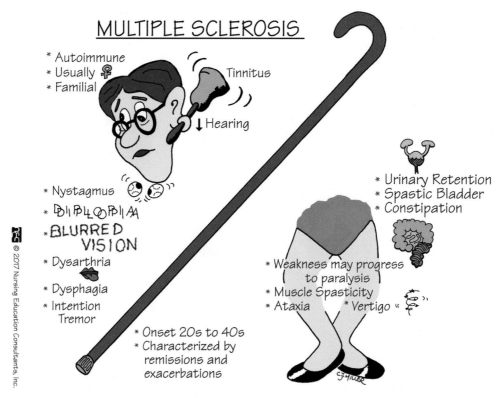

**FIGURE 22-9 Multiple Sclerosis.** (From Zerwekh, J., Garneau, A., & Miller, C. J. [2017]. *Digital collection of the memory notebooks of nursing* [4th ed.]. Chandler, AZ: Nursing Education Consultants, Inc.)

## Nursing Interventions

Client may be hospitalized for diagnostic workup or for treatment of acute exacerbation and complications.

**Goal:** To maintain homeostasis and prevent complications during an acute exacerbation of disease symptoms.

A. Maintain adequate respiratory function.
  1. Prevent respiratory tract infection.
  2. Good pulmonary hygiene.
  3. Prevent aspiration; sitting position for eating.
  4. Evaluate adequacy of cough reflex.
B. Maintain urinary tract function.
  1. Prevent urinary tract infection.
  2. Increase fluid intake, at least 2000 mL/24 hr.
  3. Evaluate voiding: assess for retention and incontinence.
C. Maintain nutrition.
  1. Evaluate coughing and swallowing reflexes.
  2. Provide food that is easy to chew.
  3. If client is experiencing difficulty swallowing, observe client closely during fluid intake.

**Goal:** To prevent complications of immobility (see Chapter 3).
**Goal:** To promote psychological well-being.

A. Focus on remaining capabilities.
B. Encourage independence and assist client to gain control over environment.
C. If impotence is a problem, initiate sexual counseling.
D. Assist client to work through the grieving process.
E. Identify community resources available.

### Home Care

A. Medical regimen and side effects of the medications.
B. Physical therapy to maintain muscle function and decrease spasticity.
C. Measures to maintain voiding; may need to perform self-catheterization.
D. Safety measures because of decreased sensation.
  1. Check bath water temperature.
  2. Wear protective clothing in the winter.
  3. Avoid heating pads and clothing that is constrictive.
E. Client should understand that relapses are frequently associated with an increase in physiologic and psychological stress. Avoid triggers if possible.

**TEST ALERT:** Determine client's ability to care for self; plan with family to assist client to meet self-care needs.

### Guillain-Barré Syndrome

**Guillain-Barré syndrome is an acute, rapidly progressing motor neuropathy involving segmental demyelination of nerve roots in the spinal cord and medulla. Demyelination causes inflammation, leading to edema, nerve root compression, decreased nerve conduction, and rapidly ascending paralysis. Both sensory and motor impairment occur. Recovery typically happens in a proximal-to-distal direction as remyelination occurs.**

A. Risk factors/etiology: cause is unknown; frequently, client has a recent history of acute illness (viral), trauma, immunizations, or surgery.

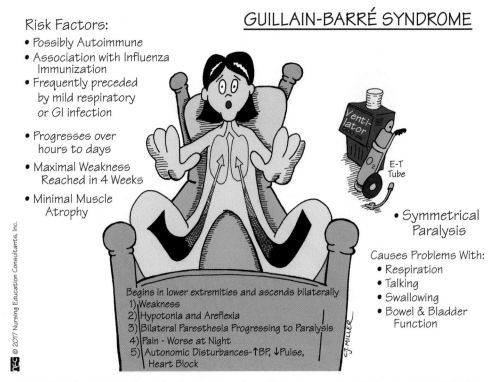

Risk Factors:
- Possibly Autoimmune
- Association with Influenza Immunization
- Frequently preceded by mild respiratory or GI infection

- Progresses over hours to days
- Maximal Weakness Reached in 4 Weeks
- Minimal Muscle Atrophy

# GUILLAIN-BARRÉ SYNDROME

Venti-lator

E-T Tube

- Symmetrical Paralysis

Causes Problems With:
- Respiration
- Talking
- Swallowing
- Bowel & Bladder Function

Begins in lower extremities and ascends bilaterally
1) Weakness
2) Hypotonia and Areflexia
3) Bilateral Paresthesia Progressing to Paralysis
4) Pain - Worse at Night
5) Autonomic Disturbances-↑BP, ↓Pulse, Heart Block

© 2017 Nursing Education Consultants, Inc.

**FIGURE 22-10  Guillain-Barré Syndrome.** (From Zerwekh, J., Garneau, A., & Miller, C. J. [2017]. *Digital collection of the memory notebooks of nursing* [4th ed.]. Chandler, AZ: Nursing Education Consultants, Inc.)

B. Clinical manifestations (Figure 22-10).
  1. Paresthesias and weakness are often first symptoms.
  2. Progressive weakness and paralysis typically begins in the lower extremities and ascends bilaterally. May cause:
    a. Paralysis of respiratory muscles.
    b. Cranial nerve involvement, can cause facial weakness, diplopia, dysphagia, and speech difficulty.
    c. Loss of sensation and function of bowel and bladder.
    d. Blood pressure lability, dysrhythmias.
    e. Decreased or absent deep tendon reflexes.
  3. Manifestations may progress rapidly over hours or may occur over 2 to 4 weeks.
  4. Muscle atrophy is minimal.
  5. Paralysis decreases as the client begins recovery; most often, there are no residual effects.

> **❗ NURSING PRIORITY:** Of the neuromuscular disorders, Guillain-Barré syndrome is the most rapidly developing and progressive condition. It is potentially fatal if unrecognized.

C. Diagnostics (see Appendix 22-1).
  1. Elevated protein concentration in CSF.
  2. Electromyogram (EMG) and nerve conduction studies.

## Treatment (Supportive)

A. Respiratory support, possibly mechanical ventilation.
B. Immunosuppressives and immunoglobulins (IV immunoglobulin G [IVIG]).
C. Plasmapheresis: plasma exchange.

## Nursing Interventions

**Goal:** To evaluate progress of paralysis and initiate actions to prevent complications.

A. Evaluate rate of progress of paralysis; carefully assess changes in respiratory pattern.
B. If ascent of paralysis is rapid, prepare for endotracheal intubation and respiratory assistance.
C. Frequent evaluation of cough and swallow reflexes.
  1. Remain with client while client is eating; have suction equipment available.
  2. Maintain NPO if gag reflex is impaired.
  3. Enteral feedings may be required; gastric emptying is delayed; monitor residual volumes.
D. Prevent complications of immobility during period of paralysis (see Chapter 3).
E. Assess for involvement of the autonomic nervous system.
  1. Orthostatic hypotension.
  2. Hypertension.
  3. Cardiac dysrhythmias.
  4. Urinary retention and paralytic ileus.

**Goal:** To prevent complications of hypoxia if respiratory muscles become involved (see Chapter 17).
**Goal:** To maintain psychological homeostasis.

A. Simple explanation of procedures.
B. Complete recovery is anticipated.
C. Provide psychological support during period of assisted ventilation.
D. Keep client and family aware of progress of disease.

## Amyotrophic Lateral Sclerosis

Amyotrophic lateral sclerosis (ALS), also known as Lou Gehrig's disease, is a progressive, invariably fatal degeneration of motor neurons. Causes are unknown and there is no cure.

### Assessment

A. Clinical manifestations.
   1. Twitching, cramping, fatigue, and muscle weakness may be early symptoms.
   2. May initially complain of "clumsiness."
   3. Dysarthria and dysphagia.
   4. Muscle spasticity, hyperreflexia, fasciculations.
   5. Muscle weakness progresses until all body is involved. Inability to breathe, speak, swallow.
   6. Intellectual functioning and all five senses are usually unaffected.
   7. Death generally from respiratory infection.
B. Diagnostics: electromyography and nerve conduction studies. Muscle biopsy may be performed to rule out other pathologies.

### Treatment

A. Riluzole slows progression; protects motor neurons from degeneration and death.
B. Supportive care.

### Nursing Interventions

**Goal:** To provide ongoing assessment in assisting client to deal with progressive symptoms.

A. Promote independence in ADLs.
   1. Conserve energy; space activities.
   2. Physical, occupational, speech therapy.
   3. Use of support devices to prolong independence in ambulation and ADLs.
B. Promote nutrition.
   1. Small frequent feedings.
   2. Have client sit upright with head slightly flexed forward while eating.
   3. Keep suction equipment easily available during meals.
C. Encourage family and client to talk about losses and the difficult choices they face.
D. Assist family and client to identify need for advanced directives and to complete them.
E. Palliative/hospice care referral.

## Muscular Dystrophy

Muscular dystrophy (MD) is a group of genetic diseases characterized by progressive weakness and skeletal muscle degeneration affecting a variety of muscle groups. The term *pseudohypertrophy* describes the characteristic muscle enlargement (caused by fatty infiltration) occurring in muscular dystrophy.

A. Duchenne muscular dystrophy (DMD) is the most common and most severe form of MD.
B. Condition is characterized by gradual degeneration of muscle fibers and progressive symmetric weakness and wasting of skeletal muscle.

### Assessment

A. Risk factors/etiology.
   1. Genetic: X-linked (recessive trait) disorder primarily affecting males.
   2. Onset generally occurs between the ages of 3 and 5 years.
B. Clinical manifestations.
   1. Normal development first year or two of life, then onset of weakness.
   2. Abnormal waddling gait and lordosis.
   3. Child falls frequently and develops characteristic manner of rising.
   4. Gower's sign: from sitting or squatting position, the child assumes a kneeling position and pushes the torso up by "walking" his or her hands up the thighs.
   5. Progressive muscle weakness, atrophy, and contractures.
      a. Ambulation is frequently impossible by 12 years of age.
      b. Progressive decline in respiratory musculature; death occurs from respiratory tract infection or cardiac failure.
C. Diagnostics.
   1. Electromyography, muscle biopsy.
   2. Serum enzymes: creatinine kinase (CK) level is increased in neonate, then gradually declines.
   3. Genetic testing – dystrophin deficiency.

### Treatment

A. Steroids administered to child older than 4 years of age.

### Nursing Interventions

Child is frequently cared for at home and hospitalized only when complications occur.
**Goal:** To maintain optimal motor function as long as possible.

A. Regular physical therapy for stretching and strengthening muscles; breathing and ROM exercises.
B. Maintain child's independence in ADLs.
C. Assist family to identify resources, adapt physiologic barriers within the home, and promote mobility of the child in a wheelchair.
D. Assist family to identify methods of preventing respiratory tract infection; assess for respiratory problems.
E. Provide braces, splints, and assistive devices as needed.

**Goal:** To assist parents and child to maintain psychological equilibrium and adapt to chronic illness.

A. Assist parents to understand importance of independence and self-help skills; frequently, parents are overprotective of the child.
B. Counseling to assist parents and family members to identify family activities that can be modified to meet child's needs.
C. Mother may feel particularly guilty because of transmission of disease to her son.
D. Identify available community resources.
E. Counseling to assist family and child with chronic illness and child's eventual death.

## Cerebral Palsy

Cerebral palsy (CP) is a group of nonprogressive, lifelong neuromuscular genetic disorders resulting from damaged motor centers of the brain causing nerve impulses to be incorrectly sent and/or received. The overall result is impairment of muscle control with poor muscle coordination.

### Assessment

A. Risk factors/etiology.
  1. Majority (80%) of CP cases linked to prenatal or neonatal brain lesion or brain development/abnormalities.
  2. Prematurity is single most important risk factor for CP, but cause is not identifiable in about 24% of cases.
B. Clinical manifestations.
  1. Delayed achievement of developmental milestones.
  2. Increased or decreased resistance to passive movement.
  3. Abnormal posture.
  4. Presence of infantile reflexes (tonic neck reflex, exaggerated Moro reflex).
  5. Associated disabilities.
     a. Intellectual impairment, seizures.
     b. Attention-deficit problems.
     c. Vision and hearing impairment.
  6. Muscle tightness and spasms.
C. Diagnostics.
  1. Diagnostic tests to rule out other neurologic dysfunction: EEG (if seizures present), magnetic resonance imaging (MRI).
  2. Frequently difficult to diagnose in early months; condition may not be evident until child attempts to sit alone or walk (up to 2 years old).
  3. Gait laboratory analysis: evaluates walking ability.

### Treatment

A. Maintain and promote mobility with orthotic/assistive devices and physical therapy.
B. Skeletal muscle relaxants.
C. Anticonvulsants, as indicated.

### Nursing Interventions

Child is frequently cared for at home and on an outpatient basis unless complications occur.
**Goal:** To assist child to become as independent and self-sufficient as possible.

A. Physical and occupational therapy designed to assist child to gain maximum function.
B. Assist child to progress according to developmental level and functional abilities; encourage crawling, sitting, and balancing appropriate to developmental level.
C. Assist child to carry out ADLs as age and capacities permit.
D. Speech therapy, as indicated.
E. Encourage play appropriate for age.
F. Encourage appropriate educational activities.
G. Bowel and bladder training may be difficult because of poor control.

**Goal:** To maintain physiologic homeostasis.

A. Maintain adequate nutrition.
  1. May experience difficulty eating because of spasticity; may drool excessively; use of manual jaw control when feeding.
  2. Encourage independence in eating and use of self-help devices.
  3. Provide a balanced diet with increased caloric intake to meet extra energy demands.
B. Maintain safety precautions to prevent injury.
C. Increased susceptibility to infections, especially respiratory tract infections because of poor control of intercostal muscles and diaphragm.
D. Increased incidence of dental problems; schedule frequent dental checkups.

**Goal:** To promote a positive self-image in the child and provide support to the family.

A. Use positive reinforcement frequently.
B. Assist parents to set realistic goals.
C. Encourage recreation and educational activities, especially those involving other children with cerebral palsy.
D. Encourage child to express feelings regarding the disorder.
E. Do not "talk down" to child; communicate at appropriate developmental level.
F. Assist parents in problem solving in home environment.
G. Identify available community resources.
H. Utilize principles in caring for chronically ill pediatric client (see Chapter 2).

## Parkinson Disease

Parkinson disease is a progressive neurodegenerative disorder with gradual onset that causes destruction and degeneration of dopamine-releasing nerve cells in the basal ganglia; results in damage to the extrapyramidal system, causing difficulty controlling or initiating voluntary movement.

### Assessment

A. Risk factors/etiology.
  1. More common in men.
  2. Exact cause unknown; genetic and environmental factors play a role.
B. Clinical manifestations (Figure 22-11).
  1. Tremor.
     a. Affects the arms and hands bilaterally; often the first sign.
     b. Tremors usually occur at rest; tremors during voluntary movement are not as common.
     c. Described as "pill-rolling" tremor.
     d. Exacerbated by emotional stress and increased concentration.
  2. Muscle rigidity.
     a. Increased resistance to passive movement.
     b. Movement may be described as "cog-wheel rigidity" because of jerky movement of extremities.

# PARKINSON'S DISEASE

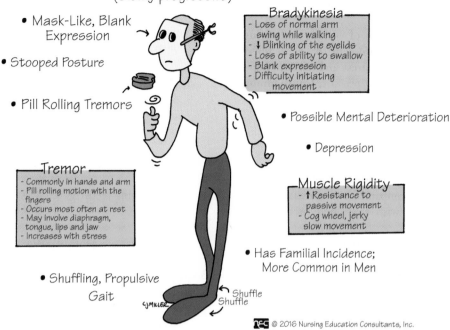

• Onset usually gradual, after age 50.
(Slowly progressive)

• Mask-Like, Blank Expression

• Stooped Posture

• Pill Rolling Tremors

**Bradykinesia**
- Loss of normal arm swing while walking
- ↓ Blinking of the eyelids
- Loss of ability to swallow
- Blank expression
- Difficulty initiating movement

• Possible Mental Deterioration

• Depression

**Tremor**
- Commonly in hands and arm
- Pill rolling motion with the fingers
- Occurs most often at rest
- May involve diaphragm, tongue, lips and jaw
- Increases with stress

**Muscle Rigidity**
- ↑ Resistance to passive movement
- Cog wheel, jerky slow movement

• Has Familial Incidence; More Common in Men

• Shuffling, Propulsive Gait

Shuffle
Shuffle

© 2016 Nursing Education Consultants, Inc.

**FIGURE 22-11 Parkinson's disease.** (From Zerwekh, J., Garneau, A., & Miller, C. J. [2017]. *Digital collection of the memory notebooks of nursing* [4th ed.]. Chandler, AZ: Nursing Education Consultants, Inc.)

3. Bradykinesia: slow movement.
   a. Decreased blinking of the eyelids.
   b. Loss of ability to swallow saliva.
   c. Facial expression is blank or "masklike."
   d. Loss of normal arm swing while walking.
   e. Difficulty initiating movement.
4. Stooped posture, shuffling propulsive gait.
5. May develop dementia as the disease progresses.
6. Mood swings, depression.
C. Diagnostics: no specific diagnostic test.

## Treatment

A. Medication to enhance dopamine secretion (see Appendix 22-2).
B. Anticholinergic medications to decrease effects of acetylcholine (see Appendix 22-2).
C. Clients frequently become tolerant to medications and require adjustments in types of medications and medication schedules.
D. Physical/occupational therapy
E. Surgical therapy: aim is to decrease symptoms.
   1. Ablation (destruction of tissue).
   2. Deep brain stimulation (DBS).

## Nursing Interventions

**Goal:** To maintain homeostasis.

A. Encourage independence in ADLs with use of assistive devices.

B. Maintain nutrition.
   1. Increase calories and protein; provide more easily chewed foods.
   2. Frequent small meals.
   3. Allow ample time for eating.
   4. Monitor weight loss.
   5. Provide pleasant atmosphere at mealtime; client frequently prefers to eat alone because of difficulty swallowing and inability to control saliva.
   6. Increase fluid intake with increased bulk in the diet to decrease problem with constipation.
C. Maintain muscle function.
   1. Full ROM to extremities to prevent contracture.
   2. Decrease effects of tremors.
   3. Exercise and stretch daily.
   4. Physical therapy, as indicated.
D. Closely monitor response to or changes in response to medications.

**TEST ALERT:** Identify situations that necessitate role changes; evaluate family involvement in health care; review necessary modifications to promote home safety.

**Goal:** To promote a positive self-image.

A. Encourage diversional activities.
B. Assist client to set realistic goals.
C. Explore reasons for depression; encourage client to discuss changes occurring in lifestyle.

D. Assist client in gaining control of ADLs and environment.

E. Assist client to identify and avoid activities that increase frustration levels.

F. Encourage good personal hygiene.

## Headache

**Headache is a common symptom of various underlying pathologic conditions in which pain-sensitive nerve fibers respond to unacceptable levels of stress and tension, muscular contraction in the upper body, pressure from a tumor, or increased ICP.**

### Assessment

A. Types of headaches.
   1. Tension headache: most common of all headaches; feeling of tightness like a band around the head; onset is gradual; may be accompanied by sensitivity to light or sound; associated with stress and premenstrual syndrome.
   2. Migraine: intracranial vessels spasm in response to a trigger. Leads to intense, throbbing pain that may begin in the eye area. Prostaglandin and other chemical mediators increase pain. May or may not have aura and visual disturbances. May have nausea, vomiting, photophobia—migraines can be seriously debilitating.
   3. Cluster headache: rare headache that is more common in men; occurs in numerous episodes or clusters; no aura; unilateral severe, nonthrobbing pain. Felt in and around eye, may radiate to temple, forehead, cheek. Often occurs at same time of day.

### Treatment

A. Migraine: sumatriptan; dihydroergotamine mesylate.

B. Nonsteroidal antiinflammatory drugs; acetaminophen.

C. Relaxation, yoga, stress management.

D. Cluster headaches may be treated with high flow oxygen.

### Nursing Interventions

A. Prevention: recognize triggers, decrease stress, adjust medications during menstrual cycle.

B. Headache can be an indicator of a serious neurologic problem. Watch for change in LOC or other indicators of increasing intracranial pressure.

C. Encourage client to keep a "headache diary" for best management and treatment.

## Trigeminal Neuralgia

**Trigeminal neuralgia is a fleeting unilateral sensory disturbance of cranial nerve V, causing recurrent stabbing, paroxysmal pain and facial spasm; also known as tic douloureux.**

### Assessment

A. Risk factors/etiology.
   1. Occurs more often in women and people after age 50.
   2. Can be caused by compression leading to injury of cranial nerve V.

B. Clinical manifestations.
   1. Abrupt onset of paroxysmal intense pain in the lower and upper jaw, cheek, forehead, and lips.
      a. Tearing of the eyes and frequent blinking.
      b. Facial twitching and grimacing.
      c. Pain is usually brief; ends as abruptly as it begins.
      d. Pain may be described as severe, stabbing, and shocklike.
   2. Recurrence of pain is unpredictable.
   3. Pain is initiated by cutaneous stimulation of the affected nerve area.
      a. Chewing.
      b. Washing the face.
      c. Extremes of temperature: either on the face or in food.
      d. Brushing teeth.

### Treatment

A. Medical management of pain (see Appendix 22-2): carbamazepine and gabapentin.

B. Surgical intervention.
   1. Local nerve block.
   2. Surgical intervention to interrupt nerve impulse transmission.
      a. Percutaneous radiofrequency rhizotomy—destroys some of the nerve fibers; assists to manage pain.
      b. Microvascular decompression (craniotomy) to relieve pain and preserve facial sensation.
      c. Acupuncture may alleviate pain.

### Nursing Interventions

**Goal:** To control pain.

A. Assess the nature of a painful attack.

B. Identify triggering factors; adjust environment to decrease factors.
   1. Keep room at an even, comfortable temperature.
   2. Avoid touching client or jarring the bed.
   3. Allow client to carry out own ADLs as necessary.

C. Administer analgesics to decrease pain.

> ⚠ **NURSING PRIORITY:** Because of the severe pain caused by the condition, clients are susceptible to severe depression and suicide.

**Goal:** To maintain nutrition.

A. Frequently, client does not eat because of reluctance to stimulate the pain.

B. Provide lukewarm food that can be easily chewed.

C. Increase protein and calories.

### Home Care

A. Identify presence of corneal reflex; provide protective eye care if reflex is absent.

B. If there is loss of sensation to the side of the face, client should:
1. Chew on the unaffected side.
2. Avoid temperature extremes in foods.
3. Check the mouth after eating to remove remaining particles of food.
4. Maintain meticulous oral hygiene.
5. Have frequent dental checkups.

## Bell Palsy (Facial Paralysis)

**Bell palsy is a transient cranial nerve disorder affecting the facial nerve (cranial nerve VII). Inflammation of CN VII causes a disruption of the motor branches on one side of the face, resulting in muscle weakness or flaccidity on the affected side.**

### Assessment
A. Clinical manifestations.
1. Lag or inability to close eyelid on affected side.
2. Drooping of the mouth, drooling, decreased taste sensation.
3. Facial drooping, flattened nasolabial fold.
4. Tinnitus.
B. Diagnostics: EMG (see Appendix 22-1).

### Treatment
A. Corticosteroids: administration should be started immediately after symptoms arise.
B. Moist heat, massage.

### Nursing Interventions
**Goal:** To assess nerve function and prevent complications.

A. Analgesics to decrease pain.
B. Evaluate ability of client to eat.
C. Meticulous oral hygiene.
D. Prevent drying of the cornea on the affected side.
1. Instill methylcellulose drops frequently during the day.
2. Ophthalmic ointment and eye patches may be required at night.
E. As function returns, active facial exercises may be performed.

**Goal:** To assist client to maintain a positive self-image.

A. Changes in physical appearance may be dramatic.
B. Tell client that the condition is usually self-limiting with minimal, if any, residual effects.
C. Client may require counseling if change in facial appearance is permanent.

## Epilepsy

**Epilepsy is a disease marked by a continuing predisposition to recurrent seizures, with neurobiologic, cognitive, psychologic, and social consequences. Incidence is higher in young children and older adults. A seizure is a paroxysmal, uncontrolled electrical discharge of neurons in the brain that interrupts normal function.**

---

**Box 22-5   Classification of Seizures**

**Simple Focal Seizures (Remains Conscious Throughout Seizure)**
• Rarely last longer than 1 minute.
• Confined to a specific area (hand, arm, leg); client may experience unusual sensations.
• Client may experience unusual feelings: anger, sadness, joy and/or see, hear, taste, or smell things that are not real.

**Complex Focal Seizures (May Have Loss of Consciousness)**
• May lose consciousness for 1 to 3 minutes.
• May produce automatisms (lip smacking, grimacing, repetitive hand movements).
• Client may be unaware of environment and wonder what is happening at the beginning of the seizure.
• In the period after the seizure, client may experience amnesia and confusion.

**Generalized Seizures (Bilaterally Symmetric and Without Local Onset)**
• No warning or aura, as client loses consciousness for a few seconds to several minutes.
• Absence (formally called petit mal): Characterized by a short period when the client is in an altered level of consciousness. Staring, blinking period (followed by resumption of normal activity) is characteristic. May occur more than 100 times per day; may go unnoticed; in general, onset is in childhood between the ages of 4 and 12 years; rarely continues past adolescence.
• Tonic–clonic seizures: May last 2 to 5 minutes. Full recovery may take several hours; client may be confused, amnesic, and irritable during this recovery period.
  • *Tonic Phase:* Loss of consciousness with stiffening and rigidity of muscles. Apnea and cyanosis are common during this period; phase generally lasts for about 1 minute.
  • *Clonic Phase:* Hyperventilation, with rapid jerking movements. Tongue biting, incontinence, and heavy salivation may occur during this period (Figure 22-11).

---

### Assessment
A. Risk factors/etiology for seizure disorder.
1. Birth to age 6 mo: severe brain injury, congenital CNS defects, infection (febrile seizure), inborn errors of metabolism.
2. Age 2 to 20: birth injury, trauma, infection, genetic factors.
3. Age 20 to 30: vascular disease, brain tumors, trauma.
4. After age 50: stroke, metastatic brain tumors.
B. Types of seizures (Box 22-5; Figure 22-12).
C. Clinical manifestations.
1. Prodromal phase: sensations or behaviors that precede a seizure.
2. Aural phase: sensory warning that is similar each time a seizure occurs.
3. Ictal phase: first symptoms to end of seizure activity.
4. Postictal phase: recovery period.
D. Complications: status epilepticus (continuous seizure activity)—it is a neurologic emergency!
E. Diagnostics: EEG, CT scan, MRI.

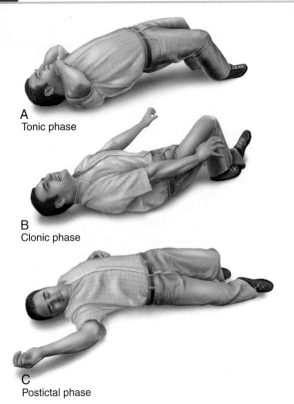

A
Tonic phase

B
Clonic phase

C
Postictal phase

**FIGURE 22-12 Tonic–Clonic Seizure Activity.** (From Black, J. M., & Hawks, J. H. [2009]. *Medical-surgical nursing: Clinical management for positive outcomes* [8th ed.]. Philadelphia: Saunders.)

### Treatment

A. Antiepileptic medication.
B. Surgery for clients unresponsive to drug therapy.

### Nursing Interventions

**Goal:** To protect client from injury (seizure precautions).

A. Monitor client's compliance with taking antiepileptic medications as prescribed.
B. Make environment safe by removing potentially unsafe objects.
C. Keep suction, bag-valve-mask resuscitator, and airway equipment at bedside.
D. Pad side rails to prevent injury during seizures.

**Goal:** To assess client during seizure.

A. Identify any activities that occurred immediately before the seizure.
B. Was the client aware a seizure was going to occur? If so, how did client know?
C. Describe type of movements that occurred and the body area affected (e.g., jaw clenched, tongue biting).
D. Presence of incontinence.
E. Period of apnea and cyanosis.
F. Presence of automatisms (lip smacking, grimacing, chewing).
G. Duration of seizure.
H. Changes in level of consciousness.
I. Condition of client after seizure: oriented, level of activity, any residual paralysis or muscle weakness.

**TEST ALERT:** Report characteristics of a client's seizure; determine changes in client's neurologic status.

**Goal:** To maintain patent airway and protect client during seizure.

A. Remain with the client who is having a seizure; note the time the seizure began and how long it lasted.
B. Turn client to the side to protect airway.
C. Do not attempt to force anything into the client's mouth if the jaws are clenched shut.
D. If the jaws are not clenched, place an airway in the client's mouth. This protects the tongue and also provides a method of suctioning the airway should the client vomit.
E. Protect the client from injury (risk for falling out of bed or striking self on bedrails, etc.).
F. Loosen any constrictive clothing.
G. Do not restrain client during seizure activity; allow seizure movements to occur, but protect client from injury.
H. Evaluate respiratory status; if vomiting occurs, be prepared to suction the client to clear the airway and prevent aspiration.
I. Maintain calm atmosphere and provide for privacy after the seizure activity.
J. Reorient client.

**❗ NURSING PRIORITY:** Airway management and ventilation cannot be performed on a client who is experiencing a tonic–clonic seizure. After the seizure is over, evaluate the airway and initiate ventilations as necessary.

### Home Care

A. Identify activities/events that precipitate the seizure activity.
B. Avoid alcohol intake, fatigue, and loss of sleep.
C. Take medications as directed.
D. Counseling for the family and for the client to assist them in maintaining positive coping mechanisms.
E. Wear medical alert bracelet or have identification card.

## CRITICAL CARE NURSING

### PRIORITY CONCEPTS

Functional Ability, Intracranial Regulation, Safety

 **Increased Intracranial Pressure**

**An increase in ICP occurs when there is an increase in the size or amount of intracranial contents.**

A. The cranial vault is rigid, and there is minimal room for expansion of the intracranial components. The components are brain tissue, blood, and cerebral spinal fluid.

B. An increase in any one of the components necessitates a reciprocal change in other cranial contents; this frequently results in ischemia of brain tissue. An increase in ICP results from one of the following:
   1. Increased intracranial blood volume (vasodilation).
   2. Increased CSF.
   3. Increase in the bulk of the brain tissue (edema).
C. Types of cerebral edema.
   1. Vasogenic edema occurs when there is disruption to the blood–brain barrier allowing protein-rich fluid to leak into the extracellular space causing an increase in the volume of brain tissue. Vasogenic edema is most often the cause of increased ICP in adults.
   2. Cytotoxic (cellular) edema occurs due to disruption of the cell membrane allowing fluid to move into cells (intracellular) with a decrease in extracellular fluid. The result is cerebral hypoxia and death of cells.
   3. Interstitial edema occurs when CSF builds up due to an increase in CSF production or decrease in CSF absorption.
D. Poor ventilation will precipitate respiratory acidosis, or an increase in the $Paco_2$.
   1. Carbon dioxide has a vasodilating effect on the cerebral arteries, which increases cerebrovascular blood flow and increases ICP.
   2. Clients should be ventilated to a normocapnic state to prevent cyclic vasodilation.
E. Regardless of the cause, increased ICP will result in progressive neurologic deterioration; the specific deficiencies seen are determined by the area and extent of compression of brain tissue.
F. If the infant's cranial suture lines are open, increased ICP will cause separation of the suture lines and an increase in the circumference of the head.

> **!! NURSING PRIORITY:** There is no single set of symptoms for all clients with increased ICP; symptoms depend on the cause and on how rapidly increased ICP develops. Vigilant assessment of the client is required!

### Assessment

A. Risk factors/etiology.
   1. Cerebral edema caused by some untoward event or trauma, including toxic exposure, blunt trauma, fluid and electrolyte imbalance.
   2. Brain tumors.
   3. Intracranial hemorrhage caused by intracerebral, epidural, or subdural bleeding (closed head injuries or ruptured blood vessels).
   4. Subarachnoid hemorrhage, hydrocephalus.
   5. Cerebral embolism, resulting in necrosis and edema of areas supplied by the involved vessel.
   6. Cerebral thrombosis, resulting in ischemia of the area and leading to edema and congestion of affected area.
   7. Encephalitis/meningitis.

# INCREASED INTRACRANIAL PRESSURE

- Changes in LOC
  - Flattening of Affect
  - ↓ Orientation & Attention
  - Coma
- Eyes
  - Papilledema
  - Pupillary Changes
  - Impaired Eye Movement
- Posturing
  - Decerebrate
  - Decorticate
  - Flaccid
- Decreased Motor Function
  - Change in Motor Ability
  - Posturing
- Headache
- Seizures
  - Impaired Sensory & Motor Function
- Changes in Vital Signs: Cushing's Triad
  - ↑ Systolic BP "Widening Pulse Pressure"
  - ↓ Pulse
  - Irregular Resp Pattern
- Vomiting
  - Not Preceded by Nausea
  - May be Projectile
- Changes in Speech
- Infants: ○ Bulging Fontanels
  - ○ Cranial Suture Separation
  - ○ ↑ Head Circumference
  - ○ High Pitched Cry

© 2018 Nursing Education Consultants, Inc.

**FIGURE 22-13 Increased Intracranial Pressure.** (From Zerwekh, J., Garneau, A., & Miller, C. J. [2017]. *Digital collection of the memory notebooks of nursing* [4th ed.]. Chandler, AZ: Nursing Education Consultants, Inc.)

B. Clinical manifestations (bedside neurologic checks) (Figure 22-13).

> **TEST ALERT:** Determine change in a client's neurologic status. Be able to rapidly evaluate the client and recognize incremental changes in the neurologic signs that indicate an increase in ICP (see Box 22-3).

   1. Assess for *changes* in level of consciousness because change is the cardinal indicator of increased intracranial pressure.
      a. Any alteration in level of consciousness (early sign for both adults and children)—irritability, restlessness, confusion, lethargy, and difficulty in arousing—may be significant.

> **!! NURSING PRIORITY:** The first sign of a change in the level of ICP is a change in level of consciousness; this may progress to a decrease in level of consciousness.

      b. Inappropriate verbal and motor response; delayed or sluggish responses.
      c. As the client loses consciousness, hearing is the last sense to be lost.
   2. Changes in vital signs.
      a. Increase in systolic blood pressure with a widening pulse pressure.
      b. Decrease in pulse rate.
      c. Alteration in respiratory pattern (Cheyne-Stokes respiration, hyperventilation).
      d. Assess temperature with regard to overall problems; temperature usually increases.

> ⚠ **NURSING PRIORITY:** Cushing's triad: increasing systolic pressure, with widening pulse pressure, decreased pulse rate, and altered respirations. Increased ICP is well established when this occurs. It is considered a neurologic emergency!

3. Pupillary response: normal pupils should be round, midline, equal in size, and equally briskly reactive to light and should accommodate to distance. Abnormal findings include:
   a. Ipsilateral: pupillary changes occurring on the same side as a cerebral lesion.
   b. Contralateral: pupillary changes occurring on the side opposite a cerebral lesion.
   c. Unilateral dilation of pupils.
   d. Sluggish or no pupillary response to light and poor or absent accommodation.
4. Motor and sensory function: normal is indicated by the ability to move all extremities with equal strength. Abnormal findings include:
   a. Unilateral or bilateral weakness or paralysis.
   b. Failure to withdraw from painful stimuli.
   c. Posturing: decorticate, decerebrate, flaccid, or opisthotonos.
   d. Seizure activity, ataxia.
5. Headache.
   a. Constant with increasing intensity.
   b. Exacerbated by movement.
   c. Photophobia.
6. Vomiting: projectile vomiting without prior nausea.
7. Infants.
   a. Tense, bulging fontanel(s).
   b. Separated cranial sutures.
   c. Increasing frontal-occipital circumference.
   d. High-pitched cry.
C. Diagnostics (see Appendix 22-1).
   1. Direct measurement of ICP using a specialized catheter or fiberoptic cable placed into a lateral ventricle, subarachnoid, subdural, or epidural space, or within brain tissue.
   2. Romberg test: measures balance. Client stands with feet together and arms at side, first with eyes open, then with eyes closed for 20 to 30 seconds.
   3. Caloric testing: test is performed at bedside by introducing cold water into the external auditory canal. If the eighth cranial nerve is stimulated, nystagmus rotates toward the irrigated ear. If no nystagmus occurs, a pathologic condition is present.
   4. Doll's eye reflex (oculocephalic reflex).
      a. Doll's eye reflex is normal when the client's head is moved from side to side and the eyes move in the direction of head movement.
      b. Doll's eye reflex is abnormal when the client's eyes remain in a fixed, midline position when the head is turned from side to side (possible brainstem involvement).
      c. Contraindicated until risk for spinal cord injury is ruled out.

5. Papilledema: edema of the optic nerve; observed by examining retina area with an ophthalmoscope.
6. Lumbar puncture is generally not performed; decrease in CSF pressure could precipitate herniation of the brainstem.

## Treatment

A. Treatment of the underlying cause of increasing pressure.
B. Neurologic checks every hour or as ordered.
   1. May involve correlation of several variables including level of consciousness, vital signs, speech, facial symmetry, grasp strength, leg strength, and pupil responses.
   2. Careful comparison to previous assessment is critical to detect incremental changes.
C. IV and oral fluids to maintain normal fluid volume status if mean arterial pressure (MAP) is low to normal. Often, normal saline solution is fluid of choice; 5% dextrose in water potentiates cerebral edema.
D. Medications.
   1. Osmotic diuretic, hypertonic saline.
   2. Corticosteroids (vasogenic edema).
   3. Anticonvulsants, antihypertensives.
E. Maintain adequate ventilation; prevent hypoxia and hypercapnia.
F. Placement of ventriculostomy drain or ventriculoperitoneal shunt.

## Complications

A. CSF leaks, especially in client with basilar skull fracture, risk for meningitis.
B. Herniation: shifting of the intracranial contents from one compartment to another; involves herniation through the tentorium cerebelli; affects area for control of vital functions.
C. Permanent brain damage or death.

## Nursing Interventions

**Goal:** To identify and decrease problem of increased ICP.

A. Neurologic checks, as indicated by client's status (Tables 22-3 and 22-4).
B. Maintain head of bed in semi-Fowler's position (15 to 30 degrees) to promote venous drainage and respiratory function.

> **TEST ALERT:** Change client's position. If the client with increased ICP develops hypovolemic shock, do not place client in Trendelenburg position.

C. Change client's position slowly; avoid extreme hip flexion and extreme rotation or flexion of neck. Maintain the head and spinal column in midline position.
D. Monitor urine osmolarity and specific gravity.
E. Evaluate intake and output.
   1. In response to diuretics.

### Table 22-3   GLASGOW COMA SCALE (GCS)

| Category of Response | Appropriate Stimulus | Response | Score |
|---|---|---|---|
| Eyes open | Approach bedside<br>Verbal command<br>Pain | Spontaneous response<br>Opening of eyes to name or command<br>Lack of opening of eyes to previous stimuli but opening to pain<br>Lack of opening of eyes to any stimulus<br>Untestable | 4<br>3<br>2<br>1<br>U |
| Best verbal response | Verbal questioning with maximum arousal | Appropriate orientation; conversant; correct identification of self, place, year, and month<br>Confusion; conversant but disorientated in one or more spheres<br>Inappropriate or disorganized use of words (e.g., cursing), lack of sustained conversation<br>Incomprehensible words, sounds (e.g., moaning)<br>Lack of sound, even with painful stimuli<br>Untestable | 5<br>4<br>3<br>2<br>1<br>U |
| Best motor response | Verbal command (e.g., "raise your arm, hold up two fingers")<br>Pain: (pressure on proximal nail bed – peripheral; trapezius pinch – central) | Obedience in response to command<br>Localization of pain, lack of obedience but presence of attempts to remove offending stimulus<br>Flexion withdrawal,[a] flexion of arm in response to pain without abnormal flexion posture<br>Abnormal flexion, flexing of arm at elbow and pronation, making a fist<br>Abnormal extension, extension of arm at elbow, usually with adduction and internal rotation of arm at shoulder<br>Lack of response<br>Untestable | 6<br>5<br>4<br>3<br>2<br>1<br>U |

[a]Added to the original scale by many centers.
From Lewis, S. L. et al. (2017). *Medical-surgical nursing: Assessment and management of clinical problems* (10th ed.). St. Louis, MO: Elsevier.

### Table 22-4   MODIFIED GLASGOW COMA SCORE FOR PEDIATRIC CLIENTS

| Activity | Score | Infant's Best Response | Children (4 years or older) |
|---|---|---|---|
| Eyes opening | 4<br>3<br>2<br>1 | Spontaneous<br>To speech<br>To pain<br>No response | Spontaneous<br>To speech<br>To pain<br>No response |
| Verbal response | 5<br>4<br>3<br>2<br>1 | Coos, babbles<br>Irritable cry<br>Cries in response to pain<br>Moans in response to pain<br>No response | Oriented; smiles, interacts, follows objects<br>Confused, disoriented, uncooperative<br>Inappropriate words, persistent cries, inconsolable, inconsistent awareness of environment<br>Incomprehensible sounds, agitated, restless, unaware of environment<br>No response |
| Motor response | 6<br>5<br>4<br>3<br>2<br>1 | Normal spontaneous movements<br>Withdraws from touch<br>Withdraws from pain<br>Abnormal flexion<br>Abnormal extension<br>No response | Normal spontaneous movements<br>Localizes pain<br>Withdraws from pain<br>Abnormal flexion<br>Abnormal extension<br>No response |

2. As correlated with changes in daily weight.
3. For complications of diabetes insipidus (see Chapter 15).
F. Suction only as necessary.
G. Sedatives and narcotics can depress respiration; use with caution because they mask symptoms of increasing ICP.

H. Client should avoid strenuous coughing, Valsalva maneuver, and isometric muscle exercises.
I. Avoid straining with stools (increases intrathoracic pressure sporadically).
J. In infants, measure frontal-occipital circumference to evaluate increase in size of the head.
K. Control hyperthermia.

**Goal:** To maintain respiratory function.

> **⚠ NURSING PRIORITY:** An obstructed airway is one of the most common problems in an unconscious client; position to maintain patent airway or use airway adjuncts.

A. Prevent respiratory problems of immobility.
B. Evaluate patency of airway frequently; as level of consciousness decreases, client is at increased risk for accumulating secretions and airway obstruction by the tongue.
C. Monitor $O_2$ saturation, ABGs; maintain $Paco_2$ levels as prescribed.
D. Maintain airway; suction only when needed. Limit suction to less than 10 seconds for adults; hyperoxygenate pre- and postsuctioning.
E. Client may require intubation and respiratory support from a ventilator (see Appendixes 17-7 and 17-8).

**Goal:** To protect client from injury.

A. Maintain seizure precautions (see Appendix 22-3).
B. Restrain client only if absolutely necessary; struggling against restraints increases ICP.
C. Do not clean the ears or nasal passages of a client with a head injury or a client who has had neurosurgery. Check for evidence of a CSF leak: CSF has glucose in it; test it with a dipstick. CSF also leaves a yellow "halo" stain.
D. Aspiration is a major problem in an unconscious client; place the client in semi-Fowler's position for tube feeding after ensuring correct tube placement.
E. Maintain quiet, nonstimulating environment.
F. Inspect eyes and prevent corneal ulceration.
   1. Protective closing of eyes, if eyes remain open.
   2. Irrigation with normal saline solution or methylcellulose drops to restore moisture.

**Goal:** To maintain psychological equilibrium.

A. Neurologic checks should be done on a continual basis to detect potential problems.
B. Encourage verbalization of fears regarding condition.
C. Give simple explanation of procedures to client and family.
D. Altered states of consciousness will cause increased anxiety and confusion; maintain reality orientation.
E. If client is unconscious, continue to talk to him or her; describe procedures and treatments; always assume client can hear.
F. Assist parents and family to work through feelings of guilt and anger.

**Goal:** To prevent complications of immobility (see Chapter 3).
**Goal:** To maintain elimination.

A. Urinary incontinence: may use condom catheter or indwelling bladder catheter.
B. Keep perineal area clean, prevent excoriation.
C. Monitor bowel function; evaluate for fecal impaction.

> **TEST ALERT:** Notify primary health care provider when client demonstrates signs of potential complications; interpret what data for a client need to be reported immediately.

 **Home Care**

A. Teach client and family signs of increased ICP.
B. Call the provider if any of the following are observed:
   1. Changes in vision.
   2. Increased drainage from incision area or clear drainage in the ears.
   3. Abrupt changes in sleeping patterns or irritability.
   4. Headache not responding to medication.
   5. Changes in coordination, disorientation.
   6. Slurred speech, unusual behavior.
   7. Seizure activity, vomiting.
C. Review care of surgical incision, wounds, or drains.

📋 **Head Injury**

**Head injury is any injury or trauma to the scalp, skull, or brain. Serious head injuries are called *traumatic brain injury* (TBI).**

A. Classification.
   1. Penetrating head injury: dura is pierced, as in stabbing or shooting.
   2. Closed head injury: blunt trauma, acceleration (whiplash), or deceleration (collision); most common head injury in civilian life.
 B. Children and infants are more capable of absorbing direct impact because of the pliability of the skull.
C. Coup–contrecoup injury: damage to the site of impact (coup) and damage on the side opposite the site of impact (contrecoup) when brain "bounces" freely inside skull (Figure 22-14).
D. Primary injury to the brain occurs by compression and/or tearing and shearing stresses on vessels and nerves.
E. Secondary injury occurs from cerebral bleeding, hypoxia, hypotension, ischemia, cerebral edema in response to the primary injury and frequently precipitates an increase in ICP.
F. Types of head injuries (Figure 22-15).
   1. Concussion: most common brain injury; injury (jolt) to brain or body shakes the brain, causing temporary interference in brain function.
      a. Usually from blunt trauma due to contact sports or falls.
      b. May cause brief loss of consciousness, headache, sensitivity to light/noise, difficulty concentrating, sleep difficulties, emotional lability.
      c. Generally short-term, but symptoms may persist for weeks to months: post-concussive syndrome.
   2. Contusion (a bruise on the brain).
      a. Multiple areas of petechial hemorrhages.
      b. Headache, pupillary changes, dizziness, unilateral weakness.
      c. Blood supply is altered in the area of injury; swelling, ischemia, and increased ICP.
      d. May last several hours to weeks.

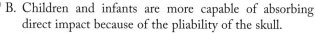

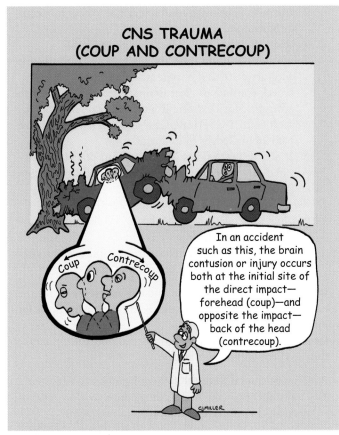

FIGURE 22-14 **CNS Trauma.** (From Zerwekh, J., Claborn, J., & Gaglione, T. [2011]. *Mosby's pathophysiology memory notecards: Visual, mnemonic, and memory aids for nurses* [2nd ed.]. St. Louis, MO: Mosby.)

b. Subdural hematoma: a collection of blood between the dura and arachnoid area filling the brain vault; usually the result of serious head injury.
   (1) May be acute (manifesting in less than 24 hours) or "chronic" (developing over days to weeks).
   (2) When neurologic compromise presents, subdural hematoma becomes an emergent event. Emergency neurosurgery may be required to relieve pressure and prevent brain herniation.
   (3) Treatment may also include diuretics and anticonvulsants.
   (4) Persistent neurologic complications—including dysarthria, unilateral weakness, memory loss, and seizures—may continue.
4. With presence of retinal hemorrhage, evaluate for "shaken baby syndrome."

### Assessment

A. Risk factors/etiology.
   1. History of trauma.
   2. Epidural hematomas are rare in children younger than 4 years.
   3. Subdural hematomas are common in infants and may result from birth trauma.
B. Clinical manifestations.
   1. Epidural hematoma: decreased LOC, signs and symptoms of rapidly increasing ICP.
   2. Subdural hematoma: headache, decreased LOC, symptoms of increased ICP, somnolence, confusion, memory loss.
C. Diagnostics (see Appendix 22-1).

### Complications

Complications include increased ICP, meningitis, diabetes insipidus, SIADH, seizures, and permanent neurologic compromise.

### Treatment

> **⊞ NURSING PRIORITY:** The primary treatment objectives for the client with a head injury are to maintain a patent airway, prevent hypoxia and hypercapnia resulting in acidosis, and identify the occurrence of increased ICP.

A. The majority of clients who experience concussion are treated at home.

3. Intracranial hemorrhage.
   a. Epidural hematoma: a blood vessel (often a meningeal artery) in the dura mater is damaged; a hematoma rapidly forms between the dura and the skull, precipitating an increase in ICP.
      (1) Momentary loss of consciousness, then free of symptoms (lucid period), and then lethargy and coma—seldom evident in children.
      (2) Symptoms of increasing ICP may develop within minutes after the lucid interval.
      (3) Tentorial herniation may occur without immediate intervention; considered a neurosurgical emergency!

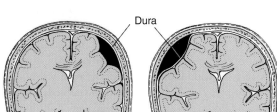
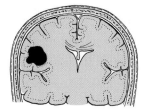

A. Subdural hematoma   B. Epidural hematoma   C. Intracerebral hematoma

FIGURE 22-15 **Formation of Head Injury after Hematoma.** (From Black, J. M., & Hawks, J. H. [2009]. *Medical-surgical nursing: Clinical management for positive outcomes* [8th ed.]. Philadelphia: Saunders.)

B. A period of unconsciousness or presence of seizures is considered a serious indication of injury.
C. Surgical intervention.
  1. Burr holes to evacuate the hematoma.
  2. Craniotomy/craniectomy.

*Nursing Interventions*

**Goal:** To provide instruction for care of the client in the home environment (Box 22-6).

A. Observe the client for increased periods of sleep; if client is asleep, awaken every 2 to 3 hours to determine whether client can be aroused normally.
B. Maintain contact with physician for reevaluation if complications occur.
C. Health care provider should be notified when any of the following are observed:
  1. Any change in level of consciousness (increased drowsiness, confusion).
  2. Inability to arouse client, seizures.
  3. Bleeding or watery drainage from the ears or nose.
  4. Loss of feeling or sensation in any extremity.
  5. Blurred vision, slurred speech, vomiting.
  6. Headache that increases in intensity.

**TEST ALERT:** Determine client and family's understanding of the discharge instructions. Written and oral instructions should be given to the client and to the family. Increased anxiety may affect comprehension of oral directions (see Box 22-6).

**Goal:** To maintain homeostasis and to monitor and identify early symptoms of increased ICP.

A. Bed rest and clear liquids initially.
B. Frequent neurologic checks for increased ICP.
  1. Change or decrease in level of consciousness is frequently the first indication.

---

**Box 22-6 DISCHARGE INSTRUCTIONS FOR CLIENTS WITH HEAD INJURY**

- Arouse the client every 3 to 4 hours for the first 24 hours.
- Anticipate complaints of dizziness, headaches.
- Do not allow client to blow his or her nose; try to prevent sneezing.
- No alcohol or sedatives for sleep.
- Administer acetaminophen for headaches.
- No exercising over next 2 to 3 days.
  Call the doctor if any of the following is noted:
  - Change in vision: blurred or diplopia
  - Poor coordination: walking, grasping
  - Drainage (serous or bloody) from the nose or ears
  - Forceful vomiting
  - Increasing sleepiness, more difficult to arouse
  - Slurred speech
  - Headache that does not respond to medication and continues to get worse
  - Occurrence of a seizure

---

2. Instruct clients with head injury not to cough, sneeze, or blow nose.
C. Evaluate drainage from nose, ears, and mouth.
  1. Do not clean out the ears: place loose cotton in the auditory canal and change when soiled.
  2. Check continuous clear drainage from the nose with a dipstick for dextrose; if glucose is present, it is indicative of a CSF leak; CSF also dries with a yellow halo around edges of drainage.
  3. If a CSF leak occurs, keep the head of the bed elevated and monitor for development of an infection (meningitis).
D. Seizure precautions (see Appendix 22-3).
E. Maintain adequate fluid intake by IV infusion or oral intake; do not overhydrate.
F. Assess for other undetected injuries; stabilize spine after head injury until spinal cord injury is ruled out.

**Goal:** To provide appropriate nursing interventions for the client experiencing an increase in ICP (see nursing goals for increased ICP).

**Goal:** To provide adequate nutritional and caloric intake for the client with a head injury.

A. Provide enteral feedings if client is unable to eat.
B. Assist client to take oral feedings once swallow reflex is normal; client is at increased risk for aspiration.

## Cerebral Aneurysm, Subarachnoid Hemorrhage

**A cerebral aneurysm occurs when a weakened saccular outpouching of the cerebral vasculature bulges from pressure on the weakened tissue. A ruptured cerebral aneurysm often results in hemorrhagic stroke.**

A. A subarachnoid hemorrhage is a potentially fatal condition in which blood accumulates below the arachnoid mater in the subarachnoid space; most often occurs secondary to aneurysmal rupture.
B. Symptoms may occur when an aneurysm enlarges. When it ruptures, blood collects in the subarachnoid space, compressing and damaging the surrounding brain tissue.
C. Complications of subarachnoid hemorrhage include rebleed, cerebral vasospasm, hydrocephalus, and death.

*Assessment*

A. Risk factors/etiology.
  1. Increased incidence with age; more prevalent in women.
  2. Atherosclerosis, connective tissue disease, cigarette smoking, hypertension, cocaine use.
  3. Head trauma and congenital vessel weakness may increase the risk.
B. Clinical manifestations.
  1. Rupture may be preceded by:
    a. Severe headache.
    b. Visual disturbances.
  2. Rupture frequently occurs without warning.
    a. Sudden, severe headache ("Worst headache of my life"), seizures.

b. Nuchal rigidity, hemiparesis.
c. Change in level of consciousness.
d. Symptoms of increasing ICP: nausea, vomiting, photophobia.

3. Severity of symptoms depends on the site and amount of bleeding.

C. Diagnostics (see Appendix 22-1).

### Treatment

A. Surgical intervention: ligation or "clipping" of the aneurysm to reduce swelling and minimize the risk for rebleeding. Coiling procedure may also be used to fill the aneurysm to reduce rebleed.
B. Calcium channel blocker, nimodipine to reduce risk of vasospasm
C. Anticonvulsants; analgesics for headache.
D. Fluids to maintain systolic blood pressure as prescribed (increase in fluid volume increases blood flow through narrowed cerebral vessels).
E. Stool softeners.
F. May require ventricular drainage for hydrocephalus.

### Nursing Interventions

**Goal:** To prevent further increase in ICP and possible rupture.

A. Bed rest; bathroom privileges may be permitted.
B. Constant monitoring of condition to identify occurrence of bleeding or vasospasm as evidenced by symptoms of increasing ICP or new or changing neurologic deficits.
C. Client should avoid straining, sneezing, pulling up in bed, and acute flexion of the neck.
D. Elevate head of the bed 30 degrees to 45 degrees to promote venous return.
E. Quiet, darkened, nonstimulating environment: disconnect telephone; limit visitors; promote relaxation.
F. Administer analgesics cautiously; the client should continue to be easily aroused so that neurologic checks can be performed.
G. No hot or cold beverages or food, no caffeine, no smoking.
H. Maintain seizure precautions.

> **NURSING PRIORITY:** If the client survives the rupture of the aneurysm and rebleeding occurs, it is most likely to occur within the next 24 to 48 hours.

**Goal:** To assess for and implement nursing measures to decrease ICP (see nursing goals for increased ICP).
**Goal:** To provide appropriate preoperative nursing interventions (see nursing goals for brain tumor).
**Goal:** To maintain homeostasis and monitor changes in ICP after craniotomy.

## Spinal Cord Injury

**Spinal cord injury (SCI) is damage to the spinal cord housed inside the spinal column and is generally a result of trauma. The degree of injury is classified as *complete*, resulting in loss of both sensory and motor function below the level of injury; or *incomplete*, with some sensation or motor function below the level of injury.**

A. Risk factors.
1. Young adult men are at highest risk.
2. Also an increased risk in older adults when falls become more common.
3. Most common causes include motor vehicle crashes, falls, violence, sports injury.

B. Initially after the injury, the nerve fibers swell, and circulation to the spinal cord is decreased; hemorrhage and edema occur, causing an increase in the ischemic process, which progresses to necrotic destruction of the spinal cord.
C. Consequences of SCI depend on the extent of damage and the level of cord injury (Figure 22-16).
1. The higher the lesion, the more severe the sequelae.
   a. Clients with lesions at C or higher require ventilatory support.
   b. Lesions between T1 and T8 often allow use of the hands.
   c. Lesions below T8 often allow upper body control.
2. Complete transection (complete cord dissolution, complete lesion): immediate loss of all sensation and voluntary movement below the level of injury; minimal, if any, return of function.
3. Incomplete injury: major syndromes.
   a. Central cord syndrome: center of cord is damaged; results primarily in impairment of upper extremities.
   b. Damage to one side of the cord (Brown-Séquard syndrome): loss of ipsilateral (same side) motor,

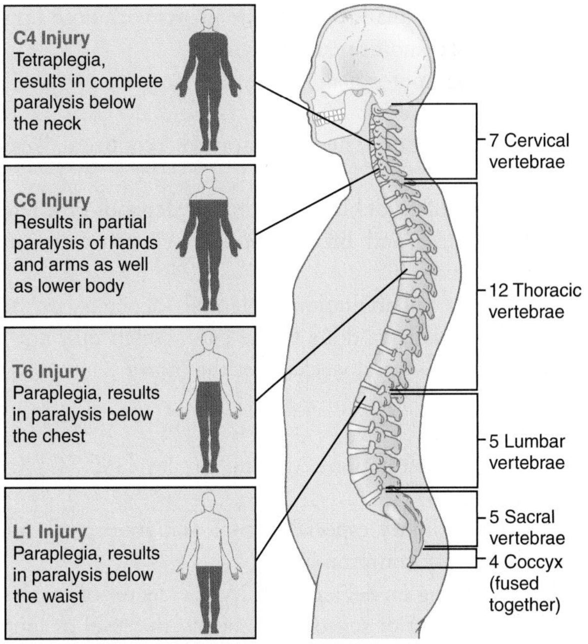


**FIGURE 22-16 Spinal Cord Injury: Areas of Paralysis.** (From Lewis, S. L., et al. [2017]. *Medical-surgical nursing: Assessment and management of clinical problems* [10th ed.]. St. Louis, MO: Mosby.)

touch, pressure, and vibration with contralateral (opposite side) loss of pain and temperature sensation.

  c. Anterior cord syndrome: disruption of blood flow results in loss of motor, pain, and temperature sensation below level of injury; touch, position, and vibration remain intact.

4. Cord edema peaks in about 2 to 3 days and subsides within about 7 days after the injury.

5. Lumbosacral injuries.

  a. Variable pattern of motor and sensory loss.

  b. Frequently result in neurogenic bowel and bladder.

D. Spinal shock: decreased reflexes, loss of sensation, flaccid paralysis below level of injury. Resolves in days to weeks; return of reflexes and development of spasticity.

E. Neurogenic shock: disruption of sympathetic nervous system causes hypotension due to peripheral vasodilation and bradycardia. Hypothermia can occur due to vasodilation. Most common in cervical and high thoracic injury (T6 and above).

F. Autonomic dysreflexia can occur in clients with an injury at T6 or higher following resolution of spinal shock.

1. A noxious stimulus below the level of injury triggers the sympathetic nervous system, which causes a release of catecholamines (epinephrine, norepinephrine).

2. Most common stimuli causing the response are a full bladder or bowel, urinary tract infection, pressure ulcers, and skin stimulation.

3. Severe hypertension (systolic may be greater than 300), nausea, pounding headache, bradycardia, restlessness, piloerection, flushing and sweating above the level of injury, and blurred vision are the most common body responses.

G. Bladder dysfunction will occur as a result of the injury; normal bladder control is dependent on the sensory and motor pathways and the lower motor neurons being intact.

1. Neurogenic bladder occurs in clients with both upper and lower motor neuron disorders.

  a. Upper motor neuron disorders produce a spastic or reflex bladder.

  b. Lower motor neuron disorders produce a flaccid bladder.

2. Management of bladder problems depends on client's preferences and lifestyle and on client's functional abilities.

H. Long-term rehabilitation potential depends on the amount of damage done to the cord, which may not be evident until several weeks after the injury.

### Assessment

A. Clinical manifestations: depend on level of SCI (see Figure 22-16).

1. Cervical injury, especially at C5 and above, will cause respiratory compromise.

2. Depending on degree of injury, the degree of paralysis and amount of sensory loss below the level of injury will vary.

3. Monitor for spinal shock and neurogenic shock.

B. Diagnostics (see Appendix 22-1).

C. Complications.

1. Respiratory stasis; pulmonary edema and emboli.

2. Cardiovascular compromise from neurogenic shock, or autonomic dysreflexia.

3. Skin breakdown resulting in localized and systemic infections.

4. Immobility issues causing renal and gastrointestinal compromise.

5. Psychological, social, and body image issues.

### Treatment

A. Emergency intervention required; manage airway, breathing, and circulation.

B. Immobilization of the vertebral column in cervical fracture.

1. Cervical tongs (Crutchfield, Gardner-Wells) for cervical immobility.

2. Halo vest/jacket traction to promote mobility.

3. Sternooccipital mandibular immobilizer (SOMI) brace worn with cervical fusion.

C. Spinal surgery to decompress spinal cord and stabilize spine.

D. Respiratory support as necessary.

### Nursing Interventions

**Goal:** To maintain stability of the vertebral column and prevent further cord damage.

A. Emergency care and treatment.

1. Suspect SCI if there is any evidence of direct trauma to the head or neck area (contact sports, diving accidents, motor vehicle accident).

2. Immobilize client and institute spinal precautions; maintain body alignment and do not allow the neck to flex.

3. Airway, status of breathing, and circulation are the primary concerns initially after injury.

4. Neurogenic shock may occur within the first 24 hours; observe for decreased blood pressure, severe bradycardia.

> **! NURSING PRIORITY:** Do not hyperextend the neck in a client with a suspected cervical injury. Airway should be opened by the jaw-lift method. Improper handling of the client often results in extension of the damaged area.

5. Maintain cervical spinal precautions and body alignment, do not remove cervical collar or spinal board until area of injury is identified.

6. Maintain patent airway at all times.

B. Maintain stability of the vertebral column as indicated by the level of injury.

1. Prescribe and maintain bed rest on firm mattress with supportive devices (sandbags, skin traction, etc.); maintain alignment in the supine position; logroll without any flexion or twisting.

2. Maintain cervical traction: tongs are inserted into the skull with traction and weights applied; do not remove weights; to turn: logroll, specialty bed or turning frame to maintain spinal alignment.
3. Halo vest/jacket traction: maintains cervical immobility but allows client to be mobile.
    a. If bolts or screws come loose, keep the client immobilized and call the health care provider.
    b. Clean pin sites according to facility policy; observe for infection.
    c. Monitor skin under vest and provide skin care.
    d. Roll client onto his or her side at the edge of the bed and allow client to push up from the mattress to a sitting position. *Never* use the halo vest frame to assist the client to turn or sit up.
    e. Correct size of wrench should be kept at bedside to remove the anterior bolts in case of emergency.
    f. Assist client to maintain balance when standing; the traction is heavy for a person who is weak, and the client is at increased risk for falling.
4. Maintain extremities in neutral, functional position.

> **TEST ALERT:** Apply, maintain, or remove orthopedic devices (e.g., traction, splints, braces, casts).

C. Perform appropriate nursing intervention when surgery is indicated to stabilize the injury.

**Goal:** To identify level of damage and changes in neurologic status.

A. Assess respiratory function: symmetric chest expansion, bilateral breath sounds, presence of retractions or dyspnea.
B. Motor and sensory evaluation.
    1. Ability to move extremities; strength of extremities.
    2. Sensory examination, including touch and pain.
    3. Presence of deep tendon reflexes.
C. Ongoing assessment and status of:
    1. Bladder, gastric, bowel function.
    2. Psychological adjustment to the injury.
D. Evaluate history of how injury occurred; obtain information regarding how client was transported.
E. Determine status of pain.

**Goal:** To maintain respiratory function.

A. Frequent assessment of respiratory function during the first 48 hours.
    1. Determine development of hypoxia.
    2. Changes in breathing pattern.
    3. Observe breathing pattern for use of sternocleidomastoid and intercostal muscles for respiration.
    4. Evaluate arterial blood gas values and pulse oximetry.
B. Maintain adequate respiratory function, as indicated.
    1. Chest physiotherapy.
    2. Incentive spirometry.
    3. Changing position within limits of injury.

4. Assess for complications of atelectasis, pulmonary emboli, and pneumonia.
5. Nasopharyngeal or endotracheal suctioning based on airway and level of injury.

**Goal:** To maintain cardiovascular stability.

A. Spinal shock.
    1. Monitor vital signs and evaluate changes.
    2. Vagal stimulation, hypothermia, and hypoxia may precipitate spinal shock.
    3. Assess deep tendon reflexes and muscle strength as resolution of shock occurs.
B. Assess for development of autonomic dysreflexia; if it occurs:
    1. Elevate the head of the bed and check the client's blood pressure.
    2. Assess for sources of stimuli: distended bladder (check urinary tubing), fecal impaction, constipation, tight clothing.
    3. Relieve the stimuli, and dysreflexia will subside.
    4. Maintain cardiovascular support during period of hypertension.
    5. A hypertensive crisis from dysreflexia will require immediate intervention.
C. Neurogenic shock
    1. Monitor blood pressure, heart rate.
    2. May require fluids to increase blood pressure; atropine to increase heart rate.
    3. Compression stocking to maintain blood pressure and prevent venous pooling.
D. Evaluate cardiovascular responses when turning or suctioning client.
E. Apply antiembolism stockings or elastic wraps to the legs to facilitate venous return. (Lack of muscle tone and loss of sympathetic tone in the peripheral vessels result in decreases in both venous tone and venous return, which predispose client to DVT.)

> **TEST ALERT:** Prevent complications of immobility; prevent venous stasis: identify symptoms of DVT, apply compression stockings, and change client's position.

**Goal:** To maintain adequate fluid and nutritional status.

A. During the first 48 hours, evaluate gastrointestinal function frequently; decrease in function may necessitate use of a nasogastric tube to decrease distention.
B. Prevent complications of nausea and vomiting.
C. Evaluate bowel sounds and client's ability to tolerate oral fluids.
D. Increase protein and calories in diet; may need to decrease calcium intake.
E. Evaluate for presence of paralytic ileus.
F. Increase fiber in diet to promote bowel function.

**Goal:** To prevent complications of immobility (see Chapter 3).

**Goal:** To promote bowel and bladder function.

A. Urine is retained as a result of the loss of autonomic and reflexive control of the bladder.
 1. Intermittent catheterization or indwelling catheter may be used initially to prevent bladder distention.
 2. Perform nursing interventions to prevent urinary tract infection; avoid urinary catheterization, if possible.
B. Determine type of bladder dysfunction based on level of injury.
C. Assess client's awareness of bladder function.
D. Initiate measures to institute bladder control.
 1. Establish a schedule for voiding; have client attempt to void every 2 hours.
 2. Use the Credé method (pressure applied over symphysis pubis) in adults for manual expression of urine.
 3. May be necessary to teach client self-catheterization.
 4. Record output and evaluate for presence of residual urine.
E. Evaluate bowel functioning.
 1. Incontinence and paralytic ileus frequently occur with spinal shock.
 2. Incontinence and impaction are common later.
F. Initiate measures to promote bowel control (after spinal shock is resolved).
 1. Identify client's bowel habits before injury.
 2. Maintain sufficient fluid intake and adequate bulk in the diet.
 3. Establish specific time each day for bowel evacuation.
 4. Assess client's awareness of need to defecate.
 5. Teach client effective use of the Valsalva maneuver to induce defecation.
 6. Induce defecation by digital stimulation, suppository, or, as a last resort, enema.

**TEST ALERT:** Assess and manage a client with alteration in elimination; initiate a toileting schedule; the client with SCI may need bowel and bladder retraining, depending on level of the injury.

**Goal:** To maintain psychological equilibrium.

A. Provide simple explanations of all procedures.
B. Anticipate outbursts of anger and hostility as client begins to work through the grieving process and adjusts to changes in body image.
C. Anticipate and accept periods of depression in client.
D. Encourage independence whenever possible; allow client to participate in decisions regarding care and to gain control over environment.

**TEST ALERT:** Plan measures to deal with client's anxiety and promote client's adjustment to changes in body image; assist client and significant others to adjust to role changes.

E. Encourage family involvement in identifying appropriate diversional activities.
F. Avoid sympathy and emphasize client's potential.
G. Initiate frank, open discussion regarding sexual functioning.
H. Assist client and family to identify community resources.
I. Assist client to set realistic short-term goals.

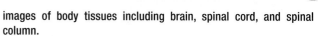 

## Appendix 22-1 NEUROLOGIC SYSTEM DIAGNOSTICS

**Skull and Spine X-Ray Studies:** Simple x-ray films are obtained to determine fractures, calcifications, etc.

**Electroencephalography (EEG):** A graphic recording of the electrical activity of the brain to assess cerebral activity; useful for diagnosing seizure disorders; used as a screening procedure for coma; also serves as an indicator for brain death. May also be used to assess sleep disorders, metabolic disorders, and encephalitis.

*Nursing Implications*
1. Explain to client that procedure is painless and there is no danger of electric shock.
2. Determine from physician if any medications should be withheld before test, especially tranquilizers and sedatives.
3. Frequently, caffeinated foods, beverages, or other stimulants are prohibited before examination.
4. Client's hair should be clean before the examination; after the examination, assist client in washing electrode paste out of hair.

**Carotid Doppler Ultrasonography:** A noninvasive ultrasound scan to estimate blood flow in carotid and cerebral vessels to assess for stenosis. No preparation is necessary.

**Magnetic Resonance Imaging (MRI):** Uses magnetic energy to align hydrogen molecules in the body and create detailed images of body tissues including brain, spinal cord, and spinal column.

*Nursing Implications*
1. Procedure will take approximately 1 hour; client must lie still during that time.
2. All metal objects should be removed from the client (dental bridges, hearing aids, hair clips, jewelry, buckles, medicine patches with foil backing).
3. Screen for implanted medical devices; may not be MRI compatible.
4. Contrast medium may be used: assess for allergy to shellfish, iodine, or contrast dye. Ensure adequate hydration.
5. Poor candidates for MRI include the following:
 a. Clients who are confused, hemodynamically unstable, or require life-supporting equipment.
 b. Clients with implanted medical devices, pins, clips, or joint replacements.
 c. Pregnant clients; if required, can be done, preferably after first trimester.
 d. Obese clients; may not fit in scanner.

**Computerized Axial Tomography (CAT)/Computed Tomography (CT) Scan:** Computer-assisted x-ray examination of thin cross-sections of the brain to identify hemorrhage, tumor, edema, infarctions, and hydrocephalus. Machine is large donut-shaped tube with table through the middle.

*Nursing Implications*

1. Explain appearance of scanner to client and explain importance of remaining absolutely still during the procedure.
2. Remove all objects from client's hair; for 4 to 6 hours before test, client receives fluids only.
3. Dye may be injected via venipuncture; assess for iodine allergy and advise the client that he or she may experience a flushing or warm sensation when the dye is injected.
4. Contrast dye may discolor urine for about 24 hours.
5. Dye may be injected into spinal cord for assessment of intervertebral disks and bone density.

**Brain Scan:** A scanner traces the uptake of radioactive dye in the brain tissue. The dye is concentrated in the damaged tissue; it will take approximately 2 hours after dye is injected for the scan to be completed.

*Nursing Implications*

1. Determine whether medications need to be withheld before procedure.
2. Client will be asked to change positions during the test to visualize the brain from different angles.
3. The client should not experience any pain.

**Caloric Testing:** Test is performed at bedside by introducing cold or warm water (or air) into the external auditory canal. It is contraindicated in the client with a ruptured tympanic membrane and is not done on the client who is awake. If the eighth cranial nerve is stimulated, nystagmus rotates toward the irrigated ear. If no nystagmus occurs, a pathologic condition is present.

**Positron Emission Tomography (PET):** See Appendix 17-1.

**Lumbar Puncture:** A needle is inserted into the lumbar area at the L3–L4 or L4–L5 level (in subarachnoid space); spinal pressure is measured and spinal fluid withdrawn; contraindicated in presence of increased intracranial pressure. Normal spinal fluid values: opening pressure, 60 to 150 mm water; specific gravity, 1.007; pH, 7.35; clear/colorless fluid; protein concentration, 15 to 45 mg/dL (0.15–0.45 g/L); glucose concentration, 45 to 75 mg/dL (2.5–4.2 mmol/L); no microorganisms present; no blood.

*Nursing Implications*

Before Test

1. Have client empty bladder and bowels.
2. Explain position (lateral recumbent with knees flexed) to client (Figure 22-17).
3. Advise physician if there is a change in the client's neurologic status before the test; increased intracranial pressure is a contraindication to a lumbar puncture.

After Test

1. Keep client flat at least 3 hours, and sometimes up to 12 hours, to decrease occurrence of headache.
2. Monitor vital signs and neurologic status.
3. Encourage high fluid intake.
4. Observe for spinal fluid leak from puncture site; if leakage occurs, it may precipitate a severe headache.

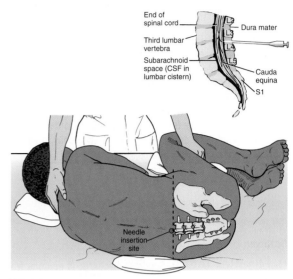

**FIGURE 22-17 Lumbar puncture.** (From Black, J. M., & Hawks, J. H. [2005]. *Medical-surgical nursing: Clinical management for positive outcomes* [7th ed.]. Philadelphia: Saunders.)

**Myelogram:** An outpatient procedure in which a lumbar puncture is performed and dye is injected into the subarachnoid space. X-ray films of the spinal cord and vertebral column are obtained to identify spinal lesions.

*Nursing Implications*

Before Test

1. Same as for lumbar puncture.
2. Check whether client has any allergies to dye.

After Test

3. Keep the head of the bed elevated 30 to 50 degrees to decrease dispersion of the dye in the CSF and to the brain.
4. Headache may occur as a result of irritation of the central nervous system.
5. Client should not receive any of the phenothiazines before or immediately after the examination with use of certain contrast material.

**Cerebral Angiogram:** Injection of contrast material into the cerebral circulation; series of x-ray films is taken to study the cerebral blood flow; dye is usually injected via a soft catheter that is inserted and threaded through the femoral artery.

*Nursing Implications*

Before Test

1. Client should be well hydrated but should receive nothing by mouth for 6 to 8 hours before the test; client should void before procedure.
2. Determine whether client has any allergies to iodine or to shellfish.
3. Inform client that he or she should remain very still during the procedure.
4. A feeling of warmth in the face and mouth and a metallic taste in the mouth are common when dye is injected.

After Test

1. Evaluate client's neurologic status; complications involve occlusion of cerebral arteries.

*Continued*

## Appendix 22-1    NEUROLOGIC SYSTEM DIAGNOSTICS—cont'd

2. Observe puncture site for bleeding and hematoma formation.
3. Check circulation distal to area of puncture.
4. Posttest complications include continuous bleeding at injection site, rash, dizziness, and tingling in an extremity.

**Electromyography (EMG):** Measures electrical discharge from a muscle. Flat electrodes or small needles are placed in the muscle. The client may be asked to move and perform simple activities; the electrical stimulus for the muscle will be recorded. Useful for diagnosis in spinal cord deformity, muscular dystrophy, myasthenia gravis, or amyotrophic lateral sclerosis.

**Nursing Implications**

**Before Test**
1. May determine pretest serum muscle determinations.
2. Explain to the client that small needles will be inserted into the skin.

**After Test**
3. Client may need something for pain because of muscle stimulation.
4. Assess needle sites for areas of hematomas; apply ice pack to prevent and/or relieve.

## Appendix 22-2    MEDICATIONS

| Medications | Side Effects | Nursing Implications |
|---|---|---|
| **Antiepileptics (AED):** Suppress discharge of neurons within a seizure focus to reduce seizure activity. | | |
| Phenobarbital: IM, PO, IV<br>Primidone: PO | Drowsiness, ataxia, excitation in children and the elderly | 1. Client should avoid potential hazardous activities requiring mental alertness.<br>2. Sudden withdrawal from chronic use may precipitate symptoms.<br>3. Closely observe response in children and elderly.<br>4. Used to treat grand mal and focal seizures.<br>5. See Appendix 22-3 for care of client with seizures. |
| Phenytoin: PO, IV<br>Fosphenytoin: IV, IM | Gingival hyperplasia, skin rash, hypoglycemia<br>Bradycardia, hypotension<br>Visual changes: nystagmus, diplopia, blurred vision | 1. Frequently used with phenobarbital for control of grand mal seizures.<br>2. IV therapeutic level: 10–20 mcg/mL<br>3. Do not mix with any other medications when administering IV solution.<br>4. Promote good oral hygiene; gum hyperplasia is a problem with long-term use.<br>5. See Appendix 22-3 for care of client with seizures.<br>6. AEDs should be withdrawn slowly over 6 weeks to several months when medication therapy is discontinued. |
| Valproic acid/ divalproex: PO, IV | GI disturbances, rash, weight loss or gain, hair loss, tremor, blood dyscrasias GI, dermatologic effects, blood dyscrasias, drowsiness | 1. Should not be given to clients with severe liver dysfunction.<br>2. Potentiates action of phenobarbital, phenytoin, diazepam.<br>3. Uses: seizures, bipolar disorder, migraine. |
| Carbamazepine: PO, suspension | Drowsiness, dizziness, headache; visual disturbances common during first few weeks of treatment | 1. Wean client from medication as soon as seizures are controlled.<br>2. Antimanic properties as well. |
| Clonazepam: PO | CNS depression, somnolence, ataxia | 1. Antianxiety effects may assist with seizure control.<br>2. Monitor results of liver function tests. |
| **Cholinergic (Anticholinesterase) Medications:** Intensify transmission of impulses throughout the CNS, where acetylcholine is necessary for transmission. | | |
| Neostigmine bromide: PO, subQ, IM, IV<br>Pyridostigmine bromide: PO, IM, IV | Edrophonium chloride: IV: Excessive salivation, increased GI motility, urinary urgency, bradycardia, visual problems | 1. Primary group of medications used for treatment of myasthenia gravis.<br>2. Atropine is the antidote for overdose.<br>3. In treatment of myasthenia gravis, medication is frequently administered 30–45 minutes before meals.<br>4. Pyridostigmine bromide is given as maintenance therapy for the client with myasthenia gravis.<br>5. Edrophonium chloride is used for diagnostic purposes (Tensilon test); not recommended for maintenance therapy.<br>6. Teach client symptoms of side effects and advise client to call the doctor if they are present. |

**Appendix 22-2    MEDICATIONS—cont'd**

| Medications | Side Effects | Nursing Implications |
| --- | --- | --- |

## Antiparkinsonism Agents

**Anticholinergics:** Inhibit action of acetylcholine at sites throughout the body and CNS. Decrease synaptic transmissions in the CNS.

| Medications | Side Effects | Nursing Implications |
| --- | --- | --- |
| Benztropine mesylate: PO, IM, IV<br>Trihexyphenidyl hydrochloride: PO | Paralytic ileus, urinary retention, cardiac palpitations, blurred vision, nausea and vomiting, sedation, dizziness<br>Minor side effects such as dry mouth, jitteriness, and nausea | 1. Administer PO preparations with meals to decrease gastric irritation.<br>2. Medications have cumulative effect.<br>3. Should not be used in clients with glaucoma, myasthenia gravis, GU or GI tract obstruction, or in children younger than 3 years.<br>4. Monitor client carefully for bowel and bladder problems.<br>5. May be used to treat side effects of chlorpromazine. |

**Dopaminergics:** Assist to restore normal transmission of nerve impulses.

| Medications | Side Effects | Nursing Implications |
| --- | --- | --- |
| Levodopa: PO (rarely used alone) | *Early:* Anorexia, nausea and vomiting, abdominal discomfort, orthostatic hypotension<br>*Long-term:* Abnormal, involuntary movements, especially involving the face, mouth, and neck; behavioral disturbances involving confusion, agitation, and euphoria | 1. Administer PO preparations with meals to decrease GI distress.<br>2. Almost all clients will experience some side effects, which are dose related; dosage gradually increased according to client's tolerance and response.<br>3. Onset of action is slow; therapeutic response may require several weeks to months.<br>4. Vitamin $B_6$ (pyridoxine) is antagonistic to the effects of the medication; decrease client's intake of multiple vitamins and fortified cereals. |
| Carbidopa/levodopa: PO | Same as for levodopa | 1. Same as for levodopa.<br>2. Use of carbidopa significantly decreases the amount of levodopa required for therapy.<br>3. Prevents inhibitory effects of levodopa on vitamin $B_6$. |
| Amantadine hydrochloride: PO | Orthostatic hypotension, dyspnea, dizziness, drowsiness, blurred vision, constipation, urinary retention (side effects are dose related) | 1. Less effective than levodopa; produces a more rapid clinical response. |

*CNS,* Central nervous system; *GI,* gastrointestinal; *GU,* genitourinary; *IM,* intramuscular; *IV,* intravenous; *PO,* by mouth (orally); *subQ,* subcutaneous.

**Appendix 22-3    APHASIA**

Aphasia is inability to comprehend or use language. Aphasia may be receptive, expressive, or global. Dysphasia is a term also used to describe impaired communication. Approximately 90% of people are left-brain dominant; the left side of the brain controls communication. That is why for most people, damage to the left side of the brain from stroke or injury causes aphasia. Clients with aphasia are often frustrated and irritable. Emotional lability is common. Accept the behavior in a manner that prevents embarrassment for the client.

| Types of Aphasia | Nursing Implications |
| --- | --- |
| *Wernicke's (fluent or receptive aphasia; left temporal lobe damage):* Cannot understand oral or written communication. Client cannot interpret or comprehend speech or read.<br>*Broca's (expressive aphasia, left frontal lobe damage):* Inability to speak or to write. However, the client can comprehend incoming speech and can read.<br>*Mixed:* Most aphasia involves both the sensory and motor aspects of speech. Rarely is aphasia only sensory or only motor.<br>*Global aphasia:* All communication and receptive function is lost.<br>*Dysarthria:* A disturbance in the muscular control of speech. Does not affect the meaning of communication or comprehension, just the mechanics of speech—pronunciation, articulation, and phonation. | 1. Stand in front of the client; speak clearly and slowly.<br>2. Do not shout or speak loudly; the client can hear.<br>3. Be patient; give the client time to respond; do not press him or her for immediate answers.<br>4. Use nonverbal communications such as touch, smiles, and gestures.<br>5. Assist the client with motor aphasia to practice repeating simple words such as yes, no, and please.<br>6. Listen carefully, try to understand, and try to communicate; this conveys to the client that you care.<br>7. Involve family members in practice and assist them to identify ways they can support the client. |

**TEST ALERT:** Assist client to communicate effectively.

## Study Questions
## Neurology: Care of Adult and Pediatric Clients

More questions on

1. The nurse is obtaining a health history from a client who reports having pain in the left arm. Which question by the nurse will elicit the most useful response from the client?
   1. "Does the pain feel like pins and needles in your arm?"
   2. "Does the pain radiate from your neck to your arms?"
   3. "Can you describe the pain you are experiencing in your arm?"
   4. "Is the numbness in your arm intermittent or constant?"

2. The nurse is assessing a client with a tentative diagnosis of a brain tumor. What primary client complaint would the nurse anticipate?
   1. Decreased appetite
   2. Frequent insomnia
   3. Recurrent headaches
   4. Peripheral edema

3. The nurse is caring for a client who has had a right-sided stroke. What would be appropriate nursing care for this client?
   1. Performing passive ROM exercises to affected side, active ROM on unaffected side
   2. Placing food on the affected side of the client's mouth
   3. Applying hot packs to the right leg to decrease muscle spasms
   4. Turning client every 2 hours and maintaining position on the right side for 2 hours

4. A client is scheduled for an electroencephalogram. What will the nurse explain to the client regarding the purpose of this test?
   1. Evaluates electrical currents of skeletal muscles
   2. Measures ultrasonic waves in the brain
   3. Determines size and location of brain activity
   4. Records brain electrical activity

5. A client who has had a stroke 1 week ago remains aphasic. The client is beginning to show functional improvement and demonstrates an ability to follow verbal directions. What will rehabilitation now include?
   1. A right-leg brace
   2. Ambulation training
   3. Speech training
   4. Vocational retraining

6. The nurse is caring for a client who is doing well after a craniotomy. What will the bowel care for this client include?
   1. An enema every other day to avoid the Valsalva maneuver
   2. High-fiber diet and stool softeners to prevent constipation
   3. Low-residue diet to decrease stool formation and prevent constipation
   4. Daily checking for impaction caused by loss of bowel innervations

7. After a tonic–clonic (formerly grand mal) seizure, what nursing action is the highest priority?
   1. Loosen or remove constricting clothing and protect client from injuring himself or herself.
   2. Maintain a patent airway by turning the client on his side and suctioning, if necessary.
   3. Remain with the client and administer anticonvulsant medications as ordered by the physician.
   4. Describe and record events before the onset of the seizure, during the seizure, and after the seizure.

8. A client with Parkinson disease is experiencing anorexia and vomiting. The client is taking levodopa. What will be the initial nursing activity?
   1. Assess client's food preferences.
   2. Monitor client's blood pressure.
   3. Hold client's medication and notify the physician.
   4. Administer client's medication with food.

9. An 8-year-old child is admitted after an accident where he sustained a closed head injury. The child is alert and oriented but very lethargic. There is clear fluid draining from the child's nose. What is the best nursing action?
   1. Gently suction the fluid from the nasal area.
   2. Turn from side to side only.
   3. Keep head of bed elevated.
   4. Encourage participation in games to play in bed.

10. When obtaining a health history, the nurse expects a client with a recent diagnosis of Parkinson disease to report which sign or symptom?
    1. Weight loss
    2. Slowness of movement
    3. Continual motor tremors
    4. Depression

11. While caring for a client who has recently been diagnosed with Parkinson disease, the nurse should understand that:
    1. Intellectual capabilities will decrease.
    2. Diversional interests may decrease.
    3. Mood fluctuations may occur.
    4. Communication skills may fluctuate.

12. Pneumonia is a common problem in children with spastic cerebral palsy. The nurse understands that this occurs because:
    1. There is an associated dysfunction of the respiratory center in the central nervous system.
    2. The immunologic system is immature and does not produce adequate antibodies to fight infection.
    3. Decreased mobility leads to stasis of secretions in the respiratory passages.
    4. There is a weakness of the voluntary muscles that control respiration.

13. The nurse is assessing a client who has just had a lumbar puncture. What nursing observation would cause the nurse the most concern?
    1. Client tells the nurse he has a headache.
    2. Nurse observes clear fluid oozing from the puncture site.
    3. Client states he has less strength in his arms.
    4. Client has difficulty voiding from supine position.

14. The nurse is caring for a client who has a temporal craniotomy, and this is the first postoperative day. What is an important nursing intervention?
    1. Take temperature orally only.
    2. Restrain the client as necessary.
    3. Suction the client every 2 hours.
    4. Maintain the client with his head elevated.

15. What will the nurse anticipate the neurologic nursing assessment of an 88-year-old client with a left cranial hemisphere hemorrhage to reveal?
    1. Spasticity, bilateral Babinski sign
    2. Right-sided flaccidity and hemiparesis
    3. Spasticity and left foot clonus
    4. Flaccidity and bilateral foot clonus

16. Which nursing observations support the identification of the early development of a chronic subdural hematoma in a 3-month-old infant?
    1. Closed posterior fontanel; open anterior fontanel
    2. Retinal hemorrhages and hemiparesis
    3. Increased irritability and vomiting
    4. Papilledema and regressive behavior

17. The nurse questions the use of which drug for the client with cerebral hemorrhage?
    1. Gemfibrozil
    2. Mannitol
    3. Enoxaparin
    4. Nitroprusside

18. The nurse is assessing a client with a tentative diagnosis of multiple sclerosis (MS). Which assessment finding would the nurse identify as characteristic of early signs of MS?
    1. Diplopia
    2. Resting tremor
    3. Flaccid paralysis
    4. Unilateral neglect

19. A client in the acute phase of Guillain-Barré syndrome is admitted with weakness and numbness of the lower extremities, along with continual pain that worsens at night. What would be a priority nursing diagnosis?
    1. Fear related to uncertain outcome and seriousness of the problem
    2. Acute pain related to paresthesias, muscle aches, and cramps
    3. Risk for ineffective breathing pattern related to progression of the disease
    4. Risk for aspiration related to dysphagia

## Answers to Study Questions

**1.** *3*

Open-ended questions are most helpful in obtaining accurate health history information because they elicit more detailed descriptions of the symptoms. Although the other options are applicable to the presenting symptom, they result in "yes" or "no" responses, and this does not encourage the client to provide detailed information about the problem. (Potter & Perry, 8 ed., p. 322)

**2.** *3*

Recurrent headaches that increase in frequency and severity are often the first complaint of a client with a brain tumor; the headaches usually correlate with the area of the brain involved. The headaches tend to be worse at night and may awaken the client. Headaches are described as dull and constant but occasionally throbbing. Nausea and vomiting can occur due to ICP. Mood and personality changes occur, especially with brain metastases. Muscle weakness, sensory losses, aphasia, and perceptual/spatial dysfunction are symptoms. Insomnia, decreased appetite, and peripheral edema are not relevant to a brain tumor. (Lewis et al., 9 ed., p. 1376)

**3.** *1*

The rehabilitation program for a client who has had a stroke includes actions that prevent deformity (passive range of motion on affected side and active ROM on the unaffected side) and prevent complications that may be associated with immobility. The client's affected side should be protected, and food should be placed on the unaffected side so that the client can control it. The client should be turned to his right (affected side) but for shorter periods of time. Hot packs would not be applied to decrease spasticity or spasms. (Lewis et al., 9 ed., p. 1393)

**4.** *4*

An electroencephalogram measures the brain's electrical activity. There are no ultrasonic waves in the brain. An electroencephalogram determines the electrical activity but not the brain activity, such as thought or cognition. The electroencephalogram has no relevance to skeletal muscle activity because this type of test would be an electromyogram (EMG), which measures skeletal muscle contraction and electrical potential of the muscle. (Lewis et al., 9 ed., p. 1352)

**5.** *3*

When a stroke occurs in the dominant hemisphere, the client experiences communication difficulties or aphasia. Speech retraining cannot begin until the client understands and can follow directions. The question is focusing on the client's ability to speak and his current problem with aphasia. Although wearing a leg brace and ambulation training will begin when the client has stabilized, the question is focusing on the client's aphasia. Vocational retraining will be part of the client's rehabilitation at a later date. (Lewis et al., 9 ed., p. 1394)

6. *2*

Straining at defecation or the use of the Valsalva maneuver may exacerbate increased ICP. The nurse promotes normal bowel movements that prevent straining by encouraging a high-fiber diet and stool softeners when needed. Enemas are discouraged, and it is important to prevent constipation so that an impaction does not occur. (Lewis et al., 9 ed., p. 1368)

7. *2*

The priority after a grand mal seizure is to maintain a patent airway. The question is asking for a nursing intervention after the seizure is over. The clothes should be loosened so that they do not constrict the client. The nurse may need to remain with the client, and the events of the seizure need to be recorded, but the priority of this question is the airway. (Lewis et al., 9 ed., p. 1426)

8. *4*

The first side effect to be noticed may be gastrointestinal problems. Taking medication with meals may alleviate these symptoms, but high-protein meals should be avoided. The client may continue to take the medication, and attempts should be made to minimize the side effects. The client's food preferences and his blood pressure are not relevant to the situation. (Lewis et al., 9 ed., p. 1435)

9. *3*

Most CSF leaks resolve spontaneously. The child should be maintained on bed rest until drainage ends. Nonsteroidal antiinflammatory drugs are not contraindicated. The child may turn and assume a position of comfort, and there are usually no dietary restrictions. (Hockenberry & Wilson, 10 ed., pp. 991–992)

10. *2*

An early symptom of Parkinson disease is slowness of movements in all normal ADLs. Tremors and weight loss may occur but are not commonly the first symptoms. Depression is a complication, along with other issues such as hallucinations, psychosis, and dementia, which can occur later in the disease process. (Lewis et al., 9 ed., p. 1434)

11. *3*

Because of the emotional stress of Parkinson disease, mood disturbances often occur. Problems with communication, intellectual skills, and diversional interest are usually not as common as mood disturbance in the early stages. (Lewis et al., 9 ed., pp. 1436–1437)

12. *3*

Decreased mobility over an extended period leads to stasis of secretions. There is no associated dysfunction in the CNS regarding the respiratory system. The immune response is mature but may become impaired as a result of the chronic illness. (Hockenberry & Wilson, 10 ed., p. 1149)

13. *2*

The spinal needle is inserted at L3–L4. If there is any oozing after the procedure, it could be spinal fluid. This would increase the risk of headache and infection. Headache is not uncommon. Remaining in the supine position should help prevent the headache. Weakness of the upper muscles is not relevant to the lumbar puncture, and many clients have difficulty voiding while confined to bed. (Lewis et al., 9 ed., pp. 1350–1351)

14. *4*

Lowering the client's head increases ICP. Restraints should not be used because pulling against restraints will increase ICP. The client should be suctioned only as necessary. The temperature monitoring depends on the equipment; if the client is prone to seizures, an oral thermometer should not be placed in the client's mouth. (Lewis et al., 9 ed, p. 1368)

15. *2*

Because the motor fibers from one side of the brain cross to the opposite side before passing down the spinal cord, hemorrhage on the brain's left side causes right-sided hemiplegia and vice versa. Spasticity is not a common occurrence, and both sides of the body are not affected. (Lewis et al., 9 ed., pp. 1392–1394)

16. *3*

Irritability and vomiting are common signs of increased ICP in the infant; the symptoms are often delayed in the infant because of the open fontanels. Retinal hemorrhage, paresis, and papilledema are indications of more acute hematoma formation. (Hockenberry & Wilson, 10 ed., p. 989)

17. *3*

Enoxaparin is a low-molecular-weight heparin. Thinning the blood of a client with cerebral hemorrhage could significantly worsen the bleed. Gemfibrozil is used to decrease cholesterol. Mannitol is an osmotic diuretic. Nitroprusside is used for a hypertensive crisis. (Lewis et al., 9 ed., pp. 1370–1373)

18. *1*

Early signs of MS include difficulty with fine motor movement, especially of the head and neck. Often, visual disturbance is the most ominous sign. Tremors, flaccid paralysis, and unilateral neglect are not seen in the client with MS. (Lewis et al., 9 ed., p. 1488)

19. *3*

Guillain-Barré is an acute and rapidly progressing condition affecting the peripheral nervous system characterized by an ascending level of paralysis leading to a serious complication of respiratory failure. This necessitates constant monitoring of the respiratory system. Although other autonomic dysfunctions can occur (requiring the other assessments), such as orthostatic hypotension, hypertension, heart block, bowel and bladder dysfunction, facial flushing, diaphoresis, and lower brainstem involvement (cranial nerves), respiratory problems are the priority. (Lewis et al., 9 ed., p. 1467)

# CHAPTER TWENTY-THREE

# Musculoskeletal: Care of Adult and Pediatric Clients

**23**

## PRIORITY CONCEPTS
Functional Ability, Mobility, Pain

## PHYSIOLOGY OF THE MUSCULOSKELETAL AND CONNECTIVE TISSUE

### Bones
A. Bone function.
1. Supporting framework allowing weight bearing.
2. Protection for underlying organs.
3. Bones act as a lever allowing movement through the attachment of tendons and muscles.
4. Bones contain hematopoietic tissue for red and white blood cell production.
5. Bones are storage units for inorganic minerals like calcium and phosphorus.
B. Bone structure.
1. Periosteum: dense fibrous membrane covering the bone.
2. Diaphysis: main shaft of the bone; marrow is in the center.
3. Metaphysis: area of cancellous bone between the epiphysis and the diaphysis.
4. Epiphysis: the widened area found at the end of a long bone.
5. Epiphyseal plate (growth zone): a cartilage area in children that provides for longitudinal growth of the bone.
C. Bone maintenance and healing.
1. Bone remodeling: removal of old bone by osteoclasts (resorption); deposition of new bone by osteoblasts (ossification).
   a. Weight-bearing stress stimulates local bone resorption and formation; in states of immobility in which weight bearing is prevented, calcium is lost from the bone.
   b. Vitamin D promotes absorption of calcium.
2. Bone healing (Figure 23-1).

**TEST ALERT:** Identify pathophysiology related to an acute or chronic condition (e.g., signs and symptoms).

### Connective Tissue: Joints and Cartilage
A. Joints.
1. A joint is a point where bones meet and facilitate body movement, which depends on cartilage for movement and flexibility. Cartilage not only covers bone for smooth movement but also acts as a shock-absorbing pad and connector.
2. The diarthrodial (synovial) joint is the most common type of joint in the body.
3. Synovial fluid is secreted and serves to decrease friction by lubricating the joint.
B. Articular cartilage is rigid, connective, avascular tissue that covers the end of each bone.
C. Ligaments and tendons are tough fibrous connective tissues that provide stability while continuing to permit movement.
1. Tendons attach muscles to the bone.
2. Ligaments attach bones to joints.

### Skeletal Muscle
A. Function: skeletal muscle move bones through contraction and relaxation; muscles also store protein for energy and metabolism.
B. Energy is consumed when skeletal muscles contract in response to a stimulus.
1. Lactic acid, a by-product of muscle metabolism, accumulates if the amount of oxygen available to the cell is not sufficient.
2. Muscle fatigue results from:
   a. Increased work of the muscle, with inadequate oxygen supply.
   b. Depletion of glycogen and energy stores.
C. Muscle contraction.
1. Flexion: bending at a joint.
2. Extension: straightening of a joint.
3. Abduction: action moving away from the body.
4. Adduction: action moving toward the body.
5. Hypertrophy (increase in muscle mass) will occur if muscle is exercised repeatedly.
6. Atrophy (decrease in muscle mass) will occur with muscle disuse.

### System Assessment
A. History.
1. History of musculoskeletal injuries, musculoskeletal surgeries, neuromuscular disabilities, inflammatory and metabolic conditions directly or indirectly affecting the musculoskeletal system.
2. Familial predisposition to orthopedic problems.
3. Level of normal activity, occupation, exercise, recreation.
4. Existence of other chronic health problems.

**515**

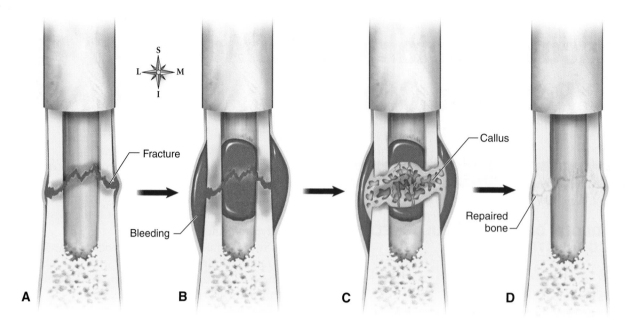

**FIGURE 23-1 Bone Repair.** (From Patton, K., & Thibodeau, G. [2014]. *The human body in health and disease* [6th ed.]. St. Louis, MO: Elsevier.)

B. Physical assessment.
   1. Initial inspection for gross deformities, asymmetry, and edema.
   2. Nutritional status: appropriateness of client's weight and body frame; 24-hour diet recall, dietary supplements.
   3. Joints.
      a. Movement: active and passive; examine active movement first; compare movement and range of motion (ROM) on one side of the body with movement and ROM on the opposite side.
      b. Inflammation and tenderness: with or without movement.
      c. Presence of joint deformities and dislocations.
      d. Palpate joints for crepitus.
   4. Evaluate limb length and circumference if hypertrophy or inconsistency in bone length is evident.
   5. Evaluate client's spinal alignment, posture, and gait.
   6. Evaluate skeletal muscle.
      a. Muscle strength bilaterally.
      b. Coordination of movement.
      c. Presence of atrophy or hypertrophy.
      d. Presence of involuntary muscle movement.
   7. Assess peripheral pulses and peripheral circulation.
   8. Assess for presence and characteristics of pain.
      a. Specific type of pain and exact location.
      b. Identify precipitating and/or alleviating factors (most musculoskeletal pain is relieved by rest).
      c. Ask about back pain and/or injury.
   9. Sensory changes: assess for decreased sensation in extremities.
   10. Body mechanics (Box 23-1).
   11. Changes in the older adult (Box 23-2).

---

**Box 23-1  BODY MECHANICS**

The wider the base of support, the greater the stability.
  • Position feet wide apart.
The lower the center of gravity, the greater the stability.
  • Flex the knees; let the strong muscles of the legs do the work.
  • Position close to client.
Face the client; keep back, pelvis, and knees aligned; avoid twisting.
Balance activity between arms and legs.
  • Avoid bending to lift; this decreases strain on the back.
Encourage client to assist.
  • Pivoting, turning, rolling, and leverage require less work.
Person with heaviest load should coordinate team efforts.
  • Obtain assistance for a lift with heavy or difficult transfers or moves.
  • Use a gait belt for all client transfers.
Teach client proper body mechanics.

**TEST ALERT:** Use ergonomic principles when providing care (assistive devices, proper lifting).

**TEST ALERT:** Perform a focused assessment and reassessment for changes in client condition. Recognize signs and symptoms of complications and intervene appropriately.

## DISORDERS OF MUSCULOSKELETAL AND CONNECTIVE TISSUE

### Developmental Dysplasia of the Hip

Developmental dysplasia of the hip (DDH) is the correct terminology for a variety of disorders related to abnormal

**Musculoskeletal Changes**
- Decreased bone density leads to more frequent fractures.
- Decrease in subcutaneous tissue results in less soft tissue over bony prominences.
- Degenerative changes in the musculoskeletal system alter posture and gait.
- Degenerative changes in cartilage and ligaments result in joint stiffness and pain.
- Range of motion of extremities decreases; older adult may need increased assistance with activities of daily living.
- Slowed movement and decreased muscle strength lead to decreased response time.
- Loss of height from disk compression, posture changes, kyphosis, dowager's hump.

development of the hip. The older term, congenital hip dysplasia, has been replaced by DDH, which includes various hip problems, such as a shallow acetabulum, subluxation, or dislocation.

### Assessment

A. Risk factors/etiology.
  1. Frequently associated with other congenital deformities.
  2. Prenatal factors.
    a. Maternal hormone secretion.
    b. Intrauterine posture, especially frank breech position.
    c. Genetic—higher incidence in siblings of affected children.
B. Clinical manifestations (newborn).
  1. Ortolani sign: infant supine, knees flexed, hips fully abducted; a click is heard or felt as the hip is reduced by abduction.

> **NURSING PRIORITY:** The Ortolani and Barlow tests should only be performed by experienced nurses trained in these tests.

  2. Asymmetric gluteal and thigh folds.
  3. Shortening of the leg on the affected side; one knee is lower than the other (Galeazzi sign).
  4. Positive Barlow maneuver—adducting the infant's hips while applying light pressure on the knee posteriorly. If the hip is dislocatable or unstable, the test is considered positive.
C. Diagnostics (see Appendix 23-1).

### Treatment

A. Treatment is initiated as soon as condition is identified.
B. For the newborn, the dislocated hip is securely held in a full abduction position. This keeps the femur in the acetabulum and stabilizes the area.
  1. Abduction devices.
    a. Pavlik harness: a fabric strap harness that is secured around the infant's shoulders and chest and is connected to straps around the lower legs. The harness acts as a brace to maintain the legs in a flexed, abducted position at the hip. The harness may be removed for bathing but should be worn 23 hours a day until the hip is stable.
    b. Hip spica cast: most often used when adduction contracture is present. After the removal of the cast, a protective abduction brace is fitted.
  2. Closed reduction: performed in older children, 6 to 24 months old.
  3. Open reduction: performed if hip is not reducible with traction or closed reduction.
C. Successful reduction becomes increasingly difficult after the age of 4 years.

### Nursing Interventions

**Goal:** To identify hip dysplasia in the newborn before discharge.

**Goal:** To assist parents to understand mechanism to maintain reduction.

A. Pavlik harness.
  1. Teach parents proper application of harness.
  2. Undershirts should be worn beneath the brace.
  3. Check skin under brace for irritation or pressure areas at least two or three times a day.
  4. No oils or lotions should be applied to skin that will be under the brace.
  5. Reposition the child frequently and lightly massage skin under straps to improve circulation at least once a day.
  6. Always place the diaper under the straps.

> **NURSING PRIORITY:** Because of rapid growth of infants, straps should be checked and adjusted every 1 to 2 weeks to prevent vascular or nerve injury.

B. Spica cast.
  1. Teach parents cast care if hip spica cast is applied (e.g., keep cast dry, do not insert foreign objects into the cast).
  2. Assess for and reduce skin irritation by maintaining cleanliness of the cast and the child.
  3. Elevate the child's head during feedings to prevent choking.
  4. If the child is being breastfed, elevating the child on pillows and using the "football" hold is recommended.

**Goal:** To facilitate developmental progress.

A. Provide stimuli and activity appropriate for developmental level.
B. Encourage parents to hold and cuddle child.
C. Maintain normal home routine.

### Congenital Clubfoot (Talipes Equinovarus)

Congenital clubfoot (talipes equinovarus) is a deformity of the ankle and foot in which adduction, plantar flexion, and inversion of the foot occur in varying degrees of severity. The unilateral form occurs more commonly than the bilateral form. *Talipes equinovarus* (TEV) involves bone deformity. Metatarsus adductus (*metatarsus varus*), which is often confused with congenital clubfoot (*talipes equinovarus*), occurs as a result of abnormal intrauterine positioning and involves medial adduction of the toes and forefoot and inversion (kidney-shaped foot); ankle ROM is normal.

## Assessment

A. Risk factors/etiology (inconclusive).
   1. Familial tendency.
   2. Arrested fetal development of the skeletal and soft tissue of the foot.
   3. Intrauterine positioning/compression.
B. Assessment.
   1. Condition is apparent at birth.
   2. In true clubfoot, there is severe limitation of ROM.
C. Diagnostics: clinical manifestations.

## Treatment

Treatment is begun immediately and most often requires three stages for correction.
A. Correction of deformity: casts are applied in series for gradual stretching and straightening; massage accompanied by special bandaging may also be used.
B. Surgical intervention followed by casting.
C. After cast(s) removal, varus prevention brace to maintain correction.
D. Maintenance of correction: orthopedic shoes.
E. Follow-up observations.

## Nursing Interventions

**Goal:** To assist parents to understand mechanism of treatment to achieve correction.

A. Appropriate care of cast or brace at home.
B. Follow-up care and importance of frequent cast changes.

**Goal:** To facilitate developmental progress and adapt nurturing activities to meet infant's and parents' needs (same as for developmental dysplasia of the hip).

## Intervertebral Disk Disease

**Intervertebral disk disease affects the cartilage disks located between the vertebrae of the spinal column. The problems may involve deterioration, herniation, or dysfunction of the intervertebral disks. Any section of the cervical, thoracic, or lumbar spine can be affected by this disease.**

## Assessment

A. Risk factors/etiology.
   1. Disease causing structural deterioration.
   2. Obesity.
   3. Injury or stress to an area of the spinal column causing a tear or weakening of the annulus fibrosus portion of an intervertebral disk allowing herniation of the disk. (The most common area for this type of injury is in the lumbar spine.)
   4. Occupations that involve heavy lifting or extended periods of sitting or driving.
B. Clinical manifestations (lumbar disk).
   1. Low back pain, commonly radiating down one buttock and posterior thigh.
   2. Coughing, straining, sneezing, bending, twisting, and lifting exacerbate the pain.
   3. Lying supine and raising the leg in an extended position will precipitate the pain.
C. Diagnostics (see Appendix 23-1).

## Treatment

A. Conservative.
   1. Analgesics, muscle relaxants, antiseizure drugs, and/or epidural corticosteroid injections.
   2. Weight reduction, if appropriate.
   3. Ice may be used for first 48 hours after injury; then moist heat is a better analgesic.
   4. Activity modification, good body mechanics, back brace.
   5. Physical and/or ultrasound therapy, transcutaneous electrical nerve stimulation (TENS), and massage.
   6. Back strengthening exercises once the pain subsides.
   7. Alternative treatment: acupuncture or acupressure.
B. Surgical.
   1. Laminectomy: removal of the herniated portion of the disk; surgery may include fusion, which involves bone grafts to stop movement between the vertebrae.
   2. Microlaminectomy (diskectomy).
   3. Intradiskal electrothermoplasty.
   4. Radiofrequency diskal nucleoplasty.
   5. Interspinous process decompression system.
   6. Diskectomy.
   7. Percutaneous laser diskectomy.
   8. Artificial disk replacement.
   9. Spinal fusion with or without instrumentation.

## Nursing Interventions for the Nonsurgical Client

**Goal:** To relieve pain by means of conservative measures and prevent recurrence of problem.

A. Decrease muscle spasm/pain with analgesics, muscle relaxants, decreased activity, and cold or heat applications.
B. Begin ambulation slowly and avoid having client bend, stoop, twist, sit, or lift.
C. Instruct the client and family regarding the principles of appropriate body mechanics.
D. The client will need a firm mattress; sleeping in the prone position, especially with a pillow, should be avoided.
E. Instruct the client and family regarding lower back (core strengthening) exercises.
F. Encourage correct posture; instruct client to avoid prolonged standing.
G. Client should sit in straight-backed chairs; avoid prolonged periods of sitting or standing.
H. Semireclining position with forward flexion of lumbar spine (recliner) may be position of comfort.

### Nursing Interventions for the Surgical Client—Laminectomy and/or Spinal Surgery

**Preoperative Goal:** To prepare client for laminectomy and/or spinal surgery.

A. Perform preoperative nursing interventions, including education as appropriate.
B. Have client practice logrolling.
C. Have client practice voiding from supine position.
D. Discuss with client postoperative pain and anticipated methods to decrease pain.
E. Evaluate bowel and bladder function.
F. Identify specific characteristics of pain to be included in database for comparison with pain after surgery.
G. Establish a baseline neurologic assessment for postoperative reference.

**Postoperative Goal:** Promote comfort and pain relief and maintain spinal alignment after laminectomy and/or spinal surgery.

A. Keep the bed in flat position.
B. Logroll client when turning.
C. Keep pillows between the legs when client is positioned on his or her side.
D. The client who has had microdisk surgery will have fewer limitations on mobility. Often, the client may assume a position of comfort.
E. Assist with application of back brace if ordered.

**Postoperative Goal:** To maintain homeostasis and assess for complications after laminectomy and/or spinal surgery.

A. Evaluate incision area for possible leakage of spinal fluid and bleeding; notify health care provider of clear fluid leaking from incisional area and for severe headache associated with the loss of spinal fluid.
B. Analgesics may be given via a patient-controlled analgesia pump or epidural catheter.
C. Assess pain and determine whether there is any pain radiation.

> **TEST ALERT:** Assess client's need for pain management and intervene as needed using pharmacologic and nonpharmacologic comfort measures.

D. Perform neurovascular checks of extremities (6 Ps; see Figure 18-1).
E. Normal bladder function returns in 24 to 48 hours; assess current status of voiding.

> **NURSING PRIORITY:** The client who has undergone laminectomy and/or spinal surgery frequently experiences difficulty voiding; this may be due to edema in the area of surgery that interferes with normal bladder sensation.

F. Ambulate as soon as indicated (frequently on first postoperative day if no fusion was done).
G. If fusion was performed, may need to apply a body brace before ambulation.

H. The client who has undergone microlaminectomy experiences less pain, is frequently out of bed on the day of surgery, and has fewer complications.
I. Paralytic ileus and constipation are common complications; assess for decreased bowel sounds and abdominal distention.

> **TEST ALERT:** Identify factors that interfere with elimination.

### Scoliosis

**Scoliosis is a lateral curvature of the spine. If it is allowed to progress without treatment, it will severely affect the shape of the thoracic cavity and impair ventilation.**

A. Idiopathic (predominant type) occurs primarily in adolescent girls.
B. Most noticeable at beginning of growth spurt, around 10 years of age.

#### Assessment

A. Clinical manifestations.
  1. Uneven hips and shoulders.
  2. Visible curvature of the spinal column; head and hips are not in alignment.
  3. When child bends forward from the waist, there is visible asymmetry of the shoulders. The ribs and shoulder are more prominent on one side.
  4. Waistline is uneven; one hip is more prominent.
B. Diagnostics.
  1. Clinical manifestations.
  2. X-ray film.

#### Treatment

A. Observation and monitoring for curvature less than 25 degrees.
B. Brace to prevent progression of the curvature (used for curvatures of 25 to 40 degrees).
  1. Milwaukee brace for high thoracic curvatures from kyphosis.
  2. Boston and Wilmington brace (underarm orthosis) for thoracic–lumbar curves.
C. Surgery (used for curvatures of more than 40 degrees): spinal fusion and placement of a rod to prevent destruction of the fused segment; the rod may be left in place permanently unless it becomes displaced or causes discomfort.

#### Nursing Interventions

**Goal:** To identify defects early and promote effective conservative therapy.

A. Promote health programs in school to identify condition.

> **TEST ALERT:** Perform targeted screening (scoliosis, vision, and hearing).

B. Assist client and parents to properly use braces.
1. Make sure brace is properly fitted and does not inadvertently rub bony prominences.
2. May put light T-shirt under brace for comfort.
3. Initially, the brace is worn 20 to 23 hours per day.
4. Brace is regularly adjusted to promote correction.
5. If progress is good, child is weaned from the brace during the daytime and wears it only at night.
6. Supplemental exercises.

**Goal:** To support normal growth and development and assist the child to develop a positive self-image.

A. Continue to encourage peer socialization.
B. Encourage independence.
C. Encourage child to participate in and be independent in scheduling of activities and other aspects of care.
D. Emphasize positive long-term outcome.

**Goal:** To maintain spinal alignment after surgical correction (see Postoperative nursing interventions for the surgical client after laminectomy and/or spinal surgery).

**Goal:** To maintain homeostasis and assess for complications after surgical correction (see Postoperative nursing interventions for the surgical client after laminectomy and/or spinal surgery).

### Fractures

**A fracture is a disruption or break in the continuity of the bone.**

A. Traumatic fractures are the most common cause of fractures and occur as a result of physical force to a bone or stress greater than the tensile strength of the bone.
B. Pathologic fractures occur as a result of a disease process, rather than excessive traumatic force, such as osteosarcoma, osteoporosis.
C. Classification of fractures (Figure 23-2).
1. Type:
    a. Complete: fracture line extends through the entire bone; the periosteum is disrupted on both sides of the bone.
    b. Incomplete: fracture line extends only partially through the bone, often the result of bending or

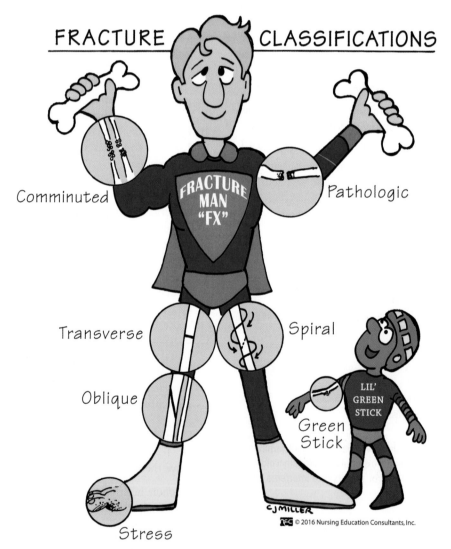

**FIGURE 23-2 Fracture Classifications.** (From Zerwekh, J., Garneau, A., & Miller, C. J. [2017]. *Digital collection of the memory notebooks of nursing* [4th ed.]. Chandler, AZ: Nursing Education Consultants, Inc.)

crushing forces applied to a bone (hairline-type fractures).

   c. Comminuted: fracture with multiple bone fragments; more common in adults.

   d. Greenstick: nondisplaced fracture in which the periosteum is intact across the fracture and the bone is still in alignment; more common in children.

   e. Impacted: complete fracture in which bone fragments are driven into each other.

2. Classified according to location on the bone: proximal, middle, or distal.

3. Stable versus unstable fracture.

   a. Stable: a portion of the periosteum usually remains intact; frequently transverse, spiral, or greenstick fractures.

   b. Unstable: bones are displaced at the time of injury, with poor approximation; frequently comminuted or impacted.

   c. Simple, closed fracture: does not produce a break in the skin.

   d. Complex, open, or compound fracture: involves an open wound through which the bone has protruded. (Figure 23-3 has more information on types of fractures.)

---

🔔 **NURSING PRIORITY:** Age, displacement of the fracture, the site of the fracture, nutritional level, medications, and blood supply to the area of injury are factors influencing time required for fracture healing, as well as complications. Be familiar with the terms used to describe fractures.

---

### Assessment

A. Risk factors/etiology.

   1. Pathologic fracture.

      a. Osteoporosis.

      b. Tumors (multiple myeloma, osteogenic sarcoma).

      c. Metabolic diseases (e.g., thyroid disorders).

   2. Trauma.

B. Clinical manifestations.

   1. Edema, swelling of soft tissue around the injured site.

   2. Pain: immediate, severe.

   3. Abnormal positioning of extremity; deformity.

   4. Loss of normal function.

   5. False movement: movement occurs at the fracture site; bone should not move except at joints.

   6. Crepitus: palpable or audible crunching as the ends of the bones rub together.

   7. Discoloration of the skin around the affected area.

   8. Sensation may be impaired if there is nerve damage.

C. Diagnostics (see Appendix 23-1).

### Treatment

A. Immediate immobilization of suspected fracture area.

B. Fracture reduction.

   1. Closed reduction: nonsurgical, manual realignment of the bones; then injured extremity is usually placed in

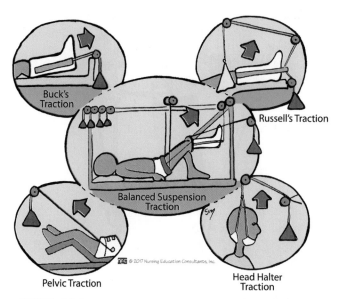

**FIGURE 23-3 Examples of Common Types of Traction.** (From Zerwekh, J., & Miller, C. J. [2017]. *NCLEX Review course.* Chandler, AZ: Nursing Education Consultants.)

a cast for continued immobilization until healing occurs.

2. Open reduction and internal fixation (ORIF): surgical correction of alignment.

C. Traction (see Figure 23-3).

   1. Purposes.

      a. Immobilization of fractures until surgical correction is done; immobilization or alignment of fracture until sufficient healing occurs to permit casting.

      b. Decrease, prevent, or correct bone or joint deformities associated with muscle diseases and bone injury.

      c. Prevent or reduce muscle spasm.

   2. Types.

      a. Skeletal: wire or metal pin is inserted into or through the bone.

      b. Skin: force of pull is applied directly to the skin and indirectly to the bone.

D. Cast application to maintain immobility of affected area.

   1. Cast applied to immobilize joints above and below the injured area.

   2. Short or long arm or leg cast.

   3. Body jacket cast for spinal injuries.

   4. Hip spica cast for femoral fractures.

E. Fixation devices.

   1. External fixation: application of a rigid external device consisting of pins placed through the bone and held in place by a metal frame; requires meticulous care of pin insertion sites (Figure 23-4).

   2. Internal fixation: done through an open incision; hardware (pins, plates, rods, screws) is placed in the bone.

   3. Both methods may be used to treat a fracture.

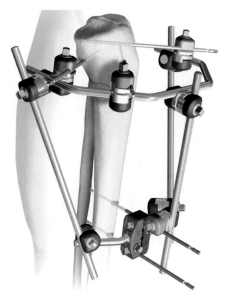

**FIGURE 23-4** **External Fixation.** (Courtesy Stryker, Kalamazoo, MI.)

### Specific Fractures

A. Colles' fracture.
  1. Fracture of the distal radius.
  2. Primary complication is compartment syndrome.
  3. Carpal tunnel syndrome may develop after the fracture has healed.
B. Fracture of humerus.
  1. Common injury of young adults.
  2. Complication is radial nerve injury.
C. Fractured pelvis.
  1. Frequently occurs in older adults and is associated with falls.
  2. May cause serious intraabdominal injuries (hemorrhage) and urinary tract injury.
  3. Bed rest is prescribed for clients with stable fractures.
  4. Combination of traction, cast, and surgical intervention may be used for the client with a complex fracture.
  5. Turn client only on specific orders.
D. Femoral shaft fracture.
  1. Common injury in young adults and children.
  2. Treatment.
    a. Immobility is achieved by means of a hip spica cast in older children.
    b. 90°-90° traction (see Figure 23-3): balanced skeletal traction for fractured femur.
    c. Older child and adult.
      (1) Internal fixation (adults).
      (2) Balanced skeletal traction for 8 to 12 weeks.
      (3) Immobilization by application of a hip spica cast alone or after balanced skeletal traction.
E. Characteristics of bones in children affecting fractures and fracture healing.
  1. Presence of epiphyseal plate; if the epiphyseal plate is damaged in the fracture, this may affect the growth of the long bone.

  2. Periosteum is thicker and stronger and has an increased blood supply, therefore healing is more rapid.
  3. Bones are more porous and allow for greater flexibility.
F. Rib fractures.
  1. Usually heal in 3 to 6 weeks with no residual impairment.
  2. Painful respirations cause client's breathing to be more shallow and coughing to be restrained; this precipitates buildup of secretions and decreased ventilation, leading to atelectasis and pneumonia.
  3. Chest taping or strapping is not usually done because it decreases thoracic excursion.
  4. Multiple rib fractures may precipitate the development of a pneumothorax or a tension pneumothorax (see Chapter 17).
G. Mandible fracture.
  1. Wiring of jaws (intermaxillary fixation) is treatment.
  2. Postoperative problems: airway obstruction and aspiration of vomitus.
    a. Wire cutters near the client at all times in case of emergency (cardiac or respiratory arrest).
    b. Suction client if vomiting.
    c. Cutting wires may complicate problem.
  3. Tracheostomy set at bedside.
  4. Oral hygiene and use of pad/pencil or picture board to communicate postop.
  5. Discharge teaching: oral care, techniques for handling secretions, how and when to use wire cutters, diet (problems with constipation and flatus due to low-bulk, high-carbohydrate liquid supplements).

### *Fracture Complications*

A. Improper healing: delayed union, nonunion, or angulation (bone heals at a distorted angle).
B. Infection: especially in injuries resulting in an open fracture and soft tissue injury.
C. Decreased neurovascular status resulting from pressure of cast and edema formation.
D. Compartment syndrome: muscle, nerves, and vessels are restricted within a confined space (myofascial compartment) within an extremity.
  1. Etiology.
    a. Decreased compartment size from cast, splints, tight bandages, tight surgical closure.
    b. Increase in compartment contents caused by hemorrhage and/or edema.
  2. Clinical manifestations of compartment syndrome.

> **TEST ALERT:** Manage a client with alteration in hemodynamics, tissue perfusion, and hemostasis (cerebral, cardiac, peripheral).

    a. Muscle ischemia occurs as a result of compression of structures in the compartment.
    b. Arterial compression may not occur; pulses may still be present.
    c. May cause permanent damage if pressure is not relieved immediately.

d. Client reports of excessive or significant increase in pain unrelieved by analgesics.

e. Loss of movement and sensation distal to injury.

f. Skin is pale and cool to the touch distal to the injury.

g. Capillary refill greater than 3 seconds.

h. Occurrence of compartment syndrome may be decreased by elevation of the extremity and application of ice packs after initial injury.

i. Treatment is directed toward immediate release of pressure: if the client has a cast, the cast may be "bivalved"—the cast is split in half, and the halves are secured around the extremity by a wrap, such as an elastic bandage.

j. Volkmann's ischemic contracture: compartment syndrome in the arms that compromises circulation; occurs most often as a result of short arm cast used to immobilize a fracture of the humerus.

k. Can result in permanent damage in a short period (6 to 8 hours).

l. Paresthesia is frequently the first sign; pulselessness is a late sign.

> **TEST ALERT:** If compartment syndrome is suspected, elevation should not be above the level of the heart.

E. Venous stasis and thrombus formation are related to immobility. Preventive measures may be initiated, such as the use of low doses of a low-molecular-weight heparin (enoxaparin).

F. Fat embolism.
   1. Associated with fractures or surgery of long bones (especially the femur); primarily occurs in adults.
   2. Clinical manifestations generally occur within 12 to 48 hours of injury.
   3. Fat embolism produces symptoms of acute respiratory distress and hypoxia.
   4. Early immobilization of fractures, especially of long bones, the best prevention of fat emboli.

G. Blisters may be associated with twisting-type fractures or compartmental syndrome.

## Fracture Immobilization–Splinting

### Nursing Interventions

**Goal:** To immobilize a fractured extremity and to provide emergency care before transporting client.

A. Evaluate circulation distal to injury.

> **! NURSING PRIORITY:** Identify orthopedic situations that can cause compromised circulation and neurologic damage; intervene and obtain assistance.

B. Splint and immobilize extremity before transfer.

C. If pulses are not present or if the extremity must be realigned to apply splint for transfer, apply just enough traction to support and immobilize the fractured extremity in

a position of proper alignment. Once the traction is initiated, do not release it until the extremity has been properly splinted.

> **TEST ALERT:** Do not apply traction to compound fractures; traction may cause more damage to tissue and vessels.

D. Elevate the affected extremity, if possible, to decrease edema.

## Fracture Immobilization–Casts

### Nursing Interventions

**Goal:** Maintain immobilization and prevent complications.

A. Plaster cast: allow cast to dry adequately before moving the client or handling the cast.
   1. Encourage drying of cast by using fans and maintaining adequate circulation.
   2. Avoid handling wet cast to prevent indentions in the cast, which may precipitate pressure areas inside the cast; support cast on plastic-covered pillows while drying.
   3. Reposition client every 2 hours to increase drying on all cast surfaces.
   4. "Petaling" a cast is done to cover the rough edges and prevent crumbling of a plaster cast; edges are covered with small strips of waterproof adhesive.
   5. Try not to get the cast wet; after the cast is dry and the initial edema is resolved, may use low setting on hair dryer after exposure to water.

> **! NURSING PRIORITY:** Teach client: DO NOT get plaster cast wet, remove any type of padding, insert any objects inside cast, bear weight on new cast for 48 hours (if weight-bearing type), or cover cast with plastic for long periods.

B. Synthetic casts (fiberglass, polyester cotton knit) are lighter and require a minimal amount of drying time.
   1. Frequently used for upper body cast.
   2. Preferable for infants and children.
   3. Cast does not crumble around the edges and does not soil as easily.
   4. Cast dries rapidly if it gets damp, and it does not disintegrate in water; some synthetic casts can be immersed for bathing.

C. Continue to assess for compromised circulation and compartment syndrome.

D. Body jacket cast and hip spica cast.
   1. Evaluate for abdominal discomfort caused by cast compression of mesenteric artery against duodenum (cast syndrome).
   2. Relief of abdominal pressure can be achieved by means of nasogastric tube and suction or cast removal and reapplication.
   3. Evaluate for pressure areas over iliac crest.

E. Elevate casted extremity, especially during the first 24 hours after application.

F. Apply ice packs over the area of injury (keeping cast dry) during the first 24 hours.

G. Encourage movement and exercise of unaffected joints.

H. Assess for infection underneath the cast.
1. Unpleasant (foul) odor and/or drainage (especially purulent) emanating from inside of cast.
2. Generalized body temperature elevation.
3. Increased warmth over outside of the cast (hot spot).

## Fracture Immobilization–Traction
(see Figure 23-3)
*Nursing Interventions*

**Goal:** To maintain immobilization and prevent complications.

A. Assume that traction is continuous unless the doctor orders otherwise.

B. Carefully assess for skin breakdown, especially under the client.

C. Do not change or remove traction weight on a client with continuous traction.

D. The traction ropes and weights should hang free from any obstructions.

E. Traction applied in one direction requires an equal countertraction to be effective.
1. Do not let the client's feet touch the end of the bed; this will cause the countertraction to be lost.
2. Do not allow the traction weights to rest on anything at the end of the bed; this negates the pull of the traction.

F. Carefully assess the pin sites in clients with skeletal traction. Osteomyelitis is a serious complication of skeletal traction.

> **TEST ALERT:** Recognize client with a condition that increases risk for insufficient vascular perfusion; monitor effective functioning of therapeutic device; prevent complications of immobility. The majority of clients with fractures will experience some level of immobility.

**Goal:** To prevent complications of immobility (see Chapter 3).

## Fracture Immobilization–External or Internal Fixation Devices

**Goal:** To maintain immobilization and prevent complications from external or internal fixation.

A. Inspect exposed skin and pin sites for infection.
B. Cleanse around pin sites using sterile technique.
C. Apply antibiotic ointment to pin sites as ordered.
D. Perform wound care on incisional area or area of trauma.
E. Observe carefully for development of an infection.
F. Evaluate for circulatory and neurosensory impairment.

### Home Care

A. Teach client what not to do.
1. Do not bear weight on the affected extremity until instructed to do so.
2. Do not allow the cast to get wet (discuss alternatives to tub baths).
3. Do not insert any objects in the cast or remove any padding.
4. Do not move or manipulate pins on an external fixator device.

B. Client should report symptoms associated with swelling or an increase in pain, especially pain unrelieved by analgesics.

C. Assess pin sites for evidence of infection.

## Fractured Hip

**Fractured hips are common in older adults, with the majority resulting from a fall. Incidence in women older than 65 years of age is increased because of loss of postural stability and loss of bone mass. The fracture involves the proximal third of the femur, which extends up to 5 cm below the lesser trochanter. It may be repaired by fixed or sliding nail plates, replacement prostheses, or hip joint replacement.**

*Assessment*

A. Types of fractures.
1. Intracapsular fracture (femoral neck): more difficult to heal; associated with osteoporosis; more likely to be associated with avascular necrosis due to interruption of blood supply.
2. Extracapsular fracture: occurs outside joint capsule; usually caused by severe direct trauma or a fall.

B. Clinical manifestations.
1. External rotation and adduction of the affected extremity.
2. Shortening of the length of the affected extremity.
Severe pain, tenderness, and muscle spasms.

C. Treatment.
1. Initially, Buck's traction to immobilize fracture and decrease muscle spasms (see Figure 23-3).
2. Surgical repair as soon as client's condition allows (permits earlier mobility and prevents complications of immobility).

D. Nursing interventions after surgery (Box 23-3).
1. Circulatory and neurologic checks distal to area of injury.
2. Position to prevent flexion, adduction, and internal rotation, which cause dislocation of the prosthesis.

> **TEST ALERT:** Position client to prevent complications.

a. Do not adduct the affected leg past the neutral position.
b. Maintain the affected leg in an abducted position with an abduction pillow or pillows between the legs.
c. Avoid flexion of the hip of more than 90 degrees, such as bending down to pick up something or tie shoes.
d. Prevent internal or external rotation by using sandbags, pillows, and trochanter rolls at the thigh.
e. Extreme external rotation accompanied by severe pain is indicative of hip prosthesis displacement.

**Musculoskeletal Nursing Implications**
- Older adults have difficulty maintaining immobility after fractures; therefore fractures are frequently repaired with surgical intervention (ORIF).
- Older adults heal more slowly, so use of extremity and weight bearing may be delayed.
- Complications of immobility occur more frequently; mobilize hospitalized clients as early as possible.
- Do not rely on fever as the primary indication of infection; decreasing mental status is more common.
- Contractures are more common in older adults.
- Encourage older adults to use assistive devices such as canes and walkers.

3. Check physician's order regarding positioning and turning.
4. Evaluate blood loss.
   a. Check the operative site for signs of hemorrhage.
   b. Measure the diameter of both thighs to evaluate the presence of internal bleeding in the affected extremity.

> **! NURSING PRIORITY:** The client is especially prone to complications of immobility (thromboembolism after hip fracture); use nursing interventions to minimize complications.

## Total Hip Arthroplasty (Total Hip Replacement)

**Total hip arthroplasty (THA) or replacement may be done because of a pathologic fracture or a disease process such as arthritis with the goal to provide relief of pain and improve function.**

### Assessment

A. History of osteoarthritis, rheumatoid arthritis, connective tissue disease, or trauma.
B. Slow loss of cartilage leads to loss of motion, chronic pain.

### Nursing Intervention

**Goal:** To provide preoperative care and pre- and postoperative instructions.

A. Encourage client to practice using either crutches or a walker, whichever is anticipated to be used after surgery.
B. Encourage client to practice moving from bed to a chair in the manner that will be necessary after surgery.
C. Help the client begin practicing the postoperative exercises so that he or she will understand and be able to do them correctly after surgery.
D. Client should discontinue use of platelet antiaggregant medications, such as nonsteroidal antiinflammatory drugs (NSAIDs); clopidogrel; anticoagulants, such as warfarin; and over-the-counter drugs and supplements, such as oral ginkgo, green tea, and ginseng for 7 days before surgery.
   1. Assess the client for other medications that may promote hemorrhage during or after surgery.

**Goal:** To provide postoperative care and prevent complications.

A. Position supine with head slightly elevated, maintain abduction of affected leg.
B. Quadriceps exercises.
C. Neurologic and circulation checks.
D. Client is mobilized on first or second postoperative day to prevent complications of immobility; may use antiembolism stockings and/or sequential compression devices on lower extremities to prevent venous stasis.
E. Low-molecular-weight heparin (see Appendix 18-2) may be given to prevent thrombophlebitis.
F. Keep client's heels off the bed to prevent skin breakdown.
G. Legs should not be crossed.

> **! NURSING PRIORITY:** After surgery, do not allow the repaired hip to flex greater than 90 degrees; avoid adduction and internal rotation of extremity. Excessive flexion and adduction may dislocate the hip prosthesis.

H. Observe for signs of possible hip dislocation.
   1. Increased hip pain.
   2. Shortening of affected leg.
   3. External leg rotation.
   4. If symptoms of possible hip dislocation are observed, contact the surgeon immediately.

## Total Knee Arthroplasty (Total Knee Replacement)

**Total knee arthroplasty (TKA) is the replacement or reconstruction of the knee joint to relieve pain and improve joint stability due to severe destruction or deterioration of the knee joint.**

### Assessment

A. History of osteoarthritis, rheumatoid arthritis, connective tissue disease, or trauma.
B. Slow loss of cartilage leads to loss of motion, chronic unremitting pain, and instability.
C. Presence of osteoporosis may necessitate bone grafting to augment defects.

### Nursing Intervention

**Goal:** To provide preoperative care (see Chapter 3).
**Goal:** To provide postoperative care and prevent complications.

A. Frequent neurovascular checks.
B. Compression dressing may be used immediately postop to immobilize knee.

C. Emphasis on physical therapy.
  1. Quadriceps exercises first day postop progressing to straight leg raises and gentle ROM to increase muscle strength and obtain 90-degree knee flexion.
  2. Continuous passive motion (CPM) machine to promote joint mobility.
  3. Full weight bearing on the info@dentistryforkidsnj.com extremity is started before discharge.

## Osteoporosis

**Osteoporosis is a chronic, progressive metabolic bone disease that involves an imbalance between new bone formation and bone resorption.**

A. Primary osteoporosis is the most common type; occurs most often in women after menopause because low levels of estrogen are associated with an increase in bone resorption. Osteoporosis can occur in men and is considered underdiagnosed; as many as one in four men over age 50 will have an osteoporosis-related fracture.
B. Bone loss occurs predominantly in the vertebral bodies of the spine, the femoral neck in the hip, and the distal radius of the arm. Bone mass declines, leaving the bones brittle and weak.

### Assessment

A. Risk factors/etiology (Figure 23-5).
  1. Age/sex/ethnicity: incidence increases in white and Asian women after the age of 50 years.
  2. Endocrine disorders of the thyroid and parathyroid glands.
  3. Nutritional deficits: insufficient intake of dietary calcium and/or vitamin D.

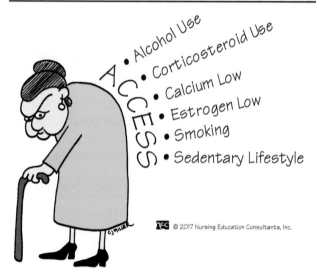

FIGURE 23-5 **Osteoporosis Risk Factors.** (From Zerwekh, J., Garneau, A., & Miller, C. J. [2017]. *Digital collection of the memory notebooks of nursing* [4th ed.]. Chandler, AZ: Nursing Education Consultants, Inc.)

B. Clinical manifestations.
  1. May be asymptomatic until x-ray films demonstrate skeletal weakening or a fracture occurs. Bone loss of 25% to 40% must occur before osteoporosis can be identified on standard x-ray films.
  2. Spinal deformity and "dowager's hump."
    a. Results from repeated pathologic, spinal vertebral fractures.
    b. Gradual loss of height (Figure 23-6).
    c. Increase in spinal curvature (kyphosis).
  3. Spinal fractures may occur spontaneously or as a result of minimal trauma.
  4. Chronic low thoracic and midline back pain.
  5. Height loss may precipitate thoracic problems, decrease in abdominal capacity, and decrease in exercise tolerance.
  6. Hip fractures and vertebral collapse are the most debilitating problems.
C. Diagnostics (see Appendix 23-1).
  1. Serum laboratory values of calcium, vitamin D, phosphorus, and alkaline phosphatase may be normal or low.
  2. Bone mineral density (BMD) measurements through quantitative ultrasound (QUS) and dual-energy x-ray absorptiometry (DEXA or DXA).
    a. DXA results are reported as T scores.
    b. Bone mineral density (BMD): 2.5 standard deviations below (22.5) mean of young adults is classified as osteoporosis.
    c. Osteopenia: T-score 5 between 21.0 and 22.5 but not at level of osteoporosis.

### Treatment

A. Dietary: increased intake of protein, calcium, and vitamin D.
B. Medications.
  1. Calcium supplements: daily intake of calcium should be approximately 1000 mg for men and 1500 mg for postmenopausal women.

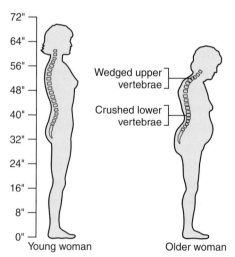

FIGURE 23-6 **Osteoporotic Changes.** (From Phillips N. [2013]. *Berry & Kohn's operating room technique* [12th ed.]. St. Louis, MO: Mosby.)

2. Vitamin D supplements (800 to 1000 IU recommended daily for postmenopausal women and older adults) to enhance utilization of calcium; spending 20 minutes daily in the sun will provide adequate vitamin D.

3. Antiresorptive medications, such as bisphosphonates and calcitonin, to facilitate increased bone density (see Appendix 23-2).

C. Exercise: activities that put moderate stress on bones by working them against gravity (walking, racquet sports, jogging).

1. Swimming and yoga may not be as beneficial because of decreased stress on bone mass.

2. Walking for 30 minutes three to five times a week is the most effective exercise in preventing osteoporosis.

3. Weight-bearing exercise decreases the development of osteoporosis and possibly increases new bone formation.

D. Compression fractures of the vertebrae usually heal without surgical intervention.

### Complications

Complications include bone fractures occurring in the vertebral bodies, distal radius, or hip.

### Nursing Interventions

**Goal:** To decrease pain and promote activities to diminish progression of disease.

A. Pain relief.
1. Bed rest initially, firm mattress.
2. Narcotic analgesics initially, followed by NSAIDs.

B. Assess bowel and bladder function; the info@dentistryfor kidsnj.com client will be prone to constipation and paralytic ileus if vertebrae are involved.

C. Regular daily exercise; encourage outdoor exercises (increases utilization of vitamin D).

D. Increased calcium and vitamin D intake and hormone replacement therapy.

### Home Care

A. Decrease falls and injury by maintaining safe home environment (Box 23-4).

B. The client should understand the need to continue taking medications, even if they do not make the client feel better. It is important for the client to understand that the calcium and vitamin D supplements are necessary to prevent further bone loss.

C. Do not exercise if pain occurs.

D. Avoid heavy lifting, stooping, and bending. Review and demonstrate good body mechanics with the client.

## Osteomyelitis

**Osteomyelitis is an infection of the bone, bone marrow, and surrounding soft tissue.**

A. The most common causative organism is *Staphylococcus aureus.*

B. Inflammatory response occurs initially, with increased vascularization and edema.

---

**Box 23-4 OLDER ADULT CARE FOCUS**

**Protecting Joints**
- If pain lasts longer than 1 hour after exercise, change the exercises that involve that joint.
- Plan activity and work that conserve energy; do important tasks first.
- Alternate activities; do not do all heavy tasks at one time.
- Minimize stress on joints; sit rather than stand, avoid prolonged repetitive movements, move around frequently, avoid stairs or prolonged grasping.
- Use largest muscles rather than smaller ones; use shoulders or arms rather than hands to push open doors; pick up items without stooping or bending; use leg muscles; women should carry purses on their shoulders rather than in their hands.
- Painful, acutely swollen inflamed joints should not be exercised beyond basic range of motion.
- Regular exercise can be done even when joints are slightly painful and stiff; swimming and bike riding maintain mobility without weight bearing.
- Expect changes in mental status after surgery.
- There may be a role change in the family due to the client's decreased mobility.

---

C. Even though the healing process occurs, the dead bone tissue frequently forms a sequestrum, which continues to retain viable bacteria; this tissue may produce recurrent abscesses for years.

D. Classified according to acute or chronic status.
1. Acute: sudden onset; may heal in 2 to 3 weeks or progress to chronic status.
2. Chronic: a problem continues for longer than 1 month; persistent problem or exacerbation of a previous problem.

### Assessment

A. Risk factors/etiology.
1. Indirect entry of organism: hematogenous.
   a. More frequently affects growing bone.
   b. Injury and infection of adjacent soft tissue in distal femur, proximal tibia, humerus, and radius.
2. Direct injury: can occur at any age.
   a. Trauma.
   b. Surgical procedures.

B. Clinical manifestations.
1. Acute.
   a. Tenderness, swelling, and warmth in affected area.
   b. Drainage from infected site.
   c. Systemic symptoms: fever, chills, nausea, night sweats.
   d. Constant pain in affected area; worsens with activity.
   e. Circulatory impairment.
2. Chronic: present longer than 1 month; failed to respond to initial course of antibiotic therapy.
   a. Drainage from wound or sinus tract.
   b. Recurrent episodes of bone pain.

c. Diminished systemic signs: low-grade fever; local signs of infection more common.
d. Remission and exacerbation of problem.
C. Diagnostics (see Appendix 23-1).
1. Bone or tissue biopsy.
2. Wound and/or blood culture.
3. Elevated white blood cell count, sedimentation rate, and C-reactive protein.
4. X-rays and radionuclide bone scan, magnetic resonance imaging (MRI), and computed tomography (CT).

### Treatment

A. Intensive intravenous (IV) antibiotics; oral antibiotic therapy for 6 to 8 weeks.
B. Immobilization of affected area.
C. Surgical debridement may be necessary.
D. Hyperbaric oxygen therapy to stimulate circulation and healing.

### Nursing Interventions

**Goal:** To decrease pain, promote comfort, and decrease spread of infection.

A. Administer IV piggyback antibiotics; frequently assess status of IV site for potential reactions to long-term, high-dose antibiotic therapy, including appropriate labs (e.g., peak and trough levels).
B. Administer analgesics and provide nonpharmacologic pain relieving interventions.
C. Maintain correct body alignment.
1. Move affected extremity gently and with support.
2. Prevent contractures, especially of affected extremity.
D. If there is an open wound, maintain wound (contact) precautions (see Chapter 9).
E. Perform sterile dressing changes. Dispose of old dressings according to hospital protocol or use "double-bag" technique to prevent cross-contamination.
F. Client is usually discharged on antibiotic therapy and instructed on the importance keeping all follow-up care appointments.

> **TEST ALERT:** Assess and document wound response to antibiotic therapy and wound care management.

## Osteosarcoma

**Osteogenic sarcoma is a malignant tumor of the bone. It is the most common primary bone cancer in children and young adults; it advances rapidly with bone destruction and metastasis to other sites throughout the body. Most commonly affects the pelvis and long bones of the lower extremities, such as the distal end of the femur, proximal tibia, or proximal humerus.**

### Assessment

A. Risk factors/etiology.
1. Peak incidence between 10 and 25 years of age.
2. Increased incidence in males during adolescence.

B. Clinical manifestations.
1. Localized pain, swelling at site of tumor, usually around knee.
2. Client may limp and be unable to function at full capacity.
C. Diagnostics (see Appendix 23-1).
1. CT scan to determine the extent of the lesion.
2. Radioisotope scans to evaluate for metastasis.
3. Lung evaluation to determine whether metastatic sites are present.
4. Results of serum laboratory studies are inconclusive; client usually has an increase in the serum alkaline phosphatase level.
5. X-ray film will reveal the tumor location and assist in determining an appropriate biopsy site.
6. Bone tissue biopsy.

### Treatment

A. Amputation of extremity and/or extensive surgical resection of bone and surrounding tissue. Limb salvage procedure more often done, often involving bone grafts, if there is a clear margin around tumor site.
B. Chemotherapy; radiation therapy.

### Nursing Interventions

**Goal:** To maintain homeostasis and prevent complications after surgery.

A. Assess for location and severity of pain; administer analgesics and provide nonpharmacologic pain relief measures as needed.
B. An extensive pressure dressing with wound drains/suction may be present; assess drainage.
C. Provide residual stump care (see Nursing Interventions of Amputations).
D. ROM is usually begun immediately; continuous passive motion may be used immediately or on first postoperative day for both upper- and lower-extremity surgery.
E. Muscle toning is important before weight bearing.
F. Frequent neurovascular assessment is necessary because of resection of nerves and vessels in area; extremity may also be casted or splinted for support.

**Goal:** To prevent complications and promote mobility after amputation.

**Goal:** To assist the client/child and family to cope with the diagnosis and build basis for rehabilitation.

A. Provide honest, straightforward information to child/client and parents regarding the situation, in language that both can comprehend.
B. Allow the family and client an opportunity to express their concerns and fears; surgery is extensive and may affect body image (see Chapter 11).
C. Anticipate sense of loss of control and anger over changes in body.
D. Encourage normal growth and developmental activities as appropriate; allow client to be as independent as possible.

**Goal:** To assist the child and the family to cope with the side effects of chemotherapy and radiation (see Chapter 11).

## Amputations

**An amputation is the removal of part of an extremity at various anatomic locations.**

### Assessment

A. Indications for amputation.
   1. Peripheral vascular disease, especially vascular disease of lower extremities.
   2. Severe trauma, congenital disorders.
   3. Acute or widespread infections (e.g., gas gangrene).
   4. Malignant tumors.
B. Diagnostic tests: dependent on underlying problem.

### Nursing Interventions

**Goal:** To prevent further loss of circulation to the extremity, promote psychological stability, promote comfort, promote optimal level of mobility.

A. Monitor circulation before surgery.
B. Provide preoperative care regarding upper-extremity exercises to promote arm strength for postoperative activities of crutch walking and gait training.
C. Discuss the phenomenon of phantom limb pain and its management in the postoperative period.

> **TEST ALERT:** Identify and prevent complications of immobility; use positioning to prevent contractures; provide support for client with unexpected alteration in body image; assist client to ambulate and move with assistive devices; promote wound healing; assist client with use of prosthesis.

**Goal:** To manage pain control and residual limb wound care postoperatively.

A. In the immediate postoperative period (24 hours), the residual limb may be elevated using one pillow to decrease edema and promote comfort. After the first 24 hours, the joint above the amputation site is kept in an extended position.
B. During the immediate postoperative period, frequently monitor vital signs and evaluate residual limb dressing for bleeding; have a surgical tourniquet available should postoperative hemorrhaging occur.

> **TEST ALERT:** Postoperative hemorrhaging requires immediate intervention and notification of the physician.

C. Administer analgesics for postoperative pain, including phantom limb pain.
D. Prevent flexion contractures, which delay the rehabilitative course of care.
   1. Avoid 45- to 90-degree flexion of residual limb. In cases involving lower limbs, do not allow client to sit

in a chair for more than 1 hour during the immediate postoperative period.
   2. Have client lie on his or her abdomen for 30 minutes three or four times per day and position the hip in extension while prone.
E. Postoperative dressing changes on residual limb are done using sterile technique to prevent infection.
F. A rigid compression dressing (plaster molded over dressing) may be applied to prevent injury and to decrease swelling. In children after an amputation, the placement of a temporary prosthesis immediately after surgery may be applied to promote functioning and psychological adaptation.
   1. Controlling the edema will enhance healing and promote comfort.
   2. Changes of the rigid dressing are necessary; as the residual limb heals, it also shrinks.
G. The compression dressing may be changed three or four times before a permanent prosthesis is fitted. The compression dressing may be formed so that it can attach to a prosthesis.
H. If the client is not fitted with a rigid compression dressing, the residual limb will be shaped with a compression bandage.
   1. Ace bandage elastic wrapping is often used for compression of this type (Figure 23-7).
I. It should be worn at all times except during physical therapy and bathing.

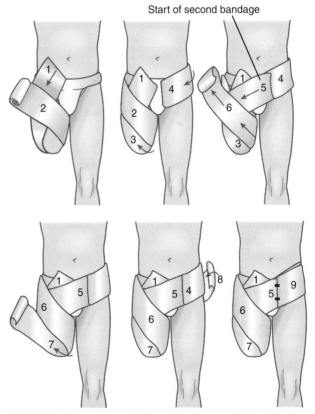

**FIGURE 23-7 Bandaging for Above-the-Knee and Below-the-Knee Amputation.** (From Ignatavicius, D. D., & Workman, M. L. [2016]. Medical-surgical nursing: *Patient-centered collaborative care* [9th ed.]. Philadelphia: Saunders.)

**Goal:** To assist the client to understand measures for residual limb care after the wound has healed.

A. Continually assess for skin breakdown; visually inspect the residual limb for redness, abrasions, or blistering.

B. The residual limb should be washed daily, carefully rinsed, and dried; residual soap and moisture contribute to skin breakdown.

C. Do not apply anything to the residual limb (alcohol increases skin dryness and cracking; lotions keep skin soft and hinder use of prosthesis).

## Home Care

A. Client should put the prosthesis on when he or she gets up and should wear it all day. The residual limb tends to swell if the prosthesis is not applied. The more the client wears the prosthesis, the less swelling will be experienced and the more comfortable and proficient the client will become in using the prosthesis.

B. Using a lower limb prosthesis requires 40% to 60% more energy for walking (Box 23-5).

C. Referral to community health nurse for instruction on ambulation, transfer techniques, prone positioning, and proper residual limb care.

## Rheumatoid Arthritis

**Rheumatoid arthritis (RA) is a chronic, progressive, systemic inflammatory disease associated with severe morbidity and functional decline caused by inflammation of connective tissue, primarily in the synovial joints.**

A. Joint involvement progresses in stages; if disease is diagnosed early, permanent joint deterioration may be prevented.
  1. The synovium becomes thickened and inflamed, and fluid accumulates in the joint space; this causes a pannus to form.
  2. The pannus tissue erodes the cartilage and destroys the joint.

B. Exacerbations and remissions occur; condition tends to be progressive with each exacerbation.

C. Rheumatoid arthritis is a problem of the connective tissue; inflammatory response may occur in organs throughout the body (heart, lungs, blood vessels, muscles).

---

### Box 23-5   OLDER ADULT FOCUS

**Older Adult Care/Considerations After Amputation**

Use of a prosthesis after amputation is dependent on the physical and mental status of the older adult client.
- Existing comorbidities (e.g., cardiac or pulmonary dysfunction)
- Physical strength and endurance abilities
- Living conditions and availability of caregiver assistance

---

### Assessment

A. Risk factors/etiology.
  1. Gender: significantly increased incidence in women.
  2. May occur at any age including childhood; peak incidence occurs between 30 and 50 years of age.
  3. Genetic predisposition.
  4. Occurs in all ethnic groups.

B. Clinical manifestations.
  1. Symmetric joint involvement (hands and feet).
    a. Swollen, warm, tender, red, painful joints; primarily affects small joints, wrists, elbows, shoulders.
    b. Decrease in ROM.
    c. Decrease in strength.
    d. Stiffness and pain are worse in the morning and decrease during the day with moderate activity.
  2. Subcutaneous nodules over bony prominences.
    a. Nodules are painless; frequently occur on the elbows and fingers.
    b. May be present for weeks to months.
  3. Systemic effects.
    a. Vasculitis, pericarditis.
    b. Pulmonary fibrosis, Sjögren's syndrome.
    c. Raynaud's phenomenon (cyanosis, pallor, coolness of the fingers).
    d. Felty's syndrome (swollen spleen, decreased white blood cell count, repeated infections).
    e. Chronic deformities develop, most often in the hands and feet.
    f. Exacerbation of symptoms may be associated with physical or emotional stress.

C. Diagnostics (see Appendix 23-1).

### Treatment

A. NSAIDs (see Appendix 23-2).

B. Corticosteroids for acute, severe exacerbations (see Appendix 9-2 and Appendix 23-2).

C. Methotrexate (see Appendix 11-1 and Appendix 23-2).

D. Disease-modifying antirheumatic drugs (DMARDs) (see Appendix 23-2).

E. Heat and/or cold applications.

F. Rest and avoidance of repetitive movements.

G. Assistive devices and splints to preserve joints and prevent deformity.

H. Physical and rehabilitative therapy.

I. Surgery: joint replacements.

### Complications

A. Musculoskeletal.
  1. Severe joint deformity, flexion contracture.
  2. Diffuse skeletal demineralization.
  3. Stress fractures.

B. Systemic involvement.

C. Decreased ability to perform self-care.

D. Depression as health declines.

*Nursing Interventions*

**Goal:** To relieve pain and preserve joint mobility and muscle strength (see Box 23-4).

A. Use warm compresses to promote relaxation and to decrease stiffness; use cold compresses to decrease inflammation.
B. If heat increases pain, cold compresses may be beneficial during an acute episode.
C. Acutely inflamed joints should be immobilized in a device that maintains a functional position.
D. Position client to maintain correct body alignment and prevent contractures, especially flexion contractures.

> **TEST ALERT:** Assess client for complications of immobility, intervene appropriately when providing care.

E. Immobility can increase pain; ROM exercises and weight bearing may help decrease pain.
F. Antiinflammatory medications should be taken before activity and with meals or food to decrease gastric upset.
G. If client is taking steroids, he or she should wear a medical identification tag.

**Goal:** To assist client to prevent joint deformity, preserve joint function, and reduce inflammation and pain.

A. Regularly scheduled rest periods (excessive fatigue is a problem); balance activities with rest.
B. For the hospitalized RA client plan care with consideration of early morning stiffness. A warm shower in the morning may decrease morning stiffness; warm blankets may also promote comfort.
C. Protect joints (see Box 23-4).
   1. Maintain functional joint alignment; avoid positions that precipitate joint contraction (sitting too long with knees bent).
   2. Warm moist or cold compresses to relieve pain and muscle spasms.
   3. Acutely inflamed joints may be splinted; splint should be removed periodically and gentle ROM exercises performed.
   4. Use large muscle groups; avoid repetitive movement of smaller joints.
D. Demonstrate ability to carry out individual exercise program.
E. Identify medications that are effective in relieving pain.
F. Chronic pain may lead to feelings of powerlessness and make the client more susceptible to false advertising regarding claims of cure and relief of chronic pain.
G. Encourage client to be independent in activities of daily living (ADLs) as long as possible.

**Home Care**

A. Encourage client to vent feelings regarding chronic progression of the disease state.

B. Evaluate family support system; help family identify measures to assist client.
C. Modify home routine to decrease stress on joints: ADLs, dressing, etc.
D. Identify measures to assist client to maintain self-esteem: What activities can client continue to participate in? Focus on what client *can* do.
E. Assist client to set realistic goals.
F. Identify available community resources.

> **TEST ALERT:** Determine client's ability to perform self-care; assist family to manage care of client with long-term care needs.

 **Osteoarthritis (Degenerative Joint Disease)**

**Osteoarthritis (OA) is a progressive, noninflammatory disease that causes a progressive degeneration of synovial joints.**

A. Primarily associated with aging; may also be caused by musculoskeletal injury or conditions that cause repetitive damage to joints.
B. The cartilage at the ends of the long bones and in the intervertebral joints of the spine deteriorates and leaves the ends of the bones or vertebrae rubbing together; this produces a painful, swollen joint or spine.

*Assessment*

A. Etiology/predisposing factors.
   1. Excessive use of a specific joint: knees in athletes, feet in dancers, etc.
   2. The hips are more commonly affected in men; in women, the hands are more commonly affected.
   3. Obesity: joints that carry excess weight are more likely to degenerate earlier.
   4. Frequently observed in older adults, especially women.
B. Clinical manifestations.
   1. Joints involved.
      a. Primarily involves weight-bearing joints; occurs as a result of mechanical stress.
      b. May also involve joints in the fingers and the vertebral column.
   2. Symptoms occurring in the joint.
      a. Pain, swelling, tenderness.
      b. Crepitation: a grating sound or feeling with movement.
      c. Instability, stiffness, and immobility.
   3. Pain occurs on motion and with weight bearing.
   4. Pain increases in severity with activity.
   5. Heberden's nodes: bony nodules on the distal finger joints.
C. Diagnostics (see Appendix 23-1).
   1. No specific laboratory test to confirm; diagnosis is made primarily on the basis of symptoms and history.
   2. CT scan, MRI, or bone scan may be prescribed to diagnose OA.

## Treatment

A. Medications for pain relief: salicylates (aspirin), acetaminophen, NSAIDs (ibuprofen), COX-2 inhibitors.
   1. Intraarticular injection of corticosteroids, methotrexate, disease-modifying antirheumatic drugs, and hyaluronic acid.
B. Activity balanced with adequate rest.
C. Weight reduction, if appropriate.
D. Physical therapy and exercise.
E. Surgical intervention with joint replacement.
F. Complementary and alternative therapies include acupuncture, oral intake of glucosamine and chondroitin, application of topical analgesics.

## Nursing Interventions

**Goal:** To relieve pain, prevent further stress on the joint, and maintain function.

A. Acutely inflamed joint should be immobilized with splint or brace.
B. Plan ADLs to prevent stress on involved joints and provide adequate rest periods.
C. Heat compresses can be used for relief of pain; cold compresses may be used if joint is inflamed.
D. It is important to maintain regular exercise program; decrease activity in acutely inflamed, painful joints.

> **! NURSING PRIORITY:** More than 4000 mg daily of acetaminophen increases client risk for liver damage in the adult. Clients taking large doses (300 to 500 mg/kg/day) of aspirin (acetylsalicylic acid) should be closely monitored for signs and symptoms of salicylism (toxicity). Aspirin poisoning is an acute medical emergency and is potentially lethal.

**Goal:** To help client understand measures to maintain health (see Box 23-4).

A. Identify activities requiring increased stress on involved joints.
B. Maintain regular exercise program (e.g., walking, swimming) to promote muscle strength and joint mobility.
C. Encourage independence in ADLs.

**Goal:** To maintain psychological equilibrium and promote positive self-esteem.

## Juvenile Idiopathic Arthritis (Juvenile Rheumatoid Arthritis)

**Juvenile idiopathic arthritis (JIA) is a new name for chronic childhood arthritis, previously called juvenile rheumatoid arthritis (JRA). It is characterized as a chronic inflammatory problem of the joints and other tissue; it involves the synovial joints. Joint destruction occurs when the synovium becomes chronically inflamed, and eventual erosive destruction of the articular cartilage of the joints causes adhesion formation between the joint surfaces, resulting in ankylosis of the joints.**

## Assessment

A. Risk factors/etiology.
   1. Possibly autoimmune and/or genetic in origin.
   2. Peak onset between 1 and 3 years and 8 and 10 years of age.
B. Clinical manifestations.
   1. Stiffness (especially in the morning or after inactivity), edema, loss of movement in affected joints.
   2. May have multiple joint involvements, both large and small joints.
   3. Joints may be tender and painful to touch.
   4. Fever, rash, and development of rheumatoid nodules on the joints or at the base of the spine.
   5. Stress such as infections/illnesses, injuries, or surgery may initiate an exacerbation of the arthritic disease.
C. Diagnostics: diagnosis is made by exclusion of other diseases; presence of antinuclear antibodies (see Appendix 23-1).
D. New classifications/categories for JIA, arthritis, oligoarthritis, rheumatoid factor (RF)-negative polyarthritis, RF-positive arthritis, psoriatic arthritis, and undifferentiated arthritis.

## Treatment

**Goal:** To provide pain relief, preserve joint function, minimize joint deformity, and promote normal growth and development.

A. Medications (see Appendix 23-1).
   1. NSAIDs, methotrexate.
   2. Tumor necrosis factor inhibitors and DMARDs.
   3. Corticosteroids in acute, severe exacerbations. Minimal doses of corticosteroids may be used prophylactically to lessen the inflammatory processes of the disease.
B. Physical and occupational therapy.
C. Moist heat is used to reduce stiffness and relieve pain.
D. Exercise, especially water exercises.
E. Regular eye examinations.
F. Splints and assistive devices.

## Complications

Complications include severe hip disease and loss of vision from iridocyclitis and/or uveitis.

## Nursing Interventions

A child is usually cared for at home except during severe exacerbations.
**Goal:** To decrease pain and promote joint mobility, normal growth and development, physiologic and psychological adaptation to chronic disease, and promote self-esteem.

A. Instruct parents and child on the use of hot/cold packs, splints, and positioning the affected joints in a neutral position and proper body alignment to promote comfort and prevent flexion contractures of affected joints.
B. Therapeutic exercises incorporated into play activities.

C. Instruct parents and child regarding importance of compliance with medication regimen; teach purpose, side effects, and measures to prevent adverse effects of medications.

D. Avoid overexercising painful joints.

E. Well-balanced diet without excessive weight gain.

F. Schedule regular exercise program appropriate to developmental level.

G. Encourage independence; allow child to participate in planning care.

H. Encourage school attendance and socialization with peers, but some modifications of some school activities may be required.

## Gout

Gout is a recurring arthritic condition causing the accumulation of uric acid crystals in one or more joints. Uric acid crystals may be found in articular, periarticular, and subcutaneous tissues. Hyperuricemia is a diagnostic finding secondary to a defect in the metabolism of uric acid.

### Assessment

A. Risk factors/etiology.
   1. Increased incidence in middle-aged men and especially men with diets high in purine-rich foods.
   2. Obesity, hypertension, diuretic use, excessive alcohol consumption, diabetes mellitus, chemotherapy, renal dysfunction, hyperlipidemia.

B. Clinical manifestations.
   1. Intense pain and inflammation of one or more small joints, especially those in the large toe.
   2. Characterized by remissions and exacerbations of acute joint pain.
   3. Onset is generally rapid with swollen, inflamed, painful joints and typically occurs at night.
   4. Presence of tophi or uric acid crystals in the area around the large toe, joints of the fingers, along tendons, and in skin and cartilage.

C. Diagnostics: serum uric acid level greater than 6 mg/dL (356.91 μmol/L).

### Treatment

A. Medications.
   1. Antigout, such as colchicine, allopurinol (see Appendix 23-2).
   2. NSAIDs for pain and to assist in preventing attacks.

B. Decrease amount of purine in diet (see Chapter 2).

### Complications

A. Uric acid kidney stones.

B. Secondary osteoarthritis.

### Nursing Interventions

**Goal:** To prevent acute attack, promote comfort, and maintain joint mobility.

A. Medications should be given early in the attack to decrease the severity of the attack.

B. Protect affected joint: immobilize, no weight bearing.

C. Cold packs may decrease pain.

D. Decrease amount of purine in diet by avoiding foods such as shellfish, lentils, red wine, asparagus, spinach, beef, chicken, and pork.

E. Encourage high fluid intake to increase excretion of uric acid and to prevent the development of uric acid stones.

F. Assist client to identify activities and aspects of lifestyle that precipitate attacks, such as decreasing alcohol consumption.

## Lyme Disease

Lyme disease is the most common vector-borne disease in the United States. An inflammatory response to bacteria *Borrelia burgdorferi;* if not treated, causes chronic arthritic pain and swelling in the large joints, carditis, and nervous system problems.

### Assessment

A. Risk factors/etiology.
   1. Caused by the bacterium *Borrelia burgdorferi* and transmitted by the bite of an infected deer tick.
   2. Residence or recreation in wooded areas of Northeastern United States from Maine to Maryland and the upper Midwestern states of Minnesota and Wisconsin.

B. Clinical manifestations (Figure 23-8).
   1. *Erythema migrans* (EM), a skin lesion (bullseye rash), anywhere on the body. EM is an expanding area of redness with a bright red border and central clearing around what looks like a small red papule that appears after the removal of a tick.
   2. Acute flulike symptoms, such as low-grade fever, chills, headache, stiff neck, fatigue, swollen lymph nodes, and migratory joint and muscle pain.
   3. Symptoms usually occur in a week but may be delayed for up to 30 days.

C. Diagnostics
   1. Serum enzyme immunoassay (EIA) followed by immunoblot (Western blot) (see Appendix 23-1).
   2. CBC and ESR are usually normal.

### Complications (if Untreated)

A. Chronic arthritis pain and joint swelling.

B. Carditis.

C. Central nervous system problems such as severe headaches or poor motor coordination.

D. Post–Lyme disease syndrome occurs in approximately 10% to 20% of persons treated with antibiotics for Lyme disease; they experience lingering fatigue or joint and muscle pain.

### Treatment

A. Medications
   1. Antibiotics: doxycycline, cefuroxime, and amoxicillin. (Erythromycin is used in clients allergic to penicillin.) (See Appendix 9-2.)
   2. NSAIDs for pain.

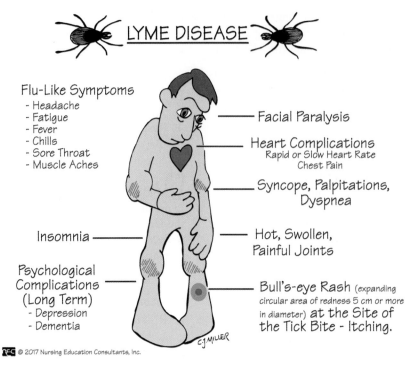

**FIGURE 23-8 Lyme Disease.** (From Zerwekh, J., Garneau, A., & Miller, C. J. [2017]. *Digital collection of the memory notebooks of nursing* [4th ed.]. Chandler, AZ: Nursing Education Consultants, Inc.)

### Nursing Interventions

**Goal:** To prevent tick bites and seek early treatment.

A. Teach people living in endemic areas on measures to prevent tick bites, inspect body thoroughly after walking in wooded areas, wear light-colored clothing, early removal of ticks using tweezers.
B. Avoid folk solutions such as painting the tick with nail polish or petroleum jelly.
C. Wash bitten area with soap and water and apply antiseptic.
D. Teach client to see a health care provider immediately if flu-like symptoms or a bullseye rash appears within 2 to 30 days after removal of tick.

### Muscular Dystrophy

**Muscular dystrophy (MD) is a group of genetic diseases characterized by progressive symmetric wasting of skeletal muscles in children without evidence of neurologic involvement. In all forms of MD an insidious loss of strength occurs with increasing disability and deformity. The types of MD differ in the groups of muscles affected, age of onset, rate of progression, and mode of genetic inheritance. The most common type of MD is Duchenne.**

### Assessment

A. Risk factors/etiology.
1. Familial history of the disease (X-linked recessive disorders).
2. Gender: male.
3. Mutation of the dystrophin gene. (Dystrophin in normal muscle cells helps skeletal muscle fibers attach to the basement membrane.)

B. Clinical manifestations.
1. Bilateral symmetric muscle wasting.
2. Ataxic or waddling gait with frequent falls.
3. Progressive weakening of muscles around the trunk.
4. Difficulty rising from the floor and climbing stairs.
5. Toe-walking children older than 3 years.
6. Lack of facial movement.
7. Difficulty raising arms over head.
C. Diagnostics (see Appendix 23-1).
1. Serum muscle enzymes (especially creatine kinase, aldolase).
2. Electromyogram (EMG) testing.
3. Muscle fiber biopsy.

### Complications

A. Contractures.
B. Disuse atrophy.
C. Infections.
D. Obesity.
E. Respiratory and cardiopulmonary problems.

### Treatment

A. No definitive therapy is available to stop the progressive wasting of MD.

### Nursing Interventions

**Goal:** To preserve mobility and independence in ADLs through physical therapy and orthopedic appliances.

A. Prevent injuries and deformities.
B. Avoid prolonged bed rest that may lead to further muscle wasting.
C. Provide psychosocial support for client and caregivers.

## Serum Diagnostics

**Anti-CCP (CCP):** Measures the presence of antibodies to cyclic citrulline protein; these antibodies are specific diagnostic markers for rheumatoid arthritis. This diagnostic test can provide early detection of RA.

**Antinuclear Antibody (ANA):** Measures the presence of antibodies that destroy the nucleus of body tissue cells (i.e., those seen in connective tissue diseases); a positive test result is associated with systemic lupus erythematosus.

**Complement:** Essential body protein to measure immune and inflammatory reactions; usually depleted in rheumatoid arthritis.

**Alkaline Phosphatase:** Enzyme produced by osteoblasts; elevated levels found in osteoporosis, healing fractures, bone cancer, osteomalacia.

**Aldolase:** Elevated levels in muscular dystrophy.

**Creatine Kinase (CK):** Elevated levels found in muscular dystrophy and traumatic skeletal muscle injury.

**Calcium, Total:** Is a cation that functions in the formation of bone and transmits nerve impulses, as well as myocardial and skeletal muscle contractions. Changes in serum calcium levels can indicate osteomalacia, thyroid, parathyroid, or renal disease, acidosis, or bone tumors. Reference range: 8.6 to 10.2 mg/dL.

**Enzyme Immunoassay (EIA):** Is the first tier of a two-tiered blood test to determine Lyme disease and is performed if the person has erythema migrans lesions. Test is considered negative if less than 1:256; if negative, no further testing is required. If positive or unequivocal, the second serum test is performed. If both serum test results are positive, the diagnosis of Lyme disease is made.

**Immunoblot Test:** Is the second tier of the two-tiered blood test to determine Lyme disease. This test is also called the Western blot test. The immunoblot is considered positive if two of the following three bands are present: 24 kDa (OspC), 39 kDa (BmpA), and 41 kDa (Fla) (1).

**Rheumatoid Factor (RF):** Used to determine presence of autoantibodies (rheumatoid factor) found in clients with connective tissue disease; if antibodies are present, it is suggestive of rheumatoid arthritis; the higher the antibody titer, the greater the degree of inflammation.

**Uric Acid:** End-product of purine metabolism. Elevation in uric acid production can be caused by alcoholism, renal disease, anemia, hyperlipidemia, and many more. Decreased levels can be caused by bronchogenic carcinoma, amyotrophic lateral sclerosis, and other diseases and by medications, both over the counter and prescribed.

Reference range adults: 2.9 mg/dL to 6.5 mg/dL (172.51–386.65 μmol/L).

## Invasive Diagnostics

**Arthroscopy:** Involves the use of an arthroscope inserted into a joint for visualization of the joint structure; preferably, procedure is conducted in the operating room with strict asepsis and performed with either local or general anesthesia; used to diagnose and/or correct structural abnormalities of the knee.

*Nursing Implications*
1. Perform preoperative nursing interventions, as appropriate with the level of anesthesia to be used.
2. After procedure, wound is covered with a sterile dressing.
3. A compression bandage may be applied for 24 hours after the procedure.
4. Teach client symptoms of vascular compromise, mobility restrictions, and sterile dressing change procedure.
5. Walking is permitted, but excessive exercise should be avoided for a few days.
6. Teach the client signs of infection (increased temperature, local inflammation at site).

**Arthrocentesis:** Incision of a joint capsule to obtain samples of synovial fluid; local anesthesia is induced, and aseptic preparation is done before fluid aspiration. Synovial fluid is examined for infection and bleeding into the joint and to confirm specific types of arthritis.

*Nursing Implications*
1. Explain procedure to client.
2. May be done at bedside or in an examination room.
3. Compression dressing is usually applied, and joint is rested for several hours after test.
4. Observe dressing for leakage of blood or fluid.
5. Assess the puncture site for evidence of infection.

**Myelogram and CT Scan:** Used to determine status of vertebral disk. See Appendix 22-1.

**Bone Biopsy:** May be performed in client's room or in a treatment room. After satisfactory local anesthesia is achieved, a long needle is inserted into the bone, or a small incision is made, to obtain bone tissue.

*Nursing Implications*
1. Plan for analgesic to be administered before procedure.
2. If an incision was made, maintain a pressure dressing over the site.
3. Extremity is elevated to decrease edema and may be immobilized for about 12 to 24 hours.
4. Assess the puncture site or incision for evidence of infection.

**Electromyelogram (EMG):** Evaluates the electric potential of the muscle with muscle contraction. Small needles are inserted into the muscle and recording of electrical activity is performed.

*Nursing Implications*
1. Explain to client that there is discomfort with procedure.
2. No stimulants (caffeine) or sedatives 24 hours before the procedure.

*Continued*

## Appendix 23-1   DIAGNOSTIC STUDIES—cont'd

### Noninvasive Diagnostics

**X-ray Films:** The most common diagnostic procedure to determine musculoskeletal problems.

1. Identify musculoskeletal problems.
2. Determine progress of disease or condition.
3. Evaluate effectiveness of treatment.

**Bone Scan:** Radioisotopes are given 2 hours before procedure. The bone is scanned to determine where the isotopes are "taken up." May be used to determine presence of malignancies, arthritis, and osteoporosis. Instruct client to empty bladder before the procedure; the procedure takes about 1 hour; the client will be lying supine during the procedure; instruct that fluid intake should be increased after the procedure to promote excretion of radioisotopes.

**Computerized Axial Tomography (CAT Scan):** See Appendix 22-1.

**Magnetic Resonance Imaging (MRI):** See Appendix 22-1.

## Appendix 23-2   MEDICATIONS

| Medications | Side Effects | Nursing Implications |
|---|---|---|
| **Antigout Agents:** Decrease the plasma uric acid levels either by inhibiting the synthesis of uric acid or increasing the excretion of uric acid. | | |
| Colchicine: PO | Nausea, vomiting, diarrhea<br>Toxic effects: bone marrow depression | 1. Take medication at earliest indication of impending gout attack.<br>2. Take medication with food.<br>3. Promote high fluid intake to promote uric acid excretion.<br>4. In acute attack, administer 1 tablet every hour until symptoms subside, until GI problems occur, or until a total of 8 mg has been taken.<br>5. Monitor serum uric acid levels. |
| Allopurinol: PO<br>Febuxostat: PO | Rash, GI distress, fever, headache | 1. Administer with food to decrease gastric upset.<br>2. Discontinue medication if rash occurs.<br>3. Use with caution in clients with renal insufficiency.<br>4. May be used to decrease serum uric acid levels in clients receiving chemotherapy.<br>5. Monitor serum uric acid levels. |
| Probenecid: PO | GI disturbances, headache, skin rash, fever | 1. Urate tophi deposits should decrease in size with therapy.<br>2. Give with food.<br>3. Avoid aspirin and aspirin-containing products; decreases drug effectiveness.<br>4. Monitor serum uric acid levels. |
| **Skeletal Muscle Relaxants:** Relax skeletal muscle by depressing synaptic pathways in the spinal cord. | | |
| Methocarbamol: PO, IM, IV<br>Cyclobenzaprine: PO<br>Carisoprodol: PO<br>Baclofen: PO | Drowsiness, dizziness, GI upset, rash, blurred vision, may turn urine brown, black, or dark green<br>Drowsiness, dizziness, blurred vision, photophobia, urinary retention, constipation, orthostatic hypotension<br>Drowsiness, weakness, fatigue, confusion<br>Drowsiness, dizziness, weakness, and fatigue | 1. Used for muscle spasms associated with multiple sclerosis and spinal cord injury.<br>2. Caution clients to avoid activities that require mental alertness for safety (e.g., driving, using power tools, etc.).<br>3. Evaluate client for postural hypotension.<br>4. Advise client to avoid CNS depressants (e.g., alcohol, opioids, antihistamines).<br>5. Administer with meals to decrease GI distress. |
| Dantrolene: PO, IV | Hepatotoxicity, muscle weakness, drowsiness | 1. Teach clients symptoms of liver dysfunction.<br>2. Acts directly to relax skeletal muscle. |

| Medications | Side Effects | Nursing Implications |
|---|---|---|

**Antiresorptive Drugs:** Decrease bone loss by limiting the activity and development of osteoclast cells.

| Medications | Side Effects | Nursing Implications |
|---|---|---|
| Calcitonin-salmon: subQ, IM, nasal spray | GI upset, local inflammation at injection site, flushing | 1. Monitor levels of serum calcium. 2. Treatment of established postmenopausal osteoporosis. |
| Bisphosphonates (the -dronates) Alendronate: PO Ibandronate: PO, IV Pamidronate: IV Risedronate: PO Tiludronate: PO Zoledronate: IV Etidronate: PO, IV | Esophagitis, GI flushing, rash, musculoskeletal pain, fever, chills, jaw pain, osteonecrosis of the jaw (rare) | 1. Have client swallow tablet whole; it should not be chewed. 2. Take in morning on an empty stomach with large glass of water (6–8 oz) and wait at least 30 minutes before eating. 3. Remain upright (sitting, standing, or walking) for at least 30 minutes after taking. 4. Make sure client has adequate intake of vitamin D. 5. Used for prevention and treatment of postmenopausal osteoporosis. 6. Client should report any signs or symptoms of gastric reflux or pain. |

**Corticosteroids:** See Appendix 9-2.

**Nonsteroidal Antiinflammatory Medications (NSAIDs):** See Appendix 3-3.

**Disease-Modifying Antirheumatic Drugs (DMARDs):** Antimetabolite, antirheumatic, and antimalarial drugs that act to decrease inflammation.

| Medications | Side Effects | Nursing Implications |
|---|---|---|
| Methotrexate: PO, IV, IM | Toxic effects: hepatotoxicity, bone marrow depression; Nausea, vomiting, stomatitis; Teratogenesis | 1. Caution women of childbearing age to avoid pregnancy; use birth control during and 3 months after treatment. 2. Monitor CBC and liver enzymes regularly. 3. Avoid alcohol during therapy. 4. Administer with food. |
| Hydroxychloroquine: PO | Toxic effects: retinopathy, skeletal muscle myopathy or neuropathy; Headache, anorexia, dizziness | 1. Recommend eye examinations every 3 months. 2. Not recommended for children. 3. Therapeutic effect may take 3–6 months. |
| Leflunomide: PO | Toxic effects: hepatotoxicity, diarrhea, teratogenesis | 1. Not recommended for women who may become pregnant. 2. May slow the progression of joint damage caused by rheumatoid arthritis and improve physical function. |

**Biologic Therapy:** Disease-modifying antirheumatic drugs (DMARDs). Agents that bind to TNF to decrease inflammatory and immune responses; used in cases of severe arthritis

| Medications | Side Effects | Nursing Implications |
|---|---|---|
| Etanercept: subQ Adalimumab; subQ Certolizumab pegol: subQ Golimumab: subQ Infliximab: IV | Increased risk for infections, injection site reactions, heart failure, headache, nausea, dizziness | 1. Use cautiously in clients with heart disease. 2. Rotate injection sites at least 1 inch apart. 3. Advise clients that injection site reaction generally decreases with continued therapy. 4. Do not administer to clients with chronic or localized infections. 5. Have clients report signs of infection, bruising, or bleeding. 6. Assess clients for infections; administer tuberculosis skin test and chest x-ray prior to starting. |
| Abatacept: IV | Not recommended for combined use with other TNF inhibitors. | 1. Indicated for clients who do not respond to TNF inhibitors and other DMARDs. |
| Tocilizumab: IV Anakinra: IV Rituximab: IV | Increased risk for infections, GI perforation, liver injury, and hematologic effects. | 1. Used for moderate to severe RA who have not responded to other DMARDs 2. Do not combine with other immunosuppressants. |

*CBC,* Complete blood count; *CNS,* central nervous system; *GI,* gastrointestinal; *IV,* intravenous; *PO,* by mouth (orally); *subQ,* subcutaneous; *TNF,* tumor necrosis factor.

## Appendix 23-3   ASSISTIVE DEVICES FOR IMMOBILITY

## Crutches

### Measuring a Client (Figure 23-9)

- Measurement may be taken with client supine or standing.
- Supine: measure the distance from the client's axilla to a point 6 inches (15 cm) lateral to the heel.
- Standing: measure the distance from the client's axilla to a point 4 to 6 inches (10–15 cm) to the side and 4 to 6 inches (10–15 cm) in front of the foot.
- Adjust hand bars so that client's elbows are flexed approximately 30 degrees.
- If client was measured while supine, assist client to stand with crutches. Check the distance between client's axilla and arm pieces. You should be able to put three of your fingers between client's axilla and the crutch bar.

### Four-Point Alternate Gait

- The four-point alternate gait is used by clients who can bear partial weight on both feet—for example, clients with arthritis or cerebral palsy. It is a particularly safe gait in that there are three points of support on the floor at all times.
- This gait provides a normal walking pattern and makes some use of the muscles of the lower extremities.

### Three-Point Alternate Gait

- For the three-point alternate gait, the client must be able to bear the total body weight on one foot; the affected foot or leg is either partially or totally non–weight bearing.
- In this gait both crutches are moved forward together with the affected leg while the weight is being borne by the client's hands on the crutches. The unaffected leg is then advanced forward.

### Crutch Walking

- Up stairs: Unaffected leg moves up first, followed by the crutches and the affected leg.
- Down stairs: Crutches and affected leg move down first, body weight is transferred to the crutches, and the unaffected leg is moved down.

> **TEST ALERT:** Assess client's use of assistive devices; evaluate correct use; assist client to ambulate with an assistive device.

## Canes (Figure 23-10)

- The cane is used on the side opposite the affected leg.
- The cane and the affected leg move together.

## Walkers

- The client takes a step, lifts the walker and moves it forward, and takes another step.
- Gain balance before moving walker forward again; balance provides stability and equal weight bearing.

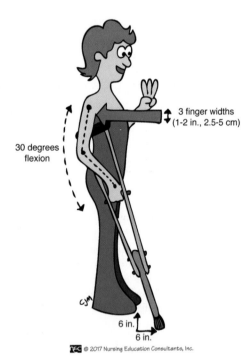

**FIGURE 23-9  Measuring a Client with Crutches.** (From Zerwekh, J., Garneau, A., & Miller, C. J. [2017]. *Digital collection of the memory notebooks of nursing* [4th ed.]. Chandler, AZ: Nursing Education Consultants, Inc.)

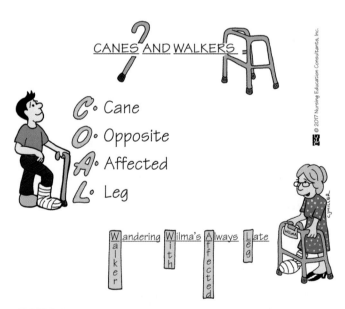

**FIGURE 23-10  Canes and Walkers.** (From Zerwekh, J., Garneau, A., & Miller, C. J. [2017]. *Digital collection of the memory notebooks of nursing* [4th ed.]. Chandler, AZ: Nursing Education Consultants, Inc.)

# Study Questions
# Musculoskeletal: Care of Adult and Pediatric Clients

More questions on

evolve

1. A week after a right knee arthroplasty, a client continues to report moderate knee pain with activity. What recommendations should the nurse make? **Select all that apply.**
   1. Rotate warm and ice packs to the incisional site around the clock.
   2. Increase the amount of narcotic pain medication.
   3. Perform isometric and active range of motion to the extremity every hour.
   4. Take pain medicine before physical therapy sessions.
   5. Progress physical activity as directed by the therapist.

2. The nurse is assessing a client who had a fractured femur repaired with an external fixator device. Which assessment findings should the nurse report to the health care provider? **Select all that apply.**
   1. Increase in pulse rate in affected leg
   2. Paresthesia distal to area of injury
   3. Toes on affected leg cool to touch and edematous
   4. Reports that pins are hurting
   5. Reports of leg pain unrelieved by analgesics or repositioning
   6. Client angry and calling loudly to the nurse every 10 minutes

3. In taking the health history of a client with severe painful osteoarthritis, which question should the nurse ask about their condition? **Select all that apply.**
   1. Do you utilize and complementary or alternative therapies for your arthritis?
   2. Do you have any joint deformities from your arthritis?
   3. Did your symptoms begin during childhood?
   4. Have you ever taken corticosteroids or immunosuppressive medication for your arthritis?
   5. Have you ever developed kidney stones from your condition?

4. The nurse is caring for a client scheduled for a bone scan. What should be included in the preprocedure teaching? **Select all that apply.**
   1. Maintain NPO (nothing by mouth) status for 8 hours before the procedure.
   2. The procedure will involve intravenous injection of radioisotopes.
   3. The procedure will involve a small incision where bone tissue is removed for biopsy.
   4. The client will have to lie supine for about an hour during the scan.
   5. Avoid stimulants such as caffeine for 24 hours before the procedure.
   6. Increase intake of fluids after the procedure is completed.

5. The nurse received handoff for a client returning from a right leg amputation. What should be included in the plan of care?
   1. Applying ice packs to the residual limb for 72 hours
   2. Having the client lie on his or her abdomen for 30 minutes three or four times a day
   3. Wrapping the residual limb with elastic bandages from proximal to distal ends
   4. Managing client's pain with antiinflammatory medications

6. The nurse is caring for a child who had a long-leg plaster cast applied for a femur fracture. What action is a priority as the cast is drying?
   1. Use only the fingertips when moving the cast.
   2. Keep the client and cast covered with blankets.
   3. Perform frequent neurovascular checks distal to fracture.
   4. Place a heat lamp directly over the cast.

7. The nurse is caring for a client is being treated with Buck's traction. What is a priority action for the nurse?
   1. Remove the traction boot every 6 hours to provide skin care.
   2. Check and clean the pin sites at least three times daily.
   3. Check the area around the hip where the traction is applied.
   4. Verify that weights are in the amounts ordered and are hanging freely.

8. For a client with severe painful osteoarthritis, a regimen of heat, massage, and exercise will:
   1. Help relax muscles and relieve pain and stiffness.
   2. Restore range of motion previously lost.
   3. Prevent the inflammatory process.
   4. Help the client cope with pain effectively.

9. A client is confined to bed with a fracture of the left femur. He begins receiving subcutaneous low-molecular-weight heparin (LMWH) injections. What is the purpose of this medication?
   1. To prevent thrombophlebitis and pulmonary emboli associated with immobility
   2. To promote vascular perfusion by preventing formation of micro emboli in the left leg
   3. To prevent venous stasis, which promotes vascular complications associated with immobility
   4. To decrease the incidence of fat emboli associated with long bone fractures

10. What is the priority assessment information to obtain from a client who is being admitted with a tentative diagnosis of fractured hip?
    1. Circulation and sensation distal to the fracture
    2. Amount of swelling around the fracture site
    3. Degree of bone healing that has occurred
    4. Amount of pain that the fracture and healing are causing

11. What evaluation is important in the preoperative nursing assessment of a client with a severely herniated lumbar disk?
    1. Movement and sensation in the lower extremities
    2. Leg pain that radiates to both lower extremities
    3. Reflexes in the upper extremities
    4. Pupillary reaction to light

12. The nursing discharge care plan for a 2-month-old infant in a Pavlik harness includes what nursing instructions?
    1. Instruct the parents how to perform the Ortolani test daily.
    2. Check at least two or three times a day for red areas under the straps.
    3. Check with the physician about using a spica cast because the harness is not effective.
    4. Adjust the harness straps if the parents think it is necessary.

13. In the immediate postoperative phase for a client with a mandibular fracture repair, what are the priority nursing concerns? **Select all that apply.**
    1. Postoperative bleeding
    2. Postoperative pain
    3. Client positioning
    4. Client's inability to speak
    5. Respiratory distress
    6. Location of scissors and wire cutters

14. The nurse is instructing a client on dietary restrictions for the management of gout. The instructions include elimination of which of the following foods? **Select all that apply.**
    1. Asparagus
    2. Almonds
    3. Chicken
    4. Grapefruit
    5. Red wine
    6. Salmon

15. The nurse is instructing a student nurse concerning the differences in the joints affected in osteoarthritis and rheumatoid arthritis. Which of the following is an important fact to include?
    1. In rheumatoid arthritis, weight-bearing joints are affected first.
    2. In osteoarthritis, only the small joints of the fingers are affected.
    3. In rheumatoid arthritis, there is usually bilateral joint involvement.
    4. In osteoarthritis, joint destruction is due to changes in the synovial fluid.

16. The nurse understands the key to managing the therapeutic regimen and client compliance for an adolescent girl recently diagnosed with scoliosis includes consideration of which of the following?
    1. The ability of the parents to afford the expenses of the braces and surgical procedures
    2. The adolescent's understanding the importance of wearing the brace
    3. The ability of the parents to control and enforce compliance with the therapeutic regimen
    4. The psychological needs and developmental stage to encourage compliance by the adolescent

17. A client with diabetes and a right below-the-knee amputation tells the nurse that he feels pain in the amputated leg, even though the leg is gone. The nurse's response is based on what information?
    1. Phantom pain is experienced by most amputees; it will resolve without pain medication.
    2. The client thinks he feels pain, but it is actually a response to his denial about the amputation.
    3. The nurse cannot adequately assess the pain, therefore medication cannot be given.
    4. Phantom pain occurs when the nerve endings have not adjusted to the loss of the extremity, and the client should be offered pain medication.

18. A client begins receiving methotrexate for severe symptoms of rheumatoid arthritis. What is the most important information for the nurse to give this client regarding the medication?
    1. Take extra fiber and fluids to counteract the constipating effect.
    2. It is important to have periodic laboratory work done.
    3. Take the drug on an empty stomach.
    4. Hirsutism and menstrual changes sometimes develop as side effects.

19. Which of the following statements by the client who has recently had a total hip replacement indicates that the client does not understand the mobility limitations?
    1. "I should not bend down to put on shoes or socks."
    2. "It is okay to cross my legs if I am sitting in a chair."
    3. "I should put a pillow between my legs when lying on my side."
    4. "I should not sit in low chairs or on toilet seats that are low."

20. A 7-year-old boy is in the emergency department with a greenstick fracture of the ulna. How will the nurse explain the fracture to the parents?
    1. The bone is broken across the growth plate.
    2. There is a splintering of the bone on one side.
    3. There is a separation of the bone at the fracture site.
    4. The bone is broken into several fragments.

# Answers to Study Questions

**1.** *3, 4, 5*
The emphasis after a knee arthroscopic surgery should be on pain management and physical therapy. Postoperative pain is reduced with movement, so it should be encouraged. Isometric and active range of motion will increase muscle strength and flexion of the joint. Pain medicine should be reduced over time to encourage activity. Increased used of narcotics will decrease the mental alertness and the activity level. (Lewis et al., 10 ed., p. 1491)

**2.** *2, 3, 5*
Paresthesia, edema, and leg pain unrelieved by analgesics are classic indicators of the development of compartmental syndrome. With a femur fracture, there is some degree of edema postoperatively that may leave the toes on the affected leg cool to touch. An increase in pulse rate is not an indication of a problem; a decrease in pulse strength is. The pins usually do not cause undue pain, and frequently the client is angry regarding the immobility and does not use effective coping measures; neither would need to be reported. (Lewis et al., 10 ed., p. 1483)

**3.** *1, 2*
Osteoarthritis has a gradual onset and affects weight-bearing joints with pain that is more pronounced after exercise. The onset of osteoarthritis is gradual, not sudden, and commonly occurs until after age 50. The client will usually complain of increased stiffness in the morning and after periods of inactivity, with improvement after activity. Joint pain generally worsens with joint use, and in the early stages of osteoarthritis, joint pain is relieved by rest. Alternative therapies are often used and need to be evaluated as to any joint deformities from the condition. The development of kidney stones would be secondary to gout, and the use of steroids and immunosuppressive medication are for rheumatoid arthritis. (Lewis et al., 10 ed., p. 1517)

**4.** *2, 4, 6*
The procedure will include an IV injection of radioisotopes that are given 2 hours before procedure; ensure client empties bladder before the procedure; the procedure takes about 1 hour; the client will lie supine during the procedure; fluid intake should be increased after the procedure to promote excretion of radioisotopes. Food or fluids are not limited before the scan, and no biopsy of the bone will be taken. (Lewis et al., 10 ed., p. 1458)

**5.** *2*
Client should lie on the abdomen for 30 minutes three or four times a day and position the hip in extension while prone. Also, to prevent flexion contractures, clients should avoid sitting in a chair for more than an hour. The residual limb is wrapped from distal to proximal. Ice packs are not used on the residual limb after surgery because the cold restricts blood flow. Antiinflammatory medications may be used for pain relief but not to prevent edema. (Lewis et al., 10 ed., p. 1488)

**6.** *3*
After cast application, observe for signs of compartment syndrome by performing neurovascular checks distal to the end of the cast. Palms of the hand should be used in turning the client. Heat should not be applied to a damp cast. (Lewis et al., 10 ed., p. 1472)

**7.** *4*
Always check the weight amounts and make sure they are not lodged against the bed or another area. There are no pin sites because Buck's traction is skin traction, not skeletal traction. The traction boot does not need to be removed as often as every 6 hours to provide skin care. (Lewis, et al., 10 ed., p. 1470)

**8.** *1*
Physical therapy relaxes muscles and relieves the aching and stiffness of the involved joints. It usually does not restore lost range of motion, and it does not prevent inflammation. Physical therapy does make the client more comfortable, but it does not assist in coping with pain. (Lewis et al., 10 ed., p. 1470)

**9.** *1*
Because of the high risk of venous thromboembolism (VTE) after a femur or hip fracture, prophylactic anticoagulant drugs such as warfarin and low-molecular-weight heparin such as enoxaparin may be ordered to prevent thromboembolic complications in the immobilized client. It is not effective in preventing fat emboli or venous stasis or promoting vascular perfusion. (Lewis et al., 10 ed., p. 1468)

**10.** *1*
Circulation and neurosensory status distal to the fracture are always priorities for clients with fractures. The amount of swelling is important, but the primary concern regarding swelling is circulatory and neurosensory deficits. The amount of bone healing cannot be assessed. There is concern regarding pain, but circulatory and neurologic checks are the priority actions. (Lewis et al., 10 ed., p. 1468)

**11.** *1*
The movement and sensation should be evaluated before surgery to serve as a baseline for comparison during the postoperative recovery period. Movement of the legs and assessment of sensation should be unchanged compared with the preoperative status. Radiating leg pain is diagnostic of the condition, and assessing it before surgery is not as beneficial as determining movement and sensation. (Lewis et al., 10 ed., p. 1504)

**12.** *2*
Check for red areas under the straps at least two or three times a day. The Ortolani test is for diagnostic purposes and should only be performed by trained health care practitioners. The success rate of the Pavlik harness is about 95% when a Pavlik harness is used on a full-time basis for 6 weeks, and spica casting is unnecessary. Adjustment of the harness is done by a health care practitioner. (Hockenberry, 10 ed., pp. 423–424)

**13.** *2, 3, 5*
Two potential life-threatening problems in the immediate postoperative period are airway obstruction and aspiration of vomitus. Because the patient cannot open the jaws, it is essential that an airway is maintained. Place the patient on the side with the head

slightly elevated immediately after surgery. The wire cutter or scissors may be used to cut the wires or elastic bands in case of an emergency. Although pain is an important consideration for any postoperative patient, it is not a life-threatening priority, nor are the patient's inability to speak or bleeding. (Lewis et al., 10 ed., p. 1468)

**14.** *1, 3, 5*
Purine-rich foods (e.g., shellfish such as crab and shrimp; vegetables such as lentils, asparagus, and spinach; meats such as beef, chicken, and pork) will not cause gout but can trigger an acute attack if a person is susceptible to gout. Other foods listed are not considered high in purine. (Lewis et al., 10 ed., p. 1532)

**15.** *3*
In rheumatoid arthritis, small joints typically first (proximal interphalangeal [PIPs], metacarpophalangeals [MCPs], metatarsophalangeals [MTPs]), wrists, elbows, shoulders, knees. Usually bilateral, symmetric joint involvement. In osteoarthritis, weight-bearing joints of knees and hips are most often affected, although small joints of the hands and feet and cervical/lumbar spine, often asymmetric, may also be involved; and joint destruction is caused by long-term use and weight bearing. (Lewis et al., 10 ed., p. 1525)

**16.** *4*
The identification of scoliosis as a "deformity," in combination with unattractive appliances and the potential of a surgical procedure, can have a negative effect on the already fragile adolescent's body image. The adolescent and family require excellent nursing care to meet not only physical needs but also psychological needs associated with a diagnosis of scoliosis. (Hockenberry, 10th ed., p. 1671)

**17.** *4*
Phantom limb pain is real pain for the client and is common in amputees. Phantom pain can best be controlled by pain medication. It is important to respect a client's interpretation of the experience of pain and offer him or her pain medication. (Lewis et al., 10 ed., p. 1487)

**18.** *2*
Laboratory work will need to be done periodically during administration to monitor for the development of anemia, leukopenia, thrombocytopenia, and/or hepatic toxicity. Hirsutism and menstrual changes occur with long-term corticosteroid use. Methotrexate should be given 1 hour before or 2 hours after meals to prevent vomiting when given by mouth (PO). Antiemetics are given concurrently with the medication. (Lewis et al., 10 ed., p. 1525)

**19.** *2*
Clients with total hip replacement should not bring their operative leg across midline, which may result in a prosthesis dislocation. Clients should maintain abduction (pillow between legs) and use elevated toilet seats. Crossing the legs is adduction, which is contraindicated for this client. (Lewis et al., 10 ed., p. 1468)

**20.** *2*
Greenstick fracture refers to splintering of the bone, not a complete fracture. The name comes from the splintering effect in attempts to break a "green stick." It is a common fracture in children. A comminuted fracture (bone is broken into several fragments) has multiple bone fragments and is more common in adults. In a nondisplaced fracture, such as the greenstick fracture, the periosteum is intact across the fracture, and the bone is still in alignment. (Lewis et al., 10 ed., p. 1468)

# TWENTY-FOUR

# Reproductive: Care of Adult and Pediatric Clients

# 24

## PRIORITY CONCEPTS

Infection, Pain, Sexuality

## PHYSIOLOGY OF THE REPRODUCTIVE SYSTEM

### Male Reproductive System

A. Penis: serves both reproductive and urinary function.
B. Scrotum: a double pouch of skin that protects the testes and sperm by maintaining temperature lower than that of the body.
C. Testes (gonads): sperm formation and production of testosterone occur here.
D. Epididymis: a tubular, coiled segment of the spermatic duct that stores spermatozoa until they are mature and then transports sperm from the testis to the vas deferens.
E. Prostate gland: produces a slightly alkalotic substance that provides both nourishment and mobility for spermatozoa.
F. Semen.
   1. Alkaline pH: 7.2 to 7.4.
   2. Average volume of ejaculate: 2.5 to 4 mL; may vary from 1 to 10 mL.
   3. Sterility: sperm count less than 20 million per milliliter (normal sperm count = 100 million per milliliter).

### Female Reproductive System

A. Vagina: a thin-walled, muscular membranous canal that has the ability to dilate and contract to facilitate giving birth and the act of intercourse.
B. Cervix: lower portion of the uterus that protrudes into the vagina.
   1. Provides an alkaline environment to shelter sperm from the acidic vagina.
   2. Cervical mucus pH increases (alkaline) and becomes clear and more viscous at ovulation, similar to egg white consistency.
C. Uterus: a hollow, pear-shaped, muscular pelvic organ; endometrium is the inner mucosal lining; undergoes cyclic changes as a result of hormonal levels.
D. Fallopian tubes: act to extract an ovum from the ovaries each month; if fertilization occurs, this takes place in the outer third of the fallopian tube.
E. Ovaries: located behind and below the fallopian tubes, produce ova, estrogen, and progesterone.

F. Breasts: function as an organ of sexual stimulation; nipple acts as a conduit for the flow of milk during breastfeeding.
G. Menstrual cycle (Figure 24-1).

### System Assessment

A. Female assessment.
   1. Obtain history data related to sexual activity, sexually transmitted infections (STIs), pregnancies, surgeries, menstrual cycle, breast abnormalities, urinary symptoms, or pain.
      a. Assess for vulvar discharge, erythema, growths, or pain.
      b. Assess breasts for lumps/masses, nipple abnormalities, or changes in the skin.
      c. Pelvic examination with Pap smear should be performed at least yearly.
      d. Breast self-examination (BSE) should be performed by patient monthly, beginning at onset of puberty.
      e. Mammogram should be performed yearly beginning at age 40 or earlier if considered high risk.
B. Male assessment.
   1. Obtain history data related to sexual activity, STDs, erectile dysfunction, urinary symptoms, surgeries, or pain.
   2. Assess penis, scrotum, and testicles for growths, masses, or ulcers.
      a. Testicular self-examination should be performed by the patient monthly beginning with onset of puberty.
      b. Digital rectal examination (DRE) and prostate-specific antigen (PSA) should be performed yearly beginning at 50 years of age or earlier if considered high risk.

## DISORDERS OF THE MALE REPRODUCTIVE SYSTEM

### Prostate Disorders

**Benign prostatic hyperplasia (BPH) or hypertrophy: enlargement of prostate gland tissue.**

**Cancer of the prostate: a malignancy of the prostate gland, which is a hormone-dependent adenocarcinoma; growth of the tumor is usually related to the presence of androgen hormone.**

**Both conditions encroach on the urethra and decrease the diameter of the bladder opening. Both can eventually cause bladder obstruction.**

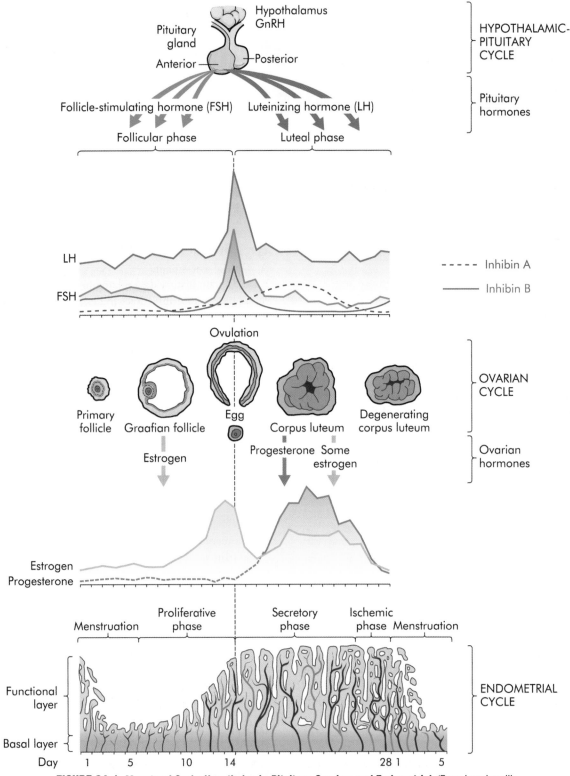

**FIGURE 24-1 Menstrual Cycle: Hypothalamic-Pituitary, Ovarian, and Endometrial.** (From Lowdermilk, D. L., et al., [2016]. *Maternity & women's health care* [11th ed.]. St. Louis, MO: Elsevier/Mosby.)

*Assessment*

A. Risk factors/etiology.
   1. BPH: very common in men older than 50 years.
   2. Prostatic carcinoma: rarely found in men younger than 60 years; usually found in the posterior lobe of the prostate gland.
B. Clinical manifestations.

**TEST ALERT:** Relate client's symptoms to adverse reactions of medication. Carefully assess the client with BPH in regard to anticholinergic medications (atropine) that cause urinary retention as a side effect.

   1. Common to both disorders.
      a. Bladder outlet obstruction.
         (1) Urinary hesitancy, frequency, urgency, and dribbling.

(2) Nocturia, hematuria, urinary retention, and a sensation of incomplete emptying of the bladder.

(3) Urinary retention may cause overflow urinary incontinence and dribbling after voiding.

  b. Acute retention may cause hydroureter and pressure in the kidney.

  c. Increased incidence of urinary tract infection due to residual urine.

2. Prostatic cancer.

  a. Tumor grows slowly and is confined to capsule; therefore prostate may appear normal, thus delaying the diagnosis.

  b. On digital rectal examination, asymmetric prostatic enlargement; prostate is described as "stony hard" and fixed.

  c. Obstruction is rare unless BPH is also present.

  d. Pain in the lumbosacral area may be presenting symptom as a result of metastasis.

C. Diagnostics.

1. Digital rectal examination.

2. Cystoscopy and bladder scan.

3. Urinalysis with culture and sensitivity.

4. Transrectal and/or transabdominal ultrasound.

5. To rule out or diagnose cancer.

  a. Prostate-specific antigen (normal PSA 0–4 mcg/L or ng/mL).

  b. Tumor markers for diagnosis, staging, and monitoring progress.

  c. Needle biopsy of prostate; definitive test for diagnosing cancer.

*Treatment*

A. Medical.

1. BPH: 5-alpha-reductase inhibitors and alpha-adrenergic blockers to shrink prostatic tissue (see Appendix 24-1).

2. "Watchful waiting" when there are mild symptoms; may include decreasing caffeine intake, avoiding decongestants and anticholinergics, and restricting fluid intake.

3. Prostate cancer: radiation, hormonal therapy, and chemotherapy for malignancy.

B. Surgical: size of prostate, presence of malignancy, and general health dictate the type of surgery.

1. Transurethral resection of the prostate (TURP): removal of prostatic tissue via a resectoscope, which is passed through the urethra (Figure 24-2).

2. Transurethral incision of the prostate (TUIP): making transurethral slits or incisions into prostate to relieve obstruction; effective with minimally enlarged prostate (BPH); indicated for clients who are poor surgical candidates.

3. Transurethral microwave therapy (TUMT) and transurethral needle ablation (TUNA): microwaves are delivered directly to the prostate; heat causes necrosis of tissue; both procedures are done on an outpatient basis.

4. Internal radiation therapy (brachytherapy) involves the placement of tiny radioactive "seeds" into the prostate for treatment of cancer.

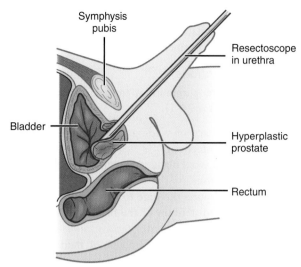

**FIGURE 24-2 Transurethral Resection of the Prostate.** (From Lewis, S. L., et al. [2017]. *Medical-surgical nursing: Assessment and management of clinical problems* [10th ed.]. St. Louis, MO: Elsevier/Mosby.)

5. Hormone therapy (antiandrogen medications—leuprorelin): depriving the cancer cells of testosterone may help slow the growth of prostatic cancer.

6. Cryotherapy (cryoablation): liquid nitrogen is applied to the prostate via a transrectal ultrasound probe; dead cells are absorbed by the body.

7. Prostatectomy: removal of the prostate via suprapubic, retropubic, or perineal approach; may be done by incision or laparoscopically; most often for removal of malignancy; robotic-assisted surgery used more frequently (less bleeding and pain and faster recovery).

*Complications*

A. BPH.

1. Preoperative.

  a. Urinary tract infection (UTI), hematuria.

  b. Acute urinary retention.

  c. Hydroureter (distention of the ureter) and hydronephrosis (enlargement of kidney caused by postrenal obstruction) with resultant renal failure.

  d. Bladder stones due to alkalinization of residual urine.

2. Postoperative.

  a. Hemorrhage: especially in the first 24 hours.

  b. Urinary incontinence, bladder spasms.

  c. Retrograde ejaculation: semen is passed back into the bladder rather than out through the penis. This causes milky or cloudy urine.

  d. Infection.

B. Prostatic cancer.

1. Preoperative.

  a. Complications are similar to BPH.

  b. Cancer may spread via the perineal lymphatic system to the regional lymph nodes. May metastasize to the pelvic bones, bladder, lungs, and liver.

2. Postoperative.

  a. Increased problems with deep venous thrombosis caused by lithotomy position during open perineal resection.

    b. Change in sexual functioning: impotence and failure to ejaculate.
    c. Urinary incontinence/dribbling.

### Nursing Interventions

**Goal:** To promote elimination, treat UTI, and provide client education (Box 24-1).

A. Evaluate adequacy of voiding and presence of urinary retention and infection.
B. Teach client to avoid bladder distention, which results in loss of muscle tone.
    1. Do not postpone the urge to void; it is important to prevent overdistention of the bladder, which further complicates the problem.
    2. Avoid drinking a large amount of fluid in a short period.
    3. Avoid alcohol and caffeine products because of the diuretic effect.
C. Encourage annual digital rectal examination of the prostate for all men older than 50 years, or earlier if at high risk.
D. Examination is recommended every 6 months for clients who have BPH or who have had a prostatectomy.

> ⚠ **NURSING PRIORITY:** Assess all male clients older than 50 years for symptoms of BPH. BPH occurs in 80% of men older than 80 years.

**Goal:** To maintain closed irrigation after surgery in the client who has undergone TURP or suprapubic prostatectomy (Figure 24-3).

A. Continuous bladder irrigation (CBI) with sterile, antibacterial, isotonic irrigating solution (also referred to as a Murphy drip or closed bladder irrigation).
    1. CBI is done with a triple-lumen catheter: one lumen for inflating the balloon (30–50 mL of water), one for

---

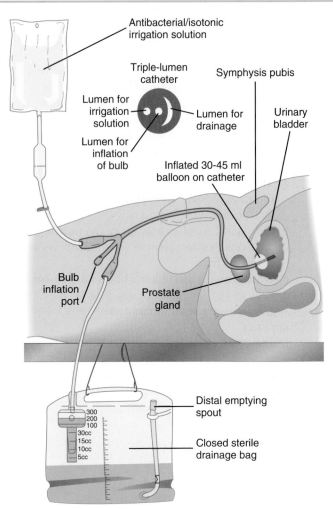

**FIGURE 24-3 Closed Bladder Irrigation (CBI).** (From Black, J. M., & Hawks, J. H. [2009]. *Medical-surgical nursing: clinical management for positive outcomes* [8th ed.]. Philadelphia: Saunders.)

---

maintaining outflow of urine, and one for the instillation of the continuous irrigating solution.
    2. Provides continuous irrigation to prevent bleeding and to flush the bladder of tissue and clots after TURP.
    3. If clots occur, the catheter may be irrigated or the rate of flow may be increased until the drainage outflow clears.
    4. Calculate intake and output carefully; amount of bladder irrigation fluid must be subtracted from total output to determine client's true urinary output.
    5. Monitor/titrate CBI so the outflow is light pink without clots; notify surgeon of any increase in bleeding.
    6. If catheter is occluded and does not drain properly, turn off the CBI until catheter patency is reestablished.
B. Blood clots and tissue are normal for the first 24 hours after TURP.
C. If client has excessive bleeding, the physician may increase the size of the balloon on the indwelling catheter and put traction on the catheter to compress the area of bleeding.
D. Client should void within 6 hours of removal of catheter.

---

### Box 24-1    OLDER ADULT CARE FOCUS

**Benign Prostatic Hypertrophy**
*General*
- All men older than 50 years of age should be assessed for urinary retention and adequacy of bladder emptying.
- Increased problem with urinary stasis; increased straining to urinate; increased incidence of infections.

*After Surgery*
- Closely evaluate for presence of infection, especially urinary tract, respiratory.
- Assess fluid balance; confusion and agitation may be symptoms of fluid overload.
- Help the client ambulate as soon as possible—increased risk for pooling of blood in pelvic cavity and pulmonary emboli from immobility.
- Client is at increased risk for falls.
- Determine psychological response to physical stress (confusion, disorientation); orient to surroundings frequently.

**NURSING PRIORITY:** Maintain CBI for the client who has undergone TURP; prevent overdistention of the bladder. If client complains of pain, check the urinary drainage and make sure it is patent. Obstruction most commonly occurs in the first 24 hours as a result of clots in the bladder.

E. Bladder spasms: belladonna and opium suppositories or antispasmodics are administered as needed; spasms often occur because of the presence of clots in the catheter; check the catheter for patency.

F. The sensation of a full bladder is common while the irrigation is occurring. May require frequent explanation about the irrigation. Advise the client to avoid bearing down in an attempt to void.

**Goal:** To provide postoperative care (Figure 24-4).

A. After client is ambulatory, encourage walking rather than sitting or lying for prolonged periods.

B. Teach client exercises to control urinary stream and maintain continence.
   1. Have client contract perineal muscles (Kegel exercises) by squeezing buttocks together.
   2. Instruct client to practice starting and stopping the stream several times while voiding.

C. Provide an opportunity for open discussion of sexual concerns. Retrograde ejaculation or erectile dysfunction may occur as a result of nerve damage during surgery.

D. Dribbling after voiding is a common problem that often subsides within a few weeks.

E. Teach client to avoid straining during bowel movement; encourage diet high in fiber, and administer stool softeners as needed.

F. Discuss with the client the importance of maintaining a high fluid intake to prevent UTIs.

G. Encourage client to minimize use of caffeine-containing products, which may cause bladder spasms.

**Goal:** To provide postoperative care for a client after radical open prostatectomy.

A. Maintain adequate pain control, frequently with patient-controlled analgesia.

B. As a result of the surgical position and postoperative immobility, client is at high risk for venous thromboembolism (VTE).
   1. Monitor sequential compression devices.
   2. Apply antiembolism stockings.
   3. Administer low-dose prophylactic anticoagulant therapy.
   4. Monitor prothrombin time/international normalized ratio (PT/INR) while on anticoagulants. Instruct client/family regarding bleeding precautions.

**TEST ALERT:** Identify symptoms of venous thromboembolism.

C. Perineal prostatectomy and total prostatectomy for cancer frequently result in erectile dysfunction and

# TURP
## (Transurethral Resection of the Prostate)

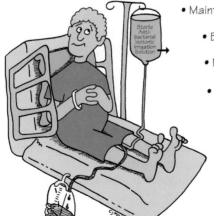

- Continuous or Intermittent Bladder Irrigation (C.B.I.)
  (Usually DC'd after 24 hours, if No Clots).   Murphy Drip

- Close observation of drainage system-
  (↑ Bladder Distention causes Pain & Bleeding).

- Maintain Catheter Patency

- Bladder Spasms

- Pain Control: Analgesics & ↓ Activity first 24 hours.

- Avoid straining with BMs. ↑ Fiber diet & Laxatives.

- Complications:
  - Hemorrhage - Bleeding should gradually ↓ to light pink in 24 hrs.
  - Urinary Incontinence - Kegel Exercises
  - Infections - ↑ Fluids
  - Prevent Deep Vein Thrombosis
  - Sequential compression stockings
  - Discourage sitting for prolonged periods

Sterile Anti-bacterial Isotonic Irrigation Solution

© 2016 Nursing Education Consultants, Inc.

**FIGURE 24-4  Transurethral Resection of the Prostate.** (From Zerwekh, J., Garneau, A., & Miller, C. J. [2017]. *Digital collection of the memory notebooks of nursing* [4th ed.]. Chandler, AZ: Nursing Education Consultants, Inc.)

urinary incontinence caused by damage to the pudendal nerves.

D. Emphasize importance of not straining against catheter to relieve bladder pressure.

E. Evaluate for urinary retention.

> **TEST ALERT:** Explain procedure to client and family. It is important to clarify for the client the information the doctor gives him, but it is the doctor's responsibility to advise the client regarding any complications he may experience with sexual functioning.

 ## Home Care

A. Teach client how to care for catheter and relieve obstruction if discharged with urinary catheter in place.

B. Avoid use of suppositories and enemas.

C. Primary care provider should be contacted if signs of UTI are noted.

D. After removal of urinary catheter, teach client Kegel exercises to increase urinary control (see BPH).

E. Adequate fluid intake, avoid strenuous exercise; avoid prolonged sitting; encourage walking.

## Inflammatory Disorders

**Prostatitis: inflammation of the prostate, usually caused by bacteria** *(Escherichia coli, Proteus, Klebsiella).*

**Epididymitis: inflammation of epididymis, often associated with prostatitis or a UTI; often develops as a complication of gonorrhea; in men younger than 35 years, the primary cause is infection with** *Chlamydia trachomatis.*

### Assessment

A. Clinical manifestations.
  1. Prostatitis.
     a. Fever and chills.
     b. Perineal, rectal, and/or back pain.
     c. Dysuria, urethral discharge.
     d. Prostate is enlarged, firm, and tender when palpated.
     e. May be acute or chronic with exacerbations.
     f. Increased risk with catheterizations, bladder infection, or alternative sexual activity.
  2. Epididymitis.
     a. Pain and tenderness in the inguinal canal.
     b. Painful swelling in the scrotum and groin.
     c. Fever and chills.
     d. Frequency, pyuria, and bacteriuria.
     e. Feeling of "heaviness" in the testicle(s).
     f. Sterile epididymitis due to increased intraabdominal pressure from physical strain or exertion; no symptoms of infection.
B. Diagnostics.
  1. Rectal examination.
  2. Complete blood count.
  3. Urine and semen culture and sensitivity.
  4. Screen for sexually transmitted infections (STIs).
  5. Doppler ultrasonography or nuclear imaging scan to rule out testicular torsion.

### Treatment

A. Prostatitis.
  1. Antibiotics.
  2. Analgesics, stool softeners, and sitz baths.
B. Epididymitis.
  1. Bed rest with elevation of the scrotum (scrotal support or scrotal bridge).
  2. Antibiotics, if indicated.
  3. Treatment of client's sexual partners (particularly if caused by gonorrhea infection).
  4. Cold compresses; nonsteroidal antiinflammatory drugs (NSAIDs).

### Complications

A. Chronic prostatitis can lead to recurrent UTIs and epididymitis.

B. May cause chronic reoccurring incapacitating infections.

### Nursing Interventions

**Goal:** To assist client to understand measures to maintain health.

A. Encourage early treatment to prevent complications.

B. For chronic prostatitis, encourage activities that drain the prostate, including intercourse, masturbation, and prostatic massage.

C. Antibiotics may not be effective because it is difficult to obtain therapeutic levels in prostatic secretion.

D. Encourage treatment of sexual partners when epididymitis is caused by chlamydia or gonorrhea.

## Undescended Testes (Cryptorchidism)

**Cryptorchidism is a condition of failure of one or both testes to descend into the scrotal sac.**

### Assessment

A. Clinical manifestations.
  1. Inability to palpate the testes in the scrotal sac.
  2. Testicle may be absent or small or may be located in the abdomen.
  3. Cremasteric reflex is normal retraction of the testes when stimulated by stroking the thigh on affected side downward; may present a problem in attempting to determine whether there is an undescended testicle or if a testicle is retractable.

### Treatment

A. Medical: condition may be observed for 1 year; most cases descend spontaneously; if undescended after 1 year, surgery may be required.

B. Surgical: testis is brought into the scrotal sac and secured (orchiopexy).
  1. Usually done between the ages of 6 and 24 months; fewer complications are encountered if repair is done before 6 years of age.
  2. Individuals with a history of cryptorchidism are at increased risk for fertility problems and development

of testicular cancer in adulthood, especially if the testes have not descended by age 6.

### Nursing Interventions

 **Home Care**

A. Long-term follow-up regarding fertility.

B. Prevent infection by careful cleansing after defecation and urination because of the close proximity of the scrotum.

C. Teach parents to show the child how to do testicular self-examinations when he is old enough.

## Testicular Tumors (Cancer)

**Tumors of the testicles are often malignant and tend to metastasize quickly.**

### Assessment

A. Risk factors/etiology.
1. Most common cancer in males ages 15 to 35 years.
2. More common in clients who have had cryptorchidism and frequent reproductive organ infections.
3. For clients 40 to 60 years of age, determine, if possible, whether mother was given diethylstilbestrol (DES) during pregnancy. There is a significant increase in the risk for testicular cancer among these clients.

B. Clinical manifestations.
1. A painless lump (typically pea sized) is palpated in the scrotum.
2. Most men experience "heaviness" in the scrotum.
3. Significant enlargement of or shrinking of one testicle.

C. Diagnostics.
1. Levels of alpha-fetoprotein (AFP) and human chorionic gonadotropin (hCG) are increased.
2. Computed tomography (CT) and magnetic resonance imaging (MRI) to identify metastases.
3. Ultrasound.
4. Biopsy is not recommended because of the risk for spreading cancer locally.

### Treatment

A. Medical.
1. Postoperative irradiation to the lymphatic drainage pathways.
2. Multiple chemotherapy medications.

B. Surgical.
1. Orchiectomy (removal of the testicle) is performed as soon as possible to remove the tumor and make a definite diagnosis.
2. If there is lymph node involvement, a retroperitoneal lymph node dissection is performed.

### Nursing Interventions

**Goal:** To detect any abnormality of the testes through client self-examination (Box 24-2).

---

| Box 24-2   **TESTICULAR SELF-EXAMINATION** |
| --- |

- Examine the testicles at same time every month to help you remember to do it.
- Visually inspect scrotum in front of a mirror, observing for swelling.
- Perform the examination after a warm bath or shower because this is when the testes are lower in the scrotal sac.
- Examine each testicle individually by placing index and middle fingers of both hands under one testicle at a time with thumbs on top of testicle. Roll the testicle between the thumbs and fingers. This should *not* cause pain. The tissue should feel smooth.
- Locate the epididymis, which is a tubular sac behind the testicle. This sac should not be confused with a lump.
- Also assess for any "heaviness" or dull ache in the groin or abdomen or significant increase or decrease in size of either testicle.
- If there is any lump or irregularity on either testicle, report it to the doctor as soon as possible.

---

**TEST ALERT:** Participate in health promotion programs. Teach men how to perform self-examinations.

A. Teach clients, especially those between the ages 15 and 35 years, to self-examine monthly while showering or bathing to detect any abnormality of the testes.

B. Emphasize importance of follow-up for clients with a history of undescended testes or a previous testicular tumor.

## Testicular Torsion

**Involves a twisting of the spermatic cord that supplies blood to the testes and epididymis.**

### Assessment

A. Risk factors/etiology.
1. Occurs in men under age 25; peak incidence 14 years of age.

B. Clinical manifestations.
1. Scrotal pain, tenderness, swelling, redness; nausea, vomiting.
2. Absent cremasteric reflex.

### Treatment

A. Surgical.
1. Emergency surgery to preserve testicle.

### Nursing Interventions

A. Provide preoperative and postoperative care if indicated (see Chapter 3).

## Hydrocele and Varicocele

**Hydrocele: a collection of fluid (cystic mass) around the testicle or along the spermatic cord.**

**Varicocele:** a cluster of dilated veins in the scrotal sac, often just above the testes; occurs most often in young adults.

A. Clinical manifestations.
1. Hydrocele usually is painless, but a chronic dull ache in the scrotal area may occur if it becomes very large.
2. May contribute to infertility because sperm temperatures may be too high, which affects sperm formation and motility.
B. Treatment.
1. Hydrocele: needle aspiration or surgical aspiration and drainage.
2. Varicocele: surgical intervention only if there are complications with fertility; otherwise, a scrotal support is used.
C. Nursing intervention.
1. Provide preoperative and postoperative care if indicated (see Chapter 3).

### Erectile Dysfunction (ED)

**Inability to attain or maintain an erection.**

*Assessment*

A. Risk factors/etiology.
1. Physiologic (organic): diabetes, hypertension, prostatectomy, trauma/tumor of the spinal cord, side effects of many medications (especially antihypertensive agents), and endocrine disorders.
2. Psychological (functional): stress, depression, low self-esteem.
B. Clinical manifestations.
1. Inability to achieve or sustain an erection.
2. Gradual onset with physiologic ED and abrupt onset with psychological ED.

*Treatment*

A. Medical.
1. ED medications (Figure 24-4 and Appendix 24-1).
2. Vacuum constriction devices (VCD): applying a suction device to the penis to pull blood up into the corporeal bodies, then placing a penile ring or constrictive band to trap the engorgement.
3. Intraurethral devices: medicated urethral system for erection (MUSE)—administration of medications as a topical gel, injection into penis, or insertion of medication pellet into urethra.
B. Surgical.
1. Penile implants: surgical insertion of an implant.

*Nursing Interventions*

**Goal:** To help the client understand the implications of the medications or devices used to treat ED and assist to obtain counseling.

A. Teach client about how ED medications can potentiate hypotensive effects of nitrates and should not be taken at the same time (Figure 24-5).

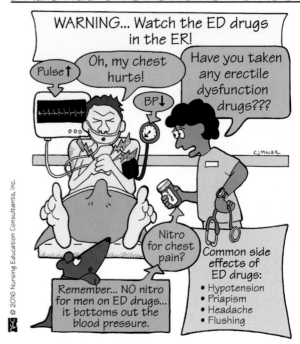

**FIGURE 24-5** **Erectile Dysfunction Drugs.** (From Zerwekh, J., Garneau, A., & Miller, C. J. [2017]. *Digital collection of the memory notebooks of nursing* [4th ed.]. Chandler, AZ: Nursing Education Consultants, Inc.)

B. Client should abstain from alcohol if taking ED medications.
C. Teach client that ED medications should only be taken once daily.

## DISORDERS OF THE FEMALE REPRODUCTIVE SYSTEM

### Cystocele and Rectocele

**Cystocele is a weakened support between the vagina and bladder allowing the bladder to bulge into the vagina. Rectocele is a weakened support between the vagina and rectum allowing the rectum to bulge into the vagina.**

*Assessment*

A. Risk factors/etiology.
1. Obesity and childbearing.
2. Genital atrophy caused by aging.
B. Clinical manifestations.
1. Cystocele: protrusion of the bladder into the vagina.
a. Stress incontinence: occurs during coughing, lifting, or sneezing.
b. Frequency and urgency.
c. Difficulty emptying bladder.
d. Recurrent UTI (especially with a large cystocele).
2. Rectocele: protrusion of the rectum through the vaginal wall.
a. Constipation.
b. Incontinence of gas or liquid feces.
C. Diagnostics: bimanual pelvic examination.

## Treatment

A. Medical.
  1. Kegel exercises for mild stress incontinence (tighten and release perineal muscles for several seconds; 10–15 times during the day).
  2. Client can also imagine that she is trying to stop passing gas in a crowded room by squeezing the muscles that would be used to stop the gas from passing.
B. Surgical.
  1. Cystocele: anterior colporrhaphy.
  2. Rectocele: posterior colporrhaphy.

## Nursing Interventions

**Goal:** To prevent wound infection and pressure on the vaginal suture line.

A. Preoperative teaching.
B. Postoperative period.
  1. Prevent wound infection.
  2. Apply ice pack locally to relieve perineal discomfort and swelling.
  3. Indwelling catheter for 4 days after anterior colporrhaphy.
  4. Monitor for excessive vaginal bleeding.
C. Frequent perineal care as well as after each voiding or defecation.

## Home Care (Postoperative)

A. Encourage the use of stool softeners to prevent straining at stool.
B. Prevent constipation.
C. Certain activities are restricted until area has healed: lifting objects heavier than 5 pounds; intercourse; prolonged standing, walking, and sitting.
D. Call the doctor if there is persistent pain or purulent, foul-smelling vaginal discharge.
E. Teach catheter care if discharged with urinary catheter.

## Vaginal Inflammatory Conditions

### Common Predisposing Factors

A. Excessive douching.
B. Oral contraceptives, steroids.
C. Antibiotics: especially broad spectrum, which wipe out normal vaginal flora (vagina is protected by an acidic pH and the presence of Döderlein's bacilli).
D. Improper cleaning after voiding and defecating.
E. Assess for recurrent chronic infection; there may be an underlying condition (prediabetic state, HIV infection) that should be further evaluated.

### Bacterial Vaginosis

A. Characteristics.
  1. Causative organisms: *E. coli, Haemophilus vaginalis,* and *Gardnerella vaginalis.*
  2. Profuse watery discharge, "fishy smell."
  3. Itching, redness, burning, and edema, which are exacerbated by voiding and defecation.
B. Treatment: antibacterial/antiprotozoal medication.
C. Complications: bacterial vaginosis may increase susceptibility to STDs and HIV infection if woman is exposed to either.
D. Factors associated with bacterial vaginosis include multiple sex partners, but may occur in non–sexually active women, douching, and smoking.

### Candidiasis

A. Characteristics.
  1. Organism: *Candida albicans* (fungus).
  2. Internal itching, beefy red irritation, inflammation of vaginal epithelium.
  3. White, cheese-like, odorless discharge that clings to the vaginal mucosa.
  4. Occurs frequently and is difficult to cure.
  5. Increased risk in women with diabetes and women taking birth control pills, during pregnancy, and after treatment with antibiotics.
  6. Clients with recurrent vaginitis should be offered HIV testing, especially if unresponsive to first-line treatment.
B. Treatment.
  1. Antifungal vaginal medication.
  2. Oral antifungals.

### Trichomoniasis

A. Characteristics.
  1. Organism: *Trichomonas vaginalis* (protozoan).
  2. May be asymptomatic.
  3. Itching, burning, dyspareunia (painful intercourse).
  4. Frothy, green-yellow, copious, malodorous vaginal discharge; strawberry spot (petechiae) on cervix.
  5. Sexual partners must be treated also because of cross-infection; men are usually asymptomatic.
B. Treatment: antibacterial/antiprotozoal medication.
C. Prevention: avoid extended time in synthetic or tight-fitting undergarments; use of condoms may reduce incidence of STIs.

### Postmenopausal Vaginitis (Atrophic Vaginitis)

A. Characteristics.
  1. Lack of estrogen (this is also the cause).
  2. Itching and burning.
  3. Loss of vaginal tissue folds and epithelial covering.
B. Treatment: estrogen vaginal cream or tablet insert.

### Nursing Interventions

**Goal:** To teach client to prevent infection by performing appropriate personal hygiene, decrease inflammation, and promote comfort.

A. Appropriate cleansing from front of vulva to back of perineal area.
B. Client should not douche; douching removes normal protective bacteria from vaginal cavity, and other bacteria are introduced.
C. If infection is chronic, it may be necessary to have sexual partner tested; partner may be reinfecting the woman.

D. Discourage use of feminine hygiene sprays because they cause increased irritation.

E. Discourage client from wearing constricting clothing and synthetic underwear (encourage use of cotton underwear).

**Goal:** To educate the woman regarding correct use of medication.

A. Vaginal tablets and creams are often used.
   1. Handwashing before and after insertion of suppository or application of cream.
   2. Remain recumbent for 30 minutes after application to promote absorption and prevent loss of the medication from the vaginal area.
   3. Wear a perineal pad to prevent soiling of clothing with vaginal drainage.

### Abnormal (Dysfunctional) Uterine Bleeding

**Bleeding that is excessive or abnormal in amount or frequency without regard to systemic conditions; occurs when the hormonal events responsible for the balance of the cycle are interrupted.**

#### Amenorrhea

A. Absence of menses.
   1. Primary: no menstruation has occurred by age 16 years.
   2. Secondary: woman previously had menses.
B. May be indicative of menopause.
C. May be first indication of pregnancy.
D. Occurs when woman has lost a critical fat percentage (e.g., athletes, clients with anorexia).

#### Menorrhagia

A. Excessive vaginal bleeding.
B. Single episode of heavy bleeding may indicate a spontaneous abortion.
C. May be associated with an intrauterine device (IUD), hypothyroidism, uterine fibroids, or hormone imbalance.

#### Metrorrhagia

A. Vaginal bleeding between periods.
B. May be normal menopause.
C. Ectopic pregnancy.
D. Breakthrough bleeding from oral contraceptives or intrauterine device (IUD).
E. Cervical polyps.

> **! NURSING PRIORITY:** Vaginal bleeding after menopause or surgical hysterectomy is a symptom of a problem that needs to be evaluated.

#### Nursing Interventions

A. Help determine cause of problem.
B. Report excessive bleeding, abdominal pain, fever.
C. Treatment.
   1. Dilation and curettage (D&C) for diagnostic purposes in older women.
   2. Endometrial ablation (balloon thermotherapy).

3. Removal of fibroids.
   a. Often done on outpatient basis with either general regional or local anesthesia.
   b. Spotting and vaginal drainage are common for several days; if amount is more than a normal period or if it lasts longer than 2 weeks, client should call the doctor.
   c. Client should report any signs of infection: fever; foul, purulent discharge; increasing abdominal pain.
   d. NSAIDs are often used for pain control.
   e. Client should avoid sexual intercourse and use of tampons for about 2 weeks.
D. Assess and treat for anemia.
   1. Encourage diet high in iron.
   2. Administer iron preparations, if required.

### Endometriosis

**Endometriosis is the presence of endometrial tissue outside of the uterus. The tissue responds to hormonal stimulation by bleeding into areas within the pelvis, causing pain and adhesions.**

#### Assessment

A. Risk factors/etiology.
   1. Cause not fully understood.
   2. Most common in women in their late 20s and early 30s who have never been pregnant.
   3. Proposed theory suggests that small pieces of endometrial tissue back up through the fallopian tubes into the abdomen during menstruation.
B. Clinical manifestations.
   1. Dysmenorrhea: deep-seated aching pain in the lower abdomen, vagina, posterior pelvis, and back occurring 1 to 2 days before menses.
   2. Abnormal excessive uterine bleeding and dyspareunia; painful defecation.
C. Diagnostics.
   1. Laparoscopy.
   2. Ultrasonography.

#### Treatment

A. Medical.
   1. Androgenic agents may be given over a 6- to 8-month period.
   2. Oral contraceptives.
   3. Condition recedes during pregnancy.
B. Surgical.
   1. Laser treatment of endometrial tissue in the extrauterine sites.
   2. Hysterectomy (usually carried out in women close to menopause).

#### Complications

A. Infertility.
B. Adhesions.
C. Bowel obstruction.

*Nursing Interventions*

**Goal:** To help client minimize the pain and discomfort associated with endometriosis.

A. Warm baths or moist heat packs may reduce discomfort.
B. Encourage client to explore alternative sexual positions that may minimize discomfort during intercourse.
C. Encourage client to discuss abstinence with her partner if intercourse is painful.

**Goal:** To assist client to understand measures to maintain health.

A. Teach client about disease process; clarify any false ideas.
B. Provide emotional reassurance; discuss potential for infertility.

## Pelvic Inflammatory Disease

**Pelvic inflammatory disease (PID) is an infectious condition of the pelvic cavity that involves the fallopian tubes, the ovaries, and/or the peritoneum.**

*Assessment*

A. Risk factors/etiology.
   1. Complication of gonorrhea and *Chlamydia trachomatis*.
   2. IUDs are correlated with an increased incidence of PID.
   3. Increased number of sexual partners.
   4. Increases risk for repeat cases after previous episode of PID.
B. Clinical manifestations.
   1. Lower abdominal pain that worsens over time.
   2. General malaise, fever, chills, nausea, and vomiting.
   3. Pain on urinating and with intercourse.
   4. Vaginal discharge that is heavy and purulent.
   5. Chronic PID: persistent pelvic pain, secondary dysmenorrhea, dysfunctional uterine bleeding, and periodic episodes of acute symptoms.
C. Diagnostics.
   1. Abdominal pain on palpation.
   2. Culture and sensitivity of drainage from the vagina, cervix, or cul-de-sac of Douglas.
   3. Ultrasonography, laparoscopy, culdocentesis.

*Treatment*

A. Medical: broad-spectrum antibiotics, analgesics.
B. Surgical: incision and drainage of abscesses with or without a laparotomy.

*Complications*

A. Sterility caused by adhesions and strictures within the fallopian tubes.
B. Ectopic pregnancy.
C. Pelvic abscess or generalized peritonitis.
D. Septic shock.

*Nursing Interventions*

**Goal:** To prevent the spread and extension of the infection.

A. Maintain semi-Fowler's position to promote drainage of the pelvic cavity by gravity.
B. Strict medical asepsis when in contact with discharge; wound and skin precautions.
C. Encourage oral fluids and maintain adequate nutrition.
D. Client should avoid sexual activity and douching during therapy.
E. Strongly encourage sexual partner(s) to seek medical treatment.

## Cervical Cancer

**Cancer of the uterine cervix that can invade the bladder, rectum, and other pelvic areas in advanced stage.**

*Assessment*

A. Risk factors/etiology.
   1. Multiple sex partners.
   2. Early sexual activity.
   3. History of STIs, herpes simplex virus type 2 (HSV-2).
   4. Genital warts (human papilloma virus [HPV]-positive), abnormal Pap smears.
B. Clinical manifestations.
   1. Clients are asymptomatic until late in disease state.
   2. Thin and watery drainage that becomes dark and foul smelling as the disease progresses.
   3. Abnormal vaginal bleeding (spotting) or discharge.
   4. Low back pain.
   5. Painful sexual intercourse.
C. Diagnostics.
   1. Pap smear.
      a. Initial Pap smear at age 21 or after first sexual intercourse.
      b. Pap smears are continued after menopause and hysterectomy.
      c. Testing for HPV-type 16 and 18. Recent research shows that testing for HPV may be better than the Pap test for screening for cervical cancer.
   2. Cervical biopsy.

**! NURSING PRIORITY:** If cancer of the cervix is identified before it becomes invasive (or in the in situ stage), there is virtually a 100% cure rate.

*Treatment*

A. Medical.
   1. Prevention through regular screening and vaccination against HPV (Gardasil).
   2. Radiation therapy, either internal (radium implant) or external for invasive cancer.
B. Surgical intervention. (Procedure depends on extent of the cancer.)
   1. Conization (cryosurgery): used for carcinoma in situ.
   2. Vaginal hysterectomy: removal of the uterus. Fallopian tubes and ovaries remain intact.

3. Hysterectomy: total abdominal hysterectomy with bilateral salpingo-oophorectomy (TAH-BSO); includes removal of fallopian tubes and ovaries.
4. Radical hysterectomy: a panhysterectomy plus a partial vaginectomy and removal of lymph nodes.
5. Pelvic exoneration: radical hysterectomy plus total vaginectomy, removal of bladder with urinary diversion, bowel resection, and colostomy.

## Nursing Interventions

**Goal:** Provide health teaching to help clients prevent and/or detect premalignant cervical dysplasia.

A. Warning signs of cancer.
B. Importance of yearly Pap smears.
C. Encourage verbalization of feelings related to the surgery and diagnosis of cancer.
D. Prevention with early immunization against HPV and safe sex education.
E. Prevention, early detection, and treatment of STIs.

**Goal:** To provide preoperative and postoperative teaching in preparation for a total abdominal hysterectomy.

A. General preoperative care.
B. After surgery, assess for complications, such as backache or decreased urine output, because these symptoms can indicate accidental ligation of the ureter.
C. Urinary retention may occur as a result of bladder atony and edema; explain to client the necessity for a urinary retention catheter.
D. Early ambulation is encouraged to prevent postoperative thrombophlebitis.
E. Determine whether hormone replacement therapy will be used and provide appropriate teaching.
F. If dyspareunia occurs, client should contact her doctor.

## Breast Cancer

**The most common malignancy in females. Second to lung cancer as a leading cause of cancer death in women in the United States.**

## Assessment

A. Risk factors/etiology.
   1. Female gender.
   2. The incidence of recurrence of breast cancer is significant.
   3. Family history of breast cancer; however, 85% of women with breast cancer have a negative family history.
   4. Inherited genetic abnormality (*BRCA1* gene).
   5. Advancing age (postmenopausal).
   6. Nulliparity or parity after the age of 30 years.
   7. Early menses, late menopause.
   8. Presence of other cancer: endometrial, ovarian, colon, rectal.
   9. Use of estrogen/progesterone hormone therapy.
B. Clinical manifestations.
   1. Asymmetry of the breasts.
   2. Skin dimpling, flattening, and nipple deviation are suggestive of a lesion.
   3. Skin coloring and thickening, large pores, sometimes called peau d'orange (orange peel appearance).
   4. Changes: retraction of the nipple; discharge from the nipple.
   5. Mass is painless, nontender, hard, irregular in shape, and nonmobile.
   6. Majority of malignant lesions are found in the upper outer quadrant of the breast (tail of Spence).
C. Diagnostics.
   1. Mammography; digital mammography; ultrasound.
   2. Breast biopsy.
   3. Serum tumor markers: carcinoembryonic antigen (CEA), human chorionic gonadotropin (hCG).
   4. Lymph node dissection.
D. Complications.
   1. Recurrence in same side or other breast.
   2. Metastases via the lymphatic system to bone, lungs, brain, and liver.
   3. Postmastectomy pain syndrome: pain persisting past 3 months.
   4. Lymphedema.
   5. Cognitive changes may occur after chemotherapy (referred to as chemobrain).

## Treatment

A. Surgical.
   1. Modified radical mastectomy (most common): removal of all breast tissue and axillary lymph nodes; the pectoralis major muscle remains intact; preservation of the muscle helps prevent the arm edema frequently associated with mastectomy; allows for breast reconstruction surgery.
   2. Local breast conserving surgery (lumpectomy): may be done to stage the malignancy and determine appropriate chemotherapy/radiation therapy, but the breast is preserved.
   3. Radical mastectomy (less common): removal of all of the breast tissue, the pectoral muscles, and the axillary lymph nodes of the surrounding tissue.
   4. Breast reconstruction: may be delayed until after radiation therapy is completed or may be done at the time of the mastectomy.
B. Radiation: combined with surgery and chemotherapy.
C. Hormonal therapy: breast cancers that are classified as "estrogen receptors" are less invasive tumors and respond to changes in estrogens; hormone therapy is being used in conjunction with surgical intervention to prevent/decrease recurrence.
D. Chemotherapy: a combination of drugs will be used to treat the malignancy; allows for use of drugs that have different mechanisms of action and work at different parts of the cell cycle.

## Nursing Interventions

**Goal:** To promote early detection of breast cancer through mammography, clinical breast examination, and BSE.

A. Screening mammography should begin at age 40 or earlier if client is at high risk.

- Evaluate risk factors; educate woman about increased risk factors.
- Woman should perform breast self-examination (BSE) on a regular basis; once a month about a week after her period or at the same time each month if the woman has no periods.
- It is important for the BSE to be done on a regular basis; this makes it easier to detect abnormalities when they occur.
- The BSE should include the following three steps:
  1. Step 1: Inspection before a mirror to determine asymmetry or changes in size. Breast should be evaluated from three positions: with the arms relaxed at the sides; with the arms over the head pressing on the back of the head; with the hands on the hips, palms pressing inward to flex the chest muscles. Look for dimpling, differences in sizes of the breast, ulcerations, enlarged pores, nipple retraction, and increased vascularity.
  2. Step 2: Breast should be palpated while lying down; flatten the right breast by placing a pillow under the right shoulder. With the fingers flat, use the sensitive pads of the middle three fingers of the left hand. Feel for lumps or changes using a rubbing motion. Press firmly enough to feel the different breast tissues. Examine the entire breast from the collarbone to area on which the base of your bra rests and the axillary area. Pay particular attention to the upper outer quadrant of each breast. Gently squeeze the nipple to determine presence of any drainage.
  3. Step 3: In the shower or bath examine your breasts; hands glide easier over wet skin.
- Women older than 40 years should have a mammogram every year; women with increased risk factors should maintain regular follow-up with a physician.
The American Cancer Society provides excellent teaching opportunities for nurses, as well as extensive information for women regarding early detection of breast cancer and rehabilitation after a mastectomy.

**TEST ALERT:** Questions regarding teaching women about breast cancer, risk factors, BSE, and preventive health care are common on the examination.

B. Teach client how to perform BSE (Box 24-3). Recent evidence from the American Cancer Society states that research has not shown a clear benefit of regular physical breast examinations done by either a health professional (clinical breast examinations) or by the client (BSE), and the recommendation is for women to be familiar with how their breasts look and feel and report any changes. See the following update: https://www.cancer.org/cancer/breast-cancer/screening-tests-and-early-detection/american-cancer-society-recommendations-for-the-early-detection-of-breast-cancer.html

C. Clinical breast examination should begin with clients in their 20s and 30s, and every year for asymptomatic woman age 40 or older.

D. American Cancer Society recommends a yearly MRI and a mammography for women age 30 or older who have a family history of breast cancer.

**Goal:** To prepare the client physiologically and psychologically for surgery (normal preoperative and postoperative care; see Chapter 3).

A. Assist woman to decrease emotional stress and anxiety; encourage use of spiritual and social resources.
B. Provide emotional support; encourage verbalization. Assist client to seek assistance from the wide variety of support groups available.
C. Anticipate concerns related to sexuality and fear of rejection by sex partner after the mastectomy (see the section on Body Image in Chapter 12).

**TEST ALERT:** Plan measures to assist client to cope with anxiety; assess client's response to illness; identify coping mechanisms of client and family.

D. Determine whether any plans for reconstructive surgery have been discussed.

**Goal:** To recognize and prevent postoperative complications (Figure 24-6).

A. There may be one or more drains in the incisional area. Jackson-Pratt drains are commonly used.

**TEST ALERT:** Empty and reestablish negative pressure of portable wound suction devices.

B. Assess wound for infection.
C. Position client in semi-Fowler's and arm on affected side so that each joint is elevated and positioned higher than the more proximal joint; this promotes gravity drainage via the lymphatic and venous circulations.
D. Do not take blood pressure or perform any injections or venipuncture on the arm of the affected side.
E. Arm exercises are usually started on the first postoperative day.
  1. Assist/teach the woman to perform flexion and extension exercises with the wrist and elbow frequently throughout the day. Squeezing a ball is good exercise at this time.
  2. The affected arm should not be abducted or externally rotated in initial exercises. Encourage movement of the arm in activities of daily living (brushing her hair, eating, washing her face).
F. Active exercises are begun after wound healing is well established.
G. Approximately 2 to 3 weeks after surgery and with good wound healing, more active exercises are initiated.
  1. Pendulum arm swings.
  2. Pulley-type rope exercise to promote forward and lateral movement of the arms.
  3. "Wall climbing" with the fingers.

# POST MASTECTOMY
## NURSING CARE

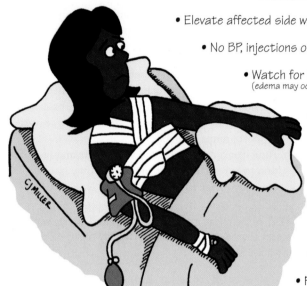

• Elevate affected side with distal joint higher than proximal joint.

• No BP, injections or venipunctures on affected side.

• Watch for S & S of edema on affected arm.
(edema may occur post op or years later)

• Lymphedema can occur any time after axillary node disection.

• Flexion and extension exercises of the hand in recovery.

• Abduction and external rotation arm exercises after wound has healed.

• Assess dressing for drainage.

• Assess wound drain for amount and color.

• Provide privacy when patient looks at incision.

• Chemotherapy, Radiation therapy.

• Monitor for Complications — hemorrhage, hematoma, lymphedema, infection, postmastectomy pain syndrome.

• Psychological concerns:
    Altered body image
    Altered sexuality
    Fear of disease outcome

© 2016 Nursing Education Consultants, Inc.

**FIGURE 24-6 Postmastectomy Nursing Care.** (From Zerwekh, J., Garneau, A., & Miller, C. J. [2017]. *Digital collection of the memory notebooks of nursing* [4th ed.]. Chandler, AZ: Nursing Education Consultants, Inc.)

**TEST ALERT:** Identify factors interfering with wound healing. The arm on the affected side will be at increased risk for developing problems of edema and infection. The arm should be protected throughout rehabilitation and during activities of daily living for an indefinite period.

 **Home Care**

**Goal:** To promote the client's return to homeostasis and to help her understand implications of modified lifestyle; to identify measures to maintain health.

A. Discuss symptoms of recurrence and importance of making regular visits to the physician to monitor recovery and to detect changes.
B. Promote a positive self-image and reintegration with family and loved ones.
C. Discuss with client plans for obtaining a breast prosthesis.
D. Encourage the woman to participate in the Reach to Recovery program through the American Cancer Society. Check with the physician to see whether representatives may visit with the client before the surgery.
E. Compression arm sleeves used to minimize swelling from lymphedema.

## SEXUALLY TRANSMITTED INFECTIONS

**STIs (previously referred to as sexually transmitted diseases [STDs]) are infectious diseases transmitted most commonly through sexual contact.**

A. Characteristics.
   1. Transmitted most commonly through sexual activity, including oral and rectal activities between people of the same or opposite sex; may also be transmitted via contaminated needles and in utero transmission to a fetus.
   2. One person can have more than one STI at a time.
   3. All sexual partners need to be evaluated.
B. Nursing role is to recognize and provide factual information.
   1. Mode of transmission.
   2. Prevention of transmission.

3. Importance of contacts being identified and treated.
4. Information provided in accepting, nonjudgmental manner.
5. Oral contraceptives do not provide any protection.
C. Clients with STIs should be tested for HIV.
D. Hepatitis B and HPV are considered STIs (see Chapter 21).

---

**■ NURSING PRIORITY:** Consider all oral, genital, and rectal lesions to contain pathologic organisms until documented otherwise.

---

## 📋 Syphilis

**Syphilis is caused by the spirochete *Treponema pallidum*, which is transmitted by direct contact with primary chancre lesion and body secretions (saliva, blood, vaginal discharge, semen) and is also transmitted transplacentally to the fetus.**

### Assessment

A. Risk factors/etiology.
1. Incubation period is 10 to 90 days, with an average of 20 to 30 days.
2. Highly infectious during the primary stage. Blood contains the spirochete during the secondary stage; usually noninfectious after 1 year during the latent stage; noninfectious in the late (tertiary) stage.
B. Clinical manifestations.
1. Primary stage.
a. Chancre: small, hard, painless lesion found on the penis, vulva, lips, vagina, or rectum.
b. Usually heals spontaneously within 2 to 3 weeks with or without treatment.
c. Highly contagious during this stage.
d. Will progress without treatment.
2. Secondary stage.
a. Usually begins anywhere from 2 weeks to 6 months after the initial chancre has healed.
b. May be asymptomatic or may have maculopapular rash on the palms of the hands and soles of the feet, sore throat, and headache; gray mucous patches in the mouth.
c. Symptoms disappear within 2 to 6 weeks.
3. Latent stage.
a. Absence of clinical symptoms.
b. Noninfectious after 1 year in the latent stage.
c. Results of serologic tests for syphilis remain positive.
d. Transmission can occur through blood contact.
e. Majority of clients remain in this stage without further symptoms.
4. Tertiary stage.
a. Gummas: chronic, destructive lesions may develop in skin, bone, and liver.
b. Causes neurologic problems from mild personality changes to tremors and major psychoses.

5. Congenital syphilis.
a. Maculopapular rash over face, genital region, palms, and soles.
b. Snuffles: a mucopurulent nasal discharge indicative of some degree of respiratory obstruction.
c. After the age of 2 years, Hutchinson's teeth appear. These are notched central incisors with deformed molars and cusps.
C. Diagnostics.
1. Serologic screening: Venereal Disease Research Laboratories (VDRL).
2. Rapid plasma reagin test (PRP & RPR) may produce false-negative results in early stages.
3. Fluorescent treponemal antibody absorption (FTA-ABS) test.
4. *T. pallidum* particle agglutination (TP-PA) test.
5. The (FTA-ABs) and (TP-PA) tests are used to confirm the diagnosis of syphilis. The VDRL and RPR are used for screening purposes.

### Treatment

A. Medical.
1. Penicillin G or aqueous procaine penicillin G.
2. May use tetracycline or doxycycline if allergic to penicillin.

### Nursing Interventions

A. If pregnant mother is treated before 18 weeks' gestation, the fetus will usually be born unaffected.
B. Education regarding means of transmission, prevention, and treatment.
C. Adequate case finding and treatment of contacts. All sexual contacts should be contacted and treated within 90 days.
D. Mandatory reporting to local public health authorities.

## 📋 Gonorrhea

**An STD that may also affect the rectum, pharynx, and eyes. Caused by the bacteria, *Neisseria gonorrheae*, and is transmitted by direct contact with exudate via sexual contact or transmission to the neonate during passage through the birth canal.**

### Assessment

A. Risk factors/etiology.
1. Incubation period is 3 to 7 days.
2. Contagious as long as organism is present.
B. Clinical manifestations.
1. In men.
a. Urethritis, epididymitis, dysuria, and purulent urethral discharge.
b. Increased evidence of asymptomatic disease or a chronic carrier state in males.
2. In women.
a. Initial urethritis or cervicitis that is often mild enough to remain undetected by client.
b. Vulvovaginitis, vaginal discharge, dysuria.

3. Both men and women experience arthralgias, joint pain from disseminated gonococcus infection (DGI).
4. Neonates may develop ophthalmia neonatorum if eyes not treated at birth. Permanent blindness occurs without treatment.

C. Diagnostics.
1. Nucleic acid amplification test (NAAT).
2. Positive gram stain smear of discharge or secretions (not as sensitive as other tests).
3. Positive culture.

### Treatment

A. Medical.
1. Dual antibiotic therapy: IM ceftriaxone plus oral azithromycin.

### Complications

A. In men: prostatitis, urethral stricture, urethritis, and sterility.
B. In women: PID, Bartholin's abscess, ectopic pregnancy, infertility.

### Nursing Interventions

A. Prophylactic antibiotic treatment to the eye in all newborns to prevent ophthalmia neonatorum.
B. Encourage follow-up cultures in 4 to 7 days after treatment and again at 6 months.
C. Teach importance of abstinence from sexual intercourse until cultures are negative.
D. Urge client to inform sexual partner so that he or she may be treated for infection. All sexual partners within 60 days of diagnosis should also be treated.
E. Importance of taking the full course of antibiotics.

## Genital Herpes

**Genital herpes is a highly contagious infection caused primarily by the herpes simplex virus 2 (HSV-2) that is characterized by recurrent outbreaks. Subsequent outbreaks are usually less severe than the original outbreak of lesions.**

### Assessment

A. Risk factors/etiology.
1. Herpes simplex virus type 2 (HSV-2) lesions generally occur below the waist (genital and perineal area), although it is possible for HSV-2 to cause oral lesions.
2. Herpes simplex virus type 1 (HSV-1) generally causes lesions above the waist, involving the gingivae, dermis, and upper respiratory tract. However, rarely, HSV-1 can cause genital lesions.
3. Transmission is by direct contact with skin or mucous membranes of an infected person.
4. Virus can be harbored for an indefinite period with no symptoms. Recurrence occurs in 50% to 80% of cases and is usually triggered by stress, fatigue, generalized illness, and immunosuppression.

B. Clinical manifestations.
1. Initial sensation of tingling and itching before appearance of the lesion; may also include local inflammation, lymphadenopathy, fever, headache, myalgia, and malaise.
2. Multiple small vesicles appear on the penis, scrotum, perineum, vagina, and cervix.
3. During asymptomatic period when there are no lesions present, there may be viral shedding, and client is infectious.
4. Symptoms of recurrent episodes are less severe, with lesions healing more quickly.
5. Common triggers of recurrence include stress, fatigue, sunburn, general illness, immunosuppression, and menses.

C. Diagnostics.
1. Tissue culture that identifies HSV-2.
2. Serologic blood tests for antibodies for HSV-2 and both immunoglobulin IgG and IgA.

### Treatment

A. Medical.
1. Oral antiviral therapy. If treatment started at first sign of outbreak, duration may be decreased.
2. Symptomatic treatment: sitz baths, wet compresses, and analgesics for relief of pain.

### Complications

A. Increased incidence of cervical cancer in women, possibly due to coinfection with HPV.
B. Lesions or positive viral culture in pregnant women should be closely monitored. Cesarean delivery may be necessary to prevent exposure to the infant during passage through the birth canal.

### Nursing Interventions

A. Teach importance of genital hygiene and avoidance of unprotected sexual contact.
B. Teach good hygiene practices. Open lesions can spread the virus through contact with the fluid from the lesion.
C. Latex condoms should always be used to prevent exposure. Sexual activity should be avoided when lesions are present.

## Cytomegalovirus

**Cytomegalovirus is a virus belonging to the herpes family that leads to mild illness but can cause a wide range of serious congenital deformities in the fetus or newborn (congenital cytomegalovirus).**

### Assessment

A. Risk factors/etiology.
1. Transmission is through human contact.
2. Prevalence: about four of five people older than 35 years of age have been infected with cytomegalovirus, usually sometime during childhood or young adulthood; symptoms are so mild that the diagnosis is frequently overlooked.

B. Clinical manifestations.
1. The mother is usually asymptomatic or has mononucleosis-type symptoms.

2. Effect on the neonate: serious hematologic and central nervous system consequences; high mortality rate in severely affected neonates.
C. Diagnostics.
   1. TORCH screening: **T**oxoplasmosis, **O**ther (hepatitis), **R**ubella, **C**ytomegalovirus infection, **H**erpes simplex.
   2. Increased lymphocyte count and abnormal liver function test results.

*Nursing Interventions*

A. Prevention is the primary goal. Pregnant women should avoid being around affected individuals and congenitally infected infants.
B. Prevention of exposure is almost impossible because the primary infection is asymptomatic.

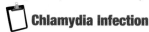

### Chlamydia Infection

**An infectious disease caused by *Chlamydia trachomatis*. Chlamydia is the most commonly reported STI in the United States.**

*Assessment*

A. Risk factors/etiology.
   1. Transmission is by sexual contact.
   2. Women and adolescents.
   3. Individuals who have multiple sex partners.
   4. Failure to use or incorrect use of a condom.
B. Clinical manifestations.
   1. Most frequently asymptomatic.
   2. In males:
      a. Urethritis, epididymitis, proctitis.
      b. Primary reservoir is the male urethra.
   3. In females:
      a. Mucopurulent cervicitis, salpingitis, vaginitis.
      b. Primary reservoir is the cervix.
   4. In newborns:
      a. Inclusion conjunctivitis.
      b. Pneumonia.
      c. Hepatomegaly and splenomegaly.
C. Diagnostics
   1. Nucleic acid amplification test (NAAT).
   2. Direct fluorescent antibody (DFA) test.
   3. Enzyme immunoassay (EIA).

*Treatment*

A. Medical.
   1. Antibiotic therapy with doxycycline and/or azithromycin.

*Complications*

A. PID, ectopic pregnancy, infertility in women.

*Nursing Interventions*

A. Urge client to have sexual partner treated.
B. Emphasize the importance of long-term drug therapy because of the pathogen's unique life cycle, which makes it difficult to eliminate.
C. Use of condoms with all sexual contacts.
D. Avoid sexual intercourse for 7 days after treatment and until all sexual partners have been treated.

### Genital Warts

**Characterized by a cluster of warts caused by the human papilloma virus (HPV); *condylomata acuminate*.**

*Assessment*

A. Risk factors/etiology.
   1. Caused by HPV, most often types 16 and 18.
   2. Highly contagious, yet most do not have symptoms.
   3. Transmission is through sexual contact with a person who has a lesion.
B. Clinical manifestations.
   1. Warts found in areas subject to trauma during sexual activity (penis, urethra, perianal area, anal canal, vulva, cervix, vaginal canal).
   2. Lesions are raised, skin-toned, damp, cauliflower-like growths.
   3. In pregnancy, the warts tend to grow rapidly and increase in size. An infected mother may transmit the condition to her newborn.
C. Diagnostics.
   1. Diagnosed by observation and serologic and cytologic testing.

*Treatment*

A. Medical.
   1. Multiple treatment of chemical or laser ablation.
   2. Podophyllin, applied topically once or twice a week for small external warts.

*Complications*

A. Cervical and/or vulvar cancer in women.
B. Rectal and/or penile cancer in men.

*Nursing Interventions*

A. Education regarding transmission.
B. Vaccination against HPV with Gardasil or Cervarix may reduce or prevent genital warts.
   1. Given before sexual activity.
   2. Can be given from age 9 through 26 years for both young women and men.
C. Close follow-up to monitor for complications.

## Appendix 24-1 MEDICATIONS USED IN REPRODUCTIVE SYSTEM DISORDERS

| Medications | Side Effects | Nursing Implications |
|---|---|---|

**Benign Prostatic Hyperplasia:** Medications decrease the size of the prostate or relax smooth muscle, therefore decreasing pressure on the urinary tract.

| Medications | Side Effects | Nursing Implications |
|---|---|---|
| **Alpha Adrenergic Antagonists**<br>Doxazosin: PO<br>Tamsulosin: PO<br>Terazosin: PO<br>Silodosin: PO<br>Alfuzosin: PO | Dizziness, fatigue, orthostatic hypotension, headaches, retrograde ejaculation, nasal stuffiness | 1. Advise client of possible problems of decreased blood pressure and orthostatic hypotension, especially 30 min to 2 hr after first dose.<br>2. Prostatic cancer should be ruled out before medications are started.<br>3. Medication should decrease problems of urination associated with BPH.<br>4. Monitor blood pressure closely if taking antihypertensive medications.<br>5. Assess for urinary hesitancy, incomplete emptying of the bladder, decreased urinary stream, and urgency before and throughout therapy. |
| **5α-Reductase Inhibitors**<br>Finasteride: PO<br>Dutasteride: PO<br>Dutasteride plus tamsulosin: PO | Erectile dysfunction, decreased libido, decreased ejaculation volume | 1. Client should take contraceptive precautions or not have sexual intercourse with women who could become pregnant.<br>2. Women who are or may become pregnant should not handle the tablets.<br>3. Client should not donate blood within 6 months after drug administration to avoid possibility of women receiving medication via blood transfusion. |

**Antifungal/Protozoal Medications:** Used to treat vaginal fungal infections.

| Medications | Side Effects | Nursing Implications |
|---|---|---|
| Clotrimazole: intravaginally (OTC)<br>Miconazole: intravaginally<br>Fluconazole: PO<br>Terconazole: intravaginally<br>Metronidazole: PO | Nausea, vomiting, headache, vaginal irritation | 1. Creams are not recommended to be used with tampons or diaphragms.<br>2. Not recommended for use during pregnancy or lactation.<br>3. Metronidazole is used to treat trichomoniasis; instruct client *to avoid alcohol* because it can lead to serious side effects of throbbing headaches, nausea, excessive vomiting, hyperventilation, and tachycardia.<br>4. Suppositories or applicators are used to place medication in the vagina.<br>5. If client does not see improvement within 3 days, she should return to her health care provider.<br>6. Fluconazole can be given orally as a single dose for vaginal candidiasis. |

**Hormone Replacement Therapy:** For treatment of symptoms of menopause.

| Medications | Side Effects | Nursing Implications |
|---|---|---|
| Conjugated estrogen: PO, intravaginally<br>Synthetic conjugated estrogen: PO, IV, IM, intravaginally<br>Micronized estradiol: PO, IM, intravaginally<br>Estradiol: transdermal patches<br>Estradiol: vaginal tablets | Nausea, vomiting, breakthrough bleeding, weight gain, swollen tender breasts, increased blood pressure | 1. Estrogen compounds should be given with progesterone combinations.<br>2. Important for menopausal women to continue with 1200–1500 mg/day calcium intake and weight-bearing exercises along with estrogen replacement to prevent osteoporosis.<br>3. Should not be used by women who have known or suspected cancer of the breast, undiagnosed vaginal bleeding, or possible pregnancy.<br>4. Used with precaution—or not at all—in women with clotting disorders or history of VTE/PE.<br>5. Report any unusual bleeding to primary care provider. |
| Medroxyprogesterone acetate: PO, IM | Menses may become more irregular (breakthrough bleeding), skin reactions (hives, acne) | 1. *Use:* for menopausal women who still have a uterus, significantly decreased risk for uterine cancer when used with estrogen therapy. Birth control injection given every 3 months, medroxyprogesterone.<br>2. Women should continue with increased calcium intake and weight-bearing exercises to prevent osteoporosis; should have yearly Pap smears, mammograms, and cholesterol series. |

## Appendix 24-1 MEDICATIONS USED IN REPRODUCTIVE SYSTEM DISORDERS—cont'd

| Medications | Side Effects | Nursing Implications |
|---|---|---|
| **Erectile Dysfunction Medications:** Cause smooth muscle relaxation and an increase in flood flow into the corpus cavernosum of the penis causing engorgement and subsequent erection. | | |
| Sildenafil: PO<br>Vardenafil: PO<br>Tadalafil: PO<br>Avanafil: PO | Hypotension can be a serious side effect<br>Headache, flushing, visual changes, priapism | 1. Should not be taken concurrently with nitrates.<br>2. Alpha blockers (used for treatment of BPH) are contraindicated in the client taking tadalafil and vardenafil; should be used with caution in client taking sildenafil.<br>3. If chest pain occurs after taking these medications, seek immediate medical care.<br>4. Primary differences in the medications are the onset and duration of action.<br>5. Priapism, painful erection, or erection lasting more than 4 hours may require medical intervention to prevent penile damage. |

❗ **NURSING PRIORITY:** Always inquire if a client is taking an ED medication before treating chest pain with any nitrate medication.

*BPH,* Benign prostatic hyperplasia; *ED,* erectile dysfunction; *HRT,* hormone replacement therapy; *IM,* intramuscular; *IV,* intravenous; *OTC,* over the counter; *PE,* pulmonary embolism; *PO,* by mouth (oral); *VTE,* venous thromboembolism.

## Study Questions
## Reproductive: Care of Adult and Pediatric Clients

More questions on

1. A client's Pap test reveals epithelial cells characteristic of adenocarcinoma of the cervix. The nurse understands that which of the following is a major risk factor for cervical cancer?
   1. Long-term use of oral contraceptives
   2. Recurrent outbreaks of human papilloma virus (HPV)
   3. Grand multiparity with history of preterm labor
   4. Alternative therapy for treatment of menopausal symptoms

2. The nurse would explain to a patient with genital herpes that he or she is most contagious at what stage?
   1. When vesicles rupture and release transudate
   2. When superficial, painful ulcers appear
   3. When yellow vaginal drainage is present
   4. When pustules become inflamed and erythematous

3. What is important to include in the discharge teaching plan for a 38-year-old client who has had a vaginal hysterectomy?
   1. Use of birth control is no longer required.
   2. Refrain from sexual intercourse for 2 months.
   3. Take hormone replacement therapy.
   4. Anticipate heavy vaginal bleeding.

4. During a well-woman physical examination, a young woman is diagnosed with a primary genital herpes lesion. When completing the client's history, the nurse would anticipate the client to report:
   1. Purulent urethral discharge
   2. Diffuse red rash
   3. Generalized abdominal pain
   4. Painful urination

5. A client had a left modified radical mastectomy 48 hours ago. What would be important for the nurse to include in a discharge teaching plan for this client? **Select all that apply.**
   1. Massage wound site with essential oils once incision has healed.
   2. Avoid needle-sticks in the left arm.
   3. Begin active exercises, such as pendulum arm swings, immediately.
   4. Avoid abduction and external rotation of the upper arm.
   5. Elevate arm on pillows to prevent edema.
   6. Take blood pressure readings from the right arm.

6. What is an important nursing action when assisting the doctor with a pelvic examination?
   1. Instruct the client to bear down and hold her breath during the procedure.
   2. Explain to the client that she will not feel any pain.
   3. Have the client empty her bladder before the examination begins.
   4. Lubricate the speculum well before handing it to the doctor.

7. A teenage boy comes to the office complaining of intense burning while urinating and gray–green discharge coming from his penis. The nurse recognizes these as symptoms of what problem?
   1. Herpes (HSV-2) with open lesions
   2. Secondary stage syphilis
   3. Urinary tract infection
   4. Gonorrhea

8. After examining a painless sore on the penile shaft, the doctor asks the nurse to order a fluorescent treponemal antibody absorption (FTA-ABS) test. The nurse knows that the purpose of this test is to diagnose what condition?
   1. Herpes simplex virus type 2 (HSV-2)
   2. Trichomoniasis
   3. Cytomegalovirus
   4. Syphilis

9. The night-shift nurse notes at the end of her shift that a client who had a mastectomy has a total of 90 mL of serosanguineous drainage from the incision over a 24-hour period. What is the best nursing action?
   1. Report amount of drainage to the physician.
   2. Start frequent blood pressure checks and observe for hemorrhage.
   3. Continue to monitor the drainage.
   4. Reinforce packing at the wound site.

10. The nurse is caring for a client who has had a mastectomy. What is important nursing care regarding the positioning of the affected arm?
    1. Hold the arm close against the side of her body.
    2. Secure the arm below the level of the heart.
    3. Wrap the arm in an elastic bandage and keep it below the heart.
    4. Elevate the arm above heart level.

11. A client is admitted because of benign prostatic hypertrophy and is scheduled to have a transurethral prostate resection. What assessment data would indicate to the nurse that a complication is developing?
    1. The client has difficulty emptying his bladder.
    2. Client states he feels like he cannot empty his bladder.
    3. The client complains of frequency and nocturia.
    4. Increasing complaints of flank pain and hematuria.

12. The nurse is discussing the importance of breast self-examination with a client who is being discharged after a vaginal hysterectomy. What is important information for the nurse to give this client?
    1. Perform breast self-examination 1 week after her normal period.
    2. Examine her breasts on a regular basis about the same time every month.
    3. Breasts should be palpated while in the sitting position.
    4. Use the tips of the fingers to palpate deeply into the breast tissue.

13. The nurse is discussing testicular self-examination with a male client. What information is important for the nurse to include in the discussion?
    1. The best time to perform the examination is 24 hours after sexual intercourse.
    2. The examination should be conducted at the same time each month.
    3. The client should perform this self-examination every 3 to 4 months.
    4. When the scrotum is pulled up tight against the body, the testes are easier to palpate.

14. The nurse is assessing a client who had a transurethral resection of the prostate (TURP) 6 hours ago. He has a urinary catheter with continuous bladder irrigation running. What nursing observations would indicate a complication is developing?
    1. Catheter drainage of 50 mL in the past hour and increase in suprapubic pain
    2. Dark, grossly bloody catheter drainage with pieces of tissue
    3. Client states that he feels like he needs to void
    4. Moderate amount of bloody discharge from around the catheter

15. A client is diagnosed with epididymitis related to bladder outlet obstruction. The nurse teaches which intervention to assist the client in recovery?
    1. Walk briskly at least 30 minutes every day.
    2. Limit oral intake to minimize nausea and vomiting.
    3. Apply scrotal support to relieve edema and discomfort.
    4. Use warm baths and compresses during acute inflammation.

16. A sexually active female 17-year-old is diagnosed with trichomoniasis through vaginal discharge analysis. The nurse explains which pharmacologic intervention to minimize symptoms and the risk for reoccurrence?
    1. Return to clinic each week for intramuscular injection of penicillin.
    2. Perform a daily vaginal douche with a weak iodine solution.
    3. Oral administration of metronidazole three times a day to client and her partner.
    4. Application of trichloroacetic acid to lesions daily for 6 to 8 weeks.

17. A client is scheduled for an abdominal hysterectomy. Preoperative teaching includes which of the following?
    1. A nasogastric tube will be left in to control vomiting after surgery.
    2. A douche and an enema may be done the evening before surgery.
    3. There will be a moderate amount of bloody vaginal drainage after surgery.
    4. Ambulation will be delayed for 48 hours because of the extensive nature of the procedure.

18. A woman has experienced an incomplete abortion. She is scheduled for a dilation and curettage (D&C). What is the purpose of this procedure?
    1. To protect the uterus and the ovaries for future pregnancies
    2. To provide a healthier uterine environment for future pregnancies
    3. To provide reinforcement for an incompetent cervix
    4. To scrape the uterine walls and remove the uterine contents

19. The nurse is teaching a client with a pelvic inflammatory disease. The nurse instructs the client to sleep with her head elevated about 45 degrees. What is the rationale behind instructing the client to sleep in this position?
    1. Assists to localize drainage in the lower abdomen
    2. Decreases abdominal muscle tension
    3. Makes coughing and deep breathing more effective
    4. Prevents scarring of the fallopian tubes

20. A young woman comes into the emergency department with menorrhagia. What is the priority concern for the nurse caring for this client?
    1. The chronic bleeding will cause anemia.
    2. The client is at a high risk for development of an infection.
    3. The woman may be pregnant and is aborting the fetus.
    4. The increased bleeding will promote later problems with infertility.

# Answers to Study Questions

**1.** *2*

Increased risk for cervical cancer is associated with a history of HPV (genital warts) infection, STDs, HSV-2, multiple sex partners, first intercourse at early age, and abnormal Pap tests. The use of alternative therapy and estrogen therapy for menopause, oral contraceptive use, and multiple pregnancies do not increase the risk. (Lewis et al., 10 ed., p. 1234)

**2.** *1*

The herpes simplex virus (HSV-2) is concentrated in the vesicles, and therefore the infection is highly contagious when this clear fluid is released. The lesions rupture and form shallow, moist ulcerations (not pustules) that eventually crust, allowing epithelialization of the erosions to occur. There is no yellow drainage. The primary infection is associated with local inflammation and pain and is often accompanied by systemic symptoms of fever, headache, malaise, myalgia, and regional lymphadenopathy. (Lewis et al., 10 ed., p. 1232)

**3.** *1*

It will no longer be possible to become pregnant, and birth control is no longer required. On her postoperative visit to the doctor, he or she will evaluate the healing of the cervical area and will advise her regarding sexual intercourse. There is no mention in the question that the client had her ovaries removed, so hormone replacement therapy is not necessary. Heavy vaginal bleeding might indicate hemorrhage. The client may experience a moderate amount of serosanguineous drainage immediately postoperative; once healed, she will not experience menses. (Ignatavicius & Workman, 7 ed., p. 1620)

**4.** *4*

The client usually seeks treatment for a variety of symptoms, including pain on urination from urine touching painful ulcerations. A purulent urethral discharge would be seen in STDs such as gonorrhea. A diffuse red rash might be caused by syphilis, and generalized abdominal pain might be caused by a variety of reproductive disorders but not genital herpes. (Lewis et al., 10 ed., p. 1232)

**5.** *2, 5, 6*

Important teaching to include in the discharge plan of care for a client who has undergone a mastectomy includes the avoidance of needle-sticks in the arm on the side of the mastectomy and having blood pressure readings taken from the opposite arm. These measures are done to avoid any type of trauma that could lead to the development of lymphedema. Begin finger, wrist, and hand exercises to facilitate muscle contraction and to help prevent edema. Active exercises, such as pendulum swings and finger wall-climbing, are started after the incision has healed. As the area heals, abduction and external rotation will help improve the range of motion. (Lewis et al., 10 ed., p. 1214)

**6.** *3*

Having the client void before the examination will make the procedure less painful and more accurate. There is no need for the patient to bear down or hold her breath. The patient should relax as much as possible during the procedure. The level of pain, if any, is highly dependent on the patient and her pain tolerance. Lubricant on the speculum may interfere with the Pap smear. The client should not douche or have intercourse before a pelvic examination, especially if any specimens are to be obtained, because changes in the normal flora and pH could occur from douching and the presence of semen. (Ignatavicius & Workman, 8 ed., p. 1454)

**7.** *4*

Gonorrhea in men is the most symptomatic, with urethritis, dysuria, and purulent drainage, but the disease can be asymptomatic. The purulent secretion should be cultured to identify the microorganism. HSV-2 infections are characterized by painful vesicles surrounded by an erythematous base that progress to shallow ulcers, which eventually crust and epithelialize as they heal. In the secondary stage of syphilis the client is often asymptomatic; however, a maculopapular rash on the palms of the hands and soles of the feet may be noted with lymphadenopathy, sore throat, headache, and condylomata lata (flat lesions appearing in moist areas—not to be confused with condylomata acuminata in genital warts). A lower urinary tract infection would be characterized by dysuria, urgency, frequency, hematuria, and possible low back pain. (Lewis et al., 10 ed., p. 1230)

**8.** *4*

The fluorescent treponemal antibody absorption test is a serum blood test used to identify the spirochete *Treponema pallidum*, which causes syphilis. HSV-2 is diagnosed by tissue culture from a specimen obtained from an active lesion and by a serologic blood test. Trichomoniasis is diagnosed by a wet mount slide obtained from vaginal or penile secretions. Cytomegalovirus is diagnosed by blood test and by urine and tissue culture. (Lewis et al., 10 ed., p. 1235)

**9.** *3*

Up to 100 mL of serosanguineous fluid would be an acceptable amount of drainage over a 24-hour period in a client who has had a mastectomy. Drains are usually removed when there is less than 25 mL in a 24-hour period. There is no indication of hemorrhage or the need to perform frequent blood pressure checks. If the nurse observes a greater amount of fluid in the drains, then it would be important to notify the physician. (Ignatavicius & Workman, 8 ed., pp. 1472–1474)

**10.** *4*

Elevating the affected arm promotes drainage of lymph from the extremity and decreases fluid from the wound site, which reduces swelling. An elastic wrap may be applied to the affected arm to reduce swelling, but it would not be positioned below the heart level. (Lewis et al., 10 ed., p. 1219)

**11.** *4*

Flank pain may be indicative of an infection or a ureteral obstruction causing increased pressure on the renal pelvis. Other options are symptoms of benign prostatic hypertrophy, for which he will be treated while he is in the hospital. (Lewis et al., 10 ed., p. 1268)

**12.** *2*

Because she no longer has regular periods, the client should pick a date and perform breast self-examination at the same time each month. Self-examination of the breast a week after the normal period is the best time for a woman who still has menstrual periods because the breast tissue is less glandular a week after the normal period. Breasts are examined lying down and standing, not sitting. The pads of the fingers are used to examine the breast using small circular motions in a spiral pattern or in an up-and-down motion. (Lewis et al., 10ed., p. 1205)

**13.** *2*
The examination should be done at the same time each month to develop a regular routine. After a shower, when the scrotum is warm and the testicles are descended away from the body, is a good time to perform the examination. (Lewis et al., 10 ed., p. 1205)

**14.** *1*
The primary complication is the obstruction of the urinary catheter with clots or tissue. There should be a large amount of drainage from the catheter because the irrigating fluid is infusing into the bladder. The catheter drainage should be closer to 300 to 400 mL/hr. It is not unusual for the drainage to be grossly bloody on the operative day, but it should begin to clear over the next 24 hours. It is common to have a feeling of needing to void with a catheter in place. (Lewis et al., 10 ed., p. 1268)

**15.** *3*
To facilitate lymphatic drainage from the inflamed epididymis, the client should be taught to use a towel roll to act as a "scrotal bridge." Cool compresses should be used in the acute phase. There is no reason to limit oral intake. Walking is extremely painful, and bed rest is usually indicated to prevent spread of infection. (Lewis et al., 10 ed., p. 1284)

**16.** *3*
Trichomoniasis is a protozoal infection transmitted through sexual intercourse. All sexual partners need to be treated with the oral administration of metronidazole, a systemic antiprotozoal. Males may be asymptomatic. Intramuscular injection of penicillin is prescribed for syphilis. Douching should be avoided because it destroys the normal vaginal flora and increases the risk for developing the problem. Trichloroacetic acid (TCA) or podophyllin is topically applied to genital warts. (Lewis et al., 10 ed., p. 1231)

**17.** *2*
Douching and some method of bowel preparation are part of the preoperative measure to cleanse the field of bacteria and pathogens. Vomiting is not a usual postoperative problem. If this occurs, it would most likely be controlled by an antiemetic. Vaginal drainage occurs with a vaginal, not an abdominal, hysterectomy. Ambulation is encouraged to prevent venous stasis. (Lewis et al., 10 ed., p. 1257)

**18.** *4*
D&C is the dilation (opening) of the cervix and curettage (scraping) of the inner walls of the uterus to remove the uterine contents to control bleeding and, in this instance, remove any products of conception that were not expelled. It does not protect the uterus or the ovaries. It is not recommended for incompetent cervical os, nor does it promote health of future pregnancies. (Lewis et al., 10 ed., p. 1246)

**19.** *1*
The nurse teaches the client to maintain a semi-Fowler's position to prevent or decrease movement of the contaminated fluid to the upper abdomen and the area of the diaphragm. (Lewis et al., 10 ed., p. 1251)

**20.** *3*
The nurse must rule out pregnancy/aborting first because of the potential for shock or damage to a fetus. Once aborting is ruled out or treated, the nurse addresses the issues of anemia and infection. Infertility would be the last concern, although it should be assessed. (Lewis et al., 10 ed., p. 1246.)

# CHAPTER TWENTY-FIVE

# Urinary-Renal: Care of Adult and Pediatric Clients

# 25

Elimination, Fluid & Electrolytes, Infection

## PHYSIOLOGY OF THE KIDNEY AND URINARY TRACT

A. Functions of the kidney.
 1. Rid the body of metabolic wastes.
  a. Regulate fluid volume; normally, 125 mL/min is filtered (glomerular filtration rate [GFR]), but only 1 mL is excreted as urine; average urine output is about 1500 to 1600 mL per day.
  b. Regulate the composition of electrolytes.
  c. Assist in maintaining acid–base balance.
 2. Regulation of blood pressure.
  a. Renin acts on angiotensin I and converts it to angiotensin II, which is a powerful vasoconstrictor. Peripheral resistance is increased; therefore blood pressure is increased.
  b. Kidneys receive 20% to 25% of total cardiac output with a renal blood flow rate of 600 to 1300 mL/min.
 3. Aldosterone production is stimulated by the increase in angiotensin I; therefore sodium and water are retained to increase circulating volume and increase blood pressure.
 4. Regulates red blood cell production through synthesis of erythropoietin; released in response to hypoxia and reduced renal blood flow.
 5. Aids in calcium metabolism by activating vitamin D, which allows for absorption of calcium from the gastrointestinal tract.
B. Nephron is functional unit of kidney.
 1. Filtration: occurs in the glomerulus via a semipermeable membrane.
  a. Pressure gradient changes occur when there is a variation in the systemic blood pressure (hypotension), a significant change in the pressure in Bowman's capsule in the glomerulus (edema), and ureteral obstruction.
  b. The kidneys' response to changes in pressures is buffered by an autoregulatory mechanism to maintain a stable range of blood pressure.

> **⚠ NURSING PRIORITY:** Determine whether client has a decreased urinary output (less than 30 mL per hour in an adult, 20 mL per hour in a child, and 1 mL/kg/hr in an infant); urinary output should be carefully evaluated regarding blood pressure level; blood pressure must provide renal perfusion to maintain adequate urinary output. The level of blood pressure to maintain renal perfusion varies greatly from one client to another.

  c. If the glomerular membrane is damaged, plasma proteins will escape. A decrease in serum proteins decreases the normal serum oncotic pressure; this results in water retention and edema formation.
 2. Tubular reabsorption: after the glomerulus has filtered the blood, the tubules separate the water and solutes by osmosis and diffusion. Only a small amount of the total water filtered out of the kidneys is excreted as urine. Solutes are also reabsorbed according to the concentration gradient.
 3. Tubular secretion: regulates the potassium level and maintains the acid–base balance with other regulatory mechanisms.
C. Urinary tract.
 1. Ureters: muscular tubes through which urine flows from the kidneys to the bladder.
 2. Bladder: in the adult, the first urge to void will occur when 200 mL to 250 mL has collected; approximately 200 mL to 250 mL of urine will initiate a feeling of bladder discomfort; bladder capacity varies from 600 mL to 1000 mL.
 3. Urethra: a small, membranous tube that conveys urine from the bladder to the exterior of the body.
  a. Female urethra is 1 to 2 inches (2.5 to 5 cm) long.
  b. Male urethra is 8 to 10 inches (20 to 25 cm) long.

## System Assessment

A. External assessment.
 1. Inspect skin for changes in color, turgor, texture (urate crystals), bruising, and excoriations.
 2. Assess face, abdomen, and extremities for edema.
 3. Determine weight gain or loss.
 4. General state: diminished alertness, lethargy.
 5. Palpate kidneys and bladder.
  a. Landmark: for kidney palpation, the landmark is the costovertebral angle, formed by the rib cage and the vertebral column.

b. Bladder is palpated just above the suprapubic area (or symphysis pubis bone).

c. Kidney and bladder should be nonpalpable with no discomfort on palpation.

6. Percuss in the flank area to determine any tenderness.

7. Auscultate (diaphragm) the renal and aortic arteries to determine the presence of bruits.

B. History.

1. Presence of renal or urologic congenital defect.

2. Determine whether client has ever been exposed to chemicals, especially carbon tetrachloride, phenol, and ethylene glycol because these are nephrotoxic. Determine smoking history: cigarette smoking is a major risk factor for kidney and bladder cancer.

3. Determine whether client has received antibiotics that may be nephrotoxic: aminoglycosides, amphotericin B, cephalosporins, vancomycin, and sulfonamides.

4. Assess dietary intake: intake of fluid is important, as dehydration may contribute to urinary tract infections (UTIs), calculi formation, and kidney failure.

a. Determine intake levels of calcium-rich and oxalate-rich food, which may predispose the client to renal calculi formation.

b. Anorexia and nausea and vomiting may cause dehydration or be the result of altered renal function.

5. Determine level of activity: immobility leads to demineralization of the bones, which can predispose to infection and calculus formation.

6. Evaluate complaints of pain: dysuria; flank, costovertebral, or suprapubic pain.

7. Assess changes in pattern of urination: frequency, nocturia, urgency, enuresis, hesitancy, slow stream, incontinence (Box 25-1).

8. Assess changes in urine output: polyuria, oliguria, anuria.

9. Assess changes in urine consistency: hematuria, pyuria, diluted, concentrated, change in color.

10. Determine whether client is taking any medications that may affect urinary or renal function.

11. Determine whether client has any chronic health care problems that affect renal and urinary tract structures (diabetes mellitus, hypertension, allergies, gout, or multiple sclerosis).

12. Assess effect of any related sexual issues (personal hygiene, fatigue during intercourse, urinary incontinence).

## DISORDERS OF THE URINARY-RENAL SYSTEM

### Urinary Incontinence

**Urinary incontinence is the client complaint of any involuntary leakage of urine.**

A. Types of incontinence.

1. **Urge:** Involuntary loss of urine associated with a strong sensation of urinary urgency.

2. **Stress:** Involuntary leakage when the urethral sphincter fails and associated with an increase in intraabdominal pressure.

---

**Box 25-1    OLDER ADULT CARE FOCUS**

**Dealing With Incontinence**

***Need to Determine:***

- Does client have difficulty initiating urinary flow?
- Is client aware of need to void?
- Can client empty bladder completely, or is there residual urine?
- Is there bladder distention and overflow dribbling?
- Is stress incontinence or urge incontinence present?
- What are usual voiding times?
- Is the client constipated or is there an impaction? Is this a chronic problem?
- When do accidental leaks occur?
- Is the client having difficulty getting to the bathroom on time?
- How often does client wear a pad or protective device?

**Nursing Interventions**

- Help the client determine when he or she needs to urinate before an accident occurs.
- Maintain adequate fluid intake but limit fluids before bedtime.
- Establish a voiding schedule: offer assistance and encourage voiding.
- Assess the client's access to the bathroom; determine need for a bedside commode.
- Assess for presence of urinary tract infection.
- Teach client how to perform Kegel exercises.

---

3. **Mixed:** Combination of different types, such as stress and urge.

4. **Overflow:** Bladder overdistention caused by poor contractility of the detrusor muscle or obstruction of the urethra.

5. **Functional:** Cognitive inability to recognize the urge to urinate or inability to reach bathroom (due to restraints, side rails, walker or cane out of reach).

6. **Neurologic or reflex:** Caused by disorders such as multiple sclerosis or spinal cord injury.

B. Older adult care focus (see Box 25-1).

*Assessment*

A. Factors contributing to urinary incontinence.

1. Unconsciousness, paralysis, urinary tract infection.

2. Interference with nerve transmission from the brain.

3. Loss of muscle tone of the bladder and sphincters.

4. Obesity, prostate surgery, endocrine problems.

5. Medications: alpha adrenergic agents, beta adrenergic agonists, and calcium channel blockers.

B. Clinical manifestations.

1. **Urge:** Loss of urine with an abrupt and strong desire to void; involuntary loss of urine (without symptoms); nocturia is common.

2. **Stress:** Small amount of urine loss during coughing, sneezing, laughing, or other physical activities; continuous leak at rest or with minimal exertion (e.g., postural changes).

3. **Mixed:** Combination of symptoms from different types, such as stress and urge.
4. **Overflow:** Frequent or constant dribbling or urge or stress incontinence symptoms, as well as urgency and frequent urination.
5. **Functional:** Residual urine after voiding is common.
6. **Neurologic or reflex:** Postmicturitional or continual incontinence; severe urgency with bladder hypersensitivity (sensory urgency).
C. Diagnostics (see Appendix 25-1).
   1. Urinalysis, postvoid residual, urodynamic studies, cystogram, cystoscopy.
   2. Client kept voiding diary.
D. Complications: infection, skin excoriation.

### Treatment

A. Medical.
   1. Pelvic floor strengthening exercises (Kegel's); biofeedback therapy.
   2. Medications: urinary antispasmodics or bladder relaxants.
B. Surgical: implanted electrical stimulation device, surgical procedures to correct anatomical position of bladder; artificial sphincter implants; sling procedure.

### Nursing Interventions

**Goal:** To assist clients to establish a toileting schedule (Box 25-2).
**Goal:** To teach clients pelvic floor strengthening exercises (Kegel's) (Box 25-3).
**Goal:** To provide dietary information.

A. Advise client to avoid caffeine, alcohol, carbonated beverages, and aspartame, as they may stimulate or irritate the bladder.
B. Encourage client to have an adequate fluid volume intake and not to restrict fluids, but to limit fluids before bedtime.

---

**Box 25-2   OLDER ADULT CARE FOCUS**

**Establishing a Toileting Schedule**
- Instruct client to keep a voiding diary.
- Help the client determine when he or she needs to urinate before an accident occurs.
- Establish a voiding schedule (use set times, such as every two hours on the even hours: 8 a.m., 10 a.m., noon, 2 p.m., etc.).
- Assess the client's access to the bathroom; determine need for a bedside commode.
- Space fluid intake and give the majority of fluids during the day.
- Encourage client to ambulate for a minimum of 10 minutes an hour or two before bedtime, because activity helps mobilize fluid.
- Assess for presence of urinary tract infection.

---

**Box 25-3   OLDER ADULT CARE FOCUS**

**Pelvic Floor Strengthening Exercise (Kegel's)**
- Explain to client how to locate the correct pelvic floor muscle by stopping the flow of urine while urinating on the toilet or by tightening the anus as if preventing a bowel movement.
- Encourage client to practice several times each time they urinate.
- Teach client while lying down to slowly count 1–2–3 while tightening the pelvic muscles. Should repeat exercise 15 times.
- Using the same counting sequence and repeating 15 times, have the client perform the exercise while sitting, then standing.
- Perform the three exercises (lying, sitting, standing) at least once a day, preferably more than once, as improvement will be noted more quickly.
- Overall improvement is often noted within 6–8 weeks following the Kegel exercise plan.

---

### Urinary Tract Infections

**Stasis of urine in the bladder and reflux of urine back into the original reservoir are the primary causes of urinary tract infections (UTIs).** *Escherichia coli* **is the most common pathogen leading to UTIs** (Figure 25-1).

A. Upper UTIs: *pyelonephritis,* an inflammation of the renal pelvis and the parenchyma of the kidney(s).
B. Lower UTI.
   1. Cystitis: inflammation/infection of the bladder.
   2. Urethritis: inflammation of the urethra.
C. The higher the infection in the urinary tract, the more serious.

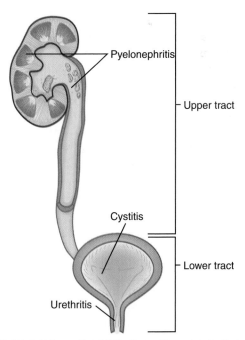

**FIGURE 25-1 Urinary Tract Infections.** (From Lewis, S. L., et al. [2017]. *Medical-surgical nursing: Assessment and management of clinical problems* [10th ed.]. St. Louis, MO: Mosby.)

## Assessment

A. Factors contributing to UTI.
   1. Adult female urethra is short, 1 to 2 inches (2.5 to 5 cm), versus 8 to 10 inches (20 to 25 cm) in men, and close to the rectum and vagina, which predisposes it to contamination from fecal material.
   2. Ureterovesical reflux: the reflux of urine from the urethra into the bladder; this causes a constant residual of urine in the bladder after voiding and precipitates UTI.
   3. Vesicoureteral reflux (ureterovesical reflux): the reflux of urine from the bladder into one or both of the ureters and possibly into the renal pelvis.
   4. Instrumentation: catheterization or cystoscopic examination.
   5. Stasis of urine in the bladder leading to urinary retention for any reason (clients with prostate disease).
   6. Obstruction of urinary flow: congenital anomalies, urethral strictures, ureteral stones, contracture of the bladder neck, tumor, fibrosis, or fecal impaction (Figure 25-2).
   7. Bladder hypotonia: mechanical compression of the ureters; hormone changes predispose pregnant and postmenopausal women to more frequent UTIs.
   8. Metabolic disorders such as diabetes.
   9. Sexual intercourse promotes development of UTI.
   10. Fecal contamination of the urethral meatus.

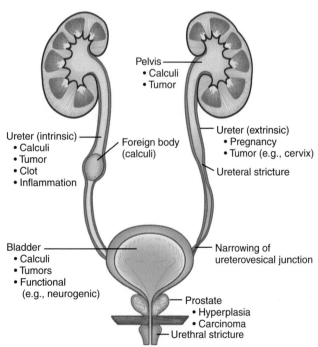

**FIGURE 25-2 Causes of Urinary Obstruction.** (From Lewis, S. L., et al. [2017]. *Medical-surgical nursing: Assessment and management of clinical problems* [10th ed.]. St. Louis, MO: Mosby.)

B. Clinical manifestations.
   1. Cystitis (lower UTI).
      a. Frequency, urgency, dysuria (classic triad of symptoms).
      b. Cloudy urine or hematuria.
      c. Nocturia, incontinence, hesitancy, weak stream.
      d. Often asymptomatic with bacteriuria.
      e. Low back pain or suprapubic pain.
   2. Pyelonephritis (upper UTI).
      a. Fever, chills, malaise, flank pain on affected side.
      b. Symptoms of cystitis.
      c. Older adults may not have a fever, and those older than 80 years may have a decrease in temperature and exhibit confusion (Box 25-4).
   3. Urosepsis: a systemic and life-threatening infection, laboratory work may show a left shift (increase in the number of band cells–immature neutrophils) in WBCs.
C. Diagnostics (see Appendix 25-1).
D. Complications.
   1. A lower UTI may progress to an upper UTI.
   2. Chronic pyelonephritis may develop after repeated bouts of acute pyelonephritis.

## Treatment

A. Medical (see Appendix 25-2).
   1. Broad-spectrum antibiotics, especially the sulfonamides for lower UTIs; fluoroquinolones for upper UTIs (see Appendix 9-2).
   2. Urinary analgesics, such as phenazopyridine.
   3. Antispasmodics.
   4. Antipyretics.
B. Dietary.
   1. Encourage fluid intake of 3000 mL per day unless contraindicated.
      a. Dilute urine causes less irritation.

### Box 25-4 OLDER ADULT CARE FOCUS

**Urinary Tract Infection**
- First symptom may be increased confusion.
- A sudden onset of incontinence or an increase in frequency of incontinence should be investigated.
- A client with fever, chills, and tachycardia in the absence of urinary tract symptoms should be evaluated for septicemia from a urinary tract origin.
- Avoid use of indwelling urinary catheters.
- Encourage clients to void every 2 hours even if they do not feel a need; this decreases residual urine and incontinence.
- Cleanse perineal area after each voiding and prevent fecal contamination of the urinary meatus by wiping from front to back in women.
- Women should wear cotton underwear and avoid tight, restrictive clothing.

b. The increase in flow of urine through the urinary tract increases the movement of bacteria down the urinary tract.

c. Discourage consumption of carbonated beverages and foods or drinks containing baking powder or baking soda. Caffeine, alcohol, citrus fruits, and highly spiced foods can cause bladder irritation.

d. Daily intake of cranberry juice or cranberry essence tablets is helpful for some clients, as it appears to decrease the ability of bacteria to adhere to the epithelial cells lining the urinary tract.

### Nursing Interventions

**Goal:** To provide relief of pain, urgency, dysuria, and fever.

A. Antibiotics need to be taken as scheduled and full course completed. Initially, therapy may be required for 1 to 3 days; if problem is recurrent, 10 to 14 days of therapy may be required. For pyelonephritis, antibiotics may be taken for 14 to 21 days; severe symptoms may require hospitalization.

B. Encourage consumption of 8 to 10 glasses of fluids daily (3000 mL).

C. Teach clients the importance of voiding every 2 to 3 hours during the day to completely empty the bladder.

D. Sitz baths may be taken to decrease irritation of urethra.

**Goal:** To prevent recurrence of infection.

A. Avoid sitting in a bathtub with added bubble bath products or other bath oils and fragrances; a warm bath will decrease symptoms, but nothing should be added to the water.

B. Explain importance of cleansing the perineal area from front to back after voiding and after each bowel movement. Avoid use of perineal sprays and powders.

C. If intercourse seems to predispose to infection, encourage voiding immediately before and after intercourse. A female client with recurrent UTIs may need to temporarily stop using a diaphragm and spermicidal creams/jelly.

D. Teach importance of long-term therapy if recurrent infections are a problem.

E. Encourage and explain the need for follow-up care to prevent complications of chronic UTIs.

F. Caffeine, alcohol, citrus juices, and carbonated beverages should be avoided.

G. Maintain adequate fluid intake.

### 📋 Urinary Calculi

**Stones may form anywhere in the urinary tract; the most common location for stones is in the pelvis of the kidney. If the stones are small, they may be passed into the bladder (see Figure 25-2).**

A. Stones in the bladder may increase in size if urinary stasis and alkaline pH are present.

B. Types of urinary calculi.
   1. Calcium oxalate or phosphate stones: tend to be small; account for 40% to 50% of all upper urinary tract calculi.

   2. Struvite stones: contain bacteria and tend to be large; more common in women than men.
   3. Uric acid stones: occur most often in clients with primary or secondary problems of uric acid metabolism (gout); high incidence in men, particularly Jewish men.
   4. Cystine stones: Autosomal recessive defect; defective absorption of cysteine in GI and kidney causing excess concentration leading to stone formation.

### Assessment

Regardless of the type of stone formed, the clinical manifestations, diagnostics, and treatment are essentially the same.

A. Risk factors/etiology.
   1. Infection, urinary stasis, immobility.
   2. Hypercalcemia and hypercalciuria (hyperparathyroidism, renal tubular acidosis).
   3. Excessive intake of dietary proteins, which increases uric acid production.
   4. Excessive consumption of foods high in oxalate, such as spinach, soy products, and peanuts.
   5. Excessive consumption of sodium, which causes the kidneys to excrete more calcium.
   6. Low fluid intake.
   7. Majority of clients are between 20 and 55 years of age, with increased incidence when family history is present. Stones occur more often in the summer months and warmer climates.
   8. Increased incidence of family history with stone formation due to inherited metabolic risk factors.

B. Clinical manifestations.
   1. Sharp, sudden, severe abdominal or flank pain.
      a. May be described as "colic," either ureteral or renal.
      b. Pain may be intermittent, depending on the movement of the stone; spasm in the ureter occurs as it attempts to move the stone toward the bladder.
      c. Pain may radiate around the flank area, down into the bladder, the genitalia, and the thigh.
   2. Hematuria may be present as a result of the traumatic effects of the stone on the ureter and the bladder.
   3. Oliguria or anuria suggest urinary obstruction and must be treated immediately.
   4. Nausea and vomiting are common.
   5. Struvite stones are associated with fever and infection.

C. Diagnostics (see Appendix 25-1).

D. Complications.
   1. Recurrent stone formation.
   2. Infection, renal failure.

### Treatment

A. Medical.
   1. Increase fluid intake to 3000 mL/day to decrease urine concentration, unless contraindicated.
   2. Medications that prevent the absorption of calcium (thiazide diuretics and phosphates).
   3. Spasmolytic agents (anticholinergics).
   4. For uric acid stones, allopurinol.

5. Opioids for pain relief.
6. Dietary.
   a. Sodium may also be restricted because sodium increases the excretion of calcium in the urine.
   b. Decrease in protein intake or an alkaline-ash diet for clients with uric acid stones.
   c. Decrease intake of cola, coffee, and tea, which tend to increase the risk for calculi formation.
   d. Maintain normal levels of calcium in diet (800 to 1000 mg) for calcium oxylate stones. Calcium binds with oxylate in the GI tract and prevents it from entering the blood and the urinary tract where it contributes to the development of calcium oxalate stones.
   e. Decrease intake of oxylate sources such as spinach, black tea, and rhubarb for calcium oxylate stones (see Table 2-4, Therapeutic Meal Plans).
B. Surgical.
   1. Nephrolithotomy: incision into the kidney and removal of the stone.
   2. Ureterolithotomy: incision into the ureter to locate a stone and remove it.
   3. Stenting: insertion of a small tube (stent) into ureter via ureteroscopy to dilate ureter to enlarge passageway for expulsion of stone or stone fragments or to temporarily bypass a stone that cannot be removed immediately.
C. Lithotripsy: cystoscopic, percutaneous ultrasonic, laser, or extracorporeal shock-wave lithotripsy (ESWL). Most often accomplished as an outpatient procedure.
   1. For ESWL, client is anesthetized and placed in a water bath. Some lithotripters do not require submersion.
      a. Sound waves travel through the water and are directed to the stone. The force of the sound wave shatters the stone, and the remains are excreted in the urine.
      b. It is essential that the client remain absolutely motionless during the procedure, which lasts about 30 to 45 minutes. Therefore some form of sedation or analgesia is necessary during the procedure.
      c. Occasionally a ureteral stent is placed after lithotripsy procedures to promote passage of stone fragments, which is left in place for 2 weeks.
   2. Hematuria is common after the procedure.
   3. Client must be able to demonstrate the ability to urinate freely before discharge.

### Nursing Interventions

**Goal:** To relieve pain.

A. Administer analgesics as prescribed: morphine or hydromorphone.
B. Hot baths or moist heat applied to flank area.
C. Encourage increased fluid intake (3000 mL/day) to prevent dehydration, if not contraindicated.

D. Strain all urine and inspect for blood clots and passage of stone.
E. If stone is passed, it should be saved and sent to the laboratory for analysis to determine the type of stone so appropriate therapy can be maintained.

**Goal:** To promote understanding of health care regimen.

A. Dietary restrictions, depending on type of stone.
B. Discuss rationale, dose, frequency, and important information relating to medication administration.
C. Teach symptoms of recurring stone formation, such as hematuria, flank pain, and signs of infection.
D. Instruct client to continue high fluid intake (3000 mL per day).
E. Promote periodic medical follow-up visits to evaluate for symptoms of infection and recurring stone formation.

## Hypospadias and Epispadias

A. **Hypospadias: the urethral opening is located behind the glans penis or along the penile shaft; this is a common congenital anomaly.**
B. **Epispadias: the urethral opening is located on the dorsal or upper side of the penis; this is a rare problem.**

### Assessment

A. Clinical manifestations.
   1. Visualization of defect.
   2. Chordee: ventral curvature of the penis, which gives it a crooked appearance (hypospadias).
   3. Stream of urine does not come out the end of the penis.
   4. Hypospadias is associated with cryptorchidism in severe cases.
   5. Bladder exstrophy is a severe form of epispadias.

### Treatment

A. Surgical correction of the defect.
   1. Hypospadias: recommended repair by 6 to 18 months of age.
   2. Epispadias is much more complex and frequently associated with other genitourinary system defects; repair may be very involved and require multi-stage surgical procedures.

### Nursing Interventions

**Goal:** To provide emotional support and to promote normal growth and development.

A. Frequently the infant is not circumcised until the repair of the hypospadias.
B. The infant with epispadias may be discharged home before repair is done.
C. The preferred time for repair is between 6 and 12 months; it is important not to delay repair of hypospadias beyond the time for toilet training.
D. A diaper and a sterile nonadherent dressing are applied over the exposed bladder when the infant has a bladder defect.

E. Teach parents signs of UTI.

F. Help parents understand realistic expectations of the outcome of surgery (epispadias and/or bladder exstrophy).

## Nephrotic Syndrome

**A problem with glomerular permeability to plasma proteins results in massive urinary protein loss. The most common type is a primary condition, minimal change nephrotic syndrome.**

A. Changes occur in the basement membrane of the glomeruli that allow the large protein molecules to pass through the membrane and be excreted. The loss of albumin from the serum decreases the oncotic pressure in the capillary bed and allows fluid to pass into the interstitial tissues and the abdominal cavity (ascites) and interstitial spaces (edema).

B. The interstitial fluid shift causes hypovolemia. The renin-angiotensin response is stimulated. Aldosterone secretion is increased, and the tubules begin to conserve sodium and water to increase the circulating volume.

C. In the majority of children with the syndrome, the cause is unknown; it may be congenital, idiopathic, or secondary to another disease; frequently, there is no evidence of renal dysfunction or systemic disease.

### Assessment

A. Risk factors/etiology.
   1. Usual history is a well child who begins to gain weight and exhibits pallor and fatigue.
   2. Majority of children affected are male and between the ages of 2 and 4 years; uncommon in infants younger than 1 year.
   3. May occur in adults secondary to systemic disease (e.g., systemic lupus erythematosus, diabetes, bacterial or viral infections), or may be idiopathic.
   4. Allergens such as bee sting or pollen.

B. Clinical manifestations.
   1. Hallmarks: edema, proteinuria, hypoalbuminemia, and hyperlipidemia in the absence of hypertension and hematuria in children.
      a. Facial edema, especially periorbital edema; may be more pronounced in the morning and subside during the day.
      b. Generalized edema of the lower extremities; may increase during the day.
      c. Labia or scrotum may become very edematous.
      d. Edema may progress to the level of severe generalized edema (anasarca).
      e. Ascites and pleural effusion.
   2. Gradual increase in weight.
   3. Volume of urine is decreased, and urine may be foamy and tea colored.
   4. Irritability, fatigue, lethargy.
   5. Malnourishment: may occur as a result of decreased intake and loss of protein in the urine but may not appear so because of edema.
   6. Infection can result in significant morbidity or mortality.

C. Diagnostics (see Appendix 25-1).
   1. Decreased serum protein levels: hypoalbuminemia.
   2. Urinalysis: increased specific gravity, massive proteinuria (greater than 31 as determined by dipstick test).
   3. Creatinine clearance may be decreased, with normal serum creatinine levels.

D. Potential complications.
   1. Compromised immune system leading to an increase in infections (e.g., pneumonia, bronchitis, peritonitis).
   2. Circulatory insufficiency caused by hypovolemia, with severe edema.
   3. Thromboembolism secondary to hypercoagulability.
   4. Hypocalcemia, hyperparathyroidism, hyperlipidemia, and osteomalacia may occur.

### Treatment

A. Medical.
   1. Corticosteroids: prednisone/prednisolone.
   2. Diuretics: used when edema progresses despite sodium restriction.
   3. Salt-poor human albumin is used for treatment of vascular insufficiency and severe edema.
   4. Prophylactic broad-spectrum antimicrobial agents.
   5. Immunosuppressant therapy is prescribed for children who are not responsive to steroid therapy.
   6. Lipid-lowering agents.

B. Dietary.
   1. Low sodium diet (2 to 3 g/day).
   2. Proteins consumed should have high biologic value (low to moderate protein diet).
   3. Fluid is usually not restricted.

### Nursing Interventions

**Goal:** To monitor disease progress and reduce edema.

A. Support edematous areas such as scrotum.

B. Provide and encourage a salt-restricted diet.

C. Administer salt-poor albumin; monitor closely for circulatory overload during and after administration.

D. Provide meticulous skin care and keep opposing skin surfaces dry; change position frequently, and monitor good body alignment.

E. Determine weight daily, maintain accurate intake and output record, measure abdominal girth daily.

F. Test urine with dipstick for protein; check specific gravity.

G. Monitor cardiac function for complications of fluid balance (marked edema but hypovolemic).

**Goal:** To prevent infection.

A. Client is susceptible to infection because of a compromised immune state as well as steroid therapy.

B. Protect from upper respiratory tract infections; provide good pulmonary hygiene; check breath sounds.

C. Prevent skin excoriation and breakdown; assess carefully for indications of infection.

**Goal:** To promote nutrition.

A. Encourage low to moderate protein intake of high biologic value.

B. Serve frequent small quantities of food to child.
C. Encourage input from client in selection of foods from prescribed diet.

 *Home Care*

A. Inform client and caregivers about medical regimen: steroids, diuretics, antibiotics.
B. Reassure client that the prognosis is good; there may be relapses that will require therapy, but few children progress to chronic disease.
C. Obtain medical assistance if relapse occurs; relapse is indicated by edema, proteinuria, fever.
D. Encourage normal growth and development activities; try to prevent social isolation.
E. Teach client/caregivers how to perform dipstick urine test for protein; may need to keep a daily diary to evaluate level of proteinuria.

## Glomerulonephritis

**Glomerulonephritis is an inflammatory reaction in the glomerulus most commonly as a result of an antigen–antibody response to beta-hemolytic streptococci. An immune complex is formed as a result of the antigen–antibody formation; the complex becomes trapped in the glomerulus. As a result of the edema in the glomeruli, the GFR is significantly decreased. It is the third leading cause of kidney failure in the United States.**

### Assessment

A. Risk factors/etiology.
  1. The stimulus of the antigen–antibody reaction is most often group A beta-hemolytic *Streptococcus* infection of the throat (tonsillitis, pharyngitis) or skin (impetigo), which ordinarily precedes the onset of the condition by about 5 to 21 days.
  2. Most common in children, but all age groups can be affected; males are affected more frequently than females.
  3. Illegal drug use, hypertension, diabetic neuropathy, and polyarteritis are other risk factors.
B. Clinical manifestations (Figure 25-3).
  1. Acute glomerulonephritis.
    a. Disease may be mild with proteinuria and/or asymptomatic hematuria.
    b. Tea- or cola-colored urine caused by hematuria.
    c. Facial and periorbital edema primarily, but edema may be generalized.
    d. Decrease in urine output (oliguria).
    e. Mild to moderate increase in blood pressure; hypertension is more severe in adults.
    f. Azotemia: presence of nitrogenous waste products in the blood.
  2. Chronic glomerulonephritis: symptoms reflect progressive renal failure; more common in adults.
C. Diagnostics (see Appendix 25-1): reduced complement (C3) levels in early stages and elevated antistreptolysin O (ASO) titer.

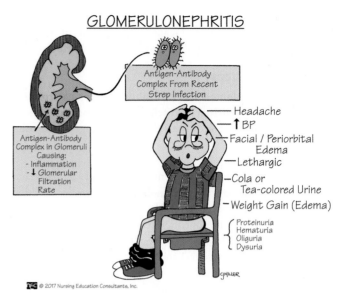

**FIGURE 25-3 Glomerulonephritis.** (From Zerwekh, J., Garneau, A., & Miller, C. J. [2017]. *Digital collection of the memory notebooks of nursing* [4th ed.]. Chandler, AZ: Nursing Education Consultants, Inc.)

D. Complications.
  1. Chronic kidney disease.
  2. Circulatory overload (pulmonary edema) and congestive heart failure (CHF).
  3. Hypertensive episodes.
  4. In children, hypertensive encephalopathy, acute renal failure, or cardiac failure may occur.

### Treatment

A. Medical.
  1. Diuretics for severe edema and fluid overload.
  2. Antihypertensives.
  3. Antibiotics if the streptococcal infection is still present.
  4. Plasmapheresis for filtering out immune complexes (antigens and antibodies).
B. Dietary.
  1. Decrease sodium intake.
  2. Protein restriction if client is azotemic; however, the anorexia that a child experiences frequently limits sufficient protein intake.
  3. Foods containing large amounts of potassium are often restricted during the oliguric phase.
C. Children with normal blood pressure, adequate urine output, and mild symptoms are cared for at home.
D. Fluid restriction may be implemented if urinary output is decreased.

### Nursing Interventions

**Goal:** To protect client's kidneys by preventing secondary infections.

A. Antibiotic therapy if cultures are positive.
B. Encourage rest until signs of glomerular inflammation (proteinuria, hematuria) and hypertension subside.
C. Avoid medications that are nephrotoxic, especially aminoglycosides.

**Goal:** To maintain fluid balance.

A. Monitor intake and output; maintain diet and fluid restrictions.
B. Monitor renal function: check proteinuria, specific gravity, and color of urine; weigh client daily; if client has hypertension, check blood pressure every 2 to 4 hours.
C. Monitor serum potassium levels.
D. Frequently, the first sign of improvement is an increase in the urine output, which may progress to profuse diuresis.

**Goal:** To prevent complications and promote comfort.

A. Encourage verbalization of fears.
B. Decrease anxiety by explaining treatments and reassuring client and family that the majority of clients recover fully.
C. Most children recover spontaneously, and recurrences are uncommon.

### Home Care

A. Teach parents or client symptoms to be reported to physician: nausea, fatigue, vomiting, decrease in urinary output, and symptoms of infection.
B. Explain the need for rest, good nutrition, and avoidance of people with respiratory tract infections.
C. Teach measures to prevent UTIs.
D. Instruct client in regard to diet, fluid needs, and medication therapy.
E. Teach client to perform dipstick urine test to monitor for protein.

## Wilms' Tumor (Nephroblastoma)

**Nephroblastoma (Wilms' tumor) is one of the most common intraabdominal tumors of childhood and is associated with congenital anomalies, especially those of the genitourinary tract. The treatment and survival rate are based on the stage of the tumor at the time it is diagnosed. Five stages are used to maximize the effectiveness of treatment protocols.**

A. Risk factors/etiology.
  1. Family history of cancer.
  2. Associated with genitourinary anomalies.
  3. Majority of children (80%) diagnosed are younger than 5 years; peak incidence at 3 years.
B. Clinical manifestations.
  1. Swelling or mass within the abdomen: firm, confined to one side of the abdomen, causing vague or no pain.
  2. Abdominal pain as tumor enlarges.
  3. Hematuria, pallor, anorexia, weight loss, and malaise occur as condition progresses.
  4. Hypertension (63%).
C. Diagnostics (see Appendix 25-1).

### Treatment

The survival rate greatly depends on the stage of the tumor at the time of diagnosis. If the tumor is diagnosed and treated in the early stages, there is a high survival rate (see Chapter 11).

A. Surgery.
  1. Surgery is frequently scheduled within 24 to 48 hours after the diagnosis.
  2. Nephrectomy: kidney is removed, but the adrenal gland may be spared, depending on the invasiveness of the tumor.
  3. If both kidneys are involved, the less affected kidney is retained, and the more involved one is removed. Bilateral nephrectomy is a last resort.
B. Medical.
  1. Preoperative and postoperative radiation therapy for large tumors.
  2. Postoperative chemotherapy.

### Nursing Interventions

**Goal:** To provide safe preoperative care.

> **NURSING PRIORITY:** Post a sign above the bed that reads "Do Not Palpate Abdomen."

A. Handle child carefully to prevent trauma to the tumor site.
B. Prepare child and family for the surgery, including anticipation of a large incision and dressing. Intensive care unit care immediately after surgery.
C. Assess vital signs, especially blood pressure, for indications of hypertension. If adrenal gland is removed, blood pressure may be labile.

**Goal:** To assess kidney function and to prevent infection.

A. Usual postoperative care for abdominal surgery.
B. Monitor for gastrointestinal (GI) complications.
C. Provide good pulmonary hygiene because child is at increased risk for pulmonary infections postoperatively.
D. Vincristine is frequently used in chemotherapy; closely observe the child for the development of a paralytic ileus. Another choice is actinomycin D, while doxorubicin and cyclophosphamide may be used in advanced-stage disease.
E. Child is at risk for intestinal obstruction from the vincristine-induced adynamic ileus, edema caused by radiation, or postsurgical adhesions.

### Home Care

A. Teach parents management of the effects of chemotherapy.
B. Child has only one kidney; teach parents how to protect renal function.
  1. Signs and symptoms of UTI and ways to prevent the occurrence.
  2. Advise all health care providers of compromised renal function.
  3. Prompt treatment of other infections.
  4. Encourage non-contact sports when older.

## Acute Kidney Injury

**Acute kidney injury (AKI) is a clinical syndrome with abrupt loss of kidney function that may occur over several hours or days, characterized by uremia. The most common causes are hypotension, prerenal hypovolemia, or exposure to a nephrotoxin.**

### Phases of Acute Kidney Injury

A. Oliguric phase (Figure 25-4).
  1. Urinary output decreases to less than 400 mL per 24 hours.
  2. Increase in blood urea nitrogen (BUN), creatinine, uric acid, potassium, and magnesium levels and presence of metabolic acidosis.
  3. Duration is 1 to 3 weeks; the longer it lasts, the less favorable the recovery.

> **⚠ OLDER ADULT PRIORITY:** The older adult client loses the ability to concentrate urine; therefore urinary output may not be significantly reduced in this stage of kidney injury.

  4. Nonoliguric acute kidney injury: urine output is greater than 400 mL/24 hr and urine is dilute.
B. Diuretic phase.
  1. Often has a sudden onset within 2 to 6 weeks after oliguric phase. Daily urine output is 1 to 3 L but may reach 5 L or more.
  2. Hypovolemia and hypotension may occur due to massive fluid losses.
  3. BUN level stops increasing. Urinary creatinine clearance stabilizes.
  4. Client must be monitored for hypokalemia and hyponatremia, as electrolytes are lost along with the urine volume.
  5. May last for 1 to 3 weeks.
C. Recovery (convalescent) phase.
  1. Begins when the GFR increases. May take up to 12 months for renal function to stabilize.
  2. There is usually some permanent loss of renal function, but remaining renal function is sufficient to maintain healthy life. The older adult is less likely to experience a return to full kidney function.
  3. Complications: secondary infection, which is the most common cause of death.

### Assessment

A. Risk factors/etiology.
  1. Prerenal (renal ischemia from factors external to the kidney).
    a. Circulatory volume depletion: caused by hemorrhage, dehydration.
    b. Decreased cardiac output: pump failure and/or CHF, especially in older adults.
    c. Decreased peripheral resistance: caused by septic shock, anaphylaxis, antihypertensives.

# ACUTE KIDNEY INJURY (AKI)
## - SIGNS & SYMPTOMS -

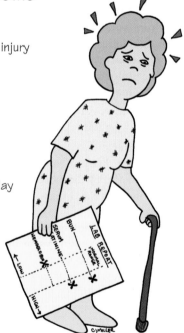

### Oliguric Phase
- Oliguria - <400mL/day; occurs within 1-7 days of kidney injury
- Urinalysis — casts, RBCs, WBCs, sp gr fixated at 1.010
- Metabolic Acidosis
- Hyperkalemia and Hyponatremia
- Elevated BUN and Creatinine
- Fatigue & Malaise

### Diuretic Phase
- Gradual ↑in urine output - 1-3 L/day; may reach 3-5 L/day
- Hypovolemia, Dehydration
- Hypotension
- BUN and Creatinine Levels Begin to Normalize

### Recovery Phase
- Begins when GFR Increases
- BUN and Creatinine Levels Plateau, then ↓

© 2016 Nursing Education Consultants, Inc.

**FIGURE 25-4 Acute Kidney Injury.** (From Zerwekh, J., Garneau, A., & Miller, C. J. [2017]. *Digital collection of the memory notebooks of nursing* [4th ed.]. Chandler, AZ: Nursing Education Consultants, Inc.)

d. Volume shifts: third spacing of fluid, gram-negative sepsis, hypoalbuminemia.
e. Vascular obstruction: renal artery occlusion, dissection abdominal aneurysm.
2. Intrarenal (kidney tissue disease).
a. Acute tubular necrosis: caused by hemolytic blood transfusion reaction, nephrotoxic chemicals (carbon tetrachloride, arsenic, lead, mercury), nephrotoxic medication (aminoglycoside antibiotics, amphotericin B, and streptomycin), radiology contrast material.
b. Infections: acute glomerulonephritis, pyelonephritis, cytomegalovirus (CMV), candidiasis.
c. Diseases that precipitate vascular changes (e.g., atherosclerosis, diabetes mellitus, hypertension).
d. Other risk factors/causes could include eclampsia of pregnancy, systemic lupus erythematosus, malignant hypertension, and thrombotic disorders.
3. Postrenal (obstructive problems restricting the outflow of urine).
a. Urinary and renal calculi.
b. Benign prostatic hypertrophy.
c. Urethral stricture.
d. Trauma (back, pelvis, perineum) resulting in obstruction.
e. Bladder cancer, neuromuscular disorders.
f. Spinal cord disease.

**NURSING PRIORITY:** Many disorders across the life span can precipitate acute kidney injury. It is important to know who is at increased risk for developing kidney injury and the initial symptoms. Kidney injury is frequently incorporated into a test question as a complication of a variety of conditions.

B. Clinical manifestations (multiple body systems affected).
1. Urinary: decreased urinary output (oliguria, less than 400 mL/day; in older adults, may be 600 to 700 mL/day).
a. Intrarenal and postrenal failure: fixed specific gravity, increased sodium in the urine; proteinuria with glomerular membrane alteration, "muddy brown" casts.
b. Prerenal failure: history of precipitating event; urine specific gravity may be high; high urinary sodium concentration and proteinuria.
2. Cardiovascular.
a. Pericarditis, pericardial effusion.
b. Arrhythmias caused by acidosis or hyperkalemia.
c. CHF, hypotension followed by hypertension.
3. Respiratory.
a. Pulmonary edema caused by fluid overload.
b. Kussmaul respiration caused by metabolic acidosis.
c. Pleural effusions.
4. Hematologic.
a. Anemia caused by impaired erythropoietin.
b. Leukocytosis, increased susceptibility to infection.
c. Altered platelet function leading to bleeding tendencies.

5. Neurologic.
a. Decreased seizure threshold caused by uremia.
b. Altered mentation, memory impairment, lethargy.
6. Fluid and electrolyte imbalances.
a. Fluid retention.
b. Hyperkalemia.
c. Hyponatremia (usually dilution).
d. Metabolic acidosis from accumulation of acid waste products.
C. Diagnostics (see Appendix 25-1).

*Treatment*

A. Medical.
1. Identify and treat precipitating cause of acute kidney injury (management varies according to whether disorder is prerenal, intrarenal, or postrenal).
2. Diuretic therapy may be used with fluid challenges.
3. Decrease serum potassium level.
a. Sodium polystyrene sulfonate: a cation exchange resin given by mouth or retention enema.
b. Sorbitol: an osmotic cathartic; may be given with exchange resins to induce diarrhea to eliminate potassium ions.
c. IV hypertonic glucose and regular insulin may be administered to move potassium into the intracellular space; used for severe hyperkalemia.
4. IV administration of sodium bicarbonate: corrects metabolic acidosis and causes electrolyte shift.
5. IV dopamine to enhance renal perfusion. **Caution:** always check for correct concentration before beginning infusion (see Appendix 18-2).
B. Dietary.
1. Fluid restriction; intake may be carefully calculated with output.
2. Intake of protein, potassium (restrict to 40 mEq/day), and sodium is regulated according to serum plasma levels.
3. Increased intake of carbohydrates and protein of high biologic value.
C. Dialysis (Box 25-5): indications are volume overload, BUN level greater than 120 mg/dL (42.84 mmol/L), metabolic acidosis, increased potassium with electrocardiographic changes, pericardial effusion, and cardiac tamponade.

*Nursing Interventions*

**Goal** To maintain client in functional homeostasis and monitor kidney function.

A. Identify and monitor high-risk clients (any client with a transient or significant decrease in blood pressure, regardless of the precipitating cause).
B. Maintain accurate intake and output record.
C. Determine weight daily (client may lose 0.2 to 0.3 kg/day during oliguric phase).
D. Assess fluid balance (hypervolemia or hypovolemia), urine specific gravity, pulmonary status, cardiac output, mental status changes (may indicate cerebral edema).

### Hemodialysis

Circulation of the client's blood through a compartment that contains an artificial semipermeable membrane surrounded by dialysate fluid, which removes excess body fluid by creating a pressure differential between the blood and the dialysate solution.

### Continuous Renal Replacement Therapy (CRRT)

An alternative measure for treating acute kidney injury. The uremic toxins are removed slowly and continuously over 24 hours. This allows for constant maintenance of acid–base and electrolyte balance in an unstable client. Can be used in conjunction with hemodialysis. There are several types: continuous venovenous hemofiltration (CVVH), slow continuous ultrafiltration (SCUF), continuous venovenous hemodialysis (CVVHD), and continuous venovenous hemodiafiltration (CVVHDF).

### Peritoneal Dialysis

Utilization of the peritoneal cavity and the peritoneum as the semipermeable membrane that removes excess fluid.

### Continuous Ambulatory Peritoneal Dialysis

The dialysate is infused into the abdomen and remains there for a specified time (2–6 hours). The dialysate is removed by gravity drainage after the prescribed time.

### Automated Peritoneal Dialysis

Uses a peritoneal dialysis cycling machine. It can be done continuously, intermittently, or nightly. Most clients prefer to have the dialysis done while sleeping.

### Wearable Artificial Kidney (WAK)

Miniaturized dialysis machine worn on the body and resembles a tool belt. The device connects to the client via a catheter. The WAK runs continuously on batteries and is not plugged into an electrical outlet or attached to a water pipe. The device weighs around 10 pounds.

E. Assess status of electrolytes and kidney parameters: serum potassium, BUN, creatinine, phosphate levels; evaluate fluctuations of serum sodium levels and GFR.

F. Evaluate for hypertension or hypotension.

G. Support involved body systems.
   1. Cardiac dysrhythmias.
   2. Pulmonary function.

H. Avoid nephrotoxic medications, including nonsteroidal antiinflammatory drugs (NSAIDs) and aminoglycosides.

**Goal:** To maintain nutrition.

A. Maintain dietary restrictions on sodium, potassium, and protein.

B. Encourage intake of carbohydrates and fats for energy source. Caloric needs are 30 to 35 kcal/kg.

C. Offer small frequent feedings; limit fluids.

D. Total parenteral or enteral nutrition may be necessary to promote healing if caloric intake cannot be maintained.

**Goal:** To prevent infection.

A. Avoid use of indwelling urinary catheter if possible.

B. Assess for development of infectious processes (local or systemic). Client is at increased risk because of compromised immune system; may not have an elevated temperature.

C. Assess for and prevent UTI.

**Goal:** To prevent skin breakdown.

A. Frequent turning and positioning; inspect the skin for problem areas.

B. Beds and protective devices are used to prevent pressure areas (see Pressure Ulcers section in Chapter 13).

C. Frequent range of motion and activities to increase circulation.

**Goal:** To provide emotional support.

A. Always explain procedures.

B. Provide honest information regarding progress of condition.

C. May take 3 to 12 months for recovery.

D. Encourage client to express fears and concerns regarding condition.

## Chronic Kidney Disease

Chronic kidney disease (CKD) is a progressive, irreversible reduction in renal function such that the kidneys are no longer able to maintain the body environment. The GFR gradually decreases as the nephrons are destroyed. The nephrons left intact are subjected to an increased workload, resulting in hypertrophy and inability to concentrate urine.

**Stages of Chronic Kidney Disease** (Table 25-1)

**Assessment**

A. Risk factors/etiology.
   1. Chronic hypertension and poorly controlled diabetes account for about 70% of cases of CKD.
   2. Chronic glomerulonephritis and pyelonephritis.
   3. Polycystic kidney disease.
   4. Kidney disease caused by nephrotoxic drugs or chemicals.
   5. Systemic lupus erythematosus (SLE).
   6. More common in African Americans and Native Americans.
   7. Age over 60.
   8. Family history of CKD.

B. Clinical manifestations (Figure 25-5).
   1. GFR is less than 60 mL/min for longer than 3 months. A GFR less than 15 mL/min indicates kidney failure.
      a. Severe azotemia, metabolic acidosis.
      b. Hyperkalemia, hypernatremia, and hyperphosphatemia.
      c. Altered renin-angiotensin system.
   2. Urinary system: specific gravity of urine fixed at 1.010; proteinuria, casts, pyuria, hematuria; oliguria eventually leads to anuria less than 100 mL/24 hr.
   3. Endocrine system.
      a. Hyperparathyroidism causes hypocalcemia and hyperphosphatemia resulting in demineralization of the bones (renal osteodystrophy).
      b. Hypothyroidism.

**Table 25-1   STAGES OF CHRONIC KIDNEY DISEASE**

| Description | GFR (mL/min/1.73 m²) | Action |
|---|---|---|
| **Stage 1**<br>Kidney damage with normal or ↑ GFR | ≥90 | Diagnosis and treatment<br>Treatment of comorbid conditions<br>CVD risk reduction<br>Slow progression |
| **Stage 2**<br>Kidney damage with mild ↓ GFR | 60–89 | Estimation of progression |
| **Stage 3a**<br>Moderate ↓ GFR | 45–59 | Evaluation and treatment of complications |
| **Stage 3b**<br>Moderate ↓ GFR | 30–44 | More aggressive treatment of complications |
| **Stage 4**<br>Severe ↓ GFR | 15–29 | Preparation for kidney replacement therapy (dialysis, kidney transplant) |
| **Stage 5**<br>Kidney failure | <15 (or dialysis) | Renal replacement therapy (if uremia present and client desires treatment) |

*CKD*, Chronic kidney disease; *CVD*, cardiovascular disease; *GFR*, glomerular filtration rate.
Source: Source: Kidney Disease: Improving Global Outcomes (KDIGO) CKD Work Group. KDIGO 2012 *Clinical Practice Guideline for the Evaluation and Management of Chronic Kidney Disease* (2013). Kidney Inter Suppl, 3(1), 1. Retrieved from https://www.kidney.org/professionals/guidelines/guidelines_commentaries http://www.kdigo.org/clinical_practice_guidelines/pdf/CKD/KDIGO_2012_CKD_GL.pdf

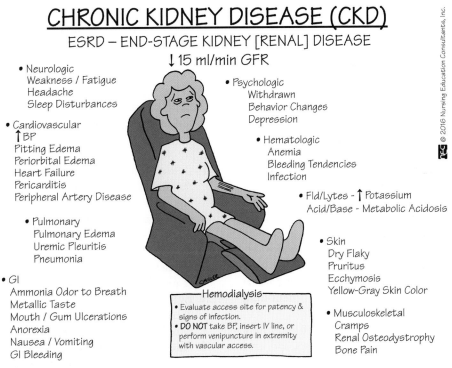

**FIGURE 25-5 Chronic Kidney Disease.** (From Zerwekh, J., Garneau, A., & Miller, C. J. [2017]. *Digital collection of the memory notebooks of nursing* [4th ed.]. Chandler, AZ: Nursing Education Consultants, Inc.)

4. Hematologic system: anemia and bleeding, infection.
5. Cardiovascular system: hypertension, HF, uremic pericarditis, pericardial effusion, atherosclerotic heart disease.
6. Gastrointestinal system: anorexia, nausea, vomiting, ammonia odor (uremic fetor) to the breath, gastrointestinal bleeding, peptic ulcer disease, gastritis.
7. Metabolic system: hyperglycemia, hyperlipidemia, gout, hypoproteinemia, carbohydrate intolerance.
8. Neurologic system: general central nervous system depression and peripheral neuropathy, headaches, seizures, sleep disturbances.
9. Musculoskeletal system: mineral and bone disorder (CKD-MBD), vascular calcification, osteomalacia.

10. Integumentary system: yellow/gray discoloration, pruritus, uremic frost, ecchymosis.
11. Psychological changes: emotional lability, withdrawal, depression, and psychosis, personality and behavioral changes.
12. Reproductive system: erectile dysfunction, amenorrhea.

C. Diagnostics (see Appendix 25-1).
 1. Urinalysis for proteinuria or microalbuminuria.
 2. Elevated blood sugar and triglyceride levels.
 3. Increased serum potassium level.
 4. Decreased hemoglobin and hematocrit.

## Treatment

A. Medical.
 1. Measures to reduce serum potassium level (see discussion under acute renal failure).
 2. Antihypertensives (see Appendix 18-2).
 3. Diuretics: thiazide and loop diuretics may be used early in the course of disease.
 4. Erythropoietin for treatment of anemia.
 5. Phosphate binders and supplemental vitamin D for CKD-MBD.
B. Dietary.
 1. Problems with the client losing body weight, both adipose tissue and muscle mass.
 2. Restricted protein intake; may vary from just a decrease in protein intake to a specific restriction of 20 to 40 g/day.
 3. Protein should be of a high biologic value (1.2 to 1.3 g/kg); this enhances the utilization of the amino acids and results in formation of fewer nitrogen waste products.
 4. Fluid restriction: 600 to 1000 mL, adjusted according to urinary output and/or dialysis.
 5. Sodium, potassium, and phosphate restriction: based on laboratory values.
C. Dialysis (see Box 25-5).
D. Surgical: kidney transplantation—the primary limiting factor in the number of transplantations done is the availability of kidneys; the average wait is 18 months to 4 years; clients with blood types B and O have the longest wait.
 1. Recipient criteria: candidates are evaluated on an individual basis as to how well they would benefit from transplantation.
    a. Candidates are usually younger than 70 years, have a life expectancy of at least 2 more years, and have reasonable expectations that the transplantation will improve the quality of life.
    b. Infection, disseminated malignancy, refractory cardiac disease, chronic respiratory failure, and unresolved psychological disorders are contraindications to transplantation; the presence of hepatitis B or C is not contraindicated if controlled.
 2. Donor criteria: living related donors provide the best possible match with a 95% 1-year graft survival; when they are not available, cadaver donors are considered; these have a 90% 1-year graft survival.

## Nursing Interventions

**Goal:** To assist the client to maintain homeostasis in early CKD.

A. Evaluate adequacy of fluid balance.
 1. Determine weight daily.
 2. Control hypertension.
 3. Discuss with the client how to monitor fluid intake and plan for the allocated amount to be distributed over the day.

> **TEST ALERT:** Monitor hydration status, identify signs of fluid and electrolyte imbalance, and identify interventions to correct any imbalance.

B. Encourage nutritional intake within dietary guidelines.
 1. Relieve gastrointestinal dysfunctions before serving meals.
 2. Plan diet according to client's preferences, if possible.
 3. Advise client that most salt substitutes contain potassium and should not be used.
C. Prevent problem of constipation.
 1. Include bran/fiber in diet.
 2. Stool softeners.
D. Avoid use of sedatives and hypnotics; increased sensitivity to these medications is caused by decreased ability of kidney to metabolize and excrete them.
E. Monitor electrolyte balance, especially levels of potassium and calcium.

> **NURSING PRIORITY:** Hypocalcemia and hyperkalemia are critical problems and may cause fatal dysrhythmias.

F. Assess cardiovascular status to determine how effectively the client's cardiovascular system is compensating for the increased fluid load and increased workload from the chronic anemic state.
G. Assess client for bleeding tendencies initially related to a decrease in production of erythropoietin and decreased platelet adhesiveness. Encourage intake of folic acid (1 mg daily) for red blood cell production and integrity.
H. Evaluate client for pruritus and assist with measures to decrease skin irritation and itching.
I. Avoid products containing magnesium (antacids).
J. Assess client's activity tolerance in relation to anemia.

**Goal:** To provide emotional support and to promote psychological equilibrium.

A. Encourage client to express concerns.
B. Recognize that the long-term management of a chronic disease may lead to anxiety and depression.
C. Encourage venting of feelings regarding lifestyle changes.
D. Encourage client and family members to seek out support groups and community resources, as well as other clients with renal failure who are undergoing the same types of treatment.

## Kidney Transplant

The transplantation of a kidney from a compatible-blood-typed deceased donor, blood relative, or a live donor. Transplanted kidney is usually placed extraperitoneally in the iliac fossa (usually right side to facilitate anastomosis and decrease occurrence of ileus), most commonly on the right lower side of the abdomen.

### Assessment

A. Recipient selection: based on a variety of factors—history of disseminated malignancies, untreated cardiac disease, chronic respiratory failure, diabetes (uncontrolled), extensive vascular disease, chronic infection, and noncompliance with medical regimens would contraindicate a transplant. Donors may be living or deceased.

B. Rejection (Figure 25-6).
   1. Hyperacute (antibody-mediated): not common.
      a. Occurs within minutes to hours after transplant.
      b. No treatment; transplanted kidney removed.
   2. Acute rejection: mediated by cytotoxic T lymphocytes.
      a. Can occur within days; 3 months is most common time but can be as late as 2 years; it is common to have at least one rejection episode.
      b. Increased white blood cell count, fever.
      c. Deteriorating renal function: increasing serum creatinine and BUN levels, increasing blood pressure.
      d. Tenderness over graft site—often an early sign, along with malaise.
      e. Hypertension.
      f. Treatment is increased immunosuppressive therapy: usually high-dose steroids, polyclonal or monoclonal antibody therapy.
   3. Chronic rejection: mediated by B cells and some T cells.
      a. Occurs over months or years and is due to gradual occlusion of the renal vasculature. It is irreversible, and the client will again require dialysis and/or be placed back on the transplant list.
      b. Hypertension, increasing serum creatinine and BUN levels, and proteinuria.
      c. Graft tenderness, malaise, and signs of early end-stage renal disease.
      d. Treatment is supportive.
         (1) Change immunosuppressive therapy or increase doses.
         (2) Add tacrolimus or mycophenolate mofetil.

### Treatment

A. Immunosuppressant medications (see Appendix 25-2).
B. Steroids (see Appendix 9-2).

### Nursing Interventions

**Goal:** To provide preoperative care for client scheduled for kidney transplantation.

A. Maintain client's metabolic state as close to homeostasis as possible; continue with dialysis.

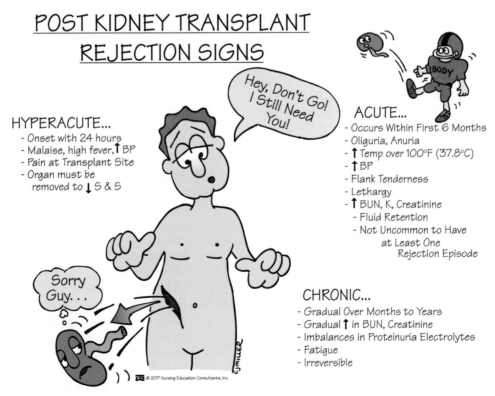

**FIGURE 25-6 Post Kidney Transplant Rejection.** (From Zerwekh, J., Garneau, A., & Miller, C. J. [2017]. *Digital collection of the memory notebooks of nursing* [4th ed.]. Chandler, AZ: Nursing Education Consultants, Inc.)

B. Tissue typing and antibody screening are conducted to determine histocompatibility of the donor and recipient.

C. Immunosuppressant drugs: may be started before surgery.

D. Conduct routine preoperative procedures, including labeling the arm with vascular access for dialysis because the client may require dialysis in the immediate postoperative period.

**Goal:** To provide postoperative care for the kidney transplant recipient.

A. Immunosuppressant therapy is continued indefinitely; the most frequent combination of maintenance therapy consists of azathioprine, cyclosporine, and prednisone.

B. Assess for renal graft function.
1. Maintain fluid and electrolyte balances because of early diuresis. Avoid dehydration.
2. Cadaveric transplant recipients may need dialysis because of acute tubular necrosis until the transplanted kidney begins to function.
3. A sudden decrease or change in urine output should be reported.

C. Monitor for rejection.

D. Prevent and monitor for infection (UTI, pneumonia, and sepsis are biggest threats in the early posttransplantation period; fungal and viral infections are also common).
1. It is important to make a distinction between infection and rejection, because impaired renal function and fever occur in both.
2. Symptoms of septicemia: infection, shaking, chills, fever, tachycardia, leukocytosis, and tachypnea.

E. Atherosclerotic cardiovascular disease is common in transplant recipients. It is the leading cause of death in these clients.

F. Promote adaptation and psychological support for the client who has undergone successful transplantation.
1. Often, there is a continual fear of possible rejection.
2. A major concern of the client and the family is related to long-term use of immunosuppressant medication, which puts tremendous psychological and financial stress on the family.
3. Refer client to community and national agencies: National Association of Patients of Hemodialysis and Transplantation, Inc. and the National Kidney Foundation.

# Dialysis

**Dialysis, also called renal replacement therapy (RRT), is the passage of particles (ions) from an area of high concentration to an area of low concentration across a semipermeable membrane.**

A. Water, by osmosis, will move toward the solution in which the ion concentration is the greatest.

B. When hemodialysis is performed, the semipermeable membrane used has pores that are large enough for waste products and water to move through but too small for blood cells and protein molecules to pass through. In peritoneal dialysis, the same process occurs, except that the client's own intraabdominal peritoneal membrane is used and protein is lost due to the pore size.

C. Indications.
1. GFR less than 15 mL/min.
2. Fluid volume overload.
3. Serum potassium level greater than 6 mEq/L (mmol/L).
4. BUN level greater than 120 mg/dL (42.84 mmol/L).
5. Uremia, uncontrolled hypertension, and metabolic acidosis.

D. ▲ Types of dialysis (see Box 25-5). Note that dialysis solutions are High-Alert Medications.

## Nursing Interventions

**Goal:** To remove waste products of metabolism and excess fluid; to maintain a safe concentration of blood components.

A. Peritoneal dialysis.
1. Prepare client for procedure: establish baseline criteria of laboratory values, weight, and vital signs; bowel and bladder should be empty.
2. Provide support and information to the client when the peritoneal catheter is first inserted.
   a. Permanent peritoneal catheters are fitted with a device to keep them in place; types of catheters—bent neck, curl, and disc.
   b. Temporary peritoneal catheters are inserted, and usually a purse-string suture holds them in place; this usually occurs in the intensive care unit.
3. Type of peritoneal dialysis being used and the physical stability of the client determine how long each cycle of dialysis will take.
   a. Cycle is initiated with the inflow of the dialysate by gravity into the abdominal cavity. The client should be carefully observed during the initial infusion to determine how well he or she will tolerate the additional fluid in the abdominal cavity. Initial infusion is usually 1 to 2 L over 10 to 20 minutes (fill time).
   b. The dialysate remains in the abdomen (dwell time) and is allowed to drain by gravity (drain time). The dwell time and drain time are specified in the doctor's orders. Seriously ill clients may receive up to 24 exchanges in a day.
   c. One exchange constitutes infusion, dwell time, and drainage.
   d. The dialysate should be warmed to body temperature before it is infused (do not use a microwave oven) to increase clearance.
   e. The procedure should be considered sterile in that masks and sterile gloves should be used when accessing the catheter to change the tubing. Remember the catheter is an open conduit to the peritoneal cavity.
4. Insufficient outflow (return of less than the amount of dialysate infused).
   a. Constipation is the primary cause of inflow and outflow problems.

b. Check the tubing for patency and keep drainage bag below the level of the abdomen.

c. Turn client from side to side or put client in semi-Fowler's position to increase abdominal pressure.

d. Gently massaging the abdomen can also help.

5. Complications: possible bowel perforation from catheter insertion, peritonitis, bleeding, hypoalbuminemia, hyperglycemia in clients with diabetes.

6. Automated peritoneal dialysis can be used while the client is sleeping. The machine provides four or more exchanges per night with 1 to 2 hours per exchange, allowing the client to be dialysis-free during waking hours.

**■ NURSING PRIORITY:** If dialysate is left in the peritoneal cavity too long, hyperglycemia may occur due to the high percentage of glucose in the dialysate fluid, which ensures hyperosmolarity. Heparin is sometimes added to the dialysate to prevent clotting of the catheter or tubing.

B. Hemodialysis.

1. Vascular access site must be established; access may be temporary or permanent (Figure 25-7).

a. External arteriovenous shunts: temporary catheters are inserted into an artery and into a vein and are connected together on the outside of the arm in a U pattern.

b. Internal arteriovenous fistula or graft: an artery and a vein in the arm are anastomosed either directly or via a synthetic graft; access is achieved via two 14- to 16-gauge needles inserted into the access site.

c. After an internal access site is created, it must heal before it can be used for dialysis.

2. Evaluate access site for patency: the appropriate method to determine patency depends on the type of vascular access used; auscultate for bruit or palpate for a thrill over site.

3. Do not take blood pressure, obtain blood samples, or infuse fluids or medications in the access site or the extremity that has a vascular access site.

4. Assess the patency of the pulses distal to the access site.

**TEST ALERT:** Provide care for client with a vascular access site before and after hemodialysis.

**Goal:** To maintain homeostasis after hemodialysis.

A. Determine whether certain medications need to be withheld before dialysis (antihypertensives); in hospitalized clients there are often standing orders for these situations.

B. Assess weight, blood pressure, peripheral edema, lung and heart sounds, and vascular access site before and after dialysis.

# HEMODIALYSIS

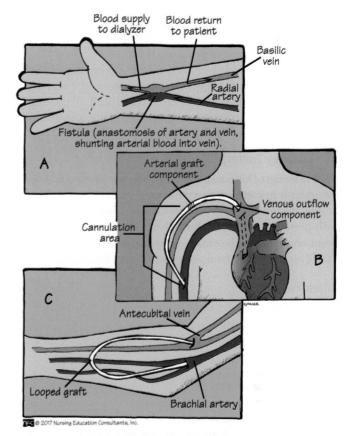

**FIGURE 25-7 Vascular Access for Hemodialysis.** (From Zerwekh, J., & Miller, C. J. [2017]. *NCLEX review course*. Chandler, AZ: Nursing Education Consultants.)

C. Most common side effects are hypotension, headache, muscle cramps, and bleeding from access site; monitor client for postural hypotension. If client has bleeding from the access site, apply pressure evenly and notify the dialysis unit.

D. Complications.

1. Dialysis disequilibrium syndrome: cerebral edema and neurologic complications (headache, nausea, vomiting, seizures); may be minimized by slower dialysis.

2. Sepsis, hepatitis B and C, blood loss, hypotension.

**Goal:** To maintain homeostasis during and after peritoneal dialysis.

A. Pain is common during first few exchanges; should gradually decrease.

B. Assess for development of peritonitis; antibiotics may be added to dialysate.

C. Dialysate should return clear to slightly yellow tinged; should not be cloudy or opaque.

D. Closely monitor blood pressure and activity after dialysis.

E. Increase protein in diet to compensate for removal of protein in dialysis; low protein level will impair tissue healing.

**Goal:** To provide emotional support and to promote psychological equilibrium.

A. Encourage client to express feelings of anger and depression. An increased rate of suicide exists among clients undergoing dialysis.
B. Encourage appropriate coping skills.
C. Clients undergoing chronic dialysis are in limbo; they know they are probably not going to get better and that they may or may not receive a transplant. Frequently, they have ambivalent feelings about dialysis; it maintains life but severely restricts lifestyle.

## Kidney Tumors

**The majority of kidney tumors are malignant and occur more frequently in men between the ages of 50 and 70 years. Most often, the tumor begins in the renal cortex, where it can actually become quite large before it begins to compress the adjacent renal tissue. The most common areas of metastasis are the liver, lungs, and bone, especially the mediastinum.**

### Risk Factors

A. Cigarette smoking is the most significant risk factor.
B. Obesity, hypertension.
C. Exposure to asbestos, cadmium, and gasoline.

### Assessment

A. Clinical manifestations.
   1. Palpable abdominal mass.
   2. Hematuria, flank pain.
   3. Weight loss, weakness, anemia, hypertension.
B. Diagnostics (see Appendix 25-1).

### Treatment

A. Medical.
   1. Palliative radiation therapy.
   2. Biologic therapy with alpha interferon and interleukin-2.
   3. Cryoablation (freezing tumor), radiofrequency ablation (tumor destroyed by radiofrequency heat).
   4. Chemotherapy in metastatic disease with 5-fluorouracil, floxuridine, and gemcitabine.
B. Surgical: radical nephrectomy (includes kidney, adrenal gland, ureter, lymph nodes, and surrounding fascia).

### Nursing Interventions

**Goal:** To provide preoperative nursing care (see Chapter 3).

A. Inform client that flank incision will be on affected side and that surgery will be performed in a hyperextended, side-lying position.
B. Often, client experiences postoperative muscle aches and discomfort as a result of surgical positioning.
C. Radiation, biologic therapy, or both after surgery.

**Goal:** To provide postoperative care.

A. Urinary output is important to assess; catheters should be labeled, and drainage should be recorded accurately.
B. Because of the level of the incision, respiratory complications are common; encourage coughing and deep breathing, as well as incentive spirometry, every 2 hours while client is awake.
C. Assess for abdominal distention and paralytic ileus.
D. Monitor for unstable blood pressure after surgery; may be caused by removal of adrenal gland.
E. Provide adequate pain control.

**Goal:** To provide supportive nursing care in relation to malignancy. See Chapter 11 for detailed nursing management.

---

| Appendix 25-1 | **DIAGNOSTICS OF THE URINARY-RENAL SYSTEM** | |
|---|---|---|
| *Laboratory Tests* | *Normal* | *Clinical and Nursing Implications* |
| BUN level | 6–20 mg/dL (2.1–7.14 mmol/L) | Common test used to diagnose renal problems; may be affected by an increase in protein intake or tissue breakdown. |
| Creatinine level | 0.6–1.3 mg/dL (53–115 umol/L) | End product of protein and muscle catabolism; more accurate determinate of renal function than the BUN level; values are higher in males. Elevated in renal disease. |
| Calcium level | 8.6–10.2 mg/dL (2.15–2.55 mmol/L) | Provides the matrix for bone and is important in muscle contraction, neurotransmission, and clotting; in chronic renal failure, low levels of calcium lead to renal osteodystrophy. |
| Phosphorus level | 2.4–4.4 mg/dL (0.78–1.42 mmol/L) | Phosphorus and calcium balances are inversely related; when phosphorus level is elevated, calcium level is decreased, which is seen in renal disease. |
| Urinalysis | Color: amber yellow<br>Ketones: none<br>Glucose: none<br>pH: 4.0–8.0 (average 6)<br>Specific gravity: (1.003–1.030) | Obtaining first-voided specimen in the morning is ideal. Presence of protein, WBC, RBC, glucose, bacteria, and hyaline casts indicates problems. Ensure specimen is examined within 1 hour of urinating.<br>Dipstick urinalysis is initially performed to determine levels of nitrites and leukocyte esterase related to infections. |

**Appendix 25-1  DIAGNOSTICS OF THE URINARY-RENAL SYSTEM—cont'd**

℞

| Laboratory Tests | Normal | Clinical and Nursing Implications |
|---|---|---|
| Urine culture and sensitivity | | Colony count of at least 100,000 colonies/mL of urine indicates infection. Use sterile container for collection of urine. After cleaning, instruct client to start urination and then continue voiding in sterile container. |
| Urinary creatinine clearance | Males: 21–26 mg/kg/24 hr<br>Females: 16–22 mg/kg/24 hr | Measure of GFR; 24-hour urine collection must be done; have client void and discard the first specimen and then begin timing the test; specimens should be kept cool or refrigerated. Decreased in renal disease. |
| Urine specific gravity | Adults: 1.003–1.030<br>Children: 1.001–1.030 | May be increased when the client is dehydrated and with glomerulonephritis. A decrease is associated with decreased tubular absorption. In renal failure, it may be fixed at 1.010–1.012. Proteinuria will increase the specific gravity. |
| 24-hour (composite) urine | | Collection of all urine over a 24-hour period, measuring levels of calcium, phosphorous, magnesium, sodium, oxylate, citrate, sulfate, potassium, uric acid, and/or total volume. Specimens may be required to be on ice during collection. |

## Laboratory Diagnostics

| Procedure | Clinical and Nursing Implications |
|---|---|
| **KUB (kidneys, ureters, bladder) x-ray examination:** a flat plate x-ray film of the abdomen and pelvis. | Bowel preparation may or may not be indicated. |
| **Intravenous urography (IVP or excretory urogram):** IV injection of radiopaque dye to visualize the urinary tract system. | 1. Client's status is NPO for 8 hours before procedure.<br>2. Cathartic or enema given the evening before procedure.<br>3. Radiocontrast medium may cause an allergic (hypersensitivity) reaction in iodine-sensitive clients.<br>4. Instruct client that he or she will need to lie still on table while serial x-ray films are taken.<br>5. Advise client that he or she may feel warm sensation and salty taste in mouth as dye is injected.<br>6. Evaluate for iodine reaction after test and force fluids after test to flush out the dye.<br>7. Be sure the older adult client is not dehydrated before the procedure; the contrast medium is nephrotoxic and can precipitate renal failure.<br>8. Force fluids (if permitted or appropriate) after to flush out contrast media. |
| **Retrograde pyelogram:** An x-ray study of the urinary tract conducted during a cystoscopic examination; ureteral catheters are inserted into the renal pelvis, and dye is injected (retrograde) into the catheters. | 1. Client's status is NPO for 8 hours before test.<br>2. Assess for sensitivity to iodine.<br>3. Explain that there may be discomfort on insertion of the cystoscope.<br>4. General anesthesia may be indicated for procedure. |
| **Renal arteriogram (angiogram):** An IV injection of radiopaque dye into the renal artery (catheter is inserted into femoral artery) to visualize the renal blood vessels. | 1. Client's status is NPO after midnight.<br>2. May have enema or cathartic the night before.<br>3. Preoperative medication is administered.<br>4. Client should be assessed for sensitivity to iodine before the procedure.<br>5. Evaluate venipuncture insertion site every 15–30 min after the procedure to assess for bleeding.<br>6. Assess pulses distal to the injection site to detect occluded blood flow. Compare pre- and postprocedure pulses.<br>7. Sandbag or pressure dressing may be applied to groin. |
| **Renogram (renal scan):** An IV injection of a radioactive nuclide (isotope) followed by use of a scanning device to detect radioactive emissions from the kidney(s); identifies renal blood flow, tubular functions, and renal excretion. | 1. No specific activity or dietary restrictions.<br>2. Explain procedure to client. |

*Continued*

**Appendix 25-1    DIAGNOSTICS OF THE URINARY-RENAL SYSTEM—cont'd**    R̥

| *Procedure* | *Clinical and Nursing Implications* |
|---|---|
| **Cystoscopy:** A direct method to visualize the urethra and bladder by use of a tubular lighted scope (cystoscope). Scope may be inserted via the urethra or percutaneously. | 1. Force fluids or administer fluids intravenously.<br>2. Explain lithotomy position that will be used.<br>3. Client may have general anesthesia or conscious sedation.<br>4. Preoperative medication is given.<br>5. Evaluate urine output after procedure; check for frequency, pink-tinged urine, and burning on urination (these are expected effects and will decrease with time). Bright red blood in urine is not normal, and health care provider should be notified.<br>6. Evaluate for orthostatic hypotension and thrombus formation after the procedure.<br>7. Provide warm sitz baths and mild analgesics to alleviate urethral discomfort. |
| **Bladder scan:** A portable ultrasound scanner used to estimate residual urine in the bladder. | 1. No specific preparation.<br>2. After client voids, apply gel to the suprapubic area, and use scanner to visualize bladder and possible retained urine.<br>3. Make certain that the crosshairs on the aiming icon on the scanner are centered on or over the bladder; if crosshairs are offset, the reading may not be accurate. |
| **Urodynamic Studies**<br>**Cystometrogram (CMG):** A procedure to determine the pressure exerted against the bladder wall by inserting a catheter and instilling water or saline solution; used to evaluate bladder capacity, bladder pressure, and voiding reflexes.<br>**Urethral pressure profile or urethral pressure profilometry (UPP):** Evaluates for urinary incontinence and retention by recording variations of pressure in the urethra.<br>**Urine stream testing:** Evaluates pelvic floor muscle strength. | 1. Assess and evaluate for UTI after procedure.<br>2. Test is often indicated for clients having difficulty with urinary control (e.g., those with spinal cord traumatic injuries, stroke, etc.). |
| **Renal biopsy:** A percutaneous needle biopsy to evaluate renal disease by obtaining a specimen of renal tissue for pathologic examination. Rarely done if client has only one kidney, uncontrolled hypertension, or a bleeding disorder. | 1. Results of blood coagulation studies should be available on the chart before the biopsy procedure.<br>2. Results of IVP or ultrasound studies should be available before the biopsy.<br>3. Immediately after the procedure, pressure dressing is applied to biopsy site and checked frequently for bleeding. Right kidney is the usual biopsy site.<br>4. Assess for gross hematuria, flank pain, or a rise or fall in blood pressure.<br>5. Report pain radiating from the flank area to the abdomen.<br>6. Encourage intake of fluids: 3000 mL per day unless the client has renal insufficiency.<br>7. Bed rest for 24 hours.<br>8. Assess for complication of hemorrhage; may necessitate emergency surgical drainage or nephrectomy.<br>9. Avoid lifting heavy objects for 5–7 days.<br>10. Follow-up with health care provider when anticoagulant drugs can be resumed. |
| **Renal ultrasound examination:** A noninvasive procedure in which ultrasound waves are used, with the aid of a computer, to record images related to tissue density. | 1. Encourage fluids because test requires a full bladder.<br>2. Place in prone position.<br>3. Skin care to remove sonographic gel after procedure. |

*BUN,* Blood urea nitrogen; *GFR,* glomerular filtration rate; *IV,* intravenous; *IVP,* intravenous pyelogram; *KUB,* kidneys, ureters, and bladder; *NPO,* nothing by mouth; *UTI,* urinary tract infection.

**Appendix 25-2 MEDICATIONS FOR THE URINARY SYSTEM**

## Renal Medications

### *General Nursing Implications*
- Encourage intake of 2000 to 3000 mL of fluid per day during treatment.
- Continue medication therapy until all medication has been taken.
- Most medications are better absorbed on an empty stomach, but if GI distress occurs, they may be taken with food.
- Monitor intake and output, as well as symptoms of increasing renal problems.
- Check drug package insert for interactions with anticoagulants.

See Appendix 9-2 for sulfonamide medications for UTI.

| Medications | Side Effects | Nursing Implications |
|---|---|---|
| **Urinary Tract Antiseptics:** These drugs concentrate in the urine and are active against common urinary tract pathogens; they do not affect infections in blood or tissue. | | |
| Nitrofurantoin: PO, IM | GI upset, blood dyscrasia, pulmonary reactions | 1. Requires adequate renal function to concentrate medication in urine. 2. Should not be administered to renal transplant recipients. 3. Will turn the urine brownish orange. 4. Avoid sunlight. |
| **Urinary Analgesics:** Pain relievers typically used on urinary tract mucosa. | | |
| Phenazopyridine hydrochloride: PO Available OTC | Headache, GI disturbances | 1. Contraindicated in renal and liver dysfunction. 2. Advise client to report any yellow discoloration of skin or eyes. 3. Urine will turn orange. 4. Administer with caution in clients with impaired renal function. 5. Can alter dipstick urine results. |
| **Voiding Dysfunction:** Drugs that assist with problems with voiding either related to inability to void or lack of voiding control | | |
| **Muscarinic Receptor Blockers:** Suppress detrusor contractions and enhance bladder storage (drugs with anticholinergic activity). | | |
| Oxybutynin: PO, transdermal | Drowsiness, dizziness, weakness, blurred vision, dry mouth, constipation | 1. Contraindicated in glaucoma, myasthenia gravis, or GI obstruction. 2. Used cautiously in older adults. 3. Can relieve bladder spasms in surgical clients. 4. Monitor intraocular pressure. |
| Tolterodine: PO Solifenacin succinate: PO | Fatigue, headache, dry mouth, dry eyes, constipation | 1. Grapefruit juice can increase blood levels. 2. Caution client to avoid use of alcohol or OTC antihistamines. |
| **Alpha Adrenergic Blockers:** Reduce urethral sphincter resistance to urinary overflow | | |
| Tamsulosin: PO | Headache, dizziness | 1. Caution client about experiencing abnormal ejaculation. 2. Associated with increased incidence of rhinitis. 3. Avoid combining with hypotensive drugs. |
| **Urinary Antispasmodics:** Reduce bladder spasm. | | |
| Belladonna and opium (B&O) suppository | Drowsiness, dry mouth, urinary retention, rapid pulse | 1. Considered a Schedule II drug. 2. Caution with clients with urinary retention issues such as BPH. 3. Contraindicated with glaucoma, hepatic or renal disease, respiratory depression, alcohol, or convulsive disorders. |
| **Glycoprotein Hormones:** Stimulate bone marrow production of RBCs. | | |
| Epoetin alfa: IV, subQ Darbepoetin alfa: IV, subQ | Hypertension, thromboembolic problems, headaches, GI disturbances | 1. Closely evaluate hemodialysis access ports for clotting. 2. Evaluate client for adequate serum iron level, hematocrit, and blood pressure; adequate levels are required for medication to be effective. 3. *Use:* Maintain hemoglobin and hematocrit values in client with renal failure and those who are HIV+ or on chemotherapy. Do not administer if Hgb is 10 (120 g/L) or greater for cancer clients or 11 for renal clients. |

*Continued*

## Immunosuppressive Medications

### General Nursing Implications

- Avoid exposure to infection; wash hands frequently.
- Wear protective clothing; use sunscreen.
- Report any sore throat, fever, or other signs of infection to health care provider.
- Take medication at the same time each day to maintain consistent blood levels.
- No live virus vaccines or immunity-conferring agents should be administered while client is immunosuppressed.
- Depending on level of immunosuppression, client may need protective isolation.

| Medications | Action | Side Effects | Nursing Implications |
|---|---|---|---|
| **Immunosuppressive Medications:** Inhibit the immunologic response. | | | |
| Azathioprine: PO, IV | Inhibits synthesis of T-cell DNA, RNA<br>Blocks metabolism of purines<br>Antiinflammatory properties<br>Used to suppress kidney transplant rejection and treat IBS and RA | Dose- and duration-dependent<br>Bone marrow suppression: leukopenia, thrombocytopenia, anemia<br>Nausea, vomiting, anorexia<br>Alopecia, rash<br>Hepatotoxicity | 1. Interacts with allopurinol, causing an increase in azathioprine toxicity.<br>2. Avoid use in pregnancy.<br>3. Take with food or milk to decrease GI upset.<br>4. Should not be given to client with active infection.<br>5. Follow-up CBC should be done at least monthly while client is taking medication.<br>6. Closely monitor client for development of infections.<br>7. Many drug interactions, including prescribed. |
| Cyclosporine: PO, IV<br>Tacrolimus: IV<br>Methotrexate: PO, IV, IM subQ<br>Cyclophosphamide: PO, IV, IM | Inhibits T-lymphocyte proliferation and function<br>See Appendix 11-1 | Dose- and duration-dependent<br>Infections, nephrotoxicity, hepatotoxicity, hypertension, hirsutism, gum hyperplasia, tremors, blood dyscrasias<br>Side effects of tacrolimus are more toxic than cyclosporine | 1. Monitor renal function because nephrotoxicity occurs frequently.<br>2. Avoid use in pregnancy.<br>3. Use the pipette supplied by manufacturer to measure dose; mix with 4–8 oz (120–236 mL) of water, milk, or juice.<br>4. Evaluate blood pressure and report elevations (especially occurs with heart transplants).<br>5. Monitor liver function studies and monitor BP in clients taking tacrolimus.<br>6. Good oral hygiene should be practiced to reduce gum problems.<br>7. Teach client that he/she should not stop taking the medication or change dosage without physician's order.<br>8. Serum blood levels and CBC are monitored at regular intervals.<br>9. Hirsutism that occurs is reversible.<br>10. Many drug interactions including prescribed and OTC herbal medicines. |
| Antilymphocyte globulin (ALG)<br>Murine monoclonal antilymphocyte therapy<br>Daclizumab | Polyclonal antibody that blocks function of T cell by reacting with T₃ antigen<br>Monoclonal antibody that binds to CD3 receptors and inhibits T-cell proliferation | Fever, chills, tachycardia, hypotension, bronchospasm<br>Aseptic meningitis (murine monoclonal antilymphocyte therapy)<br>GI toxicity (diarrhea, nausea, abdominal pain) | 1. More than 50% of clients experience a fever.<br>2. Have epinephrine and supportive emergency care available because an allergic reaction can occur at any time during therapy.<br>3. Administer slowly over 4–6 hr.<br>4. Client may be premedicated with acetaminophen, diphenhydramine HCl, or methylprednisolone. |
| Methylprednisolone sodium | See Appendix 9-2 | | |

## Appendix 25-2   MEDICATIONS FOR THE URINARY SYSTEM—cont'd

| Medications | Action | Side Effects | Nursing Implications |
|---|---|---|---|
| Tacrolimus | Inhibits T-lymphocyte production | Hepatotoxicity, nephrotoxicity, neurotoxicity, hyperglycemia, seizures, hypertension, GI effects | 1. Monitor blood pressure closely.<br>2. Increases risk for infection.<br>3. Many drug interactions, including prescribed and OTC herbal medicines |
| Sirolimus | Suppresses lymphocyte proliferation; inhibits B cells from synthesizing antibodies | GI toxicity (diarrhea, nausea, vomiting, abdominal pain) | 1. Has synergistic effect with cyclosporine and corticosteroids.<br>2. Avoid grapefruit and grapefruit juice.<br>3. Increases risk for infection.<br>4. Increases cholesterol levels.<br>5. Many drug interactions, including prescribed and OTC herbal medicines |
| Mycophenolate mofetil | Antimetabolite that inhibits DNA and RNA synthesis | Leukopenia, thrombocytopenia, GI (diarrhea, nausea, vomiting), UTI, hypertension, peripheral edema | 1. Usually used in combination with cyclosporine, tacrolimus, sirolimus, or glucocorticoids.<br>2. Give on an empty stomach.<br>3. Many drug interactions, including prescribed. |

*CBC,* Complete blood count; *DNA,* deoxyribonucleic acid; *GI,* gastrointestinal; *Hgb,* hemoglobin; *HIV+,* human immunodeficiency virus–positive; *IBS,* irritable bowel syndrome; *IL-2,* interleukin 2; *IV,* intravenous; *PO,* by mouth (orally); *RA,* rheumatoid arthritis; *RNA,* ribonucleic acid; *subQ,* subcutaneously; *UTI,* urinary tract infection.

## Appendix 25-3   URINARY DIVERSION

A urinary diversion is a means of diverting urinary output from the bladder to an external device or via a new avenue.

### Temporary Urinary Diversion

*Nephrostomy tubes (catheters):* Insertion of catheters into the renal pelvis by surgical incision or percutaneous puncture. A small catheter is inserted into the renal pelvis and attached via connecting tubing to a closed-system drainage. Nephrostomy tubes may be temporary or permanent.

#### Nursing Implications

1. Provide routine nephrostomy tube care, with sterile dressing changes and tube flushing (if ordered).
2. Complications: Infection and secondary renal calculus formation; erosion of the duct by the catheter.

*Ureteral catheters:* Small, narrow catheters placed through the ureters into the renal pelvis; drain each renal pelvis individually. Often client also has a urinary retention catheter draining the urinary bladder. The catheter splints the ureters during healing and prevents edema from occluding the ureter.

#### Nursing Implications

1. Check frequently for placement of ureteral catheters; tension should be avoided.
2. Ureteral catheter should not be clamped or irrigated.
3. Maintain accurate intake and output records and label all catheters.

### Incontinent Urinary Diversion

*Ileal conduit (ileal loop):* Transplantation of ureters into a segment of ileum or colon, which is then brought to the abdomen; a stoma is then constructed. This type of urinary diversion is permanent (Figure 25-8).

#### Nursing Implications

1. Stoma site is marked before surgery because a device must be worn continuously.

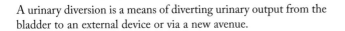

# URINARY DIVERSIONS

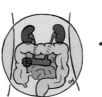 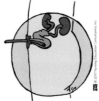

Ileal loop          Continent urinary diversion

**FIGURE 25-8   Urinary Diversions.** (From Zerwekh, J., Garneau, A., & Miller, C. J. [2017]. *Digital collection of the memory notebooks of nursing* [4th ed.]. Chandler, AZ: Nursing Education Consultants, Inc.)

2. Mucus is present in the urine after surgery when ileum segment is used; encourage a high fluid intake to flush the ileal conduit.
3. Maintain meticulous skin care and changing of appliances.
4. Provide discharge instructions in regard to symptoms of obstruction, infection, and care of the ostomy; client needs information relating to purchase of supplies, ostomy clubs, follow-up visits, enterostomal therapists, and the importance of not irrigating the ileal conduit.

### Continent Urinary Diversion

*Kock, Mainz, Indiana, or Florida pouch:* A segment of the bowel is made into a reservoir; client is taught to use a catheter to drain the pouch and maintain continence (see Figure 25-8). The main difference among the diversions is the segment of intestine utilized (ileum, ileocecal segment, or colon).

*Continued*

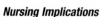

## Appendix 25-3   URINARY DIVERSION—cont'd

### Nursing Implications

1. Client will not need to wear an appliance but will need to self-catheterize every 4 to 6 hours.
2. A small bandage/pouch may be worn to collect any mucus drainage or small leaks.
3. Continuous assessment of status of skin around stoma.
4. Client should understand how to care for the stoma before he or she leaves the hospital:
   - Know continent diversion functions and how to prevent complications.

- Increase fluid intake.
- Contact health care provider if there are changes in the color of the stoma or if urine becomes dark and foul smelling.

5. A catheter will be inserted into the reservoir every 4 to 6 hours to drain urine.

## Appendix 25-4   NURSING PROCEDURE: URINE SPECIMEN COLLECTION

### ✓ KEY POINTS:  Random Sample

- May be collected at any time.
- Client may be specifically ordered to collect first voided specimen or to collect sample on second voiding.

### ✓ KEY POINTS:  Clean Catch and Midstream

- Specimen is collected for culture and sensitivity.
- Cleanse urinary meatus before specimen collection.
- For midstream collection, tell client to start the urinary stream and collect the specimen after voiding has begun. Regardless of how well the urinary meatus is cleansed, the specimen must be a midstream collection or the specimen will be contaminated with the bacteria in the urethra.

### ✓ KEY POINTS:  Catheterized Specimen

- Straight in-and-out catheterization to obtain sample for culture.

- Procedure is discouraged because of introduction of bacteria and irritation, producing a urinary tract infection. More common in infants and children and those unable to provide a midstream specimen.

### ✓ KEY POINTS:  12- to 24-Hour Collection

- When the collection time is started, have the client void, discard the urine, and start the collection with the next voiding.
- Mark the collection container and collect the urine over the prescribed time frame.
- When the time frame is completed, have the client void again, add it to the specimen collection, and send to laboratory for evaluation.

**TEST ALERT:** Collection of urine specimens is a common nursing action; be sure to know why the sample is being obtained and the type of diagnostic test for which it is being collected.

## Appendix 25-5   NURSING PROCEDURE: URINARY CATHETERIZATION

### ✓ KEY POINTS:  Insertion of a Retention Catheter

- A sterile procedure.
- Lubricate catheter with sterile lubricant provided in tray.
- Do not test balloon with fluid prior to insertion of the catheter.

**TEST ALERT:** Insert a urinary catheter.

- Cleanse the meatus:

**For a Female**
1. Cleanse the meatus with sterile cotton ball held in forceps; use one downward stroke of the forceps.
2. Repeat at least three to four times using new sterile cotton ball each time.
3. Continue to hold the labia apart until you insert the lubricated catheter.
4. When urine appears, advance the catheter another 1 to 2 inches (2.5–5 cm).

**For a Male**
1. Hold the penis upright. Hold the sides of the penis to prevent closing the urethra.

2. Cleanse the meatus in a circular motion from urinary meatus to glans with sterile cotton ball held in forceps; use one downward stroke of the forceps.
3. Repeat at least three to four times.
4. Continue to hold the penis until you insert the catheter.
5. Insert the catheter 1 to 2 inches (2.5–5 cm) beyond the point at which urine begins to flow. Inserting the catheter farther into the bladder ensures it is beyond the neck of the bladder.
6. Instill sterile water into balloon after catheter is inserted.
   - Anchor the catheter.
   *For a Female:* Anchor or tape catheter to the side of the leg.
   *For a Male:* Anchor or tape catheter to the thigh or abdomen with penis positioned toward chest, to prevent pressure on the penoscrotal angle.
- Attach drainage bag to bed frame (not side rails) so that it hangs freely and below the level of the catheter.

### ✓ KEY POINTS:  Providing Catheter Care

- Maintain external cleanliness around the catheter; wash thoroughly with mild soap and water when soiled—or two or three times every 24 hours.

**Appendix 25-5** NURSING PROCEDURE: URINARY CATHETERIZATION—cont'd

- Maintain closed system. Do not allow urine to flow from the bag or tubing back into the bladder.
- Encourage high fluid intake to maintain constant flow of urine. Increased flow of urine inhibits the upward movement of bacteria.

✓ **KEY POINT: In the home setting, intermittent catheterization may be used.**

- The correct technique is a clean technique where good hand-washing with soap and water is key to preventing infections.

✓ **KEY POINTS: Removal of a Catheter**

- Clamp catheter.
- Do not cut the catheter with a scissors. Balloon may not totally deflate if cut.
- Withdraw fluid from balloon (usually 5–10 mL water in balloon.)
- Pull gently on catheter to ensure balloon is deflated before attempting to remove. Damage to the urethra can occur if balloon is not totally deflated. If the catheter has been in place for longer than 10 days, reinflate the balloon after removal to assess for degradation.
- Record output on intake and output (I&O) bedside record.
- Wash perineum with soap and water. Dry thoroughly.
- Instruct client to drink fluids as tolerated and observe for signs and symptoms of urinary tract infection (burning, frequency, urgency).
- Offer bedpan or urinal at least every 2 to 3 hours after removing catheter, until voiding occurs. Keep accurate I&O record.

**Clinical Tips for Problem Solving**

1. If catheter is inserted in the vagina of female client:
   - Leave the catheter in place so you do not reintroduce a new catheter into the vaginal area. Obtain a new catheter and sterile gloves.
   - If sterile field has been contaminated, obtain a whole new kit.
2. If unable to insert catheter into male client:
   - Obtain a new catheter kit.
     a. Hold penis vertical to the body.
     b. Insert catheter while applying slight traction by gently pulling upward on the shaft of the penis.
     c. If you encounter resistance, rotate the catheter, increase the traction, and change the angle of the penis slightly. May consider using a Coude catheter. Problems may be noted more in older male adults or those with BPH.
     d. When urine begins to flow, lower the penis.
3. If pain occurs during inflation of balloon:
   - Remove any injected water and insert the catheter farther into the bladder.
4. If urine exceeds 1000 mL with catheterization:
   - Clamp catheter for 20 to 30 minutes and then unclamp.
5. If catheter comes out with balloon still inserted:
   - Assess client for signs of urethral trauma (i.e., bleeding, pain).
   - Obtain a new catheter and repeat the catheterization procedure, making sure that the balloon is inflated with at least 10 mL water.
   - Monitor urine output for bleeding.

## Study Questions
## Urinary-Renal: Care of Adult and Pediatric Clients

More questions on

1. The client has had a right nephrostomy tube placed after a nephrolithotomy for removal of a kidney stone. When the client returns to the room, what is a priority nursing action?
   1. Irrigate the tube with 30 mL of normal saline solution four times a day.
   2. Clamp the tube if drainage is excessive.
   3. Advance the tube 1 inch every 8 hours.
   4. Ensure that the tube is draining freely.

2. The nurse is infusing dialysate during peritoneal dialysis. What is a nursing action to make the client more comfortable at this time?
   1. Increase the rate of flow.
   2. Raise the head of the bed.
   3. Turn the client from side to side.
   4. Refrigerate the fluid before infusion.

3. A client has had a kidney stone removed, and the nurse instructs him in measures to decrease kidney stone formation in the future. Which statement by the client indicates to the nurse that he understood the teaching?
   1. "I can continue to drink soda if it is sugar free."
   2. "I should consume at least 3000 mL of fluid daily."
   3. "I should report nocturia that occurs once a night."
   4. "I will ingest megadoses of vitamins C and D daily."

4. The nurse understands that the following clinical findings are indications for dialysis. **Select all that apply.**
   1. Volume overload
   2. Blood urea nitrogen level of 18 mg/dL (6.43 mmol/L)
   3. Potassium level of 6.8 mEq/L (mmol/L)
   4. Glomerular filtration rate of 25 mL/min
   5. Metabolic acidosis
   6. Creatinine level of 5.0 mg/dL (442.0 umol/L)

5. A client in kidney failure is to have a serum blood urea nitrogen level determined. What will this diagnostic test measure?
   1. Concentration of the urine osmolarity and electrolytes
   2. Serum level of the end products of protein metabolism
   3. Ability of the kidneys to concentrate urine
   4. Levels of C-reactive protein to determine inflammation

6. A client with chronic kidney disease has an internal venous access site for hemodialysis on their left forearm. What action will the nurse take to protect this access site?
   1. Irrigate with heparin and normal saline solution every 8 hours.
   2. Apply warm moist packs to the area after hemodialysis.
   3. Do not use the left arm to take blood pressure readings.
   4. Keep the arm elevated above the level of the heart.

7. What nursing measure would be included in the plan of care for a client with acute kidney injury?
   1. Observe for signs of a secondary infection.
   2. Provide a high-protein, low-carbohydrate diet.
   3. In-and-out catheterization for residual urine
   4. Encourage fluids to 2000 mL in 24 hours.

8. What will the nurse identify as the goal of treatment for a client with chronic renal insufficiency?
   1. Increase the urine output by increasing liver and renal perfusion.
   2. Prevent the loss of electrolytes across the basement membrane.
   3. Increase the concentration of electrolytes in the urine.
   4. Maintain present renal function and decrease renal workload.

9. The nurse is discussing the prevention of urinary tract infections with a female client. What would be important to include in the discussion?
   1. Decrease fluid intake to decrease burning on urination.
   2. Take warm sitz baths with a mild bubble bath.
   3. Avoid spermicides with nonoxynol-9.
   4. Drink only acidic fluids such as orange juice.

10. At 9:00 a.m. a 24-hour (composite) urine collection is started. What instructions will the nurse provide to the client?
    1. Place the first voided specimen in the container and continue to collect the urine until 9:00 a.m. the following day.
    2. Discard the first morning specimen, collect urine for the next 24 hours, and make sure to void before the collection is completed at 9:00 a.m. the following day.
    3. Discard the first morning specimen because it may contain concentrated abnormal components.
    4. Collect all urine from 9:00 a.m. onward in separate containers that are labeled for time and amount of voiding.

11. Which nursing observations indicate that a male client with a kidney stone is experiencing renal colic?
    1. Severe flank pain radiating toward the testicles
    2. Stress incontinence with full bladder
    3. Hematuria and severe burning on urination
    4. Enuresis with hyperalbuminuria

12. The nurse is evaluating a client's response to hemodialysis. Which laboratory values will indicate the dialysis was effective? **Select all that apply.**
    1. Serum potassium level decreases from 5.4 to 4.6 mEq/L. (5.4 to 4.6 mmol/L)
    2. Serum creatinine level decreases from 1.6 to 0.8 mg/dL. (111.44-70.72 umol/L)
    3. Hemoglobin increases from 10 to 12 g/dL. (100-120 g/L)
    4. White blood cells increase from 5000 to 8000/mm3. (5.00-8.00 × 109/L)
    5. BUN decreases from 110 to 90 mg/dL. (39.27-32.13 mmol/L)

13. Which are signs and symptoms of cystitis? **Select all that apply.**
    1. Increased bladder capacity
    2. Frequency
    3. Dysuria
    4. Nocturia
    5. Urgency
    6. Polydipsia

14. A client with chronic kidney disease has been prescribed calcium carbonate. What is the rationale for this particular medication?
    1. Diminishes incidence of gastric ulcer formation
    2. Alleviates constipation
    3. Binds with phosphorus to lower concentrations
    4. Increases tubular reabsorption of sodium

15. Which is an appropriate nursing action for a child with acute glomerulonephritis?
    1. Initiating contact isolation precautions
    2. Encouraging increased fluid intake
    3. Encouraging ambulation, as tolerated
    4. Providing a fluid-restricted, low-sodium diet

16. The nurse understands that a client may experience pain during peritoneal dialysis because of which of the following? **Select all that apply.**
    1. Warming the dialysate solution before administration
    2. Too-rapid instillation of the dialysate
    3. Infiltration of solution into the bloodstream
    4. Increased intraabdominal pressure
    5. Too-rapid outflow rate of the dialysate solution

17. What is significant about the development of proteinuria in a client with type 1 diabetes mellitus?
    1. Chronic kidney disease may eventually develop.
    2. It indicates that the client's diabetes is uncontrolled.
    3. Serum creatinine will diminish as albuminuria increases.
    4. Insulin maintenance dose should be lowered.

18. A client with acute kidney injury develops severe hyperkalemia. What prescription would the nurse anticipate?
    1. Furosemide
    2. Calcium carbonate
    3. 50% glucose and regular insulin
    4. Epoetin alfa

19. During peritoneal dialysis treatment, the nurse continually evaluates the client for poor dialysate flow. How will this complication be identified?
    1. Increased urine albumin level
    2. Decreased plasma osmolality
    3. An increase in sodium transfer to serum
    4. Outflow is intermittent

20. Which client is at the highest risk for developing chronic kidney disease?
    1. Client with severe acute glomerulonephritis
    2. Client with placenta previa and hemorrhage at delivery
    3. Client with poorly controlled long-term hypertension
    4. Client who received IV aminoglycosides for an infection

## Answers to Study Questions

**1.** *4*
Failure of the tube to drain freely can result in pain, trauma, wound dehiscence, and infection. If an irrigation is ordered for a nephrostomy tube, no more than 5 mL of sterile normal saline should be gently instilled. (Lewis et al., 10 ed., p. 1062)

**2.** *3*
Movement of the client will help disseminate the fluid throughout the abdomen. The fluid should be instilled within the prescribed period of time; therefore, the dialysate flow should not be decreased. Raising the head of the bed will make the client more uncomfortable and increase intraabdominal pressure. The solutions should be infused at body temperature. (Lewis et al., 10 ed., p. 1085)

**3.** *2*
A high fluid intake will help keep solutes diluted, thus preventing kidney stone formation. Drinking soda (diet or otherwise) is not the best method of increasing urine output. Nocturia and vitamins C and D are not relevant to kidney stones. (Lewis et al., 10 ed. pp. 1045–1046)

**4.** *1, 3, 5, 6*
Indications for dialysis include volume overload, weight gain, hyperkalemia, metabolic acidosis, and rising BUN (10–20 mg/dL [3.57–7.14 mmol/L]) and serum creatinine (0.5–1.5 mg/dL [44.2–132.6 umol/L]) levels, along with decreased GFR rate (less that 15 mL/min). A potassium level of 6.8 is hyperkalemia, and a BUN of 18 mg/dL (6.43 mmol/L) is within normal range. (Lewis et al., 10 ed., p. 1084)

**5.** *2*
Urea is an end product of protein metabolism. In kidney failure, the kidneys cannot clear all of the urea from the blood, and the creatinine and BUN level will be elevated. The C-reactive protein is a diagnostic test used in assessing clients with inflammatory bowel disease, rheumatoid arthritis, autoimmune diseases, and pelvic inflammatory disease (PID). A specific gravity test of the urine would assess the ability of the kidneys to concentrate urine. The urine osmolarity (concentration of particles in urine) and electrolytes assess fluid balance. The kidneys play an important role in the balance of electrolytes and fluids. (Lewis et al., 10 ed., p. 1024)

**6.** *3*
Protect the arm with the functioning shunt. No blood pressure readings should be taken from that arm, and there should be no needlesticks. The access is not irrigated with heparin. (Lewis et al., 10 ed., p. 1087)

**7.** *1*
Secondary infections are the cause of death in 50% to 90% of clients with acute renal failure. A low-protein diet is most often offered. Catheterizations are avoided. Fluids may be limited if the client is in acute kidney injury. (Lewis et al., 10 ed., pp. 1073–1075)

**8.** *4*
The goal in chronic kidney disease is to prevent acute failure and maintain whatever function is left. This is best done by minimizing stress and the workload on the kidneys. Increasing liver perfusion does not affect renal function. Until the renal function improves, there will be increased permeability in the basement membrane and electrolyte concentration in the urine will be diminished because solutes are being retrained rather than excreted. (Lewis et al., 10 ed., p. 1083)

**9.** *3*
The use of nonoxynol-9 spermicides can be irritating to the urinary tract and lead to infections. UTIs in women can be prevented by urination before and after sexual intercourse. Fluid intake should be increased, and no soap should be added to the sitz bath. (Lewis et al., 10 ed., p. 1036)

**10.** *2*
The first specimen is discarded before the collection is started. Collection will continue until the completed time frame; the client should void before the collection is completed. (Lewis et al., 10 ed., p. 1024)

**11.** *1*
The most characteristic symptom of renal colic is sudden, severe pain. The client may also exhibit nausea and vomiting, pallor, and diaphoresis during the acute pain episode. Hematuria and burning on urination are associated with UTIs, although there may be some bleeding with the passage of the renal stone. (Lewis et al., 10 ed., p. 1045)

**12.** *1, 2, 5*
Primary action of hemodialysis is to clear nitrogenous waste products. The creatinine and BUN provide a measure of how effective the dialysate was in removing the waste products. Electrolytes are altered with a decrease in potassium. Hemoglobin, white blood cells, and sedimentation rate are not affected, these cells are too large to diffuse through the pores of the dialysate membrane. (Lewis et al., 10 ed., p. 1084)

**13.** *2, 3, 4, 5*
Classic signs of cystitis include frequency, urgency, decreased bladder capacity, nocturia, and dysuria caused by the inflammatory process. Polydipsia (excessive thirst) is associated with diabetes mellitus. (Lewis et al., 10 ed., p. 1034)

**14.** *3*
Clients with chronic kidney disease have hypocalcemia and hyperphosphatemia. Clients are prescribed calcium-based phosphate binders, such as calcium acetate or calcium carbonate to improve excretion of phosphorus. (Lewis et al., 10 ed., p. 1079)

**15.** *4*
For individuals with acute glomerulonephritis, edema is treated by restricting sodium and fluid intake and by administration of diuretics. Isolation is not required because this is an autoimmune problem. Although ambulation is not incorrect for the child, it is best to encourage rest periods and focus on ways to allow the kidneys to repair and restore themselves. (Lewis et al., 10 ed., p. 1042)

**16.** *2, 4*
Rapid instillation of dialysate fluid and accumulation of the fluid within the abdomen can lead to pain and discomfort. Warming the

dialysate solution helps in the clearance and may diminish any cold sensation of fluid entering the body. It will also assist to diminish any cold sensation of fluid entering the body. The dialysate fluid does not infiltrate and enter the circulatory system. Rapid outflow of dialysate does not cause pain. (Lewis et al., 10 ed., pp. 1084–1086)

**17.** *1*

Diabetic nephropathy is the primary cause of end-stage kidney failure. A microscopic amount of albumin in the urine is one of the earliest indications of kidney abnormality and is asymptomatic, which is the purpose of annual albumin-to-creatinine ratios being collected on random urine samples for albumin. Control of hypertension is paramount to delaying the progression of nephropathy. Serum creatinine elevates along with the increased albumin in the urine. Measure of diabetic control is the $HbA_{1c}$ laboratory test. Insulin therapy should not be altered due to proteinuria. (Lewis et al., 10 ed., p. 1079)

**18.** *3*

Hyperkalemia can develop into an emergency situation (cardiac arrest). It is important to quickly move the potassium back into the cells by administering 50% glucose and regular insulin, usually in conjunction with some type of base to correct the acidosis, such as sodium bicarbonate or calcium gluconate given intravenously. Insulin assists in the movement of potassium into the cells and helps to reduce the serum potassium level. Calcium

carbonate is used for the treatment of hyperphosphatemia that occurs with chronic kidney disease. Procrit is used for the treatment of anemia caused by a decrease in erythropoietin production by the kidneys. A diuretic, such as Lasix, may lead to a loss of potassium, but the rate is too slow. (Lewis et al., 10 ed., p. 1)

**19.** *4*

Outflow should be a continuous stream after the clamp is opened (end of dwell time). Constipation, kinked or clamped connection tubing, client's position, or catheter displacement can lead to poor dialysate flow. Sodium is often evaluated once daily but not in correlation with the outflow of the dialysate. Typically, the client does not have sufficient urine output for a fractional urine, which is a urine specimen collected that has a separate examination for different solutes (glucose, acetone, etc.). Serum plasma osmolarity does not give an indication of poor outflow. (Lewis et al., 10 ed. p. 1086)

**20.** *3*

Long-term hypertension and diabetes are the leading causes of chronic kidney disease. The client with placenta previa and hemorrhage is at risk for developing acute kidney injury. Acute glomerulonephritis may decrease renal function but seldom to the point of chronic kidney disease, as most clients recover. Aminoglycosides can be nephrotoxic and cause damage (acute kidney injury), but chronic kidney disease is not common. (Lewis et al., 10 ed., p. 1083)

# CHAPTER TWENTY-SIX

# Maternity Nursing Care

# 26

## PRIORITY CONCEPTS

Development, Reproduction, Safety, Sexuality

## ANTEPARTUM

## FAMILY PLANNING

 **Infertility**

**Infertility is the inability to conceive a child after a year or more of regular unprotected intercourse or the inability to carry a pregnancy to live birth (recurrent miscarriages).**

### Assessment

A. Causes of infertility.
  1. Male.
    a. Coital difficulties, testicular abnormalities.
    b. Semen factors—low semen, autoantibodies.
    c. Structural abnormalities.
  2. Female.
    a. Hormonal dysfunction, structural abnormalities.
    b. Coital factors: use of lubricants or douches that change the pH and may cause infection.
    c. Chronic pelvic and vaginal infections.
    d. Isoimmunization to sperm: development of antibodies.
B. Diagnostics.
  1. Male.
    a. Complete history and physical examination; laboratory studies such as thyroid function tests and other endocrine tests may be ordered.
    b. Complete semen analysis.

> **NURSING PRIORITY:** Two or more abnormal samples must be obtained before a definitive diagnosis is made. Semen collections should be repeated at least 72 hours apart to allow for new germ cell maturation.

  2. Female.
    a. Complete history and physical examination: includes routine complete blood count, urinalysis, serologic studies, thyroid function studies, sedimentation rate, chest x-ray film, and Papanicolaou (Pap) smear.
      (1) Hormonal assay of luteinizing hormone (LH; value is greatest at midcycle) or progesterone (peaks 8 days after the LH surge).

      (2) Clomiphene citrate challenge test (CCCT): determines ovarian reserves; fewer eggs means less responsiveness to follicle-stimulating hormone (FSH).
    b. Recording of basal body temperature (BBT) and cervical mucus to document ovulation.
      (1) BBT drops and then rises about 1° after ovulation.

> **NURSING PRIORITY:** Actual release of ovum occurs around 24 to 36 hours before the first temperature elevation; BBT does not predict ovulation; it only indicates that it has occurred.

      (2) A suggestion to couples for intercourse based on serial BBTs would be to recommend sexual intercourse every other day in the period beginning 3 to 4 days before and continuing for 2 to 3 days after the expected time of ovulation.
    c. Cervical mucus method.
      (1) Cervical mucus is thin, clear, profuse, watery, alkaline, and stringy at the time of ovulation.
      (2) Supplemental estrogen therapy 6 days before ovulation enhances the development of *spinnbarkeit*, which means elasticity of the cervical mucus.
      (3) *Ferning* is noted on a microscopic slide and is caused by an increase in sodium chloride that crystallizes when the mucus dries on the slide.
    d. Postcoital test.
      (1) Conducted at time of ovulation, within several hours after coitus to obtain a cervical mucus specimen; not as acceptable as in the past as a reliable test.
      (2) Purpose is to determine sperm survival and motility along with the characteristics of cervical mucus.
    e. Tubal patency tests: hysterosalpingography or hysterogram and laparoscopy.
    f. Endometrial biopsy – obtained 2 to 3 days before menses.
C. Treatment.
  1. Male.
    a. Administration of immunosuppressants, and sperm washing-dilution insemination techniques.
    b. Artificial insemination.

2. Female.
   a. Treat infections with antibiotics.
   b. Administration of fertility medications.
      (1) Clomiphene.
         (a) Administration: client takes it daily for 5 days, beginning on day 5 of the menstrual cycle; supplemental low-dose estrogen is usually given concurrently.
         (b) Side effects: vasomotor flushes, abdominal discomfort, breast tenderness, nausea, vomiting.
      (2) Human menopausal gonadotropin (hMg): used when clomiphene fails to stimulate ovulation.
         (a) Administration: given intramuscularly every day for varying periods of time during the first half of the cycle.
         (b) Couple advised to have intercourse on the day the woman receives hMg and for the next 2 days.
      (3) Metformin: an insulin-sensitizing agent may be given to women who have polycystic ovarian disease (PCOS), which induces ovulation. May be given with clomiphene.

> **⚠ NURSING PRIORITY:** The use of fertility drugs may lead to a multiple birth rate.

### Nursing Interventions

**Goal** To assist with the assessment and treatment of the couple's specific infertility problem.

A. Provide information regarding the normal functioning of the male and female reproductive systems.
B. Thoroughly explain specific examinations and diagnostic procedures to decrease anxiety and fear.

**Goal:** To provide emotional support and encourage expression of feelings connected with infertility.

A. Promote expression of feelings related to sexuality, self-esteem, and body image.
B. Assess for common reactions of surprise, denial, anger, and guilt.

C. Promote a variety of coping strategies to help deal with the uncomfortable feelings.
D. Explore alternatives such as adoption.
E. Refer to supportive community agencies.

## Contraception

**Contraception is the voluntary prevention of pregnancy. Two important factors influence the selection of the particular type of contraceptive method: acceptability and effectiveness.**

> **TEST ALERT:** Determine client's attitude toward and use of birth control methods and consider contraindications to chosen contraceptive method.

### Assessment

A. Types of contraception.
   1. Temporary contraception: methods used to delay or avoid pregnancy.
   2. Permanent: voluntary sterilization.
B. Contraceptive methods (see Appendix 26-1).

## Genetic Counseling

A. Definitions.
   1. Genetic (hereditary): describes any disorder or disease that is transmitted from generation to generation.
   2. Congenital: describes any disorder present at birth or existing before birth that is caused by genetic or environmental factors or both.
B. Patterns of inheritance (Figure 26-1).
   1. Autosomal recessive: examples are cystic fibrosis, phenylketonuria (PKU), sickle cell anemia, Tay-Sachs disease, galactosemia, maple syrup urine disease.
   2. Autosomal dominant: examples are Huntington disease, Marfan syndrome, neurofibromatosis.
   3. X-linked recessive: examples are hemophilia, Duchenne muscular dystrophy, color blindness.
   4. X-linked dominant: examples are vitamin D–resistant rickets and fragile X syndrome (FXS).

### Assessment

A. Families at risk.
   1. Maternal factors.
      a. Increased age.

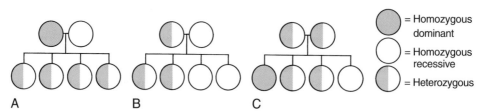

**FIGURE 26-1 Possible Offspring in Three Types of Matings. (A)** Homozygous-dominant parent and homozygous-recessive parent. Children all heterozygous, displaying dominant trait. **(B)** Heterozygous parent and homozygous-recessive parent. Children 50% heterozygous, displaying dominant trait; 50% homozygous, displaying recessive trait. **(C)** Both parents heterozygous. Children 25% homozygous, displaying dominant trait; 25% homozygous, displaying recessive trait; 50% heterozygous, displaying dominant trait. (From Lowdermilk, D. L., & Perry S. E. [2016]. *Maternity and women's health care* [11th ed.]. St. Louis, MO: Mosby.)

b. Presence of disease (e.g., diabetes mellitus, epilepsy).

c. Reproductive history of spontaneous abortions, stillbirths, or birth defects in previous children.

2. Family history (e.g., Huntington chorea, hemophilia, spina bifida).

3. Ethnicity/racial background (e.g., sickle cell trait, Tay-Sachs disease).

B. Diagnostics.

1. Prenatal detection: amniocentesis, chorionic villus sampling (CVS), percutaneous umbilical blood sampling (PUBS), maternal alpha-fetoprotein.

2. Postdelivery detection.

a. Most institutions screen for inborn errors of metabolism; these tests all use the same dried blood spot. Many states screen for inborn errors in metabolism. Examples include PKU testing, galactosemia, hypothyroidism, sickle cell anemia, maple syrup urine disease, homocystinuria, biotinidase deficiency. The list of "screenable" tests will certainly increase as technology improves.

b. Cytologic studies: detect chromosome abnormalities.

c. Dermatoglyphics.

(1) The assessment of the dermal ridges in the palm, toes, or soles of feet.

(2) Characteristic palm creases: simian line (Down syndrome).

### Nursing Interventions

**Goal:** To allow families to make informed decisions about reproduction.

A. Assist with detailed family history and pedigree chart.

B. Determine family's understanding of the information.

**Goal:** To provide information about available diagnostic tests and treatment.

A. Be precise and give detailed information.

B. Use familiar examples to illustrate probability of specific risks (e.g., flipping coins).

C. Emphasize the importance of making an informed decision.

**Goal:** To reduce incidence and impact of genetic disease by identifying families at risk and making appropriate referrals.

A. Refer to specific agencies (e.g., Cystic Fibrosis Foundation, Muscular Dystrophy Association) or a genetic counseling service.

B. Provide alternatives to childbearing such as adoption and artificial insemination.

## FETAL AND MATERNAL ASSESSMENT TESTING

### Amniocentesis

**An invasive procedure performed on the mother to obtain amniotic fluid.**

A. An outpatient procedure performed at 14 to 16 weeks of pregnancy, although it may be performed later in the

**Table 26-1  GENETIC TESTING EXAMPLES**

| *Disease* | *Test (Amniotic Fluid Sample)* |
|---|---|
| Cystic fibrosis | Decreased amounts of 4-methylumbelliferyl guanidinobenzoate (MUGB) reactive proteases |
| Neural tube defects: Anencephaly Spina bifida | Elevated maternal serum alpha-fetoprotein (MSAFP) level; decreased level may indicate Down syndrome |

pregnancy for genetic testing if an ultrasound shows an anomaly.

B. Procedure: placenta is located by ultrasound examination; a needle is inserted through the abdomen (puncture site has been anesthetized); amniotic fluid is aspirated and sent to the laboratory for testing.

1. Indications for amniocentesis: increased maternal age, history of child with a genetic defect, mother carrying an X-linked disease, or history of either parent carrying a chromosomal abnormality (Table 26-1).

2. Complications: unlikely (less than 1% of the cases), although possible; some mild discomfort at the needle site or, rarely, abdominal wall hematoma; risk for miscarriage.

a. For Rh-negative women, $Rh_o(D)$ immune globulin (also referred to as RhoGAM) is administered after the amniocentesis to prevent hemolysis of fetal blood cells.

3. Maturity studies.

a. Lecithin/sphingomyelin (L/S) ratio: the components of phospholipid protein substance that comprise surfactant; L/S ratio of 2:1 or greater is indicative of sufficient surfactant (occurs around 35 weeks' gestation).

**⊞ NURSING PRIORITY:** The fetal heart rate (FHR) is assessed before and after amniocentesis.

### Ultrasonography

**Ultrasonography is a noninvasive technique in which high-frequency pulse sound waves are transmitted by a transducer applied transvaginally or directly to the woman's abdomen.**

A. Purpose.

1. Identifies placental location for amniocentesis or to determine placenta previa.

2. Determines gestational age by crown–rump length (first trimester); later, gestational age is determined by biparietal diameter.

3. Detects fetal anomalies: hydrocephalus, myelomeningocele, anencephaly.

4. Detects multiple gestations.

5. Monitors fetal growth to assess for intrauterine growth restriction (IUGR).

6. Evaluates volume of amniotic fluid.

B. Procedure (abdominal).
1. Procedure may be done anytime during pregnancy.
2. Performed with a full bladder, except when ultrasonography is used to localize the placenta before amniocentesis.
3. Requires approximately 20 to 30 minutes to perform; client must lie flat on her back, which may be uncomfortable.
C. Transvaginal is better tolerated because client is in lithotomy position and full bladder is not required.

## Chorionic Villus Sampling

**Chorionic villus sampling is a method of obtaining fetal tissue for genetic testing.**

A. Purpose: to obtain fetal tissue to establish a genetic profile as a first-trimester alternative to amniocentesis; use is declining due to increased availability of noninvasive screening techniques.
B. Procedure.
1. An invasive procedure performed with the use of ultrasound guidance between 10 and 12 weeks' gestation; technique may be transcervical or transabdominal.
2. Allows for earlier diagnosis of genetic defects than does amniocentesis.
3. Early sampling (8 to 9 weeks' gestation) has been associated with an increased incidence of limb defects.
4. Administer $Rh_o(D)$ immune globulin to Rh-negative mothers because of possibility of fetal-maternal hemorrhage.

## Percutaneous Umbilical Blood Sampling

**An invasive procedure, also called cordocentesis, PUBS is fetal blood sampling performed during the second and third trimesters.**

A. Purpose: most widely used method for fetal blood sampling and transfusion.
B. Procedure.
1. Insertion of a needle directly into a fetal umbilical vessel under ultrasound guidance.
2. Umbilical cord is punctured 1 to 2 cm from its insertion into the placenta.
3. Continuous FHR monitoring for up to 2 hours after procedure to ensure that bleeding or hematoma formation did not occur.

## Daily Fetal Movement Count

**A simple activity performed by the mother is to count daily fetal movement, also called "kick counts."**

A. Purpose: to monitor the fetus when there may be complications affecting fetal oxygenation (e.g., preeclampsia, diabetes).
B. Procedure.
1. Count all fetal movements within a 12-hour period until a minimum of 10 movements are counted or count fetal activity 2 to 3 times daily (after meals and before bed) for 2 hours until 10 movements are counted.
2. Any change in fetal activity, either an increase or a decrease, should be reported to the health care provider.
3. *Fetal alarm signal:* no fetal movements during a 12-hour period.

> **NURSING PRIORITY:** Alcohol, depressant medications, and smoking temporarily reduce fetal movement, and obesity decreases the woman's ability to assess fetal movement. Fetal movement is not felt during fetal sleep cycle, and the movements *do not* decrease as the woman nears term.

## Nonstress Test (NST)

**This is a test to observe the response of the FHR to the stress of activity.**

A. Procedure.
1. Requires approximately 20 minutes; client is placed in semi-Fowler's position; external monitor is applied to document fetal activity; mother activates the "mark button" on the electronic fetal monitor when she feels fetal movement.
2. The client may be asked to drink orange juice or eat a light meal because an increased blood glucose level may increase fetal activity.
B. Interpretation.
1. Reactive: shows two or more fetal heart rate accelerations of 15 beats/min or more lasting at least 15 seconds for each acceleration within 20 minutes of beginning the test; indicates a healthy fetus; test may be rescheduled, as indicated by condition ($15 \times 15$ criteria is for a fetus at least 32 weeks' gestation).
2. Nonreactive: reactive criteria are not met. The accelerations are less than two in number, the accelerations are less than 15 beats/min, or there are no accelerations. If nonreactive, then the test is extended another 20 minutes; if the tracing becomes reactive, the NST is concluded. If the NST is still nonreactive after a second 20-minute trial (total of 40 minutes), then additional testing, such as a biophysical profile, is considered. If gestation is near term, a contraction stress test (CST) may be done.

> **NURSING PRIORITY:** Appearance of any decelerations of the FHR during an NST should be immediately evaluated by the physician.

C. Advantages of NST.
1. Simple; easy to perform; noninvasive.
2. Does not require hospitalization.
3. Has no contraindications.

## Biophysical Profile

**A biophysical profile is a noninvasive dynamic assessment of a fetus that is based on acute and chronic**

**markers of fetal disease. Is an accurate indicator of impending fetal death.**

A. First choice for follow-up fetal evaluation.
B. Assesses *five* fetal variables: breathing movement, fetal body movement (FBM), muscle tone, amniotic fluid volume (AFV), and FHR; the first four are assessed by ultrasonography; the fifth is assessed by NST.
C. Each area has a possible score of 2, with a maximum score of 10. A score of 4 or less indicates need for immediate delivery.
D. Contraction stress test or oxytocin challenge test and the breast self-stimulation.

## Contraction Stress Test

The test is to observe the response of FHR to the stress of oxytocin-induced uterine contractions; means of evaluating respiratory function (oxygen and carbon dioxide exchange) of the placenta as an indicator of fetal health.

> **!! NURSING PRIORITY:** Many facilities now use the breast self-stimulation contraction stress test because endogenous oxytocin is produced in response to stimulation of the breasts or nipples.

A. Indications.
   1. Preexisting maternal medical conditions: diabetes mellitus, heart disease, hypertension, sickle cell disease, hyperthyroidism, renal disease.
   2. Postmaturity, intrauterine growth restriction, nonreactive NST results, preeclampsia.
B. Contraindications.
   1. Third-trimester bleeding.
   2. Previous cesarean delivery.
   3. Risk for preterm labor because of premature rupture of the membranes, incompetent cervical os, or multiple gestations.
C. Procedure: breast self-stimulation contraction stress test.
   1. Semi-Fowler's position, with fetal monitor in place.
   2. Nipple stimulation begins with woman brushing her palm across one nipple through her shirt or gown for 2 to 3 minutes. If contractions start, nipple stimulation should stop. If contractions do not occur, one nipple should be massaged for 10 minutes.
   3. Advantages: takes less time to perform, is less expensive, and causes less discomfort because no intravenous line is used.
D. Procedure: oxytocin challenge test.
   1. Client must have nothing-by-mouth (NPO) status and be closely observed, either hospitalized or as an outpatient.
   2. Place client in semi-Fowler's position to avoid supine hypotension.
   3. Intravenous (IV) administration of oxytocin stimulates uterine contractions; uterine activity and FHR are recorded by means of external monitoring.
   4. Hypoxia is reflected in late deceleration on monitor, which indicates a diminished fetal-placental reserve. Start oxygen with a mask and reposition.
   5. IV oxytocin is delivered at a rate of 0.5 mU/min; then double the dose every 20 minutes until contractions occur at a rate of three per 10 minutes; then oxytocin is discontinued and the woman is observed until contractions stop.
E. Interpretation: oxytocin challenge test.
   1. Negative (reassuring): shows no late decelerations after any contraction; implies that placental support is adequate.
   2. Positive (nonreassuring; abnormal): shows late decelerations with at least two of the three contractions; may indicate the possibility of insufficient placental respiratory reserve.

> **!! NURSING PRIORITY:** If the CST result is positive and there is no acceleration of FHR with fetal movement (nonreactive NST result), the positive CST result is an ominous sign, often indicating late fetal hypoxia. A negative CST result with a reactive NST result is desirable.

## NORMAL PREGNANCY CYCLE: PHYSIOLOGIC CHANGES

### Uterus

A. Increase in size caused by hypertrophy of the myometrial cells is a result of the stimulating influence of estrogen and the distention caused by the growing fetus.
B. Weight of uterus increases from 50 to 1000 g.
C. Increased fibrous and connective tissues, which strengthen the elasticity of the uterine muscle wall.
D. Irregular, painless uterine contractions (Braxton Hicks) beginning after the fourth month; contraction and relaxation assist in accommodating the growing fetus.
E. Softening of the lower uterine segment (Hegar sign).

> **!! NURSING PRIORITY:** Multigravidas tend to report a greater incidence of Braxton Hicks contractions than do primigravidas.

F. Cervical changes.
   1. Softening of the cervical tip caused by increased vascularity, edema, and hyperplasia of cervical glands (Goodell sign).
   2. Formation of the mucous plug to prevent bacterial contamination from the vagina.

### Vagina

A. Influence of estrogen leads to hypertrophy and hyperplasia of the lining along with an increase in vaginal secretions.

> **!! NURSING PRIORITY:** A blue-purple hue of the vaginal walls is seen by the eighth week (Chadwick sign).

B. Vaginal secretions: acidic (pH is 3.5–6.0), thick, and white.

## Breasts

A. Increase in breast size accompanied by feelings of fullness, tingling, and heaviness.
B. Superficial veins prominent; nipples erect; darkening and increase in diameter of the areolae.
C. Thin, watery secretion, precursor to colostrum, can be expressed from the nipples by the end of the 16th week of pregnancy.

## Cardiovascular System

A. Blood volume.
   1. Increases progressively throughout pregnancy, beginning in the first trimester and peaking in the middle of the third trimester at about 40% to 50% above prepregnant levels.
   2. Normal blood pressure is maintained by peripheral vasodilation.
   3. Extra volume of blood acts as a reserve for blood loss during delivery.
B. Heart.
   1. Slight cardiac hypertrophy and systolic murmurs.
   2. Increase in heart rate by 10 to 15 beats/min by the end of the first trimester.

> **! NURSING PRIORITY:** Blood pressure falls during the second trimester and rises slightly (no more than 15 mm in either systolic or diastolic) during the last trimester. It is important to have a baseline blood pressure measurement. Pulse rate increases by 10 to 15 beats/min. Respiratory rate remains unchanged or slightly increases.

   3. Cardiac output increases 30% to 50%.
   4. Palpitations of the heart are usually due to sympathetic nervous system disturbance; later in pregnancy, palpitations are due to intraabdominal pressure of the growing uterus.
C. Red blood cells.
   1. Stimulation of the bone marrow leads to a 20% to 30% increase in total red blood cell volume.
   2. The plasma volume increase is greater than the red blood cell increase, which leads to hemodilution, typically referred to as *physiologic anemia of pregnancy* (pseudoanemia).
   3. The hematocrit, the proportion of erythrocytes in whole blood, decreases by 7%.
D. White blood cells: 10 to 11,000/mm$^3$ ($\times$ 10$^9$/L); may increase up to 25,000/mm$^3$ ($\times$ 10$^9$/L) during labor and after delivery.

## Respiratory System

A. pH slightly increases, Pco$_2$ decreases, and HCO$_3$$^-$ decreases.
B. Tidal volume increases steadily throughout pregnancy.
C. Oxygen consumption is increased by 20% to 40% between the 16th and 40th weeks.
D. Diaphragm is elevated; change from abdominal to thoracic breathing occurs around the 24th week.
E. Common complaints of nasal stuffiness and epistaxis are due to estrogen influence on nasal mucosa.

## Urinary–Renal System

A. Ureter and renal pelvis dilate (especially on the right side) as a result of the growing uterus.
B. Frequency of urination increases (first and last trimesters).
C. Decreased bladder tone (effect of progesterone); bladder capacity increases: 1300 to 1500 mL.
D. Urine contains more nutrients, leads to increased pH. Alkaline urine and increased glucose in the urine provide an ideal environment for bacteria to thrive, which leads to an increased incidence of urinary tract infections (UTIs).
E. Reduced renal threshold for sugar leads to glycosuria.
F. Because of an increased glomerular filtration rate, as much as 50%, serum blood urea nitrogen, creatinine, and uric acid levels are decreased.

## Gastrointestinal System

A. Pregnancy gingivitis: gums redden, swell, and bleed easily.
B. Increased saliva (ptyalism); decreased gastric acidity.
C. Nausea and vomiting caused by elevated human chorionic gonadotropin (hCG) level during the first trimester usually declines in second trimester related to decreasing hCG levels.
D. Cravings due to change in sense of taste: pica (craving for nonfood, which is not a normal change).
E. Decreased tone and motility of smooth muscles; decreased emptying time of stomach; slowed peristalsis caused by increased progesterone level leads to complaints of bloating, heartburn (pyrosis), and constipation.
F. Pressure of expanding uterus leads to hemorrhoidal varicosities and contributes to continuing constipation.
G. Gallbladder: decreased emptying time, slight hypercholesterolemia, and increased progesterone level may contribute to the development of gallstones during pregnancy.
H. Liver: minor changes.

## Musculoskeletal System

A. Increase in the normal lumbosacral curve leads to backward tilt of the torso.
B. Center of gravity is changed, which often leads to leg and back strain and predisposition to falling.
C. Pelvis relaxes as a result of the effects of the hormone relaxin; leads to the characteristic "duck waddling" gait.
D. Abdominal wall stretches and loses tone.
E. Increase pressure on medial nerve in the wrist causing carpal tunnel–like syndrome pain.

## Integumentary System

A. Increased skin pigmentation in various areas of the body.
   1. Facial: mask of pregnancy (chloasma).
   2. Abdomen: striae (red or purple stretch marks) and linea nigra (darkened vertical line from umbilicus to symphysis pubis).
B. Appearance of vascular spider nevi, especially on the neck, arms, and legs.

C. Acne vulgaris, dermatitis, and psoriasis usually improve during pregnancy.
D. Pruritus may occur and is common in pregnancy due to cholestasis of pregnancy.

## Endocrine

A. Placenta.
1. Functions include transport of nutrients and removal of waste products from the fetus.
2. Produces hCG and human chorionic somatomammotropin (hCS), previously called human placental lactogen.
3. Produces estrogen and progesterone after 2 months of gestation.
B. Thyroid gland.
1. May increase in size and activity.
2. Increase in basal metabolic rate.
3. Parathyroid glands: increase in activity (especially in the last half of the pregnancy) because of increased requirements for calcium and vitamin D.
C. Pituitary gland.
1. Enlargement greatest during the last month of gestation.
2. Production of anterior pituitary hormones: FSH, LH, thyrotropin, adrenotropin, and prolactin.

> **NURSING PRIORITY:** Production of posterior pituitary hormones: oxytocin promotes uterine contractility and stimulation of milk let-down reflex, which are essential changes for postpartum lactation and uterine involution.

D. Adrenal glands.
1. Minimal change in the adrenal glands.
2. An increase in aldosterone, which retains sodium, results in edema and the need to control excess salt in diet.

## Metabolism

A. Weight gain: determined by prepregnancy weight-for-height calculated by using the body mass index (BMI); BMI of 18.5 to 24.9 is considered normal.
1. Normal weight gain: recommended 11.5 to 16 kg (about 25–35 lb).
a. Underweight: 12.5 to 18 kg.
b. Overweight: 7 to 11 kg.
c. Normal for multiple gestations: 17 to 25 kg.

> **NURSING PRIORITY:** The pattern of weight gain is important. Approximately 0.4 kg/week for normal weight; 0.5 kg/week for underweight; 0.3 kg/week for overweight. Inadequate weight gain for a normal-weight woman would be less than 1 kg/month. Excessive weight gain is considered more than 3 kg/month and should be evaluated because this can indicate preeclampsia if it occurs after the 20th week of gestation.

2. Total weight gain is accounted for as follows:
a. Fetus: 7 to 8.5 lb (3175–3856 g)
b. Placenta and membranes: 2 to 2.5 lb (907–1134 g)
c. Amniotic fluid: 2 lb (907 g)
d. Uterus: 2 lb (907 g)
e. Breasts: 1 to 4 lb (455–1814 g)
f. Increased blood volume: 4 to 5 lb (1814–2268 g)
g. Remaining 4 to 9 lb (1814–4082 g) is extravascular fluid and fat reserves.
B. Nutrient metabolism.
1. Protein: positive nitrogen balance; fetus makes greatest demands during the second half of gestation as it doubles its weight in the last 6 to 8 weeks.
2. Carbohydrate: increases, especially during the last two trimesters; ketosis and glycosuria occur, along with lipidemia.
3. Fat: more completely absorbed; increase in serum lipid, lipoprotein, cholesterol, and phospholipid levels.
4. Increased intake of folic acid: 600 mcg daily (to prevent neural tube defects).
C. Mineral metabolism.
1. Increased need for calcium and phosphorus, especially during the last 1 to 2 months of gestation.
2. Iron: approximately 30 mg daily.
D. Water metabolism.
1. Increased need for water (i.e., 3 L/day): normal is 2.3 L/day, so an increase of 700 mL/day is needed.
2. Increased water retention is frequently seen as a result of the effects of hormones and the decreased plasma protein level.
3. Dehydration increases risk for cramping, contractions, and preterm labor.

> **NURSING PRIORITY:** High levels of mercury can possibly harm the fetus's developing nervous system. Teach pregnant women to avoid fish high in mercury content and limit intake to no more than 12 oz (in two meals) per week. Avoid shark, swordfish, marlin, king mackerel, albacore or white tuna, and tilefish because they have high levels of mercury.

## PRENATAL CARE

### Assessment

A. Initial visit.
1. Complete history and physical examination.
2. Obstetric history.
a. Past pregnancies (date, course of pregnancy, labor and postpartum period; information about infant and neonatal course).
b. Present pregnancy.
B. Schedule of return prenatal visits.
1. Frequency of return visits.
a. Monthly for first 32 weeks.
b. Every 2 weeks to the 36th week.
c. After the 36th week, weekly until delivery.
d. If a high-risk pregnancy, prenatal visits may be more frequent.
2. Subsequent assessment data follow-up.
a. Vital signs.
b. Urinalysis: check for protein and sugar.

   c. Monitor weight.

   d. Measurement of height of uterine fundus.

   e. Auscultation of FHR.

C. Definitions of common terms (Table 26-2).

D. Signs and symptoms of pregnancy (Table 26-3).

E. Summary of the antepartum period (Table 26-4).

## Table 26-2 DEFINITIONS OF COMMON TERMS

| Common Term | Definition |
| --- | --- |
| Gravida[a] | The number of pregnancies regardless of the duration; includes the present pregnancy. |
| Para[a] | The number of pregnancies in which the fetuses have reached 20 weeks' gestation when they are born. |
| Nulligravida | A woman who has never been pregnant. |
| Primigravida | Woman who is pregnant for the first time. |
| Multigravida | Woman who is pregnant for the second or subsequent time. |
| Nullipara (para 0) | Woman who has not completed a pregnancy with a fetus (or fetuses) who has reached 20 weeks' gestation. |
| Primipara (para I) | Woman who has completed one pregnancy with a fetus who has reached 20 weeks' gestation. |
| Multipara (para II, para III, para IV, etc.) | Woman who has completed two or more pregnancies to 20 or more weeks' gestation. |
| Parturient | A woman in labor. |

[a]The terms *gravida* and *para* refer to the number of pregnancies, not the number of fetuses. The woman who delivers twins on her first pregnancy remains a para I, despite having two infants. She is also a para I if the fetus was stillborn or died soon after birth. The most common system used to describe reproductive status is the five-digit identification system characterized by the acronym GTPAL: G = total number of pregnancies, T = number of term infants (at least 37 weeks' gestation), P = number of preterm infants (before 37 weeks' gestation), A = number of spontaneous or therapeutic abortions, L = number of living children.

## Diagnostics

A. Pregnancy tests: all tests, including over-the-counter "home pregnancy" tests, are based on the presence of hCG as the biologic marker. A false-negative test result may be due to testing too early. Whenever there is doubt about the results, further evaluation or retesting in a few days is appropriate.

B. Laboratory tests.

  1. Urinalysis and/or urine culture.

  2. Complete blood count, electrolytes, blood urea nitrogen (BUN), creatinine.

  3. Venereal Disease Research Laboratory (VDRL) test, rapid plasmin reagin (RPR) test, or fluorescent treponemal antibody-absorption (FTA-ABS) test: serologic screening for syphilis, HIV testing.

  4. Rubella antibody titer.

> **NURSING PRIORITY:** It is important to understand the rubella titer and its significance to pregnancy. The rubella vaccination is not given during pregnancy, and pregnancy should be prevented for at least 3 months after receiving the vaccination.

    a. Titer of 1:8 or less is considered serologically negative; titer 1:8 or greater indicates that woman is immune.

    b. Vaccination can be given during the postpartum period even if mother is breastfeeding.

    c. Teach pregnant woman who has not had rubella or a vaccination or who has a titer less than 1:10 to avoid contact with children who have rubella or who have received a recent vaccination.

  5. Blood type and Rh status.

    a. Administration of $Rh_o(D)$ immune globulin (RhIG), also called RhoGAM, to prevent Rh sensitization in the pregnant woman.

      (1) $Rh_o(D)$ immune globulin is given at 28 weeks' gestation to an Rh-negative mother, as a prophylactic measure.

## Table 26-3 SIGNS AND SYMPTOMS OF PREGNANCY

| Presumptive/Subjective | Probable/Objective | Positive/Diagnostic |
| --- | --- | --- |
| 1. Amenorrhea. | 1. Positive pregnancy test result. | 1. Fetal heart rate—6th to 12th week: Doppler ultrasonography; 18th to 20th week: fetal stethoscope. |
| 2. Nausea and vomiting. | 2. Enlarged abdomen. | 2. Fetal movements felt by examiner. |
| 3. Excessive fatigue. | 3. Hegar sign: softening of lower uterine segment. | 3. Fetal sonography (after 16th week). |
| 4. Urinary frequency. | 4. Chadwick sign: bluish discoloration of vagina. | 4. Fetal skeleton on x-ray film (not used often). |
| 5. Breast changes: tenderness, fullness, increased pigmentation of areola, precolostrum discharge. | 5. Goodell sign: softening of cervical lip. | |
| 6. Quickening: active movements of the fetus felt by the mother. | 6. Ballottement: pushing on fetus (fourth to fifth month) and feeling it rebound back. | |
| 7. Increased pigmentation of skin and abdominal striae. | 7. Fetal outline distinguished by palpation. | |
| | 8. Braxton Hicks contractions. | |

> **TEST ALERT:** Be sure you are able to differentiate between presumptive, probable, and positive signs.

**Table 26-4 SUMMARY OF NURSING MANAGEMENT DURING THE ANTEPARTUM PERIOD**

| Weeks' Gestation | Physical Signs and Symptoms | Characteristic Behaviors | Nursing Interventions |
|---|---|---|---|
| 0–13 | Amenorrhea<br>Fatigue<br>Nausea, vomiting<br>Increased breast size and tenderness<br>Urinary frequency<br>Increased appetite | Ambivalence with mood swings.<br>Anxiety related to confirmation of pregnancy.<br>Telling selected close persons of pregnancy.<br>*Couvade syndrome* refers to the presence of physical discomforts in the father during the pregnancy that mimic his partner's symptoms. | 1. Obtain complete history, including gynecologic and obstetric histories.<br>2. Ascertain any maternal high-risk problems such as maternal age (greater than 35 years or less than 16 years), heart disease, diabetes, or potential neonatal high-risk problems such as history of congenital defects, premature births, etc. (See complete discussion in this chapter on high-risk problems.)<br>3. Identify maternal nutritional status by assessing height and weight and comparing with BMI chart.<br>4. Complete a diet history and instruction. Important to teach about necessary changes rather than all the concepts of good nutrition.<br>5. Food cravings are usually benign and may be indulged, providing a well-balanced diet is maintained. Pica is an abnormal eating pattern and requires treatment.<br>6. Encourage client to express feelings or ambivalence about pregnancy.<br>7. Anticipatory guidance and teaching (including family) related to OTC drugs, normal signs and symptoms of pregnancy, reportable signs of possible complications, and the normality of her mood swings. |
| 14–26 | Quickening<br>"Pregnant figure"<br>Increased energy<br>Feeling of well-being<br>Round ligament pain | Wears maternity clothes.<br>Tells the world she's pregnant; begins to notice other pregnant women.<br>Interested in learning about birth and babies: reads books, seeks out and questions friends and family, attends classes.<br>Increased dependency as time goes on.<br>Promote father's involvement by allowing him to watch and feel fetal movement.<br>Father needs to confront and resolve his own conflicts about the fathering he received as a child.<br>Father will make decisions about what he does or does not want to imitate based on his own father as role model. | 1. Ongoing assessment of maternal and fetal status:<br>2. FHR; vital signs; fundal height.<br>3. Urine test for glucose (mild glycosuria is usually benign), and protein.<br>4. Finger stick for hemoglobin analysis (12–14 g/dL [120–140 g/L] normal).<br>5. Balanced diet.<br>6. Prevent or minimize activity intolerance and promote adequate rest by:<br>  a. Encouraging 8 hours of sleep each day, plus one nap.<br>  b. Scheduling rest periods at place of employment.<br>  c. Napping at home while other small children are sleeping.<br>  d. Using left lateral position while resting or sleeping.<br>7. Promote adequate exercise (e.g., Kegel, pelvic rocking, modified sit-ups), sitting tailor-fashion (lotus position).<br>8. Anticipatory guidance/teaching (including family) related to libido changes, mood swings, increasing dependency, introversion, and reportable signs of possible complications. |
| 27–40 | Dependent edema<br>Pressure in lower abdomen<br>Frequent urination<br>Round ligament pain<br>Backache<br>Insomnia<br>Clumsiness<br>Fatigue<br>Varicose veins | Introversion.<br>Increased dependency (craves attention and tenderness).<br>Altered responsiveness and spontaneity, as well as abdominal bulk and fatigue, may decrease interest in genital sex.<br>Intensifies study of labor and delivery.<br>Increasingly feeling more vulnerable.<br>Prepares nursery; buys baby things.<br>Decides on feeding method for baby. | 1. Ongoing continued physical assessment at more frequent intervals.<br>2. Reassure: provide emotional support related to attractiveness and self-worth.<br>3. Anticipatory guidance and teaching (including family) related to signs and symptoms of labor, environmental modification for coming infant, providing rest for mother, teaching associated with either breastfeeding or bottle-feeding, advising client concerning birthing and anesthesia options, promoting the developing parent/child attachment (encourage family to verbalize mental picture of infant and concepts of selves as parents). |

**TEST ALERT:** Plan anticipatory guidance for developmental transitions. Pregnancy is considered a normal maturational crisis and developmental stage for the expectant couple.

*BMI,* Body mass index; *FHR,* fetal heart rate, *OTC,* over-the-counter.

(2) A second dose of Rh$_o$(D) immune globulin is given within the first 72 hours after delivery to prevent the mother from producing antibodies to the fetal blood cells that may have entered her bloodstream during labor and delivery, if the infant is Rh positive.

   (a) Has no effect against antibodies already present in maternal bloodstream.

   (b) Provides passive immunity.

   (c) Not a treatment for women who are already sensitized; recommended only for nonsensitized Rh-negative women at risk for developing Rh isoimmunization.

   (d) Administered after abortion (13+ weeks' gestation), amniocentesis, blood transfusion, trauma, abruptio placentae, or placenta previa.

(3) A microdose of Rh$_o$(D) immune globulin is administered after pregnancies that terminate before 13 weeks' gestation, after chorionic villus sampling, and after ectopic pregnancy.

6. Tuberculin skin testing.
7. Hepatitis B surface antigen (HBsAg).
8. HIV antibody with client permission.
9. Maternal serum alpha-fetoprotein (MSAFP) at 15 to 20 weeks (ideally 16 to 18 weeks).

C. Pelvic examination.
   1. Pap smear of the cervix.
   2. Pelvic measurements (pelvimetry).

D. Calculation of estimated date of birth (EDB).
   1. Nägele's rule: count back 3 calendar months from the first day of the last menstrual period (LMP) and add 7 days.
   2. Examples.
      a. LMP, April 10: EDB, January 17.
      b. LMP, September 25: EDB, July 2.

## High-Risk Pregnancy

A. Sociodemographic factors.
   1. Age: younger than 16 and older than 35.
   2. Parity: primigravida or greater than gravida 5.
   3. Low income: inability to purchase nutritional foods.
   4. Lack of prenatal care.

> **NURSING PRIORITY:** Pregnant adolescents are at risk both physiologically and psychologically. Often they do not receive prenatal care, or care is delayed because of late recognition of pregnancy. Physiologic risks include preeclampsia, iron deficiency anemia, sexually transmitted infections (15- to 19-year-old teens have the second highest incidence of sexually transmitted infections), and low-birth-weight neonates and cephalopelvic disproportion. Psychological risks include interruption of normal growth and development for both partners; adolescent parents may drop out of school.

B. Biophysical factors.
   1. Genetic considerations: chromosomal anomalies, transmissible inherited disorders (Down syndrome), previous infant with a congenital anomaly, parents with recessive disorders (hemophilia, cystic fibrosis).

2. Nutritional status: influenced by age, three pregnancies in 2 years, inadequate dietary intake, anemia.
3. Preexisting medical problems: diabetes mellitus, renal disease, hypertension, cardiovascular disease, viral infections (rubella, cytomegalovirus, herpes virus type 2, human immunodeficiency virus).
4. Obstetric factors: history of previous high-risk pregnancy, abortions, stillbirth, or maternal complications.

C. Psychosocial factors.
   1. Drug use: alcohol, nicotine, cocaine, heroin, marijuana, and other addictive drugs.
   2. Psychological status: history of child or spouse abuse, inadequate support systems, unsafe cultural, ethnic, or religious practices, situational crisis, depression.

D. Environmental factors (Figure 26-2).
   1. Occupational hazards: excessive exposure to radiation, handling of teratogenic chemicals, lead paint/contaminated water, secondhand smoke.
   2. Adverse living conditions related to low income, abuse, and nutritional deficiencies.
   3. Changing litter box (toxoplasmosis).

### Nursing Interventions

> **TEST ALERT:** Instruct client about antepartal care; modify approaches to care in accordance with client's developmental stage (adolescence).

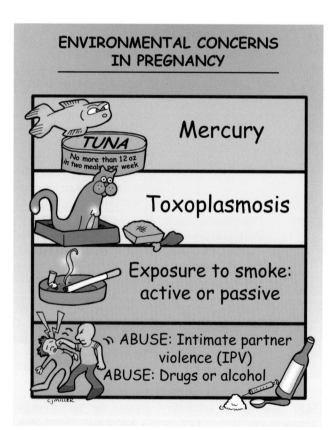

**FIGURE 26-2 Environmental Concerns of Pregnancy.** (From Zerwekh, J., & Miller, C. J. [2012]. *Mosby's OB/PEDS & women's health memory notecards: Visual, mnemonic, and memory aids for nurses.* St. Louis: Mosby.)

**Goal:** To educate families regarding general health practices.

A. Hygiene: tub baths permitted but may be awkward during later weeks of gestation.

B. Clothing: loose, comfortable clothing with supportive brassiere; low-heeled shoes.

C. Breast and nipple care: client should avoid using excessive amounts of soap or rubbing the nipples with a towel because this dries the nipple area and removes natural secretions; creams, lotions, and ointments are not needed on the nipple or areola and should be avoided.

D. Employment: no severe physical straining, heavy lifting, or prolonged periods of sitting or standing; wear support stockings.

E. Travel: client should avoid travel during the last month of pregnancy; when client is traveling by car or airplane, frequent walking and stretching are advised; seat belts (both lap and shoulder) should be used, with the lap belt positioned under the abdomen.

F. Rest and exercise: adequate amounts of exercise such as walking or swimming; client should stop exercising when she begins to feel tired; moderation is key.

G. Sexual activity: coital position may need to be altered to provide greater comfort; there is no contraindication to intercourse or any activity leading to orgasm, providing that membranes are intact, no vaginal bleeding exists,

and there is no history of threatened abortion or premature labor.

H. Smoking: not advised; associated with infants who are small for gestational age.

I. Alcohol: recommended that the pregnant woman not consume any alcohol; the more consumed, the greater the risk for fetal alcohol syndrome.

J. Dental care: regular prophylactic care is encouraged; a soft-bristled toothbrush may be needed because of bleeding gums; x-ray examinations should be postponed, if possible.

K. Immunization: live, attenuated virus immunizations (e.g., measles–mumps–rubella vaccine) are contraindicated during pregnancy; client is cautioned against getting pregnant for at least 3 months after receiving this type of immunization.

L. Medications: client is advised to avoid medications, especially during the first trimester, because of possible teratogenic effects.

**Goal:** To promote relief of common discomforts through client education regarding self-care measures (Table 26-5).

**Goal:** To promote adequate nutrition.

A. Obtain a complete diet history (see Chapter 3).
1. Assess normal food intake.
2. Determine prepregnant nutritional status (existence of deficiency state; severity and time at gestation in which it occurs).

### Table 26-5   SUMMARY OF COMMON DISCOMFORTS AND RELIEF MEASURES

| Discomfort | Relief Measures |
|---|---|
| **First Trimester** | |
| Nausea and vomiting (morning sickness) | Frequent small meals; avoid empty stomach; between meals eat crackers without fluid; take vitamin $B_6$ supplement. |
| Urinary frequency and urgency | Void frequently; decrease fluids before bedtime; avoid caffeinated or carbonated beverages; use perineal pads for leakage; perform Kegel exercises; report any pain or burning. |
| Breast tenderness | Wear a well-fitting supportive bra; alter sleep positions; avoid using soap on the nipple and areola area. |
| Increased vaginal discharge | Good hygiene; use perineal or panty liner pads; cotton underwear; no douching unless prescribed; report any pruritus, foul odor, or change in character or color. |
| **Second and Third Trimesters** | |
| Heartburn (pyrosis or acid indigestion) | Avoid fat and fried, spicy foods; eat small, frequent meals; maintain good posture; sit upright. |
| Ankle edema | Need ample fluid intake; avoid prolonged sitting or standing; support stockings should be applied before rising; elevate feet while sitting. |
| Varicose veins | Avoid prolonged periods of standing; apply support hose before rising; elevate feet while sitting; do not cross legs at knees. |
| Hemorrhoids | Avoid constipation, do not strain; use ointments, bulk-producing laxatives, anesthetic suppositories as prescribed. |
| Constipation | Increase fluid intake (6–8 glasses/day); eat food and fruits high in roughage; exercise moderately; use stool softeners as prescribed. |
| Backache | Maintain correct posture; wear low-heeled shoes; perform pelvic tilt exercises. |
| Leg cramps | Stretch affected muscle and hold until it subsides; dorsiflex foot; apply warm packs; maintain adequate calcium intake; wear support hose. |
| Faintness | Sit or lie down; avoid sudden changes in position; avoid prolonged standing. |
| Shortness of breath | Maintain correct posture; rest periods throughout the day; sleep with head elevated by several pillows. |

**TEST ALERT:** Instruct client on antepartum care.

B. Identify nutritional risk factors.
   1. Age: adolescents and older gravidas.
   2. Maternal weight variations.
   3. Abnormal dietary patterns: pica; fad diets; excessive use of alcohol, drugs, or tobacco.
   4. Socioeconomic status: low income, insufficient money to buy food.
   5. Preexisting medical problems: diabetes mellitus, anemia.
C. Dietary instructions and nutrient requirements (Figure 26-3).
   1. Increase calories for pregnancy (an additional 300 calories per day).
   2. Increase calories for lactation (an additional 500 calories per day over prepregnant intake).
   3. Increase protein (an additional 10 g per day for pregnancy; an additional 5 g per day for lactation); because the protein intake of many nonpregnant women is quite high, there may be little or no need to increase the protein intake during pregnancy.
   4. Increase vitamins (generally, intake of all vitamins is increased, especially folic acid).
   5. Increase amount of minerals (especially iron, calcium, and phosphorous).
   6. Additional calories and protein may be recommended for the pregnant adolescent.

**Goal:** To educate expectant family with regard to danger signs and symptoms requiring immediate attention.

A. Vaginal discharge: blood or amniotic fluid.

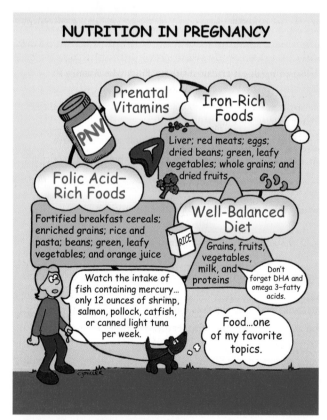

**FIGURE 26-3 Nutrition in Pregnancy.** (From Zerwekh, J., & Miller, C. J. [2012]. *Mosby's OB/PEDS & women's health memory notecards: Visual, mnemonic, and memory aids for nurses.* St. Louis, MO: Mosby.)

B. Visual disturbances: dimness or blurring of vision, flashes of light or dots before the eyes.
C. Swelling of the face or fingers.
D. Fever and chills.
E. Severe or continuous headache.
F. Pain in the abdomen.
G. Persistent vomiting; heartburn.
H. Absence of fetal movement after quickening.

**Goal:** To provide education and preparation for childbirth.

A. Childbirth programs aim to erase previous negative impressions of pregnancy, labor, and delivery; promote a positive, healthy attitude; and teach students physical exercises and relaxation techniques.
B. Points about breathing recommendations during labor.
   1. Slow abdominal breathing or chest breathing is practiced for the first stage of labor; woman concentrates on making abdominal muscles rise.
   2. Rapid shallow chest breathing is for the active and transitional phases of labor.
   3. Panting is used to prevent pushing.

## FETAL DEVELOPMENT

### Developmental Stages

A. Preembryonic stage: stage of the ovum.
   1. Conception to day 14.
   2. Fertilized ovum grows and differentiates, implants in the endometrial tissue.
   3. Formation of the three primary germ layers: endoderm, mesoderm, ectoderm.
B. Embryonic stage.
   1. Day 15 to end of eighth week.
   2. Period of organogenesis: differentiation of cells, organs, and organ systems.
   3. Highly vulnerable time; congenital anomalies are likely to occur during this period.
   4. At the end of this period of development, embryo has features of the human body.
C. Fetal stage.
   1. Nine weeks to the time of birth.
   2. Characterized by growth and development of organs and organ systems.

### Summary of Growth and Development

A. 6 weeks: heart begins beating.
B. 8 weeks: brain activity begins; fetus moves in response to touch; 1 inch (2.5 cm) long.
C. 16 weeks: sucking response begins; fetus is 3.5 inches (8.9 cm) long; sex clearly identifiable.
D. 20 weeks: hearing begins to develop; fetus can respond to external sounds in environment; 10 inches (25.4 cm) long.
E. 28 weeks: fetus can perceive light; senses are functional; sleep–wake periods; brown fat has formed; 16 inches (40.6 cm) long; viable.
F. 30 to 40 weeks: increase in subcutaneous fat and weight.

!**NURSING PRIORITY:** At week 34 or 35, the L/S ratio reaches 2:1 and surfactant production is sufficient and lungs are considered mature.

## Multifetal Pregnancy

A. Incidence.
   1. One in 430 pregnancies results in twins.
   2. Steady rise in multifetal pregnancies due to delayed childbearing and use of ovulation-enhancing drugs.
B. Dizygotic or fraternal twins.
   1. Fertilization of two separate ova.
   2. There are two placentas, but they may be fused.
   3. Fraternal twin can be either the same sex or a different sex; fraternal twins may also have different gestational ages.
   4. Increased incidence in African American women.
C. Monozygotic or identical twins.
   1. One ovum and one sperm; cells of the zygote separate and form two embryos.
   2. Same sex: resemble each other in appearance and structure.
   3. Usually one placenta, one chorion, and two amnions are present, but two placentas may be present if cell division occurs soon after fertilization.

## Placenta

A. Function.
   1. Transfer of oxygen, nutrients, and metabolites.
   2. Elimination of waste products from the fetus.
   3. Production of hormones: hCG, human placental lactogen, estrogen, and progesterone.
B. Development of the placenta.
   1. Formed from the chorionic villi lying over the decidua basalis.
   2. Formed by the end of the third month of gestation.
   3. Separated by 15 to 30 sections: cotyledons.
   4. At term, the placenta weighs one-sixth of the weight of the fetus (e.g., 6 lb [2722 g] fetus: 1 lb [454 g] placenta).
   5. Fetal surface is shiny and slightly grayish: *Schultze* (often called shiny Schultze).
   6. Maternal side is rough and beefy red: *Duncan* (often called dirty Duncan).
C. Placental circulation.
   1. Maternal and fetal bloodstreams are in close relationship to each other, but the circulations do not mix.
   2. Approximately 500 to 700 mL of maternal blood circulates through the placenta every minute.

## Fetal Circulation

A. Fetal lungs do not participate in respiratory gas exchange.
B. There are special fetal structures to bypass blood supply to the lungs.
   1. Placenta.

2. Umbilical cord: length, 55 cm (22 inches); diameter, 1.25 to 2.5 cm (½ to 1 inch).
   a. One umbilical vein carries oxygenated blood from maternal circulation to fetus.
   b. Two umbilical arteries carry unoxygenated (venous) blood from fetus to placenta.
   c. Wharton's jelly is a gelatinous substance that surrounds the three blood vessels, providing support.
3. Foramen ovale: an opening between the right atrium and the left atrium of the heart.
4. Ductus arteriosus: connects the pulmonary artery and the aorta.
5. Ductus venosus: connects the umbilical vein and the inferior vena cava.
C. At the time of birth, fetal circulation begins the transition to the adult pattern of circulation; a functional closure occurs within a few days; however, anatomic closure of the fetal vessels is not complete for several weeks or months.

!**PEDIATRIC NURSING PRIORITY:** A newborn heart murmur may not be significant because of incomplete closure of the ductus arteriosus.

## COMPLICATIONS ASSOCIATED WITH PREGNANCY

**TEST ALERT:** Identify signs of potential prenatal complications.

###  Abortion

**Abortion is termination of pregnancy before 20 weeks' gestation; abortions can be spontaneous (miscarriage) or induced (therapeutic or elective); approximately 75% to 80% of all spontaneous abortions occur during the second and third months of gestation.**

### Assessment

A. Risk factors.
   1. Maternal: chronic infections, fibroid tumors, structural uterine anomalies, chromosomal abnormalities.
   2. Endocrine disturbance: progesterone and thyroid hormone (hypothyroidism) dysfunction.
   3. Exposure to teratogens, evidence of malnutrition, and psychological factors.
B. Diagnostics.
   1. Decreased hemoglobin (less than 10.5 mg/dL [105 g/L] if bleeding has been significant).
C. Clinical manifestations (types of spontaneous abortions).
   1. Threatened abortion: slight bleeding, mild back and lower abdominal cramping, no cervical dilation, no passage of the products of conception.
   2. Inevitable abortion: moderate amount of bleeding and cramping; internal cervical os dilates, and membranes may rupture.
   3. Incomplete abortion: only some of the products of conception are expelled.
   4. Complete abortion: all the products of conception are expelled.

5. Missed abortion: fetus dies in utero, and the products of conception are retained from 4 to 8 weeks; symptoms of pregnancy subside; if fetus is retained past 6 weeks, complications of disseminated intravascular coagulation (DIC) may develop as a result of the release of thromboplastin from the fetal autolysis process.
6. Recurrent or habitual abortion: three or more successive, spontaneous abortions.

### Treatment

Treatment varies according to type of abortion.

A. Threatened abortion: bed rest and sedation; sometimes progesterone therapy is tried (may cause congenital anomalies).
B. Inevitable and incomplete abortion.
   1. Fluid replacement: IVs, type and cross-match for possible blood transfusion.
   2. Administration of oxytocin.
   3. Dilation and curettage (D&C) or suction evacuation to remove products of conception.
   4. Administration of $Rh_o(D)$ immune globulin if mother is Rh negative (given within 72 hours).
C. Missed abortion.
   1. If abortion does not occur spontaneously after 6 weeks, suction evacuation or D&C will be performed.
   2. Pregnancy beyond 12 weeks' gestation: induction of labor by IV oxytocin, prostaglandin.
D. Recurrent or habitual abortion: determination of cause, then specific therapy to correct.

### Nursing Interventions

**Goal:** To assess or control hemorrhage.

A. Monitoring of vital signs.
B. Accurate determination of number of pads used to assess bleeding.
C. Assist in medical treatment: IV therapy, preparation for D&C.

**Goal:** To prevent complications.

A. Observe for shock, hypofibrinogenemia, and DIC.
B. Prevent isoimmunization by administration of $Rh_o(D)$ immune globulin.
C. Assess for infection and anemia.
D. Encourage foods rich in iron to promote tissue repair.

**Goal:** To provide emotional support to the couple experiencing the loss of pregnancy.

A. Encourage verbalization of feelings.
B. Be available and actively listen.
C. Refer to community support groups.

> **! NURSING PRIORITY:** Be sure to know the policy and procedure at your agency for the disposition of the fetal remains.

### Ectopic Pregnancy

An ectopic pregnancy is any pregnancy in which the gestational sac is implanted outside of the uterine cavity. Most (95%) ectopic pregnancies are tubal; they are more common on the right side (Figure 26-4).

### Assessment

A. Risk factors: any condition that causes scarring or obstruction of the fallopian tubes (e.g., pelvic inflammatory disease, gonorrheal infections, postabortion salpingitis).
B. Diagnostics.
   1. Ultrasonography: abdominal or transvaginal
   2. β-hCG levels: greater than 1500 to 2000 mIU/mL (IU/L).
C. Clinical manifestations.
   1. If tube is unruptured, slow, chronic bleeding usually occurs, and the abdomen gradually becomes rigid and tender.

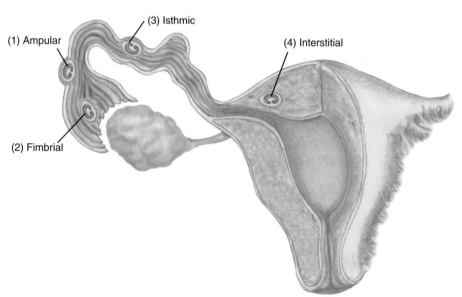

**FIGURE 26-4  Sites of Tubal Ectopic Pregnancy.** (From McKinney, E., et al. [2013]. *Maternal-child nursing* [4th ed.]. St. Louis, MO: Saunders.)

2. If a tube ruptures, sudden excruciating pain is felt in the lower abdomen, usually over the mass; referred shoulder pain is possible as the abdomen fills with blood; vaginal bleeding and shock may also occur.

**! NURSING PRIORITY:** When a woman of childbearing age has extreme sudden abdominal pain, an ectopic pregnancy should be considered, even if the woman reports that there is no risk of her being pregnant.

### Treatment

A. Surgical: laparoscopy, laparotomy, salpingectomy.
B. Medical: methotrexate used to dissolve residual tissue or as a one-time treatment for unruptured pregnancies.

**! NURSING PRIORITY:** If the woman has been on methotrexate and drugs, alcohol, or takes vitamins with folic acid (prenatal vitamins), her risk of having side effects or exacerbating the ectopic rupture may occur.

### Nursing Interventions

**Goal:** To prevent and detect early complications.

A. Provision of nursing care for shock, as indicated.
B. Prepare for surgery (IVs, oxygen, blood, etc.).
C. Administer $Rh_o(D)$ immune globulin if mother is Rh negative.

**Goal:** To provide emotional support (loss of pregnancy and reproductive organ).

A. Follow up with β-hCG levels; if they do not drop, an additional dose of methotrexate may be given.
B. Use a contraceptive method for 3 months to allow body to heal.

### Incompetent Cervical Os (Recurrent Premature Dilation of the Cervix)

An incompetent cervical os is a defect related to trauma of the cervix or a congenitally short cervix, which leads to habitual abortion and premature labor.

### Assessment

A. Risk factors: cervical trauma related to D&C, conization, cervical lacerations from previous deliveries.
B. Clinical manifestations.
  1. Cervical dilation or cervical effacement without painful uterine contractions.
  2. Membranes rupture, labor begins, and premature fetus is delivered.

### Treatment

A. Medical.
  1. Bed rest, pessaries, antibiotics, and tocolytic agents.
B. Surgical.
  1. Reinforcement of the weakened cervix by a purse-string suture, which encircles the internal os.

2. McDonald cerclage: left in place until term, then removed around 37 weeks or left in place if a cesarean birth is anticipated.

### Nursing Interventions

**Goal:** To provide client education regarding presence of purse-string suture or cerclage.

A. Advise client that some vaginal spotting may occur for several days after placement of suture.
B. Client should abstain from intercourse and douching and should reduce activity levels for 2 weeks after surgery.
C. Stress the importance of monitoring signs and symptoms of preterm labor.
D. During labor, the suture will be removed for a vaginal delivery, or it may be left in place for a cesarean delivery.

### Hydatidiform Mole (Molar Pregnancy)

Gestational trophoblastic disease (GTD) is a spectrum of diseases resulting from abnormal proliferation of the placenta—for example, hydatidiform mole, gestational trophoblastic neoplasia, or choriocarcinoma.

### Assessment

A. Risk factors.
  1. Ovulation simulation with clomiphene.
  2. Increased incidence in early teens and age over 40 years.
B. Diagnostics.
  1. Ultrasonography reveals no fetal skeleton.
  2. Elevated hCG level.
C. Clinical manifestations.
  1. Exaggerated symptoms of pregnancy: uterus large for week of pregnancy, excessive nausea and vomiting, early symptoms of preeclampsia.
  2. Discharge of brownish red fluid (like prune juice) from vagina around 12 weeks; fluid may contain vesicles.
  3. Anemia caused by loss of blood.
  4. Absence of FHR.
D. Complications.
  1. Preeclampsia, hyperthyroidism.
  2. Induction of labor is not recommended due to trophoblastic embolization occurring after evacuation of molar pregnancy.
  3. Possible choriocarcinoma.

### Treatment

A. Surgical: D&C to empty uterus.
B. Medical: follow-up supervision for 1 year.
  1. Obtain hCG levels weekly until the level decreases to normal and remains normal for 3 consecutive months; then monthly measurements are taken for 6 months; this lasts for 1 year.
  2. Rising titers of hCG indicate disease: choriocarcinoma.

> **⚠ NURSING PRIORITY:** The chemotherapeutic agent methotrexate is given for the treatment of increasing or rising hCG levels, which often indicate choriocarcinoma.

3. Pregnancy should be avoided for at least 1 year during the follow-up assessment period.
4. Oral contraceptive is preferred for birth control—no IUD.

### Nursing Interventions

**Goal:** To assess for complications associated with hemorrhage and the possibility of uterine rupture.

**Goal:** To provide emotional support and assist in selection of a contraceptive method.

A. Provide simple explanations and determine understanding of course of treatment.
B. Encourage the venting of fears associated with molar pregnancy and increased incidence of choriocarcinoma.

> **TEST ALERT:** Molar pregnancy and ectopic pregnancy are situations in which nurses must integrate care of the client with an obstetric problem and use of chemotherapeutic medications.

## 📋 Hyperemesis Gravidarum

**Hyperemesis gravidarum is intractable vomiting during pregnancy that results in dehydration, electrolyte imbalance, nutritional deficiencies, and significant weight loss. It occurs in less than 0.5% of pregnancies. The cause is uncertain.**

### Assessment

A. Risk factors: none known.
B. Diagnostic: by symptoms.
C. Clinical manifestations.
   1. Severe, persistent vomiting, dehydration.
   2. Weight loss and nutritional deficiency; progresses to fluid electrolyte imbalance and alkalosis from loss of hydrochloric acid.
   3. Monitor for complications of ketoacidosis (from loss of intestinal juices), hypovolemia, hypokalemia, jaundice, and hemorrhage that may occur.
   4. Hypothrombinemia and decreased urine output.

### Treatment

A. Medical: replacement of fluids, electrolytes, and vitamin $B_6$ (pyridoxine), along with an antiemetic.
B. Dietary: client receives nothing by mouth (NPO status) for first 48 hours; after condition improves, six small feedings are alternated with liquid nourishment in small amounts every 1 to 2 hours; if vomiting recurs, NPO status is resumed, and administration of IV fluids is restarted.
C. Most cases are managed at home, even if requiring IV or enteral therapy.

### Nursing Interventions

**Goal:** To assist with medical and dietary management.

A. Accurate recording of volume of vomitus.
B. Daily weight checks and maintenance of intake and output.
C. Desired urine output is 1000 mL in 24 hours; usually, administration of IV fluids at 3000 mL/hr in first 24 hours after admission to correct hypovolemia.
D. Oral hygiene measures.
E. Clear liquids with gradual progression to small meals that are low fat and high protein.

**Goal:** To detect and treat complications.

A. Initial acid–base imbalance is alkalosis from the loss of hydrochloric acid, but with prolonged vomiting and loss of alkaline intestinal juices, a ketoacidotic state occurs.
B. Esophageal rupture and deficiencies of vitamin K and thiamine resulting in Wernicke encephalopathy can occur in severe cases.

## 📋 Hypertensive Disorders

**Hypertensive disorders are common medical complications of pregnancy occurring in about 5% to 10% of pregnancies and the second leading cause of maternal and perinatal morbidity and mortality. Cause is unknown.**

### Pathophysiology

A. Synthesis of prostaglandin $E_2$ and prostacyclin is decreased. Both prostaglandin $E_2$ and prostacyclin are potent vasodilators. Possible decreases in these factors may lead to increased sensitivity to angiotensin II and may be responsible for most of the pathophysiology associated with preeclampsia.
B. Arteriolar vasospasm and hypovolemia: renal glomerular lesions lead to loss of serum protein (e.g., albumin and globulin); sodium reabsorption is elevated, and water is retained.
C. Oliguria results from decreased glomerular filtration rate and renal blood flow.
D. Coagulation disorder: decreased platelet count, increased intravascular coagulation, and fibrinogen deposits.
E. Central nervous system effects (hyperactivity): headaches, cerebral edema, hyperreflexia, and convulsions.

### Assessment

A. Risk factors.
   1. Diabetes mellitus, hypertension.
   2. Renal disease, hydatidiform mole.
   3. Multiple gestations, polyhydramnios.
   4. Age (younger than 20 or older than 40 years).
   5. Primarily a disease of the primigravida.
B. Clinical manifestations of preeclampsia (Table 26-6).

> **⚠ NURSING PRIORITY:** The hallmark symptoms of preeclampsia are hypertension and proteinuria.

**Table 26-6   CLINICAL MANIFESTATIONS OF PREECLAMPSIA AND ECLAMPSIA**

| Mild Preeclampsia | Severe Preeclampsia | Eclampsia |
|---|---|---|
| Elevated BP: systolic increase to 140 mmHg and diastolic increase of 90 mmHg × 2 readings, 4–6 hours apart, no more than 1 week apart | Increased hypertension: systolic at 160 mmHg; diastolic at 110 mmHg or more on 2 separate occasions 6 hours apart; pregnant woman is on bed rest | Convulsions appear suddenly and without warning. Increased hypertension and tonic contraction of all body muscles (arms flexed, hands clenched, legs inverted) precede the tonic-clonic convulsions. Hypotension follows and then coma. Nystagmus and muscular twitching persist for a time. |
| Proteinuria: greater than 0.3 g (30 mg)/24 hr (1+ to 2+ proteinuria) | Proteinuria: greater than 5 g (50 mg)/24 hr (3+ to 4+ proteinuria) Elevated BUN, serum creatinine, uric acid levels, LDH, ALT, AST Oliguria: less than 500 mL/24 hr Cerebral or visual disturbances Severe headache Vomiting Epigastric pain (due to edema of liver capsule, usually indicative of impending seizure) | Coma (lasts from few minutes to several hours). |

*ALT,* Alanine aminotransferase; *AST,* aspartate aminotransferase; *BP,* blood pressure; *BUN,* blood urea nitrogen; *LDH,* lactate dehydrogenase.

C. Complications (severe preeclampsia): *maternal.*
  1. Retinal arteriolar spasm leads to scotoma (blind spots) and blurring.
  2. Cerebral edema and hemorrhages with increased irritability (headache, hyperreflexia, positive ankle clonus, and seizures).
  3. HELLP (**H**emolysis, **E**levated **L**iver function tests, **L**ow **P**latelet count) syndrome (Figure 26-5).
     a. Associated with severe preeclampsia and hepatic dysfunction: epigastric pain, right upper quadrant pain.
     b. Complications of HELLP syndrome include renal failure, pulmonary edema, ruptured liver hematoma, placental abruption, DIC.
  4. Thrombocytopenia, hemolytic anemia, pulmonary edema.

> ⚠ **NURSING PRIORITY:** Women with HELLP syndrome may or may not have signs or symptoms of severe preeclampsia. They may have hypertension but not proteinuria.

D. Complications: *fetal.*
  1. Usually small for gestational age; born prematurely.
  2. May be born oversedated because of medications given to mother.
  3. May have hypermagnesemia because of maternal treatment with magnesium sulfate.

**Treatment**

A. Medical.
  1. Mild preeclampsia: restricted activity with periods of rest in left lateral recumbent position.
  2. Severe preeclampsia or HELLP syndrome: admitted to hospital, complete bed rest, antihypertensives (hydralazine, labetalol, or nifedipine), anticonvulsants (magnesium sulfate); prepare for preterm delivery via cesarean delivery if HELLP syndrome begins.

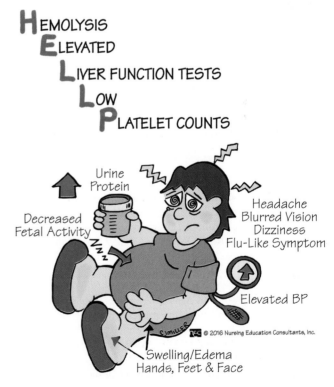

**HELLP SYNDROME**

**H**EMOLYSIS
**E**LEVATED
**L**IVER FUNCTION TESTS
**L**OW
**P**LATELET COUNTS

Urine Protein
Decreased Fetal Activity
Headache
Blurred Vision
Dizziness
Flu-Like Symptom
Elevated BP
Swelling/Edema Hands, Feet & Face
© 2016 Nursing Education Consultants, Inc.

**FIGURE 26-5 HELLP.** (From Zerwekh, J., Garneau, A., & Miller, C. J. [2017]. *Digital collection of the memory notebooks of nursing* [4th ed.]. Chandler, AZ: Nursing Education Consultants, Inc.)

> ⚠ **NURSING PRIORITY:** Monitor for magnesium toxicity characterized by loss of patellar reflexes, respiratory depression, oliguria, decreased level of consciousness. Magnesium may increase the duration of labor, requiring the client to have oxytocin to augment labor; usually requires more than a client not receiving magnesium. When administering antihypertensives in preeclampsia that is associated with a contracted intravascular volume, give medications with caution and monitor client closely.

3. Eclampsia: seizure precautions (vital signs, oxygen, suction, positioning).
B. Dietary: high-protein diet, no added salt intake, and fluid intake of six to eight glasses of water per day.

### Nursing Interventions

**Goal:** Mild preeclampsia—to initiate preventative measures.

A. Instruction for home care: encourage bed rest, provide dietary instruction, schedule regular prenatal checkups, teach symptoms of worsening of condition, provide meaningful activities to prevent boredom while on bed rest.

B. Tests to evaluate fetal status (e.g., fetal movement record, ultrasonography, NST, determination of estriol and creatinine levels).
C. Goals and nursing intervention for clients with severe preeclampsia and eclampsia are outlined in Box 26-1.

## 📋 Hydramnios

Polyhydramnios is an excessive amount of amniotic fluid that frequently develops during the third trimester in women with diabetes. Any amount greater than 2000 mL is considered excessive. Oligohydramnios is having less than 300 mL of amniotic fluid. A normal amount of fluid is 500 to 1200 mL.

### Assessment

A. Risk factors (increased incidence occurs).
  1. Diabetes, erythroblastosis fetalis.
  2. Presence of congenital anomalies.
  3. Twins, preeclampsia.
B. Diagnostics.
  1. Observation of abdomen (excessive enlargement).
  2. Ultrasonography for measurement of amniotic fluid index (AFI).
     a. AFI value greater than 25 cm suggests polyhydramnios.

---

**Box 26-1    NURSING MANAGEMENT OF CLIENTS WITH GESTATIONAL HYPERTENSION AND PREECLAMPSIA**

**Goal:** To recognize the early signs of gestational hypertension and increased BP.
1. Check BP and record Korotkoff phase V (disappearance of sound) for diastolic reading. Take BP in left lateral recumbent position or seated. Allow 10 minutes of quiet rest before taking BP to encourage relaxation. No caffeine or nicotine use 30 minutes before taking BP.
2. Monitor urine for proteinuria.
3. Monitor for nondependent pathologic edema (e.g., periorbital area and hands).

> ⚠ **NURSING PRIORITY:** Systolic increase of 30 mmHg and a diastolic BP increase of 15 mmHg warrant close observation if the BP elevation occurs with proteinuria.

**Goal:** To recognize progression of gestational hypertension symptoms and minimize or control their sequelae.
1. Institute weight controls. Check for sudden increases of more than 2 lb (0.9 kg)/week or 6 lb (2.7 kg)/month.
2. Increase protein intake in the diet. Maintain normal sodium intake; avoid use of diuretics.
3. Institute bed rest.
4. Monitor for ominous signs of deteriorating condition: headache, visual disturbances, hyperreflexia, markedly decreased urine output, epigastric or right upper quadrant pain, dyspnea, vaginal bleeding (abruptio placentae), or any change in fetal activity.
5. Administer antihypertensives, as ordered, check maternal BP, pulse and FHR.

**Goal:** To prevent or control seizures.
1. Administer IV magnesium sulfate. (Have calcium gluconate available as antidote for possible respiratory/neurologic depression.)
2. Have emergency equipment readily available (e.g., oxygen, suction, airway, sedatives).
3. Modify environment to ensure rest and quiet.
   a. Eliminate noise, bright lights, and other harsh stimuli.
   b. Minimize number of personnel giving care.
   c. Initiate painful and/or intrusive procedures after sedation.
   d. Promote comfort and total bed rest.
4. Monitor I&O, edema, and weight for evidence of vasodilation and increased tissue perfusion.

**Goal:** To recognize alterations in fetal well-being and promote safe delivery of the infant.
1. Auscultate and record FHR pattern, noting presence of variability or accelerations, and report decelerations.
2. Instruct and support client during amniocentesis.
3. Collect specimen for estriol determination.
4. Assist with NST and/or oxytocin challenge test (contraction stress test).
5. Give instructions about induction of labor and electronic FHR monitoring.
6. Instruct client on the need for intravenous magnesium sulfate for 24 hours after delivery to prevent seizures.

*BP,* Blood pressure; *FHR,* fetal heart rate; *IV,* intravenous; *NST,* nonstress test; *OCT,* oxytocin challenge test.

C. Clinical manifestations.
   1. Shortness of breath, pedal edema.
   2. Generalized abdominal discomfort.

### Treatment

A. Amniocentesis.

### Nursing Interventions

**Goal:** To anticipate, detect, and prevent complications associated with polyhydramnios.

A. Assess for history of risk factors: monitor for infection (monilial vaginitis, UTIs).
B. Anticipate premature labor.
C. Provide comfort measures.

## INTRAPARTUM AND POSTPARTUM

## LABOR AND DELIVERY

### Intrapartal Factors

A. The passenger (fetus).
   1. Fetal head.
      a. Bones of the skull: two frontal, two parietal, two temporal, and one occipital.
      b. Suture: membranous tissues between the bones.
      c. Fontanel.
         (1) Anterior, large fontanel (bregma) is located at the juncture of the coronal suture, sagittal suture, and frontal suture; diamond-shaped; closes by 18 months.

         (2) Posterior, or small, fontanel: triangular space located at the junction of the sagittal and lambdoidal sutures; closes at approximately 6 to 8 weeks after birth.
      d. Areas of the skull.
         (1) Occiput: lies behind small fontanel.
         (2) Vertex: lies between the anterior and posterior fontanels.
         (3) Bregma: area of the large fontanel.
         (4) Sinciput: the brow area.
   2. Fetal attitude: relationship of the various parts of the fetal body to one another in utero; characteristic uterine posture is one of moderate flexion of the head, extremities on the abdomen and chest.
   3. Fetal lie: relationship of the fetal axis to the maternal axis—longitudinal or transverse.
   4. Presentation and presenting parts: that part of the fetus that lies close to or has entered the true pelvis.
      a. Cephalic: most common (96%).
      b. Breech: buttocks or feet first (Figure 26-6).
      c. Shoulder: most commonly seen with transverse lie.
   5. Position: relationship of the landmark on the presenting part to a specific part of the maternal pelvis.
      a. Maternal pelvis divided into six segments: anterior, transverse, and posterior segments on the right side; anterior, transverse, and posterior segments on the left side.
      b. Fetal landmarks: occipital (O) vertex presentation, mentum (M) in a face presentation, sacrum (S) in breech presentation, acromion process of the scapula (SC) in a shoulder presentation.

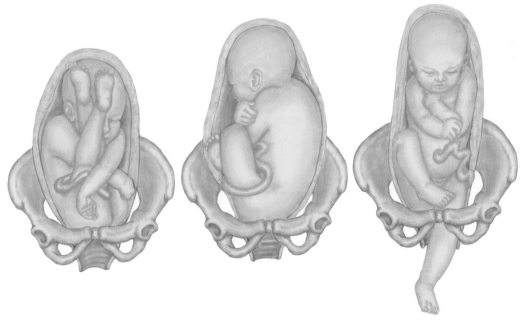

Frank breech                Full breech                Single footling breech

**FIGURE 26-6  Breech Presentations.** (From Murray, S., & McKinney, E. [2014]. *Foundations of maternal-newborn and women's health* [6th ed.]. St. Louis, MO: Elsevier/Saunders.)

## FETAL STATION
(Relationship of Fetal Head to Mother's Pelvis)

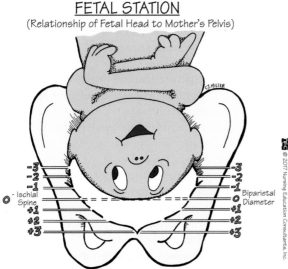

I'm At Zero... From Here It's All Positive... I'm On My Way Out!!!

**FIGURE 26-7 Stations of Presenting Part, or Degree of Descent.** (From Zerwekh, J., Garneau, A., & Miller, C. J. [2017]. *Digital collection of the memory notebooks of nursing* [4th ed.]. Chandler, AZ: Nursing Education Consultants, Inc.)

*Example:* LOA, left occiput anterior (very common); LSP, left sacrum posterior (frank breech); LSCA, left scapula anterior (shoulder presentation, transverse lie).

6. Station of the presenting part: the relationship between the presenting part and the maternal ischial spines (Figure 26-7).

> **! NURSING PRIORITY:** If presenting part is higher than the ischial spines (floating), a negative number is assigned, indicating the number of centimeters above 0 station. As labor progresses, the presenting part moves from the negative stations to the midpelvis at 0 station (engagement) into the positive stations (sequence as follows: −5, −4, −3, −2, −1, 0, +1, +2, +3, +4, +5).

B. The passage.
1. Types of pelvis.
   a. Gynecoid: normal female pelvis; inlet is rounded.
   b. Android: normal male pelvis; inlet is heart shaped.
   c. Anthropoid: inlet is oval.
   d. Platypelloid: flat female pelvis; inlet is transverse oval.
2. Soft tissues.
   a. Ability of the lower uterine segment to dilate and efface.
   b. Ability of the vaginal canal to distend for delivery.
C. The powers: involuntary, intermittent contractions of the uterine muscle (Figure 26-8).
1. **Duration** of the contraction: the time between the first tightening sensation of the muscle and its subsequent complete relaxation.
2. **Frequency** of the contraction: time interval from the beginning of one contraction to the beginning of the next.
3. **Intensity** of the contraction: firmness of the uterine muscle during the contraction.
   a. Mild: slightly tense; easy to indent with fingertips (feels like touching finger to tip of nose).
   b. Moderate: firm fundus; difficult to indent with fingertips (feels like touching finger to chin).
   c. Strong: rigid, boardlike fundus; almost impossible to indent with fingertips (feels like touching finger to forehead).
4. **Resting tone:** tension in the uterine muscle between contractions.
5. Abdominal muscle contractions are the second power; during the second stage of labor, they push the fetus to the outside.

### Assessment of the Labor Process

*Maternal Assessment*

A. Differentiate *true* labor from *false* labor (Box 26-2; Figure 26-9).
B. Mechanism of labor: sequence of passive movements of the presenting part as it moves through the birth canal.
C. Engagement → Descent → Flexion → Internal rotation → Extension → External rotation *(restitution)* → Expulsion.
D. Stages of labor (Table 26-7).

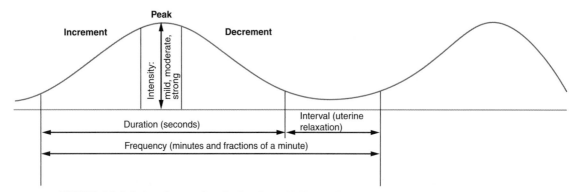

**FIGURE 26-8 Labor Contraction Cycle.** (From McKinney, E., et al. [2013]. *Maternal-child nursing* [4th ed.]. St. Louis, MO: Saunders.)

## Box 26-2 DIFFERENCE BETWEEN *TRUE* LABOR AND *FALSE* LABOR

### True Labor
- Cervical dilation and effacement.
- Contractions occur at regular intervals and increase in duration and intensity; intensity usually increases with walking.
- Pain in the back that radiates around to the abdomen.
- Bloody show: expulsion of the mucous plug: bloody show may be observed at the onset of labor.

**❗ NURSING PRIORITY:** The two most important signs of *true labor* are cervical dilation and effacement (see Figure 26-9).

### False Labor
- Lightening: descent of the fetal head into the pelvis; experienced as "dropping" of the baby.
- Increased vaginal mucus discharge.
- Softening of the cervix.
- Braxton Hicks contractions may become uncomfortable, especially at night; discomfort is usually located in the abdomen.
- Sudden burst of energy.
- Weight loss of 1 to 3 lb (0.45–1.36 kg); sometimes client has diarrhea, indigestion, or nausea and vomiting.
- Rupture of membranes.
  - If rupture occurs before onset of labor, it is called *premature rupture of the membranes.*
  - Delivery should occur within 24 hours to decrease incidence of infection.
  - Test with phenaphthazine (Nitrazine) paper; amniotic fluid is alkaline; phenaphthazine paper turns blue; normal vaginal and urinary secretions are acidic and turn the paper yellow.

### Fetal Assessment

A. Determining fetal position by performing Leopold maneuvers (Figure 26-10).
1. First maneuver: upper abdominal palpation to discover contents of uterine fundus.
2. Second maneuver: location of fetal back in relationship to right and left sides of mother; accomplished by sliding the hands down to a slightly lower position on sides of the abdomen. *FHR heard best through fetal back.*
3. Third maneuver: location of presenting part at pelvic inlet and determination as to whether the presenting part is floating or has engaged; spread hand is applied to the abdomen above the symphysis pubis; gentle palpation of the part of the fetus that lies between thumb and fingers.
4. Fourth maneuver: palpation in a downward and slightly inward direction toward the pelvic inlet; done to determine how far the presenting part has descended into the pelvis.
B. FHR monitoring.

**TEST ALERT:** Monitor fetal heart rate pattern.

1. Intermittent auscultation (IA).
   a. Very common, inexpensive, easy-to-use method using either a fetoscope or ultrasound fetoscope by counting the FHR for 30 to 60 seconds between contractions to obtain the baseline rate.
   b. Auscultate the FHR during a contraction and for 30 seconds after a contraction to identify any increases or decreases in FHR in response to the contraction.
   c. If ultrasound device is used; FHR can be heard as early as 10 to 12 weeks.

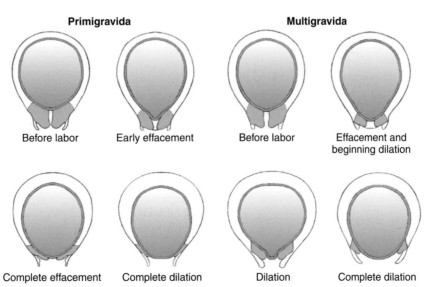

**Primigravida**

Before labor     Early effacement

Complete effacement     Complete dilation

**Multigravida**

Before labor     Effacement and beginning dilation

Dilation     Complete dilation

**FIGURE 26-9 Cervical Dilation and Effacement.** (From McKinney, E., et al. [2013]. *Maternal-child nursing* [4th ed.]. St. Louis, MO: Saunders.)

**Table 26-7 SUMMARY OF OBSERVATIONS AND NURSING CARE DURING LABOR**

| *Physical Findings* | *Nursing Interventions* |
|---|---|
| **Stage 1—Cervical Dilation:** | |
| Begins with onset of regular contractions and ends with complete cervical dilation and effacement; divided into phases—latent, active, and transition | |

| **Latent Phase** | |
|---|---|
| Cervical dilation: 0–3 cm | 1. Orient to hospital environment and personnel. |
| Cervical effacement in primipara is usually complete before dilation; in multipara, it occurs with dilation | 2. Assess history and physical status. |
| | 3. Assess attitudes, past experiences, expectations. |
| Duration of latent phase: 6–8 hours | 4. Teach about labor. |
| Uterine contractions are mild to moderate, 5–30 minutes apart, and last 30–45 seconds | 5. Practice breathing and relaxation techniques. |
| | 6. Monitor physical status: obtain vital signs including FHR. |
| Membranes ruptured or intact | 7. Monitor urine output. |
| Scant brown or pink vaginal discharge or mucous plug | 8. Amount and character of vaginal discharge. |
| Station: primipara, usually 0; multipara, 0 to +2 | 9. Provide comfort measures, oral hygiene. |
| FHR: clearest at level of or below umbilicus, dependent on fetal position | |

| **Active Phase** | |
|---|---|
| Cervical dilation: 4–7 cm | 1. Anticipate needs: |
| Duration of active phase: approximately 3–6 hours | • Sponge face; brush or braid hair per client's wishes. |
| Uterine contractions are moderate to strong, 3–5 minutes apart, and last 40–70 seconds | • Keep bed clean and dry. |
| | • Care for dry, cracked mouth. |
| Scant to moderate bloody mucus | • Check bladder for fullness. |
| Station: +1 to +2 | 2. Stay at bedside, working through each contraction with client; praise woman's efforts; point out progress. |
| FHR: heard slightly below umbilicus or lower abdomen | 3. Reinforce supportive efforts of the father. |
| | 4. Use touch to soothe, relax, comfort. |
| | 5. Check FHR every 15 minutes and BP every 30 minutes. |
| | 6. Observe for hyperventilation. |
| | 7. Client may need analgesia to enhance coping. |
| | 8. Monitor IV and fluid status: increased risk for hypervolemia as a result of fluid retention. |
| | 9. Encourage ambulation if membranes are intact. Lateral position is preferred when in bed, as it increases uteroplacental blood flow. |

| **Transition Phase** | |
|---|---|
| Cervical dilation: 8–10 cm | 1. Continue physical and supportive care. |
| Duration of transition phase: 20–40 minutes | 2. Use palpation or uterine contraction monitor to help client define contractions and rest periods. |
| Uterine contractions of transition phase: strong, 2–3 minutes apart, and last 45–90 seconds | 3. Observe perineum for bulging. |
| Copious bloody mucus | |
| Station: +2 to +3 | |
| FHR: clearest directly about symphysis pubis | |

| **Stage 2—Expulsion of Fetus:** | |
|---|---|
| Begins with complete cervical dilation and ends with delivery of the fetus | |

| | |
|---|---|
| Cervical dilation complete at 10 cm | 1. Direct pushing efforts with assistance and support from father or birthing coach for each contraction. |
| Cervical effacement 100% | |
| Duration of stage 2: 20–50 minutes | 2. Provide comfort measures and facilitate rest between contractions: |
| Uterine contractions are strong, 2–3 minutes apart and last 60–90 seconds; fetal bradycardia may occur during contraction | • Apply cool cloth to face. |
| Membranes may rupture; copious bloody mucus | • Keep perineum clean and dry. |
| Station: fetal descent continues at a rate of 1 cm/hr in primiparas and 2 cm/hr or more in multiparas until perineal floor is reached | 3. Encourage efforts; point out progress. |
| | 4. Explain preparations being made for delivery. |
| Urge to push begins | 5. Check FHR with each contraction. |
| Perineum flattens, bulges | 6. Help with panting for delivery of head and shoulders. |
| Crowning occurs | |
| Infant is born | |

**TEST ALERT:** Monitor client in labor.

**Table 26-7    SUMMARY OF OBSERVATIONS AND NURSING CARE DURING LABOR—cont'd**

| *Physical Findings* | *Nursing Interventions* |
|---|---|
| **Stage 3—Expulsion of Placenta:** | |
| Begins immediately after the infant is delivered and ends when the placenta is delivered | |
| Usually within 5–10 min of delivery | 1. Congratulate. |
| Uterine shape is globular, usually firmer; fundus rises | 2. Initiate maternal contact with infant. |
| Dark vaginal bleeding: gush or trickle | 3. Coach in relaxation for delivery of placenta and perineal repair. |
| Umbilical cord protrudes further from introitus | 4. Watch for signs of placental separation: discoid to globular shape of uterus, gush of blood, lengthening of umbilical cord, and rise of uterine fundus. |
| Placenta intact: Shiny presentation of fetal side of placental separation occurs from inner to outer margins (Schultze mechanism); rough presentation of maternal side of placental separation occurs from outer margins inward (Duncan mechanism) | 5. May administer oxytocics after placenta has been delivered (see Appendix 26-2). |
| **Stage 4—Maternal Homeostatic Stabilization:** | |
| Begins after the delivery of the placenta and continues for 1–4 hours after delivery | |
| Fundus firm or becomes firm when massaged, in midline at level of umbilicus | 1. Facilitation of attachment: ensure that parents have time with newborn; mother may initiate breastfeeding. |
| Moderate lochia rubra | 2. Ongoing assessment (every 15 minutes for 1 hour, then every 30 minutes for 2 hours) of vital signs, fundus, lochia, episiotomy, and bladder function. |
| Episiotomy or laceration repair clean without ecchymosis or discharge, minimal edema; tenderness commensurate with analgesia, usually mild; edges well approximated | 3. Encourage rest for both parents. |
| Possible extrusion of hemorrhoids | |

*BP,* Blood pressure; *FHR,* fetal heart rate.

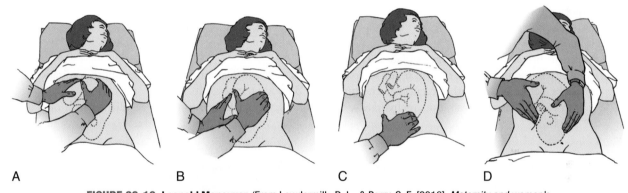

A     B     C     D

**FIGURE 26-10  Leopold Maneuver.** (From Lowdermilk, D. L., & Perry, S. E. [2016]. *Maternity and women's health care* [11th ed.]. St. Louis, MO: Mosby.)

2. Electronic fetal monitoring (EFM).
   a. **External monitoring:** noninvasive procedure that uses two external transducers placed on the maternal abdomen—the *ultrasound transducer* uses high-frequency sound waves to detect FHR, and the *tocotransducer* monitors frequency and duration of contractions by a pressure-sensing device.
      (1) Advantage is its noninvasiveness.
      (2) Does not require rupture of the membranes or cervical dilation.
   b. **Internal monitoring:** invasive procedure that provides accurate, continuous information through use of a *spiral electrode* applied to the fetal presenting part to assess FHR and an *intrauterine pressure catheter (IUPC)* to assess uterine activity (frequency, duration, and intensity of contractions) and pressure.
      (1) Spiral electrode picks up electrical impulses from the fetal ECG.
      (2) Membranes must be ruptured and cervix sufficiently dilated.
   C. Fetal scalp sampling: blood sample is drawn from fetal scalp to assess acid–base status; pH 7.25 or greater is considered normal.

**Nursing Interventions During Labor and Delivery**

*Maternal*

**Goal:** To monitor changes during each stage of labor (see Table 26-7).

**Goal:** To provide relief from pain and discomfort.

A. Administer analgesic medication.
   1. Butorphanol tartrate or nalbuphine hydrochloride.
      a. Widely used and results in good analgesia.
      b. Has less respiratory depression and nausea and vomiting.
      c. Should not be given to women with opioid dependency as may cause withdrawal symptoms.
   2. Fentanyl: used with local anesthetic for induction of spinal block or epidural anesthesia.
   3. Sedatives: hydroxyzine and promethazine.
      a. Are often given as adjuncts to analgesia to relieve tension and anxiety.
      b. Benzodiazepines should not be used during labor due to amnesic effects they have on the mother; also impair body temperature regulation in the newborn.
B. Assist with regional or general anesthesia (see Table 3-3 for nursing care).
   1. Pudendal: administered late in second stage of labor.
      a. Perineal anesthesia of short duration (30 minutes).
      b. Does not cause central nervous system depression in the fetus.
      c. May eliminate bearing-down reflex.
      d. Indicated for woman receiving an episiotomy or requiring forceps or a vacuum extractor during the birthing process.
   2. Epidural.
      a. Given in first and second stages of labor (can be administered with dilation of 4 to 6 cm in active phase or before if the mother requests); intermittent or continuous administration; prehydrate with IV fluids.
      b. May cause maternal hypotension, labor dysfunction, and inability to push effectively.
      c. Patient-controlled epidural anesthesia (PCEA): enables mother to have sense of control of pain management.
   3. Spinal anesthesia (block).
      a. Used for delivery (vaginal or cesarean), not suitable for labor pain control.
      b. May cause marked hypotension, impaired placental perfusion, and ineffective breathing pattern.
      c. Postdural puncture headache (PDPH) can occur due to leakage of CSF from site of puncture of the dura mater.
      d. Epidural blood patch: most rapid way to relieve a PDPH; inject 10 to 20 mL of woman's blood into lumbar epidural space, creating a clot.

> **⊞ NURSING PRIORITY:** To reduce the risk for postpartum infection due to the transmission of pathogens, it is recommended that masks be worn during the induction of intrathecal and epidural anesthesia/analgesia.

### Fetal

**Goal:** To monitor fetal status and detect early complications (Table 26-8).

**Goal:** To provide immediate care to the healthy newborn.

> **TEST ALERT:** Assess a newborn.

A. Airway: clear air passages to establish respirations.
B. Body temperature.
   1. Maintain warmth with a radiant heater or warm environment during initial newborn assessment.

### Table 26-8    SUMMARY OF FETAL HEART RATE: CHARACTERISTICS AND PATTERNS

| Term | Definition | Therapeutic Interventions |
|---|---|---|
| *Baseline rate:* Approximate mean FHR rounded to increments of 5 beats/min during a 10-minute segment, excluding periodic and episodic changes, periods of marked variability, and segments of baseline that differ by greater than 25 beats/min. During the 10-minute time frame, the minimum baseline duration must be at least 2 minutes, otherwise the baseline for that period is undetermined. Normal range at term is 110–160 beats/min. | | |
| *Variability:* Irregular fluctuations in the baseline FHR of two cycles per minute or greater. It is considered reassuring to have variability. | | |
| **Baseline Changes** | | |
| Tachycardia | Baseline rate greater than 160 beats/min for 10 minutes or more<br>*Pathophysiology:*<br>Mild fetal hypoxia<br>Maternal fever<br>Maternal tachycardia<br>Fetal neurologic immaturity | 1. Monitor maternal vital signs.<br>2. Change maternal position.<br>3. Continue to watch closely. |
| Bradycardia | Baseline less than 110 beats/min<br>*Pathophysiology:*<br>Later sign of fetal hypoxia<br>Known to occur before fetal death | 1. Inform neonatal personnel.<br>2. Change maternal position.<br>3. Administer oxygen to mother.<br>4. Prepare for immediate delivery. |

**Table 26-8  SUMMARY OF FETAL HEART RATE: CHARACTERISTICS AND PATTERNS—cont'd**

| Term | Definition | Therapeutic Interventions |
|---|---|---|
| Loss of variability | Smooth baseline as recorded by fetal monitor<br>Can be:<br>Absent—amplitude range undetectable<br>Minimal—amplitude range detectable but less than or equal to 5 beats/min<br>Moderate—amplitude range 6–25 beats/min<br>Marked—amplitude range greater than 25 beats/min<br>*Pathophysiology:*<br>Maternal medication<br>Fetal acidosis (especially if accompanied by late decelerations)<br>Fetal neurologic immaturity | 1. Note time and dose of medication on record.<br>2. See "late deceleration."<br>3. Change maternal position.<br>4. Temporary decrease in variability can occur when fetus is in a sleep state. |
| **Periodic Changes**<br>Acceleration | Abrupt increase in FHR above the baseline rate of 15 beats/min or greater and lasting 15 seconds or more<br>*Pathophysiology:*<br>Breech presentations; occur during fetal movement and are indications of fetal well-being | 1. No specific intervention required. |
| Early deceleration | Visually apparent gradual decrease of the FHR with return to baseline associated with contractions<br>Onset, maximal fall, and recovery coincide with onset, peak, and end of contraction, respectively<br>*Pathophysiology:*<br>Head compression | 1. Distinguish from late deceleration.<br>2. Observe mother for progress in labor because these changes are usually indicative of cervical dilation of 4–6 cm or more.<br>3. Considered a reassuring pattern not associated with fetal hypoxemia, acidosis, or low Apgar. |
| Late deceleration | Visually apparent gradual decrease (onset to lowest point [nadir] greater than or equal to 30 seconds) of FHR below the baseline<br>Generally, the onset, nadir, and recovery of the deceleration occur after the onset, peak, and recovery of the contractions<br>*Pathophysiology:*<br>Uteroplacental insufficiency | 1. Correct underlying cause—examples:<br>• Supine hypotension—change maternal position.<br>• Conduction anesthesia—elevate legs, increase hydration with IV fluids.<br>• Uterine hyperactivity—reduce or discontinue dosage of oxytocin.<br>2. Considered a nonreassuring pattern.<br>3. Left lateral position during labor.<br>4. Administer oxygen to mother.<br>5. Fetal scalp sampling.<br>6. Be prepared for operative delivery if fetal condition warrants. |
| Variable deceleration | Visually apparent abrupt decrease (onset of nadir less than 30 seconds) of the FHR below baseline<br>Decrease is greater than or equal to 15 seconds and less than 2 minutes<br>*Pathophysiology:*<br>Umbilical cord compression | 1. Change maternal position.<br>2. If severe, lasting more than 1 minute, attempt upward displacement of presenting part; help mother into knee–chest or Trendelenburg position; prepare for immediate delivery if pattern does not improve.<br>3. Administer oxygen to mother. |

**NURSING PRIORITY:** Reassuring FHR characterized by 110–160 beats/min with no periodic decelerations and moderate baseline variability; accelerations with fetal movement. Nonreassuring FHR is associated with fetal hypoxemia and include increase or decrease in baseline rate, tachycardia (greater than 160 beats/min), decrease in baseline variability, severe variable decelerations, late decelerations, absence of FHR variability, prolonged deceleration (greater than 60 to 90 seconds), and severe bradycardia (less than 70 beats/min).

*FHR,* Fetal heart rate; *IV,* intravenous.

**Table 26-9   APGAR SCORING SYSTEM**

| Sign | 0 | 1 | 2 |
|---|---|---|---|
| Heart rate | Not detectable | Slow (less than 100) | Greater than 100 |
| Respiratory effort | Absent | Slow, weak cry | Good crying |
| Muscle tone | Flaccid, limp | Some flexion of extremities | Well flexed |
| Reflex irritability | No response | Grimace | Cough, sneeze, or cry |
| Color | Blue, pale | Body pink, extremities blue | Completely pink |

2. Dry, then wrap the newborn snugly in warm blankets for the parents to hold the infant; if infant is placed on mother's chest for skin contact, cover infant with a warm blanket.
3. Place a stocking cap on the infant to decrease loss of heat by evaporation from infant's head.
C. Apgar scoring: immediate appraisal of newborn's condition taken at 1 minute and again at 5 minutes (Table 26-9).

**TEST ALERT: Determine Apgar score of newborn.**

D. Care of the umbilical cord: clamped after pulsation ceases; examine for number of vessels and record (one umbilical artery indicates increased incidence of congenital anomalies, especially renal and genitourinary); no dressing is applied to cord.
E. Care of the eyes: prophylaxis against ophthalmia neonatorum (gonorrhea and chlamydia); ophthalmic tetracycline or erythromycin; silver nitrate is not effective against chlamydia.
F. Identification: wristbands fastened to both infant and mother; appropriate footprints and fingerprints are obtained.
G. Administration of vitamin K: phytonadione: 0.5 to 1.0 mg injected intramuscularly for prevention of neonatal hemorrhagic disease caused by lack of *Escherichia coli*, necessary for the synthesis of vitamin K in the intestines.
H. Inspection for gross abnormalities: clubfoot, imperforate anus, birthmarks, etc.
I. Attachment: ensure contact between newborn and mother as soon as possible after birth.

### Induction of Labor
*Indications*
A. Presence of preexisting maternal disease (e.g., diabetes mellitus, hypertension, and renal disease).
B. Premature rupture of membranes, postterm pregnancy.

C. Hemolytic disease, fetal death, congenital anomaly (e.g., anencephaly).
D. Elective (usually only performed at 39 weeks' gestation).

*Procedure*
A. Prostaglandin E$_2$ gel (dinoprostone) is inserted vaginally to soften or ripen the cervix.
B. Amniotomy: artificial rupture of membranes ("bag of water"); labor often begins spontaneously; reassure her that it is a painless procedure.

**NURSING PRIORITY: FHR is assessed before and immediately after an amniotomy.**

C. Oxytocin is administered intravenously with a physician in attendance and a physician order. ▲ **High-Alert Medication.**
1. Oxytocin is always piggybacked and hooked up to an infusion pump along with a primary intravenous (IV) line in case it needs to be discontinued.
2. Nursing management and information regarding oxytocin is covered in Appendix 26-2.

*Assessment*
A. Careful assessment of uterine contractions is a priority; tetanic contractions could result in uterine rupture, premature separation of the placenta, and fetal hypoxia.
B. FHR: check every 15 minutes along with mother's vital signs.

*Nursing Interventions*
**Goal:** To monitor and evaluate uterine response and fetal response to induction of labor.

A. Frequent vital sign checks and determination of FHR (every 15 minutes); electronic fetal monitoring may be used.
B. Discontinue oxytocin infusion if:
1. Contractions are more frequent than every 2 minutes.
2. Contraction duration lasting greater than 90 seconds.
3. Uterus does not relax; remains contracted and tetanic.
4. Nonreassuring FHR pattern occurs; absent variability; abnormal baseline rate.
5. Repeated late decelerations or prolonged decelerations.

**Goal:** To provide basic intrapartal nursing care as outlined in Table 26-7.

### Emergency Delivery by the Nurse
A. The most important aspect of nursing care is for the nurse to remain calm and support the mother; the delivery process *cannot* be stopped.
B. *Never* force or hold back the oncoming fetal head.
C. As the head appears in the vaginal introitus, the nurse should apply gentle, even pressure with the hand on the emerging head to slow down the baby's process through

the birth canal and to protect the mother's perineum from lacerations.

D. If the membranes have not ruptured when the head is delivered, they should be broken immediately to minimize aspiration of amniotic fluid.

E. Support the head after it is delivered; it will drop toward the mother's rectum, and external rotation (restitution) will take place.

F. Check around the infant's neck for the umbilical cord; if it is found around the infant's neck, gently slip it over the head.

G. Hold infant's head between the palms of both hands and, with a gentle downward motion, bring the anterior shoulder under the symphysis pubis. Then, with a gentle upward motion, the posterior shoulder can be delivered.

H. The rest of the body follows easily.

I. Immediately position with head dependent to facilitate clearing of the airway passages; if there is no spontaneous cry or respirations, dry infant to stimulate respirations, if needed.

J. Keep infant warm by placing on mother's abdomen, skin to skin; then cover both with a warm dry blanket.

K. Palpate the uterus and assist in the delivery of the placenta.

L. Transfer both mother and infant as soon as possible to a hospital facility; it is *not* necessary to cut and tie the umbilical cord, although it may be done if sterile equipment is available.

## OPERATIVE OBSTETRICS

###  Episiotomy

**An episiotomy is an incision through the perineal body to facilitate delivery by enlarging the vaginal orifice. Episiotomy is no longer routinely performed because of evidence regarding harmful effects related to postpartum pain, blood loss, and risk for infection. Practice now is to support perineum and allow the perineum to tear rather than perform an episiotomy.**

#### *Types*

A. Median: midline.
   1. Easy to repair; heals well.
   2. Increased chance of extension through the rectal sphincter muscle (third-, fourth-degree laceration).

B. Mediolateral: made at a 45-degree angle on either right or left side.
   1. More painful healing; increased blood loss.
   2. Less risk for extension into sphincter ani muscle, increased risk of infection.

#### *Assessment*

A. Observe perineal site for bleeding, swelling, redness, or any discharge.

B. Evaluate for pain and discomfort; should be minimal discomfort related to episiotomy; pain may indicate hematoma or abscess formation.

#### *Nursing Interventions*

**Goal:** To alleviate pain and swelling and to promote comfort.

A. Ice pack (first 2 to 24 hours, then as needed for pain relief); later followed by warm or cool sitz baths as needed for perineal discomfort.

B. Analgesic sprays, ointments, or foam, as ordered.

C. Teach importance of perineal cleansing (i.e., use of the squeeze spray bottle; direct flow from front to back; and change perineal pad after each elimination—apply perineal from front to back to avoid contamination).

### Forceps Delivery

**Forceps delivery is the use of an instrument (forceps) with two curved blades to extract the fetal head during delivery.**

#### *Types*

A. Outlet forceps: used if fetal scalp is visible on the perineum without manually separating the labia.

B. Low forceps: application of forceps to the fetal head that is at least 12 cm station.

C. Midforceps: fetal head is at or below the level of the ischial spine.

D. Piper forceps: used in breech deliveries.

#### *Indications*

A. Fetal conditions: nonreassuring fetal heart rate pattern, abnormal presentation.

B. Maternal conditions: to prevent worsening of dangerous conditions (e.g., heart disease), exhaustion, infection, and dystocia.

#### *Assessment*

A. Determine criteria for forceps delivery.
   1. Head fully engaged.
   2. Complete dilation of the cervix.
   3. Membranes have ruptured.
   4. Bowel and bladder should be empty.
   5. Arrest of rotation or delivery of head in a breech position.

B. Monitor FHR, because forceps may compress umbilical cord.

#### *Nursing Interventions*

**Goal:** To assist with forceps delivery.

A. Provide physician with type of forceps required.

B. Assess for conditions necessitating forceps application.

**Goal:** To briefly explain procedure to couple.

A. Monitor FHR.

B. Provide emotional support.

**Goal:** To detect complications from forceps application.

A. Maternal: lacerations to birth canal and rectum.

B. Fetal: cephalhematoma, lacerations and bruising to face, facial paralysis, skull fracture, umbilical cord compression, brain damage.

## Vacuum-Assisted Birth or Vacuum Extraction

**Vacuum-assisted birth or a vacuum extraction is a birth method involving the attachment of a vacuum cup to the fetal head using negative pressure to assist in the birth of the fetal head.**

### Indications

A. Fetal: nonreassuring fetal heart rate pattern; abnormal presentation.
B. Maternal: prevent worsening of dangerous condition (e.g., heart disease), exhaustion, infection.

### Assessment

Same as forceps delivery.
A. Determine criteria for vacuum delivery.
 1. Head fully engaged.
 2. Complete dilation of the cervix.
 3. Membranes have ruptured.
 4. Bowel and bladder should be empty.
 5. Arrest of rotation.

### Nursing Interventions

**Goal:** To assist with vacuum delivery.

A. Provide physician with vacuum and vacuum cup.
B. Assess for conditions necessitating vacuum application.

**Goal:** To briefly explain procedure to couple.

A. Monitor FHR.
B. Provide emotional support.

**Goal:** To detect complications from vacuum application.

A. Maternal: lacerations to birth canal and rectum.
B. Fetal: cephalhematoma, scalp lacerations, and subdural hematoma.

## Cesarean Delivery

**In cesarean delivery, an incision is made in the abdominal and uterine walls to remove the fetus.**

### Types

A. Low-segment transverse incision.
 1. Preferred and most common method.
 2. Decreased blood loss; less chance of uterine rupture with subsequent pregnancy because incision is made into lower uterine segment.
 3. Fewer complications (e.g., peritonitis and postoperative adhesions).
B. Classic cesarean incision: rarely performed.
 1. Used in cases of placenta previa when there are adhesions in the lower uterine segment, transverse fetal lie, or in cases of severe prematurity.
 2. Vertical incision is made between the umbilicus and symphysis pubis.

### Indications

A. Maternal.
 1. Uterine dystocia.
 2. Preexisting maternal disease: heart disease, diabetes, genital herpes, gonorrhea.
 3. Severe preeclampsia and eclampsia.
 4. Previous cesarean delivery or surgery on the uterus.
 5. Tumors of the uterus; postterm pregnancy.
 6. Placenta previa and abruptio placentae.
B. Fetal.
 1. Nonreassuring fetal heart rate pattern.
 2. Prolapsed cord; placental abnormalities.
 3. Fetal abnormalities (e.g., hydrocephalus).
 4. Malpresentation; multiple gestations.

### Assessment

A. Assess for possible indication for cesarean delivery.
B. Trend is that once a cesarean birth occurs, it is highly likely that subsequent births will also be cesarean.
C. Cesarean delivery may be planned for a specific date or may occur as an emergency procedure; common elective reasons are previous cesarean delivery, breech presentation, and cephalopelvic disproportion, along with medical risk factors of hypertension, active genital herpes, positive HIV status, and diabetes.

### Nursing Interventions

**Goal:** To provide preoperative care.
 Preparation is similar to that for any abdominal operation (see Chapter 3).
**Goal:** To provide postoperative care.
 Cesarean delivery includes both normal abdominal postoperative care and postpartum care (see Chapter 3).

## COMPLICATIONS ASSOCIATED WITH LABOR AND DELIVERY

## Preterm Labor

**Preterm labor is defined as cervical changes and uterine contractions occurring between 20 and 37 weeks' gestation.**

### Assessment

A. Risk factors.
 1. Maternal infection; multiple gestations.
 2. Hydramnios; third-trimester bleeding.
 3. Premature rupture of the membranes: bag of water ruptures before the onset of labor.
 4. Incompetent cervical os; previous preterm labor or birth.
 5. Medical complications (e.g., diabetes, hypertension, anemia, periodontal disease).
B. Clinical manifestations.
 1. Contractions occurring with increasing frequency and intensity.
 2. Premature rupture of the membranes.
 3. Cervical dilation; cervical effacement.
 4. Cervical shortening in length.

### Treatment

A. Medications (see Appendix 26-2).
 1. Tocolytics: beta-adrenergic agonist, prostaglandin synthetase inhibitors, and calcium channel blockers.
 2. Antenatal glucocorticoids: betamethasone or dexamethasone.

## Nursing Interventions

**Goal:** To assist in delivery if maternal complications are present.

A. Maternal complications: diabetes, pregnancy-induced hypertension, hemorrhage.
B. Prepare for delivery of premature infant: if indicated, administer betamethasone to minimize/prevent respiratory distress syndrome in the newborn.

> **⚠ NURSING PRIORITY:** Any woman admitted to the hospital who is 24 to 34 weeks pregnant should receive antenatal glucocorticoids to promote fetal lung maturity, unless she has chorioamnionitis. The drug requires a 24- to 48-hour period to become effective.

1. Most effective if delivery is delayed 48 hours after administration.
2. Do not administer glucocorticoids if lecithin/sphingomyelin ratio is adequate; if the mother has diabetes, an infection, or hypertension; or if gestational age is greater than 34 weeks.
3. Administered intramuscularly; watch for pulmonary edema.

**Goal:** To provide emotional support.

A. Encourage expression of feelings related to anxiety and guilt.
B. Identify and support coping mechanisms for couple.

**Goal:** To minimize fetal complications.

A. Promote fetal oxygenation.
   1. Avoid supine position during labor: associated with risk for vena cava syndrome.

> **⚠ NURSING PRIORITY:** Encourage left lateral Sims' position because it promotes placental perfusion.

   2. Avoid maternal hyperventilation: leads to maternal alkalosis, which may decrease oxygen to fetus.
B. Avoid respiratory distress in the newborn.
   1. Conduct labor with minimal analgesia or anesthesia.
   2. Assist with breathing techniques and provide support to the laboring woman.

## 📋 Dysfunctional Labor (Dystocia)

**Dysfunctional labor (dystocia) is a long, difficult, or abnormal labor.**

### Assessment

A. Dysfunctional labor.
   1. Hypotonic contractions: slow, infrequent, weak contractions occurring more than 3 minutes apart and lasting less than 40 seconds.
      a. Causes: uterine overdistention caused by large fetus or twins, polyhydramnios, and grand multiparity.
      b. Complications: relate to prolonged or arrested labor.

   2. Hypertonic contractions: frequent, strong, painful contractions occurring 2 to 3 minutes apart, lasting 60 seconds or more.
      a. Occur more frequently in latent phase of labor.
      b. Cause: cephalopelvic disproportion (CPD) or abnormal fetal position.
      c. Tetanic contractions: uterus stays contracted for more than 90 seconds; may be caused by misuse of oxytocin or mechanical obstruction.
      d. Maternal complications: exhaustion, excessive pain, and uterine rupture.
      e. Fetal complications: fetal distress.
B. Abnormal labor patterns.
   1. Cephalopelvic disproportion (CPD): also called fetopelvic disproportion (FPD); related to excessive fetal size (4000 g or more).
      a. Fetal macrosomia occurring in women with diabetes and cases of postmaturity.
      b. Hydrocephalus.
      c. Fetal malformations: abdominal distention, incomplete twinning.
      d. Maternal pelvis may be too small or abnormally shaped.
   2. Abnormal fetal presentation: breech is most common.
   3. Prolonged or arrested labor: labor lasting for more than 24 hours after onset of regular contractions.
      a. Maternal complications: intrauterine infection, postpartum hemorrhage, fatigue, exhaustion, and dehydration.
      b. Fetal complications: fetal distress and infection.
   4. Precipitous delivery: a very rapid, intense labor lasting less than 3 hours from onset of contraction to time of birth.
      a. Maternal complications: trauma to the soft tissues of the cervix, vagina, and perineum; hemorrhage; loss of self-control.
      b. Fetal complications: fetal hypoxia.

### Treatment

A. Dysfunctional labor (dystocia) relating to CPD or faulty presentation may be treated by a cesarean delivery.
B. Prolonged labor or hypotonic uterine contractions are treated by IV administration of oxytocin.
C. Hypertonic uterine contractions are treated by sedation and rest.

### Nursing Interventions

**Goal:** To monitor level of fatigue and ability to cope with pain.

A. Provide basic comfort measures, back rubs, change of position, clean dry linen.
B. Provide emotional support to mother and significant other.
C. Give reassurance and stay with client continually.

**Goal:** To assist in the medical management of dysfunctional labor.

A. Explain procedures used to rule out cause of dystocia: sonogram, x-ray studies, etc.
B. Monitor oxytocin administration if indicated for hypotonic dysfunction or prolonged labor.

C. Prepare client for cesarean delivery (indicated in cases of CPD and/or faulty presentation).

D. Administer broad-spectrum antibiotics to decrease incidence of infection.

E. Maintain hydration, monitor intake and output, and administer oxygen as needed.

**Goal:** To detect early complications associated with dysfunctional labor.

A. Monitor maternal vital signs.

B. Assess mother for signs of exhaustion, dehydration, increasing temperature, and acidosis.

C. Assess fetal heart tones frequently through fetal electronic monitoring.

## Supine Hypotensive Syndrome

Supine hypotensive syndrome, or vena cava syndrome, occurs when the weight of the uterus causes partial occlusion of the vena cava, leading to decreased venous return to the heart.

### Assessment

A. Shocklike symptoms seen when pregnant woman assumes a supine position.

B. Clients at greatest risk: nulliparas with strong abdominal muscles, gravidas with polyhydramnios or multiple gestations, and obese women.

### Nursing Interventions

**Goal:** To decrease the duration of an episode of supine hypotensive syndrome.

A. Educate mother to turn to either right or left side with knees slightly flexed; preferred position because pressure is removed from vena cava.

B. Administer oxygen as necessary.

C. Assess FHR.

## Placenta Previa

Placenta previa is the abnormal implantation of placenta in the lower uterine segment near or over the internal cervical os.

### Assessment

A. Types of placenta previa.
1. Complete: placenta totally covers internal cervical os.
2. Marginal edge of the placenta is 2.5 cm or closer to the margin of the internal os.
3. Low-lying: placenta is implanted in the lower uterine segment but does not reach the cervical os.

B. Diagnostics.
1. Ultrasonography, especially transvaginal ultrasound, ascertains position of placenta.

C. Clinical manifestations.
1. Painless, bright-red vaginal bleeding occurring after 24 weeks' gestation.
2. Bleeding may stop spontaneously and reoccur without warning during labor and delivery.

### Treatment

A. Medical: if gestation is less than 37 weeks, conservative management of rest and monitoring of hematocrit and hemoglobin values.

B. Surgical: if fetus is mature, delivery via cesarean delivery (possible vaginal delivery for marginal placenta previa if bleeding is not excessive).

### Nursing Interventions

**Goal:** To provide nursing care associated with hemorrhage (Table 26-10).

**Goal:** To detect complications associated with placenta previa: hemorrhage, preterm labor.

**TEST ALERT:** Recognize occurrence of a hemorrhage. It is important to be able to plan nursing management for the pregnant client who has bleeding or hemorrhage (see Table 26-10).

## Abruptio Placentae

Abruptio placentae is the premature separation of part or all of a normally implanted placenta, leading to hemorrhage.

### Assessment

A. Types of abruptio placentae (Figure 26-11).
1. External: blood escapes from the vagina with separation of the placenta.
2. Concealed or internal: hemorrhage occurs within the uterine cavity.
3. Partial separation: may occur with external bleeding or be associated with concealed bleeding.
4. Complete separation: most severe, with profound symptoms of shock.

B. Risk factors.
1. Maternal hypertension; previous abruptio.
2. Cocaine use; smoking history; blunt trauma to abdomen.
3. Multiple gestations.

C. Clinical manifestations.
1. Hemorrhage; hypovolemic shock.
2. Boardlike abdomen.
3. Cramplike abdominal pain.
4. Coagulation problems: hypofibrinogenemia, DIC.

### Treatment

A. Medical: treatment of blood loss and shock; before surgery, type and cross-match for blood transfusion.

B. Surgical: emergency cesarean delivery.

### Nursing Interventions

**Goal:** To provide nursing management associated with hemorrhage (see Table 26-10).

**Goal:** To detect early complications.

A. Disseminated intravascular coagulation (DIC): may occur as a result of concealed uterine hemorrhage and damage to the uterine wall, leading to large amounts of

**Table 26-10  NURSING MANAGEMENT OF HEMORRHAGE IN THE PREGNANT CLIENT**

| Causes and Sources | Symptoms | Nursing Interventions |
|---|---|---|
| **Antepartal Period**<br>Abortion<br>Placenta previa<br>Abruptio placentae | Vaginal bleeding<br>Intermittent uterine contractions<br>Rupture of the membranes<br>**Painless vaginal bleeding**<br>Vaginal bleeding<br>Extreme tenderness in abdomen<br>Rigid, boardlike abdomen<br>**Increase in size of abdomen** | 1. Obtain history of onset, duration, amount of bleeding, and associated symptoms.<br>2. Observe perineal pads for amount of bleeding (blood loss can be measured by weighing perineal pads, approximately 1 g = 1 mL of blood).<br>3. Monitor vital signs of mother and fetus (frequency is determined by severity of clinical symptoms). |

> **TEST ALERT:** Recognize the occurrence of hemorrhage and assess mother for complications.

| | | |
|---|---|---|
| **Intrapartal Period**<br>Placenta previa<br>Abruptio placentae<br>Uterine atony in stage 3 | Bright, painless vaginal bleeding<br>Bright red vaginal bleeding<br>Ineffectual contractility | 1. Start IV and provide volume replacement.<br>2. Request type and cross-match for blood.<br>3. Administer fluids and blood as prescribed.<br>4. Monitor intake and output.<br>5. Minimize chances for further bleeding.<br>6. *NO* vaginal or rectal examinations.<br>7. Bed rest in position of comfort.<br>8. Anticipate cesarean delivery. |
| **Postpartal Period**<br>Uterine atony<br>Retained placental fragments<br>Lacerations of cervix or vagina | Boggy uterus<br>Dark vaginal bleeding<br>Presence of clots<br>Firm uterus<br>Bright red blood | 1. Massage fundus of uterus.<br>2. Assess bladder status.<br>3. Anticipate administration of oxytocin for client with uterine atony.<br>4. Reduce anxiety.<br>5. Keep woman and family advised of treatment plan.<br>6. Record amount of bleeding in a specific amount of time.<br>7. Monitor vital signs: overt hypotension and shock will not be seen until the woman has lost almost one-third of her blood volume (1500–2000 mL); watch for tachycardia and orthostatic BP changes first. |

> ❗ **NURSING PRIORITY:** Frequent, accurate assessment and documentation of blood loss are priorities in postpartum care; two-thirds of cases of postpartum hemorrhage occur without any predisposing risk factors.

*BP,* Blood pressure; *IV,* intravenous.

thromboplastin released into the maternal bloodstream, which leads to hypofibrinogenemia.
1. Assess for indications of DIC: bleeding from injection sites, epistaxis, bleeding gums, purpura, and petechiae.
2. For decreased platelet and fibrinogen levels: administer packed red cells, frozen plasma, and cryoprecipitate.
B. Hypovolemic shock: fluid volume loss caused by hemorrhage, concealed or apparent; monitor vital signs and perineal area.
C. Couvelaire uterus: bleeding into the myometrium, which causes the uterine muscle to lose its power to contract; hysterectomy may be indicated.

### 📋 Ruptured Uterus

**A ruptured uterus is characterized by a tearing or splitting of the uterine wall during labor; it is usually a result of a thinned or weakened area that cannot withstand the strain and force of uterine contractions.**

### Assessment
A. Risk factors.
 1. Multiparity; large fetus.
 2. Obstructive labor; multifetal gestation.
 3. Excessive use of oxytocin.
 4. Weakened, old cesarean delivery scar.
 5. External forces such as trauma.

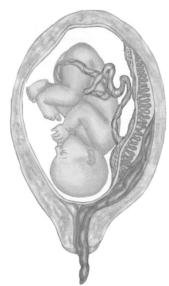

**Marginal abruption**
with external bleeding

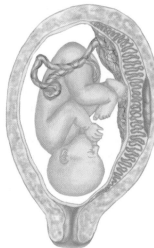

**Partial abruption**
with concealed bleeding

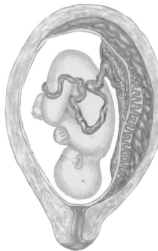

**Complete abruption**
with concealed bleeding

**FIGURE 26-11 Types of Abruptio Placentae.** (From McKinney, E., et al. [2013]. *Maternal-child nursing* [4th ed.]. St. Louis, MO: Elsevier/Saunders.)

B. Clinical manifestations.

> **❗ NURSING PRIORITY:** Monitor the following warning signs of impending uterine rupture: restlessness and anxiety, no indication of labor progress, ballooning out of the lower uterine segment (which simulates a full bladder), appearance of a pathologic retraction ring (an indentation across the lower abdominal wall with acute tenderness above the symphysis pubis).

1. Pain above the symphysis pubis.
2. Sudden, acute abdominal pain during a contraction.
3. Vaginal bleeding, shock; fetal distress.

*Treatment*

A. Surgical: laparotomy to remove fetus, possibly followed by a hysterectomy.

B. Medical.
   1. Blood transfusions.
   2. Prophylactic antibiotics.

*Nursing Interventions*

**Goal:** To provide nursing management associated with hemorrhage (see Table 26-10).
**Goal:** To assess for early diagnosis.

A. Maternal mortality rate is high.
B. Prognosis for fetus is poor; fetus usually dies as a result of anoxia caused by placental separation.

## 📋 Anaphylactoid Syndrome of Pregnancy (Amniotic Fluid Embolism)

An amniotic fluid embolism occurs when amniotic fluid, which may contain fetal debris (e.g., hair, vernix, or meconium), enters the maternal circulation through open venous sinuses in the placenta, at an area of placental separation, or through cervical tears under pressure from the contracting uterus. The fluid travels to the maternal pulmonary arterioles, and the pulmonary vessels become obstructed; prognosis is poor, and the maternal mortality rate is high.

*Assessment*

A. Risk factors.
   1. Increased incidence in multiparas.
   2. Increased incidence in a difficult, rapid labor.
B. Clinical manifestations.
   1. Sudden respiratory distress (dyspnea, cyanosis, pulmonary edema).
   2. Profound shock and vascular collapse.
   3. Decreased fibrinogen (hypofibrinogenemia) and DIC.

*Treatment*

A. Medical: management is similar to that for pulmonary embolism or respiratory distress.
   1. Administer oxygen by nonrebreather facemask (8 to 10 L/min).
   2. Medications: fibrinogen replacement and IV heparin.
   3. Insertion of central venous pressure line, blood transfusions, and cardiopulmonary resuscitation, as indicated.

*Nursing Management*

> **❗ NURSING PRIORITY:** The nurse needs to be particularly observant for symptoms of amniotic fluid embolism in any client who has had a short or difficult labor.

**Goal:** To assist in emergency resuscitation and provide critical care.

A. Assist with ventilation.
B. Prepare for central venous pressure line insertion.
C. Administer medications and blood to treat DIC and shock.

**Goal:** To provide emotional support to father and significant others.

## Abnormal Fetal Position

**This is an unfavorable fetal presentation or position that may interfere with cervical dilation or fetal descent.**

### Assessment
A. Occiput: posterior position (most common).
   1. Dysfunctional labor pattern.
   2. Prolonged active phase of labor.
   3. Intense back pain.
B. Breech presentation.
   1. Increased incidence with premature birth, placenta previa, polyhydramnios, multiple pregnancies, and grand multiparity.
   2. FHR is usually auscultated above the umbilicus.
   3. Passage of meconium is often seen.
   4. Increased danger of prolapsed umbilical cord, especially in incomplete breech presentation.
C. Transverse lie (shoulder presentation).
   1. Increased incidence with placenta previa, neoplasms, fetal anomalies, and preterm labor.
   2. Dysfunctional labor patterns are seen.

### Treatment
A. Occiput: posterior position.
   1. Vaginal delivery is possible; forceps may be needed.
   2. If CPD is present, cesarean delivery is necessary.
B. Breech presentation.
   1. Cesarean delivery is most often performed.
   2. Vaginal delivery: for a frank breech presentation, Piper forceps are used to assist in the extraction of the after-coming head.
C. Transverse lie (shoulder presentation).
   1. Cesarean delivery is the treatment of choice.
   2. External version and extraction may be attempted.
      a. No presence of CPD.
      b. Bag of waters is intact.
      c. Fetus is moveable and contractions are mild.

### Nursing Interventions
**Goal:** To provide reassurance and explanations of procedures, as indicated.

A. Explanation of possible cesarean delivery.
B. When fetus is in occiput-posterior position, encourage positioning of mother on the side or in a modified knee–chest position to decrease pressure on the sacral nerves.
C. Assess for complications related to prolonged labor and possible infection.

## Multiple (Multifetal) Pregnancy

**The term multifetal gestation or pregnancy refers to more than one fetus in the uterus and can include twins (most common), triplets, and higher-order or number of fetuses, e.g., quadruplets (4), quintuplets (5), sextuplets (6), etc.**

### Assessment
A. Risk factors.
   1. Increased incidence of dizygotic twins (fraternal twins) is dependent on race, heredity, advanced maternal age, use of fertility drugs, and parity.
   2. Maternal risks.
      a. Spontaneous abortions are more common.
      b. Anemia occurs.
      c. Increased incidence of pregnancy-induced hypertension, abruptio placentae, placenta previa, and polyhydramnios.
B. Diagnostics.
   1. Auscultation of two or more fetal heart rates.
   2. Measurement of fundal height exceeds gestational age.
   3. Ultrasound.
C. Clinical manifestations.
   1. Increased experience of more physical discomfort: shortness of breath, dyspnea on exertion, backaches, and leg edema caused by excessive size of uterus.
   2. Complications occurring during labor.
      a. Uterine dysfunction caused by overstretched uterus.
      b. Abnormal fetal presentations.
      c. Preterm labor.

### Treatment
A. Medical.
   1. Bed rest in lateral position to promote uteroplacental perfusion.
   2. Antiemetic for nausea and vomiting after the first trimester.
B. Dietary: increase of 300 calories, along with increased protein, iron, folic acid, and vitamin supplements.
C. Serial ultrasound examinations to evaluate for intrauterine growth restriction.
D. Nonstress tests, starting at 30 to 34 weeks' gestation; usually done every 3 to 7 days until delivery.

### Nursing Interventions
**Goal:** To provide anticipatory guidance during the antepartal period.

A. Second trimester: prenatal visits every 2 weeks.
B. Third trimester: weekly visits if there are no complications.
C. Discourage travel because labor may begin without warning.

**Goal:** To provide psychological support.

A. Provide assistance and advice regarding care of twins at home.
B. Because twins are apt to be small, anticipate nursing care for premature neonates.
C. Assess for maternal complications (e.g., postpartum hemorrhage).
D. Ensure correct identification: Baby A and Baby B.

## Prolapsed Cord

**A prolapsed cord occurs when the cord is washed down in front of the presenting part.**

## Assessment

A. Risk factors.
1. Malpresentations: breech.
2. Transverse lie; unengaged presenting part.
3. Increased incidence with prematurity (because of small size of fetus).
B. Clinical manifestations.
1. Commonly occurs after rupture of the membranes.
2. Cord is washed through the birth canal with a gush of amniotic fluid.
3. Visualization of the cord: FHR is decreased, with variable decelerations noted.

## Treatment

A. Surgical.
1. If dilation is incomplete, cesarean delivery is necessary.
2. Occasionally, if dilation is complete, vaginal delivery is possible.

## Nursing Interventions

**Goal:** To maintain fetal oxygenation and assist with immediate delivery.

A. Continuing assessment of FHR.
B. Insert a gloved finger into the vagina and lift the fetal head off the cord to relieve the pressure.
C. Administer oxygen to the mother; start an IV.
D. Place mother in modified Sims' position, knee–chest position, or in Trendelenburg position (head of bed or table is lowered).
E. Any prolapsed cord outside the vagina should be kept moistened with sterile towel soaked in warm saline solution.
F. Offer emotional support to the couple.

## Severely Depressed Neonate

**A neonate with hypoxia and significant acidosis is a severely depressed neonate (Apgar score is 0–6).**

## Assessment

A. Risk factors.
1. Preexisting maternal disease: diabetes, hypertension, preeclampsia.
2. Placental insufficiency caused by:
   a. Maternal hypotension, hypertension, or hemorrhage.
   b. Umbilical cord compression.
   c. Polyhydramnios.
   d. Postmaturity.
3. Rh isoimmunization disease.
4. Uterine dystocia.
B. Clinical manifestations.

> **NURSING PRIORITY:** Initiate actions in response to signs and symptoms of fetal distress. During fetal monitoring, indications of fetal distress are often late or severe variable decelerations, lack of variability, and increase in baseline rate.

1. Severe hypoxia and acidosis.
2. Pale, flaccid, apneic neonate.

3. Heart rate less than 100 beats/min.
4. Slightly reactive or unresponsive to stimulation.

## Treatment

A. Medical.
1. Administration of oxygen, and possibly naloxone, to reverse narcotic respiratory depression.
2. Laryngoscopy and airway suctioning; administration of oxygen.
3. Cardiopulmonary resuscitation, as indicated.
4. Insertion of an umbilical artery catheter; administration of glucose to alleviate hypoglycemia and calcium gluconate to alleviate hypocalcemia.

## Nursing Interventions

**Goal:** To identify appropriate treatment and initiate it quickly for the severely depressed neonate.

A. Assess for fetus at risk and be prepared for emergency measures at birth.
B. Initiate resuscitation procedures.

## Intrauterine Fetal Death

**Intrauterine fetal death is also called fetal demise.**

## Assessment

A. Absence of FHR and fetal movement.
B. Decreased maternal estriol level.
C. Diagnosis: ultrasound examination determines absence of FHR and occurrence of fetal skull collapse.
D. Monitor for complications: hypofibrinogenemia from fetal breakdown products.

## Nursing Interventions

**Goal:** To support the couple through the grieving process.

A. Objectively listen; encourage expression of feelings; do not minimize the situation or event.
B. Anticipate the steps of the grieving process (denial, anger, bargaining, depression, and acceptance).
C. Provide an opportunity for the couple to spend time with the stillborn infant, if they so desire.
D. Prepare the parents to return home by providing ways to inform the siblings, other family members, and friends about the death.
E. Offer information regarding resource or support groups for parents who have lost an infant.
F. Monitor for complications.

## POSTPARTAL ASSESSMENT

> **TEST ALERT:** Assess client for postpartal complications. The puerperium is the period of time spanning the first 6 weeks after delivery. It is the period of time in which the body adjusts both physically and psychologically to the process of childbearing.

### Physiologic Changes

A. Uterus.
1. Uterine involution: process by which the uterus returns to its normal prepregnant condition (Figure 26-12).

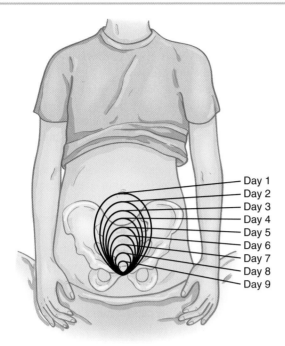

**FIGURE 26-12 Involution of Uterus.** (From Murray, S., & McKinney, E. [2014]. *Foundations of maternal-newborn and women's health* [6th ed.]. St. Louis, MO: Elsevier/Saunders)

2. Immediately after delivery, top of fundus is several finger breadths above the umbilicus.
3. At 12 hours after delivery, the fundus of the uterus is one finger breadth above the umbilicus.
4. Fundus recedes/descends into the pelvis approximately one finger breadth per day.
5. The uterus should not be palpable abdominally after 2 weeks.
6. Afterpains: alternating contractions and relaxations of the uterine muscle.
   a. Occur primarily in multiparas.
   b. May be severe, requiring analgesics.
   c. Usually subside in 48 hours.
7. Lochia.

> ❗ **NURSING PRIORITY:** Always chart the amount first, followed by the character (e.g., moderate amount of lochia rubra).

   a. Lochia rubra: dark red discharge; occurs the first 3 days.
   b. Lochia serosa: pinkish, serosanguineous discharge; lasts approximately 3 to 10 days.
   c. Lochia alba: creamy or yellowish discharge; occurs after day 10 and may last a week or two.
   d. When lochia subsides, uterus is considered closed; postpartal infection is less likely.
B. Cervix.
   1. May be stretched and swollen.
   2. Small lacerations may be apparent.
   3. External os closes slowly; at the end of the first week after delivery, the opening is fingertip size.

C. Vagina.
   1. Does not return to its original prepregnant state.
   2. Rugae reappear in 3 weeks but not as prominent.
   3. Labia majora and minora are more flabby.
D. Perineum.
   1. May be bruised and tender.
   2. Pelvic floor and ligaments are stretched.
   3. Muscle tone is restored by Kegel exercises.
E. Ovulation and menstruation.
   1. Nonbreastfeeding women.
      a. Menstruation resumes in 6 weeks.
      b. Ovulation: 50% may ovulate during the first cycle.
   2. Lactating women.
      a. Varies.
      b. Forty-five percent resume menstruation within 12 weeks after delivery.
F. Abdomen.
   1. Soft and flabby.
   2. Possible separation of the abdominal wall: diastasis recti.
   3. Muscle tone can be restored within 2 to 3 months with exercise.
G. Breasts.
   1. Anterior pituitary releases prolactin, which stimulates secretion of milk.
   2. Engorgement may occur approximately 36 to 48 hours after delivery.
   3. Colostrum (thin, yellowish fluid) is released.
      a. Contains antibodies (immunoglobulin A is 90% of the immunoglobulin present) along with more protein, fat-soluble vitamins (E, A, K), and more minerals such as sodium and zinc.
      b. Colostrum has a laxative effect on the newborn; promotes expulsion of bilirubin-laden meconium.
      c. Also encourages the colonization of the intestine with *Lactobacillus bifidus*, bacteria that inhibit the growth of pathogenic bacteria, fungi, and parasites.
H. Gastrointestinal system.
   1. Immediately after delivery, hunger is common.
   2. Gastrointestinal tract is sluggish and hypoactive because of decreased muscle tone and peristalsis.
   3. Constipation may be a problem.
I. Urinary tract.
   1. Risk for urinary tract infection is increased if client was catheterized during labor and delivery.
   2. May have bruising and swelling caused by trauma around the urinary meatus.
   3. Increased bladder capacity, along with decreased sensitivity to pressure, leads to urinary retention.
   4. Assess for bladder distension, which displaces the uterus leading to a "boggy" uterus and increased bleeding.
   5. To promote voiding, assist woman to the bathroom or with using a bedpan; to prevent excessive blood loss, catheterize the woman if she is unable to void and her bladder is distended.
   6. Diuresis occurs during the first 2 days after delivery.

J. Integumentary system.
 1. Chloasma usually disappears at the end of pregnancy.
 2. Spider nevi, darker pigmentation of areolae and linea nigra, may persist. Dark-red stitch lines gradually fade.
 3. Fingernails return to normal.
 4. Profuse diaphoresis occurs immediately postpartum.
K. Vital signs.
 1. Temperature may be slightly elevated (100.4°F) (38°C) after a long labor; should return to normal within 24 hours.
 2. Blood pressure may be slightly decreased after delivery, but it should remain stable.
 3. Pulse rate slows after delivery.
L. Blood values.
 1. Leukocytosis is present: white blood cell count of 20,000 to 25,000/mm³ (20 to 25 × 10⁹/L) is common.
 2. Hemoglobin and hematocrit values and red blood cell count return to normal within 2 to 6 weeks.
 3. Rule of thumb: 4-point (0.04 proportion of 1.0) drop in hematocrit equals 1 pint (473 mL) of blood loss.
 4. Pregnancy-induced increase in coagulation factors during the first week after delivery leads to increased risk for development of thrombophlebitis and thromboembolism.
M. Weight loss.
 1. Initial 10- to 12-lb (4–5 kg) loss is from the weight of the infant, placenta, and amniotic fluid.
 2. Diuresis leads to an additional 5-lb (2-kg) weight loss.
 3. Six to eight weeks after delivery: return to prepregnant weight if an average of 25 to 30 lb (11–13 kg) was gained.

## Attachment: Psychosocial Response

A. Phases.
 1. Dependent: taking-in phase.
  a. First 1 to 2 days after delivery.
  b. Characterized by passiveness and dependency.
  c. Mother is preoccupied with her own needs: food, attention, and physical comforts and care.
  d. Talkative.
 2. Dependent–independent: taking-hold phase.
  a. Occurs about 2 to 3 days after delivery; characterized by increase in physical well-being.
  b. Emphasis on the present; woman takes hold of the task of mothering; requires reassurance.
  c. Very receptive to teaching.
 3. Interdependent: letting-go phase.
  a. Begins 10 days to several weeks after birth.
  b. Focus is on family unit moving forward: spouse, siblings.
B. Attachment behaviors.
 1. Exploration and identification pattern.
  a. Touch: begins by stroking the extremities and the outline of the head with the fingertips; gradually moves toward using the entire surface of the hand; touches and observes first at arm's length, then on

lap, or slightly away from the body; finally enfolds infant close to body with both arms.
  b. Eye-to-eye contact: *en face position* (gazing into the eyes of the infant).
 2. Factors influencing maternal–infant attachment.
  a. Relationship with own parents.
  b. Previous experience with infants.
  c. Social, economic, and developmental levels of mother.
  d. Acceptance of pregnancy as a positive event.
  e. Anesthetic/analgesic used in labor; type of delivery.
  f. Support of significant others.
  g. Amount of time of initial contact between mother and infant.
  h. Health and responsiveness of infant.
C. Postpartum blues.
 1. Transient period of depression (occurring during the puerperium).
 2. Complaints of anorexia; insomnia; tearfulness; a general let-down, sad feeling.
 3. Thought to be caused by fatigue, discomfort, sensory overload or deprivation, and hormonal changes.
 4. Woman needs support and reassurance that it is a transient and self-limiting experience.
 5. A very small percentage of new mothers are at risk for developing severe postpartum depression, leading in the extreme to postpartum psychosis, both of which require hospitalization. Safety of both the mother and baby is a critically important priority if either of these conditions develops.

## POSTPARTUM NURSING CARE

**TEST ALERT:** Perform postpartum assessments and instruct client on postpartum care.

**Goal:** To initiate routine postpartum assessment.

A. General observations of mood, activity level, and feelings of wellness; routine vital sign assessment.
B. Inspection of breasts: check for beginning engorgement and presence of cracks in nipples, any pain or tenderness, and progress of breastfeeding.
C. Check uterine fundus: determine height of fundus in relation to umbilicus; should feel firm and globular (Figure 26-13).
D. Assess for bladder distention, especially during the first 24 to 48 hours after delivery.
E. Perineal area.
 1. Observe episiotomy site.
  a. Evaluate healing status of episiotomy.
  b. Apply anesthetic sprays or ointments to decrease pain.
 2. Determine whether hemorrhoids are present, and if so, provide relief measures.
F. Lochia: record color, odor, and amount of discharge.
G. Lower extremities: assess for thrombophlebitis; encourage ambulation as soon as possible to decrease venous stasis.

# FUNDAL MASSAGE TECHNIQUE

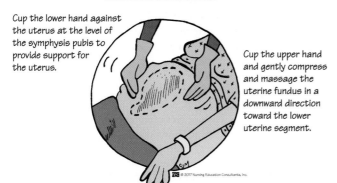

Cup the lower hand against the uterus at the level of the symphysis pubis to provide support for the uterus.

Cup the upper hand and gently compress and massage the uterine fundus in a downward direction toward the lower uterine segment.

**FIGURE 26-13 Fundal Massage Technique.** (From Zerwekh, J., Garneau, A., & Miller, C. J. [2017]. *Digital collection of the memory notebooks of nursing* [4th ed.]. Chandler, AZ: Nursing Education Consultants, Inc.)

H. Abdomen and perineum.
  1. Initiate strengthening exercises for both abdominal wall and perineum (e.g., leg lifts and isometric Kegel exercises for strengthening pelvic floor).
  2. Kegel exercises: practice trying to stop the passing of gas or the flow of urine midstream, which replicates the sensation of the pelvic muscles drawing upward and inward.

**Goal:** To provide comfort and relief of pain.

A. Episiotomy: ice packs for first 24 hours; sitz baths.
B. Perineal care: use of "peri bottles" to squirt warm water over perineum (front to back) to prevent contamination and avoid use of toilet tissue.
C. Afterpains: use of analgesics (preferably 1 hour before feeding, especially for breastfeeding mothers).
D. Hemorrhoidal pain.
  1. Sitz baths, anesthetic ointments, rectal suppositories, astringent wipes.
  2. Encourage lying on side and avoidance of prolonged sitting.
  3. Stool softeners or laxatives may be indicated; client usually has normal bowel movement by second or third day after delivery.
E. Breast engorgement (during lactation): well-fitting bra should be worn to provide support.
F. Lactation suppression: well-fitting bra or breast binder, ice packs to breasts; application of fresh cold cabbage leaves inside of bra.

**Goal:** To promote maternal–infant attachment and facilitate integration of the newborn into the family unit.

**TEST ALERT:** Facilitate parental bonding with newborn.

A. Use infant's name when talking about him or her.
B. Serve as a role model; be cautious not to appear too expert in handling the infant because it may lead to feelings of discouragement in the mother.

C. Assist parents in problem solving and meeting their infant's needs. Explain ways to distinguish different types of cries—those related to hunger, illness, discomfort, etc.
D. Encourage parents to provide as much of the care to the infant as possible while still in the hospital.
E. Accept parents' emotions; encourage expression of feelings.
F. Help parents understand sibling behavior and planning for the arrival of the new family member.

**Goal:** To establish successful infant feeding patterns.

A. Nonlactating mother.
  1. Provide supportive bra.
  2. Explain and demonstrate proper position for feeding.
  3. Formulas: review formula recommended and how it is supplied.
B. Lactating mothers.
  1. Teach mother to refrain from using sunlamps or hair dryers to dry nipples or applying breast creams.
  2. Application of expressed breast milk to nipples after each feeding has a bacteriostatic effect and may provide protection to damaged skin.
  3. On first postpartum checkup, assess breasts for engorgement, nipple inversion, cracking, inflammation, or pain.
  4. Explain process of lactation and refer mother to community resources such as a lactation consultant or La Leche League.

**Goal:** To prevent infection and detect potential complications.

A. Recognition of significant postpartum risk factors in the new mother (Box 26-3).
B. Encourage a postpartum checkup visit to take place 4 to 6 weeks after delivery.
C. If symptoms of excessive bleeding, temperature elevation, pain in the calves, foul-smelling vaginal discharge, swollen breasts, or general feelings of malaise and illness occur, woman should contact her health care provider immediately.

**Goal:** To prepare and plan for discharge.

**TEST ALERT:** Assist client with infant feeding.

A. Determine whether mother will need household help (especially important in birth of twins or after cesarean delivery).

| Box 26-3 POSTPARTUM HIGH-RISK FACTORS |
| --- |
| Preeclampsia |
| Diabetes |
| Cardiac disease |
| Cesarean delivery |
| Overdistention of uterus (multiple gestations) |
| Abruptio placentae and placenta previa |
| Precipitous or prolonged labor |
| Difficult delivery |
| Extended period in lithotomy position (legs in stirrups) |
| Retained placenta |

B. Explain and teach the following infant care skills.
1. Infant feeding (Box 26-4 and Figure 26-14).
   a. Hold bottle so that air does not get into nipple.
   b. Method of making or preparing formula.
   c. How to break the infant's suction on the nipple.
   d. Positioning for burping and bubbling.
   e. Teach how to determine whether infant is getting enough milk (Box 26-5).
2. Diapering.
   a. Frequent changing to prevent diaper rash.
   b. Protective ointment can be used to prevent irritation.
   c. Keep diaper below umbilical area.

---

### Box 26-4 BREASTFEEDING

**Types of Feeding Positions**
- Cradle position, side-lying, football or clutch position, and modified clutch position.

**Teach Mother to:**
- Bring infant to level of the breast: do not lean over.
- Turn infant completely on side with arms embracing the breast on either side.
- Bring infant in as close as possible with legs wrapped around the mother's waist and the tip of the nose touching the breast.
- Bring infant's lips to nipple; when infant opens mouth to its widest point, draw the infant the rest of the way onto the nipple for him or her to latch on (see Figure 26-14).
- Break the suction by placing a clean finger in the side of the infant's mouth before removing the infant from the breast.
- Put infant to breast 8 to 12 times per day.
- Avoid the use of nipple shields or bottle nipples.
- Avoid use of pacifier until infant is well established on breastfeeding, usually around 4 to 6 weeks of age.

---

### Box 26-5 EVALUATING BREASTFEEDING

**How Do You Know That an Infant Is Getting Enough Breast Milk?**
- Hear infant swallow and make soft "ka" or "ah" sounds.
- Observe for smooth nutritive suckling—the smooth series of sucking and swallowing with occasional rest periods (not the short, choppy sucks that occur when the baby is falling asleep).
- Breast gets softer during the feeding.
- Infant is breastfeeding 8 to 12 times per day; more milk is produced with frequent breastfeeding.
- Infant has at least two to six wet diapers per day for first 2 days after birth; six to eight diapers per day by the fifth day.
- Infant has at least three bowel movements daily during the first month and often more.
- Infant is gaining weight and is satisfied after feedings.

---

3. Bathing.
   a. Use of a mild soap.
   b. Kitchen sink is often a good place to bathe infant.
   c. Non–alcohol-based lotions can be applied; best advice is to avoid use of powders.
4. Umbilical cord.
   a. Wash with soap daily and after every diaper change.
   b. Stump usually falls off in 7 to 10 days.
5. Nonnutritive sucking.
   a. Pacifiers may be used to meet infant's sucking need.
   b. Evidence that pacifiers help prevent sudden infant death syndrome (SIDS).
   c. May be used up to age 4 years or when permanent teeth erupt.
6. Sleeping.
   a. Usually sleeps through the night at around 2 to 3 months of age.
   b. Encourage mother to sleep while infant is sleeping to avoid sleep deprivation.
7. Illness.
   a. Common behavior changes are irritability, crying, loss of appetite, and fever.
   b. Explain how to take an infant's temperature.
8. Taking the infant outside.
   a. Dress infant as you would dress yourself; do not overdress infant or "bundle up."
   b. Traveling: use a car seat.
9. Explain importance of follow-up well-baby checkup visits with health care provider, usually scheduled within a week of discharge.

**TEST ALERT:** Assess new mother for postpartum complications.

## COMPLICATIONS OF THE PUERPERIUM

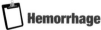

### Hemorrhage

**Postpartum hemorrhage is defined as the loss of 500 mL or more of blood after vaginal birth and 1000 mL or more after cesarean birth.**

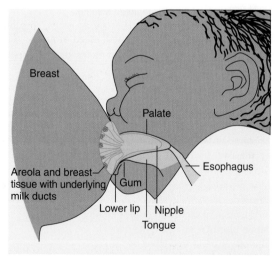

**FIGURE 26-14 Correct Attachment (Latch on) of Infant at Breast.** (From Perry, S., Hockenberry, M., Lowdermilk, D., et al. [2014]. *Maternal child nursing care* [5th ed.]. St. Louis, MO: Elsevier/Mosby.)

*Assessment*

A. Risk factors.
 1. Precipitous labor, dystocia.
 2. Premature separation of placenta.
  a. Abruptio placentae.
  b. Placenta previa.
 3. Forceps delivery, multiple pregnancy.
 4. Large fetus, polyhydramnios, prolonged labor.
B. Causes.
 1. Uterine atony.
 2. Lacerations.
 3. Retained placental tissue.
C. Clinical manifestations.
 1. Early postpartal hemorrhage: occurs within the first 24 hours after delivery.
 2. Late postpartal hemorrhage: occurs after the first 24 hours.
 3. Uterine fundus difficult to locate or feels soft, "boggy" when located.
 4. Bright red lochia, excessive clots expelled (with or without uterine massage).
 5. Symptoms of shock: weak, rapid pulse; low blood pressure; pallor; restlessness; etc.

*Treatment*

A. Medical.
 1. Uterine atony.
  a. Oxytocic medications.
  b. Bimanual compression of the uterus.
  c. Fluid and blood replacement.

> **⚠ NURSING PRIORITY:** The key to successful management of hemorrhage is prevention, which includes adequate nutrition, good prenatal care, early diagnosis and management of any complications as they arise, and avoidance of traumatic procedures.

B. Surgical.
 1. Lacerations: suturing the bleeding edges.
 2. Retained placenta: dilation and curettage (D&C) to remove retained fragment(s).

*Nursing Interventions*

**Goal:** To control and correct the cause of the hemorrhage.

A. Uterine atony.
 1. Massage uterus to stimulate contractions; make sure bladder is empty.
 2. Administer oxytocic medications.
B. Lacerations.
 1. Inspect perineal area.
 2. Hematoma formation.
  a. Vulvar hematoma may appear as a discoloration of the perineal area.
  b. Any complaint of pain in the perineal area should prompt careful inspection.
 3. Do not administer rectal suppositories/enemas or perform rectal examinations.

> **⚠ NURSING PRIORITY:** Careful observation of vaginal bleeding, by doing a pad count or weighing the perineal pads, is very important. Always check under client's buttocks, as blood may flow between buttocks onto linens under the client.

C. Retained placenta.
 1. Inspect placenta at the time of delivery for intactness.
 2. Never force the expulsion of the placenta.

**Goal:** To maintain adequate circulating blood volume to prevent shock and anemia.

A. Type and cross-match blood for women at high risk for development of postpartum hemorrhage.
B. Anticipate replacement of IV fluids and blood.
C. Check hematocrit and hemoglobin values.
D. Monitor for development of hypovolemic shock.
E. Monitor vital signs and amount of lochia.

**Goal:** To prevent postpartal infection.

A. Maintain aseptic technique.
B. Administer prophylactic antibiotics.
C. Monitor vital signs.

**Goal:** To prevent postpartal hemorrhage.

A. Identify women at increased risk.
B. Monitor hematocrit levels throughout pregnancy.
C. Encourage use of supplemental iron to prevent anemia.
D. Promote good nutrition.
E. Instruct client to palpate uterus for firmness, and teach client how to massage fundus.

## 📋 Postpartum Infection (Puerperal Infection)

**Postpartum infection is any clinical infection of the genital canal that occurs within 28 days after miscarriage, abortion, or childbirth.**

*Assessment*

A. Predisposing factors.
 1. Antepartal infection.
 2. Premature rupture of the membranes, prolonged labor.
 3. Laceration.
 4. Anemia; postpartum hemorrhage.
 5. Poor aseptic technique.
B. Clinical manifestations.
 1. Temperature elevation 38°C (100.4°F) if taken at least four times daily on any 2 of the first 10 postpartum days, with the exception of the first 24 hours after birth.
 2. Symptoms vary depending on the system involved.
 3. Area of involvement is characterized by five cardinal symptoms of inflammation (redness, pain, heat, edema, and loss of function).
 4. Tachycardia, chills, and abdominal tenderness are common.
 5. Headache, malaise, deep pelvic pain.
 6. Profuse, foul-smelling lochia.

C. Area involved.
 1. Uterus is most often affected: endometritis.
 2. May have localized wound infection of the perineum, vulva, and vagina.
 3. Local infection may extend via the lymphatics into the pelvic organs.
 4. Urinary system: urinary tract infection (UTI).

### Treatment

A. Medications: antibiotics, antipyretics.
B. Dietary.
 1. High-protein, high-calorie, high-vitamin diet.
 2. Encourage intake of 3000 to 4000 mL of fluid per day.

### Nursing Interventions

**Goal:** To prevent puerperal infection.

A. Maintain meticulous aseptic technique during labor and delivery.
B. Assess and treat antepartum infection.
C. Detect anemia: check hematocrit during prenatal visits.
D. Avoid prolonged labor.

**Goal:** To promote mother's resistance to infection.

> **! NURSING PRIORITY:** The pathophysiology related to maintaining semi-Fowler's position to localize infection is important to remember not only for clients with obstetric complications but also for others with contaminated drainage.

A. Administer antibiotic, antipyretic, and oxytocic medications.
B. Encourage good nutrition.
C. Isolate client from other maternity clients.
D. Use semi-Fowler's position to promote free drainage of lochia and prevent upward extension of infection into pelvis.

### Mastitis

**Mastitis is the invasion of the breast tissue by pathogenic organisms. It is usually unilateral and develops after the flow of milk is established.**

### Assessment

A. Predisposing factors.
 1. Fissured nipples, erosion of the areola.
 2. Mastitis is most frequently caused by *Staphylococcus*, which is transmitted from the nasopharynx of the nursing infant.
B. Clinical manifestations.
 1. Occurs most during the first 6 weeks of breastfeeding.
 2. Chills, malaise, and tachycardia.
 3. Red, swollen, painful breast(s); axillary adenopathy.
 4. Fever of 39.4°C (103°F) or 40°C (104°F).

### Treatment

A. Medication.
 1. Antibiotics for 10 to 14 days.
 2. Antipyretics, analgesics.

### Nursing Interventions

**Goal:** To prevent the complication of mastitis.

A. Teach mother how to care for breasts and nipples.

> **! NURSING PRIORITY:** Mother should continue to breastfeed on the affected side because failure to do so increases the risk for abscess formation and relapse.

B. Explain the importance of wearing a bra that provides adequate support.

**Goal:** To promote comfort and maintain lactation.

A. Frequent breastfeeding, starting on the affected side.
B. Breast massage before and during each feeding to thoroughly drain any blockages (a breast pump may be used if the infant is unable to do this).
C. Encourage good nutrition and adequate rest.
D. Application of moist heat; warm showers; increased intake of fluids and vitamin C.
E. Administer antibiotics, as ordered.

### Postpartum Mood Disorders

**This is the predominant mental health disorder during the postpartum period and includes postpartum blues (baby blues; most common), postpartum depression, and postpartum psychosis.**

### Assessment

A. Postpartum blues ("baby blues").
 1. Normal functioning is not impaired.
 2. Mood swings, feelings of sadness and anxiety, crying, difficulty sleeping, and loss of appetite.
 3. Resolves within a few days.
 4. Treatment: none.
B. Postpartum depression.
 1. Meets criteria for major depressive episode (MDE) with onset in pregnancy or within 4 weeks of child birth.
 2. Eventually cannot care for themselves or their newborn; often rejection of the infant occurs.
 3. Severe, labile mood swings.
 4. Intense fears, anger, anxiety, irritability, despondency.
 5. Difficulty falling asleep.
 6. Obsessive thoughts about harming the infant.
 7. The natural course is one of gradual improvement over the 6 months after birth.
 8. Treatment: antidepressant medication (SSRI).
C. Postpartum psychosis.
 1. Rare condition that has an onset within 2 weeks postpartum.
 2. Presence of one or more episodes of abnormally elevated energy levels, cognition, and mood and one or more depressive episodes; associated with bipolar disorder.
 3. Delusions, hallucinations, extreme deficits in judgment.
 4. Fatigue, insomnia, restlessness, tearfulness, emotional lability.

5. Complaints regarding the inability to move, stand, or work.
6. Suspiciousness, confusion, incoherence, irrational statements, obsessive concerns about infant.
7. Treatment: possible inpatient psychiatric care, antipsychotic and mood-stabilizing medications.
D. Nursing Interventions are outlined in Chapter 12.

> **! NURSING PRIORITY:** Mothers who have postpartum depression with psychotic symptoms may harm their infants, so early assessment and intervention are safety concerns.

## Thrombophlebitis

There is an increased risk (five times) for thrombophlebitis and pulmonary embolism during the postpartum period. The reason for the increased incidence is a change in blood coagulation during pregnancy and a decrease in partial thromboplastin time, along with engorgement of the veins of the lower extremities and pelvis, which leads to pooling of blood and venous stasis. Assessment and nursing interventions are discussed in Chapter 18.

## Cystitis and Pyelonephritis

Cystitis and pyelonephritis occur as a result of trauma to the bladder mucosa, the temporary loss of bladder tone, and an increased bladder capacity. All three lead to distention and incomplete emptying of urine, predisposing the postpartum client to cystitis and pyelonephritis (see Chapter 25).

## Parents' Reaction to Preterm Infant, Ill Newborn, or Infant With Congenital Anomaly

### Assessment

A. Period of disorganization.
   1. Grief reaction characterized by guilt, anger, and sorrow.
   2. Feelings of exhaustion, emptiness, and frequent crying.
B. Period of information seeking and resource utilization.
   1. Anxiety decreases; problem-solving begins.
   2. Begins to resolve the crisis.
   3. Often information seeking leads to further anger and sorrow, followed by a period of denial or disbelief.
C. Resolution of the crisis situation.
   1. Development of new coping strategies.
   2. Acceptance and coming to terms with the situation.

### Nursing Interventions

**Goal:** To provide emotional support to the parents.

A. Encourage verbalization of feelings and expression of grief.
B. Promote maternal–infant contact; point out normal characteristics.
C. Encourage parents to visit, touch, and care for their infant as much as possible.
D. Refer parents to social and community agencies.

---

| Appendix 26-1  CONTRACEPTIVE METHODS |  |
|---|---|

| Methods/Description | Nursing Implications/Client Teaching |
|---|---|
| **Natural Family Planning Methods** | |
| Calendar (rhythm) or Standard Days Method (SDM) | *Client Teaching*<br>1. Calendar (rhythm) method: calculate the days of fertility; considered to be days 10–17 of a 28-day menstrual cycle.<br>2. CycleBeads: red beads mark first day of menstrual cycle; white beads are fertile days; brown beads are when ovulation is unlikely.<br>3. BBT method: a slight decrease (0.5°) at ovulation, then an increase of about 0.2° to 0.5° in temperature after ovulation occurs; fertile period day the temperature drops through 3 consecutive days of temperature elevation; need a special BBT thermometer.<br>4. Cervical mucus method: before ovulation, mucus becomes clear and stringy; nonfertile period occurs when mucus becomes thick, cloudy, and sticky or when no mucus is apparent.<br>5. Symptothermal method: combines two methods, usually cervical mucus and BBT.<br>6. Home predictor test kits: urine test is used to determine ovulation; test monitors and identifies an LH surge via a color change. |

*Continued*

| *Methods/Description* | *Nursing Implications/Client Teaching* |
| --- | --- |
| **IUD** | |
| Hormonal intrauterine system IUD; Copper T 380A IUD | *Client Teaching*<br>1. Discuss the technique and the experience of IUD insertion and removal.<br>2. Emphasize the need for yearly Pap smears.<br>3. Encourage client to check IUD string, especially after each period.<br>4. Make sure the woman understands which type of IUD she has and when to return to have it checked or replaced. Copper IUD is approved for 10 years. The hormonal intrauterine system IUD is effective for up to 5 years, and uterine cramping and bleeding are diminished compared with the copper IUD.<br>5. Review common side effects and serious complications. Report any of the following symptoms (PAINS) (Figure 26-15). |

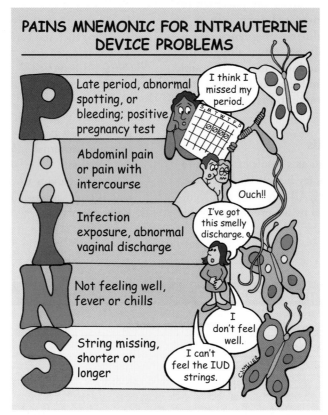

**FIGURE 26-15 PAINS Mnemonic for Intrauterine Device.** (From Zerwekh, J., Garneau, A., & Miller, C. J. [2017]. *Digital collection of the memory notebooks of nursing* [4th ed.]. Chandler, AZ: Nursing Education Consultants, Inc.)

| *Methods/Description* | *Nursing Implications/Client Teaching* |
|---|---|

### Hormonal Methods

Combined oral contraceptive: the "pill" is a combination of estrogen and progestin

Progestin only: norethindrone; medroxyprogesterone

Transdermal contraceptive patch: applied once a week; has both hormones

Vaginal contraceptive ring: a ring inserted into the vagina for 3 weeks; removed for 1 week, then new ring inserted

*Client Teaching*

1. Instruct as to correct use of medication, the need for follow-up in 3 months, and importance of taking the pill at same time each day; effectiveness is close to 100% when used correctly.
2. If using a 28-day cycle product (21 active pills and 7 inactive pills) (except Natazia), provide the following instructions regarding missed doses.
   - If *one or more pills* are missed in the *first* week, take one pill as soon as possible and then continue with the pack. Use an additional form of contraception for 7 days.
   - If *one or two pills* are missed during the *second* or *third week*, take one pill as soon as possible and then continue with the active pills in the pack—but skip the inactive pills and go straight to a new pack once all the active pills have been taken.
   - If *three or more pills* are missed during the *second* or *third week*, follow the same instructions given for missing one or two pills, but use an additional form of contraception for 7 days.*
3. Review common side effects and serious complications. Report any of the following symptoms (ACHES) (Figure 26-16).
4. Progestin-only pill causes more menstrual irregularity (breakthrough bleeding, variation in blood flow, etc.).

*Burchum, J. R., & Rosenthal., L. D. (2016). *Lehne's pharmacology for nursing care* (9 ed.). St. Louis, MO: Elsevier/Saunders, p. 766.

*Continued*

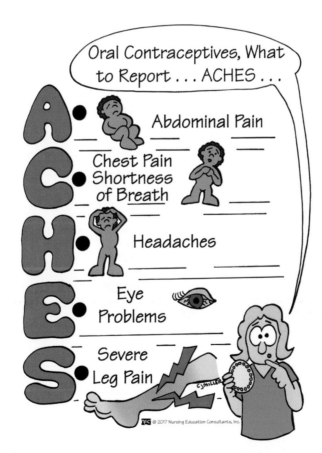

**FIGURE 26-16 ACHES Mnemonic for Oral Contraceptive Complications.** (From Zerwekh, J., Garneau, A., & Miller, C. J. [2017]. *Digital collection of the memory notebooks of nursing* [4th ed.]. Chandler, AZ: Nursing Education Consultants, Inc.)

## Appendix 26-1   CONTRACEPTIVE METHODS—cont'd

| *Methods/Description* | *Nursing Implications/Client Teaching* |
|---|---|

### Injectable/Implantable Progestins

| Injectable (Depot medroxyprogesterone acetate: IM or subQ) | *Client Teaching*<br>1. Started during the first 5 days of menstrual cycle and requires injections only four times per year (every 11–13 weeks).<br><br>**■ NURSING PRIORITY:** *Do not massage* the site after the injection because it may speed up absorption and decrease duration of effectiveness; effectiveness rate is comparable to that of oral contraceptives.<br><br>2. Disadvantages include weight gain, prolonged amenorrhea, and breakthrough uterine bleeding. Long-term use may decrease bone density; need to encourage calcium intake and exercise.<br>3. Because of loss of bone mineral density, women should be advised to have adequate calcium intake and exercise regularly. |
| Implantable: single rod implant | 1. Requires a small incision in the inner aspect of the nondominant upper arm with a local anesthetic; provides up to 3 years of contraception.<br>2. The most common side effect is irregular menstrual bleeding. |

### Barrier Methods

| Diaphragm: a dome-shaped rubber device that fits over the cervix<br>Cervical caps: a rubber or latex–silicone cap that fits snugly over the cervix | *Client Teaching*<br>1. Should be refitted after every pregnancy or when there is a weight gain or loss of 10–20 lb (4.54–9.09 kg) or a 20% weight fluctuation; replaced every 2 years.<br>2. Instruct client to use spermicidal jelly or cream around diaphragm rim and in the dome.<br>3. Instruct client to inspect diaphragm before use for any holes or punctures and leave diaphragm in place 6–8 hours after intercourse.<br>4. Explain the proper method for cleansing (use mild soap only), storing (dry thoroughly and dust with cornstarch, not baby powder), and checking for defects or holes in the diaphragm.<br>5. Allow for sufficient practice of insertion/removal techniques and use with a spermicide, such as nonoxynol-9 (N-9).<br>6. Risk of toxic shock syndrome with both devices if left in place longer than 8 hours. |
| Condoms are thin sheaths of rubber that fit over an erect penis<br>Female condom: disposable | 1. Advise client to apply condom to erect penis by rolling the sheath along the entire shaft and leaving enough slack at the end of the penis to receive the semen.<br>2. Explain importance of holding the condom in place while withdrawing the penis to prevent emptying of sperm into the vagina.<br>3. Condom should be applied before any penetration because the preejaculatory seminal fluid may contain sperm.<br>4. Ask client about allergy to latex.<br><br>**■ NURSING PRIORITY:** Use of nonoxynol-9 with diaphragms or condoms is not a recommended method for preventing STDs or HIV. |

### Unreliable Practices

| Withdrawal (coitus interruptus): withdrawal of penis before ejaculation | *Nursing Implications*<br>1. Requires absolute cooperation and control of partner.<br>2. Good choice for couples who do not have any other contraceptive methods available. |
| Douching: the act of cleansing washing the semen out of the vagina | Client Teaching<br>1. Douching may actually move the sperm upward in the vagina.<br>2. Encourage use of a more reliable contraceptive practice. |

## Appendix 26-1 CONTRACEPTIVE METHODS—cont'd

| Methods/Description | Nursing Implications/Client Teaching |
|---|---|
| **Emergency Contraception** | |
| Plan B: One-step dose of high-dose progestin<br>Other options:<br>High-dose oral estrogen<br>Insertion of copper IUD | *Client Teaching*<br>1. Available without a prescription; prescription required if under age 18.<br>2. Should be taken within 72 hours of unprotected intercourse; may be effective up to 5 days after intercourse.<br>3. Plan B will not terminate an existing pregnancy or harm a fetus; hence, it does not cause abortion because it acts prior to fertilization and implantation.<br>4. To prevent nausea with high-dose estrogen, take an over-the-counter antiemetic 1 hour before each dose.<br>5. IUD must be inserted within 5 days of unprotected intercourse. |
| **Permanent Sterilization** | |
| Tubal ligation (minilaparotomy) | *Client Teaching*<br>1. Discuss the permanence of the sterilization procedure with the couple—informed consent required for all procedures.<br>2. Explain that the woman may experience sensation of tugging but not pain during procedure, which is carried out via local anesthetic. |
| Essure system (transcervical sterilization) | 1. Insertion of an occlusive agent (small metallic implants) into the uterine tubes, which stimulate scar tissue formation that occludes the tubes.<br>2. Procedure does not provide immediate contraception—need to use another form of contraception until tubal blockage is proven, which may take up to 3 months.<br>3. Instruct client to report any unusual vaginal bleeding, spotting, purulent drainage, persistent abdominal pain, fever, or chills to health care provider. |
| Vasectomy: surgical ligation and resection bilaterally of the vas deferens | 1. Discuss with couple the permanence of vasectomy (informed consent required); even if the vas deferens is reconnected, fertility varies between 5% and 60%.<br>2. Activity level should be moderate for 2 days; skin sutures are usually removed within a week.<br>3. Encourage the use of a scrotal support and application of ice for scrotal pain or swelling.<br>4. Follow-up visit for sperm sample is usually done in 4–6 weeks.<br>5. Advise couple to use another form of birth control until it is verified that two ejaculate sperm counts contain no sperm. |

*BBT,* Basal body temperature; *IUD,* intrauterine device.

## Appendix 26-2 MEDICATIONS

### ▲ Magnesium Sulfate

| Medications | Side Effects | Nursing Implications |
|---|---|---|
| **Anticonvulsant** | | |
| IV: Given via an IV pump, piggybacked to primary infusion. A bolus dose (4–6 g over 15–20 minutes) is routinely given, followed by a maintenance infusion (1–4 g/hr). | *Maternal:* Sweating, flushing, muscle weakness, depressed or absent reflexes, oliguria, respiratory paralysis<br>*Fetal:* Crosses placenta; lethargy, hypotonia, and weakness<br>*Contraindications:* Maternal—impaired renal function | 1. Criteria for continuing administration:<br>  a. Respirations: greater than 12 breaths/min.<br>  b. Presence of patellar knee-jerk movement.<br>  c. Urinary output: greater than 30 mL/hr.<br>2. Check BP frequently for symptoms of hypotension.<br>3. Antidote for magnesium sulfate is *calcium gluconate;* should be available at bedside in case of respiratory paralysis.<br>4. Monitor FHR and serum magnesium levels.<br>5. Administration of magnesium sulfate is continued at least 24 hours after delivery to reduce risk for seizure activity.<br>6. Never abbreviate magnesium sulfate in the medical record as $MgSO_4$.<br>7. *Uses:* Prevention or control of eclampsia and as a tocolytic. |

*Continued*

| Medications | Side Effects | Nursing Implications |
|---|---|---|

## Oxytocic Medications and Prostaglandins to Cause Uterine Contractions

**Oxytocic Medications:** Stimulate contraction of uterine muscle fibers; have a mild antidiuretic effect; stimulate postpartum milk flow but do not affect amount

| Medications | Side Effects | Nursing Implications |
|---|---|---|
| ▲ Oxytocin: IM, IV, intranasal<br>Ergonovine: PO, IM, IV<br>Methylergonovine: PO, IM, IV | *Maternal:* Tetanic uterine contractions, hypertension, tachycardia<br>*Fetal:* Hypoxia, irregularity and decrease in FHR, possible hyperbilirubinemia<br>*Contraindications:*<br>Severe preeclampsia or eclampsia<br>Predisposition to uterine rupture or CPD<br>Preterm infant or presence of fetal distress | 1. Apply fetal monitor: assess FHR pattern throughout oxytocin administration.<br>2. Assess maternal vital signs before increasing oxytocin infusion rate.<br>3. Discontinue IV oxytocin and turn on primary IV solution if any of the following occur:<br>  a. Nonreassuring fetal heart rate pattern; absent variability; abnormal baseline rate.<br>  b. Sustained uterine contractions lasting more than 90 seconds.<br>  c. Insufficient relaxation of the uterus between contractions.<br>  d. Contractions occurring more often than every 2 minutes.<br>  e. Repeated late decelerations or prolonged decelerations.<br>4. Oxytocin is the only oxytocic used to induce labor; others (ergonovine and methylergonovine) are used after delivery to control bleeding.<br>5. *Uses:* Uterine dystocia; induction of labor, control of hemorrhage and uterine atony: uterine involution. |
| Prostaglandin F2α: IM | *Contraindications:* Asthma | 1. Used to contract the uterus in situations of postpartum hemorrhage. |

## Tocolytic Agents to Suppress Labor

**Tocolytic Agents:** Relax myometrial cells of the uterus leading to inhibition of labor. Also result in bronchial dilation and cardiac output.

| Medications | Side Effects | Nursing Implications |
|---|---|---|
| Beta-adrenergic agonists (betamimetics): terbutaline | *Rarely used and are being replaced by safer medications because of adverse reactions related to stimulation of beta-receptors.*<br>Maternal: Tachycardia (very little effect on BP), nervousness and tremors, headache, and possible pulmonary edema<br>*Fetal:* Tachycardia, hypoglycemia | If used:<br>1. Assess maternal (especially pulse) and fetal vital signs frequently; fetal monitoring is necessary; notify physician if maternal pulse is greater than 120 beats/min or FHR is greater than *180 beats/min.* Obtain baseline maternal ECG.<br>2. Strict I&O, daily weight.<br>3. Encourage lateral position (Sims') to decrease hypotension and increase placental perfusion.<br>4. IV: Use a pump for continuous infusion; infusion is continued for 12 hours after labor has stopped.<br>5. *Use:* Premature labor.<br><br>❗ **NURSING PRIORITY:** Watch carefully when administering IV fluids to women in preterm labor because there is an increased risk for tocolytic-induced pulmonary edema, especially when a beta-adrenergic agonist or magnesium sulfate is used. It is recommended that infusion be restricted to 1500 to 2400 mL in 24 hours. |
| Calcium channel blockers<br>Nifedipine: PO, sublingual | *Maternal:* Facial flushing, mild hypotension, reflex tachycardia, headache, nausea<br>*Fetal:* Rare problems | 1. No reported fetal side effects.<br>2. Not commonly used as a tocolytic agent.<br>3. Monitor blood pressure for hypotension.<br>4. Do not use sublingual route. |
| Prostaglandin synthesis inhibitors<br>Indomethacin: PO or rectally | *Maternal:* Nausea, vomiting, dyspepsia<br>*Fetal:* Oligohydramnios, premature closure of the ductus arteriosus in utero syndrome, respiratory distress syndrome | 1. Used when other methods fail and gestational age is less than 30 weeks.<br>2. Administer for 48–72 hours or less as may close the fetal patent ductus.<br>3. Administer with food or use rectal route to decrease gastrointestinal distress. |
| Magnesium sulfate | *Maternal:* Promotes relaxation of smooth muscles<br>Watch for other maternal and fetal side effects listed in Appendix 26-2<br>*Fetal:* Nonreactive NST, decreased breathing, reduced FHR variability | 1. *Most commonly used tocolytic agent* because maternal and fetal/neonatal adverse reactions are less common than with the other tocolytic agents, especially the beta-adrenergic agonist (terbutaline).<br>2. Monitor serum magnesium levels.<br>3. Have antidote of calcium gluconate available. |

*BP,* Blood pressure; *CPD,* cephalopelvic disproportion; *FHR,* fetal heart rate; *NST,* nonstress test; *I&O,* intake and output; *IM,* intramuscularly; *IV,* intravenously; *NSAIDs,* nonsteroidal antiinflammatory drugs; *PO,* by mouth (orally); *subQ,* subcutaneously.
▲ High Alert Medication

# Study Questions
## Maternity Nursing Care

More questions on

1. A primigravida client is experiencing Braxton Hicks contractions. Which statement is true concerning these contractions?
   1. They are intensified by walking about.
   2. They are confined to the low back.
   3. They do not increase in intensity or frequency.
   4. They result in cervical effacement and dilation.

2. A primigravida client at 26 weeks' gestation has been administered a glucose tolerance test. What would the nurse anticipate as a normal finding?
   1. Glycosylated hemoglobin A1c of 5.0% (0.05 proportion of hemoglobin)
   2. Blood glucose of 200 mg/L at 60 minutes (11.1 mmol/L)
   3. 24-hour urine glucose level of 5 mg/dL (0.28 mmol/L)
   4. Blood glucose level of 110 mg/L (6.11 mmol/L) at 3 hours

3. Which statement about the results of a contraction stress test (oxytocin challenge test) is considered accurate?
   1. Negative if no fetal heart rate accelerations occur with accompanying fetal movements
   2. Nonreactive if no late decelerations occur in more than half of the contractions
   3. Positive if late decelerations occur in more than half of the contractions
   4. Reactive if the fetal heart rate accelerates with accompanying fetal movement

4. The nurse is encouraging a pregnant woman to eat a diet rich in folic acid. Which of the following food sources would provide the most folic acid?
   1. Meat and dark green, leafy vegetables
   2. Dairy products
   3. Carrots and raisins
   4. Shellfish

5. The nurse is assessing a primigravida client who is at 26 weeks' gestation; the client's blood type is AB negative, her serology is negative, and she has a history of one miscarriage at 20 weeks. On the basis of this information, what will the nurse anticipate being ordered for this client?
   1. An amniocentesis at 30 weeks' gestation
   2. Administration of $Rh_o(D)$ immune globulin at 28 weeks' gestation
   3. A blood test on the father to determine his blood type
   4. Fetal blood sampling to determine fetal blood type

6. A client reports that her last menstrual period was November 10. She asks the nurse, "When will my baby be due?" What is the best answer?
   1. July 3
   2. August 30
   3. Around the middle of September
   4. Around the third week of August

7. The nurse is assessing a client who is at 36 weeks' gestation; this client has type 2 diabetes. The client says she is extremely upset that she will not be able to breastfeed her infant. The best nursing response would be based on what information?
   1. There are no contraindications to diabetic mothers' breastfeeding their infants; it will be important for the mother to carefully monitor her blood glucose levels and insulin needs.
   2. Because the mother's blood sugar level will be controlled by oral hypoglycemics, the medications are excreted in breast milk and would not be good for the baby.
   3. Breastfeeding puts increased carbohydrate metabolism demands on the mother and makes it unrealistic to control her blood glucose level.
   4. Offer the mother reassurance that there are some very good, nutritious infant formulas that are very close to breast milk and her infant should do well with them.

8. The labor monitor tracing shows variable decelerations. What complication would the nurse anticipate is occurring?
   1. Cord compression
   2. Fetal hypoxia
   3. Placental insufficiency
   4. Head compression

9. The nurse is assessing a client 12 hours after a prolonged labor and delivery. What assessment data would cause the nurse the most concern?
   1. Oral temperature of 100.6°F (38.1°C)
   2. Moderate amount of dark red lochia
   3. Episiotomy area bruised with small amount of dark bloody drainage
   4. Uterine fundus palpated to the right of the umbilicus

10. The nurse is caring for a client in labor. How are contractions timed?
    1. End of one to the beginning of the next
    2. Beginning of one to the end of the next
    3. End of one to the end of the next
    4. Beginning of one to the beginning of the next

11. A client is 37 weeks' gestation and is admitted to the hospital with bright red vaginal bleeding, complaining of abdominal discomfort but no contractions. After assessing the client's vital signs and determining the fetal heart rate, which is 105, what is the most important information to obtain?
    1. The amount of cervical dilation that is present
    2. The exact location of her abdominal discomfort
    3. The station of the presenting part
    4. Assess urinary output.

12. A multigravida client comes into the emergency department complaining of abdominal pain. She is at 30 weeks' gestation. On assessment, the nurse observes complete dilation and effacement of the cervix with the perineal area bulging and the infant's head crowning. The mother states she is feeling a strong urge to push. What is the best nursing action?
    1. Prepare the client for an emergency cesarean delivery.
    2. Place even gentle pressure on infant's head and support it through the birth canal.
    3. Have the client hold her legs together and take her to the labor and delivery unit.
    4. Have the client take two deep breaths and push hard with the next contraction.

13. The nurse encourages a client in labor to assume a side-lying position. What is the purpose of this position?
    1. Prevents prolapse of the cord
    2. Enhances venous return
    3. Relaxes the pelvic musculature
    4. Promotes crowning

14. The nurse is caring for a client who is at the beginning of her third trimester of pregnancy. The client has been admitted in preterm labor, and magnesium sulfate is being used. Contractions are occurring about every 4 to 5 minutes and lasting 1 to 1½ minutes; blood pressure is 130/88 mmHg; respirations are 22 breaths/min; pulse is 98 beats/min. What nursing observation would cause the nurse the most concern?
    1. Urinary output of a total of 240 mL for the past 8 hours
    2. Presence of active 2+ deep tendon reflexes
    3. Complaints of hot flashes, nausea, and a headache
    4. Blood pressure increase to 145/92 mmHg

15. A client is receiving magnesium sulfate to help suppress preterm labor. The nurse should watch for which sign of magnesium toxicity?
    1. Headache
    2. Loss of deep tendon reflexes
    3. Palpitations
    4. Dyspepsia

16. Which of the following circumstances is most likely to cause uterine atony leading to postpartum hemorrhage?
    1. Hypertension
    2. Cervical and vaginal tears
    3. Urine retention
    4. Endometritis

17. A pregnant client had an abruptio placentae after a hemorrhagic episode; an emergency delivery was completed. The client is stable, and the cesarean delivery was performed 2 days ago. During the postoperative period, the nurse is observing for potential complications. What would be important for the nurse to assess regarding the development of complications?
    1. Check the blood sugar level every 2 hours.
    2. Assess vital signs hourly.
    3. Place client in side-lying position.
    4. Monitor fibrinogen and coagulation studies.

18. Ten days after delivery, a client is diagnosed with mastitis. The nurse would anticipate what assessment findings?
    1. Tender, hard, inflamed area on the breast
    2. Dimpled skin on the upper outer quadrant of the breast
    3. Lack of milk production
    4. Nipple burning during feeding

## Answers to Study Questions

1. *3*
False labor contractions decrease when the client is walking, are not concentrated in one part of the uterus, and do not increase in intensity and frequency. True labor is characterized by cervical effacement or dilation. (Lowdermilk et al., 11 ed., p. 287)

2. *4*
In the oral glucose tolerance test (OGTT), the blood glucose level is evaluated before the test (a fasting blood glucose), 1 hour after a 100 g glucose load, 2 hours after the glucose load, and 3 hours after the glucose load. The normal value for 1 hour is less than 180 mg/L (10.0 mmol/L), the normal value for 2 hours is less than 155 mg/L (8.6 mmol/L), and the normal value for 3 hours is less than 140 mg/L (7.8 mmol/L). The glycosylated hemoglobin value reflects blood glucose control for the past 120 days, and the urine glucose level is not as reliable an indicator of control as the serum glucose level. (Lowdermilk et al., 11 ed., p. 700)

3. *3*
An oxytocin challenge test, or contraction stress test, is conducted by giving an infusion of oxytocin to the mother and evaluating the fetal response to subsequent uterine contractions as plotted on a fetal monitor. The test result is negative if there are no late decelerations; it is positive if there are late decelerations in more than one-half of the contractions. If the CST result is positive and there is no acceleration of FHR with fetal movement (nonreactive

NST result), the positive CST (nonreassuring; abnormal) result is an ominous sign, often indicating late fetal hypoxia. A negative CST (reassuring) result with a reactive NST result is desirable. (Lowdermilk et al., 11 ed., p. 649)

4. *1*
Rich dietary sources of folate are dark green, leafy vegetables, whole wheat bread, lightly cooked beans and peas, nuts and seeds, sprouts, oranges and grapefruits, liver and other organ meats, poultry, fortified breakfast cereals, and enriched grain products. Shellfish is rich in iodine. Dairy products are rich in calcium. (Lowdermilk et al., 11 ed., p. 345)

5. *2*
Rh₀(D) immune globin is given to all Rh-negative women in the 28th week of gestation. The blood type of the father may be determined, but paternity is not an important issue in this situation. An amniocentesis is not necessary at this time, and obtaining fetal blood to determine blood type is more risky than administering the medication to the mother. (Lowdermilk et al., 11 ed., p. 494)

6. *4*
According to Näegele's rule, count back 3 months from the date of the last menstrual period and add 7 days to determine the estimated date of conception. About 35% of all women deliver within 5 days of (either before or after) this date. (Lowdermilk et al., 11 ed., p. 302)

7. *1*

Mothers with diabetes can breastfeed, but they must frequently check their blood glucose levels, and insulin is recommended to maintain good blood glucose control. Oral hypoglycemics are not usually recommended for breastfeeding mothers. Breastfeeding does put an increased demand on the mother's metabolism, but this can be controlled with careful monitoring of blood glucose levels. Multiple formulas are available, but if the mother can breastfeed, that option should be made available to her. (Lowdermilk et al., 11 ed., p. 698)

8. *1*

Variable decelerations most commonly occur during the transition phase of the first or second stage of labor as a result of umbilical cord compression or stretching during fetal descent and are correctable. Fetal hypoxia and uteroplacental insufficiency are associated with late decelerations. Head compression is associated with early decelerations. (Lowdermilk et al., 11 ed., p. 420)

9. *4*

Uterus palpated to right of umbilicus may indicate a full bladder. The fundus should be at the level of the midline. The temperature, lochia, and episiotomy assessment findings are within normal limits. (Lowdermilk et al., 11 ed., p. 476)

10. *4*

The correct method of timing contractions is from the beginning of one contraction to the beginning of the next. The point at which the contraction ends is of concern only when the nurse needs to know the duration of the contraction, not the frequency or timing of the contractions. (Lowdermilk et al., 11 ed., p. 440)

11. *4*

The bright red bleeding may be an indication of placenta previa or abruptio placentae, and the client is more than 36 weeks' gestation, so the nurse should anticipate and plan for an emergency cesarean delivery. Vital signs may be normal even with heavy blood loss. Decreasing urinary output may be better indicator of acute blood loss than vital signs alone. The other options are appropriate to check, but they are not of any assistance in the woman's current situation, which could progress to hemorrhage and the need for emergency surgery. (Lowdermilk et al., 11 ed., p. 681)

12. *2*

The birth of this infant is imminent. The infant is probably small because of prematurity, the mother is multigravida, and the mother has not received any analgesics. The nurse should place hands at the perineum to apply light pressure to the fetal head to prevent rapid expulsion. Do not attempt to take the mother to labor and delivery; notify labor and delivery and newborn nursery units of the impending birth of premature infant. If the mother pushes hard with the next contraction, the infant may progress too rapidly. There is no need for a cesarean delivery; no attempt should be made to slow or prevent the delivery because this would put the infant in further jeopardy. (Lowdermilk et al., 11 ed., p. 462)

13. *2*

The weight and pressure of the uterus on the vena cava decreases the venous return to the mother's heart. This will precipitate a drop in blood pressure and decreased blood supply to the fetus. In a side-lying position, pressure is reduced and adequate cardiac output is promoted. (Lowdermilk et al., 11 ed., p. 440)

14. *1*

Monitoring during the administration of magnesium sulfate includes urine output, which should be greater than 30 mL per hour, respiratory rate should be greater than 12 breaths/min, and deep tendon reflexes should be 2+. The medication should be held or decreased if the urinary output drops to or below 30 mL per hour, as magnesium sulfate is excreted through the urine and toxicity can develop if urine output is not sufficient. Deep tendon reflexes are present, and the respiratory rate is normal. Hot flashes may occur after the medication is started, but it is not a primary concern at this time; however, the blood pressure is. The urine output is the priority. Magnesium sulfate will reduce the blood pressure once administration is started. (Lowdermilk et al., 11 ed., p.664)

15. *2*

Magnesium toxicity causes central nervous system depression; this would be observed as loss of deep tendon reflexes, paralysis, respiratory depression, drowsiness, lethargy, blurred vision, slurred speech, and confusion. Headache may be an adverse effect of calcium channel blockers, which are sometimes used to treat preterm labor. Palpitations are an adverse effect of terbutaline, which is also used to treat preterm labor. Dyspepsia may occur as an adverse effect of indomethacin, a prostaglandin synthetase inhibitor used to suppress preterm labor. (Lowdermilk et al., 11 ed., p. 664)

16. *3*

Urine retention is a common cause of uterine atony and can lead to postpartum hemorrhage. Urine retention causes a distended bladder to displace the uterus above the umbilicus and to the side, which prevents the uterus from contracting. The uterus needs to continue contracting if bleeding is to stay within normal limits. Cervical and vaginal tears can cause postpartum hemorrhage, but in the postpartum period, a full bladder is the most common cause of uterine bleeding. Neither endometritis, an infection of the inner lining of the endometrium, nor maternal hypertension causes postpartum hemorrhage. (Lowdermilk et al., 11 ed., p. 486)

17. *4*

Clients with abruptio placentae are prone to the development of disseminated intravascular coagulation after delivery, which is characterized by abnormal fibrinogen and coagulation studies. Although checking vital signs is important to continue to monitor, the delivery and hemorrhagic episode has occurred. Checking blood sugar would be appropriate for a client with gestational diabetes. Side-lying position would improve placental perfusion. (Lowdermilk et al., 11 ed., p. 683)

18. *1*

Swelling, erythema, and pain are found most often in the upper, outer quadrant of the breast. Dimpled skin (orange peel appearance) is a potential sign of breast cancer. Nipple burning is related to positioning and initiation of the let-down reflex during feeding. Milk production starts about 4 days after delivery and is not related to the development of mastitis. (Lowdermilk et al., 11 ed., p. 625)

# 27 Newborn Nursing Care

## ❦ HEALTHY NEWBORN

### ❦ Biologic Adaptations in the Neonatal Period

*Assessment*

A. Respiratory system.
1. Lung maturation process.
   a. Development of functioning lungs does not occur until at least 26 weeks' gestation.
   b. Pulmonary surfactant is usually of sufficient quantity at 35 weeks' gestation; acts to stabilize respirations and prevent atelectasis.
2. Respiratory effort.
   a. Respirations are usually established within 1 minute after birth, often within the first few seconds.
   b. Strong cry usually accompanies good respiratory effort.
   c. Newborn respiration should be quiet; no dyspnea or cyanosis.
   d. Cyanosis may be apparent in the hands and feet (acrocyanosis); circumoral cyanosis (around the mouth) may persist for an hour or two after birth but should subside.
   e. Average respiratory rate: 30 to 60 breaths/min.
   f. Respiratory movements: diaphragmatic and abdominal muscles are used; little thoracic movement.
   g. Neonate breathes through the nose (obligate nose-breather); consequently, nasal obstruction with mucus will lead to respiratory distress.

> **⚠ NURSING PRIORITY:** Oxygen transport in the newborn is significantly affected by the presence of greater amounts of HbF (fetal hemoglobin) than HbA (adult hemoglobin), which holds oxygen easier but releases it to the body tissues only at low $Po_2$ levels.

B. Circulatory system.
1. Cessation of blood flow through the umbilical vessels and placenta.
2. Closure of the ductus arteriosus, the foramen ovale, and the ductus venosus.
3. Increase in and shift to pulmonary circulation.
4. Circulatory changes are not always immediate and complete: usually complete in a few days; often this period is called *transitional circulation.*
5. Anatomic closing of the fetal blood vessels may not be complete for weeks or months; functional closure is usually adequate to produce normal circulation.

6. Heart.
   a. May hear transitory heart murmurs. Murmurs with accompanying signs such as poor feeding, apnea, or cyanosis should be investigated.
   b. Assess for dextrocardia: auscultated heart sounds are louder on the right side of the chest.
   c. Pulse rate: 100 to 160 beats/min.
   d. Obtain baseline pulse oximetry before discharge.
7. Blood pressure (BP).
   a. Measured using oscillometric monitor: need correctly sized cuff.
      (1) Blood pressure varies with size and age; usually not measured in normal term infants.
      (2) Normal BP at birth: systolic 60 to 80 mmHg; diastolic 40 to 50 mmHg.
      (3) Normal BP at 10 days: systolic 95 to 100 mmHg; diastolic 45 to 75 mmHg.
C. Body temperature and heat production.
1. Loss of body heat.
   a. Evaporation: heat loss as water evaporates from skin and from lungs; occurs when infant's body is wet with amniotic fluid at birth and during bath. Dry infant quickly.
   b. Convection: movement of body heat to cool air; infant loses heat to the cool air in the delivery room. Keep infant wrapped in blanket while in bassinette.
   c. Conduction: direct transfer of heat to a surface on which the infant is lying; infant loses heat to a cool sheet or blanket. Prewarm warmer and bassinette.
   d. Radiation: heat is lost from the infant's warm body as it travels through the air to cooler objects in the room; occurs when an unclothed infant is placed in an open crib or isolette. Avoid drafts.

> **⚠ NURSING PRIORITY:** Excessive heat loss occurs from radiation and convection because of the newborn's larger surface area compared with body weight. It is important to remember that conduction loss occurs as a result of the marked difference between core body temperature and skin temperature.

   e. Body temperature changes.
      (1) Body temperature at birth is 0.5°C higher than mother's.
      (2) Body temperature may drop to 94°F (34.4°C) or even as low as 92°F (33.3°C) after birth unless the infant is adequately protected.

2. Production of body heat.
   a. Heat is generated immediately by *shivering;* infant shivering is characterized by increased muscular activity, restlessness, and crying.
   b. Infant shivering activity is not as apparent as adult shivering activity.
   c. Metabolism of brown fat (brown adipose tissue).
      (1) Functions to produce heat under the stress of cooling.
      (2) Brown fat is located in the intrascapular region, in the posterior triangle of the neck, in the axillae, behind the sternum, and around the kidneys.
      (3) Brown fat is metabolized and utilized within several weeks after birth.
   d. Increase in metabolic rate.
      (1) Stimulation of the thyroid gland leads to increased general metabolism; usually takes 12 to 24 hours.
      (2) Metabolic rate remains elevated for 7 to 10 days, even after warming.
      (3) Effect of chilling on the neonate.
         (a) Increased heat production leads to increased oxygen consumption.
         (b) Increased oxygen consumption utilizes glucose and brown fat.
         (c) When heat production is high, caloric need is high.
         (d) Tendency to develop metabolic acidosis occurs.
         (e) Production of surfactant is inhibited by cooling, and respiratory distress syndrome may occur.
         (f) Increased risk with smaller infants because they have low reserve of glycogen and low reserve for increasing ventilation; leads to tendency to become more acidotic.

## 🍦 General Characteristics

> ❗ **NURSING PRIORITY:** Assess a newborn; monitor a newborn for complications.

A. Length.
   1. Average length of term neonate: 48 to 53 cm (19 to 21 inches).
   2. To measure: infant is placed flat on the back on paper; a pencil is used to mark the locations of the infant's head and heels; after infant is removed from the paper, the distance between the two pencil marks is measured.
B. Weight.
   1. Average birth weight for a term neonate: 3400 g (7 lb 8 oz); average range is 2700 to 4000 g (6 to 9 lb).
   2. Low birth weight: 2500 g (5 lb 8 oz).
   3. Excessive weight: 4000 g (9 lb).
   4. Weight loss: between 5% and 10% of birth weight within the first few days of life; infant usually regains weight within 10 to 14 days.
C. Head.
   1. Molding.
      a. Head may appear elongated at birth; molding usually disappears within 24 to 48 hours.
      b. Occurs as a result of abnormal fetal posture in utero and pressure during passage through the birth canal.
   2. Caput succedaneum (Figure 27-1).
      a. Edema of the scalp caused by the pressure occurring at the time of delivery.
      b. Disappears within 3 to 4 days.
      c. Edema goes across the cranial suture lines.
   3. Cephalhematoma (see Figure 27-1).
      a. A collection of blood between the periosteum and the skull.
      b. Usually results from trauma during labor and delivery.
      c. Absorbed in a few weeks.
      d. Does not cross cranial suture lines.
   4. Head measurement.
      a. Average head circumference of the term neonate: 34.2 cm; usual variation ranges from 33 to 35 cm (13 to 14 inches).
      b. Head circumference is approximately 2 to 3 cm greater than the chest circumference; extremes in

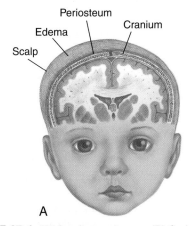
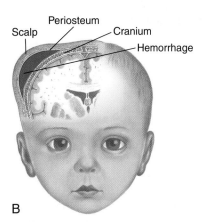

A                B

**FIGURE 27-1 (A)** Caput succedaneum. **(B)** Cephalhematoma. (From Seidel, H. M., et. al. [2006]. *Mosby's guide to physical examination* [6th ed.]. St. Louis, MO: Mosby.)

**Anterior**
- Diamond shape about 3 cm × 2 cm.
- Will increase as molding resolves.
- Closes by 18 months of age.

**Posterior**
- Triangular shape about 1 cm × 2 cm.
- Closes by 6 to 8 weeks; may be closed at birth.

***Nursing Interventions***
- Palpate for size and tension.
- Increase in tension may indicate tumor, hemorrhage, infection, or congenital anomaly.
- Decrease in tension (sunken fontanel) may indicate dehydration.

size may indicate microcephaly, hydrocephaly, or increased intracranial pressure.

    5. Fontanels (Box 27-1).

D. Umbilical cord.

    1. Determine number of blood vessels; there should be two arteries and one vein surrounded by Wharton's jelly.

    2. Cord atrophies and sloughs off in about 10 to 14 days.

    3. Should be no bleeding or oozing.

## Behavioral Characteristics

A. Sleep and awake states.

    1. Newborn sleeps an average of 16 to 20 hours a day during the first 2 weeks of life, with an average of 4 hours at a time.

    2. May vary from a drowsy or semidozing state to an alert state to a crying state.

B. Infants vary a great deal in how they respond to stimuli.

    1. Infants move easily from one state of sleep to another state of consciousness.

    2. As the infant develops, he or she will reduce the total amount of sleeping time; wakeful periods will lengthen; sleeping will shift from daytime to nighttime.

## Specific Body System Clinical Findings

A. Nervous system.

    1. Nervous system is relatively immature and characterized by the following:

        a. Poor nervous control; easily startled.

        b. Quivering chin.

        c. Tremors of the lower extremities of short duration.

    2. Reflex activity: the presence or absence of certain reflexes is indicative of ongoing normal development.

    3. Presence of positive Babinski sign.

        a. Normal finding until the age of 1 year.

        b. Dorsiflexion of big toe and fanning of the other toes.

    4. Neonatal reflexes (Table 27-1).

> **! NURSING PRIORITY:** Intactness of the neonate's nervous system is indicated by the state of alertness, resting posture, cry, and quality of muscle tone and motor activity.

B. Hematologic system.

    1. Initially at birth.

        a. Increased number of red blood cells (RBCs): $4,800,000/mm^3$ ($4.8 \times 10^{12}$/L) of blood.

        b. Hemoglobin: 14 to 24 g/dL (140 to 240 g/L) of blood.

        c. Hematocrit: 44% to 64% (0.440 to 0.640).

**Table 27-1 MAJOR NEONATAL REFLEXES**

| Reflex | Disappears | How to Elicit | Response |
|---|---|---|---|
| Rooting | 3–4 months; may persist during sleep until 7–8 months | Stroke cheek. | Head turns toward side that is touched. |
| Babinski | 1 year | Lightly stroke lateral side of foot from heel to big toe across the ball of the foot. | Infant's toes fan, with dorsiflexion of great toe. |
| Sucking | 10–12 months | Touch or stroke lips. | Infant sucks. |
| Moro (startle) | 3–4 months | Make a loud noise or suddenly disturb infant's equilibrium. | Infant stiffens, briskly abducts, and extends arms with hands open and fingers extended to C shape. Infant's legs flex and abduct, and arms return to an embracing posture. Crying is usual. |
| Grasp palmar | 3–4 months | Press a finger against infant's palm. | Infant's fingers momentarily close around object. |
| Asymmetric tonic neck (fencer's position) | 3–4 months | Turn supine infant's head over the shoulder to one side. | Infant's arm and leg partially or completely extend on side to which head is turned; opposite arm and leg flex. |

2. Leukocytosis is present at birth (white blood cell count of 9000 to 30,000 mm³) (9.00 to 30.00 × 10⁹/L).
   a. Considerable decrease in white blood cell count occurs within a few days after birth.
   b. Shift in the type of cells occurs: neutrophils decrease, and lymphocytes increase until they predominate by the end of the first week.
3. Anemia.
   a. Fetal hemoglobin has short life span; maternal/fetal iron stores sustain normal RBC production 4 to 5 months.
   b. *Physiologic anemia of the newborn* occurs as a result.
   c. Breastfed infants need iron supplements; formula should be iron fortified.
4. Jaundice.
   a. Physiologic jaundice; increased incidence in breastfed infants; occurs on the second or third day of life as a result of an increase in the serum bilirubin level.
   b. Pathologic jaundice occurs within 24 hours of birth (see hemolytic disease of the newborn).
   c. Pathophysiology (physiologic).
      (1) Inability of the liver to clear bilirubin from the plasma.
      (2) Increased level of RBCs from the maternal circulation at birth leads to increased breakdown and bilirubin production.
   d. Criteria for physiologic jaundice.
      (1) Does not appear until after 24 hours after birth.
      (2) Total serum bilirubin level is less than 12 mg/100 mL (205.05 umol/L).
      (3) Infant does not show any sign of illness or cardiac decompensation.
      (4) Serum indirect bilirubin level does not increase more than 5 mg/100 mL (85.52 umol/L) per 24 hours.
      (5) Clinical evidence of jaundice disappears within 1 week in the term infant and by the end of the second week in the premature infant. Bilirubin peaks around day 3, plateaus for 12 to 14 days, and then steadily decreases.
   e. Treatment: phototherapy.
      (1) Converts unconjugated bilirubin into conjugated (water-soluble) form, which can be excreted.
      (2) Indication for phototherapy varies according to the maturity of the fetus and presence of disease; treatment may be started earlier for premature infants.
      (3) If bili lights are used, expose all areas to the light except for eyes and genitalia; cover infant's eyes with an opaque mask or eye patch and cover genitalia with a diaper or a disposable face mask (string bikini to expose more skin).

(4) Hour specific serum bilirubin levels are recommended to predict rapid rising levels in the high-risk newborn.
(5) Noninvasive transcutaneous bilirubinometry (TcB): allows for repetitive estimation of bilirubin level; cannot be used after phototherapy has been initiated.

**NURSING PRIORITY:** If a face mask is used to cover genitalia, remove the metal nose strip to prevent burning the infant.

(6) If a fiber-optic blanket is used, infant's eyes do not need to be covered; should have a covering pad between the infant's skin and the fiber-optic blanket; with this method, the infant may remain in the room with the mother or the fiber-optic blanket may be used at home.
(7) Monitor skin temperature: treatment may increase temperature.
(8) Reposition infant every 2 hours to expose as much body surface as possible.
(9) Chart pertinent information: time phototherapy was started and stopped, maintenance of shielding of the eyes from bili light, type and intensity of lamp used, distance of light from infant, whether used in combination with an isolette or an open bassinet, and any side effects.
(10) Remove infant from light treatment for feedings; encourage parents to hold and feed infant.
(11) Effects.
   (a) Vasodilation of the skin.
   (b) Increased insensible water loss: encourage intake of fluids to maintain adequate hydration.
   (c) Decreased gastrointestinal (GI) transit time: frequent loose, green stools.
   (d) Skin discoloration: skin may become grayish brown; color is transient with no complications.
(12) Phototherapy may be used as an adjunct to treatment of pathologic jaundice.
(13) Effectiveness is determined by:
   (a) A decrease of 3 to 4 mg/100 mL (51.31 to 68.42 umol/L) of blood in the serum bilirubin after 8 to 12 hours of therapy.
   (b) A gradual diminishing of jaundice.
5. Transitory coagulation defects.
   a. Occur between the second and fifth postnatal days.
   b. Result from the lack of intestinal synthesis of vitamin K because of insufficient bacterial flora in the GI tract.
   c. Vitamin K (0.5 to 1.0 mg) is administered intramuscularly immediately after birth to prevent complications.

C. GI tract.
1. Able to absorb proteins and simple carbohydrates.
2. Stomach produces hydrochloric acid immediately after birth.
3. Digestive enzymes are present except for pancreatic amylase and lipase; this results in the inability to absorb fat adequately.
4. Stools.

> **⚠ NURSING PRIORITY:** Monitor the passage of the first meconium stool.

    a. Meconium: sticky, black, odorless, sterile stool that is passed within the first 24 to 48 hours after birth; if no stool is passed, further assessment is needed.
    b. Stools change according to type and number of feedings.
       (1) Transitional stools: occur during period between second and fourth days; consist of meconium and milk; greenish brown or greenish yellow; loose and often contain mucus.
       (2) Milk stools: usually occur by the fourth day; stools of formula-fed infant are drier, more formed, paler, and occur once or twice daily or one stool every 2 to 3 days.
       (3) Stools of breastfed infants are golden yellow, have a pasty consistency, and occur more frequently than stools of formula-fed infants, three to four stools in 24 hours.

D. Genitourinary system.
1. Urinary.
    a. Urinary output is low during the first few days of life or until fluid intake increases.

> **⚠ NURSING PRIORITY:** Most newborns void within the first 24 to 48 hours after birth. Weigh dry diaper before applying; then weigh wet diaper after infant voiding. Each gram of added weight equals 1 mL of urine.

    b. About 30 to 60 mL are voided per day during the first 2 days of life, followed by 200 mL per day by the end of the first week.
    c. Frequency of voiding: average of two to six times per day, increasing up to 10 to 15 times per day.
2. Genitalia.
    a. Female: labia majora are hypertrophied; small amount of bloody discharge from the vagina may be seen as a result of the presence of maternal hormones.
    b. Male: scrotum may be edematous; testes should have descended; assess the urethral opening.

E. Integumentary system.
1. Vernix caseosa: a white, cheesy-like material covers the skin at birth, particularly noted in the folds and creases.
2. Petechiae: pinpoint bluish discolorations primarily on the skin and face as a result of pressure from delivery; bruising of tissues may be seen.
3. Lanugo: downy, fine covering of hair that may be present on the shoulders, back, earlobes, and forehead; disappears during the first week.
4. Milia: sebaceous gland hyperplasia appears as pinpoint white bumps seen over the bridge of the nose and on the cheeks during the first 2 weeks of life.
5. Erythema toxicum: splotchy pink papular rash appearing anywhere on the body; disappears within the first few weeks of life; no treatment is necessary.
6. Mongolian spots: dark bluish pigmented areas seen on the back or buttocks of dark-skinned infants; usually disappear by school age.

F. Endocrine system.
1. Because of the presence of maternal hormones in the bloodstream, neonate may have breast enlargement or vulvar or prostatic enlargement.
2. Thymus gland is normally large; grows rapidly until age of 5 years; remains the same until about age of 10 years, then finally diminishes.

G. Sensory system.
1. Vision: visual acuity of 20/100 to 20/400; retinal development is advanced.
    a. Eyes appear large, and pupils appear small.
    b. All infants' eyes are blue, slate gray, or brown at birth; eyes become permanent color about 6 to 12 months of age.
    c. Tears do not develop until 2 to 4 weeks of age.
    d. Eyes close in response to bright light; red reflex is present; pupils react to light.
    e. Visual preferences: yellow, green, pink, and black and white patterns.
2. Hearing.
    a. Sudden loud noises may elicit startle response.
    b. Usually able to locate the general direction of sounds.
    c. Hearing of all infants is screened before discharge from birthing facility.
3. Sense of smell is present at birth; infants react to strong odors, especially mother's breast milk.
4. Taste.
    a. Differentiates between pleasant and unpleasant tastes.
    b. Rejects especially salty, sour, or bitter tastes by grimacing; also stops sucking.
5. Tactile senses.
    a. Most sensitive area is around the mouth.
    b. Searches for food when cheek is touched or begins sucking movements when lips are touched.
    c. Touch and motion are essential to attachment and normal growth.

H. Musculoskeletal system.
1. Assumes the position of comfort, which is usually the position assumed in utero.
2. Normal palmar crease is present (simian crease is indicative of Down syndrome).

3. Spine is straight and flat when in prone position.
4. Creases and fat pads are present on the soles of the feet.
5. Five digits should be present on each hand and foot; polydactyly (extra digits), syndactyly (fused digits), and oligodactyly (missing digits) should be assessed; fingernails are present.
6. Examine hips for developmental dysplasia; hips should be stable; thigh creases symmetric.

### Nursing Interventions

**TEST ALERT: Provide newborn care and education.**

**Goal:** To establish and maintain a patent airway and promote oxygenation.

A. Position infant with head slightly lower than chest; may use postural drainage or side-lying position.
B. Suction nostrils and oropharynx with bulb syringe.
C. Observe for periods of apnea lasting greater than 20 seconds, cyanosis, and mucus collection and be ready to use oropharyngeal suctioning, stimulation, oxygen administration, or resuscitative procedures, if necessary.

**! NURSING PRIORITY:** During first 4 hours after birth, the priority nursing goals are to maintain a clear airway, prevent heat loss, prevent hemorrhage and infection, and monitor transition. Bathing will be initiated when infant's temperature is stabilized; feeding may begin immediately if infant is interested.

**Goal:** To protect against heat loss (Figure 27-2).

A. Immediately after birth, wrap infant in warm blanket and dry off amniotic fluid.
B. Replace wet blanket with warm dry blanket.

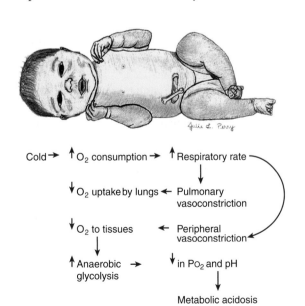

Cold → ↑O$_2$ consumption → ↑Respiratory rate
↓O$_2$ uptake by lungs ← Pulmonary vasoconstriction
↓O$_2$ to tissues ← Peripheral vasoconstriction
↑Anaerobic glycolysis → ↓in Po$_2$ and pH
Metabolic acidosis

**FIGURE 27-2  Effects of Cold Stress.** (From Lowdermilk, D., & Perry, S. [2016]. *Maternity and women's health care* [11th ed.]. St. Louis, MO: Mosby.)

C. Cover wet hair and head with a blanket or cap.
D. Immediately after birth, may provide for skin-to-skin contact with the mother; cover infant with warm blanket.
E. For initial physical assessment, place baby on a warm padded surface, preferably under a radiant heater.
F. Wrap infant securely in a warm blanket and give him or her to parents to cuddle and observe.
G. Avoid any unnecessary procedures until body temperature is stable.

**Goal:** To perform a newborn physical assessment and collect data on behavior (Box 27-2).

A. Determine Apgar score at 1 minute and again at 5 minutes (see Table 26-9 for Apgar scoring).

**! NURSING PRIORITY:** Assess a newborn and determine Apgar scores.

1. The 1-minute Apgar score is a rapid evaluation of the status of the neonate's intrauterine oxygenation.
2. The 5-minute Apgar score is an evaluation of the neonate's response to cardiorespiratory adaptation after birth.
B. Gestational age assessment within 2 hours of birth.
C. Comprehensive physical assessment completed within 24 hours of birth.
D. Determine special needs and whether any significant risk factors are present.

**Goal:** To assess periods of reactivity.

A. First period of reactivity.
1. Lasts approximately 30 minutes.
2. Newborn is alert, awake, and usually hungry.

**! NURSING PRIORITY:** Periods of reactivity are excellent opportunities for promoting attachment response.

**Box 27-2   GUIDELINES FOR PHYSICAL ASSESSMENT OF THE NEWBORN**

- Perform procedures that require quiet first, such as auscultating the lungs, heart, and abdomen.
- Perform procedures that may cause crying last, such as testing reflexes.
- Measure head, chest, and length at the same time to compare results.
- Obtain an axillary temperature (rectal thermometer may perforate mucosa).
- Monitor vital signs every 15 minutes to 1 hour until infant's temperature stabilizes (usually in about 4 hours).
- Perform glucose checks for hypoglycemia on an infant of a mother with diabetes or on a newborn with complications.

B. Sleep phase.
   1. First sleep usually occurs an average of 3 to 4 hours after birth and may last from a few minutes to several hours.
   2. Newborn is difficult to awaken during this phase.
C. Second period of reactivity.
   1. Infant is alert and awake (good time to feed infant).
   2. Lasts approximately 2 to 4 hours.

> ⚠ **NURSING PRIORITY:** It is important to monitor the infant closely because apnea, decreased heart rate, gagging, choking, and regurgitation may occur and require nursing intervention.

**Goal:** To protect against infection.

A. Follow guidelines for proper hand hygiene before handling infant.
B. Prevent ophthalmia neonatorum.
   1. Administer prophylactic treatment to eyes soon after birth.
   2. Place ophthalmic ointment or solution in the conjunctival sac.
C. Avoid exposure to people with possible upper respiratory tract, skin, or GI infections.

**Goal:** To prevent hemorrhagic disease.

A. Administer 0.5 to 1 mg of vitamin K intramuscularly into the upper third of the lateral aspect of the thigh.

**Goal:** To properly identify infant.

A. Secure identification bands to wrist or ankle of infant and wrist of mother in the delivery room. Father may be banded as well.
B. Prints of infant's foot, palms, or fingers may be obtained according to hospital policy; mother's palm prints or fingerprints may also be obtained.
C. Advise parents not to release the infant to anyone who does not have proper unit identification.

> ⚠ **NURSING PRIORITY:** Always check the infant's ID band with the mother's ID band every time the infant and mother have been separated; monitor area for anyone who does not have a security clearance to be in the newborn area; security of the newborn is a priority! Electronic tags may be placed on the infant that ring when the infant is carried out of the newborn area. Teach mothers to carefully monitor identification badges of individuals/nursing staff who come in contact with their newborn, especially if they are wanting to remove the infant from her, so that the mother does not give the infant to anyone without proper identification.

**Goal:** To promote parental attachment to infant immediately after birth.

A. Wrap infant snugly in warm blanket and encourage parents to hold infant. Do not allow chilling to occur.
B. Encourage touching and holding during periods of reactivity.

**Goal:** To initiate feeding and to evaluate parents' ability to feed infant and provide nutrition.

A. Encourage breastfeeding, if desired, immediately after delivery or in recovery area; breast milk is bacteriologically safe.
B. Assess infant's ability to feed; assess for active bowel sounds, absence of abdominal distention; rooting, sucking, swallowing reflexes, and alertness.
C. First formula feeding or test feeding: administer 10 to 15 mL of sterile water to assess GI tract patency, followed by formula.
D. Considerations in infant feeding.
   1. An infant should always be placed on the right side after feeding to avoid aspiration and prevent regurgitation and distention.
   2. Infant will require more frequent feedings initially; will generally establish a routine of feeding every 3 to 4 hours.
      a. Breastfed infants feed 8 to 12 times per 24 hours (every 2 to 3 hours).
      b. Formula-fed infants feed six to eight times per 24 hours.
E. Infant needs approximately 50 kcal/lb or 108 kcal/kg of body weight for first 3 months, then 100 kcal/kg for 3 to 6 months.
   *Example:* An infant weighing 8 lb 8 oz (240 mL) would need 50 kcal × 8 lb = 400 kcal plus 25 calories for 8 oz (240 mL) (½ lb) = 425 kcal. Most formulas contain 20 kcal/oz. Divide 425 kcal by 20 = 21.25 oz (637.5 mL) of formula per day.

**Goal:** To provide daily general care.

A. Ongoing assessment and observation of vital signs, activity, appearance, color, and bowel and bladder function.
B. Care of the umbilical cord stump.
   1. Hospital protocol directs routine cord care; initial cleaning with sterile water; subsequent cleaning with plain water is recommended.
   2. Clean the umbilical cord stump several times a day with plain water, especially after infant voids.
   3. To encourage drying of the cord, expose umbilical area to air frequently and position diaper below umbilicus.
   4. Observe for bleeding, oozing, or foul odor. Average cord separation time is 10 to 14 days.
C. Circumcision care.
   1. Keep area clean; change diaper frequently.
   2. Observe for bleeding: check site hourly for 12 hours postprocedure.
   3. A small sterile petrolatum gauze dressing may be applied to the area during the first 2 to 3 days (if Gomco or Mogen clamp are used for procedure).
   4. If a PlastiBell was used, keep area clean; application of petrolatum jelly is not necessary; plastic ring will dislodge when area has healed (5–7 days).

**! NURSING PRIORITY:** Teach the parents that a whitish yellow exudate around the glans is granulation tissue and is normal and not indicative of infection. It may be observed for 2 to 3 days and should not be removed.

D. Neonate's bath.
1. Bath is delayed until vital signs and temperature stabilize.
2. Warm water is used for the first 4 days; do not immerse infant in water until umbilical cord stump has been released.
3. When bathing neonate, apply principles of clean-to-dirty areas; wash areas in the following order: eyes, face, ears, head, body, genitals, buttocks.
4. Head is an area of significant heat loss; keep it covered.
E. Determine weight loss over first 24 hours after birth—monitor wet diapers.
F. Assess stools.
1. Meconium stools.
2. Transitional stools.

**Goal:** To detect complications and provide early treatment (Box 27-3).

A. If infant is discharged before 24 hours, explain to parents the importance of returning to health care provider for newborn checkup and screening tests. A newborn screen for phenylketonuria (PKU) should be done after the first 24 hours for a formula-fed infant; if mother is breastfeeding, the newborn screen should be done when infant is 1 week old. National newborn screening requires PKU and thyroid screens. Many states require additional newborn screens.

---

**Box 27-3 NEWBORN DISCHARGE CRITERIA**

- Newborn completed 37 to 41 weeks' gestation.
- Vital signs normal for 12 hours preceding discharge.
- Regular urination (minimum of 1 wet diaper per day for each day of life; day 2 = 2 wet diapers; day 3 = 3 wet diapers; until day 5 or 6, then approximately 5 to 6 wet diapers up to 14 days, then 6 to 10 or more per day).
- Passed meconium stool.
- Completed two successful feedings (audible swallowing; easily aroused for feeding).
- No bleeding at circumcision site.
- Initial hepatitis B vaccine administered.
- Mother and infant laboratory tests have been reviewed.
- Hearing screening, metabolic, and congenital heart disease screening (per state regulations).
- Mother's knowledge of infant care assessed for competency (bathing, feeding, umbilical cord care, cord kept above diaper line, circumcision care, position on back for sleep).
- If discharged sooner than 48 hours, then need to see health care provider within 48 hours of discharge.

Resource adapted from American Academy of Pediatrics. (2010). Policy statement: Hospital stay for healthy term newborns. *Pediatrics* 125(2): 405–409.

B. Administration of first hepatitis B vaccine before discharge; also, if mother is a hepatitis B carrier, hepatitis B immune globulin is given intramuscularly.
1. Encourage follow-up visits for second and third doses of hepatitis B vaccine and other immunizations.
2. Infants are tested at 9 months for hepatitis B surface antigen (HBsAg) and anti-HBsAg.

**! NURSING PRIORITY:** Explain to parents the importance of returning for a well-baby check when the infant is 2 to 4 weeks old.

**Goal:** To promote infant feeding.

A. Breastfeeding.
1. First feeding should occur immediately or within a few hours after birth.
2. Stimulates release of prolactin to initiate milk production.
3. Assess the mother's knowledge of breastfeeding during the first feeding and provide teaching (see Chapter 26 for further discussion of breastfeeding).
4. Frequent feedings are important initially to establish milk production, often every 1½ to 2 hours.
5. One of the primary reasons mothers stop breastfeeding is the perception that their milk supply is not sufficient.
6. Encourage mother not to offer the infant a bottle until lactation is well established, generally after about 4 weeks.
7. Engorgement and nipple soreness are the most common problems the mother experiences.
B. Bottle-feeding.
1. It is not necessary to sterilize the water used to reconstitute infant's formula.
2. The infant should be placed in a semiupright position for feeding.
3. Never prop the bottle; always hold the infant.
4. Mother should not coax infant to finish all of the bottle every time; any unused formula should be discarded.
5. Do not warm bottles or any food for infants in the microwave because formula or food gets excessively hot and the temperature is not uniform.

**! NURSING PRIORITY:** Proportions of formula must not be altered. Teach mother not to dilute or expand the amount of formula or concentrate it to provide more calories.

# ♣ HIGH-RISK NEWBORN

## ♣ Gestational Age Variation
### *Assessment*

A. Gestational age assessment (Table 27-2).
B. Clinical estimation of gestational age assessed by using visual Ballard scale (Figure 27-3).

**Table 27-2** **GESTATIONAL AGE ASSESSMENT**

| By Weight | By Age |
|---|---|
| Large for gestational age (LGA): Above the 90th percentile for estimated weeks of gestation; weight of 4000 g or more at birth. | Postmature/postterm: Born after completion of 42 weeks' gestation. |
| Appropriate for gestational age (AGA): Weight between 10th and 90th percentile for infant's age. | |
| Small for gestational age (SGA) or small for date (SFD): Weight below the 10th percentile for estimated weeks of gestation. | Full term: Born between the beginning of week 38 and the end of week 42 of gestation. |
| Low birth weight (LBW): Weight less than 2500 g (5.5 lb) regardless of gestational age. | |
| Very low birth weight (VLBW): Weight of 1500 g (3.3 lb) or less at birth. | Late preterm: Born between 34 and 36 weeks' gestation. |
| Extremely low birth weight (ELBW): Weight less than 1000 g (2.2 lb) | |
| Intrauterine growth restriction (IUGR): Growth of fetus does not meet expected norms. | Preterm or premature: Born before completion of 37 weeks' gestation, regardless of birth weight. |

## NEUROMUSCULAR MATURITY

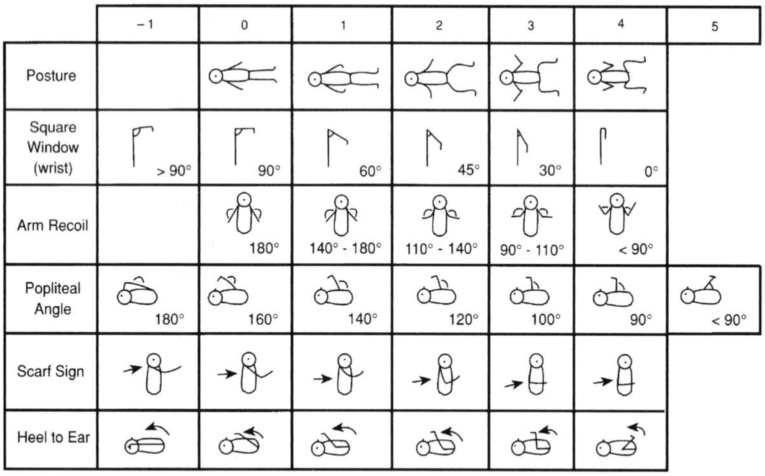

| | −1 | 0 | 1 | 2 | 3 | 4 | 5 |
|---|---|---|---|---|---|---|---|
| Posture | | | | | | | |
| Square Window (wrist) | > 90° | 90° | 60° | 45° | 30° | 0° | |
| Arm Recoil | | 180° | 140° - 180° | 110° - 140° | 90° - 110° | < 90° | |
| Popliteal Angle | 180° | 160° | 140° | 120° | 100° | 90° | < 90° |
| Scarf Sign | | | | | | | |
| Heel to Ear | | | | | | | |

## PHYSICAL MATURITY

| | | | | | | | |
|---|---|---|---|---|---|---|---|
| Skin | sticky friable transparent | gelatinous red, translucent | smooth pink, visible veins | superficial peeling or rash, few veins | cracking pale areas rare veins | parchment deep cracking no vessels | leathery cracked wrinkled |
| Lanugo | none | sparse | abundant | thinning | bald areas | mostly bald | |
| Plantar Surface | heel-toe 40-50 mm: -1 <40 mm: -2 | >50 mm no crease | faint red marks | anterior transverse crease only | creases ant. 2/3 | creases over entire sole | |
| Breast | imperceptible | barely perceptible | flat areola no bud | stippled areola 1-2 mm bud | raised areola 3-4 mm bud | full areola 5-10 mm bud | |
| Eye/Ear | lids fused loosely: -1 tightly: -2 | lids open pinna flat stays folded | sl. curved pinna; soft; slow recoil | well-curved pinna; soft but ready recoil | formed & firm instant recoil | thick cartilage ear stiff | |
| Genitals (male) | scrotum flat, smooth | scrotum empty faint rugae | testes in upper canal rare rugae | testes descending few rugae | testes down good rugae | testes pendulous deep rugae | |
| Genitals (female) | clitoris prominent labia flat | prominent clitoris small labia minora | prominent clitoris enlarging minora | majora & minora equally prominent | majora large minora small | majora cover clitoris & minora | |

## MATURITY RATING

| score | weeks |
|---|---|
| -10 | 20 |
| -5 | 22 |
| 0 | 24 |
| 5 | 26 |
| 10 | 28 |
| 15 | 30 |
| 20 | 32 |
| 25 | 34 |
| 30 | 36 |
| 35 | 38 |
| 40 | 40 |
| 45 | 42 |
| 50 | 44 |

**FIGURE 27-3** **Estimation of Gestational Age.** (From Lowdermilk, D., & Perry, S. [2016]. *Maternity and women's health care* [11th ed.]. St. Louis, MO: Mosby.)

C. Respiratory parameters.
  1. Observe respiratory rate, rhythm, and depth.
     a. Initially, rate increases without a change in rhythm.
     b. Flaring of nares and expiratory grunting are early signs of respiratory distress.
  2. Increase in apical pulse rate.
  3. Subcostal and xiphoid retractions progress to intercostal, substernal, and clavicular retractions.
  4. Color.
     a. Progresses from pink to circumoral pallor to circumoral cyanosis to generalized cyanosis.
     b. Increased intensity of acrocyanosis.
  5. Progressive respiratory distress.
     a. Respiratory rate increases 80 to 120 breaths/min; accessory muscles of respiration are used; nasal flaring.
     b. Abdominal seesaw breathing patterns; central cyanosis.
     c. Distinguish between apneic episodes (15 seconds or longer) and periodic breathing (cessation of breathing for 5 to 10 seconds, followed by 10 to 15 seconds of compensatory rapid respirations).
  6. Progressing anoxia leading to cardiac decompensation and failure.
  7. Increased muscle flaccidity: froglike position.
D. Nutrition.
  1. Assess readiness and ability to feed: swallowing, gag reflexes.
  2. Screen for hypoglycemia.
  3. Observe for congenital dysfunction and anomalies related to tracheoesophageal fistula, anal atresia, and metabolic disorders.
  4. Check amount and frequency of elimination.
  5. Assess for vomiting or regurgitation; a preterm infant's stomach capacity is small, and overfeeding can occur.
  6. Check mucous membranes, urine output, and skin turgor to identify fluid and electrolyte imbalances.
     a. Skin turgor over abdomen and inner thighs.
     b. Sunken fontanel.
     c. Urinary output of less than 30 mL/day.
E. Temperature regulation (see Figure 27-2).
  1. Assess infant's temperature: frequently done with a skin probe for continuous monitoring of temperature in infants at high risk for complications.
  2. Check coolness or warmth of body and extremities.
  3. Detect early signs of cold stress.
     a. Increased physical activity and crying.
     b. Increased respiratory rate.
     c. Increased acrocyanosis or generalized cyanosis along with mottling of the skin (cutis marmorata).
     d. Male with descended testes: presence of cremasteric reflex (testes are pulled back up into the inguinal canal on exposure to cold).
  4. Monitor infant's temperature.
     a. Axillary temperature: 36.5° to 37.2°C (Average: 37°C or 97.7°F).
     b. Place a temperature skin probe on infant while he or she is in the radiant warmer or isolette.

> **! NURSING PRIORITY:** Maintain desired temperature of newborn by using external devices.

*Nursing Interventions*

**Goal:** To maintain respiratory functioning.

A. Provide gentle physical stimulation to remind infant to breathe.
  1. Gently rub the infant's back.
  2. Lightly tap the infant's feet.

> **! NURSING PRIORITY:** Physically stimulate a newborn to breathe; administer oxygen; monitor newborn's gas exchange by obtaining arterial blood gas values, pulse oximetry readings, etc.

B. Ensure patency of respiratory tract.
  1. Maintain open airway by means of nasal, oral, or pharyngeal suctioning.
  2. Position to promote oxygenation.
     a. Elevate head 10 degrees with neck slightly extended by placement of a small folded towel under the shoulders.
     b. Flex and abduct infant's arms and place at sides.
     c. Avoid diapers or adhere them loosely.
     d. Turn side to side every 1 to 2 hours.
     e. Do not place in prone position.
C. Assist infant's respiratory efforts.
  1. Monitor oxygen pressure.
     a. Anywhere from 21% to 100% oxygen is administered to maintain the $P_{O_2}$ around 50 to 80 mmHg.
     b. Avoid high concentrations of oxygen for prolonged periods; may lead to complication of bronchopulmonary dysplasia.
  2. Positive end-expiratory pressure helps keep alveoli open at the end of expiration by providing positive pressure.
  3. Continuous positive airway pressure (CPAP) counteracts the tendency of the alveoli to collapse by providing continuous distending airway pressure.
     a. CPAP is administered either by endotracheal tube or nasal prongs.
     b. CPAP must be regulated with regard to humidification, temperature, and pressure; 6 to 10 cm of water pressure is the therapeutic range for keeping the alveoli open.
D. Monitor oxygen therapy.
  1. Transcutaneous oxygen tension monitoring: measures oxygen diffusion across the skin.
  2. Pulse oximeter: monitors beat-to-beat arterial saturation; less dependent on perfusion than transcutaneous oxygen tension or carbon dioxide tension monitoring; gives a more rapid "real-time" reading.

**Goal:** To provide adequate nutrition.

A. Detect hypoglycemia and treat immediately: administer 5% dextrose in water intravenously if infant is unable to tolerate oral feeding.

B. Oral feeding: initial feeding.
1. Use sterile water: 1 to 2 mL for a small infant.
2. Use preemie nipple to conserve infant's energy.
3. Because of small size of infant's stomach, feedings are small in amount and increased in frequency.
C. Orogastric tube feedings.
1. Usually administered by continuous flow of formula with an infusion pump (kangaroo pump) when the infant is:
   a. Having severe respiratory distress.
   b. Too immature and weak to suck.
   c. Tired and fatigues easily when a preemie nipple is used.
2. Placement and insertion of orogastric feeding tube.
   a. Position infant on the back or toward the right side with the head and chest slightly elevated.
   b. Measure correct length of insertion by marking on the catheter the distance from the tip of the nose to the ear lobe to the tip of the sternum.
   c. Lubricate tube with sterile water and slowly insert catheter into mouth and down the esophagus into the stomach.
   d. Test for placement of the tube by aspirating stomach contents or injecting 0.5 to 1.0 mL of air for the premature infant (up to 5 mL for larger infants) and auscultating the abdomen for the sound.
   e. Before infusing a feeding by gravity into the stomach, check for residual; this is done by aspirating and measuring amount left in stomach from previous feeding; feeding is usually held if residual is greater than 50% of feeding.
   f. If feeding is not continuous, remove tubing by pinching or clamping it and withdrawing it rapidly.
   g. Burp infant after feeding by turning head or positioning him or her on the right side.
   h. Check to see whether mother wants to pump her breast to provide the milk supply to the infant for gavage.
D. Total parenteral nutrition may be ordered to provide complete nutrition.
E. Detect complications that arise with feeding the preterm infant as a result of:
1. Weak or absent sucking and swallowing reflexes.
2. A very small stomach capacity, which necessitates the use of high-calorie food.
3. Poor gag reflex, leading to aspiration.
4. Incompetent esophageal cardiac sphincter.
5. Increased incidence of vomiting and development of abdominal distention.
6. Inability to absorb essential nutrients.
7. Excessive loss of water through evaporation from the skin and respiratory tract.

**Goal:** To maintain warmth and temperature control (see maintaining temperature of healthy newborn).

A. Oxygen and air should be warmed and humidified.
B. Maintain abdominal skin temperature at 36.1° to 36.7°C (97°–98°F); axillary temperature 36.5° to 37.2°C (97.7°–99.0°F).

C. Monitor infant's temperature continuously; make sure that temperature probe is set on control panel, probe is on infant's abdomen, and all safety precautions are maintained.
D. Prevent rapid warming or cooling because this may cause apnea and acidosis; warming process is increased gradually over a period of 2 to 4 hours.
E. Infant may need extra clothing or need to be wrapped in an extra blanket for additional warmth.

> **TEST ALERT:** Provide care and education that meets the special needs of the infant client 1 month to 1 year.

## Respiratory Distress

**Neonates can experience respiratory distress from a variety of factors.**

A. Types of respiratory distress.
1. Respiratory distress syndrome (RDS) occurs as a result of the deficiency of surfactant, which lines the alveoli; alveoli collapse at the end of each expiration, retaining little or no residual air, leading to generalized atelectasis.
2. Meconium aspiration syndrome.
   a. A fetus may pass meconium in utero.
   b. Associated with fetal growth retardation (small for gestational age) and postmaturity.
   c. Meconium can enter the lungs in utero and plug small air passages; this leads to inflammation of the lung tissues; areas of atelectasis occur because of obstruction and consolidation of the meconium; secondary infection frequently occurs in the lungs.
3. Pneumonia: often associated with premature rupture of the membranes or a prolonged labor.
4. Central nervous system depression: often associated with excessive maternal analgesia or anesthesia.

### Assessment

A. Usually appears within 6 hours after birth.
B. Tachypnea: more than 60 breaths/min.
C. Apneic spells (in excess of 15 seconds).
D. Abnormal breath sounds: rales and rhonchi.
E. Chest retraction.
1. Indicative of increased respiratory work.
2. Begins as a mild sinking of the intercostal spaces or xiphoid retraction on each inspiration.
3. Severe distress characterized by seesaw breathing: abdomen rises and chest sinks on inspiration; abdomen falls and chest expands on expiration.
F. Flaring of the nares.
G. Expiratory grunting.

> **NURSING PRIORITY:** Grunting is an ominous sign and indicates impending need for respiratory assistance; most often, mucus needs to be cleared from airway.

1. Protective reflex mechanism that prolongs end expiration, which increases oxygenation.

2. Grunting sound occurs as a result of air pushing past a partially closed glottis.

3. Often, it is accompanied by a whining or moaning sound.

H. Prolonged expiration: air flows in easier than it flows out.

I. Cough caused by excessive secretions in the respiratory tract.

J. Generalized cyanosis: usually not observed until $Po_2$ is less than 42 mmHg.

K. Diagnostics
   1. Chest x-ray film, echocardiogram.
   2. Blood gas values and pulse oximetry.
   3. Possible lumbar puncture (to rule out infection).
   4. Determine the lecithin/sphingomyelin ratio.

### Complications

A. Hypoxia continues to increase, leading to decreased lung compliance.

B. Respiratory acidosis caused by alveolar hypoventilation.

C. Metabolic acidosis occurs as a result of hypoxia, which leads to anaerobic metabolism, which leads to increased lactate levels and results in base deficit.

D. Retinopathy of prematurity caused by high levels of oxygen and immature blood vessels.

E. Bronchopulmonary dysplasia: chronic stiff, noncompliant lungs.

### Treatment

A. Respiratory distress syndrome.
   1. Treatment is supportive; adequate ventilation and perfusion.
   2. Monitor ABGs.
   3. Constant passive airway pressure is the primary treatment (see Appendix 15-8).
   4. Administration of surfactant through the airway into the infant's lungs.

B. Meconium aspiration.
   1. Administration of oxygen with humidification.
   2. Postural drainage and percussion.
   3. Antibiotic therapy.
   4. Correction of acid–base imbalance.

### Nursing Interventions

**Goal:** To promote oxygenation and respiratory functioning.

A. Administer antenatal steroids to mothers between 24 and 34 weeks if preterm birth is threatened and administer surfactant to neonate after delivery to stimulate surfactant production.

B. Refer to nursing intervention for the high-risk newborn.

**Goal:** To prevent respiratory distress.

A. Assess for infants at high risk because of gestational age and predisposing factors.

### 🍦 Cleft Lip

**Cleft lip is a fissure of the upper lip to the side of the midline, which may vary from a slight notch to a complete separation extending into the nostril; may be unilateral or bilateral. It is caused by failure of the maxillary process to close in early fetal life; usually occurs during the sixth week of gestation.**

### Assessment

A. Increased incidence in males; occurs in about 1:600 live births.

B. Visible at birth on an incompletely formed lip.

### Treatment

Surgical: closure of lip defect is usually done between 2 and 3 months after birth.

### Nursing Interventions

**Goal:** To provide preoperative care.

A. Maintain nutrition.
   1. Use modified nipple to increase infant's ability to obtain milk without sucking and allow feeder to provide assistance (e.g., Haberman feeder).
   2. Feed slowly.
   3. Bubble and burp frequently (after every 15 to 30 mL).
   4. Feed with infant's head in an upright position.

B. Prepare parents for newborn's surgery.
   1. Address psychosocial needs of the parents.
   2. Encourage parents to position infant flat on back in upright position or on side to accustom infant to the postoperative positioning.
   3. Encourage parents to place infant in arm restraints periodically before hospital admission, so infant becomes familiar with the necessary restriction of arm motion after surgery.
   4. Encourage parents to feed infant with the same method that will be used after surgery.

**Goal:** To provide postoperative care.

A. Prevent trauma to suture line.
   1. Position infant on back or side and elevate head (infant seat).
   2. Restrain arms with soft elbow restraints.
   3. Cleanse suture line gently after each feeding; use cotton-tipped applicator with prescribed solution and roll along the suture line; may apply antibiotic ointment.
   4. Prevent any crust or scab formation on lip and suture line.

B. Maintain a patent airway and facilitate breathing.
   1. Assess for respiratory distress.
   2. Observe for swelling of the nose, tongue, and lips.

C. Provide adequate nutrition.
   1. Feed in an upright, sitting position using modified nipple.
   2. Feed slowly and burp/bubble at frequent intervals.

D. Provide discharge teaching to parents.
   1. Encourage parents to cuddle and play with infant to decrease crying and prevent trauma to suture line.
   2. Teach feeding, cleansing, and restraining procedures.
   3. Refer to local community agencies for continued support.
   4. Long-term follow-up: dental/orthodontic needs.

# Cleft Palate

**Cleft palate is a failure of fusion of the secondary palate; may involve the soft and hard palates along with the alveolar (dental) ridge. It is important to determine whether defect is isolated or if it is part of a broader syndrome. Problem is associated with increased incidence of other malformations, especially GI tract defects.**

## Assessment

A. Opening in roof of mouth; may be isolated or associated with a cleft lip.
B. Sucking difficulties.
C. Breathing problems.
D. Later problems include increased incidence of upper respiratory tract infection and otitis media.
E. Later problems are related to speech and hearing difficulties and self-esteem issues.

## Treatment

A. Surgical.
 1. Surgery may be done in stages; closure of palate defect typically performed between 6 to 12 months of age.
B. Long-term care management.
 1. Extensive orthodontics to correct problems of malpositioned teeth and maxillary arches.
 2. Speech therapy.
 3. Hearing problems related to chronic, recurrent otitis media; varying degrees of hearing loss may occur.

## Nursing Interventions

**Goal:** To provide preoperative care.

A. Maintain nutrition.
 1. Use a modified nipple for feeding.
 2. Encourage toddler to drink from a cup.
 3. Feed child in upright position.
B. Prevent infection.
 1. Teach parents symptoms of otitis media.
C. Provide support and teaching to parents.
 1. Determine type of restraints that may be used postoperatively; parents may begin to use restraints preoperatively to promote adaptation postoperatively.
 2. Teach about various methods to meet infant's sucking needs.

**Goal:** To provide postoperative care.

A. Maintain patent airway.
 1. Observe for respiratory distress and have emergency equipment available at bedside (endotracheal tube, suction, and laryngoscope).
 2. Immediate postoperatively position on side to provide for drainage of mucus.
B. Prevent injury and trauma to the suture line.
 1. Maintain age-appropriate restraints: elbow restraints for infants, jackets for older children.
 2. Avoid use of any objects in the mouth (e.g., straws, suction catheters, tongue depressors, pacifiers, spoons, or certain toys).

3. Decrease crying by providing attention and affection or diversional activities if child is older.
C. Maintain nutrition.
 1. Give fluids initially; then advance to appropriate diet based on age.
 2. Child (even an older one) is not allowed to eat hard items such as toast, crackers, potato chips, etc.
 3. Cleanse suture line after each feeding by rinsing mouth with water.
D. Provide guidance to parents regarding long-term rehabilitation.
 1. Provide for emotional support.
 2. Encourage verbalization of feelings regarding infant with defect.
 3. Refer to appropriate community resources.
 4. Long-term follow-up: speech therapy; dental/orthodontics; ear examinations.

> **! NURSING PRIORITY:** Provide surgical wound care.

# Esophageal Atresia and Tracheoesophageal Fistula

**Esophageal atresia (EA) and tracheoesophageal fistula (TEF) are rare malformations that represent a failure of the esophagus to develop as a continuous passage and a failure of the trachea and esophagus to separate into distinct structures.**

## Assessment

A. Risk factors.
 1. Prematurity.
 2. History of maternal hydramnios.
 3. Associated with other anomalies, especially congenital heart defects, anorectal problems (imperforate anus), and genital anomalies (exstrophy of the bladder).
 4. Incidence 1:4000 births; slightly higher incidence in males.
B. Types.
 1. Esophageal atresia and tracheoesophageal fistula.
  a. Most common form of cases.
  b. Proximal end of esophagus ends in a blind pouch, and the lower segment connects to the trachea.
  c. Characterized by the classic three Cs: *choking, coughing,* and *cyanosis.*
  d. Excessive frothy saliva and constant drooling.
  e. Aspiration is a complication, especially during feeding.
C. Diagnostics.
 1. Inability to pass a catheter into the stomach.
 2. Chest x-ray films with use of radiopaque catheter.

## Treatment

A. Surgical correction (for esophageal atresia with tracheoesophageal fistula).
 1. Thoracotomy with ligation of the tracheoesophageal fistula and an end-to-end anastomosis of the esophagus.

2. If infant is in poor condition or premature, a temporary gastrostomy may be performed to allow for adequate nutrition, and the defect will be repaired at a later date.
3. A colon transplant may be done if a segment of the esophagus is too short for anastomosis.
4. Surgical repair is done in stages.

*Nursing Interventions*

**⚠ PEDIATRIC NURSING PRIORITY:** When there is any suspicion of possible esophageal problems, infant should receive nothing by mouth (have NPO status) until further evaluation can be done.

**Goal:** To provide preoperative care.

A. Maintain patent airway.
   1. Supine position with head elevated on an inclined plane of at least 30 degrees.
   2. Suction nasopharynx.
   3. Observe for symptoms of respiratory distress.
   4. Maintain NPO status.
B. Early recognition of defect is important.
   1. Assess for the classic *three Cs: choking, coughing,* and *cyanosis.*
   2. Excessive salivation and drooling may occur along with gastric distention.
C. Prepare parents for infant's surgery.

**Goal:** To provide postoperative care.

A. Maintain respirations and prevent respiratory complications.
   1. Pneumonia, atelectasis, pneumothorax, and laryngeal edema are common complications.
   2. Administer oxygen.
   3. Oral suction of secretions and position for optimum ventilation.
   4. Maintain care of chest tubes.
   5. Administer antibiotics.
   6. Place in warm, high-humidity isolette.
   7. Maintain nasogastric suctioning.
B. Provide adequate nutrition.
   1. Gastrostomy feedings may be started on the second or third postoperative day.
   2. Oral feedings are frequently delayed after surgery or until the esophageal anastomosis is healed.
   3. Meet oral sucking needs by offering infant a pacifier.
C. Prepare parents for discharge.
   1. Teach techniques such as suctioning, gastrostomy tube feeding, and progression of diet.
   2. Explain signs of respiratory difficulty and indicators of esophageal constriction (e.g., difficulty in swallowing, coughing).

## Imperforate Anus

**Imperforate anus is a type of anorectal malformation caused by abnormal development.**

A. Types.
   1. A membrane over the anal opening, with a normal anus just above the membrane.

2. Complete absence of anus (anal agenesis), with the rectal pouch ending some distance above.
3. Rectum may end blindly or have a fistula connection to the perineum, urethra, bladder, or vagina.

*Assessment*

A. No anal opening.
B. Absence of meconium or meconium in urine.
C. Gradual increase in abdominal distention.
D. Often associated with neurologic defects; approximately 1:5000 births
E. Diagnostics.
   1. Abdominal ultrasound examination.
   2. Voiding cystourethrogram: identifies any urinary fistula malformation.

*Treatment*

A. Surgery.
   1. Anoplasty: reconstruction of the anus.
   2. Posterior sagittal anorectoplasty (PSARP) or abdominal–perineal pull-through with colostomy.
   3. Colostomy (often done initially until full repair is done at 1 to 2 months of age for more complicated types).

*Nursing Interventions*

**Goal:** To identify anal malformation.

A. Detect increasing abdominal distention.
B. Inspect anal area for opening.

**⚠ NURSING PRIORITY:** Record the first passage of meconium stool. If infant does not pass stool within 24 hours, further assessment is required.

**Goal:** To provide postoperative care.

A. Prevent infection by maintaining good perineal care and keeping operative site clean and dry, especially after passage of stool and urine.
B. Instruct parents in care of colostomy (e.g., frequent dressing changes, meticulous skin care, placement of collection device, avoidance of tight diapers and clothes around stoma).
C. Anal dilations may be necessary; observe stooling patterns.

## Neural Tube Defects

**A neural tube defect (spina bifida) results in midline defects and closure of the spinal cord (may be noncystic or cystic); most common site is lumbosacral area.**

*Assessment*

A. Types.
   1. Spina bifida occulta.
      a. Noncystic spina bifida, which results in failure of the spinous processes to join posteriorly in the lumbosacral area, usually around L5 and S1.

b. Neuromuscular disturbances may be apparent with lower-extremity weakness, bowel and bladder sphincter disturbance, and numbness and tingling of the extremities.

c. Infant may have no apparent clinical manifestations.

2. Spina bifida cystica.

a. Meningocele: a saclike cyst of meninges filled with spinal fluid that protrudes through a defect in the bony part of the spine.

b. Myelomeningocele: a saclike cyst containing meninges, spinal fluid, and a portion of the spinal cord with its nerves that protrudes through a defect in the vertebral column; other defect most frequently associated with this is hydrocephalus.

B. Diagnostics.

1. Ultrasound examination.

2. Computed tomography; magnetic resonance imaging.

3. Prenatal diagnosis: ultrasound examination and elevated alpha-fetoprotein level (determined from amniotic fluid sample; performed at 16 to 18 weeks).

### Treatment

A. Surgical: closure of defect within 24 to 48 hours to decrease risk for infection, relieve pressure, repair sac, and possibly insert a shunt; closure at 12 to 18 hours if sac is leaking.

B. Prophylactic: a decrease in the incidence of neural tube defects is associated with an increase in folic acid intake during pregnancy.

### Nursing Interventions

> **! NURSING PRIORITY:** Correct positioning of the infant is critical in preventing damage to the sac and in providing nursing care after surgery.

**Goal:** To provide preoperative care.

A. Prevent and protect sac from drying, rupturing, and infection.

1. Position infant prone on abdomen.

2. Avoid touching sac.

3. Provide meticulous skin care after voiding and bowel movements.

4. Often, sterile, normal saline soaks on a nonadherent dressing may be used to prevent drying.

B. Detect early development of hydrocephalus.

1. Measure head and check circumference frequently.

2. Check fontanels for bulging and separation of suture line.

C. Monitor elimination function.

1. Note whether urine is dripping or is retained.

2. Indwelling catheter may be inserted or intermittent catheterization may be used at regular intervals to ensure regular bladder emptying.

3. Assess for bowel function: glycerin suppository may be ordered to stimulate meconium passage.

**Goal:** To provide postoperative care.

A. Prevent trauma and infection at the surgical site.

1. Place infant in same position (prone on abdomen) as before surgery.

2. Continue to provide scrupulous skin care as described under preoperative goal.

3. Good perineal care because there is frequent continuous urinary drainage.

B. Assess neurologic status frequently for indications of increasing intracranial pressure, development of hydrocephalus, or early signs of infection.

1. Continue to measure head circumference daily.

2. Perform frequent neurologic checks.

C. Provide parents with education in regard to positioning, feeding, skin care, elimination procedures, and range-of-motion exercises.

1. Encourage and facilitate parental bonding.

2. Refer to community and social agencies for financial and social support.

3. Encourage long-range planning and support of parents for long-term rehabilitation of infant.

**Goal:** To provide management and resources for long-term care.

A. Physical therapy and musculoskeletal management will be needed due to possible spasticity and progressive paralysis, along with the potential for deformity based on severity of spinal cord lesion.

B. Urinary incontinence is a chronic problem most often due to a neuropathic (neurogenic) bladder.

C. Bowel control can be achieved with dietary fiber, laxatives, suppositories, or enemas to prevent constipation and impaction.

## 🍦 Necrotizing Enterocolitis

**The condition is an acute inflammatory disease of the bowel; increased incidence in preterm infants; cause is unknown. It is characterized by ischemic necrosis of the GI tract, which leads to perforation.**

A. Bowel is often dilated, and surface is hemorrhagic.

B. Ileus often develops, and bowel may perforate.

C. Peritonitis and neonatal sepsis ensue.

### Assessment

A. Problems occur within 4 to 10 days of initiating feeding but may be evident as early as 4 hours of age, and in preterm infants may be delayed for up to 30 days; first 10 days of life in full-term infants is when it usually occurs.

B. Abdominal distention and rigidity may be seen.

C. Bowel is often dilated, and surface is hemorrhagic.

D. Bowel sounds may be absent.

E. Bile-stained emesis and blood-streaked diarrhea or guaiac-positive stool.

F. Other symptoms include episodes of apnea, temperature instability, jaundice, and shocklike symptoms.

G. Ileus often develops and the bowel may perforate; peritonitis and neonatal sepsis ensue.

H. Diagnostics: abdominal x-ray film.

### Treatment

A. Medical.
1. All enteric feedings are discontinued.
2. Nasogastric suctioning is initiated.
3. Intravenous therapy and total parenteral nutrition.

B. Medications: antibiotics.

C. Abdominal x-ray films to check for peritonitis, obstruction, or pneumoperitoneum (free air in peritoneum).

D. If condition is severe, surgery is indicated for intestinal perforation, obstruction, and peritonitis; temporary or permanent colostomy may be required.

### Nursing Interventions

**Goal:** To assist with the medical and surgical management.

A. Maintain nasogastric suctioning; keep infant NPO.

B. Administer antibiotics, IV fluids, and total parenteral nutrition.

C. Promote ventilation; prevent respiratory complications.

**Goal:** To detect early complications.

A. Assess vital signs.

B. Check for bowel sounds; absence may indicate obstruction.

C. Measure abdominal girth at regular intervals to detect abdominal distention.

D. Avoid pressure on abdomen by not diapering the infant; do not place in prone position.

**Goal:** To provide support and education to the family.

A. Explanation of treatment and, if surgery is done, postoperative management.

B. Assist in teaching parents how to care for infant's ileostomy or colostomy, as necessary.

## Neonatal Sepsis

**Infection that occurs during or after birth may result in neonatal sepsis, a systemic infection from bacteria in the bloodstream.**

### Assessment

**NURSING PRIORITY:** Neonate often has very subtle behavioral changes, which makes it more difficult to assess a gradual onset of sepsis.

A. Risk factors.
1. Predisposing factors are prematurity, invasive procedures, and nosocomial exposure to infection.
2. Immature immunologic system.
3. Maternal antepartum infection: toxoplasmosis, cytomegalic inclusion disease (cytomegalovirus).
4. Intrapartum maternal infections: amnionitis, premature rupture of membranes, bacterial (*beta-hemolytic*

*streptococci, gonococci, staphylococci*), fungal (*Candida albicans*), or direct contact with maternal GI or urinary tract organisms.

B. Clinical manifestations.
1. Apathy, lethargy, poor temperature control.
2. Poor feeding, abdominal distention, diarrhea.
3. Cyanosis, irregular respirations, apnea.
4. Hyperbilirubinemia.
5. Infant often described as "not acting right"; may be irritable.

C. Diagnostics.
1. Cultures of blood, urine, feces, and mucosa.
2. Lumbar puncture and spinal fluid for culture and sensitivity.
3. Complete blood count, chest x-ray film, and viral studies (Table 27-3).

### Treatment

A. Medications: antibiotic, antiviral, antifungal.

B. Supportive: may include oxygen, IV therapy, regulation of fluids and electrolytes.

### Nursing Interventions

**Goal:** To prevent neonatal sepsis by prenatal prevention; maternal screening for sexually transmitted infections and assessment of rubella titers.

A. TORCH (toxoplasmosis, other [congenital syphilis and viruses], rubella, cytomegalovirus, and herpes simplex virus) syndrome.

**Goal:** To prevent infection during the intrapartal period.

A. Maintenance of sterile technique.

B. Prophylactic antibiotic treatment.

## Phenylketonuria

**Phenylketonuria is inherited as an autosomal recessive trait and is an inborn error of metabolism characterized by an absence of the enzyme necessary to metabolize phenylalanine (an essential amino acid). Excessive phenylalanine leads to intellectual impairment.**

### Assessment

A. Musty urine odor.

B. Typical physical characteristics: blond hair, blue eyes, fair skin (caused by a lack of melanin).

C. Vomiting, irritability.

D. Diagnostics
1. Screening is mandatory in all states.
2. Guthrie blood test, blood obtained via heel stick.
   a. Obtain sample after ingestion of protein; done as close to discharge as possible and no later than 7 days after birth.
   b. Obtain an additional blood sample at 2 weeks if original sample was collected before infant was 24 hours old.
   c. Concern that all infants are not rescreened for PKU after early discharge.

**Table 27-3  DISORDERS ACQUIRED DURING AND AFTER BIRTH**

|  | Trauma | Peripheral Nerve Injuries | Neonatal Sepsis |
|---|---|---|---|
| Assessment | Soft-tissue injury<br>Caput succedaneum | Temporary paralysis of the facial nerve is the most common. | Apathy, lethargy, low-grade temperature |
|  | Cephalhematoma | Affected side of the face is smooth. | Poor feeding, abdominal distention, diarrhea |
|  | Injury to bone: fractured clavicle is the most common; often occurs with a large-sized infant | Eye may stay open.<br>Mouth droops at the corner.<br>Forehead cannot be wrinkled.<br>Possible difficulty sucking. | Cyanosis, irregular respirations, apnea<br>Hyperbilirubinemia |
|  |  | Brachial palsy: A partial or complete paralysis of the nerve fibers of the brachial plexus. | Infant often described as "not acting right" |
|  |  | Cannot elevate or abduct the arm. | CBC, chest x-ray film, and viral studies TORCH syndrome blood screening |
|  |  | Abnormal arm position or diminished arm movements. |  |
| Nursing interventions | Fractured clavicle<br>1. Place affected arm against chest wall with hand lying across chest.<br>2. Position is held by a figure 8 stockinette around the arm and chest.<br>3. Pick infant up carefully; shoulder should not be pressed toward middle of body.<br>4. Affected side should not be placed in gown or undershirt. | Facial nerve palsy<br>1. Apply eye patch; may use artificial tears to prevent corneal irritation.<br>2. Provide support during feeding; infant may not latch on to nipple well.<br>Brachial nerve palsy<br>1. Keep arm abducted and externally rotated with elbow flexed.<br>2. Arm is raised to shoulder height, and elbow is flexed 90 degrees. | 1. Prenatal prevention, maternal screening for STDs, and assessment of rubella titers<br>2. Maintenance of sterile technique<br>3. Prophylactic antibiotic treatment<br>4. Possible cesarean delivery for mother with genital herpes |

*CBC,* Complete blood count; *STDs,* sexually transmitted diseases; *TORCH,* **t**oxoplasmosis, **o**ther (congenital syphilis and viruses) **r**ubella, **c**ytomegalovirus, and **h**erpes virus.

---

**⚠ NURSING PRIORITY:** The newborn must be fed protein (breast milk or formula) before screening test.

### Treatment
A. Dietary: initiated as soon as possible (7 to 10 days of age).
B. Breastfeeding is preferred, but formula with low phenylalanine content may be used.
C. Phenylalanine-restricted diet required for life.

### Nursing Interventions
**Goal:** To identify infants at risk.

A. Assess newborns for clinical manifestations.
B. Proper use of the Guthrie blood test (avoid layering of blood).
C. Discuss importance of returning for a second blood test.

**Goal:** To prevent mental retardation.

A. Teach parents the dietary restrictions.
B. Encourage breastfeeding.
C. Provide family support.

## DISORDERS OF MATERNAL ORIGIN

### 🍦 Hemolytic Disease of the Newborn
**Hemolytic disease of the newborn is an antigen–antibody response causing destruction of fetal RBCs as a result of maternal sensitization of fetal RBC antigens and subsequent transfer of the resulting antibodies to the fetus.**

### Assessment
A. Types.
  1. ABO incompatibility: most frequently occurs when the mother's blood group is type O (contains anti-A and anti-B antibodies) and the fetus's blood group is type A or B.
     a. Milder form of hemolytic disease.
     b. Can occur in the first pregnancy.
     c. Does not necessarily increase in severity with each subsequent pregnancy.
  2. Rh incompatibility: Rh antigens from an Rh-positive fetus enter the blood of an Rh-negative mother, and the mother produces Rh antibodies; these cross the

placenta back into the fetal circulation; if the fetus is Rh positive, the antibodies destroy the fetal RBCs.
   a. Occurs with an Rh-negative mother who is carrying an Rh-positive fetus.
   b. Affects the second or subsequent pregnancies; rarely affects the first pregnancy.
   c. Severity of disorder progresses with each pregnancy if prophylactic treatment with Rh₀(D) immune globulin (also referred to as RhIg or RhoGAM) is not administered.
   d. The hemolysis of fetal RBCs can vary in severity from anemia to erythroblastosis fetalis; the most severe form is hydrops fetalis.
B. Clinical manifestations: ABO incompatibility.
   1. Hyperbilirubinemia.
   2. Rarely causes hemolysis that results in severe anemia of the newborn.
C. Clinical manifestations: Rh incompatibility.
   1. Hyperbilirubinemia and usually jaundice within first 24 hours.
      a. Jaundice occurs in a cephalocaudal direction: begins at the face, advances downward on the body to trunk and extremities, and finally reaches the palms and the soles of the feet.

> **⬛ NURSING PRIORITY:** Press skin against a bony prominence (e.g., chin, nose) to detect early color change.

      b. Bilirubin level rises above 12 mg/100 mL (205.25 umol/L) of blood; may reach 30 to 40 mg/100 mL (513.12 to 684.16 umol/L) within a few days if treatment is not initiated immediately.
   2. Anemia: usually evident within 12 hours; increased number of immature RBCs.
   3. Placental enlargement.
   4. Enlarged liver and spleen.
D. Diagnostics.
   1. Prenatal screening and prevention: Rh incompatibility.
      a. Administration of Rh₀(D) immune globulin to prevent Rh sensitization in first pregnancy of Rh-negative mother (see prenatal care).
         (1) Given intramuscularly to mother.
         (2) Has no effect against antibodies already present in maternal bloodstream.
         (3) Provides passive immunity.
         (4) Not a treatment for women who are already sensitized; recommended only for nonsensitized Rh-negative women at risk for development of Rh isoimmunization complications.
      b. Indirect Coombs test: performed on the mother's serum to measure the number of Rh-positive antibodies; critical level is usually defined as a titer greater than 1:8.
      c. Antibody rescreening is usually done at 24, 28, and 34 weeks' gestation to detect any developing sensitization during pregnancy.

   2. Obtain prenatal history regarding Rh incompatibility.
      a. Check to see whether mother has been pregnant before or has received a blood transfusion.
      b. Determine whether mother received Rh₀(D) immune globulin after previous pregnancies or blood transfusions.
   3. Postdelivery detection (Rh incompatibility).
      a. Direct Coombs test on cord blood: reveals presence of maternal antibodies attached to the RBCs of an Rh-positive infant.
      b. Rh₀(D) immune globulin is administered within 72 hours of an Rh-negative mother's first delivery of an Rh-positive infant, miscarriage, or abortion; repeated after subsequent pregnancies.
      c. Rh₀(D) immune globulin is also given after invasive procedures such as amniocentesis or chorionic villus sampling.
   4. Other tests.
      a. Hemoglobin and hematocrit values may be decreased.
      b. Increased reticulocyte count.
      c. Elevated bilirubin level.

*Treatment (of Affected Infants)*

A. Phototherapy for hyperbilirubinemia (see previous discussion of healthy newborn and hyperbilirubinemia).
B. Intrauterine blood transfusion (Rh incompatibility).
   1. Fetus transfused with Rh-negative type O packed RBCs to improve oxygenation and decrease anemia.
   2. May be done until fetal lung maturity is achieved and delivery can occur.
   3. Rarely done because problem is usually prevented by administration of Rh₀(D) immune globulin.
C. Exchange transfusion.
   1. Purpose.
      a. Decrease serum bilirubin levels.
      b. Correct anemia.
      c. Remove the antibodies that are responsible for hemolysis.
      d. Prevent cardiac failure and erythroblastosis fetalis.
   2. Not a common procedure because of decreased incidence of condition with prophylactic administration of Rh₀(D) immune globulin.

*Nursing Interventions*

> **⬛ NURSING PRIORITY:** It is important for the nurse to differentiate between pathologic and physiologic jaundice to detect early problems.

**Goal:** To recognize jaundice and distinguish the physiologic type (which occurs within 48 to 72 hours) from the pathologic type (which occurs within 24 hours).

A. Prenatal monitoring of maternal–fetal status.
B. Identify high-risk mother.
C. Monitor bilirubin levels in the newborn.

**Goal:** To assist with medical treatment.

A. Phototherapy (see discussion of healthy newborn).
B. Exchange transfusion.

## Infant of a Mother With Diabetes

**An infant born to a mother who has diabetes mellitus.**

> **TEST ALERT:** Identify signs of hyperglycemia and hypoglycemia.

### Assessment

A. Perinatal hazards.
1. Infant may be large for gestational age as a result of receiving a great deal of glucose (maternal hyperglycemia), or infant may be small for gestational age because of insufficient placental perfusion.
2. Size is inconsistent with gestational age; usually less mature.
3. Maternal hyperglycemia stimulates increased fetal insulin production. The fetus is left with excessive insulin during the neonatal period after maternal blood glucose has been withdrawn.
B. Clinical manifestations.
1. Puffy, cushingoid appearance, with round cheeks and stocky neck (macrosomia).
2. Enlarged heart, liver, and spleen.
3. Rapid, irregular respirations.
4. Increased Moro reflex and irritability on slight stimulation or lethargy at times.
C. Common complications.
1. Hypoglycemia: blood glucose level less than 40 mg/dL (2.2 mmol/L) within 1½ to 4 hours after birth.
   a. Lethargy, irritability, hypocalcemia.
   b. Twitching, jitteriness, seizures, high-pitched cry.
   c. Apneic spells and abdominal distention.
2. Respiratory distress syndrome, polycythemia.
3. Birth trauma caused by excessive size.
4. Congenital defects: cardiac (coarctation of the aorta, transposition of the great arteries, ASD/VSD), central nervous system (anencephaly, myelomeningocele, and hydrocephalus), renal, gastrointestinal, and musculoskeletal.

> **NURSING PRIORITY:** Prolonged hypoglycemia can cause irreversible brain damage.

### Treatment

A. Administration of glucose intravenously or 10% dextrose solution orally, depending on severity of hypoglycemia.
B. Hydration.
C. Blood glucose determinations on cord blood are done on samples obtained from infant at 30 minutes, 1 hour, 2 hours, and 4 hours after birth.
D. Maintaining glucose levels above 45 mg/dL (2.5 mmol/L)

### Nursing Interventions

**Goal:** To identify infant at risk.

A. Careful antepartal assessment of maternal diabetic status.
B. Treat infant as high risk and monitor continuously.

**Goal:** To monitor glucose levels.

A. Blood glucose levels.
B. Minimize trauma to heel site by performing heel stick correctly (Figure 27-4).
   1. Warm heel for 5 to 10 minutes before sticking.
   2. Cleanse site with alcohol and dry before sticking.
   3. The lateral heel is the site of choice.

## Drug-Exposed Infants (Neonatal Abstinence Syndrome)

**Infants born to mothers dependent on opioids exhibit neonatal abstinence syndrome. Many of the mothers often use several drugs, such as tranquilizers, nicotine, sedatives, narcotics, amphetamines, phencyclidine (PCP), marijuana, and other psychotropic agents.**

### Assessment

A. Clinical manifestations.
1. Signs of withdrawal within 12 to 24 hours after birth, depending on the substance and pattern of mother's use; symptoms more pronounced at 48 to 72 hours and may last from 6 days to 8 weeks.
2. If mother is on methadone, withdrawal lasts from 1 to 2 days to 2 to 3 weeks after birth.
3. Increased muscle tone, increased respiratory rate, disturbed sleep, fever, excessive sucking, and loose,

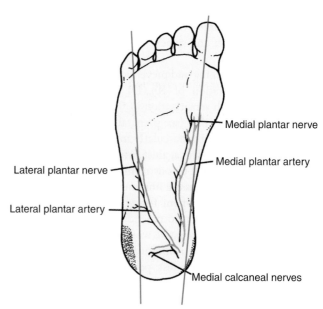

**FIGURE 27-4 Heel Stick Sites.** Use shaded areas on infant's foot for obtaining capillary blood. (From Lowdermilk, D., & Perry, S. [2016]. *Maternity and women's health care* [11th ed.]. St. Louis, MO: Mosby.)

watery stools, generalized perspiring (unusual in newborns).
4. Projectile vomiting, mottling, crying, nasal stuffiness, hyperactive Moro reflex, tremors.

## Treatment
A. Determine drugs in infant's system.
B. Appropriate withdrawal medications and support based on the particular drug.

*Nursing Interventions*

**Goal:** To reduce external stimuli to avoid triggering hyperactivity and irritability.

A. Dim lights and decrease noise.
B. Swaddle infant; rocking and holding the infant tightly limits his or her ability to self-stimulate.
C. Provide adequate nutrition and hydration.
D. Monitor with various scoring tools to evaluate level and severity of withdrawal.

## Study Questions
## Newborn Nursing Care

More questions on
evolve

1. The nursing assessment of an infant reveals expiratory grunting, substernal retractions, and a temperature of 99°F (37.2°C). What is the first nursing action?
   1. Place the infant in Trendelenburg position.
   2. Begin administration of 40% humidified oxygen via hood.
   3. Increase the temperature of the environment.
   4. Perform a complete assessment for congenital anomalies.

2. To meet the goal of promoting infant feeding in a breastfed baby, the nurse should teach the mother to do which of the following? **Select all that apply.**
   1. Feed the baby on a 3- to 4-hour schedule.
   2. Alternate breast milk and formula for each feeding.
   3. Stop breastfeeding if her nipples get sore.
   4. Maintain on-demand breastfeeding for the first 4 weeks.
   5. Drink lots of fluids and get adequate rest.
   6. Offer a pacifier between feedings to satisfy sucking needs.

3. Which statement best describes the problem of regulation of body temperature in a 3-lb (1361-g) premature infant?
   1. The surface area of the premature infant is relatively smaller than that of a healthy term infant.
   2. There is a lack of subcutaneous fat, which furnishes insulation.
   3. There are frequent episodes of diaphoresis, causing loss of body heat.
   4. There is a limited ability to produce body proteins.

4. The nurse is caring for an infant with an unrepaired tracheoesophageal fistula. In planning care, the nurse will identify which priority nursing goal?
   1. To promote oxygen exchange
   2. To prevent lung infection
   3. To promote bonding
   4. To replace fluids and electrolytes

5. The nurse would identify which situation as an indication for the administration of Rh$_o$(D) immune globulin?
   1. A woman who has been Rh sensitized in the past two pregnancies
   2. An infant with increased hemolysis of red blood cells because of ABO incompatibility
   3. An infant with an increase in serum bilirubin levels as a result of the presence of Rh factor antibodies
   4. A primigravida who is Rh negative is pregnant with an infant who is Rh positive

6. In the recovery room, the *best* immediate postoperative position for an infant who has had a cleft lip repair is:
   1. Prone with the head turned to one side
   2. Left Sims' position
   3. Supine with the head turned to the side
   4. Trendelenburg position to facilitate drainage

7. An infant born at 28 weeks' gestation weighs 4 lb 3 oz (1950 g). What does the initial nursing care of this infant include?
   1. Place the infant in protective isolation because of the underdeveloped immune system.
   2. Feed him a low-phenylalanine formula to increase digestion and utilization of calories.
   3. Provide gavage feedings every 2 hours because of an inadequate sucking and swallow reflex.
   4. Place the infant under a radiant heater to maintain regulation of body temperature.

8. The nurse is providing discharge teaching to a 20-year-old mother who has had her first male child. Which statement by the mother demonstrates that she understands the discharge teaching regarding his circumcision?
   1. "I will observe the whitish yellow drainage on his penis, but I will not remove it."
   2. "I will bring him back to the clinic in 3 days to have the drainage removed."
   3. "I will use antibiotic ointment on his penis with every diaper change."
   4. "I will rub the area briskly with a washcloth to remove the discharge."

9. The clinic nurse observes that a 3-day-old baby girl is jaundiced. A bilirubin level is 11.4 mg/dL (194.99 umol/L). What causes this bilirubin level?
   1. Physiologic jaundice
   2. Hemolytic disease of the newborn
   3. Erythroblastosis fetalis
   4. Sepsis

10. A neonate is being discharged home with a fiber-optic blanket for treatment of physiologic jaundice. What is important for the nurse to include in the discharge instructions?
   1. Cover the infant's eyes during the treatment.
   2. Reduce the daily number of formula feedings.
   3. Encourage frequent feeding to increase intake.
   4. Expect a constipated stool until jaundice clears.

11. The nurse assigned to the care of newborn infants understands the importance of keeping these infants swaddled in a warm blanket to prevent heat loss. Why is this important in the care of the newborn?
   1. Chilling leads to increased heat production and greater oxygen needs.
   2. The newborn's metabolic rate is decreased.
   3. Evaporation will affect the newborn's ability to feed.
   4. The newborn will sleep more comfortably.

12. The newborn's mother is concerned about the shape of the baby's head after delivery. She states that the baby looks like a "cone head." What is the most appropriate response by the nurse?
   1. "You don't need to worry about it. It is perfectly normal after birth."
   2. "It is molding caused by the pressure during birth and will disappear in a few days."
   3. "I will report it to the physician and recommend a diagnostic scan."
   4. "It is a collection of blood related to the trauma of delivery and will absorb in a few weeks."

13. The nurse is responsible for documenting the first meconium stool the newborn passes. If the newborn does not have a stool in the first 24 hours of life, the nurse should first:
   1. Insert a rectal thermometer to facilitate the process.
   2. Inspect the anal area for an opening.
   3. Monitor the vital signs for a rise in temperature.
   4. Increase oral feeding to stimulate passage of stool.

14. The best way for the nurse to maintain the safety of the newborn in the hospital is to:
   1. Have the mother come to the nursery to pick up the baby for feedings.
   2. Take the baby to the mother's room for rooming-in.
   3. Ask the mother her name and social security number.
   4. Compare the name band information of the mother and baby.

15. A 10-lb (4536-g) newborn of a mother with diabetes is admitted to the intensive care unit because of hypoglycemia. The baby's mother is concerned that he will have diabetes. The most appropriate response by the nurse is that the baby:
   1. May have an increased risk of acquiring metabolic syndrome in childhood or early adulthood
   2. Will not be at risk for developing diabetes
   3. Will have to follow a diabetic diet to avoid complications
   4. Will not need to be monitored closely during his early childhood years

16. A newborn is suspected of having esophageal atresia with a tracheal esophageal fistula. What nursing assessment information would assist in validating the presence of a fistula?
   1. Clammy skin and a croupy cough
   2. Crying and chest retractions
   3. Choking and coughing
   4. Chin tug and circumoral pallor

17. The nurse is caring for a newborn with an unrepaired meningocele. What is the highest priority goal for care?
   1. Maintaining a patent airway
   2. Preventing trauma to the sac
   3. Providing nourishment to prepare for surgery
   4. Encouraging long-term rehabilitation planning

18. Each newborn should be screened before discharge for phenylketonuria (PKU), which can lead to mental retardation if not treated. The nurse knows that the blood screening test will have the most reliable results if the baby:
   1. Is kept NPO for 6 hours before the blood is drawn
   2. Has the heel wrapped in a warm towel for 30 minutes
   3. Has been fed breast milk or formula at least 24 hours before the test
   4. Is held by the mother and remains perfectly still

19. The nurse would anticipate that $Rh_o(D)$ immune globulin would be administered in which of the following situations? **Select all that apply.**
   1. After chorionic villus sampling
   2. History of Rh exchange transfusion in a previous pregnancy
   3. Following a spontaneous abortion
   4. Current pregnancy of an Rh-negative infant
   5. Positive indirect Coombs' test at 28 weeks
   6. Following delivery of an Rh-positive infant

20. After delivery, a neonate is transferred to the nursery. The nurse is planning interventions to prevent hypothermia. What is the common source of radiant heat loss?
   1. Low room humidity
   2. Cold weight scale
   3. Cool bassinette walls
   4. Variable room temperature

# Answers to Study Questions

1. *2*

The priority here is the respiratory distress. The first nursing action is to increase the inspired oxygen; it would be appropriate to determine whether the infant has any mucus in the airway. Do a quick but thorough assessment of the infant and advise the supervisor or doctor regarding the infant's status. Trendelenburg position would be contraindicated because it would make breathing more difficult. Although performing an assessment is important, respiratory distress is a priority. Increasing the temperature of the neonate's environment could lead to an increased pulse rate and may lead to more oxygen consumption as an attempt of the body to cool itself. (Hockenberry & Wilson, 10 ed., p. 373)

2. *4, 5, 6*

The mother should be taught to feed the baby on demand for at least the first 4 weeks until lactation is well established. Feeding only breast milk frequently stimulates milk production. Nipple soreness is one of the most common problems, but the use of a cream to soften the nipples is often helpful, as is offering a pacifier to satisfy sucking needs of the infant between feedings after breastfeeding has been established. Adequate rest and good fluid intake help promote milk production. (Hockenberry & Wilson, 10 ed., p. 279)

3. *2*

The premature infant's temperature-regulating mechanism is poorly developed at birth. Heat production is low, and heat loss is high because of the greater body surface area relative to weight and the infant's lack of subcutaneous fat. No diaphoresis should be occurring, and the question has nothing to do with protein metabolism. The statement "The surface area of the premature infant is relatively smaller than that of a healthy term infant" describes the body surface area of the infant, and although true, it does not have any implication for maintaining temperature. (Hockenberry & Wilson, 10 ed., p. 341)

4. *1*

Promoting life-saving oxygen exchange is a priority measure at this time. Prevention of infection will be appropriate after surgical repair. It is important to prevent pulmonary infection, especially aspiration, but oxygen exchange is still a priority. (Hockenberry & Wilson, 10 ed., p. 1110)

5. *4*

The medication Rh₀(D) immune globulin is given to prevent maternal sensitization to the Rh antibodies to women who are Rh negative. Rh₀(D) immune globulin will not prevent or treat the problem if it has already occurred. Rh₀(D) immune globulin is not given to the infant. (Hockenberry & Wilson, 10 ed., p. 322)

6. *3*

It is important that the child be positioned in such a manner that he does not traumatize the incisional area and that the airway is maintained, which would be supine with the head turned to the side. Trendelenburg position would compromise respiration. The prone position would cause trauma to the incisional area and is to be avoided in infants. Sims' position is not appropriate for an infant because the infant should rest in a supine position. (Hockenberry & Wilson, 10 ed., pp. 307)

7. *4*

The premature infant is at greater risk for chilling. A premature infant has less brown fat than does a term neonate, as well as a lower reserve of glycogen and lower reserve for breathing. A lower body temperature leads to greater oxygen consumption, a decrease in surfactant production, and a tendency to develop acidosis. The infant does not need to be in protective isolation due to an underdeveloped immune system. There is no indication in the stem of the question that the infant has PKU, for which a low-phenylalanine diet would be indicated. Gavage feedings provide nourishment to the neonate who is compromised by respiratory distress or who is too immature to have coordinated suck–swallow reflexes, or who is easily fatigued by sucking. (Hockenberry & Wilson, 10 ed., p. 341)

8. *1*

The whitish yellowish exudate around the glans penis is granulation tissue and is normal. It will usually disappear within 2 to 3 days. It is not an infection; therefore antibiotic ointment is not appropriate. Soap and water cleansing after each diaper change is appropriate. A small sterile petrolatum gauze dressing may be applied to the area during the first 2 to 3 days (Gomco and Mogen clamp). If a PlastiBell was used, keep area clean; application of petrolatum jelly is not necessary; plastic ring will dislodge when area has healed (5 to 7 days). (Hockenberry & Wilson, 10 ed., p. 274)

9. *1*

Approximately 40% to 60% of all term babies develop jaundice between the second and fourth days of life. In the absence of disease or a specific cause, it is referred to as physiologic jaundice. It is most often due to the breakdown of excessive red blood cells and increased destruction of immature red cells. Hemolytic disease of the newborn caused by maternal/newborn blood group incompatibility is the most common cause of pathologic jaundice. Erythroblastosis fetalis and kernicterus are associated with pathologic jaundice. Sepsis does not normally cause an elevated bilirubin level. (Hockenberry & Wilson, 10 ed., p. 315)

10. *3*

Feedings and fluids should be encouraged to promote excretion of the bilirubin. It is not necessary to cover the neonate's eyes with use of the fiber-optic blanket, but there should be a covering pad between the infant's skin and the fiber-optic blanket. The stool would be loose, rather than constipated, while the jaundice is resolving. (Hockenberry & Wilson, 10 ed., p. 322)

11. *1*

The priority is to prevent chilling, which leads to greater oxygen consumption and to an increased utilization of glucose and brown fat. Chilling also increases caloric needs, decreases surfactant production, and promotes a tendency to develop acidosis. Evaporation occurs when the newborn is wet with amniotic fluid. (Hockenberry & Wilson, 10 ed., p. 244)

12. *2*

Explaining that the "cone-head" appearance is molding caused by pressure during birth and that it will disappear in a few days provides the most appropriate response. The nurse reassures the mother that molding is normal and caused by the pressure during delivery and will disappear in 1 to 2 days. The nurse should not tell a concerned mother not to worry, which is a type of false reassurance. The condition does not require a diagnostic scan. The collection of blood related to trauma that will take several weeks to absorb describes cephalhematoma. (Hockenberry & Wilson, 10 ed., p. 253)

**13.** *2*

The lack of passage of a meconium stool requires further assessment; it may be a sign of imperforate anus. The first assessment the nurse should perform is to visually inspect the anal area for an opening. Inserting a rectal thermometer could tear the anal mucosa, and if an imperforate anus is present, all oral feedings will be stopped. (Hockenberry & Wilson, 10 ed., p. 253)

**14.** *4*

The mother and baby have identification bands secured to a wrist or ankle in the delivery room. The nurse should compare these every time the baby is returned to the mother and when the infant is prepared for discharge. The other options are incomplete and will not ensure the safety of the baby. (Hockenberry & Wilson, 10 ed., p. 268)

**15.** *1*

There is evidence of an increased risk of acquiring metabolic syndrome (i.e., obesity, hypertension, dyslipidemia, and glucose intolerance) in childhood or early adulthood. Nursing care should focus on healthy lifestyle and prevention later in life. The hypoglycemia is transient. Hypoglycemia is a rebound response because the maternal hyperglycemia stimulates insulin production in the fetus, and the newborn is left with excessive insulin after the maternal glucose supply is ended at birth. The infant does have an increased chance of becoming diabetic during childhood, especially of symptoms of metabolic syndrome appear. (Hockenberry & Wilson, 10 ed., p. 396)

**16.** *3*

The classic three Cs—choking, coughing, and cyanosis—plus frothy saliva and constant drooling are the characteristic signs of esophageal atresia with a tracheoesophageal fistula. The other options are an incomplete description of the signs and symptoms. (Hockenberry & Wilson, 10 ed., p. 1108)

**17.** *2*

A meningocele is a saclike cyst of meninges filled with spinal fluid that protrudes through a defect in the bony part of the spine. Trauma and/or infection could lead to permanent central nervous system damage. The other responses are important, but preventing trauma to the sac is the highest priority. (Hockenberry & Wilson, 10 ed., p. 1638)

**18.** *3*

The Guthrie blood-screening test measures the amount of phenylalanine in the blood. It is most reliable if blood is drawn at least 24 hours after the newborn has ingested a source of protein. Breast milk and formula are both sources of protein. The heel stick is usually how the screening test is collected, so warming the extremity may increase blood flow. The infant would be held by a health care person, not the mother, for the blood collection. (Hockenberry & Wilson, 10 ed., p. 269)

**19.** *1, 3, 6*

$Rh_o(D)$ immune globulin is administered to Rh-negative women whose indirect Coombs tests are negative. Women who are sensitized are not given $Rh_o(D)$ immune globulin; this would be a woman with a history of Rh exchange transfusion in a previous pregnancy and a positive indirect Coombs' test at 28 weeks' gestation (a negative indirect Coombs test means sensitization has not occurred). Also, it is not necessary to give $Rh_o(D)$ immune globulin if the infant is Rh negative. It is given within 72 hours of an Rh-negative mother's delivery of an Rh-positive infant, after amniocentesis, chorionic villus sampling, ectopic pregnancy, miscarriage, elective abortion, abruptio placentae, placenta previa, or trauma at 28 weeks' gestation (with a negative indirect Coombs' test result). (Hockenberry & Wilson, 10 ed., p. 325)

**20.** *3*

The nurse understands that the common sources of radiant heat loss include cool bassinettes and bassinettes placed close to windows or areas of drafts. Low room humidity promotes evaporative heat loss. When the infant's skin has direct contact with a cooler object, such as a cold weight scale, conductive heat loss may occur. Convective heat loss occurs with a cool room temperature. (Hockenberry & Wilson, 10 ed., p. 343)

# Normal Laboratory Data

| Test | Normal Adult Values |
|---|---|
| **Blood Serum Values** | |
| Activated partial thromboplastin time (aPTT) | 30–45 sec |
| Alanine aminotransferase (ALT) | 10–40 units/L (0.17–0.68 μkat/L) |
| Albumin | 3.4–5.0 g/dL (35–50 g/L) |
| Alkaline phosphatase | 30–120 units/L (0.5–2.0 μkat/L) |
| Ammonia | 15–45 mcgN/dL (11–32 μmol N/L) |
| Amylase | 30–122 U/L [method dependent] (0.51–2.07 μkat/L) |
| Aspartate aminotransferase (AST) | 10–30 units/L (0.17–0.51 ukat/L) |
| **Bilirubin** | |
| Direct bilirubin | 0.1–0.3 mg/dL(1.7–5.1 μmol/L) |
| Indirect bilirubin | 0.1–1.0 mg/dL (1.7–17.10 μmol/L) |
| Total bilirubin | 0.2–1.2 mg/dL (3–21 μmol/L) |
| Bleeding time | Ivy method: 2–7 minutes |
| Blood platelets | 150–400 × $10^3$ units/L (150–350 × $10^9$/L) |
| Blood urea nitrogen (BUN) | 10–20 mg/dL (3.57–7.14 mmol/L) |
| Carbon dioxide (venous $CO_2$) | 20–30 mEq/L (20–30 mmol/L) |
| Calcium (ionized) serum | 4.5–5.5 mg/dL (1.13–1.38 mmol/L) |
| Calcium, total serum | 8.6–10.2 mg/dL (2.15–2.55 mmol/L) |
| Chloride (serum) | 95–105 mEq/L (95–105 mmol/L) |
| Cholesterol HDL, LDL, Triglycerides *(see Vascular chapter)* | <200mg/dL |
| Complete white blood cell (WBC) count | 4.0–11 $10^3$/mcL (× $10^9$/L) |
| Differential WBC count | Expressed as a percentage of total WBCs |
| Segmented neutrophils | 50%–70% |
| Band neutrophils | 0%–8% |
| Eosinophils | 0%–4% |
| Basophils | 0%–2% |
| Monocytes | 4%–8% |
| Lymphocytes | 20%–40% |
| C-reactive protein (highly sensitive-hs-CRP) | Less than 1.0 mg/dL (<9.52 nmol/L) |

| Test | Normal Adult Values |
|---|---|
| Creatinine (serum) | 0.2–1.0 mg/dL (7.63–76.25 umol/L) |
| Creatinine kinase (CK) | Men: 20–200 U/L (20–200 U/L ) Women: 20–180 U/L (20–180 U/L) |
| D-Dimer | <250 ng/mL (<250 mcg/L) |
| Erythrocyte sedimentation rate (ESR) | <30 mm/hr (some gender variation) |
| Fibrin split-products (FSP) | Less than 10 mcg/mL (<10 mg/L) |
| Fibrinogen | Quantitative: 200–400 mg/dL (2–4 g/L) |
| Glucose (baseline fasting) | 70–99 mg/dL (3.9–5.5 mmol/L) |
| Glucose 2-hour postprandial | Less than 140 mg/dL (7.77 mmol/L) |
| Glycosylated hemoglobin assay (A1C) | 4%–6% |
| Hematocrit | Men: 39%–50% (0.39–0.54) Women: 35%–47% (0.35–0.47) |
| Hemoglobin | Men: 13.2–17.3g/dL (132–173g/L) Women: 11.7–15.5g/dL (117–155g/L) |
| International normalized ratio (INR) | 2–3 prophylaxis for deep venous thrombosis 2.5–3.5 prosthetic cardiac valves |
| Iron binding capacity | 250–425 mcg/dL (44.8–76.1 μmol/L) |
| Iron, total serum | 50–175 mcg/dL (9.0–31.3 μmol/L) |
| Lactic acid dehydrogenase (LDH) | 140–280 units/L (0.83–2.5 ukat/L) |
| Magnesium (serum) | 1.5–2.5 mEq/L (0.75–1.25 mmol/L) |
| Partial thromboplastin time (PTT) | 60–70 sec |
| Phosphorus serum | 2.8–4.5 mg/dL (0.9–1.45 mmol/L) |
| Potassium (plasma) | 3.5–5.0 mEq/L (3.5–5.0 mmol/L) |
| Prostate specific antigen | Less than 4 ng/mL (4 ug/L) |
| Prothrombin time | 11–16 sec |
| Red blood cell (RBC) count | Men: 4.3–5.7 × $10^6$/mcL (4.3–5.7 × $10^{12}$/L) Women: 3.8–5.1 × $10^6$/mcL (3.8–5.1 × $10^{12}$/L) |

*Continued*

| Test | Normal Adult Values |
|---|---|
| Serum osmolarity | 275–295 mOsm/kg (275–295 mmol/kg) |
| Sodium (serum or plasma) | 135–145 mEq/L (135–145 mmol/L) |
| T4 (thyroxine), total | 4.6–11.0 mcg/dL (59–142 nmo/L) |
| T4 (thyroxine), free | 0.8–2.7 ng/dL (10–35 pmol/L) |
| T3 uptake | 24%–34% (0.24–0.34) |
| T3 (triiodothyronine), total | Age 20–50: 70–204 ng/dL (1.08–3.14 nmol/L) Age >50: 40–181 ng/dL (0.62–2.79 nmol/L) |
| Thyroid-stimulating hormone (TSH) | 0.4–4.2 µU/mL (0.4–4.2 mU/L) |
| Uric acid (serum) | Men: 4.0–8.5 mg/dL (240–505.62 µmol/L) Women: 2.7–7.3 mg/dL (160.61–434.24 µmol/L) |

## Normal Arterial Blood Gas Values

| Test | Normal Adult Values |
|---|---|
| Acidity index (pH) | 7.35–7.45 |
| Bicarbonate ($HCO_3-$) | 22–26 mEq/L (mmol/L) |
| Partial pressure of dissolved carbon dioxide ($Paco_2$) | 35–45 mm Hg |
| Partial pressure of dissolved oxygen ($Pao_2$) | 80–100 mm Hg |
| Percentage of hemoglobin saturated with oxygen ($O_2$ saturation) | 95% or above |

## Urine Values

| Test | Normal Adult Values |
|---|---|
| Creatinine clearance (24-hour urine collection) | 59–137 mL/min (59–137 mL/s/m²) |
| Microscopic urinalysis | |
| Bacteria | Negative |
| Casts | None present |
| Crystals | Negative |
| RBCs | Less than 2 |
| WBCs | 0–4 per low-power field |

| Test | Normal Adult Values |
|---|---|
| Specific gravity | Adult: 1.005–1.030 |
| Ketones | Older adult: values decrease 24-hr specimen—20–50 mg/dL |
| Uric acid (urine) | 250–750 mg/24 hr (1.48–4.43 mmol/day) |
| Urinalysis | |
| Microalbumin | 0.2–1.9 mg/dL |
| Bilirubin | (2.0–19.0 mcg/24 hr) |
| Color | Negative |
| Glucose | Clear, golden yellow Negative |
| Urine electrolytes (24-hour urine collection) | |
| Sodium | 40–250 mEq/24 hr (mmol/day) (varies with dietary intake) |
| Calcium | 100–250 mg/day (2.5–6.3 mmol/day) |
| Urine osmolarity | 300–1300 mOsm/kg $H_2O$ (mmol/kg $H_2O$) (random sample) |

## Cerebral Spinal Fluid (CSF) Analysis

| Test | Normal Adult Values |
|---|---|
| Albumin | 56%–76% |
| Blood | None |
| Color | Clear and colorless |
| Glucose | 40–70 mg/dL (2.2–3.9 mmol/L) |
| Pressure | Less than 20 cm $H_2O$ |
| Protein | 15–45 mg/dL (0.15–0.45 g/L) (higher in older adults and children) (up to 0.7 g/L in older adults and children) |
| White blood cells | Adults: 0–5 cells/µ/L (0–5 cells × 10⁶ WBCs/L) Children: 0–10 (0–10 cells × 10⁶ WBCs/L) |

# References and Resources

Burchum, J. R., Rosenthal, L., Jones, B. O., & Neumiller, J. J. (2016). *Lehne's Pharmacology for Nursing Care* (9th ed.). St. Louis, MO: Saunders.

Commission on Graduates of Foreign Nursing Schools (CGFNS). 3600 Market St., Suite 400, Philadelphia, PA 19104.

Halter, M. J. (2014). *Varcarolis' Foundations of Psychiatric Mental Health Nursing* (7th ed.). St. Louis, MO: Saunders.

Hockenberry, M. J., & Wilson, D. (2015). *Wong's Nursing Care of Infants and Children* (10th ed.). St. Louis, MO: Mosby.

Ignatavicius, D. D., Workman, M. L., Blair, M., Rebar, C., & Winkelman, C. (2016). *Medical-Surgical Nursing: Patient-Centered Collaborative Care* (8th ed.). St. Louis, MO: Saunders.

Keltner, N. L., & Steele, D. (2015). *Psychiatric Nursing* (7th ed.). St. Louis: Mosby.

Lewis, S. L., Bucher, L., Heitkemper, M. M., Harding, M.M., Kwong, J., & Roberts, D. (2017). *Medical-Surgical Nursing: Assessment and Management of Clinical Problems* (10th ed.). St. Louis, MO: Mosby.

Lilley, L. L., Collins, S. R., & Snyder, J. S. (2017). *Pharmacology and the Nursing Process* (8th ed.). St. Louis, MO: Mosby.

Lowdermilk, D. D., Perry, S. E., Cashion, K., Alden, K. R., & Olshansky, E. F. (2016). *Maternity & Women's Health Care* (11th ed.). St. Louis, MO: Mosby.

National Council of State Boards of Nursing. (2018). *NCLEX Examination Candidate Bulletin.* <https://www.ncsbn.org/089900_2018_Bulletin_Proof2.pdf.pdf>. *Note: this changes yearly; navigate to* https://www.ncsbn.org/1213.htm *for current bulletin.*

National Council of State Boards of Nursing. (2018). *Frequently Asked Questions About NCLEX.* <https://www.ncsbn.org/nclex-faqs.htm>.

National Council of State Boards of Nursing. (2018). *2019 RN Practice Analysis: Linking the NCLEX-RN Examination to Practice:* Vol. 72. <https://www.ncsbn.org/17_RN_US_Canada_Practice_Analysis.pdf>.

National Council of State Boards of Nursing. (2018, August). *Proposed 2019 NCLEX-RN Test Plan.* National Council of State Boards of Nursing Annual Meeting, Chicago, IL.

Nies, M. A., & McEwen, M. (2015). *Community/Public Health Nursing: Promoting the Health of Populations* (6th ed.). St. Louis, MO: Saunders.

Pagana, K. D., Pagana, T. J., & Pagana, T. N. (2015). *Mosby's Diagnostic and Laboratory Test Reference* (12th ed.). St Louis, MO: Mosby.

Potter, P. A., Perry, A. G., Stockert, P. A., Hall, A. M., & Ostendorf, W. R. (2017). *Fundamentals of Nursing* (9th ed.). St. Louis, MO: Mosby.

Stanhope, M., & Lancaster, J. (2014). *Foundations of Nursing in the Community* (4th ed.). St. Louis, MO: Mosby.

The Joint Commission, One Renaissance Blvd. Oakbrook Terrace, IL 60181. https://www.jointcommission.org/

Zerwekh, J., & Garneau, A. (2018). *Nursing Today: Transitions and Trends* (9th ed.). St. Louis, MO: Saunders.

# Index